Exercise
in
Rehabilitation
Medicine

Exercise in Rehabilitation Medicine

Editor in Chief
Walter R. Frontera, MD, PhD
*Chairman and Earle P. and Ida S. Charlton Associate Professor, Department of Physical
Medicine and Rehabilitation, Harvard Medical School
Chief, Physical Medicine and Rehabilitation, Spaulding Rehabilitation Hospital
Chief, Physical Medicine and Rehabilitation Service, Massachusetts General Hospital*

Associate Editors
David M. Dawson, MD
*Professor of Neurology and Associate Director, Division of Rehabilitation Medicine,
Harvard Medical School
Director of Residency Training in Neurology, Brigham and Women's Hospital*

David M. Slovik, MD
*Assistant Professor of Medicine and Associate Director, Division of Rehabilitation
Medicine, Harvard Medical School
Chief of Medicine, Spaulding Rehabilitation Hospital
Endocrine Unit, Massachusetts General Hospital*

Human Kinetics

Library of Congress Cataloging-in-Publication Data

Exercise in rehabilitation medicine / Walter R. Frontera, editor :
    David M. Dawson, David M. Slovik, associate editor[s].
        p. cm.
    Includes bibliographical references and index.
    ISBN 0-88011-839-3
    1. Exercise therapy. 2. Medical rehabilitation. I. Frontera,
Walter R., 1955-   . II. Dawson, D.M. (David Michael), 1930-   .
III. Slovik, David M., 1945-   .
        [DNLM: 1. Exercise. WB 541 E9541 1999]
    RM725.E926   1999
    615.8'2--dc21
    DNLM/DLC   98-53986
    for Library of Congress   CIP

ISBN: 0-88011-839-3

Part I opening illustration by Peter Paul Rubens, *Study for the Figure of Christ on the Cross*. Circa 1614-1615. London, British Museum. Part II opening illustration by Peter Paul Rubens, *A figure posed as the 'Crouching Venus' of Doidalsas*. About 1606. Berlin, Kupferstichkabinett. Part III opening illustration by Peter Paul Rubens, *A Nude Man, Kneeling*. Circa 1690. Rotterdam, Museum Boymans-van Beuingen. Part IV opening illustration by Peter Paul Rubens, *Study for a Man raising the Cross*. About 1601. Oxford, Ashmolean Museum.

Acquisition Editor: Loarn D. Robertson, PhD; **Develpmental Editor:** Elaine Mustain; **Assistant Editor:** Melissa Feld; **Copyeditor:** Brian Mustain; **Proofreader:** Sue Fetters; **Indexer:** Marie Rizzo; **Graphic Designer:** George Amaya; **Graphic Artist:** Yvonne Winsor; **Photo Editor:** Clark Brooks; **Cover Designer:** Jack Davis; **Photographer:** Tom Roberts, unless otherwise noted; **Illustrator:** George Amaya; **Printer:** Edwards Brothers

Printed in the United States of America

10 9 8 7 6 5 4 3 2 1

Human Kinetics
Web site: http://www.humankinetics.com/

United States: Human Kinetics, P.O. Box 5076, Champaign, IL 61825-5076
1-800-747-4457
e-mail: humank@hkusa.com

Canada: Human Kinetics, 475 Devonshire Road Unit 100, Windsor, ON N8Y 2L5
1-800-465-7301 (in Canada only)
e-mail: humank@hkcanada.com

Europe: Human Kinetics, P.O. Box IW14, Leeds LS16 6TR, United Kingdom
+44 (0)113-278 1708
e-mail: humank@hkeurope.com

Australia: Human Kinetics, 57A Price Avenue, Lower Mitcham, South Australia 5062
(08) 82771555
e-mail: humank@hkaustralia.com

New Zealand: Human Kinetics, P.O. Box 105-231, Auckland Central
09-523-3462
e-mail: humank@hknewz.com

To my wife and daughters, Lizie, Mara, and Natasha
  Walter R. Frontera

To my wife, Beth
  David M. Dawson

To my parents Rosalind and Arthur, and my wife and
children Lois, Elissa, and Matthew
  David M. Slovik

Contents

Foreword

You should get more exercise! This is perhaps the advice patients most frequently hear from their physicians—as well as from friends, spouses, and their own "inner voices." Yet, without greater specificity, a recommendation for "exercise" is as useless as advice to "take some pills" or "try a little surgery." What kind of exercise? For how long? At what intensity? Which technique? What apparatus? Without these and a host of other details, few will perform well or be motivated to persevere.

Although exercise as a medical intervention suffers from neglect, an "exercise craze" has swept over the general public in recent years. In the United States, concern about poor physical fitness began to grow in the 1950s, when the Krause-Weber Test of school children evidenced dismal performance on the part of American children compared to European. Both Presidents Eisenhower (1952-1960) and Kennedy (1960-1963) brought physical fitness to the forefront as a national concern.

Educators, fitness writers, and exercise crusaders such as Bonnie Prudden and Kenneth Cooper began to offer specific exercise and fitness guidelines for lay readers. Cooper's "Aerobics" exercise program became immensely popular. Health clubs and fitness centers grew in number and popularity as the "baby boom" generation came of age in the 1960s and 1970s.

Meanwhile, medically supervised exercise regimens introduced in the 1940s and 1950s for war injuries and polio epidemics expanded to serve patients with stroke, cardiac, pulmonary, and many other disabilities. Today, we find a large network of medical rehabilitation facilities, an equally vibrant health club and fitness center industry, as well as a worldwide sports medicine movement. Yet many health care providers outside these fields remain either uninformed or misinformed about how to prescribe exercise as part of a treatment plan.

The beginnings of research on physical exercise date back to the late 1700s. In 1784, the illustrious French chemist, Antoine Lavoissier, published a study on respiratory exchange during one-legged exercise. Lavoissier's methodology for estimating energy cost became standard practice, and present-day laboratory techniques follow his basic principles. However, concerted efforts to investigate acute responses and chronic adaptations to physical exercise did not begin until the early 1900s, and gathered significant impetus only in midcentury. Probably more than 99% of all exercise physiology research in the history of the world has been published since 1960.

During the last 40 years, "exercise science" has generated an impressive but still growing scientific base of objective data on the methods and outcomes of therapeutic exercise. Research has confirmed the important role of regular physical exercise in health development and health maintenance. A carefully prescribed exercise program has emerged as the most important modality employed in rehabilitation medicine. Yet the link between published research and medical practice has developed slowly and remained weak. *Exercise in Rehabilitation Medicine* organizes the application of this science to physical medicine and rehabilitation in a form that all health care providers can use in their daily patient care.

Drs. Frontera, Dawson, and Slovik have assembled a distinguished group of chapter authors who have summarized the basic science, reviewed the overall clinical considerations, and detailed the proper use of exercise therapy in 10 specific categories of disability as well as for two special groups. This book will prove indispensable for practitioners of rehabilitation and primary care medicine, as well as for individuals in many other medical and allied health specialty areas.

Paul J. Corcoran, MD
Lecturer on Physical Medicine and Rehabilitation
Harvard Medical School

Howard G. Knuttgen, PhD
Lecturer on Physical Medicine and Rehabilitation
Harvard Medical School
Professor Emeritus of Applied Physiology
Pennsylvania State University

Preface

Broadly defined, rehabilitation is the development of a person to the fullest physical, psychological, social, vocational, avocational, and educational potential, within his or her physiological or anatomic impairments and environmental limitations (DeLisa et al. 1998). That approximately 50 million Americans live with a disability demonstrates the importance of rehabilitation.

Clinicians design rehabilitation programs to prevent complications, to compensate for loss of anatomic or physiologic capacity, and to optimize function. It is appropriate that exercise is one of the most frequently used strategies to achieve these goals, since nearly 70% of disabling conditions limit mobility by interfering with the function of skeletal muscles,

joints, bones, heart, and lungs. It is therefore of utmost importance that rehabilitation professionals have a comprehensive knowledge of the physiology of exercise and its application in the clinical environment.

Many excellent publications have addressed important aspects of the basic science of exercise. Others have discussed various clinical aspects of rehabilitation. However, recent advances in both fields—exercise science and rehabilitation medicine—require an amalgamation of this knowledge. Our objective is to present, in a single volume, an organized and in-depth discussion of the basic science and the clinical correlates of exercise as a therapeutic and rehabilitative intervention strategy.

Proper use of exercise in rehabilitating patients with a wide variety of disabling illnesses requires understanding of both the basic physiological adaptations to exercise and the important biomechanical correlates of movement. Only by understanding the nature of the adaptations to training with various kinds of exercise (strength, endurance, and flexibility) can a health professional properly match a training program with the impairment, disability, or handicap in need of rehabilitation. The first part of this book takes a detailed look at these basic facts.

Rehabilitation professionals should have a working knowledge of the various testing devices and protocols used to evaluate a patient's functional capacity. They must understand the relevance of these tests for appropriate exercise prescription. The second part of this book discusses the principles of exercise testing and exercise prescription, ending with discussion of the importance of exercise in the primary prevention of disease.

In part III, specialists discuss the scientific rationale and the clinical importance of exercise in the rehabilitation of patients with a wide variety of disabling conditions, and address the factors that must be weighed when prescribing exercise for these conditions. The authors discuss diseases that impair the function of the heart, circulation, lungs, joints, endocrine system, bones, neuromuscular system, and mental function. Tables summarize published training studies; and authors provide the details of exercise prescriptions for patient populations with specific disabling illnesses.

Scientific and clinical literature increasingly address the aging of the population and the benefits of exercise training in older age groups. Also, more survivors of disabling injuries are developing interest in competitive sports. Part IV considers these two special populations: the aging and elite athletes with disabilities.

This book should be useful for many different professionals: physicians practicing rehabilitation (including specialists and primary care providers), physical therapists, occupational therapists, recreational therapists, nurses, and exercise physiologists with an interest in clinical applications of exercise. Theoretical, practical, and clinical information exist under one cover. Extensive reference lists serve as additional sources of information. The text is clearly written, so even those with little technical expertise should be able to follow it; yet it is sufficiently advanced that those who are not beginners will significantly improve their understanding.

Walter R. Frontera, MD, PhD
David M. Dawson, MD, and David M. Slovik, MD

References

DeLisa, J., G. Martin, and D. Currie. 1998. Rehabilitation medicine: past, present, and future. In *Rehabilitation medicine—principles and practice*, ed. J. DeLisa and B. Gans, 3. Philadelphia: Lippincott.

Part I

Biological Considerations

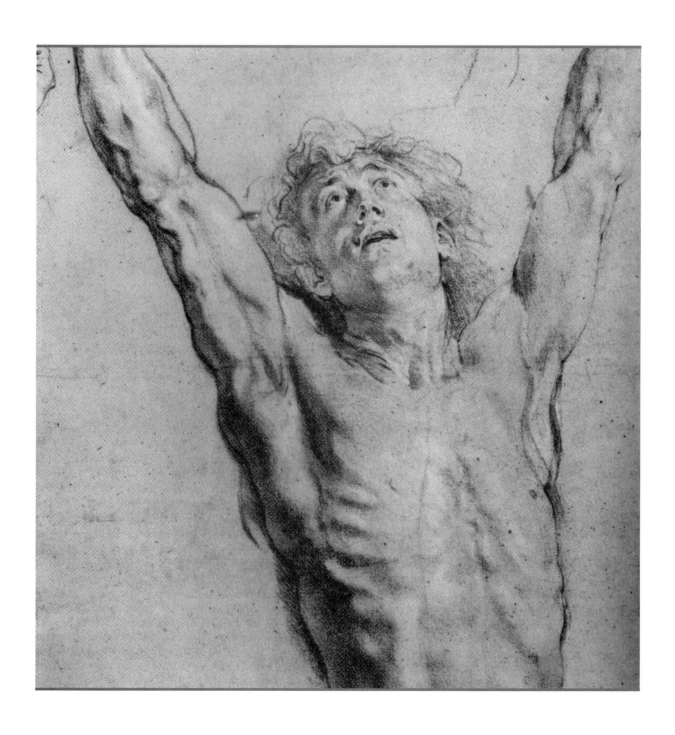

Chapter 1

Energy Balance for Muscle Function

Principles of Bioenergetics

Michael L. Blei, MD, Allison M. Fall, MD, and Martin J. Kushmerick, MD, PhD

Skeletal muscle performance requires that the muscle's synthesis of ATP must balance the demand for energy (i.e., for ATP) from contractile processes. Contracting muscle uses ATP to change chemical energy into mechanical output (via myosin ATPase) and to power ion transport (e.g., calcium uptake, sodium-potassium exchange). This demand for ATP is met by synthesis from various metabolic pathways. The requirement to balance energy demand with energy production is as important for the elite athlete as for a person afflicted with a skeletal muscle disease or with limitations of muscle mass. Across all conditions, maximization of human motor performance is a principle goal of training or rehabilitation—and a firm understanding of skeletal muscle bioenergetics, and its relationship to sustainable function, is essential for intelligent prescription of rehabilitation programs.

We begin this chapter by outlining the central concepts of energy balance for skeletal muscle bioenergetics. After reviewing the heterogeneity of fiber types and their energy characteristics, we apply the concept of energy balance to the energy utilization and synthesis of individual motor units. We discuss substrate utilization, skeletal muscle performance, and energy recovery. Finally, we show how the physiological properties directly relate to clinical practice.

A Paradigm for Energy Balance in Muscle Function

The concept of biochemical energy balance proposes that there must be functional integration of the major metabolic pathways in order to achieve a chemical energy balance within the cell, and that maintaining a chemical energy balance is central to cell energetic regulation (Kushmerick 1977). Lipmann (1941) was the first to postulate how this might be accomplished. In spite of all the intricacies of known metabolic pathways, only a small set of common biochemical molecules, containing "high-energy phosphate bonds," is involved in energy-transducing mechanisms. Adenosine triphosphate (ATP) is the molecule primarily relevant to muscle activity.

Energy transductions in skeletal muscle couple the energy of ATP to the metabolic, electrical, osmotic, and mechanical work required to maintain cell function. However, human skeletal muscle cells maintain only a small amount (8 mM) of ATP (Harris et al. 1974). With rates of ATP utilization in active muscle typically on the order of 1mM/sec or greater, the chemical potential energy in the ATP stores would be exhausted in a very short time without replenishment. The cells must therefore produce ATP concurrently with work performance. **Energy balance** describes those properties of energy-using and -generating metabolic pathways and their controls that enable the supply of chemical energy to match the demands of the chemical-transducing machines. The following four tenets provide a relatively simple scheme to integrate the diverse mechanisms of bioenergetic systems (Kushmerick 1995).

- ATP provides the energy for all forms of skeletal muscle work.
- Phosphocreatine is a biochemical capacitor.
- The sum of the coupled ATPases sets the demand of the energy balance and defines the energetic state.
- The coupled ATPases provide control signals for regulation of energy balance.

ATP Provides the Energy for All Forms of Skeletal Muscle Work

The enzyme-mediated splitting (i.e., hydrolysis) of a phosphate group from ATP produces all the free energy used by the "actin-myosin motor" to produce mechanical force and by the cell's ion pumps to do electrical and osmotic work.

Phosphocreatine (PCr) Is a Biochemical Capacitor

Certain forms of chemical potential energy are biochemically interconvertible by near equilibrium reactions. Both the forward and reverse rates of a **near equilibrium reaction** surpass the rates of any other reactions that use the same products or reactants. Perhaps the best known example is the creatine kinase reaction that catalyses the interconversion between ATP and PCr. Because both the forward and reverse rates of the creatine kinase reaction are an order of magnitude greater than measured maximal rates for ATP utilization and synthesis (Meyer et al. 1984), ATP and PCr can remain at equilibrium no matter what contractile state the muscle is in.

$$PCr^- + MgADP^- + H^+ \leftrightarrow MgATP^- + Cr$$

This reaction defines a **chemical energy capacitance**, because the content of PCr represents a readily available store of chemical potential energy (by the nature of its near equilibrium with ATP and ADP) previously synthesized by metabolism. Although PCr exists in muscle cells in higher concentrations than ATP, it is not used directly to produce mechanical work. PCr is a substrate for only one enzyme, creatine kinase. Because the stored PCr creates a kind of energy buffer or chemical storage battery, the cell can temporarily couple energy-requiring processes to ATP hydrolysis *without* the need to quickly synthesize more ATP—whatever additional ATP is needed can be drawn from the stored PCr, which is converted to ATP through the simple step described in the equation above. This scenario applies as long as the available supply of PCr is not exceeded. Phosphocreatine concentrations in resting human skeletal muscle are on the order of 30 mM. There is a slightly (10%) lower PCr concentration in human type I fibers than in type II fibers (Edstrom et al. 1982)—a difference much less pronounced than the approximately 50% difference across fiber types in other mammalian species (Kushmerick et al. 1992).

The Sum of the Coupled ATPases Sets the Demand of the Balance and Defines the Energetic State

The overall metabolic synthesis rate of a cell changes as its ATPase rates change. The only way the overall metabolic rate can increase is if the steady-state sum of the ATPase activities increases, since it is energy use that drives all the cell's metabolic activity. Hence the rate of the coupled free energy of ATP utilization is the primary and causal mechanism in bioenergetics. However, the signals that activate the coupling between ATP utilization and work performance—i.e., the intracellular release of calcium by membrane excitation—are external to the molecular motor. Neither the chemical potential of ATP nor additional availability of substrates can control the motor any more than the level of fuel in a gas tank controls how fast the engine runs. *Only* a change in the rate of ATPase activity can increase the metabolic rate.

The Coupled ATPases Provide Control Signals for Regulation of Energy Balance

Although the *in vivo* control of cellular respiration is not fully established, it is well understood that the muscle cell can maintain remarkably constant concentrations of cellular energy metabolites no matter what the levels of demand. Perhaps the signals that activate the utilization of ATP also provide information to the ATP-synthesizing pathways, in a feedforward mechanism of regulation. In this way a common external signal could create energy balance by acting in parallel on both the ATP-utilizing and -synthesizing mechanisms—a role similar to that envisioned for calcium in its activation of mitochondrial dehydrogenases (McCormack et al. 1990). Although such feed-forward mechanisms are known to exist, it seems theoretically necessary that a signal(s) derived from the coupled chemomechanical machines themselves must provide feedback regulation of ATP synthesis. The primary signal molecule presumably is one or more of the following products of ATP-coupled molecular machines: inorganic phosphate (P_i), adenosine diphosphate (ADP), hydrogen ion (H^+), or creatine. The simplest possible mechanism, feedback by ADP, sufficiently explains regulation in skeletal muscle (Jeneson et al. 1996). For further discussion of the control mechanisms of cellular respiration, see recent reviews on this topic (Jeneson et al. 1996; McCormack et al. 1990; Meyer and Foley 1996; Tamura et al. 1989; Wilson 1994).

Skeletal Muscle Fiber Types

A heterogeneous population of fiber types comprise mammalian skeletal muscles. Classical fiber typing, as displayed in table 1.1, categorizes muscle fibers according to their ATPase characteristics (type I vs. II, or slow vs. fast myosin), their aerobic capacity (oxidative vs. glycolytic), or their functional (fatigability) properties (Saltin and Gollnick 1983). Classical fiber typing has helped to clarify the basic biochemistry and physiology of skeletal muscle performance, and to explain how muscle structure and function adapt to training and to pathological states.

While each motor unit contains muscle fibers of similar phenotypic characteristics, the motor unit populations of human skeletal muscles are heterogeneous. The fiber type distribution of individual muscles varies significantly within a given individual; and the phenotypic distribution of the same muscle differs within the human population (Edgerton et al. 1975; Johnson et al. 1973). Fiber type evaluations of human skeletal muscle biopsies historically have utilized the staining properties of the myosin heavy-chain ATPase phenotype to classify fibers into

Table 1.1	Correlation of Histochemical and Physiologic Skeletal Muscle Nomenclature		
Histochemical	**Physiologic nomenclature**		
Type	**(Barnard et al. 1971)**	**(Peter et al. 1972)**	**(Burke et al. 1971)**
I	Slow twitch, intermediate	Slow twitch, oxidative (SO)	Slow twitch (S)
IIa	Fast twitch, red	Fast twitch, oxidative glycolytic (FOG)	Fast twitch, fatigue resistant (FR)
IIb	Fast twitch, white	Fast twitch, glycolytic (FG)	Fast twitch, fatigue sensitive (FF)

Reprinted, by permission, from V. Dubowitz, 1985, *Muscle biopsy: A practical approach,* 2nd ed. (London: Bailliere Tindall), 64.

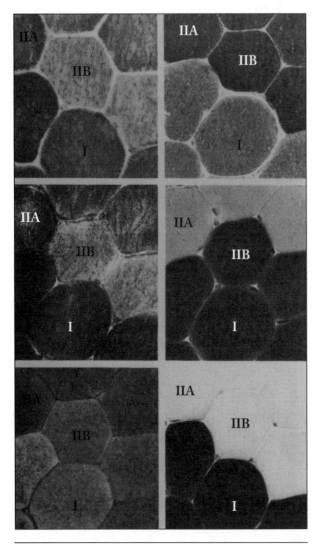

Figure 1.1 Serial sections from normal human muscle. Identical fibers are shown so that various histochemical reactions can be compared. (× 440). NADH-TR (upper left); ATPase pH 9.4 (upper right); SDH (middle left); ATPase pH 4.6 (middle right); PAS (lower left); ATPase pH 4.3 (lower right).

Reprinted, by permission, from V. Dubowitz, 1985, *Muscle biopsy: A practical approach*, 2nd ed. (London: Bailliere Tindall), 65.

type I, IIa, or IIb fibers (Dubowitz 1985)(figure 1.1). Methods used to quantitate the energy synthesis capacity of human skeletal muscle have included both enzymatic analysis (to classify biopsied muscle fibers according to activities of glycolytic or oxidative phosphorylation enzymes) and measures of mitochondrial volume densities (because it is in the mitochondria that energy generation occurs).

Energy Utilization Distribution

Individual human skeletal muscle fibers appear to express a continuum of energy demands rather than three distinct populations. The maximum shortening velocity of a single fiber correlates with its maximal ATP utilization rate (Barany 1967). The shortening velocities of fiber types I, IIa, IIa/b, and IIb exhibit overlapping distributions (Larsson and Moss 1993)(figure 1.2). Type IIa/b fibers express both type IIa and type IIb myosin heavy chains (Pette and Staron 1990). Note that there is almost a tenfold range between the mean maximum shortening velocities of human skeletal muscle type I and type IIb fibers and a many-fold range within the individual fiber type classifications (Larsson and Moss 1993).

Myosin light chain, myosin heavy chain, and calcium reuptake protein isoforms are primarily responsible for the economy of energy transduction (Pette and Staron 1990), the myosin heavy chain isoform content being the most significant determinant (Lowey et al. 1993). Fluorescent antibody staining has demonstrated that an individual fiber can coexpress differing myosin heavy chain isoforms along with varying combinations of light chains isoforms (Pette and Staron 1990). The potential number of protein combinations is more than able to produce a full spectrum of fiber characteristics with respect to energy economy during contraction.

Several research groups have measured actual energy costs of muscle contraction—both in isolated whole mammalian muscle preparations at near physiologic temperatures, and *in vivo* using human skeletal muscle (Blei et al. 1993; Boska 1991; Harkema et al. 1997). The predominant slow oxidative cat soleus muscle (>92% SO by cross-sectional area) uses 1.16 mM ATP/sec for a brief isometric tetanus; whereas the predominantly fast glycolytic biceps brachii muscle (>75% FG and <5% SO) uses 7.9 mM ATP/sec. These measurements demonstrate an approximate sevenfold difference in whole-muscle energy utilization rates depending on the fiber type predominance—results that compare favorably with data on maximum shortening velocities of individual human muscle fibers. Boska (1994) measured utilization rates of at least 1.3 mM ATP/sec in the human gastrocnemius/soleus, with presumed near maximum static voluntary contractions. On average, the human gastrocnemius comprises 52% SO, 16% FOG, and 32% FG fibers (Edgerton et al. 1975).

Energy Synthesis Distribution

Energy synthesis capacity also varies within and among fiber types. Estimates of mitochondrial volume in human skeletal muscle fibers have shown

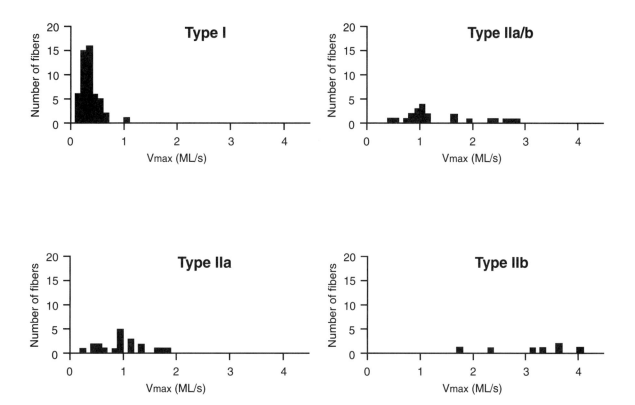

Figure 1.2 Distributions of maximum shortening velocities (Vmax) from single human quadriceps and soleus muscle fibers classified according to myosin heavy chain type.
Reprinted, by permission, from L. Larsson and R. Moss, 1993, "Maximum velocity of shortening in relation to myosin isoform composition in single fibers from human skeletal muscles," *Journal of Physiology* 472: 606.

a greater than fivefold range across fiber types (Howald et al. 1985). Since isolated mitochondria have relatively similar energy production capacities irrespective of fiber type, the primary determinant of aerobic capacity (in non-oxygen-limited conditions) appears to be the total mitochondrial volume in normal tissue (Hoppeler 1986). Based on the typical oxygen utilization rate of isolated mitochondria of 3.1 ml O_2/min/ml mitochondria, these mitochondrial volume estimates represent a 0.2 to 1.0 mM ATP/sec range in energy production capacity across human fiber types (Howald et al. 1985; Schwerzmann et al. 1989). Each fiber type demonstrates a distribution of mitochondrial volumes with significant overlap among fiber types, creating a continuous distribution of fibers with respect to mitochondrial volumes (figure 1.3).

Mitochondrial volume—more specifically, the total inner membrane surface areas of mitochondria—correlates well with estimates of maximum rates of aerobic energy synthesis (Vmax) within human skeletal muscles. Phosphorus magnetic resonance spectroscopy (P[31] MRS) can noninvasively and serially quantitate, with very high time resolution, the chang-

ing relative concentrations of phosphocreatine, ATP, inorganic phosphate, and pH. This allows for the quantitation of *in vivo* human muscle ATP utilization and synthesis rates (Blei et al. 1993). The flexor digitorum superficialis of the human forearm is composed of 40% ± 10% (mean ± SD) type I fibers (Mizuno et al. 1994). According to a simple monoexponential model of respiratory control by ADP, the Vmax of the flexor digitorum superficialis is about 0.4 mM ATP/sec (Blei et al. 1993). Compare this with the gastrocnemius, which contains 52% ± 7% type I fibers (Edgerton et al. 1975). An estimated Vmax of 0.6-1.0 mM ATP/sec was obtained from the initial phosphorylation rate of phosphocreatine recovery in the gastrocnemius (Boska 1991; Boska 1994). These values, when extrapolated to account for the variation in fiber type distributions, correlate well with estimates of the maximum rate of energy synthesis predicted from mitochondrial volumes. However, since the *in vivo* control of cellular respiration is a current area of investigation, calculations extrapolating data to obtain Vmax are at this time only model determinants subject to potentially high error factors.

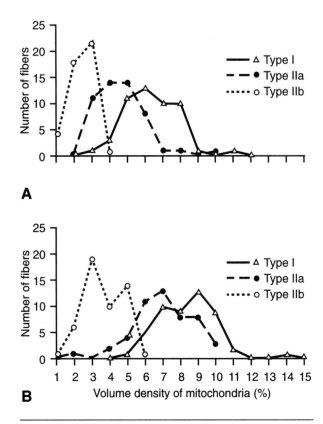

A

B

Figure 1.3 Line histograms of the volume density of mitochondria in individual human vastus lateralis fiber types, (A) before training and (B) after six weeks of endurance exercise.
Reprinted, by permission, from H. Hoppeler, 1986, "Exercise in rehabilitation medicine," *International Journal of Sports Medicine* 7: 194.

Energy Utilization and Synthesis in Human Movement

Most functional movements occur repetitively, with different muscles performing different types and intensities of contractions. For example, normal walking requires the anterior tibialis to begin with a shortening contraction during initiation of the swing phase, progressing to a relatively static contraction until heel strike, at which time there is a higher-intensity lengthening contraction. During the stance phase, the anterior tibialis is relatively inactive. This repetitive activation of individual motor units establishes their energy demand, which in turn regulates energy production to maintain an energy balance.

Determinants of Energy Demand

The energy demand for a specific motor unit during repetitive movement is dictated not only by the energy economy of its fibers as described above, but also by the intensity and type of contraction (i.e., static, shortening, lengthening). The relationship between the firing rate of a motor unit and its subsequent force generation depends on the calcium kinetics of the twitch response and on the muscle fibers' protein contractile and relaxation properties (Kernell et al. 1983). During most human movement, the recruited motor units operate well below their maximum force generation capacity—i.e., well below their maximum energy utilization rate. Energy economy also varies with the type of contraction. Shortening contractions require a rapid cycling of actin-myosin in and out of the strongly bound state. Active shortening at peak mechanical power output increases the rate of ATP hydrolysis by over 100% compared to the rate during a maximum static contraction (Kushmerick and Davies 1969). Lengthening contractions, in contrast, by increasing the time that actin-myosin are in the strongly bound state, are more economical. Lengthening contractions, in addition, rely upon the mechanical properties of the protein and collagen matrix for resistance. These factors together reduce ATP hydrolysis rates to as little as 30% of that seen in static conditions (Rall 1985; Woledge et al. 1985). Thus for a maximal contraction, the type of contraction can create over a fivefold difference in energy utilization.

As with the anterior tibialis during normal gait, muscles in most repetitive movements have a natural duty cycle. A **duty cycle** is the ratio of contraction time to the relaxation time. The combined properties of the motor units' energy properties, the type and intensity of contraction, and the duty cycle combine to establish the energy demand for repetitive movements.

Sources and Regulation of Energy Synthesis

To meet any energy demand, energy production must have sufficient substrate for the energy-producing metabolic pathways. Some substrates are stored as internal reserves (e.g., glycogen and triglycerides); vascular perfusion delivers others (mainly oxygen, glucose, and fatty acids). The substrate used for energy production depends on the energy utilization rate, the availability of substrate, and the synthesis capacities of the individual motor unit's fibers.

Phosphocreatine and Anaerobic Metabolism

The initiation of contraction turns on full energy utilization within milliseconds. Human aerobic metabolism, however, does not reach steady-state production for several minutes, with a half time to steady-state of 18-30 seconds (Connett and Sahlin 1996). Available internal energy stores therefore must temporarily buffer the immediate energy demand. Phosphocreatine is immediately available to buffer ATP concentrations through the near equilibrium creatine kinase reaction. After about 40% of the phosphocreatine supply is gone, significant anaerobic glycolytic production of new ATP begins (Conley et al. 1997). While the *in vivo* controls of glycogenolysis and glycolysis are not fully established, the combined energy production rate is apparently regulated to match the energy utilization requirements. Free calcium, which increases during contraction, appears to act as the primary activation regulator for glycogenolysis and glycolysis (Conley et al. 1997). Allosteric feedback regulation of anaerobic metabolism has also been implicated (Connett and Sahlin 1996). With the elevated glycolytic flux, the excess pyruvate not utilized for aerobic metabolism undergoes reduction to form lactate. As aerobic synthesis increases, there is a progressive decline in PCr buffering and energy production from anaerobic glycolysis.

Theoretically, if each of the recruited motor units is able to sustain an energy balance from aerobic metabolism, the glycolytic flux decreases to a rate needed to supply the necessary substrate for aerobic metabolism. Lactic acid production then essentially ceases and phosphocreatine depletion stabilizes to steady-state concentrations. However, if aerobic metabolism cannot satisfy the energy demand, the glycolytic flux must remain elevated in order to continue anaerobic ATP production (Conley et al. 1997; Connett and Sahlin 1996).

Aerobic Metabolism

The regulatory mechanisms for aerobic metabolism in skeletal muscle remain under investigation. It currently appears that the metabolic products provide feedback and primary control for regulation over the full aerobic capacity (Jeneson et al. 1996; Meyer and Foley 1996; Wilson 1994). There are instances when oxygen or substrate delivery limits energy production; but in low to moderate submaximal exercise, delivery of oxygen and substrate usually closely match the individual fiber's metabolic capacity (Taylor et al. 1996; Weibel 1984)—for most normal activities of daily living in healthy individuals, delivery of oxygen and other substrates is nonlimiting. This issue is nevertheless relevant to rehabilitation. Certain conditions and pathological states (e.g., diabetes mellitus, peripheral vascular disease, genetic metabolic disorders) decrease capacities for diffusion and substrate delivery (Engel and Franzini-Armstrong 1994). In addition, static contractions, by generating sufficient pressure gradients within muscle compartments, can limit vascular perfusion and oxygen delivery—thereby limiting aerobic performance.

The primary fuel for aerobic metabolism is acetyl-CoA, which is metabolized within the mitochondria via the tricarboxylic acid cycle. The electron transport chain uses the resultant reducing equivalents (i.e., NADH) to produce ATP. Acetyl-CoA forms either through the metabolism of pyruvate generated from glycolysis (by pyruvate dehydrogenase) or through the beta oxidation of fatty acids (FA). Glycolytic substrate can be provided from intracellular glycogen stores or from facilitated glucose uptake from the extracellular space. Oxidation of amino acids normally represents only a very small fraction of energy metabolism during contractile activities. Figure 1.4 further delineates the metabolic pathways for energy synthesis (Weibel 1979).

For decades, researchers have studied the regulation of substrates that supply acetyl-CoA for aerobic metabolism; yet the exact mechanisms controlling *in vivo* substrate utilization remain unclear. For a comprehensive discussion of this topic, see extensive reviews concerning integrative exercise physiology (Rowell and Shepherd 1996; Taylor et al. 1996). Substrate utilization studies in humans typically refer to percentages of whole-body maximal oxygen utilization rates, or $\dot{V}O_2$max. It is difficult to extrapolate these findings to substrate use in individual motor units, because the exact muscle mass activated is unknown. Nonetheless, when correlating percent $\dot{V}O_2$max with fiber type glycogen depletion during bicycle ergometry, researchers often consider histochemical and biochemical data from the vastus lateralis to be representative of the motor unit populations recruited (the vastus lateralis is one of the primary movers for this activity). Figure 1.5 depicts the estimated percentages of muscle fiber types recruited at the initiation of cycling (70 rpm) at varying

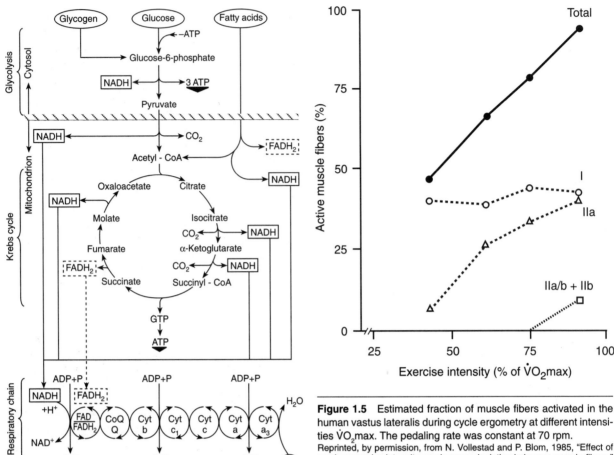

Figure 1.4 The three stages of oxidative metabolism: glycolysis, Krebs tricarboxylic acid cycle, and respiratory chain.
Reprinted, by permission, from E. Weibel, 1979, Oxygen demand and the size of respiratory structures in mammals. In *Evolution of respiratory processes*, edited by S. Wood and C. Lenfant (New York: Marcel Dekker Inc.), 310.

Figure 1.5 Estimated fraction of muscle fibers activated in the human vastus lateralis during cycle ergometry at different intensities $\dot{V}O_2$max. The pedaling rate was constant at 70 rpm.
Reprinted, by permission, from N. Vollestad and P. Blom, 1985, "Effect of varying exercise intensity on glycogen depletion in human muscle fibers," *Acta Physiologica Scandinavica* 125 (3): 402.

percentages of $\dot{V}O_2$max. As predicted, there is a progressive recruitment of type II fibers with increasing intensity. The difficult question is whether motor unit recruitment remains constant. Vollestad and Blom (1985) reported evidence suggestive that a slowly increasing percentage of the vastus lateralis's type IIa fiber population decreased their glycogen stores during a 60-minute protocol at 40% $\dot{V}O_2$max; this pattern was much more prominent at 60% $\dot{V}O_2$max. Meanwhile, the entire type I fiber population was exhibiting a fairly uniform but slower rate of glycogen depletion—implying that recruitment of additional type IIa motor units occurs even during bicycle ergometry protocols of such limited duration and intensity. This potential for changing motor unit recruitment patterns further complicates the interpretation of studies that measure whole-body energy

substrate utilization (Gollnick et al. 1974; Romijn et al. 1993; Vollestad and Blom 1985).

Figure 1.6 illustrates substrate contribution to energy expenditure at varying percentages of $\dot{V}O_2$max, for the first 30 minutes of cycle ergometry. Note the progressive dependence upon muscle glycogen as exercise intensity (i.e., energy utilization rate) increases and also the relatively stable contribution from total calories from plasma glucose and FFAs. As exercise intensity increases, there is greater activation (temporal recruitment) of the initially recruited motor units, as well as additional (spatial) recruitment of less economical and less aerobic motor units (Kernell et al. 1983; Vollestad and Blom 1985).

While the type I fibers recruited at 25% $\dot{V}O_2$max utilize trivial amounts of glycogen, glycogen depletion rates progressively increase as effort increases from 40% to 95% of $\dot{V}O_2$max (see figures 1.5 and 1.6). During bicycle ergometry at 65% of $\dot{V}O_2$max, total glycogen depletion in a portion of type I fibers begins to appear at approximately 60 minutes—with near complete depletion of the type I fiber population of the vastus lateralis by 120 minutes (Gollnick

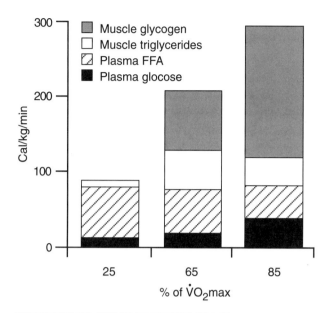

Figure 1.6 Maximal contribution to energy expenditure derived from glucose and FFA taken up from the blood, and minimal contribution of muscle triglyceride and glycogen stores after 30 minutes of cycle ergometry, expressed as a function of exercise intensity.

Reprinted, by permission, from J. Romjin et al., 1993, "Regulation of endogenous fat and carbohydrate metabolism in relation to exercise intensity and duration," *American Journal of Physiology* 266 (3 Pt 1): E387.

et al. 1974). Whole-body measures of glycogen utilization, however, do not remain constant during more prolonged aerobic activity. At moderate intensities, utilization of fatty acids and plasma glucose increases gradually, with a corresponding decrease in glycogen utilization (Coyle 1995; Hargreaves 1997). These changes occur during a period of probable additional type IIa (less economical) fiber recruitment as discussed earlier.

The overall utilization of fatty acids for aerobic metabolism substrate is limited. The traditional view is that beta oxidation is limited by the activity of carnitine palmitoyltransferase (CPT), which transports fatty acids across the mitochondrial membrane (Coyle 1995). CPT activity is inhibited by malonyl-CoA, a precursor for fatty acid synthesis; and since malonyl-CoA concentrations increase in direct proportion to glucose availability (Coyle 1995; Van der Vusse and Reneman 1996), as long as there is adequate glucose there will be relatively limited availability of fatty acids in the mitochondria. Furthermore, free fatty acid binding proteins facilitate the transport of fatty acids through the interstitium as well as the sarcoplasm. Thus, both the delivery and transport of fatty acids may be important in regulating their utilization (Van der Vusse and Reneman 1996).

Since there is some limit to the amount of fatty acids used for aerobic substrate, metabolism of carbohydrate—either glycogen or glucose—must increase as the percentage of $\dot{V}O_2$max increases. Anything that increases use of plasma glucose rather than glycogen would prolong the time to cellular glycogen depletion. During exercise, any one of three factors—supply, transport, and metabolism—may limit glucose uptake. For maximal plasma glucose utilization to occur, all three factors must increase simultaneously (Richter 1996). Changes in levels of hormones that assist aerobic metabolism lead to systemic metabolic responses to exercise. The net effect of these hormonal changes is to increase the local and systemic supply of substrates to feed the aerobic demand of the active skeletal muscle (Wasserman and Cherrington 1996). Later chapters will further delineate these events.

Motor Unit Performance

This section presents a model that integrates energetic characteristics and substrate utilization at the single muscle fiber level with sustainable performance—i.e., the continuous matching of new energy synthesis to the energy demand of contraction. The level of demand is important in both the cell's choice of metabolic substrate and the time until substrate (especially glycogen) depletion. If the demand is beyond the maximum aerobic synthesis capacity of the cell, additional anaerobic energy production must supplement aerobic synthesis in order to maintain energy balance.

As stated earlier, human skeletal muscle fiber types represent a continuum with respect to their energetic characteristics. In order to simplify the discussion, we use the mean energetic and substrate utilization characteristics of the human type I, IIa, and IIb fiber populations. The following tables delineating these characteristics are based primarily upon human skeletal muscle data. While containing some crude extrapolations, the tables represent a fairly realistic picture of the average cellular properties of human fibers. After a brief review of the data within the tables, we discuss what may be occurring within the individual fiber during performance at a set level of demand.

First, compare the energy demands to the energy synthesis capacities for both maximal and submaximal static contractions in the different fiber types. The data for human skeletal muscle in table 1.2 are based on maximum unloaded shortening velocities and on mitochondrial volumes (Hoppeler 1986; Larsson and Moss 1993). Given an absence of definitive

Table 1.2		Energy Utilization and Synthesis Rates During Static Contractions		
Fiber type	Energy demand during maximal static contraction (MVC)	Energy demand at 50% (MVC), 1:1 duty cycle	Maximal aerobic energy synthesis capacity	% synthesis capacity utilized by the 50% MVC, 1:1 duty cycle contraction
I	1 mM ATP/sec	0.25 mM ATP/sec	1.1 mM ATP/sec	23
IIa	3 mM ATP/sec	0.75 mM ATP/sec	0.8 mM ATP/sec	94
IIb	10 mM ATP/sec	2.50 mM ATP/sec	0.4 mM ATP/sec	625

The energy demand estimations used the mean maximum shortening velocity across fiber types (Larsson and Moss 1993) referenced to 1.0 mM/sec tetanic ATP utilization of the cat soleus (Harkema et al. 1997). Mean mitochondrial volumes were used to calculate estimates of maximum aerobic synthesis capacity (Hoppeler 1986).

measurements from human tissue, we referenced the maximum energy utilization rates to the cat soleus (>92% SO) tetanic energy utilization rate at physiologic temperature (Harkema et al. 1997).

The maximal energy demand during static maximal contractions (MVC) for the type I fiber can be matched by its aerobic synthesis capacity. The type IIa and IIb fibers' energy use during maximal static contractions well surpass their maximal ability to aerobically synthesize ATP. Yet rarely does a human muscle work at maximum capacity. During a submaximal static contraction at 50% of MVC and with a 1:1 duty cycle, type I fibers can aerobically synthesize abundantly more ATP than they need; type IIa fibers are approximately balanced between utilization and maximal aerobic production; and type IIb fibers are using more than six times more energy than they can aerobically synthesize. Thus even during a more economical static (vs. shortening) contraction of this limited intensity, only a minority of type IIa and probably no type IIb fibers would be likely to sustain energy balance from purely aerobic metabolism.

Earlier, we looked at whole body substrate utilization during aerobic exercise. But how might the fiber types differ in their individual use of glycogen, fatty acids, and plasma glucose? Table 1.3 depicts the maximal limit for ATP aerobic production capacity from each of these substrates as a function of fiber type (estimated from whole muscle biopsies of the human vastus lateralis) (Hultman and Harris 1988). The individual fiber type data are extrapolations based on the fiber type distribution of the human vastus lateralis and on enzyme characteristics of isolated mammalian fibers (Edgerton et al. 1975; Saltin and Gollnick 1983).

Comparison of the maximal rates in table 1.3 with maximal aerobic synthesis capacities in table 1.2 will reinforce the point that neither plasma glucose nor fatty acids alone can supply the full aerobic energy needs of muscle fiber, regardless of type. Thus as intensity or energy use increases during exercise, the limitation in maximal energy production from glucose and/or fatty acids at the cell level requires an increase in glycogen use. This relationship corresponds well to the direct link between exercise intensity and whole body glycogen substrate use discussed earlier.

Finally, if demand for energy surpasses a cell's capacity for aerobic synthesis during prolonged exercise, anaerobic metabolism must synthesize additional energy simultaneously with aerobic metabolism in order to continue to maintain energy balance. Table 1.4 presents glycogen concentration and total anaerobic ATP production capacity as a function of fiber type. While glycogen concentrations in an individual muscle can vary widely in the rested state, there is little variation across fiber types (Connett and Sahlin 1996). Thus, both the variable cellular concentration of glycogen and its utilization rates from aerobic and anaerobic metabolism are major determinants of the time to glycogen depletion within a skeletal muscle fiber.

Type I Fiber Performance

In the submaximal static contraction under consideration (50% MVC at a 1:1 duty cycle), the type I fiber's energy demand is only 23% of its $\dot{V}O_2$max and can easily maintain an energy balance via aerobic metabolism (table 1.2). Arbitrarily assuming that a

Table 1.3	Maximal Aerobic ATP Production Capacity by Metabolic Substrate		
Fiber type	**Muscle glycogen**	**Plasma glucose**	**Fatty acid**
Whole muscle	0.87 mM ATP/sec	0.32 mM ATP/sec	0.35 mM ATP/sec
I	1.20 mM ATP/sec	0.38 mM ATP/sec	0.45 mM ATP/sec
IIa	0.86 mM ATP/sec	0.38 mM ATP/sec	0.35 mM ATP/sec
IIb	0.43 mM ATP/sec	0.19 mM ATP/sec	0.22 mM ATP/sec

The calculated production capacities were based upon whole muscle ATP utilization rates by substrate per Hultman and Harris (1988). Fiber type estimates used a threefold range for glycogen ATP-based production, a twofold range for plasma glucose-based ATP production between fiber types with no difference between type I and IIa fibers (Richter 1996), and a twofold range for FA-based ATP production (Saltin and Gollnick 1983), combined with the fiber type distribution of vastus lateralis (Edgerton et al. 1975).

Table 1.4	Anaerobic ATP Production Capacity From Glycogen		
Fiber type	**Millimole glycosyl units/kg wet weight**	**Millimolar (mM) glycosyl units**	**Anaerobic ATP production capacity**
I	78	116	348 mM ATP
IIa	83	124	372 mM ATP
IIb	89	133	399 mM ATP

Conversion calculations utilized 0.67 liters of intracellular water/kg skeletal muscle wet weight and 3 ATP per glycosyl unit anaerobic glycolytic energy production. Fiber type specific glycogen content was obtained from Saltin and Gollnick (1983).

constant 40% of the energy production results from glycogen-based aerobic ATP production, there would be 0.1 mM ATP/sec synthesis from glycogen metabolism (see table 1.2: 40% of 0.25 mM ATP/sec = 0.1 mM/sec). With 38 mM ATP aerobically generated per mM glycosyl unit (Weibel 1979), it would take approximately 12 hours for a type I fiber to deplete itself of the 116 mM of the glycosyl units derivable from its glycogen stores (see table 1.4: 38 mM ATP/mM glycosyl unit × 116 mM glycosyl units/0.1 mM ATP/sec). By increasing plasma glucose and fatty acid substrate utilization, the cell could even further prolong the time to glycogen depletion. This correlates well with data that show minimal glycogen depletion in type I fibers at lower levels of aerobic exercise. Even after glycogen depletion, sufficient flux of substrate (plasma glucose and fatty acids) into the Krebs cycle could theoretically match the energy demand at this intensity (see tables 1.2 and 1.3). Clearly, greater energy and glycogen utilization rates must be occurring during the shortening contractions of human cycle ergometry at 60% of $\dot{V}O_2$max in or-

der to deplete the glycogen stores of the type I fiber population within a couple of hours (Vollestad and Blom 1985).

Type IIa Fiber Performance

In comparison, the type IIa fiber is nearly at its maximum capacity for aerobic energy synthesis during the submaximal static contraction depicted in table 1.2, reflecting its decreased economy and aerobic capacity. The result is an increased rate of glycogen utilization. Assuming again that 40% of the aerobic energy production is derived from glycogen substrate (table 1.2: 40% of 0.8 mM/sec = 0.32 mM/sec), the calculated rate of aerobic energy production from glycogen would be about 0.3 mM ATP/sec, which would deplete its glycogen stores in approximately four hours (table 1.4: 38 mM ATP/glycosyl unit × 124 glycosyl units /0.3 mM ATP/sec). Theoretically, as the glycogen stores become depleted, even the combined potential maximal ATP production from plasma glucose

(0.38 mM/sec according to table 1.3) and fatty acid oxidation (0.35 mM/sec) would not quite be able to meet the energy demand of 0.75 mM ATP/sec (0.38 + 0.35 = 0.73).

Type IIb Fiber Performance

The type IIb fiber has an extremely limited capacity for aerobic metabolism (table 1.2). Coupled with its decreased economy (10 times higher energy demand compared to type I fibers), this results in an inability to achieve energy balance via aerobic metabolism alone in our model (50% of MVC, 1:1 duty cycle static contraction). If aerobic and anaerobic metabolism were able to use the entire glycogen supply to support this contraction intensity, glycogen would be depleted in a matter of a few minutes. Assuming the fiber is using its maximal aerobic energy synthesis of 0.4 mM ATP/sec, another 2.1 mM ATP/sec must come from anaerobic metabolism to balance the energy demand of 2.5 mM/sec (table 1.2). At these rates, glycogen stores would be depleted at a rate as high as 0.01 mM glycosyl units/sec for aerobic substrate (arbitrarily assuming greater than 50%-90% of the aerobic substrate is glycogen, 90% $\times$ 0.4 mM ATP/sec / 38 mM ATP/mM glycosyl unit = 0.01 mM glycosyl units/sec) and 0.7 mM glycosyl units/sec for anaerobic substrate (2.1 mM ATP/sec/3 mM ATP/mM glycosyl unit = 0.7 mM glycosyl units/sec). This would deplete the cell's glycogen stores in approximately 3 minutes: 0.01 mM/sec (aerobic) + 0.7 mM/sec (anaerobic) = 0.71 mM/sec, which uses up all the 133 mM of glycosyl units (see table 1.4) in 187 seconds. These calculations vividly demonstrate the inefficiency associated with anaerobic energy production.

It is unclear to what degree the cell might be able to utilize the additional reducing equivalents generated by the increased glycolytic flux to generate ATP through the respiratory chain (see figure 1.4). This potential could reduce the rate of glycogen use by over 50%. These estimates of the human type IIb fiber's energetic characteristics correlate well with *in vivo* human studies. For example, the human flexor digitorum profundus (ulnar division) cannot maintain a steady-state energy balance solely from aerobic metabolism beyond an approximate 0.3 mM ATP/sec energy utilization rate during twitch stimulation (Blei et al. 1993; Jeneson et al. 1997). Thus, type IIb fibers have an extremely limited capacity for sustaining any repetitive functional activity. At the intensity of the submaximal static contraction (table 1.2), a duty cycle of approximately 1:6 would be necessary to maintain an energy balance via aerobic me-

tabolism alone—yet such a duty cycle is hardly realistic for functional movement.

If aerobic metabolism cannot meet the energy demand, glycolytic flux can increase to meet the demand by anaerobically synthesizing ATP as was presented for the type IIb fiber above. The maximum achievable anaerobic glycolytic flux varies with the fiber type, the highest rates being in the type IIb fibers (Connett and Sahlin 1996). However, anaerobic energy production cannot continue indefinitely. Glycogen supplies are limited, and the excess pyruvate is metabolized to lactic acid. The extent and rate of cellular acidification depends upon the rate of glycolytic flux, the buffering capacity, hydrogen ion exchange systems, and local perfusion (Juel 1997; Kemp et al. 1993). For reasons that are not entirely clear, skeletal muscle performance deteriorates during progressive acidification.

Glycogen depletion does occur in human skeletal muscle, potentially reducing the cell's maximal aerobic energy synthesis capacity if it is relying solely on aerobic synthesis from available glucose and FA substrate. Without glycogen, however, the cell's capacity for anaerobic energy production would be dramatically reduced—limited by the capacity for glucose transport. Energy balance may not be maintained; any remaining supply of PCr would be quickly depleted; and continued ATP utilization would quickly lead to depletion of cellular ATP. But this depletion has not been observed to a significant degree. Energy use or performance must therefore be curtailed prior to cellular depletion of ATP, as will be discussed in the next section.

Skeletal Muscle Fatigue

Fatigue is an acute impairment of performance that includes both an increase in the perceived effort necessary to exert a desired force and an eventual inability to produce this force (Enoka and Stuart 1992). We will discuss only events occurring at the level of the skeletal muscle, particularly with respect to its cellular energetics—actin-myosin cross-bridge function, calcium activation of the contractile process, and excitation-contraction coupling failure have all been implicated. For more detailed discussions on the current understanding of neuromuscular fatigue, see recent reviews (Fitts 1994; Gandevia et al. 1995; Williams and Klug 1995).

Contractile activity leads to the buildup of hydrogen ion (H^+), inorganic phosphate (Pi), ADP, and creatine. Researchers have extensively studied how these metabolic products interact with actin-myosin cross-bridge function. Isolated single glycerinated fiber studies initially showed that H$^+$ and Pi (but not ADP or creatine) strongly inhibit maximal force production at physiologic concentrations (Fitts 1994). In order to maintain preparation stability, however, researchers have used temperatures lower than *in vivo*; and recent experiments have shown that the single fiber inhibition by H$^+$ is temperature dependent—H$^+$ has little or no effect on maximal force generation or speed of shortening at physiologic temperatures (Pate et al. 1995; Wiseman et al. 1996). Inhibition of maximal force production by Pi is well attested in isolated single glycerinated fibers, but also at less than physiologic temperatures. Initiation of the powerstroke releases inorganic phosphate from the actin-myosin complex. The increasing Pi concentration increases the fraction of actin-myosin cross

bridges in the weakly bound prepowerstroke state, thus decreasing force production (Fitts 1994). These studies have yet to be performed at physiologic temperatures. Adams and colleagues (1991) investigated metabolic inhibition by H$^+$ and Pi *in vitro*, using an isolated perfused whole muscle preparation during normocapnic or hypercapnic perfusion. Hypercapnic perfusion leads to passive acidification of the preparation. The experiment demonstrated no direct relationship between maximum force and Pi concentrations over the vast majority of the physiologic range at near-physiologic temperature (see figure 1.7A). The dramatic decrease in force occurs at the point where Pi concentrations are approaching the resting Pi plus PCr concentration—i.e., when PCr has been nearly depleted. While there is a strong linear correlation between force and intracellular pH in figure 1.7B during stimulated contraction, acidification of

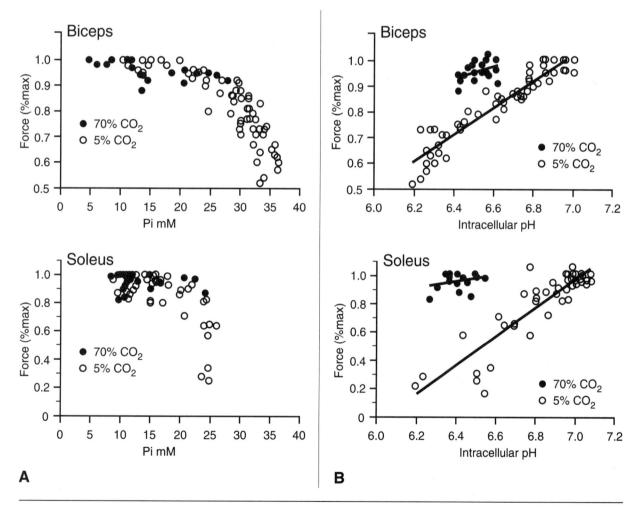

A   **B**

Figure 1.7 Relationships between the metabolic products, Pi and H$^+$ (expressed as pH), and peak tetanic force in the isolated cat biceps brachii and soleus during normocapnic ($\bigcirc$) or hypercapnic ($\bullet$) perfusion. Pooled results from four muscles are shown.
Reprinted, by permission, from G. Adams, M. Fisher, and R. Meyer, 1991, "Hypercapnic acidosis and increased H2PO4- concentration do not decrease force in cat skeletal muscle," *American Journal of Physiology* 260 (4 Pt 1): C810.

the cell with hypercapnic perfusion has minimal effects on *maximal* force production in either muscle. There are no conclusive data to suggest a difference in proton handling by the cell during acidification induced by normal contraction vs. by hypercapnic perfusion. Emerging from these studies is the general conclusion that metabolic products might have a more limited role in the direct *in vivo* inhibition of cross-bridge function than previously proposed, particularly with respect to effects on maximal force generation and speed of shortening.

Products of metabolism have also been strongly implicated in altering cellular calcium sensitivity and kinetics, in two ways. (1) The extent of activation of the actin-myosin interaction is directly dependent upon the free intracellular calcium concentration—and single fiber studies have shown that both H^+ and P_i decrease the sensitivity of calcium in contractile activation (Fitts 1994; Westerblad and Allen 1993).

Thus, at least during submaximal exercise, metabolic product accumulation may decrease performance and require additional temporal and spatial recruitment of motor units in order to achieve the same force output. Increasing concentrations of H^+ also correlate with increasing the time to achieve relaxation of the muscle postcontraction—significantly influencing dynamic performance (Enoka and Stuart 1992; Westerblad et al. 1991). (2) Failure of excitation-contraction coupling may be a major mechanism of skeletal muscle fatigue. Much of the evidence for this comes from a classic series of *in vitro* experiments using single intact muscle fibers. Figure 1.8 demonstrates the essential features of these experiments in a single mouse muscle fiber. The fiber is undergoing an intense intermittent progressive tetanic stimulation protocol (at 20° Celsius) designed to produce significant force failure in fibers of different metabolic properties (Westerblad and Allen 1991). In figure 1.8A, the

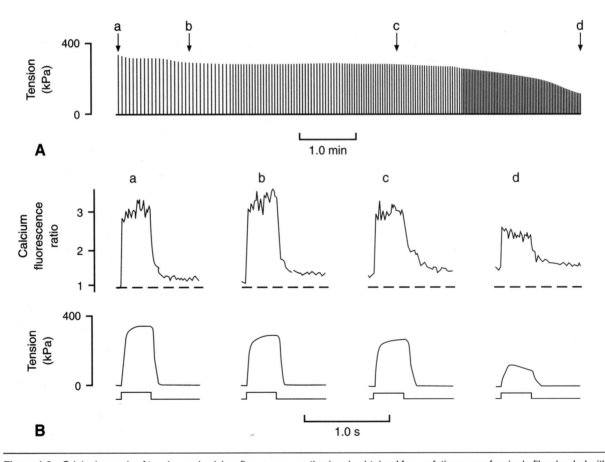

Figure 1.8 Original records of tension and calcium fluorescence ratio signals obtained from a fatigue run of a single fiber loaded with fura-2 AM (a fluorescence emitting cation indicator). (A) Continuous tension record: each tetanus appearing as a vertical line. (B) Tension and fluorescence ratio signals from specific contractions indicated above the continuous tension record in (A). The dashed lines in (B) represent the resting calcium fluorescence ratio before fatiguing stimulation. Stimulation periods are shown below the tension records.

Reprinted, by permission, from H. Westerblad and D. Allen, 1991, "Changes of myoplasmic calcium concentration during fatigue in single mouse muscle fibers," *Journal of General Physiology* 98 (3): 622.

fiber begins to develop significant tension failure 6-7 minutes into the protocol (about halfway between c and d). Note the significant decline both in free intracellular calcium-dependent fluorescence ratio and in tension (figure 1.8B) at the point of prominent force failure as depicted by contraction d in figure 1.8A. With addition of caffeine to the perfusate during this time of force failure, force generation returns to baseline levels (not shown). Caffeine stimulates the direct release of calcium from the sarcoplasmic reticulum, thereby bypassing the excitation-contraction mechanism. These experiments directly imply failure of the excitation-contraction coupling process. Recovery of this altered excitation-contraction function does not occur for many hours—possibly beyond 24 hours (Edwards et al. 1977; Westerblad et al. 1993). Recovery has not been shown to be temporally related to energetic metabolite recovery—suggesting a more structural source of the dysfunction.

No experimental data have yet fully explained the mechanism(s) of activity-induced failure of excitation-contraction coupling (both acute and prolonged) or of alterations in cellular calcium kinetics. Both of these processes appear to be very important in human skeletal muscle fatigue—however this is growing evidence that both progressive accumulation of metabolic products and energy balance failure are involved in regulating both the release/reuptake of intracellular calcium and the sensitivity of the activation of contraction to free calcium (Fitts 1994; Gandevia et al. 1995; Williams and Klug 1995).

Energy Recovery

The time required for energy recovery depends on the extent of cellular energy depletion, the metabolites involved, and the fiber types involved.

Phosphocreatine

The creatine kinase reaction (a near equilibrium reaction) breaks down and synthesizes phosphocreatine (Meyer et al. 1984). By mass action, the hydrogen ion concentration will influence the concentration of ADP (where k is the equilibrium constant).

$$[ADP] = [ATP][creatine]/k[H^+][PCr]$$

While the exact mechanism of mitochondrial regulation has yet to be established, it seems certain that

the ADP concentration is important and varies directly with the rate of mitochondrial respiration. Increased H^+ concentration results in a decreased ADP concentration—which potentially provides a mechanism for the slowed energy recovery seen with cellular acidosis.

The actual time constant of PCr recovery varies among fiber types, depending upon their mitochondrial density. In the average human muscle at a neutral pH of 7.0-7.1, the time constant of recovery for type I fibers is about 15-20 seconds; the type IIb time constant is just over 1 minute (Blei et al. 1993). As discussed previously, aerobic energy production (and thus PCr recovery) slows with cellular acidification, resulting in a nearly 30% lengthening of the initial time constant of PCr recovery for every 0.1 pH unit acidification (Bendahan et al. 1990).

pH

Cellular pH regulation and cellular recovery from acidification are complex processes (Juel 1997; Kemp et al. 1993). The cytosol has a fairly powerful acid/base buffering system, composed primarily of intracellular proteins, inorganic phosphates, and sugar phosphates. This buffering system decreases the change in pH for a given H^+ load. Human skeletal muscle has an apparent buffer capacity of approximately 20 mmol/L/1.0 pH unit at rest (Conley et al. 1997; Kemp et al. 1993). A rise in inorganic phosphate and sugar phosphate concentrations during contraction will lead to a significant increase in the cell's buffer capacity. In addition, the dissociation constant of inorganic phosphate depends on cellular pH. Thus, the buffer capacity is quite dynamic during and following a muscular contraction (Conley et al. 1997). In addition to the buffering capacity, pH equilibrium is maintained by lactate/H^+ cotransport, HCO_3^-/Cl^-, and Na^+/H^+ exchange (Juel 1997; Kemp et al. 1993). Along with the postcontraction increase in vascular perfusion and its equilibrium with the extracellular space, these mechanisms combine to achieve a near linear recovery of 0.06 pH units/minute for *in vivo* human muscle (Arnold et al. 1984). While there are few data on human fiber type differences, Juel (1997) reported that the total capacity for pH regulation is greater in slow-twitch than in fast-twitch mammalian muscle fibers.

Glycogen

Prolonged or high-intensity exercise can deplete intracellular glycogen stores. Glycogen synthesis capacity is only one-tenth the glycogenolysis capacity in human skeletal muscle (Connett and Sahlin 1996). The intracellular glycogen concentration, the phosphorylation of glycogen synthase, concentrations of glucose-6-phosphate and UDP-glucose, and even dietary intake combine to control the glycogen synthesis rate (Connett and Sahlin 1996). Recovery to basal conditions occurs over 24 hours, with the highest rates of resynthesis in the first hour of recovery. Following prominent depletion, diet manipulations can actually boost the intracellular glycogen concentration to more than twice pre-exercise levels over a two- to three-day period (Coyle 1995) in all human fiber types.

Clinical Considerations

The basic paradigm of chemical energy balance applies to all skeletal muscle in both health and disease. To sustain force production in any motor unit, there must be a balance between energy use and energy synthesis. Clinical symptoms of fatigue or signs of skeletal muscle force generation failure occur when energy balance cannot be maintained. To maximize movement, clinicians must understand the current energy state of muscle fibers, the intensity of muscle contractions with respect to motor unit recruitment, and the time required for energy recovery. By keeping these considerations in mind, health care professionals can prescribe appropriate durations of effort, as well as rest between bouts of exercise, to restore functional movement or achieve therapeutic goals.

Over the past decade, P^{31} MRS has proved very useful in bioenergetic studies of human muscle diseases. Pathologic disorders of human skeletal muscle almost always have identifiable alterations in their bioenergetic state, with the majority having a decreased capacity for energy production (Argov and Bank 1991; Bendahan et al. 1993; Radda and Taylor 1985; Radda et al. 1989). A striking example of such studies is one that evaluated carriers of the Beckers and Duchenne muscular dystrophy genetic defects. Although these muscles appear clinically normal—in bedside exams, with routine histochemical analyses, and with electrodiagnostic analyses—Barbiroli et al. (1992) found their energetic states to be abnormal. Specific muscle diseases and genetic defects in energy metabolism are relatively rare, however, in comparison with either the sarcopenia seen in aging populations or with normal adaptation to disuse. Clinically relevant muscle atrophy is common. Yet the basic clinical issue remains the same. What is the capacity of the least economical motor unit recruited to maintain energy balance? When it cannot maintain balance, the motor unit experiences force failure and overall performance begins to deteriorate. Deteriorating functional capacity of the muscle increases the risk of injury, and eventually the patient loses the capacity to maintain the desired function.

Most rehabilitative efforts require submaximal levels of the whole-body aerobic capacity. Yet even though an activity may require only a small portion of the total body exercise capacity, biomechanical inefficiency and/or loss of muscle mass (or neuronal supply limitation) can make even a basic activity of daily living into an intense effort for individual muscle groups. For example, walking at 3.5 mph would require intense effort from the gluteus maximus in patients with proximal muscular atrophy and a forward center of gravity.

Intense effort at the individual muscle level uses motor units of lower aerobic capacity and economy. Thus, only a few seconds of net muscular contraction time can evoke anaerobic glycolytic flux to synthesize new ATP in order to maintain energy balance (Conley et al. 1997). In repetitive activities, muscular contraction time depends on the duty cycle of the activity. If the activity is terminated prior to substantial acidification, 95% recovery of the cell's energetic perturbation will occur in approximately 3-4 minutes in normal skeletal muscle—although this level of recovery may take 3-4 times longer for mitochondrial disorders involving skeletal muscle (Radda and Taylor 1985). If time for full recovery is allowed, this repetitive contractile effort can continue almost indefinitely for functional or therapeutic activities. If, however, the muscle contraction causes net muscle acidification at a rate greater than approximately 0.06 pH units/min (greater than approximately a net 0.1 mM ATP/sec produced from anaerobic metabolism), progressive cellular acidosis occurs. With prominent cellular acidification or activity to fatigue, recovery of phosphocreatine is prolonged up to 2-3 times; and full pH recovery occurs over approximately 20 minutes under normal local perfusion characteristics (Arnold et al. 1984; Bendahan et al. 1990). When allowed full recovery, therefore, normal muscle can complete only 2-3 bouts of high-intensity activity per hour—with even fewer bouts possible in states involving muscle pathology or limitations for oxygen delivery.

Skeletal muscle performance declines during intense exercise from several sources. Submaximal performance likely deteriorates because metabolic byproducts (Pi and H^+) competitively inhibit free calcium activation of cross-bridge cycling (Westerblad and Allen 1993).

On the other hand, deterioration in maximum performance at the muscle level is being strongly linked to failure of excitation-contraction coupling (Meyer and Foley 1996; Williams and Klug 1995). It is clinically important to appreciate that full recovery after extremes of fatigue, thought related to the excitation-contraction coupling failure, may take many hours and possibly even a day or more to occur (Edwards et al. 1977; Westerblad et al. 1993). In addition, intense exercise bouts repeated frequently throughout the day can deplete cell glycogen. Its depletion decreases the cell's capacity for both aerobic and anaerobic energy production and thus the cell's capacity to sustain energy balance throughout an intermittent intense contractile activity. With energy balance failure, performance must decline.

Thus with activities requiring intense efforts, you as a clinician must first determine your patient's primary therapeutic or functional goal. Short-term goals often revolve around strategies to attain or preserve functional movement at a given physiologic state, whereas longer-term goals focus upon skeletal muscle's plasticity for adaptation. When attaining the therapeutic goal requires that your patient perform intense effort (even for basic functions of daily living) several times per hour, you must consider the energetic constraints. First, establish the appropriate frequency and duration for the repetitive activity. Then, create a structure that maximizes functional performance while limiting the risk of injury and the development of excitation-contraction coupling failure. You often must educate and enlist the help of allied support staff and the patient's family.

During prolonged endurance activities, energy balance maintenance relies primarily on aerobic metabolism. When the energetics of skeletal muscle limits endurance, you can use different approaches to achieve an energy balance in the recruited musculature. For example, use interval training to exercise the recruited motor units at the intensity required for full functional movement, then have the patient rest until energy recovery. This establishes a repeatable work/rest duty cycle. Relate the intensity of effort to the duration of each movement, and either end it or reduce the intensity just short of energy failure. This technique has the probable advantage of giving the greatest number of signals for adaptation.

It is possible, however, that other strategies might be more functional for a given patient, or that the skeletal muscle's adaptation capacity is limited or already maximized. For example, a function requiring sustained repetitive movements (e.g., shoulder stabilization during eating) may not lend itself to the interrupted activity described above. Or, as in many

muscle diseases, muscle economy may already be maximized with near complete phenotypic expression of type I fibers. As an alternative to the repeatable work/rest duty cycle, increase the rest phase of each cycle to the point where all recruited motor units can maintain energy balance (unless the full duty cycle would take so long as to be impractical). Another potential strategy is to limit the force requirement of the maneuver by, for example, lowering the resistance or decreasing the body weight being borne. This decreases the energy demand and uses more economical and aerobic motor units. This approach, however, promotes muscular adaptation only in the recruited motor units.

Unfortunately, it is often difficult at the bedside to fully ascertain a patient's degree of muscle atrophy and the corresponding intensity of contraction that will be required for any specific muscle during prescribed activities. However, with an understanding of the kinesiology and the energetics involved, you can learn to appreciate limitations imposed by energetic constraints during therapeutic activities and to adapt the patient's treatments accordingly. The clinician should also realize that the adaptation capacity of the components of energy balance—energy utilization and energy synthesis—appear to be independently regulated, with different time courses of expression (Booth and Baldwin 1996; Williams and Neufer 1996).

Summary

Energy balance is essential to maintain skeletal muscle performance in both health and disease. Pathological states often amplify the limitations of the energy system or require increased intensity of effort for a muscle, often beyond its metabolic capacity for energy balance. The skeletal muscle cell's energy demand during contraction depends on its phenotypic economy, the intensity and type of contraction, and the duty cycle of repetition. The energy demand, in turn, sets the rate of the cell's energy synthesis. The duration of sustainable effort for a motor unit or muscle fiber depends on the ability to maintain sufficient energy synthesis to match the energy utilization or demand. Rehabilitation strategies should use the principles of energy balance to optimize current function and cellular adaptation.

References

Adams, G.R., M.J. Fisher, and R.A. Meyer. 1991. Hypercapnic acidosis and increased $H_2PO_4^-$ concentration do not decrease force in cat skeletal muscle. *Am J Physiol* 260(4 Pt 1):C805-12.

Argov, Z., and W.J. Bank. 1991. Phosphorus magnetic resonance spectroscopy (31P MRS) in neuromuscular disorders. *Ann Neurol* 30:90-97.

Arnold, D.L., P.M. Matthews, and G.K. Radda. 1984. Metabolic recovery after exercise and the assessment of mitochondrial function in vivo in human skeletal muscle by means of 31P NMR. *Magn Reson Med* 1:307-15.

Barany, M. 1967. ATPase activity of myosin correlated with speed of muscle shortening. *J Gen Physiol* 50(Suppl.):197-218.

Barbiroli, B., R. Funicello, A. Ferlini, P. Montagna, and P. Zaniol. 1992. Muscle energy metabolism in female DMD/BMD carriers: a 31P-MR spectroscopy study. *Muscle Nerve* 15:344-48.

Barnard, R.J., V.R. Edgerton, T. Furukawa, and J.B. Peter. 1971. Histochemical, biochemical and contractile properties of red, white, and intermediate fibers. *Am J Physiol* 220:410-14.

Bendahan, D., S. Confort-Gouny, G. Kozak-Reiss, and P.J. Cozzone. 1990. Heterogeneity of metabolic response to muscular exercise in humans. New criteria of invariance defined by in vivo phosphorus-31 NMR spectroscopy. *FEBS Lett* 272:155-58.

Bendahan, D., S. Confort-Gouny, G. Kosak-Ribbens, and P.J. Cozzone. 1993. Investigation of metabolic myopathies by P-31 MRS using a standardized rest-exercise-recovery protocol: a survey of 800 explorations. *MAGMA* 1:91-104.

Blei, M.L., K.E. Conley, and M.J. Kushmerick. 1993. Separate measures of ATP utilization and recovery in human skeletal muscle. *J Physiol (Lond)* 465:203-22.

Booth, F.W., and K.M. Baldwin. 1996. Muscle plasticity: energy demand and supply processes. In *Handbook of physiology*, section 12, *Exercise: Regulation and integration of multiple systems*, ed. L.B. Rowell and J.T. Shepherd, 1098-1123. Bethesda, MD: American Physiological Society.

Boska, M. 1991. Estimating the ATP cost of force production in the human gastrocnemius/soleus muscle group using 31P MRS and 1H MRI. *NMR Biomed* 4:173-81.

Boska, M. 1994. ATP production rates as a function of force level in the human gastrocnemius/soleus using 31P MRS. *Magn Reson Med* 32:1-10.

Burke, R.E., D.N. Levine, P. Tsairis, and F.E. Zajac. 1973. Physiological types and histochemical profiles in motor units of cat gastrocnemius. *J Physiol (Lond)* 234:723-48.

Burke, R.E., D.N. Levine, F.E. Zajac, P. Tsairis, and W. K. Engel. 1971. Mammalian motor units: physiological-histochemical correlation in three types in cat gastrocnemius. *Science* 174:709-12.

Conley, K.E., M.L. Blei, T.L. Richards, M.J. Kushmerick, and S.A. Jubrias. 1997. Activation of glycolysis in human muscle in vivo. *Am J Physiol* 273(1 Pt 1):C306-15.

Connett, R.J., and K. Sahlin. 1996. Control of glycolysis and glycogen metabolism. In *Handbook of physiology*, section 12, *Exercise: Regulation and integration of multiple systems*, ed. L.B.

Rowell and J.T. Shepherd, 870-911. Bethesda, MD: American Physiological Society.

Coyle, E.F. 1995. Substrate utilization during exercise in active people. *Am J Clin Nutr* 61(4 Suppl):968S-979S.

Dubowitz, V. 1985. *Muscle biopsy: A practical approach*. 2d ed. London: Bailliere Tindall.

Edgerton, V.R., J.L. Smith, and D.R. Simpson. 1975. Muscle fibre type populations of human leg muscles. *Histochem J* 7:259-66.

Edstrom, L., E. Hultman, K. Sahlin, and H. Sjoholm. 1982. The contents of high-energy phosphates in different fibre types in skeletal muscles from rat, guinea-pig and man. *J Physiol (Lond)* 332:47-58.

Edwards, R.H.T., D.K. Hill, D.A. Jones, and P.A. Merton. 1977. Fatigue of long duration in human skeletal muscle after exercise. *J Physiol (Lond)* 272:769-78.

Engel, A.G., and C. Franzini-Armstrong. 1994. *Myology*. 2d ed. New York: McGraw-Hill.

Enoka, R.M., and D.G. Stuart. 1992. Neurobiology of muscle fatigue. *J Appl Physiol* 72:1631-48.

Fitts, R.H. 1994. Cellular mechanisms of muscle fatigue. *Physiol Rev* 74:49-94.

Gandevia, S.C., R.M. Enoka, A.J. McComas, D.G. Stuart, and C.K. Thomas, eds. 1995. *Fatigue: Neural and muscular mechanisms*. Vol. 384, *Advances in experimental medicine and biology*. New York: Plenum Press.

Gollnick, P.D., K. Piehl, and B. Saltin. 1974. Selective glycogen depletion pattern in human muscle fibres after exercise of varying intensity and at varying pedalling rates. *J Physiol (Lond)* 241:45-57.

Hargreaves, M. 1997. Interactions between muscle glycogen and blood glucose during exercise. *Exerc Sport Sci Rev* 25:21-39.

Harkema, S.J., G.R. Adams, and R.A. Meyer. 1997. Acidosis has no effect on the ATP cost of contraction in cat fast- and slow-twitch skeletal muscles. *Am J Physiol* 272(2 Pt 1):C485-90.

Harris, R., E. Hultman, and L.O. Nordesjo. 1974. Glycogen, glycolytic intermediates and high energy phosphates determined in biopsy samples of musculus quadriceps femoris of man at rest. Methods and variance of values. *Scand Clin Lab Invest* 33:109-20.

Hoppeler, H. 1986. Exercise-induced ultrastructural changes in skeletal muscle. *Intl J Sports Med* 7:187-204.

Howald, H., H. Hoppeler, H. Claassen, O. Mathieu, and R. Straub. 1985. Influences of endurance training on the ultrastructural composition of the different muscle fiber types in humans. *Pflugers Arch (Lond)* 403:369-76.

Hultman, E., and R.C. Harris. 1988. Carbohydrate metabolism. In *Principles of exercise biochemistry*, ed. J.R. Poortman, 78-119. Basel: Karger.

Jeneson, J.A., R.W. Wiseman, and M.J. Kushmerick. 1997. Non-invasive quantitative 31P MRS assay of mitochondrial function in skeletal muscle in situ. *Mol Cell Biochem* 174:17-22.

Jeneson, J.A.L., R.W. Wiseman, H.V. Westerhoff, and M.J. Kushmerick. 1996. The signal transduction function for oxidative phosphorylation is at least second order in ADP. *J Biol Chem* 271:27995-98.

Johnson, M.A., J. Polgar, D. Weightman, and D. Appleton. 1973. Data on the distribution of fibre types in thirty-six human muscles. An autopsy study. *J Neurol Sci* 18:111-29.

Juel, C. 1997. Lactate-proton cotransport in skeletal muscle. *Physiol Rev* 77:321-58.

Kemp, G.J., D. Taylor, P. Styles, and G.K. Radda. 1993. The production, buffering and efflux of protons in human skeletal muscle during exercise and recovery. *NMR Biomed* 6:73-83.

Kernell, D., O. Eerbeek, and B.A. Verhey. 1983. Relation between isometric force and stimulus rate in cat's hindlimb motor units of different twitch contraction time. *Exp Brain Res* 50:220-27.

Kushmerick, M.J. 1977. Energy balance in muscle contraction: a biochemical approach. In *Current topics in bioenergetics*, ed. R. Sanadi. New York: Academic Press.

Kushmerick, M.J. 1995. Bioenergetics and muscle cell types. In *Fatigue: Neural and muscular mechanisms*, ed. S.C. Gandevia, R.M. Enoka, A.J. McComas, D.G. Stuart, and C.K. Thomas. New York: Plenum Press.

Kushmerick, M.J., and R.E. Davies. 1969. The chemical energetics of muscle contraction. II. The chemistry, efficiency and power of maximally working sartorius muscles. Appendix. Free energy and enthalpy of ATP hydrolysis in the sarcoplasm. *Proc R Soc B Biol* 174:315-53.

Kushmerick, M.J., T.S. Moerland, and R.W. Wiseman. 1992. Mammalian skeletal muscle fibers distinguished by contents of PCr, ATP and Pi. *Proc Natl Acad Sci U S A* 89:7521-25.

Larsson, L., and R.L. Moss. 1993. Maximum velocity of shortening in relation to myosin isoform composition in single fibres from human skeletal muscles. *J Physiol (Lond)* 472:595-614.

Lipmann, F. 1941. Metabolic generation and utilization of phosphate bond energy. In *Advances in enzymology*, vol. 1, ed. F.F. Nord and C.H. Werkman, 99-162. New York: Intersciences.

Lowey, S., G.S. Waller, and K.M. Trybus. 1993. Function of skeletal muscle myosin heavy and light chain isoforms by an in vitro motility assay. *J Biol Chem* 268:20414-18.

McCormack, J.G., A.P. Halestrap, and R.M. Denton. 1990. Role of calcium ions in regulation of mammalian intramitochondrial metabolism. *Physiol Rev* 70:391-425.

Meyer, R., and J Foley. 1996. Cellular processes integrating the metabolic response to exercise. In *Handbook of physiology*, section 12, *Exercise: Regulation and integration of multiple systems*, ed. L.B. Rowell and J.T. Shepherd, 841-69. Bethesda, MD: American Physiological Society.

Meyer, R.A., H.L. Sweeney, and M.J. Kushmerick. 1984. A simple analysis of the "phosphocreatine shuttle". *Am J Physiol* 246(5 Pt 1):C365-77.

Mizuno, M., N.H. Secher, and B. Quistorff. 1994. 31P-NMR spectroscopy, rsEMG, and histochemical fiber types of human wrist flexor muscles. *J Appl Physiol* 76:531-38.

Pate, E., M. Bhimani, K. Franks-Skiba, and R. Cooke. 1995. Reduced effect of pH on skinned rabbit psoas muscle mechanics at high temperatures: implications for fatigue. *J Physiol (Lond)* 486(Pt 3):689-94.

Peter, J.B., R.J. Barnard, V.R. Edgerton, C.A. Gilespie, and K.E. Stempel. 1972. Metabolic profiles of three fiber types of skeletal muscles in guinea pigs and rabbits. *Biochemistry* 11:2627-33.

Pette, D., and R.S. Staron. 1990. Cellular and molecular diversity of mammalian skeletal muscle fibers. *Rev Physiol Biochem Pharmacol* 116:1-76.

Radda, G.K., B. Rajagopalan, and D.J. Taylor. 1989. Biochemistry in vivo: an appraisal of clinical magnetic resonance spectroscopy. *Magn Reson Q* 5:22-51.

Radda, G.K., and D.J. Taylor. 1985. Applications of nuclear magnetic resonance spectroscopy in pathology. *Int Rev Exp Path* 27:1-58.

Rall, J.A. 1985. Energetic aspects of skeletal muscle contraction: implications of fiber types. *Exerc Sport Sci Rev* 13:33-74.

Richter, E.A. 1996. Glucose utilization. In *Handbook of physiology*, section 12, *Exercise: Regulation and integration of multiple systems*, ed. L.B. Rowell and J.T. Shepherd, 912-951. Bethesda, MD: American Physiological Society.

Romijn, J.A., E.F. Coyle, L.S. Sidossis, A. Gastaldelli, J.F. Horowitz, E. Endert, and R.R. Wolfe. 1993. Regulation of endogenous fat and carbohydrate metabolism in relation to exercise intensity and duration. *Am J Physiol* 265(3 Pt 1): E380-91.

Rowell, L.B., and J.T. Shepherd, eds. 1996. In *Handbook of physiology*, section 12, *Exercise: Regulation and integration of multiple systems*. Bethesda, MD: American Physiological Society.

Saltin, B., and P.D. Gollnick. 1983. Skeletal muscle adaptability: significance for metabolism and performance. In *Handbook of physiology*, section 10, *Skeletal muscle*, ed. L.D. Peachey, R.H. Adrian, and S.R. Geiger, 555-631. Bethesda, MD: American Physiological Society.

Schwerzmann, K., H. Hoppeler, S.R. Kayar, and E.R. Weibel. 1989. Oxidative capacity of muscle and mitochondria: correlation of physiological, biochemical, and morphometric characteristics. *Proc Intl Acad Sci U S A* 86:1583-87.

Tamura, M., O. Hazeki, S. Nioka, and B. Chance. 1989. In vivo study of tissue oxygen metabolism using optical and nuclear magnetic resonance spectroscopies. *Annu Rev Physiol* 51:813-34.

Taylor, C.R., E.R. Weibel, J.M. Weber, R. Vock, H. Hoppeler, T.J. Roberts, and G. Brichon. 1996. Design of the oxygen and substrate pathways. I. Model and strategy to test symmorphosis in a network structure. *J Exp Biol* 199(Pt 8):1643-49.

Van der Vusse, G.J., and R.S. Reneman. 1996. Lipid metabolism in muscle. In *Handbook of physiology*, section 12, *Exercise:*

Regulation and integration of multiple systems. Bethesda, MD: American Physiological Society.

Vollestad, N.K., and P.C. Blom. 1985. Effect of varying exercise intensity on glycogen depletion in human muscle fibres. *Acta Physiol Scand* 125:395-405.

Wasserman, D.H., and A.D. Cherrington. 1996. Regulation of extramuscular fuel sources during exercise. In *Handbook of physiology,* section 12, *Exercise: Regulation and integration of multiple systems,* ed. L.B. Rowell and J.T. Shepherd, 1036-1074. Bethesda, MD: American Physiological Society.

Weibel, E.R. 1979. Oxygen demand and the size of respiratory structures in mammals. In *Evolution of respiratory processes,* ed. S.C. Wood and C. Lenfant. New York: Marcel Dekker.

Weibel, E.R. 1984. *The pathway for oxygen: Structure and function in the mammalian respiratory system.* Cambridge, Massachusetts: Harvard University Press.

Westerblad, H., and D.G. Allen. 1991. Changes of myoplasmic calcium concentration during fatigue in single mouse muscle fibers. *J Gen Physiol* 98:615-35.

Westerblad, H., and D.G. Allen. 1993. The influence of intracellular pH on contraction, relaxation and [Ca2+]i in intact single fibres from mouse muscle. *J Physiol (Lond)* 466:611-28.

Westerblad, H., S. Duty, and D.G. Allen. 1993. Intracellular calcium concentration during low-frequency fatigue in iso-lated single fibers of mouse skeletal muscle. *J Appl Physiol* 75:382-88.

Westerblad, H., J. Lee, J. Lannergren, and D.G. Allen. 1991. Cellular mechanisms of fatigue in skeletal muscle. *Am J Physiol* 261:C195-C209.

Williams, J.H., and G.A. Klug. 1995. Calcium exchange hypothesis of skeletal muscle fatigue: a brief review. *Muscle Nerve* 18:421-34.

Williams, R.S., and P.D. Neufer. 1996. Regulation of gene expression in skeletal muscle by contractile activity. In *Handbook of physiology,* section 12, *Exercise: Regulation and integration of multiple systems,* ed. L.B. Rowell and J.T. Shepherd, 1124-50. Bethesda, MD: American Physiological Society.

Wilson, D.F. 1994. Factors affecting the rate and energetics of mitochondrial oxidative phosphorylation. *Med Sci Sports Exerc* 26:37-43.

Wiseman, R.W., T.W. Beck, and P.B. Chase. 1996. Effect of intracellular pH on force development depends on temperature in intact skeletal muscle from mouse. *Am J Physiol* 271(3 Pt 1):C878-86.

Woledge, R.C., N.A. Curtin, and E. Homsher. 1985. Energetic aspects of muscle contraction. *Monographs of the Physiological Society* 41:1-357.

Chapter 2

Biomechanical Correlates of Movement

Principles of Gait

D. Casey Kerrigan, MD, MS,
and Thiru M. Annaswamy, MD, MA

We often prescribe exercises to improve the performance of a specific functional activity such as gait. In order for these exercises to be effective, we need a thorough understanding of the biomechanical components of that functional activity, such as which muscle groups are necessary to achieve it and the amount of strength necessary in each muscle group to perform it. Understanding the biomechanics is essential to formulating an effective exercise prescription.

The study of human biomechanics is largely an application of basic concepts of Newtonian mechanics to the human body. This chapter reviews these concepts, which are then applied to basic functional activities; discusses current state-of-the-art ways to measure the biomechanics of various activities; and

applies the concepts in detail to one of the most fundamental human activities: walking, or gait.

Basic Terminology

An understanding of biomechanical correlates of human movement requires familiarity with both currently accepted terminology and simple concepts from Newtonian physics. Tables 2.1 and 2.2 identify the most common terms, as well as the units in which they are measured and the symbols used to denote them. Refer to these tables if any symbols used in the chapter are unfamiliar to you. Of note, we often use the term **center of mass (COM)** interchangeably with the term **center of gravity (COG)** since, typically, gravity is the primary force acting on the human body. The COG is located just anterior to the second sacral vertebra in the average human lying in the anatomical position (Dempster 1955). The concept of **ground reaction force (GRF)**, defined as the equal and opposite force exerted by the ground at the point of contact, is used often to understand biomechanical principles involved in various activities and exercising techniques. The magnitude of the GRF in the static setting is basically the weight of the body and the direction is pointing upward, acting from the point of contact of the foot.

Concept of Static Equilibrium: The Foundation of Biomechanics

Much of biomechanics relies on a few basic principles pertaining to equilibrium at rest, or **static equilibrium**. These principles are derived from **Newton's first law**—a body remains in a state of rest or in constant motion unless acted upon by an external force; and from **Newton's third law**—every action has an equal

Table 2.1	Definition of Terms			
Term	**Synonyms**	**Definition**	**Symbol**	**Units**
Displacement	Length Distance	Length through which a movement is made	x	meters (m)
Velocity	Speed	Rate of change of displacement with time	v	m/second (m/s)
Acceleration		Rate of change of velocity with time	a	m/s^2
Angular displacement	Angle Arc	Angle through which the rotation is made	θ	degrees radians
Angular velocity	Rotational speed	Rate of change of angular displacement with time	ω	degrees/sec radians/sec
Angular acceleration		Rate of change of angular velocity with time	α	deg/s^2 rad/s^2
Gravity		The acceleration imparted by earth's gravitational force	g	approx. 10 m/s^2
Mass		Amount of matter in a body	m	kilogram (kg)
Moment of inertia		Angular equivalent of mass (the distribution of mass about a radius of gyration)	$I = mr^2$	$kg \cdot m^2$
Weight		Quantity of matter including grativational force (i.e., mass times the gravitational acceleration)	mg	Newton (N)
Force		The cause of all motion (the product of mass and acceleration imparted to it)	$F = ma$	N, $kg \cdot m/s^2$
Lever arm	Moment arm	Perpendicular distance between the line of action of a force and the axis of rotation		m
Torque	Moment	Product of a force and its lever arm or rotational equivalent of force	T $I\alpha$	$N \cdot m$
Work	Energy	Product of force and the distance moved	W	joules (J)
			E	$kg \cdot m^2/s^2$
Power		Rate of change of work with time	P	watt (W) J/s

Table 2.2	Description of Commonly Used Terms
Term	**Definition**
Statics	Study of properties of body at rest
Dynamics	Study of properties of body in motion
Kinematics	Description of spatial motions of a body or its segments
Kinetics	Description of forces and torques that cause motion
Translation	Motion occurring along a straight line
Rotation	Motion occurring about an axis
Center of mass (COM)	Imaginary point representing the whole body through which a force can be considered to act
Center of gravity (COG)	Imaginary point representing the whole body through which gravity can be considered to act
Ground reaction force (GRF)	The equal and opposite force exerted by the ground at the point of contact
Lever system	Specialized force system in which forces act to cause rotation about a fulcrum (axis of rotation)

and opposite reaction. Consider a 10-kg object on a table (figure 2.1). For the object to remain at rest, there must be no external force acting on it, and the vertical line passing through its center of gravity (COG), representing the gravitational force exerted on it, should pass between the legs of the table. Now consider a person carrying a 10-kg object on a string suspended from his hand (figure 2.2). In order for the object to be in static equilibrium with the hand, the

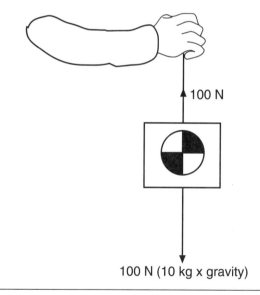

100 N

100 N (10 kg x gravity)

Figure 2.2 An example of Newton's third law of motion. The force in the string is equal and opposite to the weight of the object.

weight of the object should be equal and opposite to the force exerted by the hand on the string. The above two scenarios are examples of **linear force systems**, where the relevant forces are along the same line.

The following is an example of a **concurrent force system**. Persons A and B are carrying the same 50-kg object by means of two strings attached to it. Figure 2.3 shows the angles that the strings make with the

COG

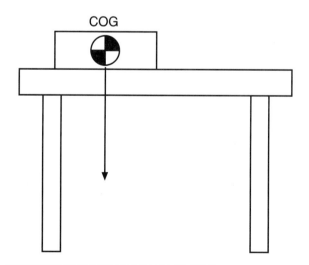

Figure 2.1 A body at rest with the vertical line through its COG falling within the base of support.

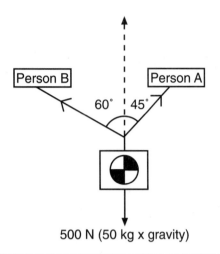

Figure 2.3 An example of a concurrent force system. Persons A and B are pulling on a 50-kg object.

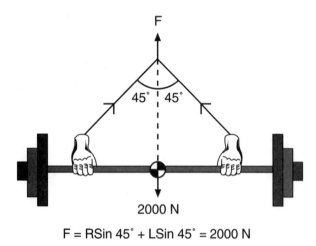

$$F = RSin\ 45° + LSin\ 45° = 2000\ N$$

Figure 2.4 An example of a concurrent force system. A weightlifter is performing a dead lift of 2000 N. Note: Rsin 45° and Lsin 45° are the vertical components of the force through the right hand and left hand, respectively.

horizontal and vertical axes. To be in static equilibrium, the sum of the vertical components of the forces exerted should be equal to the weight of the object. The same principle can be applied to a weightlifter performing a dead lift (figure 2.4). Here, the vertical components of the force exerted through each hand add up to the weight of the barbell. Pulley systems are commonly used in weight training to change the line of action of forces without significantly altering their magnitude. In figure 2.5, the force exerted in the direction indicated by the arrow should be equal to the total sum of the weights attached to the other end.

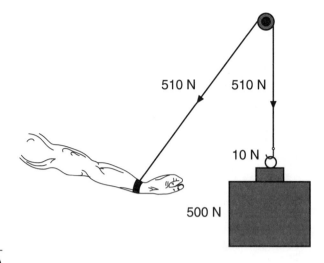

Figure 2.5 A pulley system.

Lever Systems

In biomechanics, the human body can be considered a series of rigid body segments linked to each other at joints (Winter 1990). Human movement can be broken down, in most instances, into simple **lever systems** (specialized force systems whereby forces act to cause rotation about a fulcrum) in which the joints are the fulcrums. Both external and internal forces affect these lever systems. Examples of **external forces** include the weight of an object and the ground reaction force (GRF). **Skeletal muscles** act as the primary source of **internal forces** that affect movement.

For a lever system to be in static equilibrium, the torques about the fulcrum should add to zero. Consider a 10-kg object held in the palm of the hand at a distance of 0.5 m from the elbow joint (figure 2.6). For ease of calculation, assume the weight of the arm to be 10 kg and its COG to be 0.25 m from the elbow joint. For the object and arm to be stable, we need a force, F, from the elbow flexors. Let us also assume that the biceps humerus is the only elbow flexor that is active, and that the insertion of the biceps is 0.025 m from the elbow joint. We can now calculate the force in Newtons required from the biceps to prevent rotation about the elbow:

$\Sigma\ T = 0$, where T = torque

$F(0.025\text{m}) - 100\text{N}(0.25\text{m}) - 100\text{N}(0.5\text{m}) = 0$, where F = biceps force

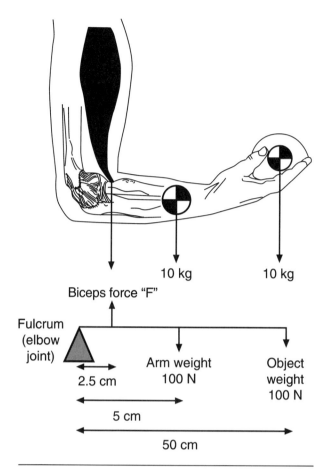

Figure 2.6 A class III lever system in static equilibrium. A schematic representation with measurements is shown below the arm.

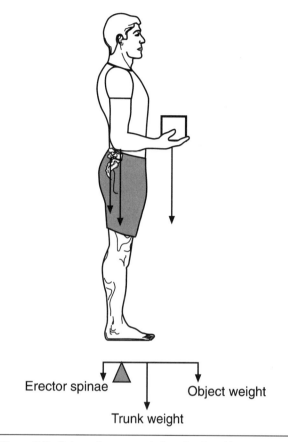

Figure 2.7 Schematic representation of a class I lever.

Solving for *F*, we find:

F = 3000N

There are three different classes of levers. In a **class I** lever the fulcrum is between the internal and external forces. An example is the low back (figure 2.7). With the lumbosacral joint as the fulcrum, both a hand-held weight and the COG of the head, arms, and trunk are external forces; the back extensor muscles (erector spinae) produce the internal force necessary to stabilize the joint. In a **class II** lever, the external force is between the fulcrum and the internal force. There is no known example of a class II lever in the human body. The previous paragraph and figure 2.6 describe a **class III** lever, a common system in the human body, where the internal force (biceps) acts between the fulcrum and the external force (force from the weight of the object and arm).

Examples of Static Biomechanical Principles

A number of daily activities and exercise techniques employ various static biomechanical principles. Here are some examples:

1. Consider again the force through the biceps muscle when carrying an external force of 10 kg in the hand (figure 2.6). The distance is constant between the insertion point of the biceps tendon on the radius and the elbow joint, but the length of the lever arm changes with different elbow angles (figure 2.8). For the system to be in static equilibrium at each of the joint positions, the force generated by the biceps muscle in each case will be different.

2. The patella increases the lever arm of the quadriceps by increasing the perpendicular distance between the quadriceps tendon and the knee joint (figure 2.9)—thus increasing the torque around

the knee joint for a given level of force generated by the quadriceps muscle. There are practical considerations. After a patellectomy, a person must produce more force through the quadriceps muscle to produce a similar torque around the knee joint as before the surgery. In weighing the need for such a procedure (e.g., in the case of a comminuted fracture or severe degenerative changes in the patellofemoral joint), a surgeon

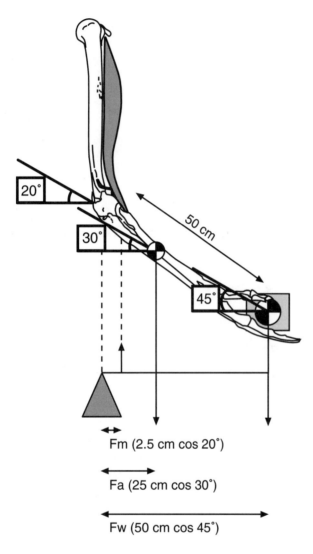

Fm (2.5 cm cos 20°)

Fa (25 cm cos 30°)

Fw (50 cm cos 45°)

Fm (2.5 cm cos 20°) = Fa (25 cm cos 30°) + Fw (50 cm cos 45°)

Fm = Force of the muscle
Fa = Force of the arm
Fw = Force of the object weight

Figure 2.8 Schematic representation of the arm-forearm segment at a different elbow angle with equations. Note: Multiplying by cosine of the angle gives the horizontal component of the forces.

actually could quantify the levels of forces and torques involved and predict the biomechanical results of the procedure.

3. The human body has many pulley systems. An example: around the long flexor tendons of the fingers and toes, tendon sheaths tightly hold down the tendons to the underlying bones to help transmit forces with minimal dissipation (figure 2.10). An ideal pulley system should have the same amount of force on both ends of the pulley. In many athletic programs, athletes try to artificially increase the efficiency of these pulley systems by applying tape around their fingers; in theory, the tape helps to hold the tendons as close to the bone as possible, aiding a more efficient transfer of forces.

4. To test the strength of a muscle group, clinicians use various static positions while performing manual muscle tests on patients. While this technique, if used consistently, would give a good clinical assessment of a patient's strength over time, it would give an incorrect estimate of strength if performed differently by different clinicians. Consider the manual muscle test for the shoulder abductors (figure 2.11). Clinician A tests by pressing down at the elbow on an arm held at 90 degrees of abduction; clinician B presses down at the wrist. The length of the lever arm in each case is different. In order to maintain static equilibrium, the force produced by the abductors in scenario B would be greater than in scenario A. Use of different joint angles in testing a muscle group also can lead to inconsistent results. Different angles not only result in different lever arm lengths (thereby requiring different muscle forces to resist the torque exerted by the examiner), but also challenge muscles at different positions along their force-length curves.

The Complete Approach to Analyzing Biomechanics

A biomechanical system can remain in static equilibrium only when all the translational and rotational forces (torques) acting on it add to zero. This principle can be represented as follows:

$\Sigma F = 0$, where F = translational force and

$\Sigma T = 0$, where T = torque

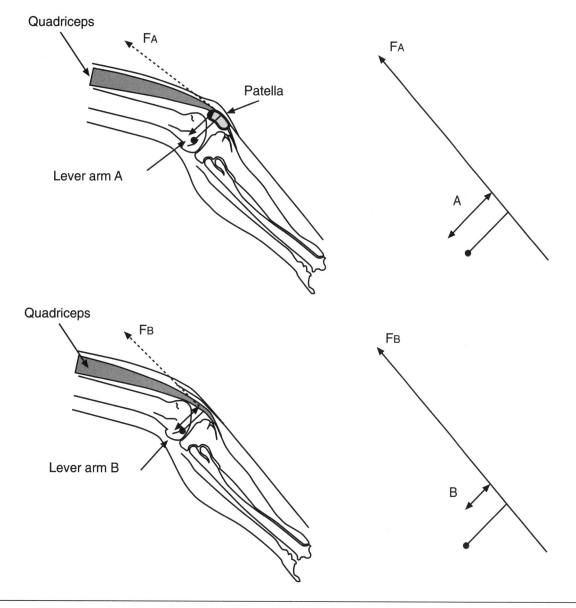

Figure 2.9 Lever arms of the quadriceps muscle with and without the patella. Schematic representations are shown alongside. Note: Presence of the patella makes lever arm A longer than lever arm B.

A biomechanical system is commonly represented schematically by a free-body diagram or a linked-segment model. The model assumes the following:

1. Each segment behaves as a rigid body and has a fixed COG.
2. The length of each segment remains constant.
3. The locations of the joint centers and COGs of limb segments remain fixed with respect to each other.
4. The moment of inertia of each segment about its COG is constant during the movement (Winter 1990).

The free-body diagram of the leg segment in figure 2.12 would have the knee joint at its proximal end and the ankle joint at its distal end. The forces acting on this segment would be

1. gravitational force—this acts downward through the COG and is equal to the mass (of the segment) times gravitational acceleration;
2. ground reaction force—in this case the leg segment is not in direct contact with the ground, and therefore the ground reaction force is transmitted to it through the ankle and is represented by ankle joint reaction force;

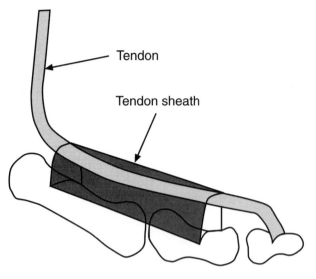

Tendon

Tendon sheath

Figure 2.10 Flexor tendon sheath of a finger acting as a biological pulley system. Note: The direction in the tendon changes due to the pulley-like effect of the tendon sheath.

IM: Moment of inertia

JKY: Vertical component of joint reaction force at knee

JKX: Horizontal component of joint reaction force at knee

JAX: Horizontal component of joint reaction force at ankle

JAY: Vertical component of joint reaction force at ankle

TX: Net muscle torque at the knee

TA: Net muscle torque at the ankle

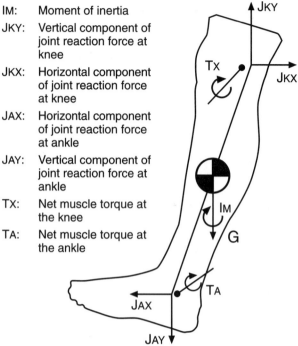

Figure 2.12 Free-body diagram of the leg segment.

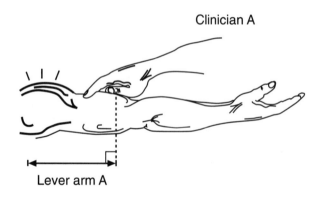

Clinician A

Lever arm A

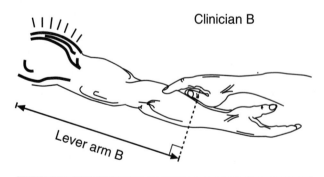

Clinician B

Lever arm B

Figure 2.11 Manual muscle testing of the shoulder abductors, performed at different lever arms.

3. the knee joint reaction force—the force, transmitted through the knee, that represents the body weight above the knee and the net resultant of all other proximal forces; and

4. muscle and ligament forces.

Ligaments, tendons, and other passive structures that might contribute to internal forces generally come into play only at the extremes of joint range of motion. Within the normal range of a joint, therefore, the net torque is largely represented by muscles. Remember that this is the "resultant" torque, which represents only the net torque; if there is co-contraction, individual muscular torques may cancel each other out if they act in opposite directions. For a segment to be in static equilibrium, all torques and forces must sum to zero. Thus, if you can measure all the external forces and their associated lever arm lengths, you can calculate the necessary internal torques and forces.

Dynamic Equilibrium

The same principles that govern static equilibrium also apply to dynamic equilibrium, with a few additional requirements. A dynamic condition basically implies that the body is in motion so that:

$$\sum F = ma \text{ and/or}$$

$$\sum T = I\alpha$$

where

a = net linear acceleration of the segment and

α = net angular acceleration of the segment

The above equations and principles can provide an estimate of the *net* muscle force and torque around a joint. Estimating *individual* muscle forces still remains a problem. For example, around the knee there are ten major muscles—semitendinosus, semimembranosus, biceps femoris, sartorius, gracilis, rectus femoris, the three vastii, and the gastrocnemius—all of which contribute to the net muscle torque in the sagittal plane. The lines of action and lever arms for each of these muscles are different, and change continuously with time. Detailed assessment of individual muscle forces would require more detailed muscle and joint models, involving highly complex calculations and analysis of huge amounts of data. This is an area in need of research.

As defined in table 2.1, **work** is performed when a body is moved a distance by a force, and **power** is the rate at which work is performed. The concept of **joint power** derives from the angular kinematics and kinetics of joint motion (see table 2.2 for descriptions of these terms). Joint power can be positive (power generation), resulting from concentric muscle actions, or negative (power absorption), resulting from eccentric muscle actions. The direction of movement at a joint determines whether a muscle action is concentric or eccentric. During the final stages of throwing a baseball, for example, the forearm is extending and the triceps humerus (elbow extensor) is active; thus the triceps is acting concentrically, since the limb segment is moving in the same direction as the action of the muscle. There is net joint power generation at the elbow during this stage. Shortly after the burst of activity in the triceps, and while the forearm is still extending, the biceps muscle begins to slow the forearm from its peak extensor velocity (the unopposed force from the triceps would abnormally and injuriously hyperextend the forearm). The elbow absorbs net joint power during this stage, and the biceps muscle is acting eccentrically.

Measurement Tools in Biomechanics

Tools to analyze the components of human movement have evolved significantly over the last ten years. Advanced instrumentation and technology have improved the sensitivity and accuracy of measurements. Moreover, the time necessary to perform the measurements has declined dramatically, so that these tools are much more feasible to use in routine clinical settings. Table 2.3 summarizes the three measurements commonly used to assess biomechanics: kinematics, kinetics, and dynamic electromyography. Figure 2.13 provides an overview of the equipment used to assess all three of these parameters, including two (out of four) optoelectronic cameras, the two force plates, and the EMG equipment.

Kinematics

Although a simple instrumented **goniometer** can measure joint angles, joint angle information is only one kinematic variable—and it is therefore important to use more sophisticated equipment to obtain more useful measurements. Computerized **electrogoniometers** use one or more potentiometers placed between two bars, with one bar strapped to the proximal limb segment and the other strapped to the distal limb segment. The potentiometer lies over the joint and provides continuously varying electrical impulses, depending on the instantaneous joint angle. The internal computer plots joint angle information over time. One drawback of current electrogoniometers is that, because they are difficult to place over certain joints like the hip and the ankle, they are relatively inaccurate. The most important drawback is that they provide only limited kinematic information. To calculate torques and associated joint forces as described previously, it is also necessary to measure the limb segment and the absolute joint positions.

Markers placed over various anatomic landmarks can help identify all important kinematic variables, including the location and orientation of limb segments and joints. Camera systems can record the instantaneous location of markers in a two-dimensional plane. Historically, such information was collected using cinematography and then manually digitized frame by frame to determine the coordinates of each

Table 2.3		Biomechanical Measurements
Measurement	**Variables**	**Instruments**
Kinematics	Joint angle Joint position Limb segment position	Optoelectronic motion analysis system (electro-goniometers only measure joint angle)
Kinetics	Ground reaction force Joint torque Joint power	Force plates (and an optoelectronic motion analysis system to measure joint torque and power)
EMG	Electrical muscle activity	Dynamic electromyography (surface or fine-wire electrodes)

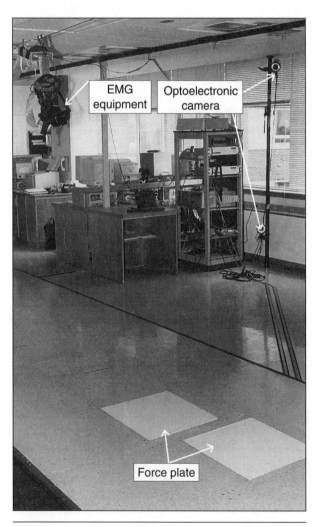

Figure 2.13 Picture of our gait laboratory showing two (out of four) optoelectronic cameras, force plates, and the dynamic EMG equipment.
Photograph by SRH Publications.

marker position. Use of two cameras and a technique called triangulation can provide information about three-dimensional marker positions similar to what our brains (analogous to the computer) use to interpret information provided by our two eyes (the cameras) to assess the depth of an object.

Contemporary camera systems typically involve a sophisticated computerized video camera apparatus, referred to as **optoelectronic motion analysis systems**. These systems automatically digitize and triangulate information obtained from markers to instantaneously locate three-dimensional markers. Two currently available varieties of such systems are

1. **active marker systems**, where the markers are actively illuminated by a computerized power supply; and

2. **passive marker systems**, which use light passively reflected from the markers.

The main disadvantage of active marker systems is that the markers require wires attached to a power source, which might encumber the subject performing the movement. Although passive marker systems require no such cumbersome wires, in the past they were less desirable because (unlike active marker systems) they did not already have information about marker identity stored in the computer. It was therefore more difficult to identify markers recorded by the camera system with passive than with active marker systems. Fortunately, recent software developments permit automatic marker identification, making passive marker systems, in general, the currently preferred motion analysis system.

To facilitate accurate estimates of joint motion from marker placement, data obtained with the above systems must be coupled with biomechanical or mathematical models. Such models vary in complexity—from simple, straight lines connecting two markers representing a limb segment, to complex multidimensional models allowing many degrees of freedom at joints (Murray et al. 1964; Kadaba et al. 1990). The nature of the model used in a system frequently determines the placement of markers on anatomic landmarks.

Kinetics

Analysis of the kinetic parameters of a movement requires measurement of the forces in the segments. Such measurements are often made at one end of a linked-segment model, and forces and torques are computed at the various joints linking the segments, using the equations of dynamic equilibrium as described on page 31. Measurement of such forces must be synchronized with the recording of kinematic variables such as limb segment, joint position, and joint angle to enable precise application of the equations. In addition, the mass and COG position of each limb segment must be determined and are usually estimated on the basis of anthropometric information collected from cadavers, and approximated to individuals based on their demographic characteristics (Dempster 1955; Zatsiorsky and Seluyanov 1983).

Force transducers measure reaction forces at one end of the segment. Ground reaction forces are measured by **force plates**—instruments composed of piezoelectric or strain-gauge transducers. One or more force plates are typically embedded in the ground of a walkway in a gait laboratory. During other activities that are not related to gait, reaction forces are recorded by similar devices composed of force transducers or torque motors. In these cases, one end of the limb must be attached to the device. For example, in the case of a throwing motion (e.g., a baseball pitch), force transducers placed in the baseball record the reaction forces at the end of the hand.

Dynamic Electromyography

Dynamic electromyography (EMG) is the study of electrical muscle activity. When a muscle is activated, it generates electrical signals that can be recorded by means of electrodes. Dynamic EMG is the recording of muscle activity during movement. For example, in quantitative gait analysis, dynamic EMG is frequently used in conjunction with kinematic and kinetic measurements, providing useful information about the timing and duration of specific muscle activity during a movement. Since muscle activity does not correlate linearly with the magnitude of force generated, merely quantifying the amplitude of activity does not provide useful information for routine biomechanical analysis. Normalizing EMG activity to the peak activity (commonly defined as activity during isometric maximum voluntary contraction) can improve the clinical utility of the data (Perry 1992).

EMG activity is recorded using either surface electrodes affixed to the skin or fine-wire electrodes inserted into the muscles. Surface EMG is typically recorded using disposable, gelled bipolar electrodes attached to the skin overlying the subject's muscle. Fine-wire EMG is often recorded using a bipolar wire electrode consisting of two thin, insulated wires with bared tips that are inserted into the muscle using a needle carrying the wires in its lumen (Kerrigan et al. 1997). The recorded signal is the potential difference between the two poles of the electrode.

Noninvasive surface electrodes are adequate for recording EMG activity from large superficial muscle groups, and can record activity from many more motor units than can fine-wire electrodes. Fine-wire electrodes, on the other hand, are not as prone as surface electrodes to interference from neighboring muscles (i.e., "crosstalk") and are useful for recording EMG activity from deeper, smaller muscles such as the iliopsoas and posterior tibialis (Basmajian and DeLuca 1985).

EMG signals are recorded, preamplified, and transmitted by cable or radio wave telemetry to a receiver connected to a computer system. They are filtered to remove noise and then synchronized with the kinematics of the performed movement. For example, in quantitative gait analysis, the EMG signals are routinely synchronized with the events of the gait cycle to enable meaningful interpretation of muscle activity. Optimally, EMG activity, in patients with gait disorders, is assessed in conjunction with kinetics to help distinguish primary impairment from compensatory action. The following section discusses inappropriate versus compensatory EMG activity in relation to gait.

Gait

Gait, which commonly refers to walking and running in humans, is of the most fundamental activities in life. Understanding the basic biomechanical principles of gait enables one to better appreciate the enormous complexities of what is usually assumed to be a simple, automatic activity.

The functional unit of gait is the **gait cycle** or stride, consisting of the stance period and the swing period. Functionally, the **stance period** can be divided into weight acceptance and single limb support tasks; **limb advancement** occurs during the swing period (Perry 1992). **Weight acceptance** consists of the **initial contact** phase and the **loading response** phase. **Single limb support** comprises the **midstance** and **terminal stance** phases. Limb advancement actually commences in the final phase of stance (**pre-swing**) and continues through the **initial swing, midswing,** and **terminal swing** phases to complete the gait cycle. Figure 2.14 summarizes the chief actions in each phase with a visual representation of the limb and joint positions, the ground reaction force vector, and the muscles active during that phase.

While exercise prescriptions may aim to improve a subject's overall walking efficiency and energy costs,

it is important to understand the biomechanical effects that such prescriptions might have on various limb segments (Corcoran 1971). Frequently, an exercise prescription includes some form of muscle strengthening. It is therefore important to understand the interplay between muscle behavior, various joint and segmental forces and torques, and overall power and energy exchanges that occur during gait.

During walking, various limb segments and joints are in a continuous state of dynamic equilibrium. **External forces** include gravity, the body's ground reaction force, and inertial forces from limb segments. **Internal forces** include muscle and ligament forces, inertial forces, and joint forces (Perry 1992). In the stance period of the gait cycle, the predominant external force is the ground reaction force; during the swing period, when there is no ground reaction force, there are only gravitational and inertial forces.

The importance of knowing the direction of the ground reaction force vector, and its relationship with

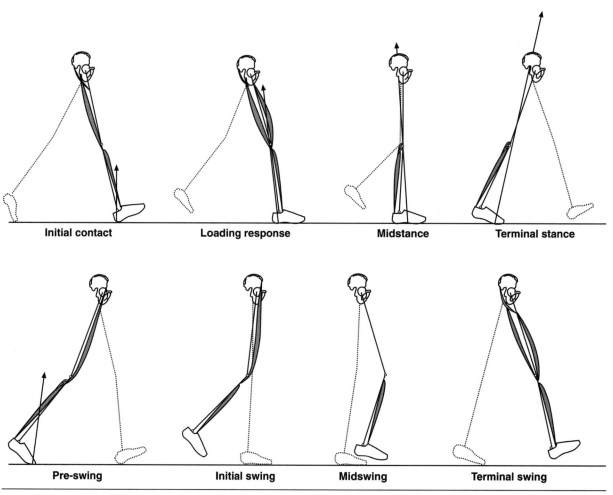

| Initial contact | Loading response | Midstance | Terminal stance |

| Pre-swing | Initial swing | Midswing | Terminal swing |

Figure 2.14 Summary of the phases of the gait cycle with a visual representation of the limb and joint positions, the ground reaction force vector, and the muscles active during each phase.

Reprinted, by permission, from D.C. Kerrigan, 1998, "Gait analysis". In *Rehabilitation medicine,* edited by J. DeLisa (Philadelphia: Lippincott-Raven).

muscle behavior and maintenance of equilibrium, is best illustrated by the example of quiet standing. In quiet standing, the ground reaction force vector extends from the ground through the midfoot, passing anterior to the ankle and knee joints and posterior to the hip joints. At the hip, passive ligamentous forces transmitted through the iliofemoral ligaments usually are sufficient to counter the external extensor torque. Similarly, at the knee, the external knee extensor torque is countered by the passive forces transmitted through the posterior capsule and ligaments of the knee joint. At the ankle joint, the external dorsiflexion torque is usually countered with an internal ankle plantar flexor torque provided by the ankle plantar flexors. Thus, the only lower extremity muscles that are usually consistently active during quiet standing are the plantar flexors—namely, the gastrocnemius and soleus. This activity can be verified with dynamic electromyographic measurement.

During comfortable walking, initial contact normally occurs with the heel. The ground reaction force vector is anterior to the hip and the knee and is posterior to the ankle. Predictably, the hip extensors, hamstrings, and ankle dorsiflexors are active.

Weight acceptance and shock absorption occur during the loading response phase. The ground reaction force vector remains anterior to the hip, and the hip extensors are acting concentrically. The knee extensors are now active eccentrically as the knee is flexing, with the ground reaction force vector posterior to it. Eccentric action of the dorsiflexors slowly lowers the ankle into about 10 degrees plantar flexion.

During midstance the ground reaction force vector passes through the hip and knee joints; predictably, very little muscle activity takes place around these joints. The ankle plantar flexors are now acting eccentrically to counter the external dorsiflexor torque being created by an anteriorly oriented ground reaction force.

During terminal stance, the extensor torque created by the ground reaction force at the hip is countered passively by the iliofemoral ligaments. The ankle plantar flexors continue to act as the ground reaction force vector progresses further anteriorly on the foot. However, now they are concentrically acting as the ankle is actively plantarflexing. This continues into pre-swing, during which phase the hip flexors (iliopsoas, adductors, and rectus femoris) are also concentrically acting to flex the hip. The knee is flexing while possibly being controlled by eccentric action of the rectus femoris at the knee.

The ground reaction force exerts no influence during the swing period, since the foot is not in contact with the ground. The first phase of the swing period is initial swing, during which the hip and knee continue to flex with the momentum generated previously. The ankle is dorsiflexing due to the concentric activity of the dorsiflexors. Inertial forces continue to act during midswing, making the hip flex passively while the knee begins to extend due to the additional effect of gravity. At terminal swing, stabilizing internal forces (primarily generated by the muscles) begin acting to prepare the limb for the weight acceptance phase. At the hip and knee, strong eccentric action of the hamstrings decelerate hip flexion and knee extension. The ankle dorsiflexors remain active to ensure a neutral position at initial contact. Figure 2.15 displays the mean kinematics and kinetics data collected during level walking from nondisabled subjects in our laboratory. Figure 2.16 gives typical dynamic electromyographic data from major lower extremity muscle groups.

Biomechanical Assessment of Gait Disability

The above was a description of gait in an average nondisabled person. When prescribing for a patient with an atypical gait, be sure to make a detailed biomechanical assessment of the patient's gait pattern, to understand the spectrum of abnormalities occurring at each segment and in the body as a whole. Such analysis is essential for anyone hoping to improve gait by prescribing exercises for targeted muscle groups. Other physiatric treatments frequently prescribed to improve gait include intramuscular neurolytic techniques, bracing, functional electrical stimulation, stretching, application of ice or heat, and other treatment paradigms aimed at improving or mimicking strength, stretching a contracture, or reducing tone in a spastic muscle. It is an axiom in medical practice that proper prescription requires proper diagnosis: the outcomes of physiatric treatments ultimately rely on proper determination of the biomechanical bases of the gait disabilities they are designed to overcome.

A number of atypical gait patterns have been described, generally based on observational, kinematic abnormalities (Hirschberg and Nathanson 1947; Peat et al. 1976; Knutsson and Richards 1979; Shiavi et al. 1987; Winters et al. 1987). Table 2.4, page 38, lists the associated causes and distinguishing features of stiff-legged gait, knee recurvatum, equinus gait, and crouched gait. Although a stereotypical description of a gait pattern might be sufficient for initial evaluation, it is often imprecise for determining

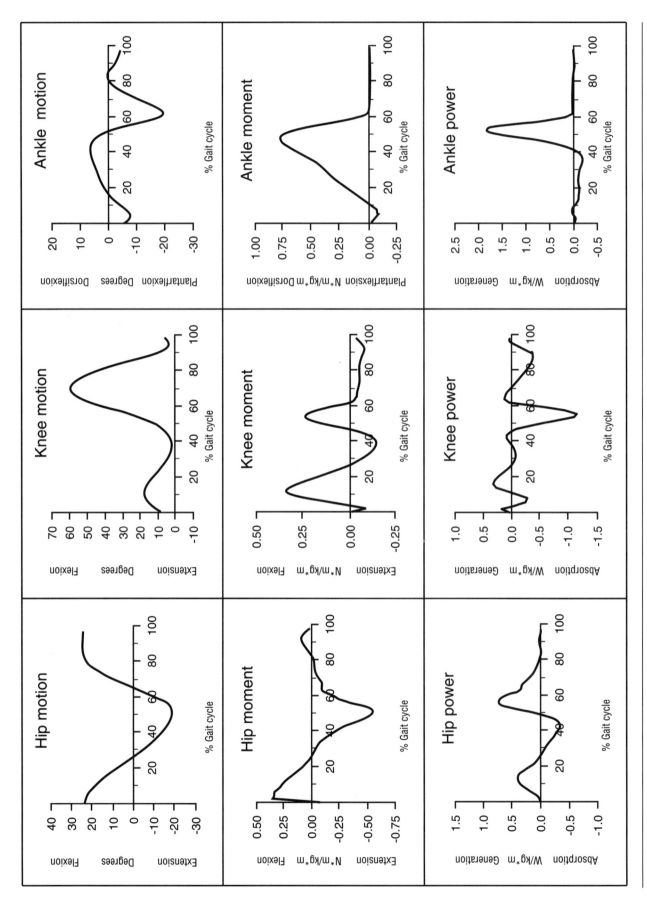

Figure 2.15 Graphic representation of the averaged kinematics and kinetics data collected during level walking from nondisabled subjects in our laboratory.

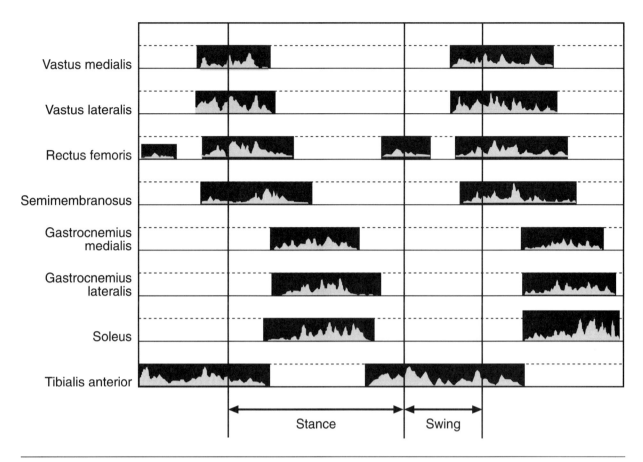

Figure 2.16   Typical dynamic electromyographic data from major lower extremity muscle groups during level walking.

the mechanisms of impairment, functional limitation, compensation, and disability in an individual.

Evaluate any atypical gait pattern to determine if it is functionally significant. Consider it functionally significant if it substantially alters energy requirement, risk of falling, risk of biomechanical injury, or cosmesis. Pursue an exercise prescription only if a gait pattern is functionally significant. For example, knee recurvatum may be associated with increased biomechanical forces across the posterior capsule and ligaments of the knee, increasing the risk of biomechanical injury to these structures. For every individual with knee recurvatum, attempt to determine quantitatively whether these forces are present. One person with knee recurvatum may experience increased knee extensor torque, implying an increased risk for biomechanical injury; another may have normal knee extensor torque (Kerrigan et al. 1996). Only for the first person would knee recurvatum be functionally significant and indicate the need for a rehabilitation program.

Clinicians commonly record and analyze dynamic EMG during biomechanical assessment of gait, first comparing the EMG data to normative data. **Ab-normal EMG** activity is defined as activity observed in a muscle during a phase when the muscle is normally inactive (Kerrigan and Annaswamy 1997). **Inappropriate EMG** activity is defined as abnormal EMG activity that is not compensating for a primary kinetic abnormality. In other words, *inappropriate abnormal* muscle activity creates an internal muscular force large enough to be the major factor responsible for the abnormal kinetics; *appropriate abnormal* muscle activity occurs to compensate for the primary kinetic abnormality. It is necessary to assess muscle firing patterns in conjunction with kinetics to distinguish between primary impairment and compensatory action.

Kinetics provides information about net muscular torque about each joint. With the help of dynamic EMG, it is possible to determine if one muscle group is responsible for the generation of the torque or whether co-contraction is taking place. Based on normative data, we can now determine if there is sufficient power generation or absorption about a joint, and if the net muscular torque is within normal range. Lack of adequate power generation and decreased muscle torque point to decreased muscle group strength.

Table 2.4   Common Atypical Gait Patterns and Associated Possible Causes

Gait pattern	Possible causes	Distinguishing features
Stiff-legged gait (reduced knee flexion in swing)	• Inappropriate quadriceps activity • Weak hip flexors • Poor ankle mechanics	• Inappropriate quadriceps EMG activity in pre- or initial swing • Reduced hip power generation • Reduced ankle torque and power
Knee recurvatum (hyperextension)	• Inappropriate ankle plantarflexor activity • Ankle plantarflexor contracture • Weak ankle dorsiflexors • Weak ankle plantarflexors	• Inappropriately early gastrocnemius or soleus activity • Reduced initial knee flexor moment • Reduced peak ankle moment
Equinus gait (ankle equinus in swing)	• Inappropriate ankle plantarflexor activity • Ankle plantarflexor contracture • Weak ankle dorsiflexors	• Inappropriate gastrocnemius, soleus, or posterior tibialis EMG activity in swing • Limited ankle dorsiflexion motion per static testing
Crouched gait (excessive knee flexion in stance)	• Inappropriate hamstring activity • Hamstring contracture • Knee flexion contracture • Hip flexion contracture	• Inappropriate hamstring activity in mid or terminal stance • Limited knee or hip extension range per static testing

Consider, for example, spastic paretic stiff-legged gait. A clinician might initially suspect inappropriate activity in the quadriceps during pre- or initial swing—a common cause (Treanor 1969; Waters et al. 1979; Sutherland et al. 1990; Kerrigan et al. 1991). However, gait analysis may point to dynamically significant, weak hip flexors, as indicated by slow progression into hip flexion and poor hip power generation. Routine clinical examination, using static analysis, may or may not reveal hip flexor weakness; but this information would be somewhat irrelevant in any case, since static hip flexor weakness is not always correlated with dynamic weakness (Kerrigan and Sheffler 1995). What if, on the other hand, gait analysis revealed a different problem, perhaps reduced internal plantarflexor ankle torque during stance, indicating insufficient ankle plantarflexor muscle action—which indirectly, through foot-ankle mechanics, limits knee flexion? Again, mere static analysis might miss the diagnosis, since plantarflexor strength or spasticity measured by static testing is not correlated with the same problems as determined by gait analysis. Only a detailed biomechanical assessment will reveal the correct diagnosis.

Proper exercise prescription for spastic paretic stiff-legged gait depends on the proper determination of the primary cause for the problem:

• Inappropriate quadriceps activity during pre- or initial swing, if limited to just one head, may be treated with an intramuscular neurolytic procedure, icing, inhibitive casting, or stretching exercises.

• Dynamically weak hip flexors may be treated by specific strengthening exercises.

• Poor ankle mechanics may be treated by strengthening exercises for the ankle plantarflexors.

Consider another example. Knee recurvatum during stance is another kinematic gait abnormality (Simon et al. 1978; Perry 1992). There could be several causes: (1) inappropriately early activity in the ankle plantarflexors; (2) dynamic weakness of the ankle plantarflexors, as revealed by a reduction in the peak ankle torque (in this case, recurvatum occurs because the tibia does not progress forward—tibial progression requires sufficient eccentric ankle plantarflexor action to prevent rapid collapse into dorsiflexion); (3) dynamically weak quadriceps, as revealed by a reduction in the initial knee flexor torque. Only a correct diagnosis would lead to a correct prescription—EMG biofeedback or stretching exercises in the case of inappropriate muscle activity, strengthening exercises for dynamically weak muscles.

Summary

You must understand the biomechanics of an activity before you can formulate an effective exercise prescription to improve the performance of that activity. In this chapter, we reviewed basic Newtonian principles and applied them to a number of basic activities to understand the necessary biomechanical functions for that activity. In addition to discussing underlying biomechanical principles, we reviewed current state-of-the-art tools for assessing the biomechanics of activities. We discussed the application of both principles and measurement techniques to the analysis of gait so as to formulate a proper prescription. You can perform similarly detailed biomechanical analysis for many other activities, permitting prescription of exercise programs tailored to individual subjects.

Acknowledgments

This work is supported, in part, by Public Health Service Grant NIH HD01071-04 and by the Ellison Foundation.

References

Basmajian, J.V., and C.J. De Luca. 1985. *Muscles alive: Their functions revealed by electromyography*. Baltimore: Williams & Wilkins.

Corcoran, P.J. 1971. Energy expenditure during ambulation. In *Physiological basis of rehabilitation medicine*, ed. J.A. Downey and R.D. Darling, 185-198. Philadelphia: W.B. Saunders.

Dempster, W.T. 1955. *Space requirements of the seated operator*. Ph.D. diss., University of Michigan.

Hirschberg, G.G., and M. Nathanson. 1947. Electromyographic recordings of muscular activity in normal and spastic gaits. *Arch Phys Med Rehabil* 33:217-224.

Kadaba, M.P., H.K. Ramakrishnan, and M.E. Wootten. 1990. Measurement of lower extremity kinematics during level walking. *J Orthop Res* 8:383-392.

Kerrigan, D.C., and T.M. Annaswamy. 1997. The functional significance of spasticity as assessed by gait analysis. *J Head Trauma Rehabil* 12:29-39.

Kerrigan, D.C., L.C. Deming, and M.K. Holden. 1996. Knee recurvatum in gait: a study of associated knee biomechanics. *Arch Phys Med Rehabil* 77: 645-650.

Kerrigan, D.C., J. Gronley, and J. Perry. 1991. Stiff-legged gait in spastic paresis: a study of quadriceps and hamstrings muscle activity. *Am J Phys Med Rehabil* 70:294-300.

Kerrigan, D.C., M. Meister, and T.A. Ribaudo. 1997. A modified technique for preparing disposable fine-wire electrodes. *Am J Phys Med Rehabil* 76:107-108.

Kerrigan, D.C., and L.R. Sheffler. 1995. Spastic paretic gait. *Critical Reviews in Physical Medicine & Rehabilitation* 7:253-268.

Knutsson, E., and C. Richards. 1979. Different types of disturbed motor control in gait of hemiparetic patients. *Brain* 102:405-430.

Murray, M.P., A.B. Drought, and R.C. Kory. 1964. Walking patterns of normal men. *J Bone Joint Surg Am* 46A:335-360.

Peat, M., H.I. Dubo, D.A. Winter, A.O. Quanbury, T. Steinke, and R. Grahame. 1976. Electromyographic temporal analysis of gait: hemiplegic locomotion. *Arch Phys Med Rehabil* 57:421-425.

Perry, J. 1992. *Gait analysis: Normal and pathological function*. Thorofare, NJ: Slack, Inc.

Shiavi, R., H.J. Bugle, and T. Limbird. 1987. Electromyographic gait assessment, Part 2: Preliminary assessment of hemiparetic synergy patterns. *J Rehabil Res Dev* 24:24-30.

Simon, S.R., S.D. Deutsch, and R.M. Nuzzo. 1978. Genu recurvatum in spastic cerebral palsy. Report on findings by gait analysis. *J Bone Joint Surg Am* 60:882-894.

Sutherland, D.H., M. Santi, and M.F. Abel. 1990. Treatment of stiff-knee gait in cerebral palsy: a comparison by gait analysis of distal rectus femoris transfer versus proximal rectus release. *J Pediatr Orthop* 10:433-441.

Treanor, W.J. 1969. The role of physical medicine in stroke rehabilitation. *Clin Orthop* 63:14-22.

Waters, R.L., D.E. Garland, J. Perry, T. Habig, and P. Slabaugh. 1979. Stiff-legged gait in hemiplegia: surgical correction. *J Bone Joint Surg* 61:927-933.

Winter, D.A. 1990. *Biomechanics and motor control of human movement*. New York: Wiley.

Winters Jr., T.F., J.R. Gage, and R. Hicks. 1987. Gait patterns in spastic hemiplegia in children and young adults. *J Bone Joint Surg Am* 69:437-441.

Zatsiorsky, V.M., and V.N. Seluyanov. 1983. *The mass and inertia characteristics of the main segments of the human body*, ed. H. Matsui and K. Kobayashi, 1152-1159. Champaign, IL: Human Kinetics.

Chapter 3

Physiological Adaptations to Dynamic Exercise

Roger A. Fielding, PhD, and Jonathan Bean, MD, MS

Exercise and increased physical activity improve cardiovascular fitness (Saltin 1985) and, according to several recent epidemiological studies, decrease mortality from all causes (Blair et al. 1989; Lee et al. 1992; Paffenbarger et al. 1986). Nearly all providers within medical rehabilitation use exercise as an important therapeutic intervention. This chapter reviews acute cardiorespiratory and metabolic responses to dynamic exercise, focusing particularly on the coordination of these responses throughout the body by alterations in specific regulatory processes. We also briefly discuss the roles of exercise training and detraining as they influence physiological responses to acute exercise. At the end of each section, we discuss a specific pathophysiological process that relates to perturbations in the physiological response to exercise.

During dynamic exercise, different organ systems interact to maximize the resynthesis of ATP within active muscle in order to perform physical work. For the purposes of this chapter, we define **dynamic exercise** as muscular activity that induces an increase in oxygen uptake and cardiac output. In explaining the relationships among whole-body measures of oxygen consumption, energy expenditure during exercise, and cellular energy metabolism, we explore the connections between the cardiorespiratory system and peripheral factors linked to oxygen extraction and substrate utilization.

Cardiorespiratory Response to Dynamic Exercise

Whole-body oxygen consumption is the product of maximal cardiac output and maximal peripheral O_2 extraction. These two terms are usually considered the central and peripheral links in the oxygen transport chain, respectively. Oxygen is the final electron acceptor during oxidative phosphorylation. Because researchers cannot conveniently measure rates of **adenosine triphosphate (ATP)** turnover through direct means, they have traditionally used whole-body oxygen consumption to indirectly estimate energy expenditure during exercise (Åstrand 1960).

Maximal Oxygen Uptake

Hill and Lupton (1923) first described **maximal oxygen uptake ($\dot{V}O_2$max)** as an upper physiological limit for aerobic exercise; Taylor and colleagues (1955) validated the concept. These studies demonstrated a direct relationship between whole-body oxygen consumption and exercise intensity (figure 3.1). Oxygen consumption increases linearly with the intensity of exercise, until it plateaus at or near the $\dot{V}O_2$max. Across a wide span of individuals, $\dot{V}O_2$max is a reproducible estimate of aerobic exercise capacity and cardiovascular fitness (Rowell 1974).

The Fick equation describes $\dot{V}O_2$max as the product of **maximal cardiac output (CO)** centrally and maximal peripheral arterial-venous oxygen difference (arterial O_2 − venous O_2) (see table 3.1). The Fick equation illustrates the partitioning of the components of $\dot{V}O_2$max into central and peripheral factors (Saltin and Rowell 1980). In healthy individuals, the central and peripheral processes work in tandem to facilitate oxygen delivery and utilization within active skeletal muscle. Cardiac output and peripheral oxygen uptake are coupled in a tight physiological relationship. Differences in maximal cardiac output explain most of the variance in $\dot{V}O_2$max among individuals (Åstrand et al. 1964; Saltin and Strange 1992)—differences that appear to result solely from differences in maximal stroke volume in individuals with a wide range of aerobic capacities (Blackmon et al. 1967). This exceptional linkage of oxygen supply and demand to active muscle occurs through virtually all intensities and conditions of exercise, and represents a remarkable example of the integration of central and peripheral responses during aerobic exercise.

$\dot{V}O_2$max and the Cardiovascular System

Cardiac output is the product of heart rate and stroke volume. Factors that regulate heart rate include intrinsic autonomic input via sympathetic and parasympathetic pathways, and extrinsic hormonal factors such as circulating catecholamines. Heart rate increases under conditions of sympathetic activation. Conversely, elevated parasympathetic input decreases heart rate. At all exercise intensities, elevations in sympathetic input and release of circulating catecholamines result in increased heart rate (Seals et al. 1988). These same intrinsic and extrinsic neurohormonal factors regulate cardiac function, influencing both heart rate and stroke volume under conditions of stress or relaxation (Stone et al. 1985). Factors that determine stroke volume include venous return and ventricular compliance (related to ventricular filling), plus ventricular contractility and total peripheral resistance (related to ventricular emptying). Elevations in stroke volume with exercise are due to improved filling and emptying of the ventricles (Polinar et al. 1980). Improved filling increases stroke volume via the Frank-Starling mechanism. With increased filling, there is greater ventricular stretch and therefore a stronger resultant contraction of the myocardium. Greater emptying occurs with a larger myocardial contraction regardless of the ventricular volume of blood (Polinar et al. 1980).

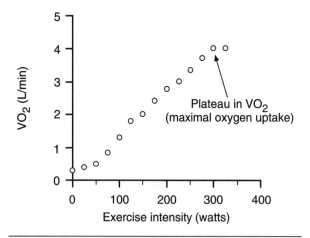

Figure 3.1   Plot of oxygen uptake versus exercise intensity (watts) during an incremental cycling test in a young sedentary individual. Note the linear relationship between power output and $\dot{V}O_2$ up to the plateau and achievement of $\dot{V}O_2$max.
Source: Fielding, 1997, unpublished data.

Table 3.1	Fick Equation		
$\dot{V}O_2$max	= Cardiac output max	$\times$	Arterial-venous oxygen difference
Influenced by:	• Stroke volume maximum		• Blood flow
			• Muscle capillarization
	• Heart rate maximum		• Skeletal muscle oxidative capacity

$\dot{V}O_2$max and the Arterial-Venous Oxygen Difference

Peripheral factors are those that affect extraction of oxygen from the blood by the metabolically active skeletal muscle (Holloszy 1967). These factors can be intrinsic (intracellular) or extrinsic (extracellular). **Intrinsic factors** within muscle fibers include the absolute quantity and the respiratory capacity of the mitochondria. **Extrinsic factors** include the quality and quantity of capillarization, red blood cell transit time, and blood flow to active muscle (Saltin 1985). Exercise training can modify these factors, which contribute to $\dot{V}O_2$max and submaximal exercise capacity (Holloszy and Coyle 1984).

Pulmonary System and Oxygen Transport

The lungs are the interface between the central and peripheral factors. They serve the central role of oxygenating the blood under all conditions; yet if arterial O_2 concentration is low, they can profoundly influence peripheral O_2 extraction. Fortunately, in individuals with normal pulmonary functioning this essentially does not occur (Dempsey and Fregosi 1985). The products of metabolism mediate much of the respiratory response to exercise, and the lungs serve as a gateway for metabolism: oxygen enters the body, and carbon dioxide and water (the products of metabolism) exit. **Ventilation (VE)** is quantified in liters of air exchanged per minute. Like cardiac output, it is the product of rate (ventilatory rate) and volume (tidal volume). **Tidal volume** is the volume of air moved in and out of the lungs with a single breath (Guyton 1991).

The brain stem regulates pulmonary ventilation at centers that control both inspiration and expiration. The centers control both the rate and volume of breathing. The primary factors that mediate this control in normal individuals are changes in body temperature, circulating pH, and concentrations of O_2 and CO_2. Stretch receptors within the diaphragm, lung, and intercostal muscles also can modulate inspiration and expiration by feedback through autonomic pathways. CO_2 and pH act centrally within the brain stem through direct means. More peripherally, receptors within the carotid bifurcation and the aortic arch respond primarily to the **partial pressure of oxygen (pO_2)** along with the **partial pressure of carbon dioxide (pCO_2)** and pH (Dempsey et al. 1985). At these sites pO_2 exerts the strongest influence, causing ventilation to increase under conditions of low oxygenation and decrease when pO_2 levels are high. Centrally, it appears that pCO_2 exerts the greatest influence, causing ventilation to increase with rising blood concentrations and to decrease under opposite conditions. Increased temperature increases ventilation through direct central stimulation (Dempsey et al. 1985).

Ventilation is the mechanism by which hemoglobin is saturated with oxygen. **Hemoglobin (Hb)** is the carrier protein for oxygen within the blood. Factors that control ventilatory function will influence Hb saturation. Optimal physiologic functioning during exercise requires maximal binding of oxygen within pulmonary capillaries and release of oxygen within skeletal muscle capillaries. Under such conditions the alveolar environment is characterized by elevated pH, low pCO_2, and reduced temperature; active skeletal muscle exchange sites have a low pH, high pCO_2, and elevated temperature. Under conditions that mirror the chemical environment of alveolar capillaries in exercising lungs, the oxygen dissociation curve for hemoglobin favors higher hemoglobin saturation levels. In contrast, conditions that reflect the environment of the exercising muscle favor oxygen release from hemoglobin (Guyton 1991). This remarkable phenomenon, known as the **Bohr**

effect, maintains the strong coupling between central supply and peripheral extraction of oxygen.

To summarize what we have discussed thus far:

- Whole-body oxygen consumption is correlated with exercise intensity.
- Both central and peripheral factors determine oxygen consumption.
- These central supply functions and peripheral demand functions work together. Some processes, such as those in the exercising lung, affect both functions.
- Chemical mechanisms, such as the Bohr effect on Hb saturation, underlie the coupling of oxygen supply and metabolic demand.

Cardiovascular Response to Dynamic Exercise

In untrained individuals, resting heart rate is generally 60-100 beats per minute; it increases directly and proportionally with exercise intensity, and, like oxygen consumption, plateaus at maximal exercise intensities (Ekelund and Holmgren 1967). Heart rate and work rate are so intimately linked that, within an individual with known $\dot{V}O_2$max, one can closely predict oxygen uptake at a given submaximal heart rate. Clinicians often use heart rate as an indirect measure of exercise intensity (ACSM 1995). Maximal heart rate varies within individuals and declines with age, typical maximal rates being 190-200 in young adults and 140-160 in older adults. Because the variance increases significantly as the population ages, however, heart rate is a poor predictor of exercise intensity in the geriatric population (Shephard 1990). Regulation of heart rate occurs via neurohormonal input. The elevation in heart rate with dynamic exercise is mediated intrinsically via elevated sympathetic

input and extrinsically via stimulation from circulating catecholamines (Stone et al. 1985).

Although stroke volume also increases with rising exercise intensity, it tends to plateau prior to maximal work loads—at approximately 40%-60% $\dot{V}O_2$max (Crawford et al. 1985; Hermansen et al. 1970). Therefore, whereas heart rate is closely linked to intensity of exercise, stroke volume is more loosely associated. Body position and the form of exercise testing can influence stroke volume, accounting in part for some of the variability researchers have found with stroke volume response (Crawford et al. 1985; Polinar et al. 1980). A number of factors mediate changes in stroke volume. Sympathetic input and circulating catecholamines influence stroke volume through a direct effect on cardiac contractility and compliance (Stone et al. 1985). Increased activity through pumping action of the active skeletal muscle augments venous return, while redistribution of blood to the active muscle reduces total peripheral resistance. These factors increase with heavier levels of exercise (see table 3.2). Together, these changes in heart rate and stroke volume can increase cardiac output two to four times with heavy exercise (Dowell 1983).

Along with the elevation in cardiac output during dynamic exercise, there are dramatic changes in blood flow distribution. In order to maximize delivery of oxygen-rich blood to active skeletal muscle, flow is shunted away from inactive tissues (see table 3.3): active skeletal muscle blood flow increases to 20 times normal levels, and circulation to inactive skeletal muscle declines by approximately one-third. Coronary circulation increases by 400% in order to support the increased myocardial demands; splanchnic blood flow, however, declines by as much as 50%, slowing gastrointestinal transit time. Although blood flow to the skin varies with the ambient temperature, overall it increases in order to maximize heat exchange and slow the rise in core body temperature during

Table 3.2	Cardiovascular Reponses During Dynamic Exercise		
	Rest	**Moderate exercise**	**Maximal exercise**
Cardiac output (L/min)	5.0	17.0	25.0
Stroke volume (ml)	71	117	131
Heart rate (beats/min)	70	145	190
Oxygen uptake (L/min)	0.3	2.0	3.4

Human Cardiovascular Control by Rowell, L.B. © 1993 by Oxford University Press, Inc. Reprinted by permission.

Table 3.3	Typical Distribution of Cardiac Output at Rest (CO = 5 L/min)		
Tissue	**L/min**	**%**	
Heart	0.2	4	
Skin	0.3	6	
Brain	0.7	14	
Liver	1.3	27	
Kidneys	1.1	22	
Skeletal muscle	1.0	20	
Other	0.4	7	

Typical Distribution of Cardiac Output During Maximal Exercise (CO = 25 L/min)

Tissue	**L/min**	**%**
Heart	1.0	4
Skin	0.6	2
Brain	0.9	4
Liver	0.5	2
Kidneys	1.1	3
Skeletal muscle	21.0	83
Other	0.8	2

Human Cardiovascular Control by Rowell, L.B. © 1993 by Oxford University Press, Inc. Reprinted by permission.

exercise (Rowell 1986). Lastly, with dynamic exercise, circulation to the brain needs to remain constant and thus does not change appreciably. The combination of input from circulating catecholamines and local metabolites mediates all the above-mentioned changes. Vascular changes influence central factors through a reduction in total peripheral resistance (TPR) and through increased delivery of oxygen-rich arterial blood to the exercising muscle (Blomquist and Saltin 1983; Saltin 1985).

Respiratory Response to Dynamic Exercise

At rest, normal respiratory rate is 8-20 breaths per minute. It increases with increasing effort, as does tidal volume, in an effort to maximize ventilation. Like heart rate, pulmonary ventilation increases linearly with oxygen consumption. Again there is close linkage between central supply of oxygen and peripheral demand. In all but highly trained individuals, arterial pO_2 remains at resting levels even with heavy exercise. This is accomplished through three mechanisms:

1. In the resting state there is a large functional reserve of both alveolar and capillary surface area. These underutilized surfaces for diffusion serve as added sources for oxygen exchange.

2. Pulmonary capillary blood flow increases three times with maximal exercise, and lymphatic drainage is optimized. These mechanisms slow red blood cell transit time and reduce diffusion distance, respectively.

3. The ratio of ventilation to perfusion increases four to five times over resting levels, maintaining a high gradient for diffusion.

Together, these factors maximize arterial oxygenation (Dempsey et al. 1985). By maximizing oxygenation of hemoglobin during exercise, the lungs balance the increased peripheral extraction of oxygen.

Cardiorespiratory Response to Exercise in Patients With Spinal Cord Injury

Exercise response in spinal cord injury (SCI) patients is particularly interesting. It is the level of spinal injury that dictates the major physiologic differences between individuals who are labeled as SCI and those who are able-bodied. The two most significant factors that influence the exercise response are reductions in active muscle mass and reductions in circulating blood volume. Since large segments of the body are paralyzed in SCI, the amount of active muscle mass declines—thereby reducing $\dot{V}O_2$max, since less muscle is available to consume oxygen (Glaser 1989; Lasko-McCarthey and Davis 1991). This fact significantly limits overall endurance and influences the substrates used for metabolism. For a given task such as propelling a wheelchair, the same level of work represents a much higher percentage of $\dot{V}O_2$max in an SCI patient. Thus, with more challenging tasks, the ratio of anaerobic to aerobic metabolism is higher, leading to early fatigue and reduced endurance.

Reductions in circulating blood volume also impair work capacity in patients with spinal cord injury (Figoni et al. 1991; King et al. 1994), for two reasons: (1) There is a considerably smaller active muscle mass with SCI, resulting in a large increase in venous pooling during exercise and thus reducing venous return. (2) Changes in autonomic control of blood flow also increase venous pooling in SCI. With SCI (especially lesions at higher thoracic levels), cortical control of autonomic pathways is either reduced or absent, preventing the normal redistribution of blood to active muscle (Glaser 1989; Sawka et al. 1989). There is a qualitative reduction in substrate delivery and in disposal of metabolic end products. The reduced venous return due to excessive pooling also reduces cardiac output. In fact, a challenge in prescribing cardiovascular exercises for individuals with SCI is providing exercises that generate large increases in cardiac output. Researchers have explored a variety of exercise techniques to maximize the exercise stimulus in SCI patients—including supine positioning and use of electrical stimulation to inactive muscle (Glaser 1989; Rodgers et al. 1991). Given the physiological circumstances of spinal cord injury, it is not surprising that a leading source of morbidity and mortality in such individuals is cardiac disease (DiTunno and Formal 1994).

Metabolic Response During Dynamic Exercise

Physical exercise profoundly challenges homeostasis of fuel in normal humans. Whole-body energy expenditure can increase ten- to twentyfold from rest to maximal exercise (Taylor et al. 1955). Since quantities of high-energy phosphate compounds such as **creatine phosphate (CP)** and ATP within muscle are relatively limited (26 mM/kg wet wt. for CP; 8 mM/kg wet wt. for ATP), metabolic machinery and oxidizable substrate are necessary for sustained muscular activity. Enzymes in human skeletal muscle produce energy by oxidizing carbohydrate (in the forms of glucose and glycogen), nonesterified fatty acids (transported from adipocytes and derived from intramuscular triglycerides), and, to a small extent, amino acids (Newsholme and Start 1973) (see table 3.4). In order to meet the requirements of exercise and at the same time maintain the fuel supply to vital organs, the body must make major metabolic, hormonal, and cardiovascular adjustments.

Carbohydrate Metabolism

Glucose uptake in skeletal muscle is a carrier-mediated process initiated by the pancreatic hormone **insulin** (Berger et al. 1976; Ivy et al. 1983). Minimum levels of insulin are necessary for glucose uptake to occur at rest; but during exercise, glucose uptake increases despite declining circulating insulin concentrations (Felig et al. 1982; Felig and Wahren 1975), apparently because of non-insulin-dependent signaling mechanisms (Goodyear et al. 1996). Blood glucose may account for up to 40% of the total oxidizable substrate during prolonged submaximal exercise (i.e., 40% to 50% $\dot{V}O_2$max). The decline in blood glucose concentrations at the end of prolonged exercise may be a possible cause of fatigue (Coyle et al. 1983; Coyle et al. 1986; Felig et al. 1982).

Under resting conditions, catecholamines, glucagon, cortisol, and growth hormone stimulate hepatic glucose production, balancing the stimulatory action of insulin on glucose uptake. The result is **euglycemia,** in which glucose production matches glucose utilization (Kemmer and Berger 1986). During exercise, skeletal muscle glucose uptake can increase up to 28-fold, depending on the intensity of the exercise (Katz

Table 3.4	Fuel Reserves and Rates of Utilization Under Different Conditions in Humans		
	Approximate total fuel reserve		**Estimated period for which fuel store would provide energy**
Tissue	**g**	**kcal**	**Minutes of marathon running**
Adipose tissue triacylglycerol	16,000	144,000	7,143
Liver glycogen	90	360	18
Muscle glycogen	350	1,400	71
Blood and extra fluids	20	80	4

Adapted, by permission, from E.A. Newsholme and C. Start, 1973, *Regulation in metabolism* (New York: Wiley), 255.

et al. 1986), despite a decrease in insulin secretion by the pancreas. It appears that catecholamines released from the adrenal medulla, and/or from nerve endings in the liver and pancreas, may suppress both insulin secretion and stimulate hepatic glucose production (Galbo et al. 1977; Wasserman 1995). In addition to the effects of sympathetic nerve endings in the liver, a state of hypoinsulinemia (coupled with relative hyperglucagonemia in the portal blood) further increases hepatic glucose output during exercise (Vranic et al. 1976). The result of these hormonal alterations is that blood glucose levels remain unchanged during exercise of relatively short duration.

Skeletal muscle glucose uptake increases linearly with increasing exercise intensity (Katz et al. 1986). Despite this dramatic increase in glucose uptake by active muscle, plasma glucose concentration remains notably level in normal humans during exercise of low to moderate intensity. Feedback signals from plasma glucose sensors appear to elicit changes in neuroendocrine function that increase hepatic glucose production (Richter et al. 1992). Decreases in plasma glucose may also directly stimulate hepatic glucose production. Feedback mechanisms are less involved during intense exercise as plasma glucose concentrations increase initially, then fall as hepatic glycogen stores are depleted (Richter et al. 1992). Instead, the glycemic response during periods of intense exercise may be subject to a feed-forward regulation elicited by the central command—it changes neuroendocrine function, causing an initial overshoot in hepatic glucose production. For example, at the onset of exercise, impulses from the working muscles

and motor centers increase neuroendocrine activity in an intensity-dependent manner (Galbo 1983).

As happens with blood glucose supply, intramuscular stores of glycogen are broken down to enable resynthesis of high-energy phosphate compounds. Muscle glycogen's direct availability to the contractile tissue eliminates the need for a circulatory response for its mobilization. Muscle glycogen utilization appears greatest at the onset of exercise; as other substrates become available, the rate of muscle glycogen utilization slows (Hermansen et al. 1967) (figure 3.2). As with blood glucose uptake, the rate of muscle glycogen utilization increases with exercise intensity, reaching maximal rates well above the maximal oxygen uptake (Hermansen et al. 1967). Animal studies have shown a close relationship between intramuscular availability of glycogen and its rate of utilization during contractile activity (Richter and Galbo 1986). Several researchers have noted a relationship between pre-exercise muscle glycogen concentrations and time to exhaustion during submaximal endurance exercise (Bergstrom et al. 1967; Hermansen et al. 1967). Fatigue during intermittent high-intensity exercise also appears to coincide with low intramuscular glycogen concentrations (Jacobs 1980; Maughan and Poole 1981). It is possible that with the depletion of muscle glycogen, selected muscle fibers may no longer be able to generate the necessary force to maintain a given power output. Sedentary untrained individuals have lower baseline muscle glycogen levels than do active trained people (Costill et al. 1985); reduced substrate availability may be a significant cause of fatigue in patients undergoing exercise training in rehabilitation.

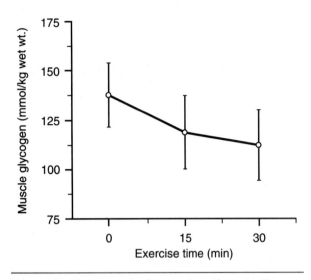

Figure 3.2 Plot of muscle glycogen (mmol/kg wet wt.) versus exercise time during 30 min of treadmill running (70% V̇O₂max) in well-trained runners.

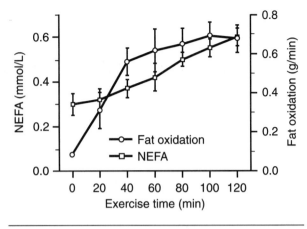

Figure 3.3 Plot of serum NEFA (non-esterified fatty acids) concentration and rates of fat oxidation during 2 hour of cycling exercise (70% V̇O₂max).
Source: Fielding, 1995, unpublished observations.

Fatty Acid Metabolism

Skeletal muscle can derive energy from blood-borne nonesterified fatty acids and intramuscular stores of triglyceride. In an individual of normal body mass and composition, the total body stores of carbohydrate and fat account, respectively, for 2,000 and 140,000 kcal of energy (Newsholme and Start 1973). Because of the enormous difference in the amounts of these substrates available for energy metabolism, a coordinated process of carbohydrate and fat metabolism is essential for prolonged muscular activity. During prolonged exercise and the resultant hypoinsulinemia and increased catecholamine release, **free fatty acids (FFAs)** mobilized from adipose tissue become a more important energy-yielding substrate. The process of **lipolysis** in adipose tissue results in the breakdown of triglycerides to FFA and glycerol. In addition to its stimulatory effect on hepatic glucose output, epinephrine further stimulates lipolysis in an effort to preserve circulating glucose (Zinman et al. 1977). Transported in the plasma bound to albumin, FFAs are then taken up by contractile tissue independent of insulin, but not necessarily by simple diffusion (Richter et al. 1992). Sorrentino et al. (1988) and Stremmel (1988) have isolated FFA-binding proteins from plasma membranes of adipocytes, hepatocytes, and cardiac myocytes. Because antibodies to these proteins inhibit FFA uptake, it is possible that FFA transport across the plasma membrane is in fact carrier-mediated.

Fatty acid oxidation rates increase progressively during prolonged exercise. The increase appears to be related to increases in circulating nonesterified fatty acid (NEFA) concentrations; however, there appears to be some dissociation between the rate of fatty acid lipolysis from adipose tissue and the increased rates of skeletal muscle fatty acid oxidation (figure 3.3). Interestingly, despite similar increases in adipose tissue lipolysis and fatty acid uptake, rates of fatty acid oxidation are higher during low-intensity exercise in exercise-trained than in untrained men (Klein et al. 1994)—an effect possibly related to increased oxidation of fatty acids derived from intramuscular triglycerides (Hurley et al. 1986) and enhanced fatty acid extraction during exercise by the more trained muscle (Turcotte 1992).

Protein and Amino Acid Metabolism

Oxidation of specific amino acids (e.g., the branched-chain amino acids leucine, isoleucine, and valine) increases during exercise to a smaller extent than oxidation of fat and carbohydrate (10% to 15% of total oxidized substrate) (Rennie et al. 1981). Several researchers have reported that increased amino acid oxidation during prolonged exercise increases the dietary requirement for protein in physically active individuals (Meredith et al. 1989; Tarnopolsky et al. 1992).

Several variables can significantly modify the sequence of metabolic fuel mobilization outlined above; these include the duration of exercise, its intensity, the fitness of the individual, and the previous nutritional state. Carbohydrate and fatty acid oxidation appear to be inversely related: carbohydrate (as muscle glycogen and blood glucose) tends to be preferred early during exercise, and at higher exercise intensi-

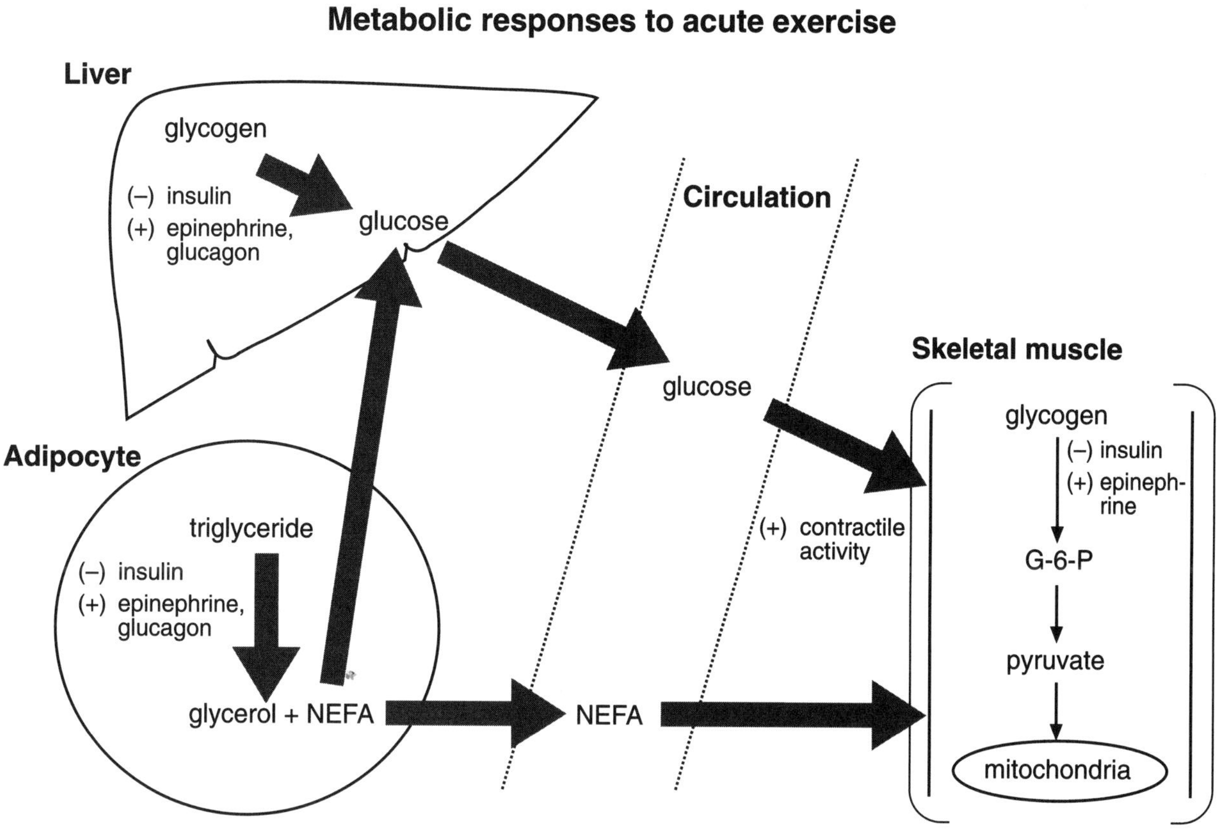

Metabolic responses to acute exercise

Figure 3.4 Overview of the metabolic response to dynamic exercise: (+) indicates activator, (–) indicates inhibitor. NEFA (non-esterified fatty acids), G-6-P (glucose-6-phosphate).

ties; fat becomes the primary substrate toward the end of prolonged exercise (see figure 3.4).

Acute Exercise Response in Diabetes Mellitus

Exercise-induced changes in glucose homeostasis in patients with insulin-dependent diabetes mellitus (IDDM) are quite complex (Vitug et al. 1988; Zinman et al. 1984). The metabolic perturbations caused by exercise in diabetic individuals superimpose additional challenges to the normal metabolic response to exercise.

The method of insulin replacement in patients with IDDM does not duplicate the normal secretion of insulin from the pancreas. Yet insulin and contractile activity constitute the two most instrumental stimulators for membrane transport of glucose in skeletal muscle (Arvill 1967; Helmreich and Cori 1957).

Average whole-body measures of aerobic fitness appear to be reduced in the IDDM population, pri-

marily as a result of a characteristically sedentary lifestyle (Kemmer and Berger 1986). Interestingly, $\dot{V}O_2$max in physically active individuals with IDDM generally is no different from that in nondiabetic individuals; only if individuals with IDDM also have clinical manifestations of autonomic neuropathy will their $\dot{V}O_2$max be lower than in nondiabetic individuals (Veves et al. 1997). The metabolic alterations commonly associated with diabetes have a profound effect on the metabolic response to exercise. Diabetic patients commonly oscillate between states of insulin excess and insulin deficiency—and their metabolic responses to exercise correlate with the metabolic state at the onset of exercise (Giacca et al. 1991; Hilsted 1982; Kawamori and Vranic 1977; Vranic et al. 1990; Vranic and Wrenshall 1969). The most familiar disturbance of glucose homeostasis during exercise in IDDM is hypoglycemia. Hypoglycemia most often occurs during a relatively prolonged session of moderately intense exercise, when hepatic glucose production cannot keep pace with the increased use of glucose by exercising muscle. There is unrestrained peripheral glucose utilization, while portal hyperinsulinemia suppresses an appropriate rise in hepatic glucose output (Kawamori and Vranic 1977; Zinman et al. 1977). Conversely, patients in a state of chronic, moderate insulin deficiency have decreased glycogen stores in the liver and, to a lesser extent, in skeletal muscle (Wasserman and Zinman 1995). Insulin deficiency results in impaired aerobic exercise endurance; more rapid switch of fuels (during prolonged activity) to the utilization of free fatty acids; hyperglycemia; and accelerated formation of ketone bodies by the liver (Wasserman and Zinman 1995). Already increased levels of plasma glucose are further elevated by an exaggerated increase in hepatic glucose production caused by insulin deficiency (Vranic et al. 1976; Vranic and Wrenshall 1969). Elevated muscle glycogen concentrations, along with a rapid rate of glycogen breakdown, lead to high intramuscular concentrations of glucose-6-phosphate, which inhibits hexokinase (Newsholme and Leech 1983). As intracellular muscle glucose concentrations increase, the gradient of glucose from the interstitial space to the cytoplasm decreases; in turn, cells reduce their net uptake of glucose (Hespel and Richter 1990; Richter and Galbo 1986). Furthermore, lactate production is higher when glycogen concentrations are elevated than when they are low. Thus, the metabolic profile of an exercising individual with hyperglycemia after 40 minutes mirrors that of a normal human who has been performing aerobic exercise for 4 hours. This is known as the **accelerated adaptation to exercise** (Wahren et al. 1984).

In non-insulin dependent diabetes mellitus (NIDDM), the diabetic state (i.e., hyperglycemia concomitant with either insulin deficiency or hyperinsulinemia) causes metabolic changes that affect skeletal muscle glucose transport (Olefsky et al. 1988). Exercise-induced changes in glucose homeostasis in NIDDM result from a positive impact on peripheral insulin action. Insulin resistance in the periphery occurs primarily in the skeletal muscle (the body's largest insulin-sensitive tissue) and therefore significantly affects overall glucose homeostasis in type II diabetic patients (Wallberg-Henriksson 1987).

Cardiorespiratory Changes With Activity and Inactivity

Cardiorespiratory fitness varies across different populations of healthy individuals. Generally, $\dot{V}O_2$max is higher in trained than in untrained individuals of both genders (although higher differences tend to be found in men). Yet because considerable variability exists

among the four groups (Drinkwater 1984; Hermansen and Anderson 1965), overall means can be misleading when $\dot{V}O_2$max and levels of conditioning are measured across gender lines. As one might expect, $\dot{V}O_2$ values are larger in adults than in children. When controlled for variations is body size, however, these differences tend to diminish (Rowland et al. 1997). Many of the differences noted by gender, age, and training level correlate to increases in cardiac output and body size; increases in cardiac output, in turn, are directly related to elevated levels of stroke volume; and stroke volume is a function of increased cardiac size, left ventricular volume, and blood volume (Dowell 1983). Body size also contributes to differences in $\dot{V}O_2$max, since a larger mass of muscle consumes a larger absolute volume of oxygen—one must account for this factor when drawing comparisons across populations.

It is well known among rehabilitation professionals that training improves fitness and can reverse changes induced by inactivity or immobilization. Improvements in $\dot{V}O_2$max vary with initial level of conditioning and intensity of training, but range on average between 10% and 30% (Pollack 1973). Central effects of training include increased cardiac size (specifically, elevated left ventricular wall thickness) and left ventricular volume (Dowell 1983). Both circulating blood volume and red blood cell number increase in endurance-trained athletes. These factors collectively contribute to increased cardiac output. Peripherally, training increases levels of oxidative enzymes and positively influences the quantity and concentration of capillaries (Andersen 1975; Hermansen and Wachlova 1971). The net result is that skeletal muscle increases its capacity to utilize oxygen (Saltin and Rowell 1980), paralleling the body's increased capacity for oxygen delivery.

For over a century, physicians have prescribed immobility and bed rest for a variety of medical conditions. The adverse effects of immobility are a common comorbidity in patients with chronic disease. In large part, exercise rehabilitation aims to reverse the negative effects of prolonged inactivity (DeLisa 1993). Not surprisingly, debility is now a recognized diagnosis for admission to inpatient rehabilitation units (CFAR 1996). Immobility (specifically, bed rest) has detrimental effects on $\dot{V}O_2$max. Saltin and colleagues (1968) demonstrated these effects in a classic study using healthy young males. Twenty-one days of complete bed rest decreased $\dot{V}O_2$max by 25%, and reduced stroke volume, cardiac output, and plasma volume by similar levels. Both resting and maximal heart rates increased. Reduced cardiac output appears primarily to be a function of reduced cardiac size and reduced plasma volume (Convertino 1997). The latter, along with changes in stroke volume, reduces cardiac output largely via the Frank-Starling mechanism. Increases in heart rate may represent a physiologic attempt to maintain cardiac output. Peripherally, there is a concomitant reduction in levels of oxidative enzymes and alterations in capillarization. With inactivity or complete cessation of training, the reductions in skeletal muscle oxidative capacity appear to occur sooner than the absolute declines in VO_2max (Costill et al. 1985; Henriksson and Reitman 1977). All of these changes contribute to impaired extraction of oxygen within active skeletal muscle (Bloomfield 1997; Convertino et al. 1997). The coupling of these central and peripheral factors leads to decline in work capacity (Convertino et al. 1997; Saltin and Rowell 1980). Again, note the close linkage of these physiologic adjustments to decreased physical activity.

Physiological Adjustments to Isometric Exercise

Isometric exercise presents unique physiological demands. Hettenger and Muller first popularized it in the 1950s, describing it as muscle contraction against an immovable object. More specifically, active muscle contraction occurs with an absence of any limb movement or change in muscle length. Isometric muscle actions occur during normal human activity. For example, an individual waiting in line or leaning against a post or wall can have low-level isometric muscle activity within his paraspinal muscles as well as his lower extremity musculature. For people with slight hip and knee contractures, even quiet standing requires extensive isometric activity within lower extremity extensor musculature. All rehabilitation professionals—especially those who work with the elderly and debilitated populations—should understand the physiologic effects of isometric muscular activity.

Significant cardiovascular effects can occur with isometric exercise, including marked elevation of both systolic and diastolic blood pressure. There also can be greatly elevated stress to the left ventricular wall. Patients with hypertension, congestive heart failure, and other forms of cardiovascular disease should perform isometric exercise with caution (Atkins et al. 1976). Blood pressure increases in proportion to the effort exerted: as little as 15% of maximal voluntary contraction can produce changes in blood pressure (Coote et al. 1971). We do not know the specific mechanism by which this occurs; but apparently it is mediated in part through peripheral reflexes, since the phenomenon occurs in both large and small muscle groups (Buck et al. 1980). Heart rate accelerates, compromising diastolic filling time and in turn reducing stroke volume. Total peripheral resistance remains unchanged. The net effect is an elevation in blood pressure (Donald et al. 1967).

Supervision and feedback on technique and breathing can temper these potentially adverse effects (Goldberg et al. 1982; O'Connor et al. 1989)—in fact, even at high levels of isometric contraction, blood pressure response can be indistinguishable from that seen in other forms of strength training (Greer et al. 1984). Isometric exercise programs in appropriate patient populations can even lower resting blood pressure Wiley et al. 1992).

Not only are isometric training effects generally specific to the joint angles at which they occur (Graves et al. 1989)—pure isometric exercise can reduce maximal limb velocity. Despite these apparent adverse effects, isometric exercise can be very beneficial in many cases. Under conditions where limited limb motion is required, such as acute arthritis or joint injury, isometric exercise can maintain strength and muscle bulk. Depending on the technique, clinicians have reported strength gains of as much as 5% per week in such patients (DeLisa 1993).

Summary

This chapter has introduced several key components of the physiological response to dynamic exercise, including the relationships between oxygen transport and peripheral oxygen extraction. We have highlighted the tight coupling of metabolism to its substrate delivery mechanisms. By illustrating the exercise response to several disease states, we have also illustrated the abundant overriding and compensatory mechanisms that these diverse pathologies call into play. Because exercise is a key component of many treatments in rehabilitation, these fundamental principles underlie nearly every procedure and treatment plan in modern physical rehabilitation. Understanding normal and abnormal responses to exercise may stimulate new and innovative thinking about future roles of exercise and physical activity in the prevention and treatment of chronic diseases.

References

American College of Sports Medicine. 1995. *ACSM's guidelines for exercise testing and prescription*. 5th ed. Media, PA: Williams & Wilkins.

Andersen, P. 1975. Capillary density in skeletal muscle of man. *Acta Physiol Scand* 95:203-205.

Arvill, A. 1967. Relationship between the effects of contraction and insulin on the metabolism of the isolated levator ani muscle of the rat. *Acta Endocr* 56(Suppl. 122):27.

Åstrand, I. 1960. Aerobic work capacity in men and women with special reference to age. *J Appl Physiol* 169:1-92.

Åstrand, P.O., T.E. Cuddy, B. Saltin, and J. Stenberg. 1964. Cardiac output during maximal and submaximal work. *Acta Physiol Scand* 19:268-272.

Atkins, J.M., O.A. Matthews, C.G. Blomquist, and C.B. Mullins. 1976. Incidence of arrhythmias induced by isometric and dynamic exercise. *Br Heart J* 38:465-471.

Berger, M., S. Hagg, M.N. Goodman, and N.B. Ruderman. 1976. Glucose metabolism in perfused skeletal muscle: effects of starvation, diabetes, fatty acids, acetoacetate, insulin, and exercise on glucose uptake and disposition. *Biochem J* 158:191-202.

Bergstrom, J., L. Hermansen, E. Hultman, and B. Saltin. 1967. Diet, muscle glycogen and physical performance. *Acta Physiol Scand* 71:140-150.

Blackmon, J.R., L.B. Rowell, J.W. Kennedy, R.D. Twiss, and R.D. Conn. 1967. Physiological significance of maximal oxygen uptake in "pure" mitral stenosis. *Circulation* 36:497-510.

Blair, S.N., H.W. Kohl, R.S. Paffenbarger, D.G. Clark, K.H. Cooper, and L.W. Gibbons. 1989. Physical fitness and all-cause mortality: a prospective study of healthy men and women. *JAMA* 262:2395-2401.

Blomqvist, C.G., and B. Saltin. 1983. Cardiovascular adaptations to physical training. *Ann Rev Physiol* 45:169-189.

Bloomfield, S.A. 1997. Changes in musculoskeletal structure and function with prolonged bed rest. *Med Sci Sports Exerc* 29:197-206.

Buck, J.A., L.R. Amundsen, and D.H. Nielsen. 1980. Systolic blood pressure responses during isometric contractions of large and small muscle groups. *Med Sci Sports Exerc* 12:145-147.

Center for Functional Assessment Research. 1996. *Guide for uniform data set for medical rehabilitation*, Version 5. Buffalo: School of Medicine and Biomedical Sciences, State University of New York at Buffalo.

Convertino, V.A. 1997. Cardiovascular consequences of bed rest: effect on maximal oxygen uptake. *Med Sci Sports Exerc* 29:191-196.

Convertino, V.A., S.A. Bloomfield, and J.E. Greenleaf. 1997. An overview of the issues: physiological effects of bed rest and restricted physical activity. *Med Sci Sports Exerc* 29:187-190.

Coote, J.H., S.M. Hilton, and J.F. Perez-Gonzalez. 1971. The reflex nature of the pressor response to muscular exercise. *J Physiol* 215:789-804.

Costill, D.L., W.J. Fink, M. Hargreaves, D.S. King, R. Thomas, and R.A. Fielding. 1985. Metabolic characteristics of skeletal muscle during detraining from competitive swimming. *Med Sci Sports Exerc* 17:339-343.

Coyle, E.F., A.R. Coggan, M.K. Hemmert, and J.L. Ivy. 1986. Muscle glycogen utilization during prolonged exercise when fed carbohydrate. *J Appl Physiol* 61:165-172.

Coyle, E.F., J.M. Hagberg, B.F. Hurley, W.H. Martin, A.H. Ehsani, and J.O. Holloszy. 1983. Carbohydrate feeding during prolonged strenuous exercise can delay fatigue. *J Appl Physiol* 55:230-235.

Crawford, M.H., M.A. Petru, and C. Rabinowitz. 1985. Effect of isotonic exercise training on left ventricular volume during upright exercise. *Circulation* 72:1237-1243.

DeLisa, J.A. 1993. *Rehabilitation medicine: Principles and practice.* 2d ed. Philadelphia: J.P. Lippincott.

Dempsey, J.A., and R.F. Fregosi. 1985. Adaptability of the pulmonary system to changing metabolic requirements. *Am J Cardiol* 55:55D-59D.

Dempsey, J.A., B.D. Johnson, and K.W. Saupe. 1990. Adaptations and limitations in the pulmonary system during exercise. *Chest* 97:81S-87S.

Dempsey, J.A., E.H. Vidruk, and G.S. Mitchell. 1985. Pulmonary control systems in exercise: update. *Fed Proc* 44:2260-2270.

DiTunno, J.F., and C.S. Formal. 1994. Chronic spinal cord injury. *New Engl J Med* 330:550-556.

Donald, K.W., A.R. Lind, and G.W. McNichol. 1967. Cardiovascular response to sustained [static] contractions. *Circ Res* XX-XXI Suppl. 1:15-32.

Dowell, R.T. 1983. Cardiac adaptations to exercise. *Exerc Sport Sci Rev* 11:99-117.

Drinkwater, B.L. 1984. Women and exercise: physiologic aspects. *Exerc Sport Sci Rev* 12:12-51.

Ekelund, L.G., and A. Holmgren. 1967. Central hemodynamics during exercise. *Circ Res* (Suppl.) 20:33-43.

Felig, P., A. Cherif, A. Minigawa, and J. Wahren. 1982. Hypoglycemia during prolonged exercise in normal men. *N Engl J Med* 302:895-900.

Felig, P., and J. Wahren. 1975. Fuel homeostasis in exercise. *N Engl J Med* 293:1078-1084.

Fielding, R.A., D.L. Costill, W.J. Fink, D.S. King, J.E. Kovaleski, and J.P. Kirwan. 1986. Effect of pre-exercise carbohydrate feedings on muscle glycogen use during exercise in well-trained runners. *Eur J Appl Physiol* 56:225-229.

Figoni, S.F., R.M. Glaser, M.M. Rodgers, S.P. Hooker, B.N. Ezenwa, S.R. Collins, T. Matthews, A.G. Suryaprasad, and S.C. Gupta. 1991. Acute hemodynamic responses of spinal cord injured individuals to functional neuromuscular stimulation-induced knee extension exercise. *J Rehab Research* 28:9-18.

Galbo, H. 1983. *Hormonal and metabolic adaptations to exercise.* New York: Thieme Verlag.

Galbo, H., E. Richter, J. Hilsted, J. Holst, N. Christensen, and J. Henrickson. 1977. Hormonal regulation during prolonged exercise. *Ann NY Acad Sci* 301:72-80.

Giacca, A.M., J. Davidson, and H. Lickley. 1991. Exercise and stress in diabetes mellitus. In *Clinical diabetes mellitus: A problem oriented approach*, ed. J. Davidson. New York: Thieme-Stratton, Inc.

Glaser, R.M. 1989. Arm exercise training for wheelchair users. *Med Sci Sports Exerc* 21:S147-S149.

Goldberg, L.I., J. White, and K.B. Pandolf. 1982. Cardiovascular and perceptual responses to isometric exercise. *Arch Phys Med Rehabil* 63:211-216.

Goodyear, L.J., P.-Y. Chung, D. Sherwood, S.D. Dufresne, and D.E. Moller. 1996. Effects of exercise and insulin on mitogen-activated protein kinase signaling pathways in rat skeletal muscle. *Am J Physiol* 271:E403-E408.

Graves, J.E., M.L. Pollock, A.E. Jones, A.B. Colvin, and S.H. Leggett. 1989. Specificity of limited range of motion variable resistance training. *Med Sci Sports Exerc* 21:84-89.

Greer, M., S. Dimick, and S. Burns. 1984. Heart rate and blood pressure response to several methods of strength training. *Phys Ther* 64:179-183.

Guyton, A.C. 1991. *Textbook of medical physiology.* 8th ed. Philadelphia: W.B. Saunders.

Helmreich, E., and C.F. Cori. 1957. The distribution of pentoses between plasma and muscle. *J Biol Chem* 224:663.

Henriksson, J., and J.S. Reitman. 1977. Time course of changes in human skeletal muscle succinate dehydrogenase and cytochrome oxidase activities and maximal oxygen uptake with physical activity and inactivity. *Acta Physiol Scand* 99:91-97.

Hermansen, L., and K.L. Anderson. 1965. Aerobic work capacity in young Norwegian men and women. *J Appl Physiol* 20:425-431.

Hermansen, L., B. Ekblom, and B. Saltin. 1970. Cardiac output during submaximal and maximal treadmill and bicycle exercise. *J Appl Physiol* 29:82-86.

Hermansen, L., E. Hultman, and B. Saltin. 1967. Muscle glycogen during prolonged severe exercise. *Acta Physiol Scand* 71:129-137.

Hermansen, L., and M. Wachlova. 1971. Capillary density of skeletal muscle in well-trained and untrained men. *J Appl Physiol* 30:860-863.

Hespel, P., and E.A. Richter. 1990. Glucose uptake and transport in contracting, perfused rat muscle with different precontraction glycogen concentrations. *J Physiol* 427:347-359.

Hill, A.V., and H. Lupton. 1923. Muscular exercise, lactic acid, and the supply and utilization of oxygen. *Q J Med* 16:135-171.

Hilsted, J. 1982. Pathophysiology in diabetic autonomic neuropathy: cardiovascular, hormonal, and metabolic studies. *Diabetes* 31 (August):730-737.

Holloszy, J.O. 1967. Biochemical adaptations in muscle. Effects of exercise on mitochondrial oxygen uptake and respiratory enzyme activity in skeletal muscle. *J Biol Chem* 242:2278-2282.

Holloszy, J.O., and E.F. Coyle. 1984. Adaptations of skeletal muscle to endurance exercise and their metabolic consequences. *J Appl Physiol* 56:831-838.

Hurley, B.F., P.M. Nemeth, W.H. Martin, J.M. Hagberg, G.P. Dalsky, and J.O. Holloszy. 1986. Muscle triglyceride utilization during exercise: effect of training. *J Appl Physiol* 60:562-657.

Ivy, J.L., J.C. Young, J.A. McLane, R.D. Fell, and J.O. Holloszy. 1983. Exercise training and glucose uptake by skeletal muscle in rats. *J Appl Physiol* 55:1393-1396.

Jacobs, I. 1980. Lactate concentrations after short maximal exercise at various glycogen levels. *Acta Physiol Scand* 111:465-469.

Katz, A., S. Broberg, K. Sahlin, and J. Wahren. 1986. Leg glucose uptake during maximal dynamic exercise in humans. *Am J Physiol* 251:E65-E70.

Kawamori, R., and M. Vranic. 1977. Mechanism of exercise-induced hypoglycemia in depancreatized dogs maintained on long-acting insulin. *J Clin Invest* 59:331-337.

Kemmer, F., and M. Berger. 1986. Therapy and better quality of life: the dichotomous role of exercise in diabetes mellitus. *Diabetes/Metabolism Reviews* 2 (1 & 2):53-68.

King, M.L., S.W. Lichtman, J.T. Pellicone, R.J. Close, and P. Lisanti. 1994. Exertional hypotension in spinal cord injury. *Chest* 106:1166-1171.

Klein, S., E.F. Coyle, and R.R. Wolfe. 1994. Fat metabolism during low-intensity exercise in endurance-trained and untrained men. *Am J Physiol* 267:E934-E940.

Lasko-McCarthey, P., and J.A. Davis. 1991. Protocol dependency of $\dot{V}O_2$max during arm cycle ergometry in males with quadriplegia. *Med Sci Sports Exerc* 23:1097-1101.

Lee, I.M., R.S. Paffenbarger, and C.C. Hsieh. 1992. Physical activity and risk of prostatic cancer among college alumni. *Am J Epidemiol* 135:169-179.

Maughan, R.J., and D.C. Poole. 1981. The effects of a glycogen loading regimen on the capacity to perform anaerobic exercise. *Eur J Appl Physiol* 46:211-219.

Meredith, C.N., M.J. Zackin, W.R. Frontera, and W.J. Evans. 1989. Dietary protein requirements and body protein metabolism in endurance-trained men. *J Appl Physiol* 66:2850-2856.

Newsholme, E.A., and A.R. Leech. 1983. Biochemistry for the medical sciences. In *Biochemistry for the medical sciences.* New York: Wiley.

Newsholme, E.A., and C. Start. 1973. Regulation in metabolism. In *Regulation in metabolism.* New York: Wiley.

O'Connor, P.J., G.A. Sforzo, and P. Frye. 1989. Effect of breathing instruction on blood pressure responses during isometric exercise. *Phys Ther* 69:757-761.

Olefsky, J.M., W.T. Garvey, R.R. Henry, D. Brillon, S. Matthaei, and G.R. Freidenberg. 1988. Cellular mechanisms of insulin resistance in non-insulin dependent (type II) diabetes. *Am J Med* 85:86-105.

Paffenbarger, R.S., R.T. Hyde, A.L. Wing, and C.-C. Hsieh. 1986. Physical activity, all-cause mortality and longevity of college alumni. *N Engl J Med* 314:605-613.

Polinar, L.R., G.J. Dehmer, S.E. Lewis, R.W. Parkey, C.G. Blomquist, and J.T. Willerson. 1980. Left ventricular performance in normal subjects: a comparison of the responses to exercise in the upright and supine positions. *Circulation* 62:528-534.

Pollack, M.L. 1973. Quantification of endurance training programs. *Exerc Sport Sci Rev* 1:155-188.

Rennie, M.J., R.H.T. Edwards, S. Krywawych, C.T.M. Davies, D. Halliday, J.C. Waterlow, and D.J. Milward. 1981. Effect of exercise on protein turnover in man. *Clin Sci* 62:627-639.

Richter, E.A., and H. Galbo. 1986. High glycogen levels enhance glycogen breakdown in isolated contracting skeletal muscle. *J Appl Physiol* 61:827-831

Richter, E.A., L. Turcotte, P. Hespel, and B. Kiens. 1992. Metabolic responses to exercise: effects of endurance training and implications for diabetes. *Diabetes Care* 15:1767-1776..

Rodgers, M.M., R.M. Glaser, S.F. Figoni, S.P. Hooker, B.N. Ezenwa, S.R. Collins, T. Matthews, A.G. Suryaprasad, and S.C. Gupta. 1991. Musculoskeletal responses of spinal cord injured individuals to functional neuromuscular stimulation-induced knee extension exercise training. *J Rehab Research* 28:19-26.

Rowell, L.B. 1974. Human cardiovascular adjustments to exercise and thermal stress. *Physiol Rev* 54: 75-159.

Rowell, L.B. 1986. *Human circulation: Regulation during physical stress.* New York: Oxford University Press.

Rowland, T., B. Popowski, and L. Ferrone. 1997. Cardiac responses to maximal upright cycle exercise in healthy boys and men. *Med Sci Sports Exerc* 29:1146-1151.

Saltin, B. 1985. Hemodynamic adaptations to exercise. *Am J Cardiol* 55:42D-47D.

Saltin, B., G. Blomqvist, J.H. Mitchell, R.L. Johnson, K. Wildenthal, and C.B. Chapman. 1968. Response to exercise after bed rest and after training: a longitudinal study of adaptive changes in oxygen transport and body composition. *Circulation* 38(5 Suppl.):VII1-VII78.

Saltin, B., and L.B. Rowell. 1980. Functional adaptations to physical activity and inactivity. *Fed Proc* 39:1506-1513.

Saltin, B., and S. Strange. 1992. Maximal oxygen uptake: "old" and "new" arguments for a cardiovascular limitation. *Med Sci Sports Exerc* 24:30-37.

Sawka, M.N., W.A. Latzka, and K.B. Pandolf. 1989. Temperature regulation during upper body exercise: able-bodied and spinal cord injured. *Med Sci Sports Exerc* 21:132S-140S.

Seals, D.R., R.G. Victor, and A.L. Mark. 1988. Plasma norepinephrine and muscle sympathetic discharge during rhythmic exercise in humans. *J Appl Physiol* 65:940-944.

Shephard, R.J. 1990. The scientific basis of exercise prescribing for the very old. *J Am Ger Soc* 38:62-69.

Sorrentino, E., D. Stump, B.J. Potter, R.B. Robinson, R. White, C. Kiang, and P.D. Berk. 1988. Oleate uptake by cardiac myocytes is carrier mediated and involves a 40-kD plasma membrane fatty acid binding protein similar to that of liver, adipose tissue, and gut. *J Clin Invest* 82:928-935.

Stone, H.L., K.J. Dormer, R.D. Foreman, R. Thies, and R.W. Blair. 1985. Neural regulation of the cardiovascular system during exercise. *Fed Proc* 44:2271-2278.

Stremmel, W. 1988. Fatty acid uptake by isolated rat heart myocytes represents a carrier-mediated transport process. *J Clin Invest* 81:844-852.

Tarnopolsky, M.A., S.A. Atkinson, J.D. MacDougall, A. Chesley, S. Phillips, and H.P. Schwarcz. 1992. Evaluation of protein requirements for trained strength athletes. *J Appl Physiol* 73:1986-1995.

Taylor, H.L., E. Buskirk, and A. Henschel. 1955. Maximal oxygen uptake as an objective measure of cardiorespiratory performance. *Am J Physiol* 8:73-80.

Turcotte, L.P. 1992. Increased plasma FFA uptake and oxidation during prolonged exercise in humans. *Am J Physiol* 262:E791-E799.

Veves, A., R. Saouaf, V.M. Donaghue, C.A. Mullooly, J.A. Kistler, J.M. Giurini, E.S. Horton, and R.A. Fielding. 1997. Aerobic exercise capacity remains normal despite impaired endothelial function in the micro- and macrocirculation of physically active IDDM patients. *Diabetes* 46:1846-1852.

Vitug, A., S. Schneider, and N. Ruderman. 1988. Exercise and type I diabetes mellitus. *Exerc Sport Sci Rev* 16:285-304.

Vranic, M., R. Kawamori, S. Pek, N. Kovacevic, and G.A. Wrenshall. 1976. The essentiality of insulin and the role of glucagon in regulating glucose utilization and production during strenuous exercise in dogs. *J Clin Invest* 57:245-255.

Vranic, M., D. Wasserman, and L. Bukowiecki. 1990. Metabolic implications of exercise and physical fitness in physiology and diabetes. In *Diabetes mellitus: Theory and practice*, ed. H. P. Rifkin, Jr. New York: Elsevier Science.

Vranic, M., and G. Wrenshall. 1969. Exercise, insulin and glucose turnover in dogs. *Endocrinology* 85:165-171.

Wahren, J., Y. Sato, J. Ostman, L. Hagenfeldt, and P. Felig. 1984. Turnover and splanchnic metabolism of free fatty acids and ketones in insulin deficient diabetes at rest and in response to exercise. *J Clin Invest* 73:1367-1376.

Wallberg-Henriksson, H. 1987. Glucose transport into skeletal muscle. Influence of contractile activity, insulin, catecholamines on diabetes mellitus. *Acta Physiol Scand* 131:1-80.

Wasserman, D., and B. Zinman. 1995. Fuel homeostasis. In *Health professionals' guide to diabetes and exercise*, ed. N. Ruderman and J. Devlin. Alexandria, VA: American Diabetes Association.

Wasserman, D.H. 1995. Control of glucose fluxes in the postabsorptive state. *Ann Rev Physiol* 57:191-218.

Wiley, R.L., C.L. Dunn, R.H. Cox, N.A. Hueppchen, and M.S. Scott. 1992. Isometric exercise training lowers resting blood pressure. *Med Sci Sports Exerc* 24:749-754.

Zinman, B., F. Murray, M. Vranic, A. Albisser, P. McClean, and E. Marliss. 1977. Glucoregulation during moderate exercise in insulin treated diabetics. *J Clin Endocrinol* 45:641-652.

Zinman, B., S. Zuniga-Guajardo, and D. Kelly. 1984. Comparison of the acute and long term effects of exercise on glucose control in type I diabetes. *Diabetes Care* 7:515-519.

Chapter 4

Adaptations to Endurance Exercise Training

Martin D. Hoffman, MD

Aerobic or **endurance exercise** refers to dynamic contractions of large muscle groups at relatively low tensions, with sufficient oxygen present to allow continuation of the exercise for several minutes or longer. This type of exercise stimulates many systems of the body, resulting in acute **physiological responses** (see chapter 3). Endurance exercise performed regularly, at adequate intensities and durations, is referred to as **endurance exercise training**. The body responds to this training through **physiological adaptations**. Associated with the physiological adaptations are a host of **health benefits** (see chapters 10-20). This chapter focuses on the physiological adaptations that result from endurance exercise training.

It is important that rehabilitation clinicians understand the adaptations that result from endurance training, since their goals are to prevent deterioration of and to restore functional capacity. Since endurance capacity is a major determinant of functional abilities, knowledge of the factors affecting endurance is fundamental for the clinical practice of rehabilitation medicine.

Physiological Adaptations to Endurance Exercise Training

Endurance exercise training results in a wide variety of adaptations that enhance a person's ability to respond to subsequent exercise loads. Many adaptations involve improved oxygen delivery to the exercising muscles; others serve to reduce the demands on the body in other ways. A description of the most important adaptations to endurance exercise training follows.

56   HOFFMAN

Maximal Aerobic Power

An important adaptation to endurance exercise training is increased maximal aerobic power ($\dot{V}O_2$max), considered the best single indicator of the cardiorespiratory system's functional capacity. $\dot{V}O_2$max is defined as the highest rate of oxygen consumption attainable during maximal exercise. Increasing the exercise intensity beyond the point at which an individual is at $\dot{V}O_2$max induces no further increase in oxygen consumption.

The rate at which the body consumes oxygen is defined by the product of the cardiac output and the arterial-venous oxygen difference. **Cardiac output** is the rate at which blood is pumped by the heart to the tissues of the body. The **arterial-venous oxygen difference** is the difference in oxygen content between arterial and venous blood, and indicates how much oxygen has been extracted by the tissues.

Most studies indicate that sedentary people within diverse populations (age, gender, income, ethnic background, health status) experience improvements in $\dot{V}O_2$max of 15% or more within three months of starting an endurance exercise training program (Clausen 1977; Lavie and Milani 1995; NIH 1996; Sheldahl et al. 1993). This increase generally is about equally due to **peripheral adaptations** that primarily increase the arterial-venous oxygen difference and **central adaptations** that primarily raise maximal cardiac output (Rowell 1974).

Central Adaptations

Cardiac output is determined by the product of heart rate and stroke volume. Since maximal heart rate does not rise and may even be slightly lower in well-conditioned endurance athletes (Ekblom 1969;

Ekblom et al. 1968; Rowell 1986), the rise in maximal cardiac output from training results from increased stroke volume. In adapting to endurance exercise training, stroke volume increases not only during maximal exercise, but also at rest and during submaximal exercise. The mechanisms by which stroke volume increases with training appear to involve increased cardiac preload, enhanced myocardial contractility, and reduced afterload (figure 4.1).

The increased cardiac preload induced by endurance training is partly due to expanded plasma volume: during exercise, increased release of both antidiuretic hormone and aldosterone cause the kidney to retain water; and increased levels of plasma proteins, particularly albumin, raise the osmotic pressure of the blood and cause intravascular fluid retention.

Increased left ventricular filling time and volume are also important factors that increase cardiac output. Endurance exercise training induces an increase in left ventricular volume, along with some increase in the thickness of the posterior and septal walls of the left ventricle (Ehsani et al. 1991; Landry et al. 1985; Morrison et al. 1986; Rerych et al. 1980). The increased ventricular volume may be due to a chronic stretch of the myocardium at rest from the training-induced plasma volume expansion and to the greater diastolic filling time associated with a slower resting heart rate (Rowell 1986). It has been postulated that the heart adapts to the resultant increase in end-diastolic volume by increasing the left ventricle chamber size.

As a result of the increased left ventricular preload, the greater stretch on the ventricular walls produces greater elastic recoil via the Frank-Starling mechanism. This effect, coupled with the more forceful contraction that occurs from the larger ventricular muscle mass, also serves to increase stroke volume.

Another factor serving to increase maximal stroke volume after endurance exercise training is a reduc-

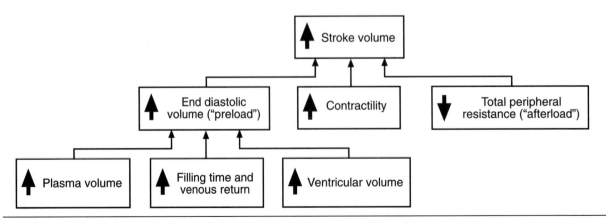

Figure 4.1 Summary of factors causing an increase in stroke volume with endurance exercise training.
Adapted, by permission of McGraw-Hill, from S. Powers and E. Howley, 1997, *Exercise physiology: Theory and application to fitness and performance*, 3rd ed. (Brown and Benchmark), 234.

tion in total peripheral resistance, or afterload. Because the increased cardiac output can maintain mean arterial blood pressure, sympathetic vasoconstrictor activity to the arterioles of the trained muscles can be reduced (Rowell 1986).

Peripheral Adaptations

About half of the training-induced improvements in $\dot{V}O_2$max result from peripheral adaptations that primarily increase the arterial-venous oxygen difference—an increase due to lower mixed venous oxygen content, reflecting both greater oxygen extraction at the tissue level and more effective distribution of total blood volume. The arterial oxygen content does not increase with training, even though total hemoglobin is increased. The increase in plasma volume is greater than the increase in hemoglobin, so the amount of hemoglobin per volume of blood is the same or slightly reduced. Since the arterial partial pressure of oxygen is usually sufficient to maintain arterial saturation of hemoglobin, the arterial oxygen content does not increase with training.

A variety of structural and metabolic changes enhance oxygen extraction within the trained muscle. An increase in the number and size of mitochondria, along with increases in their respiratory enzyme activities, enhances the capacity of trained muscle cells for aerobic energy provision from both fatty acid and carbohydrate oxidation (Holloszy and Coyle 1984). There is also an increase in capillary density and capillary-fiber ratio, which promotes efficient metabolic exchange. The increase in the number of capillaries surrounding each muscle fiber improves the

oxygen exchange between capillary and fiber by presenting a greater surface area for the diffusion of oxygen; by shortening the average distance required for oxygen to diffuse into the muscle; and by slowing the rate of blood flow, thereby increasing the length of time for diffusion to occur. The increase in muscle myoglobin observed with endurance training is also important in oxygen delivery. When oxygen enters the muscle fiber, it binds to myoglobin, which shuttles the oxygen to the mitochondria.

There appear to be rather minor changes in glycolytic enzyme activities in endurance-trained skeletal muscle (Baldwin et al. 1973; Gollnick et al. 1972; Schantz et al. 1983). There is no evidence that fast-twitch (type II) fibers are converted to slow-twitch (type I) fibers, or vice versa. However, there may be complete conversion of fast-twitch white (type IIb) fibers to fast-twitch red (type IIa) fibers in response to endurance training (Chi et al. 1983; Jansson and Kaijser 1977). Furthermore, the mitochondrial content of type II fibers tends to increase more than in type I fibers in response to very strenuous endurance training, essentially eliminating the difference in mitochondrial enzyme levels between type I and II fibers (Chi et al. 1983; Jansson and Kaijser 1977).

Figure 4.2 summarizes the factors causing an increase in $\dot{V}O_2$max. Besides increasing maximal exercise capacity, endurance training allows one to perform submaximal work with less cardiovascular stress—probably providing the broadest therapeutic value of exercise training. Table 4.1 summarizes the cardiorespiratory adaptations to endurance exercise training at rest, during submaximal exercise, and during maximal exercise.

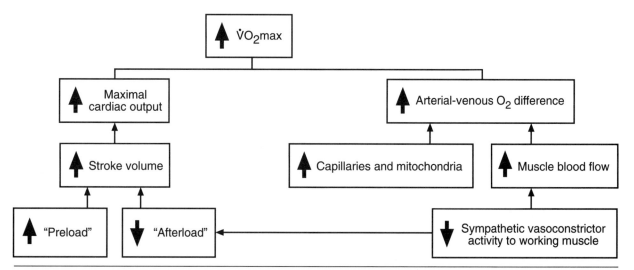

Figure 4.2 Summary of factors causing an increase in $\dot{V}O_2$max with endurance exercise training.
Adapted, by permission of McGraw-Hill, from S. Powers and E. Howley, 1997, *Exercise physiology: Theory and application to fitness and performance*, 3rd ed. (Brown and Benchmark), 235.

Table 4.1   Cardiorespiratory Adaptations to Endurance Exercise Training as Observed in Resting and Exercise States

	Rest	Submaximal exercise	Maximal exercise
Oxygen uptake	No change*	No change†	Increase
Heart rate	Decrease	Decrease	Decrease
Stroke volume	Increase	Increase	Increase
Cardiac output	No change	No change	Increase
Myocardial oxygen demand	Decrease	Decrease	No change
Ventilation	No change	Decrease	Increase
Arterial-venous oxygen difference	No change	Increase	Increase
Blood lactate concentration	No change	Decrease	Increase
Muscle blood flow	No change	Decrease	Increase
Splanchnic blood flow	No change	No change	Decrease
Systolic blood pressure	Decrease	Decrease	No change
Diastolic blood pressure	Decrease	Decrease	No change

*Or may increase slightly

†Or may decrease slightly

Respiratory Adaptations

The respiratory system usually does not limit endurance exercise capacity. As a result, adaptations to the respiratory system from endurance training have less functional importance than some of the other adaptations. Adaptations to the respiratory system are observed primarily during exercise rather than at rest.

Endurance training may slightly lower respiratory rate and tidal volume, and slightly decrease ventilation at light exercise loads (Åstrand and Rodahl 1977; Martin et al. 1979). It is thought that this small reduction in ventilation may be due to reduced sensitivity of the arterial and brain chemoreceptors that respond to carbon dioxide in the blood (Martin et al. 1979). At moderate to heavy exercise intensities, the ventilation for a fixed work rate can be reduced by 20%-30% below pretraining levels (Casaburi et al. 1987; Clanton et al. 1987). This training adaptation is thought to result from a lower accumulation of lactic acid in the blood, which causes less afferent feedback from the working muscles to stimulate breathing. Because of the greater work rates that can be produced as a result of endurance training, maximal exercise after such a program induces greater respiratory rates and tidal volumes, causing an overall increase in ventilation.

Metabolic Adaptations

Endurance training markedly changes the metabolic responses of muscles to submaximal exercise. There are smaller increases in muscle and blood lactate concentrations, reduced reliance on carbohydrate, and increased utilization of fatty acid oxidation. These interrelated metabolic adaptations are largely responsible for the increased endurance from training.

Lactate Levels

Lactate accumulation has long been suspected to be important in the development of fatigue. While the mechanisms are not clear, it is apparent that there is an association between endurance performance and the exercise intensity required to elicit a given lactate concentration (Farrell et al. 1979; LaFontaine et al. 1981; Sjodin and Jacobs 1981).

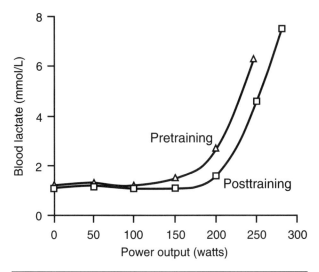

Figure 4.3 Blood lactate concentrations relative to work rate before and after an endurance exercise training program.

Endurance exercise training allows a higher work rate, and higher absolute oxygen consumption, without raising blood lactate concentrations above resting levels (figure 4.3). Intense endurance training can also lead to an increase in the percentage of $\dot{V}O_2$max at which an individual must exercise in order to induce a given blood lactate level (Hurley et al. 1984).

Decreased blood lactate concentrations after endurance exercise training may be due largely to decreased lactate production by the exercising muscles (Henriksson 1977; Saltin et al. 1976), resulting from improvements in blood flow and oxygen extraction. Increased lactate removal may also play a role in accounting for the lower blood lactate concentrations after training, possibly related to improved blood flow to the liver (a major site for lactate removal for gluconeogenesis).

Fuel Utilization

Biochemical adaptations in trained muscle have metabolic effects that improve function during prolonged exercise. The biochemical signals that accelerate metabolism during submaximal exercise are attenuated in trained muscles, reducing the rate of carbohydrate metabolism and tending to spare the use of muscle glycogen in trained individuals (Hermansen et al. 1967; Karlsson et al. 1972). A proportional increase in fatty acid oxidation compensates for the decreased utilization of carbohydrate during submaximal exercise in the trained state, even when the circulating fatty acid concentration is not elevated (Mole et al. 1971)—an effect reflected by a lower respiratory

exchange ratio at both the same absolute and the same relative exercise intensities after training compared with before training (Holloszy 1973).

There is evidence that depletion of glycogen stores can be important in the development of fatigue during prolonged exercise (Holloszy 1973). The glycogen-sparing effect probably plays a major role in the increase in endurance that occurs with training.

Oxygen Uptake

Oxygen consumption at rest is either unchanged or slightly increased following an endurance exercise training program (Poehlman et al. 1991). The oxygen consumption required for a given submaximal task, which defines the economy for performing the task (Cavanagh and Kram 1985), is either unchanged or slightly reduced after training, depending on the mode of training. For activities such as walking, running, and cycling, there is minimal or no improvement in economy with training, since individuals generally are proficient at these activities when they begin a training program. In contrast, training at activities that are more likely to require developed skills, such as swimming and cross-country skiing, results in improvements in economy at these activities, as demonstrated by a reduction in oxygen uptake and cardiac output at submaximal workloads after training. From a practical standpoint, an improved economy reduces the physiological demands on an individual in performing a given task.

Thermoregulatory Adaptations

Although full adaptation to heat requires a period of acclimatization, endurance-trained individuals show some of these adaptations without undergoing heat acclimatization (Terrados and Maughan 1995). Endurance-trained individuals therefore have a greater heat-dissipating capacity than sedentary individuals (Wyndham 1973). The beneficial effects of endurance training on heat tolerance appear more closely related to training volume than to aerobic capacity (Pandolf et al. 1988).

Endurance exercise training leads to increased sensitivity of sweating mechanisms and a lowering of the sweating threshold (Nadel et al. 1974). Increased sweating limits the rise in body temperature during exercise. And because trained individuals maintain a higher total blood volume during exercise (Convertino et al. 1983), allowing better maintenance of cardiac output, more blood can be directed to the periphery for heat transfer to the environment.

Hormonal Adaptations

Hormones are chemical messengers secreted by endocrine glands and cells throughout the body. Collectively, hormones are involved in the regulation of energy metabolism, fluid and electrolyte balance, circulation, reproductive function, growth and development, and pain perception. Because of the widespread influence of hormones on various body systems, the hormonal adaptations to endurance exercise training have a vast array of effects. In fact, it is probable that the adaptations in hormonal function play a role in many of the physiological adaptations to exercise. Selected hormones will be discussed below.

Exercise stimulates secretion of **catecholamines** (epinephrine and norepinephrine), whose plasma concentrations increase exponentially with exercise intensity (Bloom et al. 1976; Galbo et al. 1975). In addition to their effects on cardiorespiratory function and thermoregulation, catecholamines have a number of important metabolic effects, including the stimulation of lipolysis and hepatic glycogenolysis (Vander et al. 1985). Training reduces plasma epinephrine and norepinephrine concentrations at a given *absolute* exercise intensity; at the same *relative* exercise intensity, however, responses of epinephrine and norepinephrine are unchanged after training (Hartley et al. 1972a and 1972b; Peronnet et al. 1981; Winder et al. 1979). Trained individuals possess an enhanced adrenal medullary secretory capacity, as demonstrated by plasma epinephrine concentrations almost double the pretraining levels for the same relative supramaximal intensity (Kjaer et al. 1986).

Insulin and glucagon are secreted by the pancreas. **Insulin** generally increases fat and glycogen synthesis and lowers blood glucose levels, whereas **glucagon** increases the rate of glycogenolysis. Appropriately, insulin levels decrease as the duration or intensity of exercise increases, and glucagon levels increase to maintain blood glucose levels during exercise. Regular endurance exercise reduces the capacity of pancreatic beta cells to secrete insulin (Dela et al. 1987; Mikines et al. 1987); at the same time, the effect of insulin on glucose uptake from plasma is increased (Mikines et al. 1988). In other words, exercise training results in a lower need for insulin to handle a given carbohydrate load. The resting levels of glucagon decrease with training, but the exercise response increases (Galbo et al. 1977).

Growth hormone, produced by the anterior pituitary, enhances lipolysis and gluconeogenesis (Shephard and Sidney 1975). It is thought that growth hormone is important in maintaining blood levels of free fatty acids and glucose during exercise of long duration (Shephard and Sidney 1975). Although training has been reported to generally diminish the growth hormone response (Bloom et al. 1976; Sutton 1978), maintenance of peak levels during prolonged exercise durations may be enhanced in trained individuals (Hartley 1975).

Another anterior pituitary hormone that increases with exercise is **adrenocorticotropic hormone (ACTH)**, which acts on the adrenal cortex to secrete cortisol. **Cortisol** enhances free fatty acid mobilization and acts to conserve carbohydrates. Like growth hormone, cortisol may be more significant for potentiating than for initiating lipolysis. Training does not change the plasma concentrations of cortisol at the same relative exercise intensity, whereas the levels may be lower for a given absolute exercise intensity after training (Hartley et al. 1972a and 1972b; Sutton 1978; Sutton et al. 1969).

Maintenance of fluid and electrolyte balance is under hormonal control through actions on renal function. **Aldosterone** secretion from the adrenal cortex is elevated during exercise, leading to increased renal reabsorption of sodium. Sodium retention results in a higher plasma osmolarity which, in turn, stimulates **antidiuretic hormone** secretion by the posterior pituitary to increase renal retention of water. Training reduces the degree to which these hormones increase during exercise at a given absolute intensity (Convertino et al. 1981; Melin et al. 1980).

Reproductive hormones can indirectly (and possibly directly) affect fuel utilization during exercise. However, the bulk of research in recent years has focused on the responses of these hormones to exercise training and the resulting effect on reproductive function. The anterior pituitary hormone **prolactin** increases during exercise, and trained women exhibit an enhanced response (Brisson et al. 1980). It is possible that repeatedly elevated prolactin levels suppress ovarian function, which in turn contributes to menstrual dysfunction, including delayed menarche, a shortened luteal phase, and primary and secondary amenorrhea (Prior et al. 1981). While most adaptations to endurance training appear to serve a beneficial role, long-term amenorrhea from intense training has been associated with reduced bone density (Cann et al. 1984; Drinkwater et al. 1984). In men there is evidence that intense training causes a suppression of spermatogenesis and testosterone (Ayers et al. 1985; Wheeler et al. 1984), the significance of which is unclear.

Endogenous opioid peptides have been associated with many physiological processes. At least one of these peptides, **beta-endorphin**, appears to act within the central nervous system to produce analgesia

(Hosobuchi and Li 1978). Several animal studies have demonstrated that the concentration of beta-endorphin increases in specific regions of the brain following exercise (Blake et al. 1984; Christie and Chesher 1983; Hoffmann et al. 1990; Sforzo et al. 1986), and a number of human studies have shown decreased pain perception immediately after exercise (Droste et al. 1991; Janal et al. 1984; Kemppainen et al. 1990; Kemppainen et al. 1985; Koltyn et al. 1996; Olausson et al. 1986; Pertovaara et al. 1984). There appears to be good support for the presence of exercise-induced analgesia. However, the evidence is inconclusive that endogenous opioid peptides are the cause of mood alterations and the "runner's high" frequently attributed to these peptides. There is some evidence that there is an enhanced beta-endorphin output during exercise among trained individuals (Carr et al. 1981; Farrell et al. 1987; Mougin et al. 1987); the data are not consistent, however (Metzger and Stein 1984). It has been suggested that exercise may offer protection from the development of chronic pain syndromes (Moldofsky and Scarisbrick 1976), and there is some evidence that pain is reduced through endurance exercise training among individuals with chronic pain states (Goldman 1991; McCain et al. 1988; Nichols and Glenn 1994). Whether endogenous opioid peptides are involved in these phenomena is not clear.

Neurological Adaptations

Little is known about adaptations of the nervous system to exercise, since it is difficult both to measure performance and to examine tissue of the central and peripheral nervous system. Nevertheless, it is evident that adaptations occur to the nervous system from exercise training. For instance, it is recognized that resistance training can enhance recruitment of motor units through greater synchronization (Sale 1987). This adaptation theoretically enhances the power output of a muscle, independent of adaptation of the muscle tissue itself. It is also clear that exercise training can result in improved neuromuscular coordination and a reduction in the energy required to perform the activity (i.e., an improvement in economy).

Animal studies show that regular exercise may cause changes in neural tissue, including lengthening of the terminal axons to muscles; an increase in the area of the neuromuscular junctions; an increase in the activity of cholinesterase enzyme at the neuromuscular junction; and an increase in the size of the cell bodies, nuclei, and nucleoli of spinal motor neurons (Edgerton 1976). While the significance of these changes is not clear, this evidence indicates that there may be important neural adaptations to exercise.

Exercise training may also affect central motor drive. Although it is possible for highly motivated subjects to voluntarily achieve full activation of muscles, under normal conditions the strong desire to reduce the intensity of the motor drive is a limiting factor during physical exertion. It has been suggested that learning to overcome these inhibitory sensations is one of the most important adaptations of exercise training (Bigland-Ritchie 1990).

Exercise is also widely believed to improve sleep quality and reduce daytime sleepiness. While there is some scientific evidence to support these beliefs, the evidence is mixed and, as yet, inconclusive (O'Connor and Youngstedt 1995).

Adaptations of Bone and Connective Tissue

Bone and connective tissue adapt to mechanical loading. Mechanical loading, like that experienced with exercise, contributes to an increase in bone mass and can reduce the bone demineralization that occurs with aging (Aloia et al. 1987; Gleeson et al. 1990; Margulies et al. 1986; Williams et al. 1984). Furthermore, the effect on bone density from exercise during the peak bone forming years appears to remain evident years later (Kohrt et al. 1995; Ulrich et al. 1996).

Endurance exercise training strengthens ligaments and tendons, as well as the attachments of ligaments and tendons to bones (Tipton et al. 1975). Moreover, damaged ligaments regain strength at a faster rate if physical activity is performed after the injury (Tipton et al. 1975).

Adaptations in Functional Capacity

While many adaptations result from endurance exercise training, the most important change may relate to function. Since endurance capacity is a major determinant of functional abilities, it should be clear from the preceding discussion that endurance exercise training produces functional benefits. Training increases maximal work capacity and the sustainable work rate. Perhaps even more importantly, an endurance exercise training program decreases the physiological and psychological demands from an absolute work rate—in other words, the individual performs a given amount of work with less physiological stress and perceives it as being easier.

Enhancing functional capacity can especially benefit those with limited work reserve due to age, disease, or disability (Clausen and Trap-Jensen 1976; NIH 1996; Shephard 1993). Endurance exercise training enables one to be more active in normal daily routines; maintain greater independence in older age or with disabilities; and resume activities—including occupational work—after a disabling injury or illness (Fentem 1992; Fries 1996; Fries et al. 1994; Hiatt et al. 1994; Shephard 1993; Strawbridge et al. 1996; Young et al. 1995). There appears to be an obligatory decrease in $\dot{V}O_2$max of about 5% for every decade of adult life (Heath et al. 1981; Kasch et al. 1990; Rogers et al. 1990), and it has been estimated that an able-bodied person needs a $\dot{V}O_2$max of about 12-14 ml/kg/min to sustain independent living (Shephard 1991). Remaining physically active into old age may allow a person to maintain functional independence for 10 to 20 years longer than if he or she is inactive (figure 4.4).

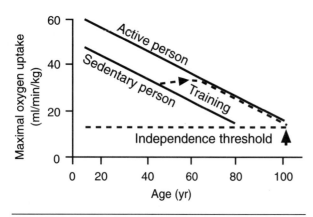

Figure 4.4 Demonstration of the effect of endurance exercise training on improving maximal aerobic power and on delaying its drop to a threshold where independent function can no longer be maintained.

Psychological Adaptations to Endurance Exercise Training

A large body of evidence indicates that regular exercise produces a variety of psychological benefits. Acutely after endurance exercise, ratings of self-esteem, depression, psychological tension, and mood are significantly improved (Farrell et al. 1987; Janal et al. 1984; Markoff et al. 1982; McCann and Holmes 1984; Sonstroem 1984). Regular physical activity improves the sense of well-being (Blumenthal et al. 1990; Lavie et al. 1993). Endurance exercise, when performed on a regular basis, is associated with acute reductions in anxiety (Morgan 1979) and muscle tension (deVries 1968) in normal individuals. Among those who are mildly or moderately anxious or depressed, positive mood changes are associated with exercise training (Simons et al. 1985).

Factors Affecting Adaptations to Endurance Exercise Training

The adaptations to endurance exercise training, as described above, can occur in all populations—young, old, able-bodied, and disabled. Several factors influence the extent and time course of the adaptations, however, including initial level of fitness, genetics, age, gender, and design and duration of the training program.

Initial Level of Fitness

In general, the extent of adaptations to training is greater among individuals who are less conditioned at the beginning of the training program (Sharkey 1970). Sedentary middle-aged men with heart disease may improve their $\dot{V}O_2$max by 50%; a similar training program in normal active adults may lead only to 10%-15% improvement (Cronan and Howley 1974; Ekblom 1969; Hickson et al. 1981; Saltin 1969). Well-conditioned athletes may increase their $\dot{V}O_2$max by only 2-3% following an increase in their training (Cronan and Howley 1974).

Intensity, Duration, and Frequency of Exercise

The extent of physiological adaptations to endurance training is highly related to the intensity, duration, and frequency of training. Figure 4.5 shows the effects of these variables on oxidative capacity of muscle. Numerous longitudinal studies have also demonstrated that the intensity, duration, and frequency of training are important determinants of the improvement in $\dot{V}O_2$max (Sharkey 1970; Shephard 1968). Figure 4.6 schematically displays the effects of these variables on $\dot{V}O_2$max. In general, optimal increases

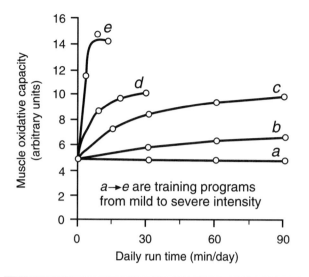

Figure 4.5 Influence of exercise bout duration and intensity on muscle oxidative capacity (as measured by cytochrome *c* concentration) in rats that underwent various treadmill training regimens for eight weeks.
Adapted, by permission, from G. Dudley, W. Abraham, and R. Terjung, 1982, "Influence of exercise intensity and duration on biochemical adaptations in skeletal muscle," *Journal of Applied Physiology* 53(4):846.

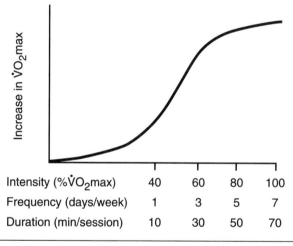

Figure 4.6 Schematic representation of the effect of exercise intensity, frequency, and duration on $\dot{V}O_2$max.

in $\dot{V}O_2$max result from training programs that are 20-60 minutes per session, 3-5 times per week, at intensities of 50%-85% $\dot{V}O_2$max (ACSM 1990). Below these levels, little or no gains in $\dot{V}O_2$max occur. Beyond these levels, the benefits become small relative to the additional demands.

Recent reports from both the Surgeon General (1996) and the NIH (1996) have emphasized the importance of regular physical activity for all Americans. These statements stress the health benefits of even moderate levels of physical activity performed on a regular basis.

Using meta-analysis, Londeree (1997) recently examined how training intensity alters the exercise intensity at which blood lactate concentration begins to rise (**lactate threshold**) or a fixed blood lactate concentration occurs. He concluded that exercise intensity near the lactate threshold is necessary to improve the threshold intensity among sedentary people. Training at higher intensities seems to have minimal benefits in sedentary individuals, but is probably necessary to increase the lactate threshold in conditioned individuals.

Genetics

The extremely high $\dot{V}O_2$max levels of elite endurance athletes have been ascribed to genetics. While training is necessary for these individuals to reach their upper limit in $\dot{V}O_2$max, genetic factors probably establish the upper boundaries. The importance of genetics in determining $\dot{V}O_2$max is rather clear: identical (monozygous) twins have very similar $\dot{V}O_2$max values, whereas the variability for fraternal (dizygous) twins is much greater (Bouchard et al. 1986; Klissourus 1971). As much as 25%-50% of variations in $\dot{V}O_2$max are thought to be related to genetic factors (Bouchard et al. 1992).

An individual's responsiveness to a training program also seems to have a genetic association (Bouchard 1990; Prud'Homme et al. 1984). Recent evidence suggests that differences in mitochondrial DNA might be responsible for individual differences in $\dot{V}O_2$max and the response to training (Dionne et al. 1989).

Age

$\dot{V}O_2$max typically peaks at 15 to 20 years of age, with women being at the lower end of this range. Cross-sectional analysis suggests that, after this age, $\dot{V}O_2$max gradually declines—typically about 10% per decade (Buskirk and Hodgson 1987). Until recently, it was difficult to determine whether the decline is related to age, disease, or just physical inactivity. It is now clear that maximal heart rate declines with aging regardless of training status (Åstrand 1960; Reeves and Sheffield 1971), and that there is an obligate decrease in $\dot{V}O_2$max of about 5% per decade (Heath et al. 1981; Kasch et al. 1990; Rogers et al. 1990). The typical age-related decline in $\dot{V}O_2$max apparently can be slowed through regular endurance training (Bortz and

Bortz 1996). Furthermore, it is well documented that the elderly have a capacity similar to that of younger individuals to adapt to endurance training (Hagberg et al. 1989; Kohrt et al. 1991; Makrides et al. 1990; Meredith et al. 1989; Saltin et al. 1969; Seals et al. 1984; Sheldahl et al. 1993).

Gender

$\dot{V}O_2$max values of females and males are similar until puberty. Beyond puberty, the average woman's $\dot{V}O_2$max is only 70%-75% that of the average man's (Åstrand 1960). The difference is smaller, but still present, among elite endurance athletes (Pollock 1977; Saltin and Åstrand 1967). The higher percentage of body fat in women accounts for a major part of the difference (Cureton and Sparling 1980). To a lesser extent, the gender difference in $\dot{V}O_2$max is related to the lower hemoglobin concentrations of women and the impact this has on oxygen delivery to active muscles (Cureton et al. 1986).

The adaptations to endurance exercise training do not appear to be gender-specific. Similar cardiorespiratory and metabolic adaptations have been found in women and men (Mitchell et al. 1992). As in men, the adaptations to training in women depend on the initial level of fitness; the intensity, duration, and frequency of training sessions; the length of the training program; and genetic factors.

Specificity of Training

Physiological adaptations to exercise training are highly specific to the type of training. Magel and coworkers (1975) examined the change in $\dot{V}O_2$max after a 10-week swim training program. Subjects performed maximal treadmill running and tethered swimming tests before and after the training program. Whereas the swimming $\dot{V}O_2$max significantly increased by 11.2%, the mean running $\dot{V}O_2$max was only 1.5% greater, an amount not statistically different from the pretraining value. Pierce and colleagues (1990) examined the lactate threshold after subjects performed either cycle or running training. Running training increased the lactate threshold by 58% and 20% for running and cycling, respectively. The cycle training increased the lactate threshold for cycling by 39%, but induced no change in the lactate threshold during running.

Both of these studies demonstrate that training adaptations are most evident with the activity used in the training. In other words, the adaptations are primarily specific to the type of training. When evidence of adaptations is confined to the exercise used in training, these adaptations are considered to be peripheral in nature; they are specific to the muscles and motor units involved in the activity.

Active Muscle Mass Involved in the Exercise Training

Physiological adaptations to exercise are dependent on the mass of muscle involved in the exercise. Endurance training with large muscle groups elicits central and peripheral adaptations; adaptations from training with small muscle groups may be limited to the periphery. In general, a training program induces central and peripheral adaptations in proportion to the degree of stress placed on both the heart and skeletal muscle—an important point to recognize when designing programs for disabled persons whose impairments may limit the muscle groups they can exercise.

Arm endurance exercise training leads to increased arm exercise capacity, according to a number of studies (Clausen et al. 1970; Clausen et al. 1973; Glaser et al. 1981; Magel et al. 1978; Pollock et al. 1974); it may not, however, strongly affect the central cardiovascular system. Magel et al. (1978) found no significant increase in running $\dot{V}O_2$max after an intensive arm training program; other researchers observed some central adaptations after arm training—including a decrease in heart rate at rest and during submaximal leg exercise (Clausen et al. 1973) and an increase in running $\dot{V}O_2$max (Pollock et al. 1974). It is likely that peripheral adaptations specific to the trained muscles account for a large component of the training adaptations from arm training. Central adaptations appear to be possible, but less pronounced, when training with small muscle groups such as the arms—presumably because lower blood flow and cardiac output requirements lessen the stimulus for central adaptations.

Although arm ergometry and wheelchair propulsion may represent reasonable exercise modes for many disabled individuals, these modes of exercise use a relatively small muscle mass. Training can be expected to induce peripheral adaptations and may improve economy, resulting in improved functional capacity (Hoffman 1986). However, because of the small muscle mass used in these modes of exercise, the potential for central cardiovascular adaptations is limited (Hoffman 1986).

Mode of Exercise Training

An important training issue is the effect of exercising muscle mass on the relationship between oxygen uptake and perceived effort. This comparison is important since most individuals set their exercise intensity by their perception of effort, while many of the benefits of endurance exercise are a function of the absolute exercise intensity. Hoffman and colleagues (1996) compared leg cycling with combined leg cycling and dynamic arm exercise in a group of young healthy subjects. Oxygen uptake at a given perceived effort was higher for the combined arm and leg exercise than for the leg-only exercise. It appears that individuals are more likely to exercise at higher oxygen uptakes with exercise modes that use a large muscle mass.

When Zeni et al. (1996) compared oxygen uptake at different levels of perceived exertion among six different modes of exercise, they found significant differences in oxygen uptake among the modes of exercise (figure 4.7). Interestingly, the amount of ex-

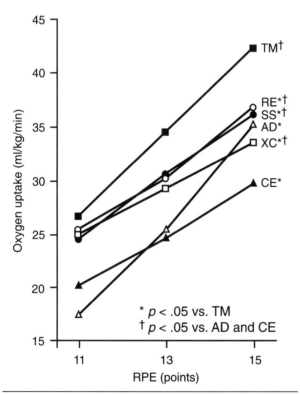

Figure 4.7 Mean oxygen uptakes as a function of rating of perceived exertion (RPE) on the 6-20 point scale (Borg 1970) for Airdyne exercise (AD), simulated cross-country skiing (XC), cycle ergometry (CE), rowing ergometry (RE), stair stepping (SS), and treadmill walking/running (TM).

Adapted, by permission, from A. Zeni, M. Hoffman, and P. Clifford, 1996, "Energy expenditure with indoor exercise machines," *Journal of the American Medical Association* 275 (18): 1426. Copyright 1996, American Medical Association.

ercising muscle could not always explain the differences between exercise modes. For example, treadmill walking and running induced higher oxygen uptakes at given levels of perceived effort than rowing ergometry and simulated cross-country skiing, both of which might be expected to engage a larger muscle mass than walking and running. Factors related to the movement pattern of the exercise may be important—such as the degree to which eccentric and isometric contractions are required, the incorporation of neural pathways for reciprocal innervation, and the familiarity with the movement pattern.

Simultaneous Strength and Endurance Exercise Training

Simultaneous performance of endurance exercise training and strength training programs can induce gains in endurance, strength, and power. However, strength training by itself creates greater gains in muscular strength and power than when the strength training is combined with endurance training (Dudley and Fleck 1987). In contrast, improvements in $\dot{V}O_2$max do not appear to be impaired by the combination of strength and endurance training (Hickson et al. 1988).

Summary

Regular endurance exercise elicits a wide variety of physiological changes that improve an individual's ability to respond to subsequent exercise demands. These adaptations allow the body to send more blood to the tissues and the muscles to extract more oxygen from the blood. The adaptations lead to improved maximal exercise capacity and reduced physiological demands during submaximal exercise, both of which favorably affect functional abilities. Adaptations to endurance exercise training can occur among all populations regardless of age or disability. However, the extent of the adaptations is influenced by a number of factors including the individual's age, gender, genetic makeup, initial level of fitness, and design and duration of the exercise training program.

References

Aloia, J., S. Cohn, J. Ostuni, R. Cane, and K. Ellis. 1987. Prevention of involutional bone loss by exercise. *Ann Intern Med* 89:356-358.

American College of Sports Medicine. 1990. Position stand: The recommended quantity and quality of exercise for developing and maintaining cardiorespiratory and muscular fitness in healthy adults. *Med Sci Sports Exerc* 22:265-274.

Åstrand, I. 1960. Aerobic work capacity in men and women with special reference to age. *Acta Physiol Scand* Supp. 169:1-92.

Åstrand, P.-O., and K. Rodahl. 1986. *Textbook of work physiology: Physiological bases of exercise.* 3d ed. New York: McGraw-Hill.

Ayers, J.W., Y. Komesu, T. Romani, and R. Ansbacher. 1985. Anthropomorphic, hormonal and psychological correlates of semen quality in endurance-trained athletes. *Fertil Steril* 43:917-921.

Baldwin, K.M., W.W. Winder, R.L. Terjung, and J.O. Holloszy. 1973. Glycolytic enzymes in different types of skeletal muscle: adaptation to exercise. *Am J Physiol* 225:962-966.

Bigland-Ritchie, B. 1990. Discussion: Nervous system and sensory adaptations. In *Exercise, fitness, and health*, ed. C. Bouchard, R.J. Shephard, T. Stephens, J.R. Sutton, and B.D. McPherson, 377-383. Champaign, IL: Human Kinetics.

Blake, M.J., E.A. Stein, and A.J. Vomachka. 1984. Effects of exercise training on brain opioid peptides and serum LH in female rats. *Peptides* 5:953-958.

Bloom, S.R., R.H. Johnson, D.M. Park, M.J. Rennie, and W.R. Sulaiman. 1976. Differences in the metabolic and hormonal responses to exercise between racing cyclists and untrained individuals. *J Appl Physiol* 48:1-18.

Blumenthal, J.A., M. Fredrikson, C.M. Kuhn, R.L. Ulmer, M. Walsh-Riddle, and M. Appelbaum. 1990. Aerobic exercise reduces levels of cardiovascular and sympathoadrenal responses to mental stress in subjects without prior evidence of myocardial ischemia. *Am J Cardiol* 65:93-98.

Borg, G. 1970. Perceived exertion as an indicator of somatic stress. *Scand J Rehabil Med* 2-3:92-98.

Bortz, W.M. IV, and W.M. Bortz II. 1996. How fast do we age? Exercise performance over time as a biomarker. *J Gerontol A Biol Sci Med Sci* 51A:M223-M225.

Bouchard, C. 1990. Discussion: heredity, fitness, and health. In *Exercise, fitness, and health*, ed. C. Bouchard, R.J. Shephard, T. Stephens, J.R. Sutton, and B.D. McPherson, 147-153. Champaign, IL: Human Kinetics.

Bouchard, C., F.T. Dionne, J.-A. Simoneau, and M.R. Boulay. 1992. Genetics of aerobic and anaerobic performances. *Exerc Sport Sci Rev* 20:27-58.

Bouchard, C., R. Lesage, G. Lortie, J.A. Simoneau, P. Hamel, M.R. Boulay, L. Perusse, G. Theriault, and C. Leblanc. 1986. Aerobic performance in brothers, dizygotic and monozygotic twins. *Med Sci Sports Exerc* 18:639-646.

Brisson, G.R., M.A. Volle, D. DeCarufel, M. Desharnais, and M. Tanaka. 1980. Exercise-induced dissociation of the blood prolactin response in young women according to their sports habits. *Horm Metab Res* 12:201-205.

Buskirk, E.R., and J.L. Hodgson. 1987. Age and aerobic power: the rate of change in men and women. *Federation Proc* 46:1824-1829.

Cann, C.E., M.C. Martin, H.K. Genant, and R.B. Jaffe. 1984. Decreased spinal mineral content in amenorrheic women. *JAMA* 251:626-629.

Carr, D.B., B.A. Bullen, G.S. Skrinar, M.A. Arnold, M. Rosenblatt, I.Z. Beitins, J.B. Martin, and J.W. McArthur. 1981. Physical conditioning facilitates the exercise-induced secretion of beta-endorphin and beta-lipotropin in women. *N Engl J Med* 305:560-563.

Casaburi, R., T.W. Storer, and K. Wasserman. 1987. Mediation of reduced ventilatory response to exercise after endurance training. *J Appl Physiol* 63:1533-1538.

Cavanagh, P.R., and R. Kram. 1985. The efficiency of human movement—a statement of the problem. *Med Sci Sports Exerc* 17:304-308.

Chi, M.M., C.S. Hintz, E.F. Coyle, W.H. Martin III, J.L. Ivy, P.M. Nemeth, J.O. Holloszy, and O.H. Lowry. 1983. Effects of detraining on enzymes of energy metabolism in individual human muscle fibers. *Am J Physiol* 244:C276-C287.

Christie, M.J., and G.B. Chesher. 1983. [³H]Leu-enkephalin binding following chronic swim-stress in mice. *Neurosci Lett* 36:323-328.

Clanton, T., G.F. Dixon, J. Drake, and J.E. Gadek. 1987. Effects of swim training on lung volumes and inspiratory muscle conditioning. *J Appl Physiol* 62:39-46.

Clausen, J.P. 1977. Effect of physical training on cardiovascular adjustments to exercise in man. *Physiol Rev* 57:779-815.

Clausen, J.P., K. Klausen, B. Rasmussen, and J. Trap-Jensen. 1973. Central and peripheral circulatory changes after training of the arms or legs. *Am J Physiol* 225:675-682.

Clausen, J.P., and J. Trap-Jensen. 1976. Heart rate and arterial blood pressure during exercise in patients with angina pectoris. Effects of training and of nitroglycerin. *Circulation* 53:436-442.

Clausen, J.P., J. Trap-Jensen, and N.A. Lassen. 1970. The effects of training on the heart rate during arm and leg exercise. *Scand J Clin Lab Invest* 26:295-301.

Convertino, V.A., L.C. Keil, E.M. Bernauer, and J.E. Greenleaf. 1981. Plasma volume, osmolality, vasopressin, and renin activity during graded exercise in man. *J Appl Physiol* 50:123-128.

Convertino, V.A., L.C. Keil, and J.E. Greenleaf. 1983. Plasma volume, renin, and vasopressin responses to graded exercise after training. *J Appl Physiol* 54:508-514.

Cronan, T.L., and E.T. Howley. 1974. The effect of training on epinephrine and norepinephrine excretion. *Med Sci Sports* 6:122-125.

Cureton, K., P. Bishop, P. Hutchinson, H. Newland, S. Vickery, and L. Zwiren. 1986. Sex differences in maximal oxygen uptake: effect of equating haemoglobin concentration. *Eur J Appl Physiol* 54:656-660.

Cureton, K.L., and P.B. Sparling. 1980. Distance running performance and metabolic responses to running in men and women with excess weight experimentally equated. *Med Sci Sports Exerc* 12:288-294.

Dela, F., K.J. Mikines, and H. Galbo. 1987. Arginine stimulated insulin response in trained and untrained man. *Diabetologia* 30:513A.

deVries, H.A. 1968. Immediate and long-term effects of exercise upon resting muscle action potential. *J Sports Med* 8:1-11.

Dionne, F.T., L. Turcotte, M.-C. Thibault, M.R. Boulay, J.S. Skinner, and C. Bouchard. 1989. Mitochondrial DNA sequence polymorphism, $\dot{V}O_2$max, and response to endurance training. *Med Sci Sports Exerc* 23:177-185.

Drinkwater, B.L., K. Nilson, C.H. Chestnut, III, W. Bremmer, S. Shainholtz, and M. Southworth. 1984. Bone mineral content of amenorrheic and eumenorrheic athletes. *N Engl J Med* 311:277-281.

Droste, C., M.W. Greenlee, M. Schreck, and H. Roskamm. 1991. Experimental pain thresholds and plasma beta-endorphin levels during exercise. *Med Sci Sports Exerc* 23:334-342.

Dudley, G.A., W.M. Abraham, and R.L. Terjung. 1982. Influence of exercise intensity and duration on biochemical adaptations in skeletal muscle. *J Appl Physiol* 53:844-850.

Dudley, G.A., and S.J. Fleck. 1987. Strength and endurance training: are they mutually exclusive? *Sports Med* 4:79-85.

Edgerton, V.R. 1976. Neuromuscular adaptation to power and endurance work. *Can J Appl Sport Sci* 1:49-58.

Ehsani, A.A., T. Ogawa, T.R. Miller, R.J. Spina, and S.M. Jilka. 1991. Exercise training improves left ventricular systolic function in older men. *Circulation* 83:96-103.

Ekblom, B. 1969. Effect of physical training on oxygen transport system in man. *Acta Physiol Scand Suppl* 328:1-45.

Ekblom, B., P.-O. Åstrand, B. Saltin, J. Stenberg, and B. Wallstrom. 1968. Effect of training on circulatory responses to exercise. *J Appl Physiol* 24:518-528.

Farrell, P.A., A.B. Gustafson, W.P. Morgan, C.B. Pert. 1987. Enkephalins, catecholamines, and psychological mood alterations: effects of prolonged exercise. *Med Sci Sports Exerc* 19:347-353.

Farrell, P.A., M. Kjaer, F.W. Bach, and H. Galbo. 1987. Beta endorphin and adrenocorticotropin responses to supramaximal treadmill exercise in trained and untrained males. *Acta Physiol Scand* 130:619-625.

Farrell, P.A., J.H. Wilmore, E.F. Coyle, J.E. Billings, and D.L. Costill. 1979. Plasma lactate accumulation and distance running performance. *Med Sci Sports* 11:338-344.

Fentem, P.H. 1992. Exercise in prevention of disease. *Br Med Bull* 48:630-650.

Fries, J.F. 1996. Physical activity, the compression of morbidity, and the health of the elderly. *J R Soc Med* 89:64-68.

Fries, J.F., G. Singh, D. Morfeld, H.B. Hubert, N.E. Lane, B.W. Brown Jr. 1994. Running and the development of disability with age. *Ann Intern Med* 121:502-509.

Galbo, H., J.J. Holst, and N.J. Christensen. 1975. Glucagon and plasma catecholamine responses to graded and prolonged exercise in man. *J Appl Physiol* 38:70-76.

Galbo, H., E.A. Richter, J. Hilsted, J.J. Holst, N.J. Christensen, and J. Henriksson. 1977. Hormonal regulation during prolonged exercise. *Ann N Y Acad Sci* 301:72-80.

Glaser, R.M., M.N. Sawka, R.J. Durbin, D.M. Foley, and A.G. Suryaprasad. 1981. Exercise program for wheelchair activity. *Am J Phys Med* 60:67-75.

Gleeson, P.B., E.J. Protas, A. Leblanc, V.S. Schneider, and H.J. Evans. 1990. Effects of weight lifting on bone mineral density in premenopausal women. *J Bone Miner Res* 5:153-158.

Goldman, J.A. 1991. Hypermobility and deconditioning: important links to fibromyalgia/fibrositis. *South Med J* 84:1192-1196.

Gollnick, P.D., R.B. Armstrong, C.W. Saubert, K. Piehl, and B. Saltin. 1972. Enzyme activity and fiber composition in skeletal muscle of untrained and trained men. *J Appl Physiol* 33:312-319.

Hagberg, J.M., J.E. Graves, M. Limacher, D.R. Woods, S.H. Leggett, C. Cononie, J.J. Gruber, and M.L. Pollock. 1989. Cardiovascular responses of 70- to 79-yr-old men and women to exercise training. *J Appl Physiol* 66:2589-2594.

Hartley, H.L. 1975. Growth hormone and catecholamine response to exercise in relation to physical training. *Med Sci Sports Exerc* 7:34-36.

Hartley, L.H., J.W. Mason, R.P. Hogan, L.G. Jones, T.A. Kotchen, E.H. Mougey, F.E. Wherry, L.L. Pennington, and P.T. Ricketts. 1972a. Multiple hormonal responses to graded exercise in relation to physical training. *J Appl Physiol* 33:602-606.

Hartley, L.H., J.W. Mason, R.P. Hogan, L.G. Jones, T.A. Kotchen, E.H. Mougey, F.E. Wherry, L.L. Pennington, and P.T. Ricketts. 1972b. Multiple hormonal responses to prolonged exercise in relation to physical training. *J Appl Physiol* 33:607-610.

Heath, G., J. Hagberg, A.A. Ehsani, and J.O. Holloszy. 1981. Physical comparison of young and old endurance athletes. *J Appl Physiol* 51:634-640.

Henriksson, J. 1977. Training induced adaptations of skeletal muscle and metabolism during submaximal exercise. *J Physiol (Lond)* 270:661-675.

Hermansen, L., E. Hultmen, and B. Saltin. 1967. Muscle glycogen during prolonged severe exercise. *Acta Physiol Scand* 71:129-139.

Hiatt, W.R., E.E. Wolfel, R.H. Meier, and J.G. Regensteiner. 1994. Superiority of treadmill walking exercise versus strength training for patients with peripheral arterial disease. Implications for the mechanism of the training response. *Circulation* 90:1866-1874.

Hickson, R.C., B.A. Dvorak, E.M. Gorostiaga, T.T. Kurowski, and C. Foster. 1988. Potential for strength and endurance training to amplify endurance performance. *J Appl Physiol* 65:2285-2290.

Hickson, R.C., J.M. Hagberg, A.A. Ehsani, and J.O. Holloszy. 1981. Time course of the adaptive responses of aerobic power and heart rate to training. *Med Sci Sports Exerc* 13:17-20.

Hoffman, M.D. 1986. Cardiorespiratory fitness and training in quadriplegics and paraplegics. *Sports Med* 3:312-330.

Hoffman, M.D., K.M. Kassay, A.I. Zeni, and P.S. Clifford. 1996. Does the amount of exercising muscle alter the aerobic demand of dynamic exercise? *Eur J Appl Physiol* 74:541-547.

Hoffmann, P., L. Terenius, and P. Thoren. 1990. Cerebrospinal fluid immunoreactive ß-endorphin concentration is increased by voluntary exercise in the spontaneously hypertensive rat. *Regul Pept* 28:233-239.

Holloszy, J.O. 1973. Biochemical adaptations to exercise: aerobic metabolism. *Exerc Sport Sci Rev* 1:45-71.

Holloszy, J.O., and E.F. Coyle. 1984. Adaptations of skeletal muscle to endurance exercise and their metabolic consequences. *J Appl Physiol* 56:831-838.

Hosobuchi, Y., and C.H. Li. 1978. The analgesic activity of human beta-endorphin in man (1,2,3). *Commun Psychopharmacol* 2:33-37.

Hurley, B.F., J.M. Hagberg, W.K. Allen, D.R. Seals, J.C. Young, R.W. Cuddihee, and J.O. Holloszy. 1984. Effect of training on blood lactate levels during submaximal exercise. *J Appl Physiol* 56:1260-1264.

Janal, M.N., E.W.D. Colt, W.C. Clark, and M. Glusman. 1984. Pain sensitivity, mood and plasma endocrine levels in man following long-distance running: effects of naloxone. *Pain* 19:13-25.

Jansson, E., and L. Kaijser. 1977. Muscle adaptation to extreme endurance training in man. *Acta Physiol Scand* 100:315-324.

Karlsson, J., L.-O. Nordesjo, L. Jorfeldt, and B. Saltin. 1972. Muscle lactate, ATP, and CP levels during exercise after physical training in man. *J Appl Physiol* 33:199-203.

Kasch, F.W., J.L. Boyer, S.P. Van Camp, L.S. Verity, and J.P. Wallace. 1990. The effect of physical activity and inactivity on aerobic power in older men (a longitudinal study). *Physician Sportsmed* 18(4):73-83.

Kemppainen, P., P. Paalasmaa, A. Pertovaara, A. Alila, and G. Johansson. 1990. Desamethasone attenuates exercise-induced dental analgesia in man. *Brain Res* 519:329-332.

Kemppainen, P., A. Pertovaara, T. Huopaniemi, G. Johansson, and S.L. Karonen. 1985. Modification of dental pain and cutaneous thermal sensitivity by physical exercise in man. *Brain Res* 360:33-44.

Kjaer, M., P.A. Farrell, N.J. Christensen, and H. Galbo. 1986. Increased epinephrine response and inaccurate glucoregulation in exercising athletes. *J Appl Physiol* 61:1693-1700.

Klissouras, V. 1971. Adaptability of genetic variation. *J Appl Physiol* 31:338-344.

Kohrt, W.M., M.T. Malley, A.R. Coggan, R.J. Spina, T. Ogawa, A.A. Ehsani, R.E. Bourey, W.H. Martin III, and J.O. Holloszy. 1991. Effects of gender, age and fitness level on response of $\dot{V}O_2$max to training in 60-71 yr olds. *J Appl Physiol* 71:2004-2011.

Kohrt, W.M., D.B. Snead, E. Slatopolsky, and S.J. Birge, Jr. 1995. Additive effects of weight-bearing exercise and estrogen on bone mineral density in older women. *J Bone Miner Res* 10:1303-1311.

Koltyn, K.F., A.W. Garvin, R.L. Gardiner, and T.F. Nelson. 1996. Perception of pain following aerobic exercise. *Med Sci Sports Exerc* 28:1418-1421.

LaFontaine, T.P., B.R. Londeree, and W.K. Spath. 1981. The maximal steady state versus selected running events. *Med Sci Sports Exerc* 13:190-192.

Landry, F.C. Bouchard, and J. Dumesnil. 1985. Cardiac dimension changes with endurance training. *JAMA* 254:77-80.

Lavie, C.J., and R.V. Milani. 1995. Effects of cardiac rehabilitation program on exercise capacity, coronary risk factors, behavioral characteristics, and quality of life in a large elderly cohort. *Am J Cardiol* 76:177-179.

Lavie, C.J., R.V. Milani, and A.B. Littman. 1993. Benefits of cardiac rehabilitation and exercise training in secondary coronary prevention in the elderly. *J Am Coll Cardiol* 22:678-683.

Londeree, B.R. 1997. Effects of training on lactate/ventilatory thresholds: a meta-analysis. *Med Sci Sports Exerc* 29:837-843.

Magel, J.R., G.F. Foglia, W.D. McArdle, B. Gutin, G.S. Pechar, and F.I. Katch. 1975. Specificity of swim training on maximal oxygen uptake. *J Appl Physiol* 38:151-155.

Magel, J.R., W.D. McArdle, M. Toner, and D.J. Delio. 1978. Metabolic and cardiovascular adjustment to arm training. *J Appl Physiol* 45:75-79.

Makrides, L., G.J.F. Heignehauser, and N.L. Jones. 1990. High-intensity endurance training in 20- to 30- and 60- to 70-yr-old healthy men. *J Appl Physiol* 69:1792-1798.

Margulies, J.Y., A. Simkin, I. Leichter, A. Bivas, R. Steinberg, M. Giladi, M. Stein, H. Kashtan, and C. Milgrom. 1986. Effect of intense physical activity on the bone-mineral content in the lower limbs of young adults. *J Bone Joint Surg Am* 68:1090-1093.

Markoff, R.A., P. Ryan, and T. Young. 1982. Endorphins and mood changes in long-distance running. *Med Sci Sports Exerc* 14:11-15.

Martin, B.J., K.E. Sparks, C.W. Zwillich, and J.V. Weil. 1979. Low exercise ventilation in endurance athletes. *Med Sci Sports* 11:181-185.

McCain, G.A., D.A. Bell, F.M. Mai, and P.D. Halliday. 1988. A controlled study of the effects of a supervised cardiovascular fitness training program on the manifestations of primary fibromyalgia. *Arthritis Rheum* 31:1135-1141.

McCann, L., and D.S. Holmes. 1984. Influence of aerobic exercise on depression. *J Pers Soc Psychol* 46:1142-1147.

Melin, B., J.P. Eclache, G. Geelen, A. Annat, A.M. Allevard, E. Jarsaillon, A. Zebidi, J.J. Legros, and C. Gharib. 1980. Plasma AVP, neurophysin, renin activity, and aldosterone during submaximal exercise performed until exhaustion in trained and untrained men. *Eur J Appl Physiol* 44:141-151.

Meredith, C.N., W.R. Frontera, E.C. Fisher, V.A. Hughes, J.C. Herland, J. Edwards, and W.J. Evans. 1989. Peripheral effects of endurance training in young and old subjects. *J Appl Physiol* 66:2844-2849.

Metzger, J.M., and E.A. Stein. 1984. Beta-endorphin and sprint training. *Life Sci* 34:1541-1547.

Mikines, K.J., F. Dela, B. Sonne, P.A. Farrell, E.A. Richter, and H. Galbo. 1987. Insulin action and secretion in man; effects of different levels of physical activity. *Can J Sport Sci* 12 (Suppl. 1):113-116.

Mikines, K.J., B. Sonne, P.A. Farrell, B. Tronier, and H. Galbo. 1988. Effect of physical exercise on sensitivity and responsiveness to insulin in man. *Am J Physiol* 17:E248-E259.

Mitchell, J.H., C. Tate, P. Raven, F. Cobb, W. Kraus, R. Moreadith, M. O'Toole, B. Saltin, and N. Wenger. 1992. Acute responses and chronic adaptations to exercise in women. *Med Sci Sports Exerc* 24:S258-S265.

Moldofsky, H., and P. Scarisbrick. 1976. Induction of neurasthetic musculoskeletal pain syndrome by selective sleep stage deprivation. *Psychosom Med* 38:35-44.

Mole, P.A., L.B. Oscai, and J.O. Holloszy. 1971. Adaptation of muscle to exercise. Increase in levels of palmityl CoA synthetase, carnitine palmityltransferase, and palmityl CoA dehydrogenase, and in the capacity to oxidize fatty acids. *J Clin Invest* 50:2323-2330.

Morgan, W.P. 1979. Anxiety reduction following acute physical activity. *Psychiatr Ann* 9:36-45.

Morrison, D.A., T.W. Boyden, R.W. Pamenter, B.J. Freund, W.A. Stini, R. Harrington, and J.H. Wilmore. 1986. Effects of aerobic training on exercise tolerance and echocardiographic dimensions in untrained postmenopausal women. *Am Heart J* 112:561-567.

Mougin, C., A. Baulay, M.T. Henriet, D. Haton, M.C. Jacquier, D. Turnill, S. Berthelay, and R.C. Gaillard. 1987. Assessment of plasma opioid peptides, beta-endorphin and met-enkephalin, at the end of an international Nordic ski race. *Eur J Appl Physiol* 56:281-286.

Nadel, E.R., K.B. Pandolf, M.F. Roberts, and J.A.J. Stolwijk. 1974. Mechanisms of thermal acclimatization to exercise and heat. *J Appl Physiol* 37:515-520.

Nichols, D.S., and T.M. Glenn. 1994. Effects of aerobic exercise on pain perception, affect, and level of disability in individuals with fibromyalgia. *Phys Ther* 74:327-332.

NIH Consensus Development Panel on Physical Activity and Cardiovascular Health. 1996. Physical activity and cardiovascular health. *JAMA* 276:241-246.

O'Connor, P.J., and S.D. Youngstedt. 1995. Influence of exercise on human sleep. *Exerc Sport Sci Rev* 23:105-134.

Olausson, B., E. Eriksson, L. Ellmarker, B. Rydenhag, B.-C. Shyu, and S.A. Anderson. 1986. Effects of naloxone on dental pain threshold following muscle exercise and low frequency transcutaneous nerve stimulation: a comparative study in man. *Acta Physiol Scand* 126:299-305.

Pandolf, K.B., B.S. Cadarette, M.N. Sawka, A.J. Young, and R.P. Francesconi. 1988. Thermoregulatory responses of middle-aged men and young men during dry heat acclimation. *J Appl Physiol* 65:65-71.

Peronnet, F., J. Cleroux, H. Perrault, D. Cousineau, J. de Champlain, and R. Nadeau. 1981. Plasma norepinephrine responses to exercise before and after training in humans. *J Appl Physiol* 51:812-815.

Pertovaara, A., T. Huopaniemi, A. Virtanen, and G. Johansson. 1984. The influence of exercise on dental pain thresholds and the release of stress hormones. *Physiol Behav* 33:923-926.

Pierce, E.F.A., A. Weltman, R.L. Seip, and D. Snead. 1990. Effects of training specificity on the lactate threshold and O_2 peak. *Int J Sports Med* 11:267-272.

Poehlman, E.T., C.L. Melby, and M.I. Goran. 1991. The impact of exercise and diet restrictions on daily energy expenditure. *Sports Med* 11:78-101.

Pollock, M.L. 1977. Submaximal and maximal working capacity of elite distance runners. Part I: Cardiorespiratory aspects. *Ann N Y Acad Sci* 301:310-322.

Pollock, M.L., H.S. Miller, A.C. Linnerud, E. Laughridge, E. Coleman, and E. Alexander. 1974. Arm pedaling as an endurance training regimen for the disabled. *Arch Phys Med Rehabil* 55:418-424.

Powers, S.K., and E.T. Howley. 1997. *Exercise physiology: Theory and application to fitness and performance.* 3d ed. Madison, WI: Brown and Benchmark Publishers.

Prior, J.C., L. Jensen, B.H. Yuen, H. Higgins, and L. Brownlie. 1981. Prolactin changes with exercise vary with breast motion: analysis of running versus cycling. *Fertil Steril* 36:268.

Prud'Homme, D., C. Bouchard, C. Leblanc, L.F. Landry, and E. Fontaine. 1984. Sensitivity of maximal aerobic power to training is genotype-dependent. *Med Sci Sports Exerc* 16:489-493.

Reeves, T.J., and L.T. Sheffield. 1971. The influence of age and athletic training on maximal heart rate during exercise. In *Coronary heart disease and physical fitness*, ed. O. Andree-Larsen and R.O. Malmborg, 209-216. Copenhagen: Munksgaard.

Rerych, S.K., P.M. Scholz, D.C. Sabiston Jr., and R.H. Jones. 1980. Effects of exercise training on left ventricular function in normal subjects: a longitudinal study by radionuclide angiography. *Am J Cardiol* 45:244-252.

Rogers, M.A., J. Hagberg, S.H. Martin, A.A. Eksani, and J.O. Holloszy. 1990. Decline in $\dot{V}O_2$ max with aging in masters athletes and sedentary men. *J Appl Physiol* 68:2195-2199.

Rowell, L.B. 1974. Human cardiovascular adjustments to exercise and thermal stress. *Physiol Rev* 54:75-159.

Rowell, L.B. 1986. *Human circulation-regulation during physical stress.* New York: Oxford University Press.

Sale, D.G. 1987. Influence of exercise and training on motor units activation. *Exerc Sport Sci Rev* 15:95-151.

Saltin, B. 1969. Physiological effects of physical conditioning. *Med Sci Sports* 1:50-56.

Saltin, B., and P.-O. Åstrand. 1967. Maximal oxygen uptake in athletes. *J Appl Physiol* 23:353-358.

Saltin, B., L.H. Hartley, A. Kilbom, and I. Åstrand. 1969. Physical training in sedentary middle-aged and older men. II. Oxygen uptake, heart rate, and blood lactate concentration at submaximal and maximal exercise. *Scand J Clin Lab Invest* 24:323-334.

Saltin, B., K. Nazar, D.L. Costill, E. Stein, E. Jansson, B. Essen, and P.D. Gollnick. 1976. The nature of the training response: peripheral and central adaptations to one-legged exercise. *Acta Physiol Scand* 96:289-305.

Schantz, P., J. Henriksson, and E. Jansson. 1983. Adaptations of human skeletal muscle to endurance training of long duration. *Clin Physiol* 3:141-151.

Seals, D.R., J.M. Hagberg, B.F. Hurley, A.A. Ehsani, and J.O. Holloszy. 1984. Endurance training in older men and women. I. Cardiovascular responses to exercise. *J Appl Physiol* 57:1024-1029.

Sforzo, G.A., T.F. Seeger, C.B. Pert, A. Pert, and C.O. Cotson. 1986. In vivo opioid receptor occupation in the rat brain following exercise. *Med Sci Sports Exerc* 18:380-384.

Sharkey, B.J. 1970. Intensity and duration of training and the development of cardiorespiratory endurance. *Med Sci Sports* 2:197-202.

Sheldahl, L.M., F.E. Tristani, J.E. Hastings, R.B. Wenzler, and S.G. Levandoski. 1993. Comparison of adaptations and compliance to exercise training between middle-aged and older men. *J Am Geriatr Soc* 41:795-801.

Shephard, R.J. 1968. Intensity, duration, and frequency of exercise as determinants of the response to a training regime. *Int Z Angew Physiol* 26:272-278.

Shephard, R.J. 1991. Benefits of sport and physical activity for the disabled: implications for the individual and for society. *Scand J Rehab Med* 23:51-59.

Shephard, R.J. 1993. Exercise and aging: extending independence in older adults. *Geriatrics* 48(5):61-64.

Shephard, R.J., and K.H. Sidney. 1975. Effects of physical exertion on plasma GH and cortisol levels in human subjects. *Exerc Sport Sci Rev* 3:1-30.

Simons, A., C.R. McGowan, L.H. Epstein, D.J. Kuper, and R.J. Robertson. 1985. Exercise as a treatment for depression: an update. *Clin Psychol Rev* 5:553-568.

Sjodin, B., and I. Jacobs. 1981. Onset of blood lactate accumulation and marathon running performance. *Int J Sports Med* 2:23-26.

Sonstroem, R.J. 1984. Exercise and self-esteem. *Exerc Sport Sci Rev* 12:123-155.

Strawbridge, W.J., R.D. Cohen, S.J. Shema, and G.A. Kaplan. 1996. Successful aging: predictors and associated activities. *Am J Epidemiol* 144:135-141.

Surgeon General of the Public Health Service. 1996. Surgeon General's report on physical activity and health (S/N 017-023-00196-5).

Sutton, J.R. 1978. Hormonal and metabolic responses to exercise in subjects of high and low work capacities. *Med Sci Sports Exerc* 10:1-6.

Sutton, J.R., J.D. Young, L. Lazarus, J.B. Hickie, and J. Maksvytis. 1969. The hormonal response to physical exercise. *Aust Ann Med* 18:84-90.

Terrados, N., and R.J. Maughan. 1995. Exercise in the heat: strategies to minimize the adverse effects on performance. *J Sports Sci* 13:S55-S62.

Tipton, C.M., R.D. Matthes, J.A. Maynard, and R.A. Carey. 1975. The influence of physical activity on ligaments and tendons. *Med Sci Sports* 7:165-175.

Ulrich, C.M., C.C. Georgiou, C.M. Snow-Harter, and D.E. Gillis. 1996. Bone mineral density in mother-daughter pairs: relations to lifetime exercise, lifetime milk consumption, and calcium supplements. *Am J Clin Nutr* 63:72-79.

Vander, A.J., J.H. Sherman, and D.S. Luciano. 1985. *Human physiology: The mechanisms of body function.* 4th ed. New York: McGraw-Hill.

Washburn, R.A., and D.R. Seals. 1984. Peak oxygen uptake during arm cranking for men and women. *J Appl Physiol* 56:954-957.

Wheeler, B.D., S.R. Wall, A.N. Belcastro, and D.C. Cumming. 1984. Reduced serum testosterone and prolactin levels in male distance runners. *JAMA* 252:514-516.

Williams, J.A., J. Wagner, R. Wasnich, and L. Heilbrum. 1984. The effect of long distance running upon appendicular bone mineral content. *Med Sci Sports Exerc* 16:223-227.

Winder, W.W., R.C. Hickson, J.M. Hagberg, A.A. Ehsani, and J.A. McLane. 1979. Training-induced changes in hormonal and metabolic responses to submaximal exercise. *J Appl Physiol* 46:766-771.

Wyndham, C.H. 1973. The physiology of exercise under heat stress. *Annu Rev Physiol* 35:193-220.

Young, D.R., K.H. Masaki, and J.D. Curb. 1995. Associations of physical activity with performance-based and self-reported physical functioning in older men: the Honolulu Heart Program. *J Am Geriatr Soc* 43:845-854.

Zeni, A.I., M.D. Hoffman, and P.S. Clifford. 1996. Energy expenditure with indoor exercise machines. *JAMA* 275:1424-1427.

Chapter 5

Adaptations to Strength Conditioning

Bette Ann Harris, PT, MS, and Mary P. Watkins, PT, MS

As an element of physical rehabilitation, strength training has a positive impact not only on skeletal muscle, but also on neuromotor excitation, on the integrity and viability of connective tissue, and even a person's sense of well-being. This chapter describes the rationale for strength training, and considers the effects of training and detraining on muscle performance. It presents the factors that affect muscle strength, and discusses how to increase that strength, especially where immobilization or pathological processes have created a decline in muscle performance. It describes how the anatomy and physiology of muscle are affected by training (or by the lack thereof).

For *conceptual* purposes, we define strength as "the ability of skeletal muscle to develop force for the pur-pose of providing stability and mobility within the musculoskeletal system, so that functional movement can take place" (Harris and Watkins 1993). There are many *operational* definitions of strength. It has been interpreted as "the magnitude of the torque exerted by a muscle or muscles in a single maximal isometric contraction of unrestricted duration" (Enoka 1994). Other definitions refer to the type of muscle contraction (e.g., concentric, eccentric, or isometric) and to velocity. These may be classified as either static or dynamic exercise conditions. Strength conditioning programs traditionally incorporate high-load, low-repetition formulas. The challenge for rehabilitation professionals is to select the most appropriate and safe form of strength training of sufficient intensity, frequency, and duration to achieve maximal benefit.

Anatomical and Physiological Factors in Strength

The rationale for strength training is based on an understanding of the structure and function of the musculoskeletal system. The following summary reviews the important anatomical and physiological factors that affect an individual's response to strengthening exercise.

The amount of force that can be generated by skeletal muscle depends on the integrity of both contractile and noncontractile structural elements, motor units, metabolic support systems, and central nervous system control mechanisms. Voluntary muscular contraction is initiated by the firing of anterior horn cells in the ventral horn of the spinal cord, as directed from the higher centers of the central nervous system. Each anterior horn cell innervates a number of individual muscle fibers. A **motor unit** comprises a single anterior horn cell and all the fibers it innervates. Motor units vary in size, reflecting the role of muscles in performance. The innervation ratio is small in muscles required for fine, precision activity, such as the small muscles of the hand; large motor units supply muscles that perform gross functions such as postural control.

Contractile Elements

Muscle fibers are the contractile elements of skeletal muscle. These cells are cylindrically shaped, multinucleated, and are encased in a plasma membrane called the **sarcolemma**. The **myofibril**, comprising repeated sarcomeres demarcated by dense Z lines, is the subcellular unit of the muscle fiber. The myosin molecules, comprising thick filaments, include projections which, when activated, form crossbridges with actin molecules, comprising thin filaments, causing bonds that result in muscle contraction. The thin and thick filaments, arranged between Z lines, give skeletal muscle its striated appearance. This series of events, from the electrical activity of depolarization to the chemical formation of actin-myosin bonds, is called excitation-contraction coupling (Åstrand and Rodahl 1986).

The magnitude of force developed in the contractile process depends not only on the number of activated motor units and frequency of motor unit firing, but also on the integrity of supporting connective tissue (Stone 1988), on metabolic support (Evans 1995), and on biomechanical factors of overall muscle length and speed of contraction.

Noncontractile Elements

The noncontractile tissues in skeletal muscle contribute to force production. The continuity of muscle is supported by the **endomysium** that covers each muscle fiber, the **perimysium** that groups fibers into bundles, and the **epimysium** that covers the entire muscle structure. These structures taken together merge at the peripheral ends of muscles to form the **myotendinous** or **aponeurotic junctions** to bone. These attachments complete the structural chain that allows for movement during muscular contraction. Muscle contraction imposes stress on this connective tissue matrix, whose elastic properties dampen the effects of contraction, resulting in smooth translation of force to accomplish functional movement.

Muscle Fiber Types

Skeletal muscle comprises different fiber types that vary structurally, histochemically, and metabolically (Åstrand and Rodahl 1986). There are two major categories. Type I (SO [slow oxidative]) fibers are best suited for sustained or repeated contractions requiring relatively low tension, such as walking, quiet standing, and most activities of daily living. These functions are well supported by a rich blood supply. The major pathway for energy production in type I fibers is oxidative phosphorylation. Type II fibers are subdivided into types IIb and IIa. Metabolic energy sources for type IIb (FG [fast glycolytic]) fibers— used for activities that require rapid, high-tension development such as heavy lifting—are primarily anaerobic, from gycolysis. The intermediate IIa (FOG [fast oxidative glycolytic]) fibers use both aerobic and anaerobic pathways. Type II fibers are more easily fatigued than type I (see chapter 1 for further details regarding muscle fiber types).

Motor Unit Recruitment

Although each fiber type occurs in all human skeletal muscles, the mix of types varies from muscle to muscle (Saltin et al. 1977; Thorstensson et al. 1976). The grouping of fiber types is directly related to the motor neurons supplying each motor unit. Small alpha motor neurons innervate small type I motor units. Larger, type II motor units are supplied by the larger alpha motor neurons (figure 5.1). The normal sequence of motor unit activation calls upon the smaller units first, because the threshold for firing within the anterior horn cell pool is lowest for the smaller motor neurons. Therefore, with weak effort, the type I motor units are recruited. As the demand for higher force levels increases, the type II motor units become active. This phenomenon, known as the "size principle of recruitment" (Henneman et al. 1965), has implications for strength training. Patients whose exercise program is limited to submaximal effort may be stressing only the type I fibers. Only when the exercise challenge increases above the threshold of the larger motor units will the type II motor units experience a training effect. Several factors affect the ability of patients to exercise at intensities effective in training the larger motor units. For example, joint pain and swelling may interfere with high-intensity levels of exercise, limiting the effectiveness of muscle-strengthening programs (Fahrer et al. 1988; Spencer et al. 1984; Young et al. 1987).

Functional Biomechanics

The mechanical factors of muscular contraction type, muscle length, and speed of contraction affect the ability of skeletal muscle to generate force.

Types of Muscle Contraction

The contraction of muscle generates force. The effect on skeletal levers varies, depending on the amount of force generated in relation to externally applied forces. A **concentric contraction** occurs when the force developed by a muscle exceeds the magnitude of the external force, resulting in shortening of the whole muscle. An **isometric contraction** occurs when the force developed by a muscle is equal to the external force. An **eccentric contraction** occurs when the external force exceeds the force developed by the muscle, resulting in a lengthening of the whole muscle. The purpose of the eccentric contraction is to control the acceleration of the moving lever as it is being subjected to external forces.

Length-Tension

Muscle length affects the binding capacity between actin and myosin molecules of the component muscle fibers. There is an optimal length at which the greatest number of crossbridges between these molecules can be formed (Åstrand and Rodahl 1986). The length-tension relationship has been documented *in situ* by maximal voluntary effort performed during isometric, concentric, or eccentric contractions (figure 5.2). Maximal force is generated at some midpoint in the range of motion, while less force is developed at either shortened or lengthened positions.

Force-Velocity

The speed of contraction also affects the binding capacity of actin and myosin. There is an optimal

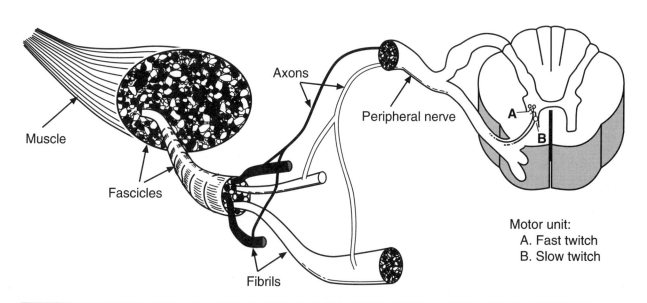

Motor unit:
A. Fast twitch
B. Slow twitch

Figure 5.1 Innervation of muscle fibers.

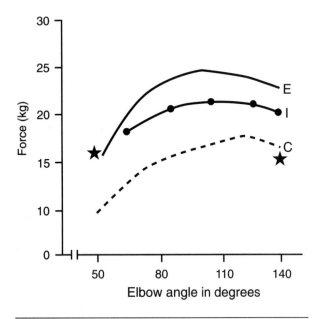

Figure 5.2 Relationship of maximal force of human elbow flexor muscles to elbow position for three types of contraction: eccentric (E), isometric (I), and concentric (C).
Source: Knuttgen 1976.

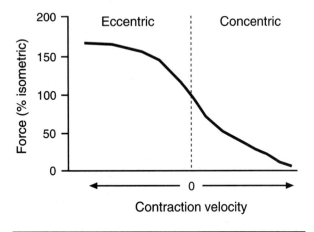

Figure 5.3 The force-velocity relationship for skeletal muscle.
Source: Newham 1993.

frequency at which the ratchet-like cycling of crossbridge formation can occur. Figure 5.3 depicts the force-velocity relationship in isolated muscle preparations. This force-velocity relationship can be demonstrated by a series of efforts using changing loads, or by controlling the speed of contraction as with "isokinetic" devices.

In *concentric* contractions, greater force is generated as the speed of shortening decreases, becoming maximal at zero velocity—which equates to a static

isometric contraction. With *eccentric* contractions, increasing speed (to the extent permitted by voluntary and neuromotor control) can generate greater force than that generated during isometric contractions. These higher forces may reflect the contribution of the passive elastic components of muscle connective tissues in addition to the contractile mechanism.

Factors Influencing Muscle Strength

Strength arises from an interaction between the musculoskeletal system and systems that provide required neurologic, metabolic, and hormonal support. Psychological well-being, lifestyle, nutrition, level of physical activity and fitness, and general health status also influence muscle performance. Rehabilitation professionals must consider all of these factors when designing a program. The effects of age, disuse, immobilization, and musculoskeletal trauma warrant primary consideration because of their immediate and direct impact on muscle function.

Age

The ability to generate force decreases with age (Hopp 1993; Thompson 1994). Muscle loses mass as it ages, because of the decline in the number of motor neurons—mainly those innervating type II muscle fibers. This selectivity is clinically supported by the fact that there is little or no change in fatigability. Edstrom and Larsson (1987) have documented, in rats, that the remaining motor units are larger because of collateral sprouting of active axons from remaining motor units. Furthermore, sensory and motor conduction velocity and axonal transport slow with aging; the decline in motor unit recruitment and frequency of action potentials slow reaction time, and lessen the ability of older persons to rapidly develop maximal force.

Many elderly individuals have chronic, debilitating diseases that contribute to diminished muscle performance. Chapter 20 provides a full discussion of the effects of aging.

Disuse and Immobilization

Muscular activity is compromised by prolonged bed rest, habitual limited physical activity, and cast immobilization. The extent of these changes depends on the duration and magnitude of inactivity; the position of limb immobilization further influences the type and extent of local muscle weakness. Much of our knowledge about the effects of inactivity comes from animal studies (St. Pierre and Gardner 1987), studies of weightlessness during space flight (Baldwin 1996), studies of patients immobilized secondary to orthopedic injuries (Gossman et al. 1982; Tardieu et al. 1982), and studies of normal healthy subjects and elderly subjects (Bloomfield 1997; Convertino et al. 1997). Decreased demand for muscular contraction causes generalized structural changes, including loss of muscle mass evidenced by decreased muscle fiber size. Metabolic changes include decreases in myofibrillar proteins, phosphocreatine, glycogen, potassium, and the enzymes necessary for glycolysis and oxidative phosphorylation. Capillary density, and therefore oxygen uptake, is diminished. Because the sarcolemma becomes thinner and other connective tissues weaken, the entire muscular unit loses elasticity. All of these factors reduce both the aerobic and anaerobic capacity of inactive muscle, resulting in compromised muscular performance (St. Pierre and Gardner 1987). Finally, diminished neuromuscular activity and sensory input impair perception, coordination, and muscle tone.

The impact of fixed immobilization depends on duration and limb position. The rate of atrophy is rapid during the first few weeks of immobilization and then progresses more slowly (Booth 1977). Muscles immobilized in a shortened position will atrophy more than those in a neutral or elongated position. In a shortened position, adult muscle loses sarcomeres, diminishing the capacity to develop tension. In a lengthened position, muscles will adapt by increasing the number of sarcomeres—apparently a response to chronic stretch. These structural alterations change the normal length-tension relationship, causing maximal force to occur at an abnormal point in the physiologic range of motion, and thereby compromising muscle performance (Gossman et al. 1982).

Whether disuse and immobilization selectively affect one muscle fiber type more than others is not clear. Loss of cross-sectional area of both type I and type II fibers has been reported (Haggmark et al. 1981; Sargeant et al. 1977). Findings of proportional losses of one or the other fiber type may have been affected by selection of muscles studied, diagnosis, length of immobilization, age, and method of analysis. In general, studies of immobilization in otherwise healthy subjects show initially diminished neural activity (Berg et al. 1997) followed by decreased type I fiber cross-sectional area and, over time, loss of both type I and type II cross-sectional area. Stud-

ies involving older subjects report a preferential loss of type II cross-sectional area—possibly a reflection of normal changes with aging, and/or of prolonged periods of inactivity (Hopp 1993; St. Pierre and Gardner 1987).

Musculoskeletal Trauma

Trauma involving connective tissue or joint structures can cause atrophy and decreased muscle performance. During the inflammatory process, pain and swelling inhibit muscle function. Activation of nociceptors inhibits the anterior horn cell pool, thereby diminishing the motor neuron outflow to muscle (Spencer et al. 1984). Mechanical deformation of tissue caused by joint effusion and abnormal afferent firing of joint receptors can inhibit muscle function. Fahrer et al. (1988) measured isometric quadriceps strength in patients with chronic knee effusions. Immediately following aspiration of fluid, quadriceps strength improved. Injecting lidocaine into the aspirated joints brought further improvement.

Events that occur during the healing process also affect muscle performance. Because immature scar tissue has decreased tensile strength, it is vulnerable to reinjury. As scar tissue matures, there is a loss of elasticity in the affected tendon, in the musculotendinous junction, or in the intramuscular connective tissue matrix. The resulting inability to store elastic energy limits production of force (Akeson et al. 1977; Hardy 1989; Williams and Goldspink 1984).

Training

Skeletal muscle and neuromotor mechanisms are extremely adaptable to the stresses of activity. The magnitude of change in the capability of muscle is directly related to the intensity, duration, and frequency of exercise. Many methods to increase strength are described in the literature and used by clinicians. In order to achieve a strength benefit, an exercise regimen must be of sufficient frequency, intensity, and duration to challenge the physiologic components of muscle. Hakkinen and Komi (1983) and Komi (1986) described that the first response to isometric strength training is an increase in neural activation, followed by hypertrophy of individual muscle fibers. Exercise increases stiffness in the noncontractile components of muscle, allowing these passive components of force production to be more efficient. In addition to these general adaptations, there may be specific adaptations based on whether concentric, isometric, or eccentric contractions are emphasized. In prescribing exercise training to increase strength, always keep the patient's functional goals in mind, with full understanding of the underlying causes of his or her strength performance deficits.

Principles of Strength Training

Several strengthening methods are available. The selection of method depends upon the clinical assessment of the magnitude of the muscle impairment, the functional goals of the patient, and the settings in which the patient will conduct the program. Factor into your treatment decisions how the patient's pathology and comorbidities will affect the exercise program. Because adherence to programs is directly linked to success, take care to design a program that the patient understands and is able to perform at the prescribed dosage. We will describe the principles of muscle strengthening based on levels of weakness. Although our descriptions focus on strength training, all rehabilitation programs should include endurance training as well. Both endurance and strength are necessary for optimal physical function, which is the primary goal of rehabilitation.

The Basic Principles

Effective strengthening programs are based on overload, specificity, cross training, and reversibility (Enoka 1994).

• **Overload.** Muscle tissue must be challenged beyond its current force capability in order to change both structurally and functionally. The intensity of the exercise program must reach a threshold that exceeds that current capability.

• **Specificity.** Training effects are specific to the mode of exercise stress imposed on the exercising muscle. For example, isometric training at a selected point in the range of motion does not necessarily carry over to concentric or eccentric demands—perhaps a reflection that the adaptations are not limited to changes in muscle (such as hypertrophy), but also include neuromotor adaptation by which the individual learns to use muscle force for specific musculoskeletal functions.

• **Cross training.** To overcome the limitations of specificity and to maximize the broad range of muscle performance, incorporate all modes of training into your programs whenever possible—i.e., include isometric, concentric, and eccentric elements as well as an endurance component.

• **Reversibility.** The benefits of training are not sustained unless muscles remain sufficiently challenged through continuous use of the strength gains. The initial changes that occur with detraining are decreased muscle recruitment, followed by muscle fiber atrophy.

Exercise Methods

Techniques of muscle re-education are useful in cases of major weakness and diminished neuromotor function, where the goal is to activate a voluntary contraction. The techniques include shortened held resisted contraction, active assisted range of motion, facilitation techniques such as quick stretch, and application of vibratory stimuli (Sullivan and Markos 1995). Ancillary techniques of biofeedback (Krebs 1990) or neuromuscular electrical stimulation (Delitto and Robinson 1989) can be useful. The functional goal in this circumstance is to encourage active voluntary motion within a specified movement pattern. For a patient on bed rest following knee surgery, for example, regaining active control of the quadriceps is a prerequisite for transferring from bed to chair, or for using crutches.

Initially, simply moving against gravity may challenge skeletal muscle. As patients gain strength, they should increase resistance through a variety of methods. Manual resistance applied by the therapist is often the first procedure. In this way, the therapist can judge the capability of muscle to safely meet externally applied forces, and can select appropriate facilitation techniques to optimize the muscle output and to provide feedback to the patient. These techniques are especially useful in postoperative orthopedic patients and in patients who have neuromotor disorders that compromise normal voluntary motor unit recruitment.

When the affected muscles are able to tolerate externally applied resistance, and the patients understand the rules of safe exercise regarding their specific condition, they can choose from several methods to increase resistance. The patients become responsible for carrying out their own programs, with guidance from the therapist. The methods and specific goals of the programs are based on the patients' functional requirements. For example, for an elderly patient who is recovering from a hip fracture and whose goal is walking and light housekeeping, a program using graded weights or resistive elastic bands through a range of motion may be adequate. Such a program would enable the patient to do what he needs to do, and would also be easy to continue at a maintenance level at home. In contrast, a college soccer player whose lower extremity was immobilized for three months following a tri-malleolar fracture would require much more intense exercise to enable her to resume athletic activity. Modes of resistance could include progressive resistance exercise using free weights or isokinetic or hydraulic machines.

The paradigm for strength conditioning programs is based on DeLorme's prescription of high load and low repetition. His technique, known as **progressive resistance exercise**, consists of establishing the maximal load a patient can lift through 10 repetitions (10 RM). The program proceeds to a regimen of 10 repetitions of 50% of that maximal value, followed by 10 repetitions at 75%, and finally 10 repetitions at 100% of the 10RM load, with one to two minutes of rest between sets. The usual frequency is three or four times a week. The spacing of sessions permits a recovery period (DeLorme and Watkins 1951). Modifications of this technique have been described, such as the "Oxford" technique (Zinovieff 1951) and the "brief maximal effort or one repetition maximum (1 RM)" (Rose et al. 1957).

Strengthening programs originally used the "open chain" method, whereby the distal segment of the extremity moves and stabilization occurs proximally. Today many programs use a "closed chain" model whereby the distal part is fixed, as in weight bearing, and muscles perform reverse action. Many consider closed chain exercises—particularly with the lower extremities—to be safer because they use normal movement patterns and sensory cues (Falkel and Cipriani 1996; Sullivan and Markos 1995). With the variety of exercise devices available, the therapist can design strengthening programs based on the type of muscle contraction, force, or speed required for optimal therapeutic response. Selecting the "best" mode of strengthening depends upon the patient's particular impairment, medical problem, and requirements for optimal functional performance. The therapist must also consider practical issues. For example, can the patient go to a facility that has a selection of exercise equipment, or is she confined to home?

Adaptations to Strength Conditioning

The most obvious result of strength conditioning is an increase in the functional capacity of muscle to generate force—an increase stemming from several alterations in morphology and physiology caused by the stresses of exercise. Many studies have described these local and systemic effects of strength training (table 5.1).

Neuromuscular Adaptation

Hakkinen and Komi (1983) elucidated the sequence of adaptation to strength training in the neuromuscular system. In the early stages of exercise, the changes as documented by electromyography include increased motor unit recruitment and synchronization of motor unit discharge. These changes reflect more effective activation of anterior horn cells, elicited by improved voluntary motor control. In addition, Deschenes et al. (1993) demonstrated (in rats) hypertrophic alteration of the neuromuscular junction—namely, a broadening of the synaptic area—in response to heavy resistance exercise. As the efficiency of neural elements improves, hypertrophy of skeletal muscle occurs when the exercise challenge is adequate. The changes that result in this increase in muscle fiber size include remodeling of muscle proteins, increase in size and number of myofibrils, and an increase in the number of sarcomeres (Åstrand and Rodahl 1986). Each of the major fiber types may be affected differentially, depending on the intensity of the imposed resistance and the type of contraction. Studies have reported increased cross-sectional area selectively for type II fibers or in both type I and type II fibers (Kraemer et al. 1996). Further, Staron et al. (1994) documented a metabolic response of fiber types with a conversion of type IIb fibers to type IIa, indicating an increase in oxidative capacity following strength training. Exercise studies of subjects who have been immobilized for long periods of time have reported initial increases in type I fiber cross-sectional area, followed by changes in type II fibers. Based on the size order of recruitment, low-intensity exercise may not challenge the large type II fibers sufficiently to cause hypertrophic changes.

Antonio and Gonyea (1993) reviewed evidence that exercise may induce hyperplasia, which is an

Table 5.1		Adaptations to Strength Conditioning	
Physiologic adaptations	**Positive changes in impairments**	**Positive changes in function**	**Quality of life**
Increased motor unit recruitment	Strength-force production	Balance and coordination	Athletic performance
Synchronization of motor unit discharge	Bone mass	Gait	Job performance
Hypertrophy increased fiber size remodeling of muscle proteins increase in size and number of myo-fibrils increase in sarcomeres	Body composition—improved fat to lean body mass ratio	Activities of daily living	Social activity
	Reaction time		Sense of well-being
Hyperplasia (from animal models, possibly in humans)	Immunologic function		
	Cardiopulmonary status		
Increased tensile strength of connective tissue	Metabolism		

increase in the number of muscle fibers. The mechanism for hyperplasia may be fiber splitting (Gonyea 1980), or perhaps activation of satellite cells (Darr and Schultz 1987). It may be caused by heavy resistance exercise and overuse (Hall-Craggs 1970) or by weight-induced prolonged stretch (Alway et al. 1989). Several animal studies have demonstrated this phenomenon. Evidence of hyperplasia in humans is less convincing at this time. However, Tesch and Larsson (1982) concluded on somewhat indirect evidence that hyperplasia does occur in humans. They described an increase in muscle mass and limb circumference in body builders in whom there was no evidence of muscle fiber hypertrophy.

The temporal relationship between neural and muscular changes depends on the interaction of several factors: the intensity, frequency, and duration of the exercise program; the age and health status of the patient; and the specific cause of the muscle weakness. With minimal impairment or in healthy subjects, strength changes during the first 6 to 12 weeks of a training program are primarily due to increased motor unit recruitment and motor learning (Komi 1986). However, in patients who have coordination problems or disuse secondary to immobilization, the

neural adaptation phase may be prolonged (Buckwalter et al. 1993; Kraemer et al. 1996).

Alterations of connective tissue within skeletal muscle also occur (Stone 1988). Application of an external load stimulates the proliferation of connective tissue and satellite cells. The resultant increase in tensile strength improves the structural and functional integrity of the skeletal muscle unit, allowing for more efficient force production.

System Benefits

Adaptations to a strength conditioning program include increased bone mass and alterations in body composition.

Bone mass increases in response to the stresses imposed during strength training (Stone 1988). The extent of this effect depends on the magnitude of skeletal loading through weight bearing and on the torque applied to bone during muscular contraction. For example, when Smith and Rutherford (1993) compared male rowers, triathletes, and sedentary men, the rowers (whose training included heavy resistive exercise and high mechanical loading) had higher bone mineral density than the triathletes (whose training emphasized lower intensities and endurance). Recent studies have addressed the effectiveness of exercise in retarding bone loss during menopause and aging. Ayalon et al. (1987) reported site-specific increases in bone mineral density in the forearm in response to dynamic resistance exercise of the forearm in postmenopausal women. In studying the effect of high-intensity strengthening in 50- to 70-year-old women, Nelson et al. (1994) found increased bone mineral density in the femoral neck and lumbar spine. Chapter 17 presents a full discussion of this topic.

Strength training increases lean tissue mass and decreases percent fat. These changes have been documented after resistance training in athletes, normal healthy subjects, and older individuals. The demands of active muscle include the utilization of fatty acids, particularly to support oxidative phosphorylation. Mobilization and utilization of free fatty acids accounts in part for the decrease in adipose tissue (Martin 1996). In highly trained athletes, the ratio of lean body mass to fat is high (Åstrand and Rodahl 1986). Treuth et al. (1995) and Nichols et al. (1993) have documented these same benefits in older women as a result of heavy resistance training.

Functional Benefits

Improvement in strength can result in improved balance and coordination, gait, ability to perform activities of daily living, and higher-level activity in athletic performance or occupational tasks. The magnitude of functional changes depends on the interaction of premorbid strength, the strength requirements to perform specific tasks, and health status factors, such as disorders of metabolism or cardiorespiratory support systems. Psychological state also affects the carryover from strength improvement to actual function.

Several recent studies have measured functional change in response to strength training in older individuals. Lord and Castell (1994) studied the effects of a 10-week strengthening and cardiovascular exercise program in 50- to 75-year-old men and women. They found improvement in the exercised lower extremity muscles, reaction time, and body sway. In a randomized placebo-controlled trial with 100 elderly subjects, Fiatarone et al. (1994) compared high-intensity exercise, nutritional supplement, a combination of both, and no intervention. The exercise regimen improved muscle strength, gait velocity, stair climbing, and the level of spontaneous physical activity. There was no change in the groups who took nutritional supplements. Ettinger et al. (1997) reported positive results in an 18-month home-based resistive exercise program for community-dwelling men and women who had osteoarthritis. Significant, though modest, improvements were noted in subjects' self-reports of physical activity, six-minute walk tests, and timed activities of lifting, stair climbing, and getting in and out of a chair. In a study by Jette et al. (1996) of a three-month home-based exercise program for older subjects, the older men reported a significant decrease in perceived anger and a significant increase in vigor.

Summary

This chapter has presented an overview of the adaptations to strength training. Over a period of time, strength training elicits significant alterations in morphology and physiology. The magnitude of these changes is affected by the type of stress imposed and the age and general health status of the patient. Specific improvements in functional performance have been demonstrated. These adaptations justify the use of strength training to ameliorate the impairments of muscle weakness and atrophy that result from disuse and immobilization, and to maximize muscle performance in conditions that create permanent dysfunction of muscle. The ultimate goal is to optimize the functional performance of the patient.

References

Akeson, W.H., D. Amiel, G.L. Mechanic, S.L. Woo, F.L. Harwood, and M.L. Hamer. 1977. Collagen cross linking adhesions in joint contractures: changes in the reducible cross-links in periarticular connective tissue collagen after nine weeks of immobilization. *Connective Tissue Res* 5:15-19.

Alway, S.E., P.K. Winchester, M.E. Davis, and W.J. Gonyea. 1989. Regionalized adaptations and muscle fiber proliferation in stretch-induced enlargement. *J Appl Physiol* 66:771-781.

Antonio, J., and W.J. Gonyea. 1993. Skeletal muscle fiber hyperplasia. *Med Sci Sports Exerc* 25:1333-1345.

Åstrand, P-O., and K. Rodahl. 1986. *Textbook of work physiology: Physiological bases of exercise.* 3d ed. New York: McGraw-Hill.

Ayalon, J., A. Simkin, I. Leichter, and S. Raifmann. 1987. Dynamic bone loading exercises for postmenopausal women: effect on density of distal radius. *Arch Phys Med Rehabil* 68:280-283.

Baldwin, K.M., T.P. White, S.B. Arnaud, V.R. Edgerton, W.J. Kraemer, R. Kram, D. Raab-Cullen, and C.M. Snow. 1996. Musculoskeletal adaptations to weightlessness and development of counter measures. *Med Sci Sports Exerc* 10:1247-1253.

Berg, H.E., L. Larsson, and P.A. Tesch. 1997. Lower limb skeletal muscle function after 6 wk of bed rest. *J Appl Physiol* 82:182-188.

Bloomfield, S.A. 1997. Changes in musculoskeletal structure and function with prolonged bed rest. *Med Sci Sports Exerc* 29:197-206.

Booth, S.W. 1977. Time course of muscular atrophy during immobilization of hind limbs of rats. *J Appl Physiol* 43:656-661.

Buckwalter, J.A., S.L. Woo, V. Goldberg, E.C. Hadley, F. Booth, T.R. Oegema, and D.R. Eyre. 1993. Current concepts review: soft-tissue aging and musculoskeletal function. *J Bone Joint Surg* 75A:1533-1547.

Clarkson, P.M., and M.E. Dedrick. 1988. Exercise-induced muscle damage, repair, and adaptation in old and young subjects. *J Gerontol* 43:M91-96.

Convertino, V.A., S.A. Bloomfield, and J.E. Greenleaf. 1997. An overview of the issues: physiological effects of bed rest and restricted physical activity. *Med Sci Sports Exerc* 29:187-190.

Darr, K.C., and E. Schultz. 1987. Exercise-induced satellite cell activation in growing and mature skeletal muscle. *J Appl Physiol* 63:1816-1821.

Delitto, A., and A.J. Robinson. 1989. Electrical stimulation of muscle: techniques and applications. In *Clinical electrophysiology: Electrotherapy and electrophysiologic testing*, ed. L. Snyder-Mackler and A.J. Robinson, 95-135. Baltimore: Williams & Wilkins.

DeLorme, T.L., and A.L. Watkins. 1951. *Progressive resistance exercise*. New York: Appleton-Century-Croft.

Deschenes, M.R., C.M. Maresh, J.F. Crivello, I.E. Armstrong, W.J. Kraemer, and J. Covault. 1993. The effects of exercise training of different intensities on neuromuscular junction morphology. *J Neurocytol* 22:603-615.

Dook, J.E., C. James, N.K. Henderson, and R.I. Price. 1997. Exercise and bone mineral density in mature female athletes. *Med Sci Sports Exerc* 29:291-296.

Edstrom, L., and L. Larsson. 1987. Effects of age on contractile and enzyme-histochemical properties of fast- and slow-twitch single motor units in the rat. *J Physiol (Lond)* 392:129-145.

Enoka, R.M. 1994. Chronic Adaptations. In *Neuromechanical basis of kinesiology*. 2d ed., ed. R.M. Enoka, 303-349. Champaign, IL: Human Kinetics.

Ettinger, W.H., R. Burns, S.P. Messier. W. Applegate, W.J. Rejeski, T. Morgan, S. Shumaker, M.J. O'Toole, J. Monu, and T. Craven. 1997. A randomized trial comparing aerobic exercise and resistance exercise with a health education program in older adults with knee osteoarthritis. The Fitness Arthritis and Seniors Trials (FAST). *JAMA* 277:25-31.

Evans, W.J. 1995. Effects of exercise on body composition and functional capacity of the elderly. *J Gerontol A Biol Sci Med Sci* 50A (Special issue):147-150.

Fahrer, H., H.U. Rentsch, N.J. Gerber, C. Beyeler, C.W. Hess, and B. Grunig. 1988. Knee effusion and reflex inhibition of the quadriceps. *J Bone Joint Surg (Br)* 70B:635-638.

Falkel, J.E., and D.J. Cipriani. 1996. Physiologic principles of resistance training and rehabilitation. In *Athletic injuries and rehabilitation*, ed. J.E. Zachazewski, D.J. Magee, and W.S. Quillen, 206-226. Philadelphia: W.B. Saunders.

Fiatarone, M.A., N.D. Ryan, K.M. Clements, G.R. Solares, M.E. Nelson, S.B. Roberts, J.J. Kehayias, L.A. Lipsitz, and W.J. Evans. 1994. Exercise training and nutritional supplementation for physical frailty in very elderly people. *N Engl J Med* 330:1769-1775.

Gonyea, W. 1980. Role of exercise in inducing increases in skeletal muscle fiber number. *J Appl Physiol* 48:421-426.

Gossman, M.E., S.A. Sahrmann, and S.J. Rose. 1982. Review of length associated changes in muscle: experimental evidence and clinical implications. *Phys Ther* 62:1799-1808.

Haggmark, T., E. Jansson, and E. Erikson. 1981. Fibre type area, metabolic potential of the thigh muscle in man after knee surgery and immobilization in man. *Int J Sports Med* 2:12-17.

Hakkinen, K., and P.V. Komi. 1983. Electromyographic changes during strength training and detraining. *Med Sci Sports Exerc* 15:455-460.

Hall-Craggs, E.C.B. 1970. The longitudinal division of fibres in overloaded rat skeletal muscle. *J Anat* 107:459-470.

Hardy, M.A. 1989. The biology of scar formation. *Phys Ther* 69:1014-1024.

Harris, B.A., and M.P. Watkins. 1993. Muscle performance: principles and general theory. In *Muscle strength*, ed. K. Harms-Ringdahl, 5-18. Edinburgh: Churchill Livingstone.

Heinonen, A., P. Kannus, H. Sievanen, P. Oja, M. Pasanen, M. Rinne, K. Uusi-Rafi, and I. Vuori. 1996. Randomized controlled trial of effect of high impact exercise on selected risk factors for osteoporotic fractures. *Lancet* 348:1343-1347.

Henneman, E., and C.B. Olson. 1965. Relations between structure and function in the design of skeletal muscle. *J Neurophysiol* 28:581-598.

Henneman, E., G. Somjen, and D.O. Carpenter. 1965. Functional significance of cell size in spinal motoneurons. *J Neurophysiol* 28:560-598.

Hopp, J.F. 1993. Effects of age and resistance training on skeletal muscle: a review. *Phys Ther* 73:361-373.

Jette, A.M., B.A. Harris, L. Sleeper, M.E. Lachman, D. Heislein, M. Giorgetti, and C. Levenson. 1996. A home-based exercise program for nondisabled older adults. *J Am Geriatr Soc* 44:644-649.

Knuttgen, H.G., ed. 1976. *Neuromuscular mechanisms for therapeutic and conditioning exercise*, 97-118. Baltimore: University Park Press.

Komi, P.V. 1986. Training of muscle strength and power: interaction of neuromotoric, hypertrophic and mechanical factors. *Int J Sports Med* 7(Suppl.):10-15.

Kraemer, W.J., S.J. Fleck, and W.J. Evans. 1996. Strength and power training: physiologic mechanisms of adaptation. *Exerc Sport Sci* 46:363-397.

Krebs, D.E. 1990. Biofeedback in therapeutic exercise. In *Therapeutic exercise*, ed. J.V. Basmajian and S. L. Wolfe, 109-124. Baltimore: Williams & Wilkins.

LaPierre, A., G. Ironson, M.H. Antoni, N. Schneiderman, N. Klimas, and M.A. Fletcher. 1994. Exercise and psychoneuroimmunology. *Med Sci Sports Exerc* 26:182-190.

Leon, A.S. 1985. Physical activities and coronary heart disease. *Med Clin North Am* 69:3-17.

Lord, S.R., and S. Castell. 1994. Physical activity program for older persons: effect on balance, strength, neuromuscular control and reaction time. *Arch Phys Med Rehabil* 75:648-652.

Martin, W.H. 1996. Effects of acute and chronic exercise on fat metabolism. *Exerc Sport Sci Rev* 24:203-231.

Nelson, M.E., M.A. Fiatarone, C.M. Morganti, I. Trice, R.A. Greenberg, and W.J. Evans. 1994. Effects of high intensity strength training on multiple risk factors for osteoporotic fractures: a randomized controlled trial. *JAMA* 272:1909-1914.

Newham, D. F. 1993. Eccentric muscle activity in theory and practice. In *Muscle strength*, ed. K. Harms-Ringdahl, 61-81. Edinburgh: Churchill Livingstone.

Nichols, J.F., D.K. Omizo, K.K. Peterson, and K.P. Nelson. 1993. Efficacy of heavy-resistance training for active women over sixty: muscular strength, body composition and program adherence. *J Am Geriatr Soc* 41:205-210.

Rose, D.L., S.F. Radzyminski, and R.R. Beatty. 1957. Effect of brief maximal exercise on the strength of the quadriceps femoris. *Arch Phys Med Rehabil* 33:157-164.

Sale, D.G. 1988. Neural adaptation to resistance training. *Med Sci Sports Exerc* 20:S135-145.

Saltin, B., J. Henriksson, and E. Nygaard. 1977. Fibre types and metabolic potentials in sedentary man and endurance runners. *Ann N Y Acad Sci* 301:3-29.

Sargeant, A.J., C.T. Davies, and R.H. Edwards. 1977. Structural and functional changes after disuse of human muscle. *Clin Sci Mol Med* 52:337-342.

Smith, R., and O.M. Rutherford. 1993. Spine and total body bone mineral density and serum testosterone levels in male athletes. *Eur J Appl Physiol* 67:330-334.

Spector, S.A., C.P. Simard, and M. Fournier. 1982. Architectural alterations of the rat hind-limb skeletal muscles immobilized at different lengths. *Exp Neurol* 76:94-110.

Spencer, J.D., K.C. Hayes, and I.J. Alexander. 1984. Knee joint effusion and quadriceps reflex inhibition in man. *Arch Phys Med Rehabil* 65:171-177.

Starkey, D.B., M.L. Pollock, Y. Ishida, M.A. Welch, W.F. Brechue, J.E. Graves, and M.S. Feigenbaum. 1996. Effect of resistance training volume on strength and muscle thickness. *Med Sci Sports Exerc* 28:1311-1320.

Staron, R.S., D.L. Karapondo, W.J. Kraemer, A.C. Fry, S.E. Gordon, J.E. Falkel, F.C. Hagerman, and R.S. Hikida. 1994. Skeletal muscle adaptations during the early phase of heavy resistance training in men and women. *J Appl Physiol* 76:1247-1255.

Stone, M.H. 1988. Implications for connective tissue and bone alterations resulting from resistance exercise training. *Med Sci Sports Exerc* 20(Suppl.):162-168.

St. Pierre, D., and P.F. Gardner. 1987. The effect of immobilization and exercise on muscle function: a review. *Physiotherapy Canada* 39:24-35.

Sullivan, P.E., and P.D. Markos. 1995. *Clinical decision making in therapeutic exercise.* Norwalk, CT: Appleton & Lange.

Tardieu, C., J.C. Tabary, C. Tabary, and G. Tardieu. 1982. Adaptation of connective tissue length to immobilization in the lengthened and shortened positions in the cat soleus muscle. *J Physiol Paris* 78:214-220.

Tardieu, C., J.C. Tabary, and G. Tardieu. 1980. Adaptation of sarcomere number to the length imposed on the muscle. *Advances in Physiologic Science* 24:99-114.

Tesch, P.A., and L. Larsson. 1982. Muscle hypertrophy in bodybuilders. *Eur J Appl Physiol* 49:301-306.

Thompson, L.V. 1994. Effects of age and training on skeletal muscle physiology and performance. *Phys Ther* 74:71-84.

Thorstensson, A., G. Grimby, and J. Karlsson. 1976. Force-velocity relations and fibre composition in human extensor muscles. *J Appl Physiol* 40:12-16.

Treuth, M.S., G.R. Hunter, T. Kekes-Szabo, R.L. Weinsier, M.I. Goran, and L. Berland. 1995. Reduction in intra-abdominal adipose tissue after strength training in older women. *J Appl Physiol* 78:1425-1431.

Williams, P., and G. Goldspink. 1984. Connective tissue changes in immobilized muscle. *J Anat* 138:343-350.

Young, A., M. Stokes, and J. Iles. 1987. Effects of joint pathology on muscle. *Clin Orthop* 219:21-27

Zinovieff, A.N. 1951. Heavy resistance exercise: the "Oxford technique". *Br J Phys Med* 14:129-132.

Chapter 6

Training Flexibility

Lisa S. Krivickas, MD

Strength, endurance, and flexibility training are integral components of any comprehensive exercise, fitness, or sport-specific training program. While researchers have extensively studied endurance and strength training, they have largely ignored flexibility training, especially in individuals with normal muscle tone. While most professionals and athletes believe that adequate or even above-average flexibility is an asset, scientific work to support this assertion is weak. In this chapter, I will summarize the current scientific literature on flexibility and suggest areas requiring further investigation. I will apply the limited results of existing literature to clinical situations. Topics addressed include the definition of flexibility; factors influencing flexibility; both cellular and macroscopic responses of muscle to stretching; methods of measuring and quantifying flexibility; the relationship between muscle stiffness and flexibility; the relationship between flexibility, ligamentous laxity, and injury; and the relationship between flexibility and activities of both daily living and athletic performance. I will also discuss stretching techniques, a prescription for developing flexibility, the effect of strength training on flexibility, and the effect of various disease processes on flexibility.

Definition of Flexibility

Flexibility is the range of motion of a joint or series of joints. Although flexibility is influenced by muscles, tendons, ligaments, bones, and bony structures, muscle is by far the greatest contributor (Anderson and Burke 1991; Corbin 1984). Tendon has very little ability to elongate because of its high collagen and low elastin content. Ligament, with its higher elastin content, is somewhat more extensible (Liebesman and Cafarelli 1994). Gajdosik (1995) has challenged the preceding definition of flexibility, suggesting that flexibility is a physiologic phenomenon requiring simultaneous measurement of the length-tension relationship of muscles as they are lengthened passively without muscle activation. According to this definition, flexibility must be measured as a ratio of change in muscle length or change in joint angle to change in force or torque; these ratios are actually measures of compliance. Gajdosik's definition does not encompass the concept of dynamic vs. static flexibility, since he requires that the muscle be lengthened without muscle activation. Because there is no consensus as to the definition of flexibility, it is best defined operationally, i.e., as either a change in length or a change in ratio of length to tension . While reviewing studies that have used both definitions, this chapter focuses primarily on the role of muscle—and to a lesser extent of ligamentous laxity—on joint range of motion and stiffness.

Factors Influencing Flexibility

Flexibility is muscle- and joint-specific and is influenced by the age, gender, and, possibly, the race of

Factors Influencing Flexibility

- Muscle and joint specificity
- Age
- Gender
- Ethnic origin
- Temperature
- Reflex activity
- Central nervous system disease processes
- Antagonist muscle strength (dynamic flexibility)

the individual. **Static flexibility** refers to the ability of a joint to move through a passive range of motion. It differs from **dynamic flexibility** in that the latter depends on the strength of antagonist muscles to move the limb *and* on the freedom of the limb to move. A ballet dancer with excellent static hamstring flexibility may perform a split on the floor with ease; however, if she has weak hip flexors or hip pain that impairs her ability to move her leg, she may have poor dynamic flexibility and be unable to lift her leg even 90 degrees when standing. Neuromuscular factors (e.g., reflex activity, and diseases affecting the central nervous system) strongly influence both static and dynamic flexibility, as does muscle temperature because of its effect on collagen extensibility. See "Factors Influencing Flexibility" above.

Case Study

An elite 17-year-old male singles figure skater trains 35 hours per week including on-ice and off-ice activities. He recently experienced a growth spurt, adding two inches to his height in nine months. He suffered from jumper's knee (patellar tendinitis) in the right (his landing) leg, and had very tight rectus femoris muscles. The flexibility of the rectus femoris is assessed by measuring the quadriceps inhibited knee flexion angle (QFA). The QFA is the difference between (1) the angle of maximal knee flexion with the ipsilateral hip flexed 80 degrees, and (2) the angle of maximal knee flexion with the ipsilateral hip fully extended. A QFA greater than 10 degrees indicates rectus femoris muscle tightness. In elite adolescent skaters, rectus

femoris tightness is associated with anterior knee pain overuse syndromes (Smith et al. 1991). When this skater initially came to us with right jumper's knee, he had a QFA of 30 degrees on the right and 38 degrees on the left. We placed him on a quadriceps muscle stretching program and a general rehabilitation program for his jumper's knee. After six months, his jumper's knee had resolved, and QFA was 0 degrees bilaterally. One year later, he presented with bilateral jumper's knee. He had discontinued his quadriceps muscle stretching program, and QFA was now 30 degrees on the right and 18 degrees on the left. This case study demonstrates the importance of flexibility training for both injury prevention and rehabilitation.

Gender, Age, and Race

Scientific literature is scant on the relationship between flexibility and gender, age, or race. No normal values have been established for flexibility of specific joints or muscles in various populations, and clinicians do not agree on what should be considered the optimal degree of muscle flexibility. Laubach and McConville (1966) explored the relationship between flexibility and somatotype in college men and found no significant association. Comparisons of hip flexion and shoulder extension in college students, and of lower extremity flexibility in male and female college athletes, have shown that women generally have greater flexibility than men (Etnyre and Lee 1988; Krivickas and Feinberg 1996). A study of children attending tennis camp found greater hamstring flexibility in girls than in boys, but no difference in soleus, adductor, or shoulder external rotator flexibility (Marshall et al. 1980). In the same study, age was negatively correlated with flexibility in shoulder external rotation ($r = -0.68$) and ankle dorsiflexion ($r = -0.26$), but was not significantly correlated with hamstring or adductor flexibility.

Before we accept any such associations, we must critically evaluate the methods by which experimenters have measured flexibility. For example, one study of male high school athletes concluded that flexibility increased with both age and sexual maturation. However, the measure used for flexibility was the sit-and-reach test, which is influenced by body proportion (both trunk-to-leg length ratio and arm length)—and body proportion changes as children grow (Pratt 1989). I will address specific methods for measuring flexibility in a later section.

Clinicians generally believe that flexibility decreases with age, but no one has systematically studied this relationship. Children tend to lose flexibility during growth spurts, because their bones elongate at a faster rate than their muscles (Micheli 1983)—a major factor in the high number of lower extremity overuse injuries in adolescent athletes. A longitudinal study performed in Sweden demonstrated a decrease in flexibility in both men and women from age 16 to 34 (Barnekow-Bergkvist et al. 1996). In the elderly, inactivity caused by medical illness, social factors, or environmental factors may contribute to loss of muscle flexibility. In addition, an age-associated cross-linking of collagen molecules may alter the properties of collagen and contribute to decreased joint range of motion in the elderly (Liebesman and Cafarelli 1994). No one has formally studied the relationship between race and muscle flexibility, but variations in ligamentous laxity in different ethnic populations have been observed. The influence of activity level has not been incorporated into any of the observed associations between age, gender, and flexibility. Training and activity may have a greater influence than genetic factors on muscle flexibility in healthy individuals.

Physiological and Neurological Factors

The cytoskeletal protein **titin** gives myofibrils their intrinsic elasticity (Waterman-Storer 1991). We may hypothesize that the quantity and quality of titin in any given muscle influences its flexibility. The third most abundant protein in the sarcomere (after actin and myosin), titin runs the entire length of the half sarcomere. Its major function is to maintain the central position of the myosin filaments in the relaxed sarcomeres. Figure 6.1 illustrates the positioning of titin within the muscle fiber. Fast-twitch muscle fibers have more titin than slow-twitch fibers and are more flexible. The degradation of titin during exercise-induced muscle damage may explain the loss of muscle flexibility sometimes reported in association with heavy resistance training and eccentric exercise.

Two spinal reflexes, initiated by the muscle spindle and the Golgi tendon organ, influence muscle flexibility (Proske 1997). The **muscle spindle** is a muscle stretch receptor composed of 2-12 thin intrafusal (within the spindle) muscle fibers arranged in parallel with the extrafusal, or main, muscle fibers. Muscle spindles are composed of three types of intrafusal fibers (dynamic nuclear bag or bag_1, static nuclear bag or bag_2, and nuclear chain), which combine to function as primary and secondary spindles. **Primary spindles** respond to rate of length change, creating a dynamic response. **Secondary spindles** respond to a static absolute length change. When muscle stretch activates the spindle reflex, the extrafusal fibers contract, shortening the muscle. The **Golgi tendon organ** is a braided structure consisting of collagenous fibers and afferent axons in series with several extrafusal muscle fibers at the muscle tendon interface. When the extrafusal fibers contract, a force is applied to the Golgi tendon organ, which sends to the spinal cord a message that results in inhibition of the agonist muscle and contraction of the antagonist. Thus, the **Golgi tendon reflex** enhances the ability of a muscle to stretch, while the **spindle reflex** attempts to prevent muscle elongation. The goal of a stretching exercise should be to enhance the Golgi tendon reflex and inhibit the spindle reflex. Figure 6.2 illustrates the complex interaction between these two spinal reflexes.

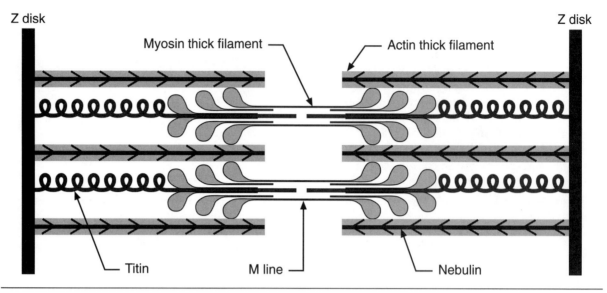

Figure 6.1 An illustration of the position of titin within the sarcomere.
From: MOLECULAR CELL BIOLOGY 3/E by Lodish, Baltimore, Berk, Zipursky, Matsudaira, Darnell © 1995 by Scientific American Library. Used with permission of W.H. Freeman and Company.

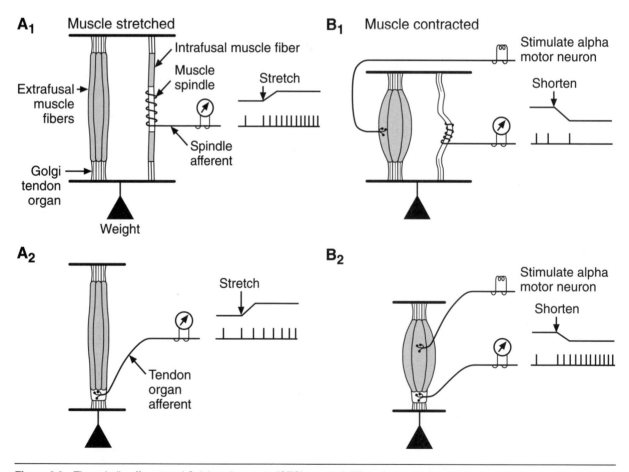

Figure 6.2 The spindle afferent and Golgi tendon organ (GTO) respond differently to muscle stretch and contraction. Both discharge when muscle is stretched (A), the GTO (A_2) less than the spindle (A_1). When the muscle contracts (B), the spindle ceases firing (B_1), and the GTO increases its firing rate (B_2).
Reprinted, by permission, from E.R. Kandel, J.H. Schwartz, and T.M. Jessell, 1991, *Principles of neural science,* 3rd ed. (Norwalk, CT: Appleton & Lange), 568.

In addition to the spinal reflexes, supraspinal reflexes and other neural pathways influence muscle flexibility. A detailed discussion of these phenomena is beyond the scope of this chapter, but damage to these neural pathways produces spasticity, rigidity, or hypotonia. **Spasticity** occurs in upper motor neuron lesions, such as cortical stroke and spinal cord injury, because the spinal reflexes are isolated from inhibitory or modulating supraspinal reflexes. Spasticity is defined by three characteristics:

1. Unidirectional resistance to passive movement
2. Velocity-dependent resistance to muscle stretch
3. Hyperactive muscle stretch reflexes

Rigidity occurs in patients, such as those with Parkinson's disease, with damage to the basal ganglia. In rigidity, resistance to muscle stretch is bidirectional and independent of velocity. In addition, muscle stretch reflexes are not hyperactive. **Hypotonia,** or lack of normal muscle resistance to stretch, is seen in patients with cerebellar lesions, because the baseline alpha motor neuron and muscle spindle activity are decreased, and the firing thresholds of both alpha and gamma motor neurons are increased.

Temperature

Muscle and joint temperature affect flexibility. Heating augments the increase in range of motion achieved by stretching, by increasing the extensibility of collagen, a major component of tendon and joint capsules (Gersten 1955; Lehman et al. 1970). Thus the increased range of motion achieved with heating is probably more related to elongation of the tendon than of the muscle. Heat also facilitates the response of the major spinal reflexes to stretch, by decreasing the sensitivity of muscle spindle reflexes and increasing the firing rate of Golgi tendon organs (Mense 1978). This is the physiologic basis of muscle spasm relaxation with heat application. Animal studies have shown that warming up muscle and tendon by preconditioning with electrically stimulated isometric contractions increases extensibility. It was hypothesized that the warm-up elevated temperature, thereby increasing the extensibility of collagen (Safran et al. 1988).

Response of Muscle to Stretch

Tabary and colleagues (1972) studied the effect of chronic stretch on cat muscle fibers. They found that chronic stretch increased the number of sarcomeres by 20%-25%, but decreased the sarcomere length by 11%-16%; the additive effect was a 5% overall increase in muscle fiber length. Presumably, increasing muscle fiber length increases joint range of motion; the extent to which this is true will depend on the architecture of each specific muscle.

Viscoelastic Muscle-Tendon Behavior

The muscle-tendon unit is **viscoelastic** in its mechanical behavior. Frequently, a spring and dash pot model is used to describe its behavior. The term **dash pot** describes a disk attached to a plunger that is immersed in a fluid, providing frictional resistance to movement. The spring represents the elastic elements, and the dash pot the viscous elements. Gottlieb (1996) has expanded the classic three-element model of muscle (figure 6.3A) into a more complex five-element model (figure 6.3B). The classic model consists of a contractile element (CE), a series elastic element (SE), and a parallel elastic element (PE) that is passive and comes into play only at longer muscle lengths. The more complex model includes a parallel elastic element (K_p), a viscous element (B), a force generator (F) controlled by neural activation, a series elastic element for muscle (K_s), and a nonlinear series elastic element for tendon (K_t). Under most physiologic conditions, muscle behaves like a spring, and the viscous element has minimal influence on its behavior.

In order to understand the **viscoelastic behavior** of muscle, one must understand several engineering terms that describe the behavior of viscoelastic substances. In general, when a pure **elastic material** is stretched, it returns to its initial length when the stretch is released. When a purely **viscous material** is stretched, its rate of deformation is proportional to the force applied, and it does not return to its original length when the stretch is released. Viscoelastic materials combine these properties such that the phenomena of **stress relaxation, creep, strain rate dependence,** and **hysteresis** occur. These behaviors are defined in table 6.1.

Studies of Viscoelastic Properties

Taylor and his colleagues at Duke University (1990) have studied the viscoelastic properties of the muscle-tendon unit, using a rabbit model consisting of muscle with an intact neurovascular supply. **Stress relaxation** was demonstrated by stretching the muscle to 10% greater than its initial length and then immediately releasing it. After 10 repetitions, the tension required to produce the stretch decreased 17%. Most of the

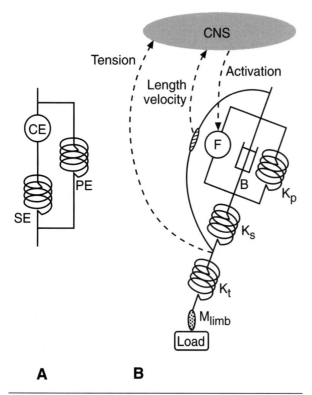

A   **B**

Figure 6.3 (A) Three-element muscle model has a complex contractile element (CE) in parallel with a passive elastic element (PE) and in series with another elastic element (SE) that has both passive (tendon/aponeurosis) and active (cross-bridge) components. (B) A more complex model of muscle contains elastic (K_s and K_p), viscous (B, a dash pot), and force-generating (F) elements. K_t is a nonlinear elastic element representing tendon and aponeurosis. These elements are modulated by length- and force-sensitive reflexes, which are in turn modulated by the central nervous system (CNS).
Reprinted, by permission, from G. Gottlieb, 1996, "Muscle compliance: Implications for the control of movement," *Exercise and Sport Sciences Reviews* 24: 4.

Table 6.1	Behavior of Viscoelastic Materials
Behavior	**Definition**
Stress relaxation	Less force is required over time to maintain a given increase in length during a sustained stretch.
Creep	A fixed force is applied to a material, and continued slow deformation occurs.
Strain rate dependence	A slower stretch (strain) produces greater elongation than a faster stretch.
Hysteresis	More energy is absorbed during a stretch than is released when the stretch is terminated; the material absorbs energy when stretched.

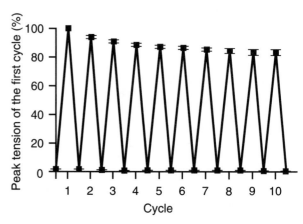

Figure 6.4 The extensor digitorum longus (EDL) muscle of rabbits is repeatedly stretched to 10% beyond its resting length. The overall tension decreases 16.6%, demonstrating the phenomenon of stress relaxation with repeated stretches.
Reprinted, by permission, from D. Taylor, J. Dalton, A. Seaber, and W. Garrett, 1990, "Viscoelastic properties of muscle-tendon units: The biomechanical effects of stretching," *American Journal of Sports Medicine* 18(3): 303.

stress relaxation occurred during the first four stretches (figure 6.4). **Creep** was demonstrated by a similar experiment in which muscle was stretched to a given tension, held at that tension for 30 seconds, and then relaxed. After this series of stretches was repeated 10 times, overall muscle length increased by 3.5%; the greatest elongation occurred with the first stretch (figure 6.5). This experiment simulates the static stretching technique. **Strain rate dependence** and **hysteresis** were demonstrated by stretching muscle to 10% greater than its initial length at four different velocities. Energy absorption and the tensile force required to achieve elongation were greatest at the highest stretch velocity. Hysteresis may occur either because of heat transfer to the muscle or because of internal changes in the muscle structure.

The experiments of Taylor et al. (1990) have several clinical implications. They demonstrate that muscle length gains achieved by stretching are not

rapidly reversible. They help explain why ballistic stretching may be harmful and ineffective—rapid stretching velocity increases tension and energy storage in muscle, which may increase both risk and severity of injury. In addition, ballistic stretches are not held long enough to allow stress relaxation or creep to occur. Most muscle lengthening occurs during the first 12-18 seconds of a stretch and during the first four stretch cycles.

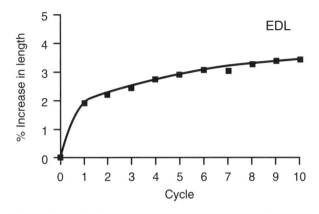

Figure 6.5 Rabbit EDL is repeatedly stretched to the same tension. The progressive increase in muscle length demonstrates the phenomenon of creep in a viscoelastic material.

Reprinted, by permission, from D. Taylor, J. Dalton, A. Seaber, and W. Garrett, 1990, "Viscoelastic properties of muscle-tendon units: The biomechanical effects of stretching," *American Journal of Sports Medicine* 18(3): 300-309.

Measuring and Quantifying Muscle Flexibility and Ligamentous Laxity

Most researchers have used goniometers to measure **static joint range of motion**. Gajdosik and Bohannon (1987) have extensively reviewed this technique's limitations, which affect both its reliability and validity. The measurements are dependent on the amount of force applied to range the joint, the stretch or pain tolerance of the subject, and any contraction of the muscle being stretched. Joint range of motion may be limited by nonmuscular structures or by the inflexibility of more than one muscle. To assess the flexibility of muscles that cross two joints (e.g., the rectus femoris and gastrocnemius), one must position both joints appropriately, properly stabilizing them to insure validity and reliability. For example, in using a passive straight leg raise with the subject supine to assess flexibility of the hamstring muscle group, one must stabilize the pelvis—pelvic rotation can increase hip flexion range of motion (figures 6.6A and B). Flexibility measurements made at two different times, such as before and after initiation of a stretching program, should be made at the same time of day, at the same environmental temperature, and following a similar level of activity (e.g., with no warm-up or after a similar warm-up).

A more valid method of measuring flexibility might be to measure a ratio of change in joint range of motion to the force applied to achieve that change (Gajdosik 1995). Although this technique can be

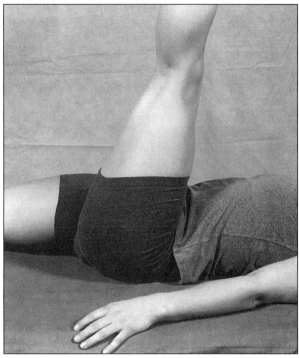

A

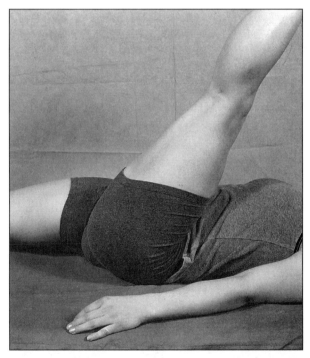

B

Figure 6.6 An athlete performing a hamstring stretch in the straight leg raise position with the pelvis squared (A). The same athlete can achieve a much greater arc of motion by rotating the pelvis during the straight leg raise (B).

applied in research settings, it is not very practical for clinicians, as it requires specialized apparatus with force transducers.

A Proposed Composite Scale

There are no widely used composite scales for clinical assessment of flexibility. We have proposed one such scale for assessing the flexibility of lower extremity muscles in which poor flexibility or tightness has been associated with overuse injuries (Krivickas and Feinberg 1996). We derive a composite **muscle tightness score** by assessing the bilateral flexibility of five muscle groups and classifying each group as either acceptably flexible or excessively tight. Since each tight muscle is given a score of 1, the total score ranges from 0 to 10—a score of 0 indicating adequate flexibility and a score of 10 indicating very poor flexibility. Muscle groups included in this scale are the iliotibial band, the rectus femoris, the hamstrings, the iliopsoas, and the gastrocsoleus; table 6.2 lists the criteria for muscle tightness. We assess flexibility of the iliotibial band with a modified version of the **Ober test** (figures 6.7A, B, and C); of the iliopsoas with the **Thomas test** (figure 6.8); and of the hamstrings by measuring **popliteal angle** (figure 6.9). For rectus femoris flexibility, we measure the difference between knee flexion with the hip flexed and with the hip extended (**Ely test**, figure 6.10). This difference is called the quadriceps inhibited knee flexion angle (QFA). Gastrocsoleus flexibility is measured by determining maximal ankle dorsiflexion with the knee

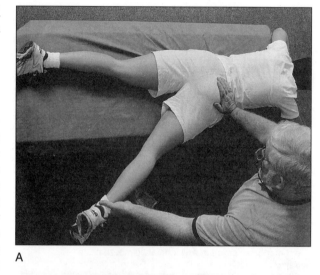

A

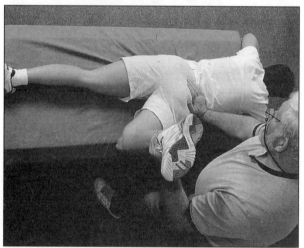

B

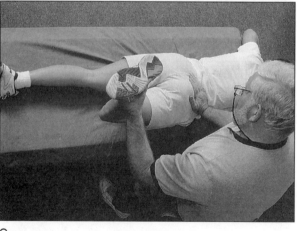

C

Table 6.2	Lower Extremity Muscle Tightness Score
Muscle	**Tightness criterion**
Iliotibial band	Positive Ober test
Rectus femoris	QFA* ≥ 10°
Iliopsoas	Positive Thomas test
Hamstrings	Popliteal angle ≥ 25°
Gastrocsoleus	Ankle dorsiflexion ≤ 5°

Evaluate each lower extremity. Score one point for each tight muscle group in each leg, yielding a score ranging from 0 (all muscles flexible) to 10 (all muscles tight).

*QFA = quadriceps inhibited knee flexion angle (see paragraph above for explanation)

Figure 6.7 The Ober test assesses iliotibial band flexibility. A modified form of the traditional test, eliminating the assistance of gravity, is depicted. The leg to be tested is abducted while the subject is prone (A). The knee of the abducted leg is flexed 90° and the hip extended (B). The leg should freely adduct to midline from the position in figure 6.7B if the iliotibial band is flexible (C).

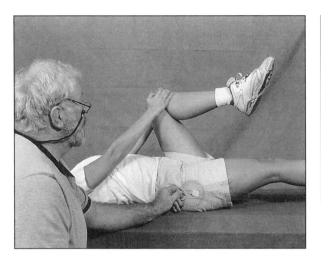

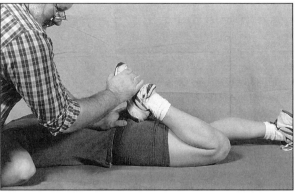

Figure 6.10 The Ely test assesses rectus femoris flexibility. With the subject prone and the pelvis stabilized against the examining table, the knee is flexed until the heel touches the buttock. If this maneuver cannot be performed without flexing the hips and/or lifting the pelvis from the examining table, the rectus femoris muscle is tight.

Figure 6.8 The Thomas test assesses iliopsoas flexibility. The subject holds one knee flexed to the chest while extending the other hip and knee. In the absence of iliopsoas tightness, the extended leg should rest comfortably on the examining table.

tion of a scoring system Carter and Wilkinson (1964) devised to study children with congenital dislocation of the hip (see table 6.3 and figure 6.11). The first four of the five elements in the scale are assessed bilaterally, for a maximum score of 2; the last element is scored either 0 or 1, giving a maximum ligamentous laxity score of 9 points (hyperlax) and a minimum of 0 (tight). Several authors have labeled Beighton scores of 0-3 as normal and scores of 4-9 as representing ligamentous laxity (Al-Rawi et al. 1985; Diaz et al. 1993; Klemp et al. 1984). The spinal forward flexion criterion (palms to floor) differs from the other criteria, in that it measures hamstring flexibility and anatomic proportions in addition to

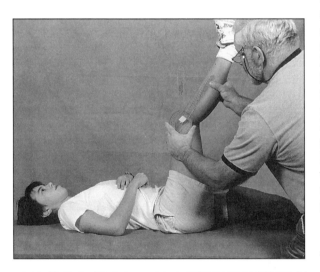

Figure 6.9 Measurement of popliteal angle assesses hamstring flexibility. With the subject supine, the hip is flexed 90° and the knee extended as much as possible. A goniometer is used to measure the angle between the lower leg and vertical.

extended—a position closer to that experienced during ambulation than the 90-degree knee flexion used in many tests. This muscle tightness scale has been used to assess flexibility in collegiate athletes, but requires studies of validity and reliability before use in other populations.

Measuring Ligamentous Laxity

Ligamentous laxity is widely assessed by using the **Beighton scale,** (Beighton et al. 1973) a modifica-

Table 6.3	Beighton Scale for Ligamentous Laxity
Test element	**Maximum score**
Thumb to forearm	2
5th MCP* extension > 90°	2
Elbow hyperextension > 10°	2
Knee hyperextension > 10°	2
Palms to floor	1
TOTAL	9

*MCP = metacarpal phalangeal joint
Adapted, by permission, from P.L. Beighton, L. Solomon, and C. Soskolone, 1973, "Articular mobility in an African population," *Ann Rheum Dis* 32: 413-418.

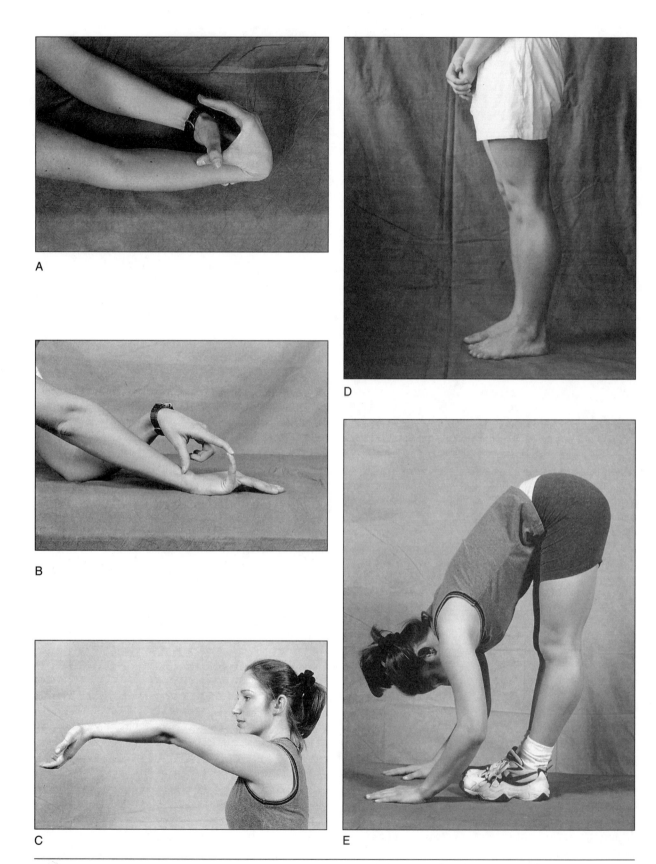

Figure 6.11 Elements of Beighton scale. Passive opposition of the thumb to the flexor aspect of the forearm (A). Passive hyperextension of the 5th metacarpal phalangeal joint beyond 90° (B). Hyperextension of the elbow by 10° or more (C). Hyperextension of the knee by 10° or more (D). Forward flexion of the trunk with the knees fully extended and palms flat on the floor (E).

ligamentous laxity (Klemp et al. 1984); some believe it should be dropped from the scale.

Relationship Between Muscle Stiffness and Flexibility

The **stiffness** of a material describes its ability to resist elongation or stretching. Engineers use **Young's modulus** (also known as the "modulus of elasticity") to describe stiffness. Young's modulus (Y) is defined as:

$$Y = \text{stress/strain} = (F/A)/(\Delta l/l_o)$$

where F = pulling force, A = cross-sectional area, $\Delta 1$ = change in length, and l_o = initial length. Since A and l_o are fixed properties of an individual muscle, Y, or stiffness, is proportional to $F/\Delta l$. It may be that muscle stiffness rather than range of motion (which we typically call flexibility) is more properly associated with risk and severity of injury.

Halbertsma and colleagues (1994, 1996) studied the effect of both a single 10-minute stretch and a 4-week stretching program on range of motion and muscle stiffness in neurologically normal individuals with short hamstring muscles. Both the single stretch and the 4-week program increased hamstring flexibility, measured by a passive straight leg raise. However, neither program altered muscle stiffness, measured by Young's modulus. In these subjects, the improvement in flexibility apparently was due to increased stretch tolerance rather than to a change in mechanical properties of the muscle. Although the authors concluded that muscle flexibility and stiffness are unrelated, their conclusion is controversial. Magnusson and colleagues (1996) used a slightly different model to study the effect of hamstring stretching on stiffness. They found that a series of five stretches decreased stiffness, but that stiffness returned to its baseline level within one hour. Gleim and McHugh (1997) recently demonstrated that stiffness in the central portion of a joint's range of motion is related to the terminal range of motion.

Wilson and his colleagues (1991, 1994) used a more complex model to study active muscle stiffness in weightlifters performing the bench press. Conceptually, it is difficult to relate this measurement of active stiffness to flexibility when the latter is defined either as range of motion or as a length:tension ratio. The model uses a damped oscillation technique in which the weightlifters hold a barbell in a static bench press position 3 cm above the chest. The experimenter manually perturbs the bar (causing it to oscillate),

while instructing the subject not to alter his muscle firing pattern. The more rapidly the oscillations are damped, the stiffer the muscles are assumed to be. According to this model, flexibility of the anterior deltoid and pectoralis muscles decreased as muscle stiffness increased. These authors also demonstrated that strength training increases muscle stiffness. A study of the relationship between power generation and muscle stiffness during the bench pressing exercise showed that increased muscle stiffness was associated with increased power generation during concentric and isometric contractions, but not during eccentric contractions. Klinge et al. (1997) recently demonstrated increased stiffness and energy storage in hamstring muscles trained isometrically.

More research is needed. With our current knowledge we can assume, at best, that changes in muscle stiffness must develop over time. We also must be careful to note how we are defining both stiffness and flexibility when we try to relate one property of muscle to the other.

Relationship Between Muscle Flexibility and Injury

Most health care professionals, athletes, and coaches believe that improving flexibility helps prevent musculoskeletal injuries—particularly overuse injuries and muscle strains. Most researchers addressing this issue have studied athletes or other "healthy," relatively young populations; and they have looked only at the relationship between *static* flexibility and injury. Ideally, of course, one would like to measure flexibility immediately before an injury occurs. Since this is not possible, investigators must measure flexibility at some point prior to the injury, such as at the beginning of an athletic season. Measuring flexibility after an injury has been sustained is not acceptable: either the injury itself or the treatment of the injury may alter flexibility. Theoretically, one can randomize subjects to stretching vs. nonstretching programs and record injuries for each group; but such a study must control many extraneous variables.

Several investigators have observed correlations between flexibility deficits and specific types of injuries. A study of adolescent elite figure skaters found an association between anterior knee pain syndromes and hamstring, rectus femoris, and gastrocsoleus muscle tightness (Smith et al. 1991). Adults with increased femoral anteversion and patellofemoral pain syndrome have tighter hamstring muscles than those with increased femoral anteversion without

| Table 6.4 | Flexibility Deficits Associated With Overuse Injuries |

	Lesser trochanter apophysitis	PFSS*	JK*	OS*	MTSS*	ITB* syndrome	Plantar fasciitis
Iliopsoas	X						
ITB*						X	
Rectus femoris		X	X	X			
Hamstrings		X	X	X			
Gastrocsoleus		X			X		X
Tibialis posterior							
Shoulder external rotators							

	Sever's	Accessory navicular	Anterior impingement
Iliopsoas			
ITB*			
Rectus femoris			
Hamstrings			
Gastrocsoleus	X	X	
Tibialis posterior		X	
Shoulder external rotators			X

*PFSS = patellofemoral stress syndrome; JK = jumper's knee; OS = Osgood Schlatter's disease; MTSS = medial tibial stress syndrome; ITB = iliotibial band

Adapted, by permission, from L.S. Krivickas, 1997, "Anatomical factors associated with overuse injuries," *Sports Med* 24(2): 132-146.

patellofemoral pain syndrome (Stroud et al. 1989). In collegiate physical education students, Lysens et al. (1989) found an association between muscle inflexibility and increased incidence of overuse injuries. Knapik et al. (1991) observed that female collegiate athletes with asymmetric lower extremity flexibility developed more lower extremity injuries than those with symmetric flexibility. Table 6.4 shows specific flexibility deficits that have been associated with particular overuse injuries (Krivickas 1997).

We studied the relationship between lower extremity muscle tightness and lower extremity injuries in college athletes using the 10-point muscle tightness scale previously described (Krivickas and Feinberg 1996). Men had significantly tighter muscles than women. For men, each additional point on the muscle tightness scale increased risk of injury by 23%; but muscle tightness was not associated with injury incidence in women. It may be that the women in this study had achieved a threshold flexibility level necessary to avoid increased risk of injury.

Hilyer and colleagues (1990) assigned municipal fire fighters either to a flexibility training program or to no training program. Those in the experimental group performed flexibility exercises for one-half hour per shift for two years. Overall flexibility improved in the trained group, and although the incidence of injury did not differ from that in the control group, those in the trained group sustained less severe and less costly injuries. This is the type of prospective study that needs to be done to further explore the relationship between flexibility and injury.

No one has specifically studied the relationship between flexibility and injury in the elderly, but one study found that elderly adults with a history of falls had decreased hip flexion and ankle dorsiflexion range of motion when compared to the "nonfallers" (Gehlsen and Whaley 1990). Falls are a major cause of injury in the elderly, and decreased lower extremity flexibility may increase the risk of injury in the elderly. Few or no clinical studies have addressed the relationship between flexibility deficits and injury in populations with various disease processes.

Relationship Between Ligamentous Laxity and Injury

The relationship between ligamentous laxity and musculoskeletal injuries is even more confusing than the relationship between flexibility deficits and injury. Some studies have shown associations between ligamentous laxity and an increased injury incidence, while others have found no association or even an association with decreased incidence of injury. Two types of studies have attempted to address this issue. One has looked at generalized ligamentous laxity, as measured by the Beighton scale, while the other type has focused on joint-specific ligamentous laxity, such as knee ligament laxity measured by a *KT-100* arthrometer.

Researchers have explored the relationship between generalized ligamentous laxity and injury in ballet dancers, soldiers, football players, and collegiate athletes (Klemp et al. 1984; Diaz et al. 1993; Godshall 1975; Grana and Moretz 1978; Kalenak and Morehouse 1975; Moretz et al. 1982; Nicholas 1970; Krivickas and Feinberg 1996). Ballet dancers with hypermobility, defined as a score of 4 or greater on the Beighton scale, sustained significantly more injuries (Klemp et al. 1984). In a group of soldiers undergoing a two-month period of intense military training, those with hypermobility sustained more ankle sprains and knee injuries but fewer muscle strains (Diaz et al. 1993). In contrast, in collegiate athletes there was no association between generalized ligamentous laxity and the incidence of ankle sprains (Baumhauer et al. 1995). Nicholas (1970) found an association between generalized ligamentous laxity and knee ligament rupture in professional football players, but Kalenak and Morehouse (1975) found no such association among collegiate football

players. The findings of Moretz et al. (1982), Grana and Moretz (1978), and Godshall (1975) agree with those of Kalenak and Morehouse.

In our study of collegiate athletes participating in a variety of sports, male athletes with tight ligaments (i.e., low scores on the Beighton scale) sustained a greater number of lower extremity injuries during a single competitive season than those with higher Beighton scores (Krivickas and Feinberg 1996). Although we saw no such relationship among the female athletes, it should be noted that they had significantly higher Beighton scores than the males (mean $\pm$ SD = 3.3 $\pm$ 2.2, vs. 1.8 $\pm$ 2.0). Because very few men had Beighton scores greater than or equal to 4, this study did not have the power to detect an association between true hypermobility and injury in men. One hypothesis that would explain the conflicting results is that either too little or too much ligamentous laxity increases the risk of injury.

Larsson et al. (1993) used the Beighton scale to assess hypermobility in 660 musicians, testing the relationship between ligamentous laxity and injury of individual joints. Unlike in previous studies, individual elements of the scale were correlated with specific injuries, and no composite ligamentous laxity score was assessed for overall injury incidence. Musicians playing instruments requiring repetitive upper extremity motion were less likely to experience hand and wrist symptoms if they had wrist hypermobility; however, hypermobility of joints *not* involved in repetitive motion was a liability rather than an asset. Those with knee and spine hypermobility suffered more frequently from knee and low back pain.

Effect of Disease Processes on Flexibility

Several categories of disease processes adversely affect joint range of motion, and when severe, may result in a **contracture**, which means that muscle cannot be passively extended to its full normal length without pain or soft tissue injury such as a muscle tear. The flexibility of muscles surrounding a joint must be lost in order for a contracture to develop. However, once a contracture has developed, it does not respond readily to a stretching program and is difficult to treat. All of the following conditions decrease flexibility and predispose to the development of contractures: upper motor neuron lesions that produce spasticity, lower motor neuron lesions that produce severe weakness, chronic pain, arthritis, and burns or orthopedic injuries whose treatment requires immobilization.

Spasticity decreases flexibility via hyperactivity of the muscle spindle reflex and of suprasegmental reflexes. If spastic muscles are not stretched regularly, contractures develop. Muscle cooling decreases the firing rate of the spindle, while heat increases its firing rate (DeLateur 1994; Eldred et al. 1960; Mense 1978; Miglietta 1973; Petajan and Watts 1962). In individuals whose weakness is related to lower motor neuron dysfunction (e.g., spinal muscular atrophy or a severe myopathy), loss of flexibility and contractures develop despite normal or decreased muscle spindle activity. Muscles are maintained in a shortened position because the patient is too weak to move the joints through a full range of motion. The most common sites for contracture are the shoulders in those with proximal upper extremity weakness, the hip and knee flexors in those who are wheelchair bound, and the ankle plantar flexors of individuals with foot drop. A daily range-of-motion program can easily prevent loss of range of motion in these cases. People requiring immobilization of a joint for a prolonged period of time also lose flexibility in muscles that are chronically shortened. For example, an elbow flexion contracture may develop after an arm has been kept in a sling for six weeks to treat a proximal humerus fracture. Similarly, pain—such as that produced by a flare of rheumatoid arthritis—can limit joint range of motion enough to promote contracture.

A few disease processes, such as pentazocine fibrous myopathy, actually cause muscle fibrosis to develop (DeLateur 1994). In these cases, the application of heat increases collagen extensibility and should be used prior to stretching the involved muscles. Burn injuries also result in formation of tissue with excessive collagen content, and heat application facilitates stretching.

A few other disease processes produce excessive flexibility. These are primarily connective tissue diseases such as Ehlers-Danlos syndrome, Marfan's syndrome, and osteogenesis imperfecta. Individuals with diseases of amino acid metabolism, such as homocystinuria and hyperlysinemia, may also have joint hypermobility.

Relationship Between Flexibility and Athletic Performance

Only a few studies have explored the relationship between flexibility and performance. In these stud-ies, researchers have measured both muscle power generation and the VO_2 required to complete a given activity, in order to assess muscle efficiency. Once again, the results conflict with one another, and it is not yet known whether increasing range of motion enhances athletic performance.

Gleim et al. (1990) assessed trunk and lower extremity flexibility in healthy men and women, and then measured VO_2 during treadmill walking and jogging. Those with the tightest muscles were the most efficient, with the lowest VO_2 at any given speed. A similar study by Craib et al. (1996) looked at the relationship between flexibility and running economy in sub-elite male distance runners. Tightness of the hip external rotators and ankle dorsiflexors was associated with lower VO_2 and accounted for 47% of the variance in running economy. An earlier study by DeVries (1963) did not find any change in VO_2 or speed when runners stretched prior to a 100-yard sprint. In contrast, a study of college students by Godges et al. (1989) demonstrated greater gait economy after a single session of stretching. The elastic recoil of muscle contributes to energy necessary for movement (Cavagna et al. 1964), and tighter muscles may have greater elastic recoil, enabling them to store more energy.

Other investigators have attempted to correlate muscle flexibility with force and power production. Wilson et al. (1994) found that weightlifters with the greatest stiffness of their upper extremity and chest muscles were able to generate more power during isometric and concentric contractions, but not during eccentric contractions. The same investigators found that flexibility training decreases muscle stiffness. According to their work, increasing flexibility appears to decrease power production. In contrast, Worrell and colleagues (1994) found that a hamstring stretching program in healthy university students increased peak eccentric and concentric hamstring torque. Theoretically, improving flexibility of a muscle should increase its ability to generate concentric force: during stretch, elastic components of muscle absorb mechanical work and store it as potential energy, which is released when the muscle shortens. By increasing muscle length, more energy can be stored and then released during the subsequent concentric contraction. Hortobagyi et al. (1985) found that a hamstring stretching program increased the power of concentric quadriceps contraction by increasing the speed of contraction without altering force production. Thus, it appears that increasing the flexibility of an antagonist muscle can also increase contraction speed of the agonist muscle.

Flexibility and Activities of Daily Living in the Elderly or Disabled

No one has scientifically studied the relationship between flexibility and performance of activities of daily living (**ADLs**) in the elderly or disabled population. Clinicians caring for the elderly or disabled realize that a certain minimal range of motion is necessary to perform ADLs. Adequate shoulder range of motion is required to reach a glass on an overhead shelf, handle garment closures behind one's back, brush one's hair, and even feed oneself. Table 6.5 shows the necessary joint range of motion for commonly performed ADLs. In a study of patients with elbow flexion contractures associated with spinal muscular atrophy or congenital myopathy, 59% of the patients reported that the contractures interfered with their ADLs, while 12% felt the contractures were beneficial (Willig et al. 1995). Research evaluating the effect of flexibility training on function in the elderly or disabled must be performed before we can draw conclusions about the benefits of flexibility training in these populations.

Stretching Techniques and Prescription of a Flexibility Training Program

The three major forms of stretching are ballistic, static, and proprioceptive neuromuscular facilitation (PNF).

Ballistic stretching utilizes rapid bouncing motions that tend to have relatively high force and velocity. Animal studies suggest that ballistic stretching should increase the risk of muscle injury (Taylor et al. 1990). Although it can be effective, ballistic stretching is not recommended. It activates the spindle reflex, which is counterproductive, and it is more likely than other stretching methods to produce muscle soreness.

Static stretching is an effective means of improving flexibility. It minimizes activation of the spindle reflex, activates the Golgi tendon reflex if held long enough, does not require a partner, and is unlikely to cause muscle soreness. A static stretch must be held for at least six seconds in order to fully activate the Golgi tendon reflex (Shellock and Prentice 1985).

Knott and Voss (1968) popularized **PNF stretching**. There are several different techniques of PNF, but they all involve isometric contraction and relaxation of the muscle being stretched. Two of the most popular PNF techniques are **contract-relax (CR)** and **contract-relax agonist-contract (CRAC)**. To stretch the hamstrings using the CR technique, the subject lies supine while a partner passively performs a straight leg raise on the subject. The subject then contracts his hamstrings while the partner resists movement of the leg; when the subject relaxes his hamstrings, the partner pushes the straight leg raise further, increasing hip range of motion. Using the CRAC technique, the subject would contract his quadriceps while the partner assisted the straight leg raise. PNF stretching techniques take advantage of neurophysiologic principles such as autogenic and reciprocal inhibition, which are believed to alter the spinal reflexes. **Autogenic inhibition** refers to stimulation of the Golgi tendon organ by contraction of the muscle that is being stretched. **Reflex inhibition**

Table 6.5	Joint Range of Motion Required for Activities of Daily Living	
Joint	**Range of motion**	**Activity**
Elbow	120° flexion	Eating, grooming, personal hygiene
Shoulder	45° flexion, 90° abduction, 20° external rotation	Eating, grooming, personal hygiene
Ankle	10° dorsiflexion, 20° plantar flexion	Walking
Knee	60° flexion 90° flexion	Walking Stair climbing
Hip	30° flexion 70° flexion	Walking Sitting

is believed to occur when the CRAC technique is used; contraction of the antagonist muscle induces relaxation in the muscle being stretched. One drawback of PNF techniques is that most require a partner, and some training is necessary for them to be performed properly.

Which Technique?

Several investigators have compared the efficacy of ballistic, static, and PNF stretching programs (DeVries 1963; Etnyre and Lee 1988; Godges et al. 1989; Lucas and Koslow 1984; Moore and Hutton 1980; Sady et al. 1982; Wallin et al. 1985). All three methods improve flexibility, but it is not clear which is most effective. Table 6.6 summarizes the studies.

Moore and Hutton (1980) compared static, CR, and CRAC hamstring stretching protocols in college-aged female gymnasts, quantifying muscle contraction by use of surface EMG recordings from the quadriceps and hamstrings. The CRAC method produced the greatest hamstring EMG activity while the hamstrings were supposed to be relaxed. It was perceived as the most painful technique, and was less effective than either static or CR stretches. Overall, the subjects perceived the static stretch as the most effective—it produced the greatest increase in range of motion and was least painful. It appears that PNF and static stretching have similar effects in healthy young adults. If a PNF technique is used, the CR may be preferable to the CRAC method because it is less painful and less likely to produce co-contraction of the muscle being stretched.

Table 6.6		Comparison Studies of Stretching Techniques			
Author	**Year**	**Population**	**Stretching techniques**	**Muscle**	**Result**
DeVries	1962	College M	1. Static 2. Ballistic	Multiple	No difference
Moore and Hutton	1980	College F gymnasts	1. PNF—CR 2. PNF—CRAC 3. Static	Hamstrings	CRAC > static > CR; only statistically significant difference between CRAC and CR; CRAC most painful
Sady et al.	1982	College M	1. PNF—CR 2. Static 3. Ballistic	Mutliple	PNF best
Lucas and Koslow	1984	College F	1. PNF—CR 2. Static 3. Ballistic	Hamstrings	No difference
Wallin et al.	1985	M, age 19-32	1. PNF—CR 2. Ballistic	Hamstrings, hip adductors, gastrocsoleus	PNF best
Etnyre and Lee	1988	College M and F	1. PNF—CR 2. PNF—CRAC 3. Static	Hamstrings, shoulder flexors	CRAC best in M; CR and CRAC equal in F but better than static
Godges et al.	1989	College M	1. PNF and soft tissue massage 2. Static	Hamstrings	Static best

M = male, F = female, PNF = proprioceptive neuromuscular facilitation, CR = contract-relax PNF technique, CRAC = contract-relax agonist-contract PNF technique

One interesting stretching technique that may hold promise is the addition of **vibratory stimulation** to a stretching protocol (Issurin et al. 1994). Issurin and colleagues (1994) devised a counterweight pulley system that provided a 44-Hz, 3-mm amplitude oscillation to the foot while the hip adductors and hamstrings were being stretched. The protocol included a series of static stretches followed by a series of ballistic stretches. One group of subjects performed the stretches using the vibratory stimulation and the other group without it. The group using the vibratory stimulation made significantly greater gains in flexibility. Possible explanations for the efficacy of vibratory stimulation include an increase in the pain threshold, increased blood flow to local muscle (producing a temperature increase), and increased stimulation of the Golgi tendon organ.

Prescription Recommendations

How long and how frequently must one stretch to increase or maintain flexibility? What is the most appropriate prescription for a flexibility training program? Bandy and Irion (1994) studied hamstring stretching programs with prescribed stretches of 15, 30, or 60 seconds. They found no improvement in flexibility with a single daily 15-second stretch, and equal flexibility improvement with a single daily 30- or 60-second stretch, suggesting that 30 seconds may be the ideal length of time to hold a static stretch. Grady and Saxena (1991) also found that a 30-second stretch is adequate to improve flexibility, with minimal additional gains when the stretch is extended to 1 or 2 minutes. The animal work of Taylor and colleagues (1990) suggests that the greatest muscle elongation occurs during the first 12-18 seconds of a static stretch, and during the first 4 static stretches in a series of 10. Wallin et al. (1985) studied the frequency with which a stretching program must be performed to improve or maintain flexibility. After flexibility had been increased through a training program, one session of stretching per week was enough to *maintain* the increases. Three sessions of stretching per week *improved* flexibility, but even greater gains in flexibility were made when stretching was performed five times per week.

Based on the few studies that have addressed the appropriate frequency, duration, and intensity of stretching programs, I recommend the following:

1. Prescribe either static, PNF, or a combination of both types of stretches.
2. Use the CRAC PNF technique with caution, as it may be more painful than other techniques and may encourage co-contraction of the muscle being stretched.
3. Do not prescribe ballistic stretching.
4. Have your patients perform stretching exercises at least three times per week to improve flexibility; daily stretching will probably result in greater, faster gains.
5. Have your patients perform each stretch at least three times and hold it for 15-30 seconds.
6. Because of most patients' tendency to exercise less than prescribed, I suggest that you instruct patients to stretch at least five days per week, hold each stretch 30 seconds, and perform each stretch five times. You will increase compliance by limiting the number of different stretches prescribed, i.e., prescribe only one stretching exercise for each tight muscle.

Effect of Strength Training on Flexibility

In the past, athletes involved in activities requiring extreme flexibility, such as gymnastics and ballet, were discouraged from performing heavy resistance training because they and their coaches believed that it would decrease their flexibility. Unfortunately, few have addressed this issue in a scientific manner. One study of healthy young men found no relationship between strength and flexibility (Laubach and McConville 1965). A nonscientific observation can be made by looking at elite male gymnasts. They represent a population with both extreme flexibility and very high strength-to-weight ratios (see figure 6.12). By combining strength and flexibility training, these athletes do not compromise their flexibility with heavy resistance training.

Studying flexibility in older men (mean age 61 years), Girouard and Hurley (1995) compared the effects of either (1) flexibility training alone, or (2) a combination of flexibility training and heavy resistance strength training. Those who performed only flexibility training increased their flexibility; while those who performed both types of training had no improvement in flexibility. Although the effect of heavy resistance training alone on flexibility was not studied, these findings suggest that resistance training without flexibility training might actually decrease flexibility in the elderly. Until further research is conducted in this area, it is prudent to incorporate stretching into any strength training program, particularly in the case of older individuals.

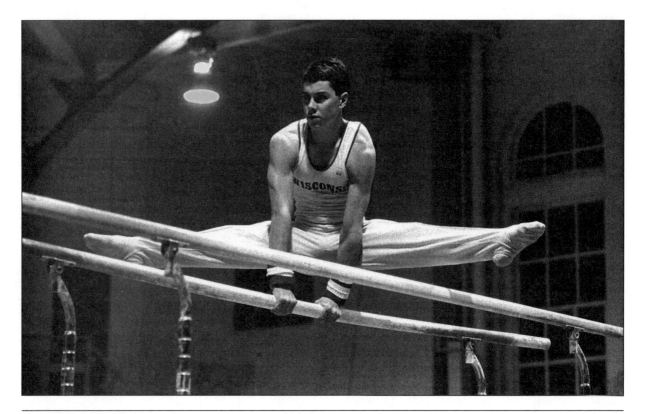

Figure 6.12   A male gymnast demonstrates both excellent flexibility and excellent strength.
Photo © Mary Langenfeld Photo.

Summary

Flexibility may be defined either as the range of motion of a joint or series of joints, or as a ratio of change in muscle length or joint angle to the force or torque required to passively elicit that change. Flexibility is joint- and muscle-specific and may differ in static and dynamic situations. Age, gender, race, training, injury history, spinal reflexes, supraspinal neural pathways, temperature, and the cellular composition of muscle all influence flexibility. The muscle-tendon unit is a viscoelastic structure that can be modeled simplistically as a spring and dash pot. It exhibits the viscoelastic properties of stress relaxation, creep, strain rate dependence, and hysteresis when stretched. There are various ways to assess the stiffness of muscle; some feel that measurement of stiffness may have more clinical relevance than measurement of flexibility.

Although there is no universal clinical scale for the measurement of muscle flexibility, many clinicians use the Beighton scale to measure ligamentous laxity. The literature concerning the relationship between flexibility deficits and injury is confusing, with some studies suggesting that flexibility deficits predispose to injury and others showing no relationship between flexibility and injury patterns. The relationship between ligamentous laxity and injury is even more controversial—some studies suggest that ligamentous laxity is beneficial, others suggest it is detrimental. Research addressing the relationship between VO_2, power production, and flexibility is also contradictory. While many disease processes affect flexibility, most research on flexibility training has focused on healthy individuals or athletes rather than on the disabled or elderly. Resistance strength training appears to influence flexibility, but the interaction between these two forms of training requires further study.

At the present time, prescription of a flexibility training program is somewhat empirical: little work has been done to determine the optimal duration, intensity, and frequency of training. Of the three major methods of stretching, it is clear that both static and PNF techniques are superior to ballistic stretching. Of the three major components of a comprehensive training and fitness program—strength, endurance, and flexibility training—flexibility training has received the least scientific attention. The unanswered questions concerning flexibility training are numerous, and opportunities for research in this area abound. What we do not know about flexibility is far greater than what we know.

References

Al-Rawi, Z.S., A.J. Al-Aszawi, and T. Al-Chalabi. 1985. Joint mobility among university students in Iraq. *Br J Rheumatol* 24:326-331.

Anderson, B., and E.R. Burke. 1991. Scientific, medical, and practical aspects of stretching. *Clin Sports Med* 10:63-86.

Bandy, W.D., and J.M. Irion. 1994. The effect of time of static stretch on the flexibility of hamstring muscles. *Phys Ther* 74:845-852.

Barnekow-Bergkvist, M., G. Hedberg, U. Janlert, and E. Jansson. 1996. Development of muscular endurance and strength from adolescence to adulthood and level of physical capacity in men and women at the age of 34 years. *Scand J Med Sci Sports* 6:145-155.

Baumhauer, J.F., D.M. Alosa, A.F. Renstrom, S. Trevino, and B. Beynnon. 1995. A prospective study of ankle injury risk factors. *Am J Sports Med* 23:564-570.

Beighton, P., L. Solomon, and C.L. Soskolone. 1973. Articular mobility in an African population. *Ann Rheum Dis* 32:413-418.

Carter, C., and J. Wilkinson. 1964. Persistent joint laxity and congenital dislocation of the hip. *J Bone Joint Surg (Br)* 46:40-45.

Cavagna, G.A., F.P. Saibene, and R. Margaria. 1964. Mechanical work in running. *J Appl Physiol* 19:249-256.

Corbin, C.B. 1984. Flexibility. *Clin Sports Med* 3:101-117.

Craib, M.W., V.A. Mitchell, K.B. Fields, T.R. Cooper, R. Hopewell, and D.W. Morgan. 1996. The association between flexibility and running economy in sub-elite male distance runners. *Med Sci Sports Exerc* 28:737-743.

DeLateur, B.J. 1994. Flexibility. *Phys Med Rehabil Clin* 5:295-307.

DeVries, H.A. 1962. Evaluation of static stretching procedures for improvement of flexibility. *Res Q* 33(2):222-229.

DeVries, H.A. 1963. The "looseness" factor in speed and O_2 consumption of an anaerobic 100 yard dash. *Res Q* 34:305-312.

Diaz, M.A., E.C. Estevez, and P.S. Guijo. 1993. Joint hyperlaxity and musculoligamentous lesions: study of a population of homogeneous age, sex and physical exertion. *Br J Rheumatol* 32:120-122.

Eldred, E., D.E. Linsley, and J.S. Buchwald. 1960. The effect of cooling on mammalian muscle spindles. *Exp Neurol* 2:144-157.

Etnyre, B.R., and E.J. Lee. 1988. Chronic and acute flexibility of men and women using three different stretching techniques. *Res Q* 59:222-228.

Gajdosik, R.L. 1995. Flexibility or muscle length? *Phys Ther* 75:238-239.

Gajdosik, R.L., and R.W. Bohannon. 1987. Clinical measurement of range of motion: review of goniometry emphasizing reliability and validity. *Phys Ther* 67:1867-1872.

Gehlsen, G.M., and M.H. Whaley. 1990. Falls in the elderly: part II. Balance, strength, and flexibility. *Arch Phys Med Rehabil* 71:739-741.

Gersten, J.W. 1955. Effect of ultrasound on tendon extensibility. *Am J Phys Med Rehabil* 34:362-369.

Girouard, C.K., and B.H. Hurley. 1995. Does strength training inhibit gains in range of motion from flexibility training in older adults? *Med Sci Sports Exerc* 27:1444-1449.

Gleim, G.W., and M.P. McHugh. 1997. Flexibility and its effects on sports injury and performance. *Sports Med* 24:289-299.

Gleim, G.W., N.S. Stachenfeld, and J.A Nicholas. 1990. The influence of flexibility on the economy of walking and jogging. *J Orthop Res* 8:814-823.

Godges, J.J., H.M. MacRae, C. Longdon, C. Tinberg, and P. MacRae. 1989. The effects of two stretching procedures on hip range of motion and gait economy. *J Orthop Sports Phys Ther* 10:350-357.

Godshall, R.W. 1975. The prediction of athletic injury: an eight year study. *J Sports Med* 3:50-54.

Gottlieb, G.L. 1996. Muscle compliance: implications for control of movement. In *Exerc Sports Sci Rev* 24: 1-34, ed. J.O. Holloszy. Philadelphia: Williams & Wilkins.

Grady, J.F., and A. Saxena. 1991. Effects of stretching the gastrocnemius muscle. *J Foot Surg* 30:465-469.

Grana, W.A., and J.A. Moretz. 1978. Ligamentous laxity in secondary school athletes. *JAMA* 240:1975-1976.

Halbertsma, J.P.K., A.I. van Bolhius, and L.N.H. Goeken. 1996. Sport stretching: effect on passive muscle stiffness of short hamstrings. *Arch Phys Med Rehabil* 77:688-692.

Halbertsma, J.P.K., and N.H. Goeken. 1994. Stretching exercises: effect on passive extensibility and stiffness in short hamstrings of healthy subjects. *Arch Phys Med Rehabil* 75:976-982.

Hilyer, J.C., K.C. Brown, A.T. Sirles, and L. Peoples. 1990. A flexibility intervention to reduce the incidence and severity of joint injuries in municipal firefighters. *J Occup Med* 32:631-637.

Hortobagyi, T., J. Faludi, J. Tihanyi, and B. Merkely. 1985. Effects of intense "stretching"—flexibility training on the mechanical profile of the knee extensors and on the range of motion of the hip joint. *Int J Sports Med* 6:317-321.

Issurin, V.B., D.G. Lieberman, and G. Tenenbaum. 1994. Effect of vibratory stimulation training on maximal force and flexibility. *J Sports Sci* 12:561-566.

Kalenak, A., and C.A. Morehouse. 1975. Knee stability and knee ligament injuries. *JAMA* 234:1143-1145.

Kandel, E.R., and J.H. Schwartz. 1991. *Principles of neural science.* Norwalk, CT: Appleton & Lange.

Klemp, P., J.E. Stevens, and S. Isaacs. 1984. A hypermobility study in ballet dancers. *J Ortho Rheumatol* 11:692-696.

Klinge, K., S.P. Magnusson, E.B. Simonsen, P. Aagaard, K. Klausen, and M. Kjaer. 1997. The effect of strength and flexibility training on skeletal muscle electromyographic activity, stiffness, and viscoelastic stress relaxation response. *Am J Sports Med* 25:710-716.

Knapik, J.J., C.L. Bauman, B.H. Jones, J.M. Harris, and L. Vaughan. 1991. Preseason strength and flexibility imbalances associated with athletic injuries in female collegiate athletes. *Am J Sports Med* 19:76-81.

Knott, M., and D.E. Voss. 1968. *Proprioceptive neuromuscular facilitation: Patterns and techniques*. 2d ed. New York: Harper & Row.

Krivickas, L.S. 1997. Anatomical factors associated with overuse sports injuries. *Sports Med* 24:132-146.

Krivickas, L.S., and J.H. Feinberg. 1996. Lower extremity injuries in college athletes: relation between ligamentous laxity and lower extremity muscle tightness. *Arch Phys Med Rehabil* 77:1139-1143.

Larsson, L., J. Baum, G.S. Mudholkar, and G.D. Kollia. 1993. Benefits and disadvantages of joint hypermobility among musicians. *N Engl J Med* 329:1079-1082.

Laubach, L.L., and J.T. McConville. 1965. Muscle strength, flexibility and body size of adult males. *Res Q* 37:384-392.

Laubach, L.L., and J.T. McConville. 1966. Relationship between flexibility, anthropometry, and the somatotype of college men. *Res Q* 37:241-251.

Lehman, J.F., A.J. Massock, C.G. Warren, and J.N. Koblanski. 1970. Effect of therapeutic temperatures on tendon extensibility. *Arch Phys Med Rehabil* 51:481-487.

Liebesman, J.L., and E. Cafarelli. 1994. Physiology of range of motion in human joints: a critical review. *Crit Rev Physican Rehabil Med* 6:131-160.

Lodish, H., D. Baltimore, and A. Berk et al. 1995. *Molecular cell biology*. New York: Scientific American Books.

Lucas, R., and R. Koslow. 1984. Comparative study of static, dynamic, and proprioceptive neuromuscular facilitation stretching techniques on flexibility. *Percept Mot Skills* 58:615-618.

Lysens, R.J., M.S. Ostyn, Y.V. Auweele, J. Lefevre, M. Vuylsteke, and L. Renson. 1989. The accident-prone and overuse-prone profiles of the young athlete. *Am J Sports Med* 17:612-619.

Magnusson, S.P., E.B. Simonsen, P. Aagaard, and M. Kjaer. 1996. Biomechanical responses to repeated stretches in human hamstring muscle in vivo. *Am J Sports Med* 24:622-627.

Marshall, J.L., N. Johanson, T.L. Wickiewicz, H.M. Tischler, B.L. Koslin, S. Zeno, and A. Meyers. 1980. Joint looseness: a function of the person and the joint. *Med Sci Sports Exerc* 12:189-194.

Mense, S. 1978. Effect of temperature on the discharges of muscle spindles and tendon organs. *Pflugers Arch* 374:159-166.

Micheli, L.J. 1983. Overuse injuries in children's sports: the growth factor. *Orthop Clin North Am* 14:337-360.

Miglietta, O. 1973. Action of cold on spasticity. *Am J Phys Med Rehabil* 52:198-205.

Moore, M.A., and R.S. Hutton. 1980. Electromyographic investigation of muscle stretching techniques. *Med Sci Sports Exerc* 12:322-329.

Moretz, J.A., R. Walters, and L. Smith. 1982. Flexibility as a predictor of knee injuries in college football players. *Physician Sports Med* 10:93-97.

Nicholas, J.A. 1970. Injuries to knee ligaments: relationship to looseness and tightness in football players. *JAMA* 21:2236-2239.

Petajan, J.H., and N. Watts. 1962. Effects of cooling on the triceps surae reflex. *Am J Phys Med Rehabil* 41:240-251.

Pratt, M. 1989. Strength, flexibility, and maturity in adolescent athletes. *Am J Dis Child* 143:560-563.

Proske, U. 1997. The mammalian muscle spindle. *News Physiol Sci* 12:37-42.

Sady, S.S., M. Wortman, and D. Blanke. 1982. Flexibility training: ballistic, static or proprioceptive neuromuscular facilitation? *Arch Phys Med Rehabil* 63:261-263.

Safran, M.R, W.E. Garrett, A.V. Seaber, R.R. Glisson, and B.M. Ribbeck. 1988. The role of warmup in muscular injury prevention. *Am J Sports Med* 16:123-129.

Shellock, F.G., and W.E. Prentice. 1985. Warming-up and stretching for improved physical performance and prevention of sports-related injuries. *Sports Med* 2:267-278.

Smith, A.D., L. Stroud, and C. McQueen. 1991. Flexibility and anterior knee pain in adolescent elite figure skaters. *J Pediatr Orthop* 11:77-82.

Stroud, L., A.D. Smith, and R. Kruse. 1989. The relationship between increased femoral anteversion in childhood and anterior knee pain in adulthood. *Orthop Trans* 13:554.

Tabary, J.C., C. Tabary, C. Tardieu, G. Tardieu, and G. Goldspink. 1972. Physiological and structural changes in the cat's soleus muscle due to immobilization by plaster casts at different lengths. *J Physiol* 224:231-244.

Taylor, D.C., J.D. Dalton, A.V. Seaber, and W.E. Garrett. 1990. Viscoelastic properties of muscle-tendon units: the biomechanical effects of stretching. *Am J Sports Med* 18:300-309.

Wallin, D., B. Ekblom, R. Grahn, and T. Nordenborg. 1985. Improvement of muscle flexibility: a comparison between two techniques. *Am J Sports Med* 13:263-268.

Waterman-Storer, C.M. 1991. The cytoskeleton of skeletal muscle: is it affected by exercise? A brief review. *Med Sci Sports Exerc* 23:1240-1249.

Willig, T.N., J.R. Bach, M.J. Rouffet, L.S. Krivickas, and C. Maquet. 1995. Correlation of flexion contractures with upper extremity function and pain for spinal muscular atrophy and congenital myopathy patients. *Am J Phys Med Rehabil* 74:33-39.

Wilson, G.J., A.J. Murphy, and J.F. Pryor. 1994. Musculotendinous stiffness: its relationship to eccentric, isometric, and concentric performance. *J Appl Physiol* 76:2714-2719.

Wilson, G.J., G.A. Wood, and B.C. Elliot. 1991. The relationship between stiffness of the musculature and static flexibility: an alternative explanation for the occurrence of muscular injury. *Int J Sports Med* 19:403-407.

Worrell, T.W., T.L. Smith, and J. Winegardner. 1994. Effect of hamstring stretching on hamstring muscle performance. *J Orthop Sports Phys Ther* 20:154-159.

Part II

Special Clinical Considerations

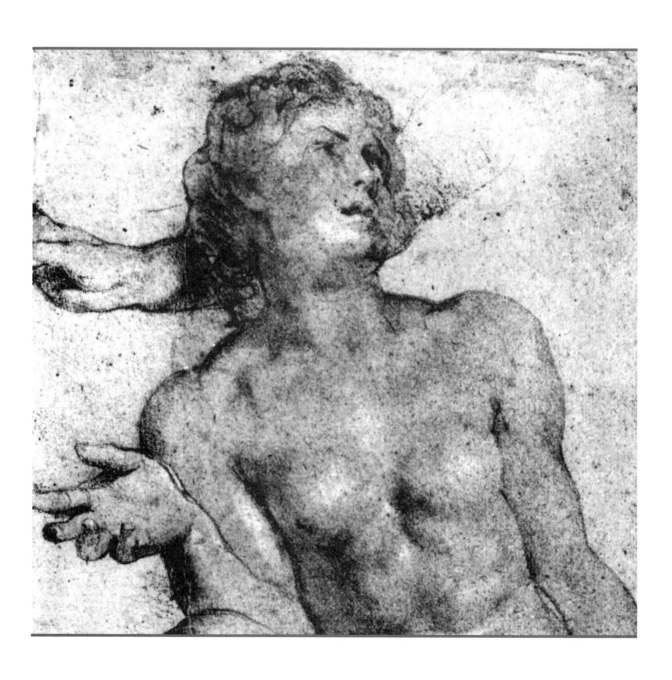

Chapter 7

Testing the Capacity to Exercise in Disabled Individuals

Cardiopulmonary and Neuromuscular Models

James C. Agre, MD, PhD

Since the time of the ancient Greeks, physical activity has been acclaimed as an adjunct to good health (Leon and Blackburn 1977). Many research studies of the past half century have confirmed the health-related benefits of regular physical activity (Åstrand and Rodahl 1986; McArdle et al. 1991). The **beneficial physiological adaptations**, resulting from regular physical activity, have been reviewed (Paffenbarger and Hyde 1984; Serfass and Gerberich 1984; Hahn et al. 1990) and include the following: reduction in heart rate and blood pressure, both at rest and during activity; morphological change in skeletal muscle, resulting in improved physical work capacity; morphological change in cardiac muscle, resulting in improved cardiovascular efficiency; in-

creased muscular endurance; reduced blood coagulability and transient increase in fibrinolysis; reduction in adiposity; increased lean body mass; increased cellular sensitivity to insulin; favorable changes in blood lipids and lipoproteins, including a reduction in plasma triglycerides and an increase in high-density lipoprotein (HDL) cholesterol; reduction in coronary artery disease risk factors; and decreased mortality and morbidity due to primary and secondary prevention. The **beneficial psychological adaptations** of regular physical activity are difficult to measure; however, it is well known that regular physical activity helps relieve muscular tension, makes one feel better and sleep better, and may aid motivation for improving other health habits including dietary changes (reduction in saturated fat consumption) and cessation of cigarette smoking (Leon and Blackburn 1977). In contrast, **limitation in physical activity** in the form of bed rest results in progressive deterioration of cardiovascular performance and efficiency, metabolic disturbances, difficulty in maintaining normal body weight, disturbed sympathetic nervous system activity, and possible emotional disturbances (Kottke 1966; Leon and Blackburn 1977; Taylor et al. 1949). Unquestionably, the physiological and psychological benefits of regular physical activity improve quality of life.

Yet physical activity carries risks. Regular physical activity increase one's risk for musculoskeletal injury (Buschbacher and Braddom 1994; Prentice 1994); and more serious consequences, such as acute myocardial infarction or cardiac arrest, can occur during the performance of physical activities (ACSM 1995; Siscovick et al. 1984; Thompson et al. 1982). Fortunately, the incidence of such adverse events is very low (Thompson et al. 1982)—the incidence of cardiac arrest during physical activity, for example, is about one event in 18,000 healthy men per year (Siscovick et al. 1984); and pre-participation screening (and appropriate testing where necessary) can lower the risk associated with physical activity (ACSM 1995).

While there is no nationally accepted standard of guidelines and policies for exercise testing and participation, the American College of Sports Medicine has published very reasonable guidelines for exercise testing and prescription. These guidelines discuss, in detail, many topics concerning exercise testing and prescription—including health screening and risk stratification, pretest evaluation, physical fitness testing, clinical testing, and interpretation of test data. Since it is beyond the scope of this chapter to cover these issues in depth, for more detailed information please refer to the *ACSM's Guidelines for Exercise Testing and Prescription, 5th Edition* (ACSM 1995).

Rationale for Health Screening and Risk Stratification

Health screening and **risk stratification** help physicians to identify individuals who are at risk from physical activity and to stratify individuals according to risk. Screening and stratification also help to determine what (if any) specific medical assessments are needed to assess an individual's response to physi-

cal activity, or what supervision (if any) an individual may require to safely participate in a physical activity program. The purposes of a **pre-participation health screen** include the following:

- Identify and exclude individuals with contraindications to physical activity.
- Identify individuals who need medical evaluation and clearance before starting an activity program.
- Identify individuals who should have medical supervision during physical activity.
- Identify people with other special needs (such as individuals with physical disabilities) (ACSM 1995).

Health screening can range from completing a simple questionnaire to undergoing very expensive medical testing. The **Physical Activity Readiness Questionnaire (PAR-Q)** (Thomas et al. 1992) sets minimal standards for adults who wish to participate in a low- to moderate-intensity physical activity program (ACSM 1995). This questionnaire helps identify adults with conditions that might require medical evaluation or advice prior to beginning a physical activity program. You may copy and used the PAR-Q, but only if you use the entire questionnaire. The revised version is in *ACSM's Guidelines for Exercise Testing and Prescription, 5th Edition* (ACSM 1995). Adults who wish to start a physical activity program should also be evaluated for signs and symptoms of coronary artery disease (see "Major Symptoms or Signs Suggestive of Cardiopulmonary Disease Risk Factors" and "Positive Coronary Artery Disease Risk Factors").

The American College of Sports Medicine has suggested that individuals be stratified into one of **three risk categories**, based on the individuals' potential risks for participation in a physical activity program:

1. **Apparently healthy**—individuals with no disease symptoms and no more than one major coronary artery disease risk factor (see "Positive Coronary Artery Disease Risk Factors")
2. **At increased risk**—individuals who have signs or symptoms suggestive of serious disease, or two or more major risk factors for coronary artery disease
3. **With known disease**—individuals with known serious medical problems (ACSM 1995)

You can make initial medical decisions after you have stratified an individual into one of the three categories. When you have a medical concern regarding an individual's risk, medically monitored exercise test-

Major Symptoms or Signs Suggestive of Cardiopulmonary Disease

1. Pain or discomfort in the chest, neck, jaw, arms, or other areas that may be ischemic in nature

2. Shortness of breath at rest or with mild exertion

3. Dizziness or syncope

4. Orthopnea or paroxysmal nocturnal dyspnea

5. Ankle edema

6. Palpitations or tachycardia

7. Intermittent claudication

8. Heart murmur

9. Unusual fatigue or shortness of breath with activities

Adapted, by permission, from American College of Sports Medicine, 1995, *ACSM's guidelines for exercise testing and prescription*, 5th ed. (Baltimore: Williams & Wilkins).

Positive Coronary Artery Disease Risk Factors

1. **Age.** Men: 45 years; women: 55 years or premature menopause without estrogen supplementation

2. **Family history.** Myocardial infarction or sudden death before 55 years in father or other first-degree male relative; or before 65 years of age in mother or other first-degree female relative

3. **Current cigarette smoker.**

4. **Hypertension.** Blood pressure > 140/90 mm Hg, confirmed by measurements on at least two separate occasions or on antihypertensive medication

5. **Hypercholesterolemia.** Total serum cholesterol > 200 mg/dl or HDL < 35 mg/dl

6. **Diabetes mellitus.** Persons with insulin-dependent diabetes mellitus (IDDM) who are 30 years of age or have had IDDM for > 15 years; persons with non-IDDM who are > 35 years of age

7. **Sedentary lifestyle.** Persons comprising the least physically active 25% of the population

Adapted, by permission, from American College of Sports Medicine, 1995, *ACSM's guidelines for exercise testing and prescription*, 5th ed. (Baltimore: Williams & Wilkins).

ing and other medical assessments can determine whether the individual can safely exercise.

For individuals with heart disease, the **American Heart Association** has developed a **special classification system** (Fletcher et al. 1990) that divides patients into one of five classes, from Class A (apparently healthy) to Class E (unstable cardiac disease with activity restrictions) (see "The American Heart Association (AHA) Risk Stratification Criteria," pages 108-109).

Once you have classified an individual's risk category, ACSM guidelines can help determine when diagnostic medical evaluation(s) and/or exercise test(s) are appropriate, and when a physician should be present for such exercise testing (see ACSM 1995, and figure 7.1).

Rationale for Exercise Testing

The following are the major reasons for both cardiopulmonary and neuromuscular exercise testing.

Class A: **Apparently healthy**

- Individuals < 40 years of age without symptoms or known presence of heart disease, no major risk factors, and normal exercise test.

  Supervision or monitoring required: none

Class B: **Documented, stable cardiovascular disease with low risk of cardiac events during vigorous exercise, but slightly greater than for apparently healthy individuals**

- CAD (including myocardial infarction, CABG, PTCA, angina pectoris, abnormal exercise test, and abnormal coronary angiograms) whose condition is stable and who have all of the following clinical characteristics:

  1. NYHA Class I or II
  2. Exercise capacity 5-6 METS
  3. No evidence of heart failure
  4. Free of ischemia or angina at rest or on the exercise test at or below 6 METS
  5. Appropriate rise in systolic blood pressure during exercise
  6. No sequential premature ventricular contractions
  7. Ability to self-monitor exercise intensity

- Valvular heart disease

- Congenital heart disease

- Cardiomyopathy

- Exercise test abnormalities that do not meet the criteria outlined in Class C or D below

  Supervision or monitoring required: medical supervision and ECG and blood pressure monitoring only during prescribed sessions; nonmedical supervision of other exercise sessions if the patient can self-monitor activity

Class C: **Documented, stable cardiovascular disease with low risk for vigorous exercise but unable to self-regulate activity or to understand recommended activity levels**

- Includes individuals with the disease states and clinical characteristics outlined above in Class B but without the ability to self-regulate activity

  Supervision or monitoring required: medical supervision and ECG and blood pressure monitoring only during prescribed sessions; nonmedical supervision of other exercise sessions to help regulate activity

Class D: **Those at moderate to high risk for cardiac complications during exercise**

CAD with:

  1. Two or more previous MIs
  2. NYHA Class III or greater

(continued)

    3. Exercise capacity < 6 METS, ischemic horizontal or down sloping ST depression ≥ 4.0 mm, or angina during exercise

    4. Fall in systolic blood pressure with exercise

    5. A medical problem that the physician believes may be life-threatening

    6. Previous episode of primary cardiac arrest

    7. Ventricular tachycardia at a workload < 6 METS

- Cardiomyopathy

- Valvular heart disease

- Exercise test abnormalities not directly related to ischemia

- Previous episode of ventricular fibrillation or cardiac arrest that did not occur in the presence of an acute ischemic event or cardiac procedure

- Patients with complex ventricular arrhythmias that are uncontrolled at mild to moderate work intensities with medication

- Individuals with 3-vessel of left main disease

- Individuals with low ejection fractions (< 30%)

    Supervision or monitoring required: Continuous ECG monitoring during rehabilitation sessions until safety is established, usually 6 to 12 sessions or more; medical supervision during all rehabilitation sessions until safety is established

Class E: **Unstable disease with activity restriction**

- Unstable angina

- Heart failure that is not compensated

- Uncontrolled arrhythmias

- Severe and symptomatic aortic stenosis

- Other conditions that could be aggravated by exercise

    No activity is recommended for conditioning purposes.

    Attention should be directed to treating the patient and restoring him or her to Class D or higher. Daily activities must be prescribed based on individual assessment by the patient's personal physician.

Adapted, by permission, from G.A. Fletcher et al., 1990, "AHA medical scientific statement. Exercise standards: a statement for health professionals from the American Heart Association," *Circulation* 82:2286.

Cardiopulmonary Exercise Testing

Most reasons for evaluating a patient's cardiorespiratory condition are related to heart disease, but such evaluation may be appropriate for anyone planning to participate in a physical activity program. There are five **general indications for clinical cardiopulmonary exercise testing** (ACSM 1995; Moldover and Bartels 1996):

1. Predischarge status after an acute cardiac event

2. Postdischarge status after a cardiac event

3. Medical diagnosis

4. Disease severity and prognosis

5. Patient's functional status

Determination of Predischarge Status After an Acute Cardiac Event

Cardiorespiratory exercise testing after an acute cardiac event (e.g., **acute myocardial infarction, percutaneous**

ACSM Recommendations for Medical Examination and Exercise Testing Prior to Participation in a Physical Activity Program

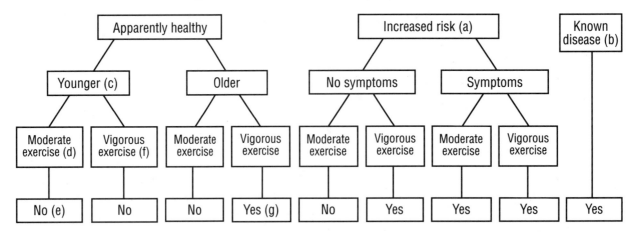

ACSM Recommendations for Physician Supervision of Exercise Tests

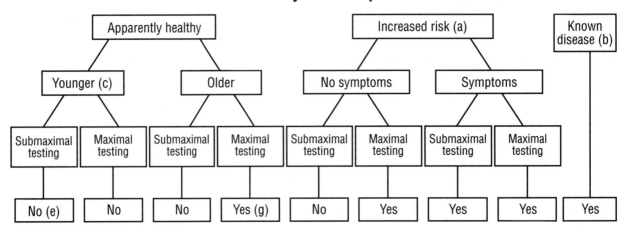

(a) Persons with two or more risk factors or one or more signs or symptoms (see page 107).

(b) Persons with known cardiac, pulmonary, or metabolic disease.

(c) Younger implies ≤ 40 years for men, ≤ 50 years for women.

(d) Moderate exercise as defined by intensity of 40% to 60% $\dot{V}O_2$max; if intensity is uncertain, moderate exercise may alternately be defined as an intensity well within the individual's current capacity; one that can be comfortably sustained for a prolonged period of time (60 minutes); that has a gradual initiation and progression; and that is generally noncompetitive.

(e) A "No" response means that an item is deemed "not necessary." The "No" response does not mean that the item should not be done.

(f) Vigorous exercise is defined by an exercise intensity > 60% $\dot{V}O_2$max; if intensity is uncertain, vigorous exercise may alternately be defined as exercise that represents a substantial cardiorespiratory challenge, or that results in fatigue within 20 minutes.

(g) A "Yes" response means that an item is recommended. For physician supervision, this suggests that a physician is in close proximity and readily available should there be an emergent need.

Figure 7.1
Source: American College of Sports Medicine 1995.

transluminal coronary angioplasty, or **coronary artery bypass graft surgery**) is based upon the patient's specific clinical situation. Some patients have undergone exercise testing—usually submaximal—as soon as three days after an uncomplicated acute myocardial infarction (Topol et al. 1988). Although used primarily to verify that the patient is stable and that the activity level does not cause cardiac ischemia or dysrhythmia, the testing can also help confirm that the patient's medications are adequately controlling the medical condition, and document the intensity of activity that the patient can safely perform during the recuperative phase (ACSM 1995; Moldover and Bartels 1996).

Determination of Postdischarge Status After a Cardiac Event

Patients usually perform postdischarge tests when it is believed they are ready to return to normal activities. This exercise test can help determine both the intensity of activity the patient can safely perform, and the response of the patient to medication (ACSM 1995; Moldover and Bartels 1996). Depending on the patient's medical condition, you can perform this test three or more weeks after the acute event (ACSM 1995).

Determination of Medical Diagnosis

Sometimes a patient's history, physical examination, and other medical evaluations do not lead to a clear medical diagnosis. When there is a concern about the possibility of cardiac ischemia, dysrhythmia, or other adverse problem related to physical activity, a standard exercise tolerance test—with monitoring of the **electrocardiogram** (ECG), blood pressure, and patient's subjective clinical status—is the best initial diagnostic test (ACSM 1995).

Determination of Disease Severity and Prognosis

Exercise testing for disease severity and prognosis is used primarily in patients with coronary artery disease. The **size of the ischemic myocardium** is *directly* proportional to the level of ST segment depression, the number of ECG electrodes that show ST segment depression, and the duration of ST segment depression after an exercise test. It is *inversely* proportional to the slope of the ST segment; the product of heart rate × systolic blood pressure (double product) at which the ST segment depression occurs; and the maximal heart rate, systolic blood pressure, and maximal exercise intensity attained (ACSM 1995).

The patient's **prognosis** depends on the magnitude of ischemia and the presence or absence of dysrhythmia. The greater the extent of ischemia and the greater the cardiac dysrhythmia, the worse the prognosis.

Determination of Functional Status

Either submaximal or maximal exercise testing can determine a patient's functional status. **Submaximal exercise testing** can help determine a safe level of exertion for a patient's physical activity program. It can also help estimate maximal exercise capacity and maximal aerobic power, by performance of several levels of submaximal exertion and use of a nomogram (Åstrand and Rodahl 1986; Morris et al. 1993). Submaximal exercise can help evaluate patients' responses to their physical activity programs. Comparison of heart rate at submaximal levels of exercise before and after an exercise program can provide an indirect assessment of improvement in cardiorespiratory fitness. **Maximal exercise testing** can determine safety for participation in rigorous physical activity programs, and can help estimate an individual's maximal aerobic power when you are unable to directly measure oxygen utilization during the test. As in the submaximal test, nomograms can provide estimates of maximal aerobic power (Åstrand and Rodahl 1986; Morris et al. 1993).

Measurement of respiratory variables permits determination of **oxygen utilization** and **carbon dioxide production**, thereby allowing for the direct measure of an individual's **peak oxygen utilization** (aerobic power) and determination of the ventilatory threshold. **Ventilatory threshold** is the point in an individual's ventilation when there is a nonlinear increase in expired carbon dioxide as compared to oxygen utilization; it can be used to estimate the maximal intensity at which an individual can be expected to exercise for prolonged periods of time without accumulating excessive amounts of lactic acid. Exercise at an intensity above the individual's ventilatory threshold will lead to lactic acidosis and fatigue. You can also use ventilatory threshold and peak oxygen utilization to determine an individual's cardiorespiratory functional impairment (see table 7.1) (Weber et al. 1987). Comparison of these variables before and after a physical activity program can determine the individual's level of cardiorespiratory fitness improvement.

Neuromuscular Exercise Testing

The ability to perform activities of daily living depends upon neuromuscular function. In order to stand up out of a chair, for example, people need sufficient

Table 7.1		Functional Classification of Patients Based on Gas Exchange Criteria	
Severity of impairment	**Functional class**	**Peak $\dot{V}O_2$ (ml/kg/min)**	**Ventilatory threshold (L/min)**
None to mild	A	>20	>14
Mild to moderate	B	16-20	11-14
Moderate to severe	C	10-15	8-10
Severe	D	<10	<8

Adapted, by permission, from K.T. Weber, J.S. Janicki, and P.A. McElroy, 1987, "Determination of aerobic capacity and the severity of chronic cardiac and circulatory failure," *Circulation* (Suppl. VI) 76: 40-46.

strength in the lower limbs and trunk to lift themselves up. To continue with activities, they need muscular endurance. Specific measures of muscular strength and endurance can help clinicians assess patients' abilities to function in general and design therapeutic exercise programs to improve their patients' capacities to function. Such measures are also useful in assessing the efficacy of a therapeutic exercise program.

Muscle strength can be defined in a number of ways. With the use of free weights, one can determine the one repetition maximum and ten repetition maximum. The **one repetition maximum** (or **1 RM**) is the maximum amount of weight a person can lift only one time using proper lifting technique. The **ten repetition maximum** (or **10 RM**) is the maximum weight he or she can lift ten times (but not more) successfully, using proper lifting technique. Special equipment can also measure muscle strength statically, or isokinetically, by measuring the force or torque generated by the muscular activity.

Although strength and endurance are separate neuromuscular factors, they are interrelated. **Muscle strength** may be defined as the maximum force generated by a muscle; **endurance** as "the ability to continue a prescribed task in the desired manner" (de Lateur 1996); **absolute endurance** as "the time that a subject can sustain a given workload, or the number of seconds a given force can be held, or the number of repetitions of a given load" (de Lateur 1996); and **relative endurance** as the time that a subject can sustain an activity at a certain percentage of maximal force, or the number of seconds a force can be maintained at a certain percentage of maximal force, or the number of repetitions that can be performed at a certain percentage of maximal force. Figure 7.2 shows the relationship between intensity of activity and endurance (defined in figure 7.2A as the total number of muscular contractions, and in figure 7.2B as time

in minutes of successful cycling). Both figures 7.2A and 7.2B are examples of absolute endurance, with the absolute units (those that define the assigned workload) recorded on the abscissa. Both the total number of muscular contractions (figure 7.2A) and endurance time (figure 7.2B) decrease as the intensity of effort increases. In figure 7.2A, the total number of muscular contractions that can be successfully repeated is inversely related to the force of contraction—i.e., the greater the force of muscular contraction, the fewer the number of successful muscular contractions. In figure 7.2B, the endurance time on a cycle ergometer is inversely related to the power of cycling—i.e., the greater the power at which the individual cycles, the shorter the endurance time. In figure 7.3, the abscissa reflects relative static force (i.e., the assigned workload is a certain percentage of the individual's maximal static force) from 20% of maximal force to 100% of maximal force. This figure, an example of relative endurance, shows that endurance time (the time that the subject can successfully statically contract the muscle at the assigned relative level of force) is inversely related to the relative workload. When the subject contracts the muscle at 20% of maximal force, the endurance time is approximately 10 minutes, while at 100% of maximal force, the endurance time is well under 1 minute.

In fact, the endurance time of a 100% maximal muscle contraction has been shown to be very short indeed: the time that an individual can hold a maximal static muscle contraction is less than one second (see figure 7.4) (Mundale 1970).

The laboratory data in figure 7.3 suggest that muscle strengthening exercise should result in improved endurance in the performance of daily activities—for improvements in strength appear to increase endurance time. Suppose that an individual, prior to an exercise program, performs an activity at an exertion level equal to 40% of her maximal

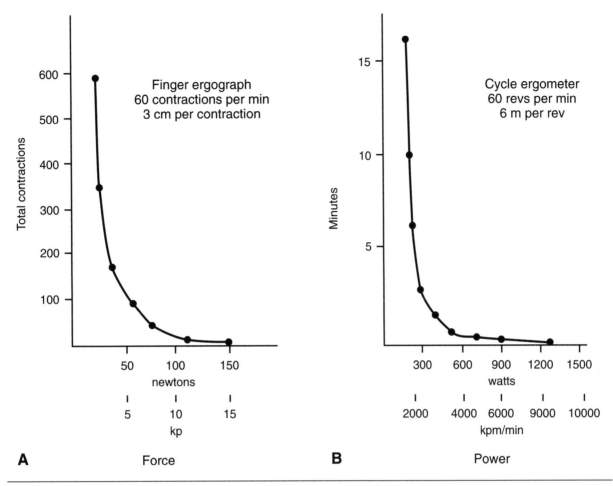

Figure 7.2   (A) Relationship of endurance (as total contractions) of repeated flexion of third digit to effective force of contraction. (B) Relationship of endurance (as minute to fatigue) of cycle ergometer exercise to external power production. In both A and B, the intercept with the abscissa represents the exercise intensity for which the maneuver could be performed only once (and, therefore, the strength of the concentric movement). In both graphs, endurance could be presented as either total contractions or minutes to fatigue, and, as the contraction rate and velocity are designated, either abscissa could be designated as force (per individual repetition) or power (work per unit time).

Reprinted, by permission, from H. Knuttgen, 1976, Development of muscular strength and endurance. In *Neuromuscular mechanisms for therapeutic and conditioning exercises*, edited by H. Knuttgen (Baltimore: University Park Press), 97.

strength. Figure 7.3 shows that the expected endurance time for this activity would be approximately 2 minutes. If this individual doubles her strength through an intensive exercise program, that previous activity would then be performed at only 20% of her maximal strength. Figure 7.3 now shows that the endurance time would now be expected to be approximately 10 minutes.

The data in figure 7.3 may also show why stronger individuals have less difficulty performing certain activities than weaker individuals. In general, the endurance of the stronger individual should be greater than that of the weaker individual when both are performing the same activity (such as a job requiring repeated lifting of 50-pound boxes), because the stronger individual would be working at a lower relative level of effort than the weaker individual.

This example has important ramifications for patients with physical disabilities. Many individuals with physical disabilities (e.g., those with postpolio syndrome) are weaker than nondisabled individuals, and therefore they may have less endurance than nondisabled individuals in performing daily activities.

Protocols for Exercise Testing, With Examples

The following section presents common protocols for both cardiopulmonary and neuromuscular exercise testing, followed by some examples.

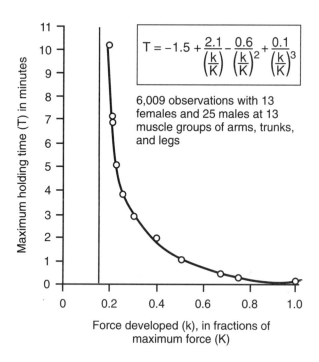

$$T = -1.5 + \frac{2.1}{\left(\frac{k}{K}\right)} - \frac{0.6}{\left(\frac{k}{K}\right)^2} + \frac{0.1}{\left(\frac{k}{K}\right)^3}$$

6,009 observations with 13 females and 25 males at 13 muscle groups of arms, trunks, and legs

Figure 7.3 Endurance and intensity of work. Static work: tension at fractions of maximum strength.

Reprinted, by permission, from E. Simonson, 1971, *Recovery and fatigue*, (Springfield, IL: Charles C Thomas), 440.

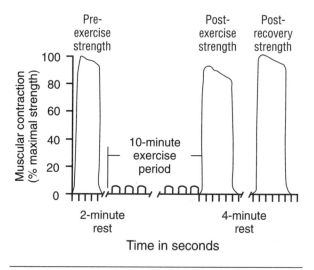

Figure 7.4 Maximal tension can be maintained during a voluntary maximal contraction of hand grip for less than 1 second before evidence of fatigue appears as the available supply of ATP is exhausted. Fatigue (unavailability of ATP) increases in proportion to the intensity of the activity but can be demonstrated following 10 minutes of intermittent contractions at 5% of maximal.

Reprinted, by permission, from M.O. Mundale, 1970, "The relationship of intermittent isometric exercise to fatigue of hand grip," *Arch Phys Med Rehabil* 51:532-539.

Cardiopulmonary Testing Protocols

The best way to test the cardiopulmonary system is with dynamic (such as treadmill or bicycle ergometry), rather than static, exercise. Dynamic exercise permits accurate control of the workload and places a *volume* load on the heart; static exercise is much more difficult to control, and it places a *pressor* load on the heart (ACSM 1995). Treadmill and bicycle ergometry are the most common methods for testing the cardiopulmonary system. Although maximal heart rate is similar in both types of testing (ACSM 1995), peak oxygen uptake is approximately 10%-15% higher with treadmill ergometry (Myers et al. 1991).

Measure heart rate and blood pressure prior to, during, and after all cardiopulmonary exercise tests; and monitor the ECG during the test and during the cooldown period until it returns to baseline values (ACSM 1995). Before the exercise test, take blood pressure and a 12-lead ECG both in the supine position and in the position in which the test will be performed. During the exercise test, continuously monitor the ECG. Record blood pressure and a 12-lead ECG during the last minute of every exercise stage (ACSM 1995). Finally, record blood pressure and a 12-lead ECG immediately after completion of the exercise and every one to two minutes thereafter, for a minimum of five minutes. If you observe changes on the ECG, continue to monitor it until it returns to the baseline level. Similarly, monitor blood pressure till it also stabilizes near the baseline level.

It is possible to evaluate an individual's subjective response to exercise by assessing the **rating of perceived exertion (RPE)** at the end of each stage (Borg 1973). The RPE is a 15-point scale with gradations beginning at 6 (level of exertion less than "very, very light") and progressing to 20 (level of exertion greater than "very, very hard"). This scale can also be of assistance in designing an individual's exercise program. The level of effort usually recommended for an aerobic program is approximately 13 (a level of exertion defined by the individual as "somewhat hard") (ACSM 1995).

In order to determine oxygen utilization, carbon dioxide production, ventilatory threshold, and **respiratory exchange ratio** (the ratio of expired carbon dioxide to oxygen used) during an exercise test, you must measure expired gases—ideally during the last minute of each exercise stage (ACSM 1995). These variables can help evaluate an individual's level of fitness. You can also use them to assess the effectiveness of an exercise program by comparing measurements made before and following the program.

Treadmill Ergometry

Treadmill exercise is the most common ergometric test performed in the United States (Moldover and Bartels 1996), and a number of different protocols have been published. Figure 7.5 shows the most commonly used protocols and the predicted oxygen utilization ($\dot{V}O_2$) for each stage. The Bruce protocol is the most commonly used, but has the disadvantage of using exercise stages that are large and unequal as the stages progress. These increments may overestimate the individual's exercise capacity (ACSM 1995). Protocols that use large increments between exercise stages (such as the Bruce protocol) are probably best suited for younger and/or more active individuals; those with smaller increments (such as the Balke-Ware) are better for testing older or more deconditioned individuals, patients with cardiovascular or respiratory disease, or individuals with physical disabilities (ACSM 1995). Another test of cardiorespiratory status is the individualized ramp protocol, in which the workload increases at a constant and continuous rate throughout the exercise test (Myers et al. 1992).

There are no published treadmill exercise protocols specifically for individuals with physical disabilities. Modifications to the above-mentioned protocols may permit testing some populations of physically disabled but ambulatory people. For some individuals with physical disabilities, discontinuous exercise testing may be necessary, with rest breaks between the exercise stages. In any case, the test protocol should be individualized, with the treadmill speed and/or inclination based on the individual's physical capabilities. Choose workload increments so that the total exercise time is between 8 and 12 minutes (ACSM 1995; Buchfuhrer et al. 1983).

Bicycle Ergometry

Bicycle ergometry is the most common alternative to treadmill exercise testing in the United States and is the most common ergometric test performed in Europe (Moldover and Bartels 1996). Figure 7.5 shows the most commonly used protocols and the predicted oxygen utilization ($\dot{V}O_2$) for each stage of bicycle ergometric testing. The initial workload is 150 kiloponds (25 watts) for healthy individuals, with increments of 150 kiloponds (25 watts) for each new stage. In deconditioned, elderly, or physically disabled individuals, the initial workload may be reduced to 60 to 90 kiloponds (10 to 15 watts), with even smaller increments for each new exercise stage. Choose workload increments so that the total exercise time is between 8 and 12 minutes (ACSM 1995).

Upper Limb Ergometry

Upper limb ergometry can be performed either with a modified bicycle ergometer or with a device specifically designed for upper limb testing. The main advantage is its suitability for patients with impairment of the lower limbs (Moldover and Bartels 1996). Since upper limb ergometry uses a smaller muscle mass than bicycle ergometry, use lower initial workloads and smaller increments than with bicycle ergometry—but still set the workload increments so that total exercise time is between 8 and 12 minutes. Upper limb ergometry has been used to assess paraplegic individuals (Lin et al. 1993), post-polio individuals (Kriz et al. 1992), and men with lower limb disabilities (spinal cord injury or lower limb fracture) (Langbein and Maki 1995).

Wheelchair Ergometry

Wheelchair ergometry is uncommon—the necessary equipment is not readily available commercially, and is often custom-made. Publications concerning wheelchair ergometry are all very individualized, depending upon the equipment available to the experimenters (Bhambhani et al. 1993; Eriksson et al. 1988; Janssen et al. 1993; Kerk et al. 1995; Pare et al. 1993; Vanlandewijck et al. 1994). The primary advantage of wheelchair ergometry is its most obvious one—it can assess cardiopulmonary fitness in those whose primary means of locomotion is the wheelchair. As in other protocols, set the initial workload as well as incremental increases according to the individual's capabilities, and prescribe increments in the workload so that total exercise time is between 8 and 12 minutes.

Other Ergometry

Other devices are occasionally used to assess the cardiopulmonary system, including rowing machine ergometers, simulated cross-country skiing ergometers,

Functional class	Clinical status	O_2 Cost ml/kg/min	METS	Bicycle ergometer (1 watt = 6 KP; For 70 kg body weight KP)	Treadmill protocols: BRUCE 3-min stages mph	BRUCE %grade	Kattus mph	Kattus %grade
Normal and I	Healthy, dependent on age, activity				5.5	20		
Normal and I	Healthy, dependent on age, activity	56.0	16		5.0	18		
Normal and I	Healthy, dependent on age, activity	52.5	15				4	22
Normal and I	Healthy, dependent on age, activity	49.0	14	1500	4.2	16		
Normal and I	Healthy, dependent on age, activity	45.5	13				4	18
Normal and I	Healthy, dependent on age, activity	42.0	12	1350			4	14
Normal and I	Healthy, dependent on age, activity	38.5	11	1200				
Normal and I	Sedentary healthy	35.0	10	1050	3.4	14	4	10
Normal and I	Sedentary healthy	31.5	9	900				
Normal and I	Sedentary healthy; Limited	28.0	8	750				
Normal and I	Sedentary healthy; Limited	24.5	7		2.5	12	3	10
II	Sedentary healthy; Limited; Symptomatic	21.0	6	600				
II	Sedentary healthy; Limited; Symptomatic	17.5	5	450	1.7	10	2	10
III	Sedentary healthy; Limited; Symptomatic	14.0	4	300				
III	Limited; Symptomatic	10.5	3		1.7	5		
III	Limited; Symptomatic	7.0	2	150	1.7	0		
IV	Symptomatic	3.5	1					

(continued)

Figure 7.5 Common bicycle and treadmill exercise testing protocols.
Reprinted, by permission, from American College of Sports Medicine, 1995, *Guidelines for exercise testing and prescription,* 5th ed. (Baltimore: Williams & Wilkins), 92-3.

and elliptical cross-training ergometers (a hybrid between treadmill and bicycle ergometers). The **simulated cross-country skiing ergometer,** which simulates the motion of diagonal stride cross-country skiing, has separate devices for the poling and kicking motions associated with cross-country skiing. The **elliptical cross-training ergometer,** with pedals that revolve in an elliptical motion, demands movements that are somewhat of a combination between walking and bicycling. The resistance for all of these ergometers can be varied in different ways from low to high. All test protocols using these ergometers must be custom-designed for each individual. As always, select workload increments so that the total exercise time is between 8 and 12 minutes.

Examples of Cardiopulmonary Testing in Physically Disabled Individuals

Below are a few examples of cardiopulmonary assessment in disabled patients. They are not exhaustive, but should help guide your thinking as you evaluate and care for such patients.

Treadmill protocols											
Balke-Ware	Ellestad		USAFSAM		"Slow" USAFSAM		McHenry		Stanford		METS
% grade at 3.3 mph 1-min stages	3/2/3–min stages mph	%grade	mph	%grade	mph	%grade	mph	%grade	% grade at 3mph	% grade at 2mph	
26											
25	6	15									
24											16
23			3.3	25							
22	5	15									15
21											14
20			3.3	20			3.3	21			
19											13
18							3.3	18	22.5		
17	5	10									12
16			3.3	15			3.3	15	20.0		11
15					2	25			17.5		
14											10
13									15.0		
12	4	10			2	20					9
11			3.3	10			3.3	12	12.5		8
10					2	15			10.0	17.5	
9	3	10					3.3	9			7
8			3.3	5	2	10			7.5	14.0	6
7							3.3	6			
6	1.7	10			2	5			5.0	10.5	5
5			3.3	0							
4									2.5	7.0	4
3							2.0	3	0	3.5	3
2											
1			2.0	0	2	0					2
											1

Figure 7.5   *(continued)*

Example 1: Treadmill Exercise Testing

A 56-year-old male is admitted to the hospital with acute right hemiparesis due to an ischemic left hemispheral cerebral infarction. The patient smoked one pack of cigarettes per day for the past 40 years, but stopped smoking two years previously; his history includes hypercholesterolemia, hypertension, one myocardial infarction four years ago, and coronary artery bypass graft surgery two years ago. Prior to his recent stroke, he complained occasionally of chest pain with exertion, which resolved with rest. You see the patient two days after admission to evaluate him for possible admission into the acute stroke rehabili-

tation program. Because the stroke has impaired the patient's walking ability, his maximal velocity is just under two miles per hour.

Given this man's cardiac status and significant past medical history, you are concerned about the safety of his participation in the stroke rehabilitation program. In consultation with the patient's cardiologist, you order a treadmill exercise test to determine (1) his pressor response to exercise, (2) if he has any dangerous arrhythmia associated with exercise, and (3) whether there is evidence of myocardial ischemia during activity.

You choose a modified Bruce protocol for the treadmill test. As the activities in the stroke rehabilitation

Stage	Blood Pressure	Heart Rate	ECG Response	RPE
1.7 mph, 0 degrees	120/82	110	Normal rhythm	15
1.7 mph, 5 degrees	140/78	130	Normal rhythm	19
1.7 mph, 10 degrees	Unable due to fatigue			

Table 7.2   Treadmill Exercise Testing Results

program will not exceed 3-4 METs (i.e., an intensity of exercise equal to 3-4 times the energy expenditure at rest), the exercise stages for this exercise test are 1.7 miles per hour at a treadmill incline of zero, five, and ten degrees, providing a maximum level of 5 METs. Blood pressure, heart rate, and ECG are obtained at rest, in supine and standing positions. The pressor response in both supine and standing positions show that the patient's blood pressure is well controlled with antihypertensive medication. The ECG shows no acute abnormalities at rest. The exercise test begins at 1.7 miles per hour at a zero percent grade. Table 7.2 summarizes the results of the exercise test including blood pressure, heart rate, ECG response, and rating of perceived exertion (RPE).

The ECG shows no dysrhythmia or ischemic change during the test and cooldown. The maximal heart rate achieved in the test is low at 130 beats per minute (quite high for the 4 MET level of exertion, but consistent with severe deconditioning). The pressure response is normal during and after the test. The patient does not complain of anginal symptoms during the testing or recovery phase, and is able to complete the second stage of the test (at the 4 MET level—the maximal exertion he would need to attain in the stroke rehabilitation program). These results indicate that the patient can safely participate in the acute stroke rehabilitation program. The RPE demonstrated, however, that he is very deconditioned.

Example 2:
Bicycle Ergometer Exercise Testing

The typical post-polio patient is very deconditioned from the cardiovascular standpoint. Owen and Jones (1985) found that the average maximal level of exertion in post-polio individuals was 5-6 METs—comparable to a patient shortly after an acute myocardial infarction. Until a few years ago there were no published guidelines for aerobic exercise programs for post-polio patients. Clinicians feared that the exercise might increase overuse weakness rather than

aerobic fitness. When Jones et al. (1989) tested this hypothesis, they found it to be without merit; their data form the basis for aerobic exercise programs for many post-polio patients.

A 55-year-old post-polio woman sees you for advice about exercise. She had acute polio at the age of five and has been sedentary for many years. However, she now wants to start an aerobic exercise program. Your initial assessment reveals no cardiovascular disease risk factors other than her age and sedentary life style (see "Positive Coronary Artery Disease Risk Factors," page 107). Her neurological examination shows weakness in both lower limbs, but her strength is antigravity or stronger in all muscle groups tested in her hips and thighs. She walks with an ankle foot orthosis on the right because of paresis of the ankle dorsiflexor muscles. You prescribe a cardiovascular exercise test to determine whether she can safely start an exercise program, and, if so, to determine the initial exercise intensity. The resting heart rate, blood pressure, and ECG in the supine and sitting positions are normal. Table 7.3 summarizes results of a bicycle ergometer exercise test (three-minute stages, with rest breaks between the stages).

The patient's blood pressure response to the exercise is normal. The ECG shows no evidence of ST segment depression or dysrhythmia. It appears safe for her to start an exercise program. Her maximal capacity, however, is very low—only 50 watts (or 300 kiloponds or approximately 4 METs; see figure 7.5). Using the exercise program described by Jones and colleagues (1989) above, she starts a bicycle ergometric exercise program. Initially, she exercises for two minutes with one-minute rest breaks, for a total exercise time of 10 minutes. As she progresses, the duration of each bout of exercise gradually increases until she is able to perform six five-minute bouts of exercise, with one-minute rest breaks between bouts (for a total exercise time of 30 minutes). After four months of exercise, a maximal exercise test measures her maximal capacity at 70 watts (or 420 kiloponds or approximately 5 METs). She has no adverse response to the exercise program and finds that she has less

Table 7.3		Bicycle Ergometer Exercise Testing Results		
Stage	**Blood Pressure**	**Heart Rate**	**ECG Response**	**RPE**
10 watts	110/70	92	Normal	11
20 watts	122/66	106	Normal	12
30 watts	132/64	122	Normal	16
40 watts	144/60	144	Normal	19
50 watts	152/56	156	Normal	20
60 watts	Unable due to fatigue			

fatigue during her daily activities. She also reports increased strength in her hip and thigh muscles; and she notes less difficulty in climbing stairs, improved endurance while walking, and less difficulty getting into and out of the bathtub.

Example 3:
Upper Limb Ergometer Exercise Testing

You are evaluating a 42-year-old insulin-dependent diabetic with a history of coronary artery disease, hypertension, and a recent below-knee amputation due to peripheral vascular disease. You question the safety of the patient's participation in rehabilitation—especially because of the exertion required for prosthetic training.

You need an appropriate exercise test. For obvious reasons, a treadmill test is ruled out; and the patient would find it difficult to use a bicycle ergometer with only one lower limb. Upper limb ergometry is the exercise test of choice—not only is

it convenient, but when the patient begins to use the preparatory prosthesis, the upper limbs will bear much of the stress.

Prior to testing, you measure resting blood pressure, heart rate, and ECG in both the supine and sitting positions. The results show no abnormalities. As the patient is very deconditioned, the exercise test begins at 10 watts, with 10-watt increases every three minutes. Table 7.4 summarizes the results.

Although the ECG shows 2 millimeters of ST segment depression, indicative of myocardial ischemia, at the 40-watt stage, the patient denies angina. At the third stage, however, with the heart rate at 124 and the RPE at 14 ("moderately hard"—Borg 1973), the ECG shows neither ST segment depression nor dysrhythmia.

These findings suggest that the patient can safely exercise up to a heart rate of approximately 120 beats per minute and a rating of perceived exertion of "moderately hard." The silent ischemia noted during higher levels of the exercise test, however, is worrisome. For safety reasons, you have the patient wear a heart

Table 7.4		Upper Limb Ergometer Exercise Testing Results		
Stage	**Blood Pressure**	**Heart Rate**	**ECG Response**	**RPE**
10 watts	132/94	98	Normal	11
20 watts	142/90	110	Normal	13
30 watts	150/84	124	Normal	14
40 watts	168/72	146	2mm ST segment depression	

monitor during therapy, and have the therapist keep the activity level at a heart rate of 120 beats per minute or less. A Holter monitor, worn during the first 24 hours after the start of therapy, reveals no ECG abnormalities (ST segment depression or dysrhythmia). The monitor also confirms that the patient is able to keep the heart rate at the desired and safe level. With these precautions, the patient safely and successfully completes the rehabilitation program.

Example 4:
Wheelchair Ergometer Exercise Testing

A 44-year-old construction worker falls two floors, sustains a fracture of T12, and becomes paraplegic. After completion of the acute rehabilitation program, he wants to join a wheelchair basketball team. The patient smokes cigarettes and has hypercholesterolemia, and his father had an acute myocardial infarction at age 52. To determine the safety of his participation in *any* regular exercise, you recommend a wheelchair ergometry test. Table 7.5 shows the results of the exercise test.

The test concludes at the completion of the 100-watt stage due to fatigue. The ECG reveals neither dysrhythmia nor ST segment abnormality. The exercise test is normal. You tell your patient that there is no contraindication for participation in the wheelchair basketball program, and encourage him to join the team after starting a wheelchair aerobic exercise program. The initial exercise is 50 watts, with an exercise heart rate of 120 (74% of his maximal heart rate) and a rating of perceived exertion of 14. You also strongly encourage him to stop smoking!

Neuromuscular Testing Protocols

Assessment of neuromuscular function can be divided into the evaluation of muscle strength and, in special circumstances, the evaluation of muscle endurance. Although muscular strength is commonly assessed, muscular endurance is rarely assessed—primarily only in research studies. The most common way to assess muscle strength in the clinical setting is with **manual muscle testing** (McPeak 1996). Manual muscle testing, however, is quite subjective and sometimes is not sufficiently accurate to be clinically useful. Clinicians instead need an objective, quantitative assessment of muscular strength that will enable them to assess the effectiveness of a patient's therapeutic program.

All normal activities entail static, concentric, or eccentric muscle contractions. A **static contraction** occurs when there is no movement of the joint(s) that the muscle crosses, but the contraction stabilizes the joint. A **dynamic contraction** occurs with movement of the joint(s) that the muscles crosses. If the muscle shortens during this dynamic contraction, the contraction is **concentric**. If the muscle lengthens during contraction, the contraction is **eccentric**. Muscles may also contract **isokinetically** using special isokinetic testing equipment—the limb is attached to an arm on the isokinetic dynamometer, which can be set at any predetermined angular velocity (such as 60 degrees per second) to assess the strength of the muscle at that specific angular velocity. Unlike static and dynamic muscular contractions, isokinetic contraction is not performed during normal daily activities.

In all assessments of muscular strength, in order to prevent injury as well as to enhance reliability of the measurements, you should provide clear instructions concerning the evaluation procedure. Have your patient practice with the device before the test, both to warm up and to be certain that she fully understands how to perform the test and that the testing procedure will not cause pain. Pain during the warm-up procedure usually indicates that the individual is not performing the effort correctly and needs further instruction. Stabilization of the patient's body is also important—not only for safety reasons (to minimize

Table 7.5	Wheelchair Ergometer Exercise Testing Results			
Stage	**Blood Pressure**	**Heart Rate**	**ECG Response**	**RPE**
25 watts	112/84	92	Normal	12
50 watts	120/78	120	Normal	14
75 watts	134/72	142	Normal	17
100 watts	142/66	166	Normal	20

the risk of injury), but also to prevent her from using substitution patterns that would result in erroneous measurements of her strength.

There are no universally accepted protocols for evaluating muscle strength. Below are some suggested guidelines. In all methods, take care to avoid injury during testing. With reasonable care, injury can be very rare; and when it does occur, it will be a minor strain.

Assessing Static Strength

Static muscle strength is usually assessed with special dynamometers (e.g., the Cybex, Kin-Com, or Biodex dynamometers for static assessment), cable tensiometry (Clarke 1952; Clarke 1973; Clarke and Clarke 1984; Andres et al. 1986), or loadcell dynamometry (Mundale 1970), which can measure either the force or the **torque** (force times the length of the lever arm) generated during muscular contraction. After properly positioning your patient on the dynamometer and setting the joint at the desired angle, be careful to instruct her in the test procedure. In assessments of static strength, the joint which the muscle crosses should not move during the muscular contraction. At first, have your subject practice with the dynamometer, performing several submaximal muscular contractions; then gradually build up to one or two maximal contractions. After she rests for a short time, she should perform three or four maximal effort contractions of the muscle (usually for three to five seconds each) with timed rest intervals between efforts.

The rest periods you prescribe depend upon whom you are evaluating. In disabled individuals, we have found one-minute rest breaks between maximal effort trials to be reasonable. The maximal force or torque generated during these efforts is defined as the **static strength** of the muscle.

Assessing Dynamic Isotonic Strength

The term *isotonic* is actually a misnomer. **Isotonic** means "equal tension," but its use in strength testing means that the individual is lifting a specific amount of weight. The most common ways to define isotonic strength are

- the determination of the amount of weight that the individual can lift only once through full range of motion with proper mechanics (the one repetition maximum, or 1 RM); or
- the amount of weight the subject can successfully lift ten times, but not more, through full

range of motion with proper mechanics (the ten repetition maximum, or 10 RM).

These determinations require spotting or the use of special frames (such as a weight frame) to protect the individual in case the weight slips or in case he cannot successfully lift the weight. As with all strength testing, always provide proper instruction, warm-up, and stabilization for safety, validity, and reliability.

Assessing Dynamic Isokinetic Strength

Special equipment such as the Cybex, Kin-Com, or Biodex dynamometers can assess isokinetic muscle strength. The manufacturers provide specific suggestions for the use of each device. These machines are rather sophisticated and are quite expensive. All isokinetic dynamometers are now computer-controlled, and allow the operator to set the maximum angular velocity at which the arm of the dynamometer moves as well as the range of motion to be tested. These devices also have mechanisms that continuously measure the torque that the individual is exerting as well as the range of motion through which he is being tested. For the dynamometer to measure maximal torque, have your patient try to move the dynamometer arm as fast and forcefully as possible throughout the range of motion you're testing. Because the dynamometer arm has a braking mechanism, and will move only as fast as the angular velocity you set, it will appear to your patient that the dynamometer is resisting his effort. By moving his arm as fast and forcefully as possible, your patient will generate maximal torque at the predetermined angular velocity. The dynamometer measures and stores in the computer the torque generated throughout the range of motion that was tested.

Ordinarily, straps will stabilize your subject on the dynamometer's chair or bench (figure 7.6). Place the fulcrum of the lever arm in the plane of the center of rotation of the joint you're testing. Pass the arm of the dynamometer through the full range of motion to be tested (this allows the dynamometer's computer to measure the weight of the limb throughout the range of motion to be tested). Set the angular velocity for the test (in most cases, between 60 and 300 degrees per second). Instruct your subject in the testing procedure. Have him warm up by moving the arm of the dynamometer gently, gradually increasing the force till he performs one or two full efforts. He should rest for a specified period of time, usually one minute. During the test, he extends and flexes the joint through a full range of motion, with maximal muscular effort, for a specified number of

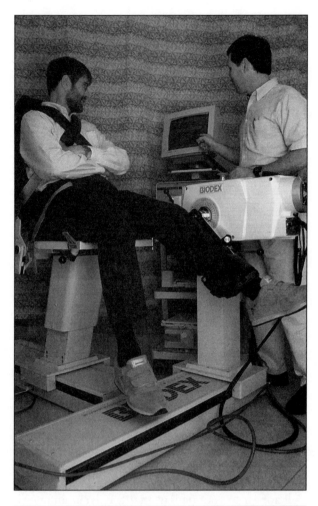

Figure 7.6 A patient on an isokinetic dynamometer during the assessment of isokinetic quadriceps femoris strength.
Photograph by Ms. Linda Bayer, Director of Public Relations, Howard Young Health Center, Woodruff, WI 54568.

contractions—often between three and six maximal efforts. Identify the maximal torque generated by the muscle during the test as the strength of the muscle at the specific angular velocity tested. In some situations, especially in clinical research, you might choose to test the muscle at several angular velocities.

Assessment of Endurance

Although often tested for research purposes, endurance is rarely assessed in the clinical setting. One can assess endurance statically, dynamically, or isokinetically.

Static Endurance

You can assess either absolute or relative static endurance. **Absolute endurance** is defined in terms of a specified workload, while **relative endurance** is defined in terms of a specific percentage of the individual's maximal capacity (see page 112).

Consider the maximum time during which an individual can statically contract a muscle at a certain specified level of effort. If that level of effort is set at 100 Newton-meters, then absolute endurance for that person is the time during which she can contract the muscle statically at 100 Newton-meters of torque. If the level of effort is defined as 40% of maximum static torque (or any other specific percentage between 0 and 100% of maximal effort), then the subject's relative endurance is determined as the time during which she can contract the muscle statically at that specific relative level of torque.

Dynamic Endurance

As with static endurance, you can assess either absolute or relative dynamic endurance. To assess **absolute dynamic endurance,** you would have the individual lift a certain amount of weight with a specific technique (such as knee extension using a table specifically designed to assess knee extension) through full range of motion at a specific cadence (such as one complete lifting motion every two seconds), until he is no longer able to successfully lift the weight. You would define the number of successful repetitions as the absolute dynamic endurance for lifting that specific amount of weight. To assess **relative dynamic endurance,** first determine the subject's 1 RM for the test to be performed. Then have him lift a certain percentage of the 1 RM through full range of motion at a specific cadence until he is no longer able to successfully lift the weight. The number of successful repetitions would be the relative endurance for the specific relative amount of weight lifted.

Isokinetic Endurance

Although they do not measure absolute or relative endurance, several useful endurance tests employ isokinetic dynamometers (Davies 1987).

- **The 50% decrement test.** The individual performs maximal effort muscle contractions at a specific angular velocity until the peak torque fails to reach 50% of the initial peak torque for a predetermined number of repetitions (usually 2-5 consecutive reps). The number of repetitions successfully performed is used as a measure of endurance.

- **The predetermined time bout endurance test.** The individual performs as many maximal repetitions as possible at a predetermined angular velocity for a predetermined period of time. Measure endurance either as the total number of repetitions performed or as the total work performed by the muscle during the activity (as calculated by the device's computer).

- **The predetermined repetitions bout endurance test** (Davies 1987). The individual performs a predetermined number of repetitions at a predetermined angular velocity. The dynamometer's computer tallies the total amount of work performed by the muscle during the contractions; use the total work performed as a measure of endurance.

- **The 50-repetition decrement test.** The individual performs 50 consecutive maximal effort isokinetic contractions at a predetermined angular velocity. Compare the average torque generated during the last three contractions with that of the first three contractions; use the percent decrement as a measure of endurance.

Examples of Neuromuscular Testing in Physically Disabled Individuals

Below are a few examples of neuromuscular assessments in patients with physical disabilities. Such assessments usually aim either to guide the care of patients or to assess the effectiveness of a therapeutic exercise program.

Example 1:
Evaluating the Effect of Strength Training on Strength, Endurance, and Work Capacity in Post-Polio Individuals

Many post-polio individuals complain of fatigue and pain (Halstead and Rossi 1985, 1987). Some are quite weak, with reduced work capacity and a deficit in strength recovery after activity (Agre and Rodriquez 1990). Reduced endurance is also a common problem (Berlly et al. 1991). Several researchers have shown that strengthening exercise can improve muscle strength in post-polio individuals (Agre et al. 1996; Einarsson and Grimby 1987; Feldman and Soskolne 1987; Fillyaw et al. 1991); but until recently, no one had tested whether the improved strength would increase the work capacity or absolute endurance time of muscle.

To investigate this question, we first assessed static strength of the quadriceps muscles of seven post-polio subjects, with the knee positioned 60 degrees from full extension. After permitting the subjects to rest for five minutes after the assessment, we gave them static endurance tests at 40% of maximal strength to the point of failure, recording the endurance time in seconds. (We verbally encouraged the subjects to perform this activity as long as possible.) We calculated the static tension time index (or "work capacity") as the product of the endurance time in seconds and the torque (40% of maximal strength) (Agre et al. 1997).

Following a 12-week home exercise program, we reassessed the subjects in the laboratory for strength, endurance, and work capacity, using the same absolute torque as was performed initially (i.e., not 40% of the new strength, but 40% of the previous strength). Table 7.6 gives pre- and postexercise program data.

The exercise program clearly led to significant increases in muscle strength, absolute endurance time, and work capacity—confirming that muscle-strengthening exercise can not only increase strength in post-polio individuals, but also increase work capacity and absolute endurance of the muscle. These findings may have important implications for individuals with weakness due to other neuromuscular diseases or disorders.

Table 7.6	Neuromuscular Variables Before and After the Exercise Program (mean ± SD)		
Variable	**Before**	**After**	**Percent change**
Strength (N · m)	98 ± 63	134 ± 65	+36%
Endurance (holding time in seconds)	142 ± 46	172 ± 50	+21%
Work capacity (N · m · sec)	6090 ± 2280	7200 ± 2240	+18%

Example 2:
Evaluating the Effect of Strength Training in an Elderly Man With Degenerative Joint Disease of the Knee

A 70-year-old man is referred to the rehabilitation clinic by his orthopedic surgeon for assessment. He has a history of severe left knee pain due to arthritis. The surgeon is contemplating total knee arthroplasty, but refers the patient to you because the patient wants to try a nonsurgical approach before considering surgery. You find that the patient has severe weakness and atrophy of the left thigh musculature, the strength being barely above antigravity. He keeps the left knee fully extended while he walks (to keep from falling due to the weakness). You believe that a strengthening exercise program might be very beneficial (as will be the use of a cane to decompress the knee). Frontera and colleagues (1988) reported that, in men aged 60 to 72, strength training significantly increased muscle strength as well as hypertrophy of the exercised muscles. You have your patient follow the same exercise program.

In the Frontera study, participants exercised three days per week for twelve weeks, performing three sets of exercise of the knee extensor and flexor muscles, with eight repetitions in each set. They used weights that were 80% of their 1 repetition maximum (1 RM). The 1 RM was measured each week. By the end of the exercise program, the 1 RM increased by over 100% in the knee extensor muscles and 200% in the knee flexors. Dynamic isokinetic assessment showed increases in the knee extensor and flexor strength of 10% and 18%, respectively. Muscle biopsies obtained before and after the program revealed increases in muscle fiber area of the vastus lateralis of over 25%.

After following the above described exercise program for three months, the patient is much stronger (with strength increases similar to those found in the research study, as measured with a dynamometer just as in the research study). He also reports that the knee pain has significantly improved: he has minimal difficulty and almost no pain with ambulation, and his gait pattern on physical examination is much improved (because of increased strength as well as use of the cane).

Example 3:
Assessing the Effect of a Work Hardening Program on the Functional Lifting Capabilities of an Injured Worker

A 40-year-old heavy manual laborer injured his lower back while lifting a 100-pound box—his third back injury within the past year that has resulted in time off from work. He has undergone several evaluations by other clinicians, but with no specific findings. Radiographs show some evidence of degenerative joint disease and degenerative disc disease. The MRI shows disc bulging at L4-L5 and L5-S1. Analgesics, muscle relaxants, rest, hot packs, and massage did not resolve the problem after six weeks. The patient came to you, a specialist in physical medicine and rehabilitation, for further assessment.

The patient's neurological examination is normal. Through manual muscle testing you observe weak trunk and lower limb musculature, which you believe to be secondary to deconditioning from the past six weeks of inactivity in addition to the inactivity associated with his previous injuries and their treatment. You order physical therapy, and have the patient start an active therapeutic exercise program including strength training. After two weeks, the physical therapist reports that the patient has made improvement in strength, but is not yet ready to return to his usual work activity. You prescribe a work hardening program, at the completion of which you order a functional capacity evaluation. The physical capacity evaluation assesses a number of factors, including the patient's 1 RM lifting strength to lift from floor to waist height, waist to shoulder height, and shoulder height to overhead. The physical therapist notes that the patient puts forth good effort during this assessment, and believes that the functional capacity accurately reflects the patient's capabilities for work. You advise the patient about his specific capacities for lifting so that he can return to gainful employment and perform his lifting tasks within these guidelines. With this specific information, based upon the functional capacity assessment, the patient successfully returns to work without recurrent injury.

Summary

Physical activity is a crucial component of healthy lifestyles. Before beginning exercise programs, subjects should be screened for relevant health factors in order to

- optimize the results from an exercise program,
- allow for the development of a sensible and effective exercise prescription, and
- determine safety of participation in an exercise program or exercise testing. There are five general indications for clinical cardiopulmonary testing:

1. The predischarge status after an acute cardiac event
2. The postdischarge status after a cardiac event
3. The medical diagnosis
4. The disease severity and prognosis
5. The patient's functional status

There are three general indications for neuromuscular testing:

1. It helps assess an individual's abilities to function.
2. It aids in the design of a patient's therapeutic exercise program.
3. It can be used to assess the effectiveness of the therapeutic exercise program.

Athough there are several ways to assess cardiopulmonary and neuromuscular function, there is no specific set of tests for individuals with physical disabilities. You must simply choose those tests that will be most useful in your patient's particular clinical situation. This chapter has provided several examples that demonstrated how this testing can be helpful in caring for patients with physical disabilities.

References

American College of Sports Medicine. 1995. *ACSM's guidelines for exercise testing and prescription.* 5th ed. Baltimore: Williams & Wilkins.

Agre, J.C., and A.A. Rodriquez. 1990. Neuromuscular function: comparison of symptomatic and asymptomatic polio subjects to control subjects. *Arch Phys Med Rehabil* 71:545-551.

Agre, J.C., A.A. Rodriquez, and T.M. Franke. 1997. Muscle strengthening exercise can increase strength, endurance, and work capacity in post-polio subjects. *Arch Phys Med Rehabil* 78:681-686.

Agre, J.C., A.A. Rodriquez, T.M. Franke, E.R. Swiggum, R.L. Harmon, and J.L. Curt. 1996. Low-intensity, alternate-day exercise improves muscle performance without apparent adverse affect in post-polio patients. *Am J Phys Med Rehabil* 75:50-58.

Andres, P.L., W. Hedlund, L. Finison, T. Conlon, M. Felmus, and T.L. Munsat. 1986. Quantitative motor assessment in amyotrophic lateral sclerosis. *Neurology* 36:937-941.

Åstrand, P.-O., and K. Rodahl. 1986. *Textbook of work physiology: Physiological bases of exercise.* 3d ed. New York: McGraw-Hill.

Berlly, M.H., W.W. Strauser, and K.M. Hall. 1991. Fatigue in postpolio syndrome. *Arch Phys Med Rehabil* 72:115-118.

Bhambhani, Y.N., L.J. Holland, and R.D. Steadward. 1993. Anaerobic threshold in wheelchair athletes with cerebral palsy: validity and reliability. *Arch Phys Med Rehabil* 74:305-311.

Borg, G.A.V. 1973. Perceived exertions: a note on 'history' and methods. *Med Sci Sports Exercise* 5:90-93.

Buchfuhrer, M.J., J.E. Hansen, T.E. Robinson, D.Y. Sue, K. Wasserman, and B.J. Whipp. 1983. Optimizing the exercise protocol for cardiopulmonary assessment. *J Appl Physiol* 55:1558-1564.

Buschbacher, R.M., and R.L. Braddom, eds. 1994. *Sports medicine and rehabilitation: A sport-specific approach.* Philadelphia: Hanley & Belfus.

Clarke, D.H. 1973. Adaptations in strength and muscular endurance resulting from exercise. In *Exercise and sports science reviews.* Vol. 1, ed. J.H. Wilmore. New York: Academic Press.

Clarke, D.H., and H.H. Clarke. 1984. *Research processes in physical education, recreation, and health.* Englewood Cliffs, NJ: Prentice-Hall.

Clarke, H.H. 1952. New objective strength tests of muscle groups by cable tension methods. *Res Quart* 23:136.

Davies, G.J. 1987. *A compendium of isokinetics in clinical usage and rehabilitation techniques.* 3d ed. Onalaska, WI: S&S Publishers.

de Lateur, B.J. 1996. Therapeutic exercise. In *Physical medicine and rehabilitation*, ed. R.L. Braddom, R.M. Buschbacher, D. Dumitru, E.W. Johnson, D. Matthews, and M. Sinaki, 401-419. Philadelphia: W.B. Saunders.

Einarsson, G., and G. Grimby. 1987. Strengthening exercise program in post-polio subjects. In *Research and clinical aspects of the late effects of poliomyelitis*, ed. L.S. Halstead and D.O. Wiechers, 275-283. White Plains, NY: March of Dimes Birth Defects Foundation.

Eriksson, P., L. Lofstrom, and B. Ekblom. 1988. Aerobic power during maximal exercise in untrained and well-trained persons with quadriplegia and paraplegia. *Scand J Rehabil Med* 20:141-147.

Feldman, R.M. and C.L. Soskolne. 1987. The use of non-fatiguing strengthening exercises in post-polio syndrome. In *Research and clinical aspects of the late effects of poliomyelitis*, ed. L.S. Halstead and D.O. Wiechers, 335-341. White Plains, NY: March of Dimes Birth Defects Foundation.

Fillyaw, M.J., G.J. Badger, G.D. Goodwin, W.G. Bradley, T.J. Fries, and A. Shukla. 1991. The effects of long-term non-fatiguing resistance exercise in subjects with post-polio syndrome. *Orthopedics* 14:1253-1256.

Fletcher, G.A., V.F. Froelicher, L.H. Hartley, W.L. Haskell, and M.L. Pollock. 1990. AHA medical scientific statement. Exercise standards: a statement for health professionals from the American Heart Association. *Circulation* 82:2286-2322.

Frontera, W.R., C.N. Meredith, K.P. O'Reilly, H.G. Knuttgen, and W.J. Evans. 1988. Strength conditioning in older men: skeletal muscle hypertrophy and improved function. *J Appl Physiol* 64:1038-1044.

Hahn, R.A., S.M. Teutsch, R.S. Paffenbarger, and J.S. Marks. 1990. Excess deaths from nine chronic diseases in the United States, 1986. *JAMA* 264:2654-2659.

Halstead, L.S., and C.D. Rossi. 1985. New problems in old polio patients: results of a survey of 539 polio survivors. *Orthopedics* 8:845-850.

Halstead, L.S., and C.D. Rossi. 1987. Post-polio syndrome: clinical experience of 132 consecutive outpatients. In *Research and clinical aspects of the late effects of poliomyelitis,* ed. L.S. Halstead and D.O. Wiechers, 13-26. White Plains, NY: March of Dimes Birth Defects Foundation.

Janssen, T.W., C.A. van Oers, A.P. Hollander, H.E. Veeger, and L.H. van der Woude. 1993. Isometric strength, sprint power, and aerobic power in individuals with a spinal cord injury. *Med Sci Sports Exerc* 25:863-870.

Jones, D.R., J. Speier, K. Canine, R. Owen, and A. Stull. 1989. Cardiorespiratory responses to aerobic training by patients with post-poliomyelitis sequelae. *JAMA* 261:3255-3258.

Kerk, J.K., P.S. Clifford, A.C. Snyder, T.E. Prieto, K.P. O'Hagan, P.K. Schot, J.B. Myklebust, and B.M. Myklebust. 1995. Effect of an abdominal binder during wheelchair exercise. *Med Sci Sports Exerc* 27:913-919.

Knuttgen, H.G. 1976. Development of muscular strength and endurance. In *Neuromuscular mechanisms for therapeutic and conditioning exercises,* ed. H.G. Knuttgen, 97-118. Baltimore: University Park Press.

Kottke, F.J. 1966. The effects of limitation of activity upon the human body. *JAMA* 196:825-830.

Kriz, J.L., J.L. Speier, J.K. Canine, R.R. Owen, and R.C. Serfass. 1992. Cardiorespiratory responses to upper extremity aerobic training in postpolio subjects. *Arch Phys Med Rehabil* 73:49-54.

Langbein, W.E., and K.C. Maki. 1995. Predicting oxygen uptake during counterclockwise arm crank ergometry in men with lower limb disabilities. *Arch Phys Med Rehabil* 76:642-646.

Leon, A.S., and H. Blackburn. 1977. The relationship of physical activity to coronary artery disease and life expectancy. *Ann NY Acad Sci* 301:561-578.

Lin, K.H., J.S. Lai, M.J. Kao, and I.N. Lien. 1993. Anaerobic threshold and maximal oxygen consumption during arm cranking exercise in paraplegia. *Arch Phys Med Rehabil* 74:515-520.

McArdle, W.D., F.I. Katch, and V.L. Katch. 1991. *Exercise physiology energy, nutrition, and human performance.* 3d ed. Philadelphia: Lea & Febiger.

McPeak, L.A. 1996. Physiatric history and examination. In *Physical medicine and rehabilitation,* ed. R.L. Braddom, R.M. Buschbacher, D. Dumitru, E.W. Johnson, D. Matthews, and M. Sinaki, pp. 3-42. Philadelphia: W.B. Saunders.

Milner-Brown, H.S., R.B. Stein, and R.G. Lee. 1975. Synchronization of human motor units: possible role of exercise and supraspinal reflexes. *EEG Clin Neurophysiol* 38:245-254.

Moldover, J.R., and M.N. Bartels. 1996. Cardiac rehabilitation. In *Physical medicine and rehabilitation,* ed. R.L. Braddom, R.M. Buschbacher, D. Dumitru, E.W. Johnson, D. Matthews, and M. Sinaki, 649-670. Philadelphia: W.B. Saunders.

Moritani, T., and H.A. de Vries. 1979. Neural factors versus hypertrophy in the tie course of muscle strength gain. *Am J Phys Med* 58:115-130.

Morris, C.K., J.N. Myers, V.F. Froelicher, T. Kawaguchi, K. Ueshima, and A. Hideg. 1993. Nomogram based on metabolic equivalents and age for assessing aerobic exercise capacity in men. *J Am Coll Cardiol* 22:175-182.

Mundale, M.O. 1970. The relationship of intermittent isometric exercise to fatigue of handgrip. *Arch Phys Med Rehabil* 51:532-539.

Myers, J., N. Buchanan, D. Smith, J. Neutel, E. Bowes, D. Walsh, and V.F. Froelicher. 1992. Individualized ramp treadmill: Observations on a new protocol. *Chest* 101:2305-2315.

Myers, J., N. Buchanan, D. Walsh, M. Kraemer, P. McAuley, M. Hamilton-Wessler, and V.F. Froelicher. 1991. Comparison of the ramp versus standard exercise protocols. *J Am Coll Cardiol* 17:1334-1342.

Owen, R.R., and D. Jones. 1985. Polio residuals clinic: conditioning exercise program. *Orthopedics* 8:882-883.

Paffenbarger, R.S., and R.T. Hyde. 1984. Exercise in the prevention of coronary heart disease. *Prev Med* 13:3-22.

Pare, G., L. Noreau, and C. Simard. 1993. Prediction of maximal aerobic power from a submaximal exercise test performed by paraplegics on a wheelchair ergometer. *Paraplegia* 31:584-592.

Prentice, W.E. 1994. The healing process and the pathophysiology of musculoskeletal injury. In *Rehabilitation techniques in sports medicine.* 2d ed., ed. W.E. Prentice, 1-26. St. Louis: Mosby.

Serfass, R.C., and S.G. Gerberich. 1984. Exercise for optimal health: strategies and motivational considerations. *Prev Med* 13:79-99.

Simonson, E. 1971. *Recovery and fatigue,* 440-458. Springfield, IL: Charles C Thomas.

Siscovick, D.S., N.S. Weiss, R.H. Fletcher, and T. Lasky. 1984. The incidence of primary cardiac arrest during vigorous exercise. *N Engl J Med* 311:874-877.

Taylor, H.L., A. Henschel,, J. Brozek, and A. Keys. 1949. Effects of bed rest on cardiovascular function and work performance. *J Appl Physiol* 2:223-239.

Thomas, S., J. Reading, and R.J. Shephard. 1992. Revision of the Physical Activity Readiness Questionnaire (PAR-Q). *Can J Sport Sci* 17:338-345.

Thompson, P.D., E.J. Funk, R.A. Carleton, and W.Q. Sturner. 1982. The incidence of death during jogging in Rhode Island from 1975 through 1980. *JAMA* 247:2535-2538.

Topol, E.J., K. Burek, W.W. O'Neill, D.G. Kewman, N.H. Kander, M.J. Shea, M.A. Schork, J. Kirscht, J.E. Juni, and B. Pitt. 1988. A randomized controlled trial of hospital discharge three days after myocardial infarction in the era of reperfusion. *N Engl J Med* 318:1083-1088.

Vanlandewijck, Y.C., A.J. Spaepen, and R.J. Lysens. 1994. Wheelchair propulsion efficiency: movement pattern adaptations to speed changes. *Med Sci Sports Exerc* 26:1373-1381.

Weber, K.T., J.S. Janicki, and P.A. McElroy. 1987. Determination of aerobic capacity and the severity of chronic cardiac and circulatory failure. *Circulation* (Suppl. VI) 76:40-46.

Chapter 8

The Quantity and Quality of Physical Activity for Health and Fitness

A Behavioral Approach to Exercise Prescription

Gregory W. Heath, DHSc, MPH

Regular physical activity increases physical working capacity, decreases body fat, increases lean body tissue and bone density, and lowers rates of coronary heart diasese (CHD), diabetes mellitus, hypertension, and cancer (Lee et al. 1991; Paffenbarger et al. 1978; Sidney et al. 1977; Smith et al. 1976; Tipton 1991; USDHHS 1996). It is also associated with greater longevity. Regular physical activity and exercise can also enhance quality of life, improve capacity for work and recreation, and alter the rate of decline in functional status (Shephard 1993).

Both health and fitness should result from exercise prescriptions, where **health** is defined as physical and emotional well-being (not merely the absence of disease), and **physical fitness** is "something that people possess or achieve such as aerobic power, muscular endurance, muscular strength, body composition, and flexibility" (Caspersen et al. 1985; USDHHS 1991). Exercise rehabilitation programs must take account of physiologic, anatomic, and behavioral factors to insure a safe, effective, and enjoyable exercise experience for the participant.

Preliminary Factors Important for Exercise Prescription

We can discuss physical activity in terms of health benefits and fitness benefits—not a true dichotomy of benefits, but a useful approach for outlining the outcome-specific nature of the exercise prescription and for providing the rationale for individualized approaches to physical activity recommendations.

Health Benefits of Physical Activity

Physical activity has been defined as any bodily movement produced by skeletal muscles that results in caloric expenditure (Pate et al. 1995). Since caloric expenditure enhances weight loss or weight maintenance, physical activity is important in the prevention and management of obesity, CHD, and diabetes mellitus. The Healthy People 2000 Physical Activity and Fitness Objective 1.3 highlights the need for every person to engage in regular—preferably daily—physical activity (USDHHS 1991). Current research suggests that light to moderate physical activity for at least 30 minutes per day significantly raises the level of caloric expenditure and confers important health benefits. For example, physical activity equivalent to a sustained walk for 30 minutes per day uses about 1050 kcal per week. Epidemiologic studies suggest that a weekly expenditure of 1000 kcal could have significant individual and public health benefits for CHD prevention, especially among those who are currently inactive.

According to the American College of Sports Medicine (ACSM) and the Centers for Disease Control and Prevention (CDC), the scientific evidence clearly demonstrates that regular, moderate-intensity physical activity provides substantial health benefits (Pate et al. 1995). After an extensive review of the physiologic, epidemiologic, and clinical evidence, the expert panel formulated the following recommendation:

> Every U.S. adult should accumulate 30 minutes or more of moderate-intensity physical activity on most, preferably all, days of the week.

Because intermittent activity confers substantial benefits, people can accumulate the recommended 30 minutes of activity in shorter bouts of 8-10 minutes spaced throughout the day. This is not the optimal amount of physical activity for health, of course, but rather a minimum standard to which people can add in order to obtain even more beneficial effects. For someone undergoing comprehensive exercise rehabilitation, the additional effects might be improved cardiorespiratory fitness, muscle endurance, muscle strength, flexibility, and enhanced body composition.

Fitness Benefits of Physical Activity

Cardiorespiratory endurance, muscular strength, muscular endurance, flexibility, and body composition are the health-related components of physical fitness (Pate et al. 1995).

Health-Related Components of Physical Fitness

- Cardiorespiratory endurance
- Muscular strength
- Muscular endurance
- Flexibility
- Body composition

Regular vigorous physical activity helps achieve and maintain higher levels of cardiorespiratory fitness than light to moderate physical activity. As outlined in HP2000, **cardiorespiratory fitness** or **aerobic capacity** describes the body's ability to perform high-intensity activity for a prolonged period of time without undue physical stress or fatigue (Caspersen et al. 1985). Having higher levels of cardiorespiratory fitness helps people carry out their daily occupational tasks and leisure pursuits more easily and with greater efficiency. Vigorous physical activities that help to achieve and maintain cardiorespiratory fitness can also contribute substantially to caloric expenditure, and probably provide more protection against CHD than do less vigorous activities. Vigorous physical activities include very brisk walking, jogging/running, swimming laps, cycling, fast dancing, skating, jumping rope, and selective competitive sports (soccer, basketball, volleyball). Individuals can achieve higher levels of cardiorespiratory fitness by increasing the frequency, duration, or intensity of activities beyond the minimum recommendation of 20 minutes per occasion, three times per week, at ≥50% of aerobic capacity (ACSM 1990).

Muscular strength is the maximal amount of force generated by a muscle or muscle group, while **muscle endurance** is the ability of a muscle or muscle group to do prolonged exercise. Muscle strength and endurance are accepted components of health-related fitness (Braith et al. 1989). Strength and endurance greatly affect one's ability to perform the tasks of daily living without undue physical stress and fatigue. Regular use of skeletal muscles helps to improve and maintain strength and endurance. Engaging in regular physical activity, such as weight training or the regular lifting and carrying of heavy objects, appears to be a sufficient stimulus to maintain necessary muscle strength and endurance for most activities of daily living (Barry and Eathorne 1994).

Musculoskeletal flexibility describes the range of motion in a joint or sequence of joints. Those with greater flexibility may have a lower risk of future back injury (Cady et al. 1979). Older adults with better joint flexibility may be able to drive an automobile more safely than less flexible individuals (West Virginia University 1988). Joint movement through the full range of motion helps to improve and maintain flexibility. Stretching exercises can help to maintain a level of flexibility that supports quality activities of daily living—as can a variety of physical activities that require one to stoop, bend, crouch, and reach.

The maintenance of an acceptable ratio of fat to lean body weight is another desired component of health-related fitness. Overweight occurs when individuals expend fewer calories than they consume (Passmore 1971). Data from weight-loss programs focused on diet alone have not been encouraging. Since physical activity burns calories, increases the proportion of lean to fat body mass (lean tissue burns more calories per unit weight than fat tissue), and raises the metabolic rate, a combination of both caloric control and increased physical activity is important for attaining and maintaining a healthy body weight.

Determinants of and Barriers to Participation in Regular Physical Activity

When designing any exercise prescription, be sure to consider physiological, behavioral, and psychological variables related to participation in physical activity (Sallis and Hovell 1990). **Self-efficacy**—a construct from social cognitive theory characterized by a person's confidence to exercise under a number of circumstances—is positively associated with greater participation in physical activity, as is **social support** from family and friends. Incorporating some mechanism of social support within the exercise prescription appears to be an important strategy for enhancing compliance.

Significant barriers to participation in physical activity are injury and a lack of time. You can minimize these barriers by encouraging people to include physical activity as part of their lifestyle, integrating not only planned exercise but also transportation and occupational and household activity into their daily routines (e.g., always choose a parking space far from the door, and use stairs rather than elevators). Emphasizing low- to moderate-intensity physical activities—which are more likely to be continued than high-intensity activities and less likely to cause injury or undue discomfort—will increase the rate of patient adherence (Pollock 1988).

A number of physical and social environmental factors can affect physical activity behavior (Sallis et al. 1992). Family and friends can be role models, provide encouragement, or be companions during physical activity. The environment often presents significant barriers to participation in physical activity—e.g., a lack of bicycle and walking paths away from vehicular traffic, inclement weather, and or unsafe neighborhoods (Sallis et al. 1989). Excessive television viewing may also deter people from being physically active.

Barriers to Assessment and Counseling for Exercise

Because physicians, therapists, nurses, and clinical exercise scientists have unique access to persons undergoing rehabilitation, they have many opportunities for physical activity assessment and counseling (Harris et al. 1989). Physicians generally believe exercise is important, but indicate that they are not well prepared to provide counseling in that area (Wells et al. 1989). The primary barriers to routine assessment and counseling about exercise in rehabilitation settings are time, reimbursement, perceived effectiveness, and a lack of training in behavioral counseling techniques. A number of programs have attempted to improve the physical activity counseling skills among primary care physicians; results have been small but generally positive, with from 7%-10% of inactive patients starting to be physically active (Calfas et al. 1996; Logsdon et al. 1989). Recently, a number of professional organizations—including the American Heart Association, the American Academy of Pediatrics, and the President's Council on Physical Fitness and Sports—have recommended routine physical activity counseling for people of all ages (American Academy of Pediatrics 1994; American Heart Association 1992; President's Council on Physical Fitness and Sports 1993; U.S. Preventive Services Task Force 1996). Rehabilitation professionals historically have studied exercise therapy and reconditioning methods as part of their training. Yet they often have targeted this information only at specific conditions, with little regard for promoting overall health and for changing their clients' long-term daily behavior. Regardless of their reasons for a clinical visit, patients typically have not responded well to general exercise advice. Often they comply well during the acute rehabilitation phase of therapy; but following a period of "restoration" they begin to discontinue their exercises, and eventually fail to maintain the reconditioning effects of their rehabilitation. This pattern is consistently observed in a number of conditions, including orthopedic, cardiac, pulmonary, and stroke rehabilitation.

We must begin to emphasize behavioral-based assessment and counseling approaches, adapting them to the rehabilitation setting and to maintenance of rehabilitation outcomes. As rehabilitation professionals, we have access to patients in multiple settings: hospitals, clinics, nursing homes, athletic departments, community health sites, and rehabilitation centers. Because of this great opportunity, we must expand our roles as providers of preventive care through physical activity and exercise.

Risk Assessment

You can approach exercise prescription in at least three different ways:

1. A program-based level that consists primarily of supervised exercise training (King et al. 1991)
2. Exercise counseling and prescription followed by a self-monitored exercise program (Kriska et al. 1986)
3. Community-based exercise programming that is self-directed and self-monitored (Young et al. 1996)

Participants in any kind of exercise program should complete a brief medical history and risk factor questionnaire (see "Medical History and Clearance: Essential Elements") (Hassman et al. 1992).

A questionnaire provides important information regarding potential limitations and restrictions for activity programs. Always encourage clients to consult their personal physicians if they have any questions about their medical status.

After gathering an appropriate medical history, give potential participants a **preprogram evaluation**

Medical History and Clearance: Essential Elements

Medical history

- Cardiovascular disease
- Degenerative joint disease
- Hypertension
- Back syndrome
- Obstructive or restrictive lung disease
- Hypothyroidism
- Diabetes mellitus
- Dizziness
- Ataxia

Risk factors

- Family history of CAD
- Cigarette smoking
- Physical inactivity
- Obesity
- Hypertension (blood pressure > 140/190)
- Elevated blood lipids (cholesterol ≥ 240 mg/dl or low-density lipoprotein cholesterol ≥ 130 mg/dl)

Medications

- Beta blockers
- Calcium channel blockers
- Other antianginal medications
- Other antiarrhythmic medications
- Digitalis preparations
- Antihypertensives
- Nonsteroidal anti-inflammatory analgesics
- Bronchodilators
- Thyroid replacement
- Hypoglycemic

to document baseline measures of flexibility, cardiorespiratory endurance, and strength. These measures not only will help you prescribe an appropriate physical activity level, but will also encourage your clients by enabling them to measure their progress. To find more information on patient assessment, please see "Read More About It" (below), and refer again to chapter 7 of this book.

Evaluation measures need not be sophisticated. You can assess flexibility with sit-and-reach tests, both on the floor and in a chair (Shephard et al. 1990). Goniometers can help determine limitations in joint flexibility and mobility. Observations of gait and movement from a seated to standing position provide insight into sensory impairment, impaired equilibrium, or orthostatic hypotension. You can measure strength by simple tests of grip strength combined with modified push-ups and sit-ups. Field tests—such as a walking-speed test for 12 minutes or the chair-step test (ACSM 1991)—can assess cardiorespiratory endurance, as can submaximal bicycle testing with pulse palpation and blood pressure measurements. These cardiorespiratory tests are intended to be functional evaluations at submaximal levels. For appropriately screened individuals they are relatively safe and effective, while providing data for exercise prescription and physical activity education.

If potential participants have documented CHD, diabetes mellitus, or known risk factors for these diseases, recommend them for diagnostic exercise tolerance testing as well as functional assessment. Chapter 7 deals with such testing in detail. The testing and evaluation should be directed by a physician trained in diagnostic exercise testing. Typical exercise tolerance testing includes graded treadmill exercise testing with continuous electrocardiographic (ECG) monitoring and simultaneous measurement of heart rate and blood pressure. Exercise tolerance testing often involves a symptom-limited testing protocol that pro-

vides an estimation of $\dot{V}O_2$max. The modified Balke and modified Bruce protocols, in which the speed and grade are initially at less than 2.5 METs with gradual increases in workload of 1 to 2 METs every 2-3 minutes, are examples of appropriate testing protocols (ACSM 1998).

An alternative to treadmill testing is bicycle ergometry. The principles of ECG, heart-rate, and blood pressure monitoring are the same. The most common reason for employing the bike is medical contraindications for use of the treadmill, including the presence of osteoarthritis or an artificial limb, an unstable gait, or severe obesity. The major disadvantage of using the bike for symptom-limited testing is localized muscle fatigue in the legs that sometimes interferes with the participant's ability to achieve heart rates high enough to be of diagnostic value.

In community-based, self-directed programs, medical clearance is left to the judgment of the individual participant. Any campaign promoting physical activity should provide precautions and recommendations for moderate and vigorous physical activity (King et al. 1995). These messages should list steps for participants to follow *before* beginning a regular moderate-to-vigorous physical activity program, including

1. awareness of pre-existing medical problems (i.e., CHD, arthritis, osteoporosis, or diabetes mellitus),

2. consultation before starting a program, with a physician or other appropriate health professional if any of the above-mentioned problems are suspected,

3. appropriate modes of activity and tips on different types of activities,

4. principles of training intensity and general guidelines as to rating of perceived exertion (RPE) and training heart rate (THR),

5. progression of activity, and with principles of starting slowly and gradually increasing activity time and intensity,

6. principles of monitoring symptoms of excessive fatigue, and

7. making exercise fun and enjoyable.

Read More About It

Vivian Heyward's *Advanced Fitness Assessment & Exercise Prescription* 3rd ed. published by Human Kinetics, Champaign, Illinois 1998, is an excellent resource on patient assessment.

Promoting Physical Activity: A Guide for Community Action (DHHS/PHS/CDC, 1999) provides guidelines for working with community physical activity promotion advocates.

General Exercise Prescription Guidelines

Exercise prescriptions include five factors that warrant definition:

• **Mode of activity.** Most people who want to participate in regular exercise programming have no significant limitations. But some, especially older persons, have one or more chronic conditions that may necessitate changing the mode of physical activity. Degenerative joint disease, including osteoarthritis, is common among older people. The mode of exercise must accommodate these participants—usually by emphasizing minimal or nonweightbearing activities such as cycling, swimming, and chair and floor exercises. For participants with difficulty in joint mobility of the knees and hips, movement down and up from the floor may initially be contraindicated.

Generally, most people will be able to engage in moderate walking activities. Individualization of the mode of activity is important, including variation of activity as well as adjustments for participant bias and preference. Prescribe calisthenics cautiously for individuals suffering from degenerative joint changes, appropriately modifying the stretching and strengthening exercises. Table 8.1 lists guidelines for prescribing activities for selected chronic conditions.

• **Frequency.** The Surgeon General's most recent recommendations call for more frequent cardiorespiratory endurance and flexibility activities (five to seven days per week) than previous recommenda-

Table 8.1	Modification of the Exercise Prescription: Selected Conditions
Condition	**Recommended modification**
Degenerative joint disease	Nonweightbearing activities such as stationary cycling, water exercises, and chair exercises. Emphasis placed on interval activity. Low-resistance, low-repetition strength training.
Coronary artery disease (CAD)	Physician oversight. Symptom-limited activities. Moderate-level endurance activities preferred (i.e., walking, slow cycling), although at physician's discretion more vigorous activities can be prescribed. Low-resistance, higher-repetition strength training.
Diabetes mellitus	Daily, moderate-endurance activities. Low-resistance, higher-repetition strength training. Flexibility exercises. Monitoring of symptoms and caloric intake. In the presence of obesity, nonweightbearing exercises.
Dizziness, ataxia	Chair exercises may be preferred. Low-resistance, low-repetition strength training. Moderate flexibility activities with minimal movement from supine or prone to standing positions.
Back syndrome	Moderate-endurance activities (i.e., walking, cycling, chair exercises). Modified flexibility exercises. Low-resistance, low-repetition strength training. Modified abdominal strengthening activities. Water activities.
Osteoporosis	Weightbearing activities with intermittent bouts of activity spaced throughout the day. Low-resistance, low-repetition strength training. Chair-level flexibility activities.
Chronic obstructive lung disease	Moderate-level endurance using an interval or intermittent approach to exercise bouts. Low-resistance, low-repetition strength training. Modified flexibility and stretching exercises.
Orthostatic hypotension	Minimize movements from standing to supine and supine to standing. Sustained moderate-endurance activities with short rest intervals. Emphasize activities that minimize the changing of body positions.
Hypertension	Emphasize dynamic large muscle endurance activities; minimize isometric work and focus on low-resistance, low-repetition isotonic strength training.

tions. Greater frequency provides for greater flexibility and more ready maintenance of endurance capacity. It also enhances compliance and increases the probability that people will assimilate physical activity into their daily routines. Strength-related activities should be done at least twice a week.

• **Duration.** An appropriate goal for most adults is 20-40 minutes of endurance activity per session. However, because of physiologic and pathophysiologic limitations, shorter exercise sessions of 10-15 minutes repeated two or three times throughout the day may be necessary for some participants. If aging-related limitations require a decrease in intensity of activities, older adults can increase the duration of the activities—preferably approaching one hour—in order to derive optimal benefits.

• **Intensity.** Because of the common medical and physiologic limitations among individuals in rehabilitation settings, intensity of activity is of critical importance. For those with a history of CHD, or who are at high risk for CHD, base the exercise prescription on the results of a recent (within three months) ECG-monitored exercise evaluation. You can use the formula of Karvonen to calculate appropriate target heart rates and MET levels, adjusted for symptoms or ECG changes noted in the exercise test (see "Use of Karvonen's Formula for the Calculation of Training Heart Rate" p. 136) (Pollock 1988). "Young-old" (≤75 years) individuals usually can have peak work capacities of 7 METs or greater, whereas the "old-old" (>75 years) frequently have peak levels that do not exceed 4 METs. Unfortunately, the medical and physical activity statuses of participants can vary considerably, making it difficult to generalize workload prescriptions. After assessing an individual's work capacity, you can use MET levels to calculate appropriate exercise intensities. Ratings of perceived exertion (RPE) are quite helpful in regulating intensity. An RPE level of 12-15 (on a scale of 6-20) is adequate for most conditioning activities. When people are well oriented to this method, it becomes a very useful self-monitoring mechanism for regulating intensity of exercise.

• **Progression of activity.** A gradual approach to increasing activity levels is best. After beginning an exercise program, most people require from four to six weeks to progress from a low- to moderate-intensity conditioning level. Another four to six weeks is of-

ten necessary to achieve an appropriate maintenance level or to progress to a more vigorous conditioning level. Individual variability in fitness and adaptation to the exercise usually dictates the appropriate progression of activity. Once someone achieves a maintenance level of fitness, varying the regimen may enhance compliance. One way to achieve variety is to alter the duration component by interchanging continuous and intermittent activities. Above all, emphasize enjoyment and purpose of the activity sessions needed for maintenance.

Theories and Models Used in Physical Activity Promotion

Historically, health professionals have observed the following sequence in prescribing exercise: assessing the individual (usually with cardiorespiratory fitness measures); formulating the exercise prescription; and counseling the patient regarding exercise mode (usually large muscle activity), frequency (3-5 sessions per week), duration (20-30 minutes per session), and intensity (assigned target heart rate based on the exercise assessment) (ACSM 1991). Often the clinicians review the plans along with the patients, and then send the patients on their way. Some professionals schedule follow-up visits for reassessment and revision of the exercise prescription, while others follow up only via telephone. Most researchers who have evaluated this traditional approach to exercise prescription have noted poor long-term compliance, and therefore few long-term benefits (Dishman 1991).

Recent Theories and Models

Exercise scientists have developed a number of theories and models of human behavior for use in exercise counseling and interventions (USDHHS 1996) (table 8.2). The approaches of different models vary in their applicability to promoting physical activity: some are intended primarily as guides to understanding behavior, not designing counseling protocols; others were constructed specifically with a view toward developing intervention protocols.

The **health belief model** suggests that health-related behavior depends on a person's perception of four critical areas:

Use of Karvonen's Formula for the Calculation of Training Heart Rate

Mrs. Kim is a 45-year-old Korean American who comes to you for a physical activity prescription. She currently is not taking any medicines, has no history of cardiovascular disease, has no known cardiovascular risk factors, and reports being in good health. She is 5' 4" and weighs 135 pounds, with resting blood pressure of 116/82. She played intercollegiate soccer and has subsequently participated in adult senior soccer leagues. Approximately 12 weeks ago she injured her right knee during a soccer match. The injury was precipitated by a quick turn to the inside, pivoting off of the right foot, but with no physical contact with another player. She underwent an MRI evaluation and arthroscopic surgery to remove the distal horn of the lateral meniscus of the right knee. She returns today after six weeks of successful physical therapy, to begin a cardiorespiratory reconditioning program.

As measured using a treadmill, Mrs. Kim's $\dot{V}O_2$max is 2.8 L/min or 45 ml O_2/kg/min, with maximal heart rate of 179 beats/minute. Her seated resting heart rate was 74 beats/minute. You set her initial exercise prescription at an intensity of 0.6 to 0.8 of $\dot{V}O_2$max (see Pollock 1988 for Karvonen's formula).

Training heart rate = (Maximum heart rate − Resting heart rate)(0.6 to 0.8) + Resting heart rate

Training heart rate = (179 beats/min − 74 beats/min) (0.6 to 0.8) + 74 beats/min

Training heart rate = 105 beats/min (0.6 to 0.8) + 74 beats/min = 137-158 beats/min

1. The severity of a potential illness
2. The person's susceptibility to that illness
3. The benefits of taking a preventive action
4. The barriers to taking that action (Rosenstock 1990)

The model incorporates cues to action as important elements in eliciting or maintaining patterns of behavior, and includes the construct of self-efficacy, or a person's confidence in his/her ability to successfully perform an action—perhaps allowing the model to better account for habitual behaviors, such as physical activity.

The **relapse prevention model** can help new exercisers anticipate problems with adhering to their programs. Factors that contribute to relapse include negative emotional or physiologic states, limited coping skills, social pressures, interpersonal conflicts, limited social support, low motivation, high-risk situations, and stress. Principles of relapse prevention include identifying situations containing high risk for relapse (e.g., changes in season) and developing appropriate solutions (e.g., finding a place to walk inside during the winter). It is thought that if exercisers understand that a lapse is not as serious as a relapse—which comprises repeated lapses and requires a more specific strategy to overcome—their adherence will improve (Marlatt and George 1990).

The **theory of reasoned action** states that individual performance of a given behavior is primarily determined by a person's intention to perform that behavior. This intention is determined by two major factors: the person's attitude toward the behavior and the influence of the person's social environment or subjective norm (i.e., beliefs about what other people think the person should do, as well as the person's motivation to comply with the opinions of others) (Ajzen and Fishbein 1980). The **theory of planned behavior** adds to the theory of reasoned action the concept of perceived control over the opportunities, resources, and skills necessary to perform a behavior (Ajzen 1988). Ajzen's concept of **perceived behavioral control** is similar to Bandura's concept of self-efficacy—i.e., that perceived control over the opportunities, resources, and skills necessary to perform a behavior is critical to the process of changing the behavioral (Bandura 1977a).

Social learning theory, later renamed **social cognitive theory**, proposes that behavior change is affected by environmental influences, personal factors, and attributes of the behavior itself (Bandura 1977b; Bandura 1986). And each factor affects the other two. Self-efficacy is a central tenet of social cognitive theory. People must believe in their ability to perform the behavior, and must perceive an incentive to do so. Additionally, they must value the consequences that they believe will occur as a result of the behavior.

Table 8.2		Summary of Theories and Models Used in Physical Activity Promotion
Theory/model	**Level**	**Key concepts**
Health belief model	Individual	Perceived susceptibility Perceived severity Perceived benefits Perceived barriers Cues to action Self-efficacy
Relapse prevention	Individual	Skills training Cognitive reframing Lifestyle rebalancing
Social cognitive theory	Interpersonal	Reciprocal determinism Behavioral capability Self-efficacy Outcome expectations Observational learning Reinforcement
Theory of planned behavior	Interpersonal	Attitude toward behavior Outcome expectations Value of outcome expectations Subjective norm Beliefs of others Motive to comply with others Perceived behavioral control
Social support	Interpersonal	Instrumental support Informational support Emotional support Appraisal support
Ecological perspective	Environmental	Multiple levels of influence Intrapersonal Interpersonal Institutional Community Public policy
Transtheoretical model	Individual	Precontemplation Contemplation Preparation Action Maintenance

Source: U.S. Department of Health and Human Services 1995.

Benefits may be immediate (e.g., feeling energized following physical activity) or long-term (e.g., improving cardiovascular health as a result of physical activity). But because these expected outcomes are filtered through a person's expectations of being able to perform the behavior in the first place, self-efficacy is believed to be the single most important characteristic that determines a person's behavior change. To increase self-efficacy in a client, provide clear instructions, provide the opportunity for skill development or training, and see that someone models the desired behavior. To be effective, models must evoke trust, admiration, and respect from the observer; they must not, however, present a level of behavior that the observer is unable to visualize attaining for himself or herself.

Social support for physical activity can be instrumental, as in giving a nondriver a ride to an exercise class; informational, as in telling someone about a walking program in the neighborhood; emotional, as in calling to see how someone is faring with a new walking program; or appraising, as in providing feedback and reinforcement in learning a new skill. Sources of support for physical activity include family members, friends, neighbors, coworkers, and exercise program leaders and participants.

A criticism of most models of behavior change is that they emphasize individual processes and pay little attention to sociocultural and physical environmental influences on behavior (McLeroy et al. 1988). Recently, interest has developed in increasing participation in physical activity through ecological approaches (Stokols 1992) that place creation of supportive environments on a par with the development of personal skills and the reorientation of health services. Examples of such environmental supports are bike paths, parks, and incentives to encourage walking or bicycling to work. An underlying theme of ecological perspectives is that the most effective interventions simultaneously influence multiple levels and multiple settings (e.g., schools, work sites, etc.).

The transtheoretical model of behavior change (Prochaska and DiClemente 1984) integrates an ecological approach with other theories and models of health behavior. In this model, which is demonstrably effective in changing physical activity behaviors (Calfas et al. 1996), behavior change consists of a five-stage process related to a person's readiness to change:

1. Precontemplation
2. Contemplation
3. Preparation
4. Action
5. Maintenance

People progress through these stages at varying rates, often moving back and forth along the continuum a number of times before attaining the goal of maintenance—the stages of change are more spiral or cyclical than linear. In this model, people use different processes of change as they move from one stage to another. Efficient self-change thus depends on doing the right thing (processes) at the right time (stages). According to this theory, tailoring interventions to match a person's readiness or stage of change

is essential. For example, for people who are not yet contemplating becoming more active, encouraging a step-by-step movement along the continuum of change may be more effective than encouraging them to move directly into action (Marcus et al. 1992).

PACE—A Behavioral Approach to Physical Activity Counseling

In collaboration with the CDC, investigators from San Diego State University developed the Physician-based Assessment and Counseling for Exercise (PACE) materials, especially for use by primary care providers in targeting apparently clinically healthy adults (Patrick et al. 1994). A number of clinicians have evaluated the materials for both acceptability and effectiveness (Long et al. 1996). The PACE protocols assume that a single counseling approach is not appropriate for all patients. Using the stages-of-change model, the PACE counseling protocols classify patients according to their readiness to become physically active, and encourage coupling the counseling approach to the patient's stage (figure 8.1). The theory is that people make behavioral changes progressively and have different counseling needs at each stage. The PACE protocols (figures 8.2-8.5) distill the five original stages of change into three functional stages: precontemplators, contemplators, and actives. Each of these stages has a corresponding counseling protocol.

The score patients receive on the assessment form ("What Is Your PACE Score?", figure 8.2) determines the stage they are in. Precontemplators are patients who have not been in nor are currently active in an exercise program, and have no interest in doing so. A score of 1 means the patient is a precontemplator, and you may use the "Getting Out of Your Chair" form (figure 8.3) as a guide in counseling him. Your goal is to get such people to consider becoming more physically active. The counseling protocol for this stage requires patients to identify potential benefits of physical activity (e.g., recovery of strength following injury or surgery), thus moving them to the point of realizing that being active is desirable. Patients identify two main reasons why they are inactive and two strategies to overcome these barriers. This sets the stage for you to suggest activities and approaches to overcome any obstacles. Success among these patients is measured by their desire to consider becoming more physically active.

Contemplators (PACE score 2-4) are patients who, although they do little or no regular physical activity, are interested in becoming more active—but usually do not have the knowledge, skills, or the right

PACE Assessment and Counseling Flow Chart

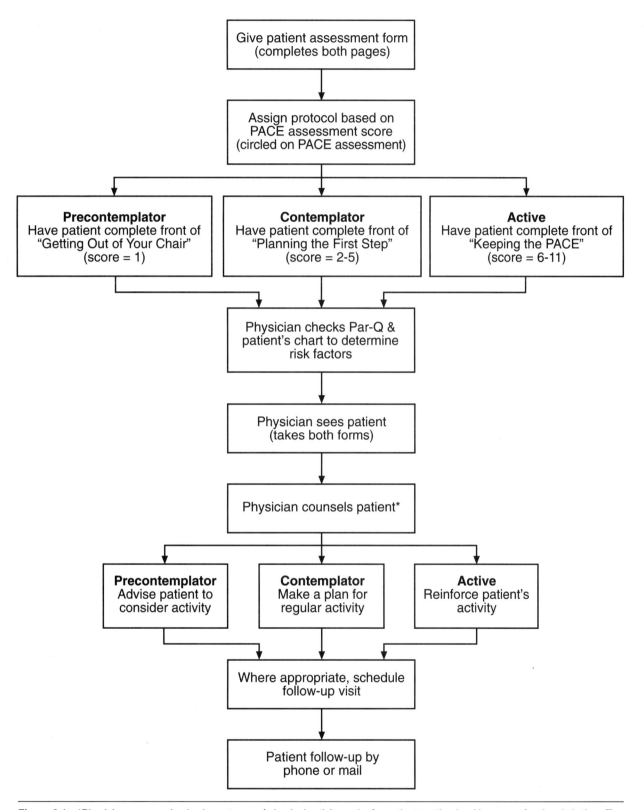

Figure 8.1 *Physician may emphasize importance of physical activity and refer patient to other health care professionals in the office for counseling.

Permission to reprint from the PACE Manual (Patient-centered Assessment and Counseling for Exercise and Nutrition) granted by the SDSU Foundation and the San Diego Center for Health Intervention.

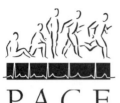

What is Your PACE Score?

This form will help your health care provider understand your level of physical activity. Please read the entire form and then choose the ONE number below that best describes your current level of physical activity or your readiness to do more physical activity. Do not include activities you do as part of your job.

"Vigorous" exercise includes activities like jogging, running, fast cycling, aerobics classes, swimming laps, singles tennis, and racquetball. Any activity that makes you work *as hard as jogging* and *lasts 20 minutes* at a time should be counted. These types of activities usually increase your heart rate, and make you sweat, and you get out of breath. *(Do not count weight lifting.)* **Regular *vigorous* exercise** is done for at least 20 minutes at a time and at least 3 days a week.

"Moderate" exercise includes activities like brisk walking, gardening, slow cycling, dancing, doubles tennis, or hard work around the house. Any activity that makes you work *as hard as brisk walking* and that lasts at least *10 minutes* at a time should be counted. **Regular *moderate* exercise** is done at least 30 minutes a day and at least 5 days a week.

CURRENT PHYSICAL ACTIVITY STATUS

Circle one number only.

1. I don't do regular vigorous or moderate exercise now, and I don't intend to start in the next 6 months.

2. I don't do regular vigorous or moderate exercise now, but I have been thinking of starting in the next 6 months.

3. I'm trying to start doing vigorous or moderate exercise, but I don't do it regularly.

4. I'm doing vigorous exercise less than 3 times per week (or) moderate exercise less than 5 times per week.

5. I've been doing 30 minutes a day of moderate exercise 5 or more days per week for the last 1-5 months.

6. I've been doing 30 minutes a day of moderate exercise 5 or more days per week for the last 6 months or more.

7. I've been doing vigorous exercise 3 or more days per week for the last 1-5 months.

8. I've been doing vigorous exercise 3 or more days per week for the last 6 months or more.

1/99

Please complete other side.

Figure 8.2
Permission to reprint from the PACE Manual (Patient-centered Assessment and Counseling for Exercise and Nutrition) granted by the SDSU Foundation and the San Diego Center for Health Interventions.

PHYSICAL ACTIVITY READINESS QUESTIONNAIRE (PAR-Q)*

A SELF-ADMINISTERED QUESTIONNAIRE FOR ADULTS

PAR-Q is designed to help you help yourself. Many health benefits are associated with regular exercise, and the completion of PAR-Q is a sensible first step to take if you are planning to increase the amount of physical activity in your life.

For most people, physical activity should not pose any problem or hazard. PAR-Q has been designed to identify the small number of adults for whom physical activity might be inappropriate or those who should have medical advice concerning the type of activity most suitable for them.

Common sense is your best guide in answering these questions. Please read them carefully and check YES or NO opposite the question as it applies to you.

YES   NO

○   ○   1. Has your doctor ever said that you have a heart condition and that you should only do physical activity recommended by a doctor?

○   ○   2. Do you feel pain in your chest when you do physical activity?

○   ○   3. In the past month, have you had chest pain when you were not doing physical activity?

○   ○   4. Do you lose your balance because of dizziness or do you ever lose consciousness?

○   ○   5. Do you have a bone or joint problem that could be made worse by a change in your physical activity?

○   ○   6. Is your doctor currently prescribing drugs (for example, water pills) for your blood pressure or heart condition?

○   ○   7. Do you know of any other reason why you should not do physical activity?

Note: If you have a temporary illness, such as a common cold, or are not feeling well at this time—Postpone.

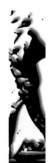

Adapted from the 1994 revised version of the Physical Activity Readiness Questionnaire PAR-Q and YOU. The PAR-Q and YOU is a copyrighted pre-exercise screen owned by the Canadian Society for Exercise Physiology.

Figure 8.2   *(continued)*

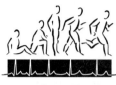

Getting Out of Your Chair

Assessment Score = 1

On your PACE Assessment you said you do not intend to start regular physical activity in the next 6 months. That is fine, because everyone makes changes at his or her own speed.

However, PACE and your health care provider want to make sure you know about the many important benefits of physical activity.

P A C E

Think About the Benefits of Physical Activity. Please list up to 10 benefits of physical activity. You may have heard these on the news, read about them, or heard about them from friends. Think about benefits you get right away and in the future.

1. _____   6. _____
2. _____   7. _____
3. _____   8. _____
4. _____   9. _____
5. _____   10. _____

If you listed 10 benefits, that's great. You are well informed. But did you know there are many more benefits? Turn this page over to see a much longer list of the benefits you can get by being physically active.

What are 4 more benefits that are important *to you* but you did not know about before? *List them here.*

1. _____   3. _____
2. _____   4. _____

Because of all these benefits, doctors now realize that being physically active is one of the most important things you can do for your health. We understand that you are not ready to increase your physical activity now, but please think about how these benefits could help you.

Good News About Moderate Physical Activity. Did you know you can enjoy many of these benefits without working up a heavy sweat? The recommendations for physical activity have changed. The new recommendations can be done by everybody, because they emphasize moderate amounts of physical activity on a daily basis. Brisk walking, bicycling, pushing a baby carriage and digging in the garden are all moderate activities. Being active can be an enjoyable part of your day, instead of a chore. Here is the current physical activity recommendation:

> *"Every adult should accumulate 30 minutes or more of moderate-intensity physical activity on most, preferably all, days of the week. An example of moderate intensity physical activity is a brisk walk."*

This means you don't even have to do all 30 minutes at once. You do not have to wear special clothes, use special equipment or spend a lot of money to get the benefits of physical activity.

PROVIDER'S USE ONLY:

⭕ As your health care provider, I strongly encourage you to plan to be more physically active. I may ask you at your next visit if you are ready to begin.

Based on your medical status and health history, the most important benefits of physical activity for you are:

_____
Provider's Signature

1/99

Figure 8.3

Permission to reprint from the PACE Manual (Patient-centered Assessment and Counseling for Exercise and Nutrition) granted by the SDSU Foundation and the San Diego Center for Health Interventions.

142

Your physician strongly encourages you to think about the benefits you could get from physical activity.

Most people can improve their health a great deal by taking a walk for 30 minutes a few times every week. If you want information on how to start doing more physical activity, ask your doctor.

Hundreds of research studies show physical activity has dozens of health benefits. It improves many systems of the body and reduces risks for important mental and physical illnesses. Here are some of the benefits of being physically active.

BENEFITS OF PHYSICAL ACTIVITY

Benefits you can get right away	*Benefits you get over the long run*
· Reduces blood sugar levels	· Increases life expectancy. Active people live up to 2 years longer.
· Increases metabolic rate after workout	· Improves overall quality of life
· Improves mental health	· Reduces heart attacks by about 50%
· Increases self-esteem and self-concept	· Reduces stokes
· Increases well-being	· Reduces blood pressure
· Increases quality of life	· Reduces risk of becoming hypertensive
· Reduces depression	· Reduces triglycerides (fats in the blood)
· Reduces anger	· Increases HDL (good) cholesterol
· Reduces anxiety	· Reduces risk of colon cancer
· Helps cope with stress	· Possibly reduces risk of breast cancer
· Improves vitality and "energy"	· Possibly reduces risk of prostate cancer
· Improves sleep	· Improves functioning of immune system
· Aids relaxation	· Reduces risk of becoming diabetic
· Can help quit smoking	· Controls body weight
· Can help stick with dietary changes	· Helps weight loss
· Builds muscle tissue	· Promotes loss of body fat
· Improves pain tolerance	· Promotes loss of dangerous abdominal fat
· Improves some hormonal functions	· Necessary for maintaining weight loss
· Improves blood flow to the brain	· Prevents depression
· May enhance cognitive functioning	· Prevents anxiety
· May aid recovery from substance abuse	· Improves immune system
· Burns calories	· Makes heart stronger
	· Reduces blood clotting
	· Can reduce falls in the elderly
	· Reduces risk of osteoporosis
	· Improves functioning in arthritis patients

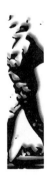

Figure 8.3 *(continued)*

kind of encouragement. Use "Planning the First Step" (figure 8.4) to counsel them, helping these patients draw up a specific plan to begin an exercise program. Begin with praise for their desire to become more physically active. Ask patients to list at least two benefits they hope to gain from their activity program and to draft a sample activity plan that they will review with you. Have them list the type of activities they enjoy doing and where and when they plan to do them. To elicit social support, ask patients to identify a family member, friend, or coworker who will support their new activity plan. Patients should be as specific as possible in their plans. If necessary you should adjust the exercise plan because of the patient's clinical and health status. The result is a plan that is both realistic and potentially beneficial. The patient agrees to the plan for a specified time period and signs an agreement—signing a contract is an effective behavioral modification technique (Marcus et al. 1994). Contemplators will require more of your time than either precontemplators or actives. It is helpful to provide these patients with additional educational materials and to arrange occasions for them to see people modeling the prescribed exercise behaviors.

Actives (PACE score of 5-8) are already participating in regular physical activity at any level of intensity. These are usually patients who, following their initial rehabilitation sessions, carry the principles of these sessions into lifetime physical activities. Use "Keeping the Pace" (figure 8.5) to counsel these patients, encouraging them to maintain an active lifestyle. Do this by developing strategies to prevent relapse, and by encouraging a return to activity after unavoidable time off (e.g., illness, work demands). Counseling these patients also begins with praise for current activities. Ask them to list at least three benefits they receive from their current activity program. Review the program, drawing attention to potential problem areas (e.g., overuse or underexercising). Occasional lapses are expected: challenge these patients to list potential barriers they may need to overcome in the future in order to maintain their programs. Focus on building self-efficacy (i.e., patients' confidence to maintain their programs in the face of certain barriers, such as weather, travel, etc.). Both you and your patient should sign the exercise plan and make a commitment to review and revise it as necessary.

To obtain the PACE forms contact the SDSU Foundation and the San Diego Center for Health Interventions, 5500 Campanile Dr., San Diego, CA 92182-4701.

Summary

Within the past decade, physical activity has emerged as a key element in preventing and managing chronic conditions. Although for decades clinicians have appreciated the role of exercise in rehabilitation medicine, recent findings regarding the mode, frequency, duration, and intensity of physical activity have modified exercise prescription practices. An important part of these modifications has been a clearer separation of the results of exercise into those related to health and those related to fitness. Most importantly, new behavioral approaches to physical activity assessment and counseling have led to documented improvements in compliance.

Behavioral theories and models of health behavior have been reexamined in light of physical activity and exercise. A set of behavioral principles and guidelines now exists to help health providers guide patients into lifelong patterns of increased levels of physical activity and improved exercise compliance. The PACE materials provide an integrated behavioral approach to exercise prescription that takes into account the providers' limited time and expertise in counseling patients about physical activity; the patients' needs and behavioral readiness for increased physical activity; and the appropriate desired outcomes for health and fitness.

Further refinement of the PACE and other protocols will be necessary for its use in rehabilitation medicine, dictated by the spectrum of patients seen. The more we learn about exercise in specific populations, the more we will be able to refine our prescriptions in terms of mode, frequency, duration, and intensity of exercise for specific classes of people. Combining more refined prescriptions with more effective behavioral paradigms will yield enhanced compliance on the part of previously unmotivated people. The net result will be healthier and more functional patients.

Acknowledgments

I would like to acknowledge my colleagues at CDC and those at San Diego State University who so profoundly influenced my thinking about "exercise prescription" and health behavior change. I trust that this chapter reflects a bit of their wisdom. Thanks to Dr. Walter Frontera for providing me with the opportunity to pen a few of the animated points from my Boston presentation. And, finally, thank you to Elaine Mustain and her editorial staff at Human Kinetics for persevering with me on this.

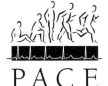

Planning the First Step

Assessment Score = 2-4

PACE

Congratulations. On your PACE Assessment you said you are ready to increase your physical activity. You are taking a big step toward improving your physical and mental health. This form can help you start an activity program you can stick with.

What are the two main benefits you hope to get from being active? Writing them down here will help you keep them in mind.

1. _____   2. _____

> *Work up to these physical activity guidelines (see example activities on back).*
> · Do moderate physical activity for 30 to 60 minutes on 5 to 7 days a week.
> · Do vigorous physical activity for 20 to 40 minutes on 3 to 5 days a week.
> · Most inactive people should start with moderate activities.

MAKE A PHYSICAL ACTIVITY PLAN

Choose an activity or two. Do you enjoy it? Can you afford the supplies, equipment, facilities, or classes? Are there family or friends to do this activity with you? Can you do it year-round? Consider a back-up activity.
Type of Activity: _____

Where will you do your activity? Can you do this activity at home or in your neighborhood? Do you have to go to a gym, a park, or a health club?
Place for Activity: _____

What is the most realistic time for you to do this activity? Do you have to reschedule other activities? Start slowly and work up to this goal.
Days and Times for Activity: _____

How long do you plan to do your activity each time? You should build up time gradually over several weeks. Start with 5-10 minutes and build up to 30-60 minutes of moderate activity or 20-40 minutes of vigorous activity.
Length of Activity: _____

Who can support you or help with your new activity program? It is ideal for someone to work out with you. You may want to ask someone to encourage you or help you to be active.
Who will help you and how? _____

PROVIDER'S USE ONLY:

Based on your health status, your doctor recommends you do the following to improve your health:

○ Before you increase your physical activity, you need to have an exercise tolerance test.*

○ You could benefit greatly by starting a program of regular walking or other moderate activity.

○ If you want to do vigorous activities like jogging, you need to have an exercise tolerance test.*

○ You appear to be able to do either moderate or vigorous physical activities.

*Call this office for an appointment or referral.

1/99

SUGGESTED PROGRAM (FITT)

Frequency   F _____ times per week

Intensity   I _____ moderate _____ vigorous activity

Type   T_____ type of physical activity

Time   T _____ minutes per session (Work up to ____minutes in ___weeks.)

I agree to try out this physical activity plan from _____ to _____

_____
Patient's Signature

_____
Provider's Signature

(continued)

Figure 8.4

Permission to reprint from the PACE Manual (Patient-centered Assessment and Counseling for Exercise and Nutrition) granted by the SDSU Foundation and the San Diego Center for Health Interventions.

EXAMPLES OF ACTIVITIES

Moderate Intensity

Walking *(at home, to work, on lunch break)*

Gardening *(must be regular)*

Hiking

Slow cycling

Folk, square, or popular dancing

Ice and roller skating

Doubles tennis

Pushing a baby carriage

Vigorous Intensity

Jogging

Aerobic dance

Basketball

Fast cycling

Cross-country skiing

Swimming laps

Singles tennis and racquet sports

Soccer

HOW TO GET PAST YOUR ROADBLOCKS

Roadblock	*How To Get Past It*
○ I do not have the time	We're talking about only three 30-minute sessions each week. Could you do without three TV shows each week?
○ I do not enjoy exercise	Do not "exercise." Start a hobby or way of playing that gets you moving.
○ I am usually too tired for exercise	Tell yourself, "This activity will give me more energy." This is what most people find.
○ The weather is too bad	There are many activities you can do in your own home, in any weather. Ask your friends for ideas.
○ Exercise is boring	Listening to music during your activity keeps your mind occupied. Walking, biking, or running can take you past lots of interesting scenery. Do activity with a friend.
○ I get sore when I exercise	Slight muscle soreness after physical activity is common when you are just starting. It should go away in 2-3 days. You can avoid this by building up gradually.

ACTIVITY LOG

Use this Activity Log to keep track of your physical activity. Write down how long you do your activity as well as positive feelings and experiences. Note any roadblocks that discourage you from doing your activity and do something about them. When this log is full, make one of your own.

DATE	ACTIVITY	MINUTES	FEELING/COMMENTS

How confident are you that you can do regular physical activity for the next 3 months?

○ Not at all confident   ○ Somewhat confident   ○ Very confident

---

Figure 8.4   *(continued)*

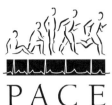

Keeping the PACE

P A C E

Assessment Score = 5-8

Congratulations. You are doing regular physical activity. You have a right to feel proud that you are doing something very positive for yourself. Sometimes you lose sight of the health and mental health benefits you are getting from physical activity.

What motivates you to stay active?

1. _____   2. _____   3. _____

REVIEW YOUR PROGRAM

By reviewing the activities you are doing now, you can see if any changes need to be made in your plan. The goal is to improve your chances of staying active.

What *type(s)* of activity do you usually do? _____

How many *times a week*? _____

How long each time? _____

Who *helps* you or does activity with you? _____

Have you had any *injuries*? _____

What parts of your activity plan are you *most satisfied* with? _____

What parts of your activity plan are you *least satisfied* with? _____

What *changes* could you make in your activity plan to make it more enjoyable, convenient, or safe? _____
_____

GETTING BACK ON TRACK

Most people who are regularly active have stopped at one time or another in the past. Sometimes they stop for a few weeks. Sometimes it is years before they start being active again. Planning ahead by answering these questions now can help you get past roadblocks later.

If you have stopped regular activity in the past, what caused you to stop? _____
_____

What could you have done differently that would have helped you stay active or what helped you get back on track quickly?

KEEPING THE PACE

How confident are you that you can do regular physical activity for the next 3 months?

○ Not at all confident   ○ Somewhat confident   ○ Very confident

PROVIDER'S USE ONLY:

SUMMARY OF CURRENT PROGRAM (FITT)	MAJOR CVD RISK FACTORS
Frequency F _____ times per week	○ Smoking ○ Physical Inactivity
Intensity I _____ moderate _____ vigorous activity	○ Hypertension ○ Positive Family History
Type T _____ type of physical activity	○ Elevated Lipids ○ Obesity
Time T _____ minutes per session	
Provider's Signature _____	

1/99

(continued)

Figure 8.5
Permission to reprint from the PACE Manual (Patient-centered Assessment and Counseling for Exercise and Nutrition) granted by the SDSU Foundation and the San Diego Center for Health Interventions.

TIPS FOR KEEPING THE PACE

Injury to muscle, joints and bones may be the *most common* cause of stopping activity. The best way to prevent injury is to avoid over-exercise. Do not do an activity that is too vigorous for you. If you are overdoing it, slow down. If you feel pain during physical activity, stop and take a rest. The *most serious* risk of physical activity is heart trouble, but it is *rare*. If you feel pain in your chest, immediately stop the activity and consult a physician.

The PACE recommendation of 30 to 60 minutes of moderate activity 5-7 days a week or 20 to 40 minutes of vigorous activity 3 to 5 days a week provides maximum benefit at low levels of risk. Exercise scientists also suggest warming up before your main activity and cooling down and stretching after your activity to lower your risk of injury. Warming up and cooling down can be slow versions of your activity, like slow walking. Gently, stretch the muscles you use during the activity. Hold each stretch 5-10 seconds and don't bounce.

There are times when you may stop your regular activity. This may be due to more demands on your time at home or work, travel, house guests, or illness. Interruptions are normal and expected. *The key is starting your regular activity again as soon as possible.*

HOW TO GET BACK ON TRACK

· Remind yourself it is OK to have a pause in your activity once in a while. Don't be hard on yourself. Feeling guilty will make it more difficult to get back on track.

· You may need some extra help to get going again. Ask family and friends to help and encourage you.

· Ask someone to be active with you.

· It may be helpful to tell everybody you know that you are restarting your activity.

· Use an Activity Log to keep track of your activity again.

· Give yourself small rewards each time you go out and do your activity. Make a chart for your refrigerator. Use stickers or gold stars to keep track of your activity. Put change in a jar as a reward. Praising yourself is an effective reward ("I did it and I'm proud of myself.")

· For variety, try new activities.

· Do whatever worked for you in the past to restart physical activity.

LOOK AHEAD FOR YOUR ROADBLOCKS

What situation is most likely to make you stop being active? _____

_____

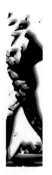

What can you do about this roadblock to prevent it or prepare for it? _____

_____

What is the best way for you to get back on track if you stop? _____

_____

Figure 8.5   *(continued)*

References

Ajzen, I. 1988. *Attitudes, personality, and behavior.* Chicago: Dorsey Press.

Ajzen, I., and M. Fishbein. 1980. *Understanding attitudes and predicting social behavior.* Englewood Cliffs, NJ: Prentice-Hall.

American Academy of Pediatrics. 1994. Assessing physical activity and fitness in the office setting. *Peds* 93:686-689.

American College of Sports Medicine. 1991. *Guidelines for exercise testing and prescription.* 4th ed. Philadelphia: Lea & Febiger.

American College of Sports Medicine. 1998. *Resource manual for guidelines for exercise testing and prescription.* 2d ed. Philadelphia: Lea & Febiger.

American Heart Association. 1992. Statement on exercise: benefits and recommendations for physical activity programs for all Americans. *Circulation* 86:340-343.

Bandura, A. 1977a. Self-efficacy: toward a unifying theory of behavioral change. *Psychol Rev* 84:191-215.

Bandura, A. 1977b. *Social learning theory.* Englewood Cliffs, NJ: Prentice-Hall.

Bandura, A. 1986. *Social foundations of thought and action: A social-cognitive theory.* Englewood Cliffs, NJ: Prentice-Hall.

Barry, H.C., and S.W. Eathorne. 1994. Exercise and aging: issues for the practitioner. *Med Clin North Am* 78:357-376.

Braith, R.W., J.E. Graves, J.L. Pollock, S.L. Leggett, D.M. Carpenter, and A.B. Colvin. 1989. Comparison of 2 vs. 3 days/week of variable resistance training during 10-and 18-week programs. *Int J Sports Med* 10: 450-454.

Cady, L.D., D.P. Bischoff, E.R. O'Connell, P.C. Thomas, and J.H. Allan. 1979. Strength and fitness and subsequent back injuries in firefighters. *J Occup Med* 21:269-272.

Calfas, K.J., B.J. Long, J.F. Sallis, W.J. Wooten, M. Pratt, and K. Patrick. 1996. A controlled trial of physician counseling to promote the adoption of physical activity. *Prev Med* 25:225-233.

Caspersen, C.J., K.E. Powell, and G.M. Christenson. 1985. Physical activity, exercise, and physical fitness: definitions and distinctions for health-related research. *Public Health Rep* 100:126-131.

Ching, P.L.Y.H., W.C. Willet, E.B. Rimm, G.A. Colditz, S.L. Gortmaker, and M.J. Stampfer. 1996. Activity level and risk of overweight in male health professionals. *Am J Public Health* 86:25-30.

Dishman, R.K. 1991. Increasing and maintaining exercise and physical activity. *Behavior Therapy* 22:345-378.

Glanz, K., and B.K. Rimer. 1995. *Theory at a glance: A guide for health promotion practice.* Bethesda, MD: U.S. Department of Health and Human Services.

Griffin, P. 1998. *Client-centered exercise prescription.* Champaign, IL: Human Kinetics.

Harris, S.S., C.J. Caspersen, G.H. DeFriese, and E.H. Estes Jr. 1989. Physical activity counseling for healthy adults as a primary prevention intervention in the clinical setting. *JAMA* 261:3590-3598.

Hassmen, P., R. Ceci, and L. Backman. 1992. Exercise for older women: a training method and its influences on physical and cognitive performance. *Eur J Appl Physiol* 64:460-466.

Kampert, J.B., S.N. Blair, C.E. Barlow, and H.W. Kohl 3rd. 1996. Physical activity, physical fitness, and all-cause and cancer mortality: a prospective study of men and women. *Ann Epidemiol* 6:452-7.

King, A.C., W.L. Haskell, C.B. Taylor, H.C. Kraemer, and R.F. DeBusk. 1991. Group- vs. home-based exercise training in healthy older men and women. *JAMA* 266:1535-1542.

King, A.C., W.L. Haskell, D.R. Young, R.K. Oka, and M.L. Stefanick. 1995. Long-term effects of varying intensities and formats of physical activity on participation rates, fitness, and lipoproteins in men and women aged 50 to 65 years. *Circulation* 91:2596-2604.

King, A.C., C.B. Taylor, and W.L. Haskell. 1993. Effects of differing intensities and formats of 12 months of exercise training on psychological outcomes in older adults. *Health Psychol* 12:292-300.

Kriska, A.M., C. Bayles, J.A. Cauley, R.E. LaPorte, R.B. Sandler, and G. Pambianco. 1986. Randomized exercise trial in older women: increased activity over two years and the factors associated with compliance. *Med Sci Sports Exerc* 18:557-562.

Lee, I.M., R.S. Paffenbarger, and C.C. Hsieh. 1991. Physical activity and risk of developing colorectal cancer among college alumni. *J Natl Cancer Inst* 83:1324-1329.

Logsdon, D.N., C.M. Lazaro, and R.V. Meier. 1989. The feasibility of behavioral risk reduction in primary medical care. *Am J Prev Med* 5:249-256.

Long, B.J., K.J. Calfas, K. Patrick, J.F. Sallis, W.J. Wooten, M. Goldstein, B. Marcus, T. Schwenck, R. Carter, T. Torez, L. Palinkas, and G. Heath. 1996. Acceptability, useability, and practicality of physician counseling for physical activity promotion: Project PACE. *Am J Prev Med* 12:73-81.

Marcus, B.H., S.W. Banspach, R.C. Lefebvre, J.S. Rossi, R.A. Carleton, and D.B. Abrams. 1992. Using the stages of change model to increase adoption of physical activity among community participants. *American Journal of Health Promotion* 6:424-429.

Marcus, B.H., B.M. Pinto, L.R. Simkin, J.E. Audrain, and E.R. Taylor. 1994. Application of theoretical models to exercise behavior among employed women. *American Journal of Health Promotion* 9:49-55.

Marcus, B.H., and A.L. Stanton. 1993. Evaluation of relapse prevention and reinforcement interventions to promote exercise adherence in sedentary females. *Res Q Exerc Sport* 64:447-452.

Marlatt, G.A., and W.H. George. 1990. Relapse prevention and the maintenance of optimal health. In *The handbook of health behavior change*, ed. S.A. Shumaker, E.B. Schron, and J. Ockene, 44-63. New York: Springer Publishing Company.

McLeroy, K.R., D. Bibeau, A. Steckler, and K. Glanz. 1988. An ecological perspective on health promotion programs. *Health Educ Q* 15:351-377.

Paffenbarger, R.S., R.T. Hyde, and A.L. Wing. 1978. Physical activity as an index of heart attack risk in college alumni. *Am J Epidemiol* 108:161-175.

Passmore, R. 1971. The regulation of body weight in man. *Proc Nutr Soc* 30:122-127.

Pate, R.R., M. Pratt, S.N. Blair, W.L. Haskell, C.A. Macera, C. Bouchard, D. Buchner, W. Ettinger, G.W. Heath, and A.C. King. 1995. Physical activity and public health: a recommendation from the Centers for Disease Control and Prevention and the American College of Sports Medicine. *JAMA* 273:402-407.

Patrick, K., J.F. Sallis, B. Long, K.J. Calfas, W. Wooten, G. Heath, and M. Pratt. 1994. A new tool for encouraging activity: Project PACE. *Physician Sportsmed* 22:45-55.

Pollock, M.L. 1988. Prescribing exercise for fitness and adherence. In *Exercise adherence*, ed. R.K. Dishman. Champaign, IL: Human Kinetics Publishers.

President's Council on Physical Fitness and Sports. 1993. *The physician's Rx: Exercise*. Washington, DC: President's Council on Physical Fitness and Sports.

Prochaska, J.O., and C.C. DiClemente. 1984. *The transtheoretical approach: Crossing traditional boundaries of change*. Homewood, IL: Dorsey Press.

Rosenstock, I.M. 1990. The health belief model: explaining health behavior through expectancies. In: *Health behavior and health education: Theory, research, and practice*. San Francisco: Jossey-Bass Publishers.

Sallis, J.F., and M.F. Hovell. 1990. Determinants of exercise behavior. *Exerc Sport Sci Rev* 18:307-330.

Sallis, J.F., M.F. Hovell, and C.R. Hofstetter. 1992. Predictors of adoption and maintenance of vigorous physical activity in men and women. *Prev Med* 21:237-251.

Sallis, J.F., M.F. Hovell, C.R. Hofstetter, P. Faucher, J.P. Elder, J. Blanchard, C.J. Caspersen, K.E. Powell, and G.M. Christenson. 1989. A multivariate study of determinants of vigorous exercise in a community sample. *Prev Med* 18:20-34.

Shephard, R.J. 1993. Exercise and aging: extending independence in older adults. *Geriatrics* 48:61-64.

Shephard, R.J., M. Berridge, and W. Montelpare. 1990. On the generality of the 'Sit and Reach' Test: an analysis of flexibility data for an aging population. *Res Q Exerc Sport* 61:326-330.

Sidney, K.H., R.J. Shephard, and J.E. Harrison. 1977. Endurance training and body composition of the elderly. *Am J Clin Nutr* 30:326-333.

Smith, D.M., M.R.A Khairi, J. Norton, and C.C. Johnston Jr. 1976. Age and activity effects on rate of bone mineral loss. *J Clin Invest* 58:716-721.

Sotile, W.M. 1998. *Psychosocial interventions for cardiopulmonary patients*. 3d ed. Champaign, IL: Human Kinetics.

Stokols, D. 1992. Establishing and maintaining healthy environments: toward a social ecology of health promotion. *Am Psychol* 47:6-22.

Tipton, C.H. 1991. Exercise, training, and hypertension: an update. *Exerc Sport Sci Rev* 19:447-505.

U.S. Department of Health and Human Services. 1991. *Healthy People 2000: National health promotion and disease prevention objectives*. Washington, DC: U.S. Department of Health and Human Services, Public Health Service Publication No. 91-50213.

U.S. Department of Health and Human Services. 1996. *Physical activity and health: A report of the Surgeon General*. Atlanta: U.S. Department of Health and Human Services, Centers for Disease Control and Prevention, National Center for Chronic Disease Prevention and Health Promotion.

U.S. Department of Health and Human Services. 1996. Chapter 6: Understanding and promoting physical activity. In *Physical activity and health: A report of the Surgeon General*. Atlanta: U.S. Department of Health and Human Services, Centers for Disease Control and Prevention, National Center for Chronic Disease Prevention and Health Promotion.

U.S. Department of Health and Human Services. 1996. Physiologic responses and long-term adaptations to exercise. In *Physical activity and health: A report of the Surgeon General*. Atlanta: U.S. Department of Health and Human Services, Centers for Disease Control and Prevention, National Center for Chronic Disease Prevention and Health Promotion.

U.S. Department of Health and Human Services, Public Health Service, Centers for Disease Control and Prevention, National Center for Chronic Disease Prevention and Health Promotion, Division of Nutrition and Physical Activity. 1999. *Promoting physical activity: A Guide for community action*. Champaign, IL: Human Kinetics.

U.S. Preventive Services Task Force. 1996. Counseling to promote physical activity. In *Guide to clinical preventive services*. 2d ed. Baltimore: Williams & Wilkins.

Wells, K.B., C.E. Lewis, B. Leake, M.K. Schleiter, and R.H. Brook. 1989. The practices of general and subspecialty internists in counseling about smoking and exercise. *Am J Public Health* 76:1009-1013.

West Virginia University, Department of Safety and Health Studies and Department of Sports and Exercise Studies. 1988. *Physical fitness and the aging driver: Phase I. AAA Foundation of Traffic Safety*, Washington, DC.

Wood, P.D., M.L. Stefanick, D.M. Dreon, D. Frey-Hewitt, B.C. Garay, P.T. Williams, H.R. Superko, S.P. Fortmann, J.J. Albers, K.M. Vranizan, N.M. Ellworth, R.B. Terry, and W.L. Haskell. 1988. Changes in plasma lipids and lipoproteins in overweight men during weight loss through dieting as compared with exercise. *New Engl J Med* 319:1173-1179.

Young, D.R., W.L. Haskell, C.B. Taylor, and S.P. Fortmann. 1996. Effect of community health education on physical activity knowledge, attitudes, and behavior: the Stanford Five-City Project. *Am J Epidemiol* 144:264-274.

Chapter 9

Exercise and the Prevention of Chronic Disabling Illness

Carlos J. Crespo, DrPH, MS

This chapter discusses the effects of physical activity or exercise in the primary prevention of selected chronic diseases. Being physically active has been associated with lower rates of coronary heart disease, stroke, certain cancers, type 2 diabetes, osteoporosis, osteoarthritis, and some mental conditions. The challenge is to differentiate among the independent effects that an active lifestyle, physical fitness, and heredity may have on the occurrence of chronic diseases (Bouchard 1993).

For many years we have observed that people who exercise experience a lower rate of chronic diseases. This relationship between physical activity and chronic disease is confounded, however: physically active individuals tend to have a genetic predisposi-

tion for high levels of physical fitness. This predisposition raises the possibility that people who exercise do so because they have a genetic advantage of better physical fitness levels than nonexercisers. Thus, people who are physically fit simply by virtue of their genes are more likely to engage in physical activity than people who are less fit genetically. It is possible that the lower prevalence of chronic diseases among exercisers may not be the result solely of their participation in physical activity, but of "healthier" genes accompanied by better fitness levels.

In one population-based study, former elite athletes—particularly those in aerobic sports—required less hospital care later in life than their nonathlete cohorts (Kujala et al. 1996). But we do not know if the athletes went less to the hospital because they were athletes earlier in life, because they continued exercising throughout their lifetime, or because their genes, which made them athletes in the first place, also protected them from illnesses later in life.

Definitions

Exercise or exercise training is a planned, structured, and repetitive bodily movement done to improve or maintain one or more components of physical fitness. **Physical activity** refers to any bodily movement, produced by contraction of skeletal muscle, that substantially increases energy expenditure (Caspersen et al. 1985; Nieman 1996). Thus, exercise is a form of physical activity. Physical activity can be occupational, or can involve housework, leisure activities, transportation (e.g., bicycling), entertainment (e.g., dancing), and, of course, sports. This chapter will use the terms "physical activity" and "exercise" interchangeably.

Physical fitness, defined as a set of attributes that relates to the ability to perform physical activity, can be health-related or skill-related. Health-related fitness has an independent effect on health. Skill-related physical fitness may predispose people to continue or to increase their level of physical activity. Even when skill-related endeavors have no direct health component, they can provide additional psychological confidence that lead people to engage in activities that do improve their health.

Participation in sports or work-related activities requires both health- and skill-related components of physical fitness. Prevention of chronic disease through exercise requires not only that people be physically active, but also that they train and improve certain health- and skill-related components of physical fitness.

Physical Activity and Physical Fitness

Improvements in one or more fitness components can help prevent chronic diseases. Maintaining a healthy body weight or improving cardiorespiratory and muscular endurance can help prevent coronary heart disease, type 2 diabetes, osteoporosis, and other chronic diseases.

Earlier longitudinal studies of the relationship between physical activity and chronic disease compared occupations with higher energy expenditure to those with lower energy expenditure (Morris et al. 1966) and found that physical activity protects against heart disease. Later studies found that leisure-time physical activity offers more protection against heart disease than work activities (Haskell 1995; USDHHS 1996)—probably because physical activity has been engineered out of most people's occupations. Unfortunately, data from the National Health Interview Survey and the Third National Health and Nutrition Examination Survey showed that more than half of American adults engage in little or no leisure-time physical activity (Crespo et al. 1996; USDHHS 1996). It is clear that America is experiencing a virtual pandemic of inactivity.

Simultaneous measurements of physical activity and physical fitness may be useful in epidemiologic studies of habitual physical activity and chronic disease. For example, physical activity and physical fitness correlate significantly and independently with different coronary heart disease risk factors in men and women. Measuring physical fitness and participation in physical activity among members of different churches in Rhode Island, Eaton et al. (1995) found that physical fitness was more related to systolic and diastolic blood pressure, body mass index, and high-density lipoprotein (HDL) cholesterol than was physical activity. Multiple regression analysis of physical fitness, physical activity, and their interaction suggested that lack of physical fitness correlates strongly with CHD risk factors. Other studies have found physical fitness to be improved by heavy or vigorous physical activity, but not by light to moderate physical activity (Knapik et al. 1993).

In summary, both exercise training and general physical activity can improve physical fitness. The physiological and metabolic changes from improved physical fitness are very likely to produce substantial benefits in the prevention of certain chronic diseases. Physical activity, especially if it is vigorous, plays a crucial role in the maintenance and improvement of acceptable levels of physical fitness.

Physical Activity and Health

Powell and Blair (1994) estimated that 20,000 to 30,000 deaths from coronary heart disease, colon cancer, and diabetes could be postponed if inactive individuals were to become regularly active. These estimates do not even take into account the additional risks that inactivity poses for people with stroke, osteoporosis, and depression; nor does it address the issue of quality of life for these and other classes of people. Abundant literature shows the benefits to overall health and quality of life from even moderate amounts of physical activity.

Figure 9.1 compares years of healthy life and life expectancy among the major race/ethnic groups in the United States. Years of healthy life are at least 11 years less than total life expectancy. The difference between total life expectancy and years of healthy life is greater among blacks and Hispanics (around 14 years) than among whites or all races combined (around 12 years). The average American life expectancy had increased to 75.8 years by 1995; yet figure 9.2 shows that physical inactivity increases as people become older (Anderson et al. 1997; Crespo et al. 1996). The ability to be independent, functional, and to perform activities of daily living is closely related to being physically active later in life.

Some chronic conditions can severely limit participation in major or outdoor activities. Figures 9.3 and 9.4 show that heart disease, asthma, arthritis, and deformities or orthopedic impairments are the primary culprits in limiting physical activities. Table 9.1 shows the top causes of death in the general population as well as in population subgroups. The remainder of this chapter examines the effect of physical activity, exercise training, or physical fitness in the primary prevention of selected chronic diseases shown in table 9.1 and figures 9.3 and 9.4.

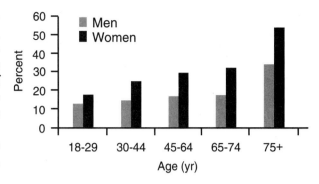

Figure 9.2 Prevalence of no leisure-time physical activity in men and women of different age groups in the United States, 1988-1991.
Source: NHANES III 1988-91.

Physical Activity and the Prevention of Heart Disease

Heart disease, sometimes referred to as cardiovascular disease, is a general name for more than 20 different diseases of the heart and its vessels. Coronary heart disease—the number one cause of death in the United States for both men and women of all racial backgrounds—is one of the most prevalent forms of heart disease and of chronic disease. It is also the chronic disease causing the second highest percent limitation in major or outside activity (see figure 9.4).

Physical Activity and Cardiovascular Disease in General

Physical inactivity is a major, independent risk factor for heart disease (USDHHS 1996; NIH 1996). The evidence that physical activity protects against coronary heart disease is dramatic, with a clear dose-response effect between physical activity and lower incidence of heart disease. A number of longitudinal, cross-sectional, clinical trials and case-control studies strongly suggest a cause-effect relationship (Blair et al. 1995; Blair et al. 1996; Leon 1991; McBride et al. 1992; USDHHS 1996).

Postmortem studies have shown that death from coronary heart disease is twice as common, and occurs at an earlier age, in men who perform light occupational tasks as in those who do heavy work.

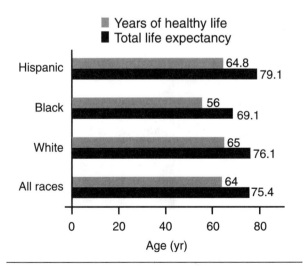

Figure 9.1 Total life expectancy and years of healthy life in the United States, 1990.
Source: Erickson, Wilson, and Shannon 1995.

Table 9.1   Age-Adjusted Death Rates From Selected Chronic Conditions by Race and Gender: United States, 1996

Cause of death	Age-adjusted rates per 100,000 population				
	All persons	Male	Female	White	Blacks
Major cardiovascular diseases	170.7	219.7	130.6	163.6	251.0
Ischemic heart disease	86.7	119.3	60.4	86.4	99.4
Hypertensive heart disease	5.2	6.1	4.3	4.0	17.2
Hypertension with or without renal disease	2.3	2.5	2.1	1.8	6.9
Malignant neoplasms	127.9	153.8	108.8	125.2	167.8
Malignant neoplasms of respiratory and intrathoracic organs	39.3	54.2	27.5	38.9	48.9
Malignant neoplasms of digestive organ	28.5	36.7	21.8	27.0	42.4
Malignant neoplasm of breast			20.2	19.8*	26.5*
Malignant neoplasm of genital organs	12.5	15.3	11.4	11.7	21.6
Cerebrovascular diseases (strokes)	26.4	28.5	24.6	24.5	44.2
Chronic obstructive pulmonary diseases	21.0	25.9	17.6	21.5	17.8
Diabetes mellitus	13.6	14.9	12.5	12.0	28.8
Suicide	10.8	18.0	4.0	11.6	6.6

*Females only

Source: Peters, Kochanek, and Murphy 1998.

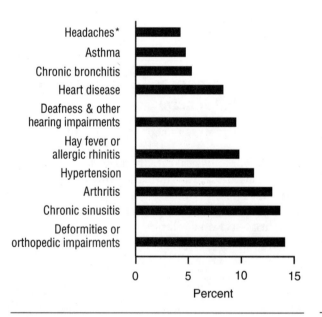

Figure 9.3 Top 10 chronic conditions with highest prevalence rate in rank order, United States, 1990-1992 (*excludes tension headaches).
Source: Collins 1997.

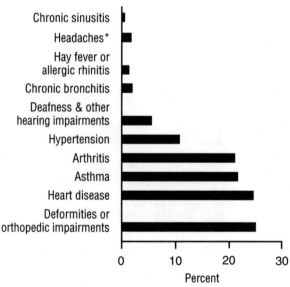

Figure 9.4 Selected reported chronic conditions with highest prevalence, by percent, causing limitation in major or outside activity, United States, 1990-1992 (*excludes tension headaches).
Source: Collins 1997.

Physically active men have significantly larger coronary artery luminal areas, less frequent complete or nearly complete coronary occlusions, and less ischemic myocardial damage than less active workers (Leon and Norstrom 1995).

To be effective in preventing coronary heart disease, exercise must be habitual, maintained, and current. Engaging in school athletics does not protect against heart disease later in life. There is good evidence that coronary atherosclerosis originates in adolescence, if not earlier. Because it is associated with a decrease in CHD, physical activity is today's best buy in public health—especially when one considers the relatively small investment of time, effort, and money that moderate-intensity physical activity requires. Physical activity also provides indirect benefits by reducing other risk factors such as hypertension, hyperlipidemia, diabetes, and obesity (Haskell 1995; Morris 1994).

Some Landmark Studies

At a 1995 National Institutes of Health conference, an expert panel agreed that the burden of cardiovascular disease (CVD) and other chronic diseases rests most heavily on the least active (NIH 1996). This association of physical inactivity with cardiovascular disease is independent of blood pressure, smoking, and blood lipid levels. Many studies have observed that physical activity has a negative association with body fat and a positive association with high-density lipoprotein. Moderately intense physical activity— that need be neither vigorous nor in a structured program—apparently provides the majority of the preventive benefits of physical activity. The greatest difference in risk is between those people who do almost nothing and those who regularly perform a moderate amount of exercise. A much smaller risk differential is observed between moderately active and the most active individuals (Bijnen et al. 1996; Haskell 1995; Lakka and Salonen 1993; NIH 1996).

A meta-analysis by Berlin and Colditz (1990) showed that the negative correlation between exercise and cardiovascular disease is generally stronger when one compares high-activity groups with sedentary groups rather than with moderately active groups—findings that support a dose-response relationship between physical activity and reduced risk of coronary heart disease.

Physical activity protects both men and women from CVD. Folsom et al. (1997) examined the relationship between physical activity and the incidence of coronary heart disease in middle-aged women and men from the Atherosclerosis Risk in Community

Study (ARIC), tracking a bir[...] aged adults over a 4- to 7-yea[...] cluded 7,852 women and 6,18[...] who were free of CHD at bas[...] ticipation in sports, leisure p[...] of work-related physical activi[...] age, race, ARIC field center[...] rette smoking, alcohol, and (i[...] placement therapy, the sports and leisure indexes were inversely related to both CHD and total mortality. Physical activity during work was not associated with a protective role against coronary heart disease. The findings also confirmed that physical activity can be effective in preventing coronary heart disease among women.

Postmenopausal women can lower their risk of nonfatal myocardial infarction by being more physically active. Lamaitre et al. (1995) compared women who had sustained a nonfatal myocardial infarction (n = 268) to a random sample of women (n = 925) enrolled in the same health maintenance organization, matched by age and calendar year between 1986 and 1991. Women who engaged in modest leisure-time energy expenditures, equivalent to 30 to 45 minutes of walking three times a week, had approximately 50% fewer myocardial infarctions.

Mechanisms of Heart Disease Prevention and Exercise

The biological mechanisms through which physical activity mediates its positive effects appear to be the following:

1. Reduction in severity of coronary atherosclerosis both directly and through favorable effects on other major coronary risk factors (body composition, blood pressure, HDLs, insulin sensitivity, and glucose tolerance)

2. Reduction in myocardial oxygen demands at rest and during submaximal physical effort, evidenced by decreased heart rate and systolic blood pressure

3. Increased myocardial oxygen supply through lengthening of diastole, slowed heart rate, and/ or increased vascularization

4. Reduction in risk of coronary thrombosis by decreased platelet adhesiveness and aggregability and by promotion of fibrinolysis

5. Reduced myocardial vulnerability to lethal ventricular arrhythmias in the presence of advanced coronary atherosclerosis, even during heavy physical exertion (Leon and Norstrom 1995; USDHHS 1996)

…e previous studies have shown that physical activity exerts an independent effect in the prevention of coronary heart disease. However, physical activity indirectly ameliorates other coronary risk factors, leading to decreased hypertension, more favorable body composition, more favorable blood lipid profile (including lowered levels of plasma triglycerides and their lipoprotein carriers), and improvements in cell insulin sensitivity and glucose tolerance (Andersen and Haraldsdottir 1995; Bijnen et al. 1996; Leon 1991).

Exercise in the Prevention of Hypertensive Disease

Moderate-intensity physical activity, such as brisk walking, 30-45 minutes most days of the week can help prevent and treat hypertension (National High Blood Pressure Education Program, JNC VI 1997). Cross-sectional data from the civilian noninstitutionalized population of the United States show a substantial reduction in the prevalence of hypertension among those who are active most days of the week, as compared with those who engage in no leisure-time physical activity (Crespo and Roccella 1997).

Studies on Blood Pressure and Exercise

Several longitudinal studies have confirmed the trend of higher hypertension among those less physically active. Paffenbarger and colleagues (1983) studied approximately 15,000 Harvard University alumni and found that those who were inactive had a 35% greater risk of developing hypertension than their more active counterparts. In a study of approximately 6,000 men and women, Blair et al. (1984) observed that people with low fitness levels were 1.52 (95% CI, 1.08-2.15) times as likely to develop hypertension than those with high fitness levels.

Folsom et al. (1990) reported on the longitudinal effect of physical activity among more than 41,000 women, ages 55-69 years. After a two-year follow-up, incidence of physician-diagnosed hypertension was inversely associated with physical activity; however, after adjustment for body mass index, waist-to-hip ratio, cigarette smoking, and age, this association disappeared. The consistent pattern among these studies is the association of physical *in*activity with higher risks of developing hypertension. Unfortunately, no longitudinal study has tested the protective role of physical activity in minority populations, who consistently exhibit a disproportionate risk of developing and dying from hypertension.

Confounding Factors

The effect of exercise on blood pressure can be confounded by changes in body composition and improvements in psychosocial behaviors. Comparing a sedentary population with 571 men and 430 women who had enrolled in a vigorous fitness program, Sedgwick and colleagues (1993) examined the effect of physical fitness on blood pressure and lipid profile over a period of four years. They observed almost no *direct* effect of exercise on either blood pressure or lipids, except for a weak correlation among the women. Almost all the positive effects could be explained by changes in body composition.

Mechanisms of Reducing Blood Pressure and Exercise

The mechanisms by which physical activity lowers blood pressure are complicated (ACSM 1993). There is consensus that physical activity not only is effective in *treating* hypertension, but also provides significant benefits in *preventing* hypertension. Some researchers believe that, in addition to its effect on body weight, chronic exercise training attenuates sympathetic nervous system activity—which in turn may decrease the activity of the renin-angiotensin system, reset baroreceptors, or promote arterial vasodilation, as thought by some researchers. Another hypothesis involves the effect of exercise on insulin sensitivity and circulating insulin levels: if exercise reduces insulin or prevents hyperinsulinemia, the kidneys presumably would reduce insulin-mediated sodium reabsorption (USDHHS 1996).

Exercise and the Prevention of Stroke

Stroke is the third leading cause of death in the United States (see table 9.1) and one of the most disabling diseases affecting working Americans. Major risk factors for ischemic stroke include cigarette smoking and high blood pressure, while for hemorrhagic stroke high blood pressure seems to be the predominant risk factor. Figure 9.5 shows the steady decline in the percent of deaths due to stroke ("cerebrovascular accidents") in the United States since 1972. We can attribute part of this decline to decreases in the number of persons with high blood pressure, and, perhaps, to the reduction

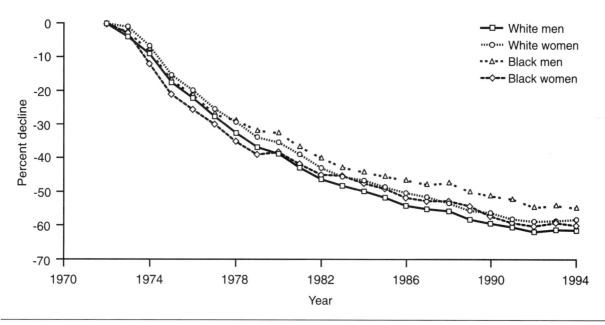

Figure 9.5   Percent decline in age-adjusted mortality rates for stroke by sex and race, United States, 1972-1994. *Source:* U.S. National Vital Statistics, 1972-1994: CDC, NCHS.

in cigarette smoking that have occurred during the same period.

Kiely and colleagues (1994) prospectively examined the effect of physical activity on the risk of stroke for participants in the Framingham Study. They performed two separate analyses involving 1,897 men and 2,299 women with mean ages of around 49 years, and again when the cohorts were around 63 years of age (1,361 men and 1,862 women), calculating a physical activity index for leisure-time and occupational physical activities. The authors concluded that increased levels of physical activity offer a unique independent protective effect in men. It is possible that the women, the majority of whom were housewives, underestimated the level of physical activity associated with their housework and related activities.

Investigators found an inverse association for all strokes and subtypes in a longitudinal study of older Japanese men (ages 55-68 years) from the Honolulu Heart Program (Abbot et al. 1994), particularly in nonsmoking men. Among smokers, however, physical activity did not appear to reduce the risk of thromboembolic stroke. The incidence of hemorrhagic stroke was three- to fourfold greater among inactive older men than among their active counterparts. Wannamethee and Shaper reported in 1992 that moderate-intensity exercise—such as frequent walking and recreational activity, or weekly sporting activity—reduces the risk of stroke and heart attacks in men both with and without pre-existing ischemic

heart disease. More vigorous activity did not confer any further protection. Lindsted et al. (1991) assessed mortality due to stroke in Seventh Day Adventists. Based on a baseline assessment of physical activity in 1960, the authors observed a nonlinear "U shape" association between physical activity and risk of stroke. This nonlinear association was based on classifications of low, moderate, and high activity levels, where the lowest risk was observed among those in the moderate category and higher risk was observed in the low and high activity categories. At the very least, these studies suggest in aggregate that moderate-intensity physical activity may confer a primary preventive effect against strokes; and that high-intensity physical activity appears to offer little more or no more benefit than moderate activity (or perhaps even can be harmful, according to the Linsted paper).

Exercise and Some Emerging Risk Factors for Heart Disease

A reduction in plasma fibrinogen is one mechanism through which physical activity may protect against coronary heart disease. Several studies have associated fibrinogen with increased risk of heart disease. In 1993, Lakka and Salonen reported the effect of conditioning leisure-time physical activity and cardiorespiratory fitness on plasma fibrinogen concentration in smokers and nonsmokers from the Kuopio

Ischemic Heart Disease Risk Factor Study. Plasma fibrinogen was lower among men whose activity intensity averaged more than 4 METs than among men with less intensive physical activity. Durations of the most intensive activities, such as jogging and skiing, were inversely associated with plasma fibrinogen, as was maximal oxygen uptake. The effect was even more pronounced among smokers. These findings suggest that moderate-intensity physical activity is sufficient, but vigorous physical activity is more effective, in reducing fibrinogen; and that physical activity vigorous enough to elevate maximal oxygen uptake has the strongest effect in decreasing plasma fibrinogen. The researchers found no relationship, however, between weekly sessions of vigorous exercise and plasma fibrinogen.

Exercise can also prevent heart disease by inducing adaptations of myocardial blood vessels, such as the development of new capillaries and coronary arterioles (Laughlin 1994; Leon and Norstrom 1995). Niebauer and Cooke (1996) suggested that exercise is associated positively with nitric oxide and prostacyclin, and eventually with reducing the generation of superoxide anions, adherence of monocytes, aggregation of platelets, and proliferation of vascular smooth muscle.

Exercise and Prevention of Peripheral Artery Disease

Peripheral artery disease, characterized by the inability of the circulatory system to deliver oxygenated blood to the limbs, limits activity by decreasing the total cross-sectional area of vascular flow. Housley et al. (1993) examined the protective effects of physical activity on peripheral arterial disease in 1,592 men and women, ages 55-74 years, from the Edinburgh Artery Study in Scotland. The authors queried the subjects about their participation in moderate and strenuous physical activity between the ages of 35 and 45, and compared those histories to physical activity habits at time of the survey. Decreasing levels of the ankle brachial pressure index were associated with increased severity of peripheral artery disease. The amount of leisure-time physical activity at 35-45 years showed good correlation with the amount of physical activity at time of the survey, although activity was slightly less at ages 55-74. In women, higher levels of exercise at ages 35-45 correlated with higher current alcohol intake and higher HDL concentrations, and with lower plasma fibrinogen and blood viscosity at ages 55-74. Similar results were observed among men, in conjunction with smoking fewer cigarettes—

a major independent risk factor for peripheral artery disease. Multiple regression analysis showed that the association of increased ankle brachial pressure index with exercise was most noticeable in men who had at some time in their lives smoked. In men and women who had never smoked, there was no significant association between leisure-time physical activity and the change in mean ankle brachial pressure index after correcting for the other risk factors. Thus, among men who had smoked, leisure-time physical activity seems to exert a protective effect against the development of peripheral artery disease later in life (Housley et al. 1993).

Exercise and the Prevention of Diabetes Mellitus

One of the most important modifiable risk factors for primary prevention of type 2 (non-insulin-dependent) diabetes is physical inactivity. Most of the direct effect of physical activity in preventing type 2 diabetes occurs because exercise normalizes blood glucose by decreasing insulin resistance and improving insulin sensitivity. Examining the effect of exercise on glucose tolerance and insulin sensitivity, Heath et al. (1983) found that active individuals had better insulin and glucose profiles than their inactive counterparts. Several studies have shown that exercise training can improve insulin action or decrease insulin resistance, especially among persons at high risk for diabetes or those with hyperinsulinemia.

Significant Studies

Considerable evidence supports the independent effect of physical inactivity in the development of type 2 diabetes. Cross-sectional, longitudinal, and retrospective studies have consistently shown that physically active individuals are less likely to develop diabetes than physically inactive people. Groups of people who migrated to societies with more sedentary lifestyles had higher prevalences of type 2 diabetes than their ethnic counterparts who remained in their native land (Hara et al. 1983; Kawate et al. 1979; Ravussin et al. 1994). Similar findings were observed among urban and rural residents (Cruz-Vidal et al. 1979; Taylor et al. 1983). In a case-control study, Kaye and colleagues (1991) found that women who reported high levels of physical activity were half as likely to develop type 2 diabetes as were women in the same age range with low levels of physical activity.

Moderately active women also enjoyed the protective effect of physical activity, but to a lesser extent.

Manson et al. (1991) reported a protective effect against type 2 diabetes among female nurses who reported being vigorously active one or more times per week, as compared to less active female nurses. Since the assessment of activity in this study consisted of only one question—about participation in *vigorous* physical activity—the authors could say nothing about *moderate* physical activity. Similar findings were observed with male physicians (Manson et al. 1992).

In another prospective study, Helmrich and colleagues (1994) expanded their assessment of leisure-time physical activity to include walking, stair climbing, and participation in sports. They observed an inverse correlation between physical activity and incidence of type 2 diabetes; the reduced likelihood of type 2 diabetes was more clearly manifested among men with a high body mass index (BMI), a history of high blood pressure, or a parental history of diabetes. For every 500 kilocalories per week of leisure-time physical activity, the authors reported a 6% reduction in the risk of developing type 2 diabetes. Furthermore, among this group of male college graduates, the protective effect of physical activity was greater among those who participated in vigorous sports than among those who obtained their physical activity mostly from climbing stairs or walking.

In these three prospective studies, two—those involving men—found a dose-response relationship. Although female nurses who participated one or more times per week in vigorous physical activity had a significantly reduced likelihood of developing type 2 diabetes, the Manson study failed to show a dose-response relationship.

Most Effective Physical Activities for Diabetes Prevention

What type of physical activity is most effective for preventing type 2 diabetes? (Aerobic activities—such as brisk walking, biking, swimming, or other activities that use large muscle mass—probably best for the general public because of their demonstrated benefits in decreasing both type 2 diabetes and cardiovascular risk factors. This recommendation, however, is based on epidemiological data that examined the specific benefits of aerobic physical activities or cardiorespiratory fitness on primary prevention of type 2 diabetes. Strength training, as part of an overall exercise training program that includes aerobic activity, can also provide acute benefits to improve glucose tolerance and insulin sensitivity in individuals with

both normal and abnormal glucose tolerance (Kriska 1997; Smutok et al. 1994). These studies suggest that high levels of physical activity or vigorous-intensity aerobic activity are more likely to effect the necessary metabolic changes to prevent type 2 diabetes than lower- or moderate-intensity exercises. Light- and moderate-intensity physical activities, however, are easier to incorporate into people's lifestyles, are less likely to result in injury, and (if the population is mostly sedentary) are more likely to be maintained for life) It is not certain if lower-intensity activities will help prevent type 2 diabetes in women, since no dose-response relationship has been observed for them. But given the dose-response data for men, one can assume that light to moderate levels of activity will at least provide some protection. In this case, more is better.

Another benefit of regular physical activity is its effect on body composition. National cross-sectional data indicate that over 60% of people with type 2 diabetes are obese at the time of diagnosis (Diabetes Data Group 1995). Obesity and (probably more importantly) central fat distribution seem to be additional primary risk factors for development of type 2 diabetes. Because increased adiposity in the abdominal (as opposed to the peripheral) area boosts the likelihood that individuals will develop insulin resistance, it is strongly involved in the pathogenesis of type 2 diabetes. Numerous studies have shown the ability of exercise to affect body weight. Physical activity appears to prevent type 2 diabetes not only by decreasing adiposity—it also acutely affects insulin resistance and glucose tolerance. Much of the effect of physical activity appears to be due to the metabolic adaptation of skeletal muscle, suggesting that exercise training helps prevent type 2 diabetes by increasing sensitivity to insulin. More specifically, it appears that physical activity is more likely to improve abnormal glucose tolerance when the abnormality is caused primarily by insulin resistance than when it is caused by deficient amounts of circulating insulin (Kriska 1997).

Exercise and Primary Prevention of Cancer

Cancer, from which deaths are increasing every year (Peters et al. 1998), is the second leading cause of death in the United States and is also responsible for many days spent in hospital care (Lee 1995). Although the etiologic factors are highly variable, certain cancers are associated with certain behaviors or lifestyles—usually identified through epidemiological studies and not because we have discovered any plausible mechanisms of action. Of course everyone is aware that lung cancer is directly associated with the cancer-causing agents found in cigarettes. Other behaviors associated with different cancers include excess alcohol consumption, diet, and physical inactivity.

Anti-Cancer Benefits of Exercise

Our immune systems largely regulate our susceptibility to cancer. We have evidence that engaging in moderately intense physical activity can enhance our immune capabilities (Nieman and Nehlsen-Cannarella 1992; Nieman et al. 1995). On the other hand, higher-intensity physical activities, such as running a marathon, appear to suppress the immune system. There seems to be a threshold in the duration and intensity of physical activity that determines whether it will enhance or compromise the immune system.

Other indirect benefits of active lifestyles in protection against site-specific cancers are reduced body fat, increased adrenergic activity, and the inverse association between smoking and aerobic activities.

Significant Studies

Physical activity has been inversely associated with cancer mortality. Wannamethee and colleagues reported in 1993 on the relationship between resting heart rate, usual physical activity, and cancer mortality in 7,735 men from the British Regional Heart Study. Men were followed for approximately 9.5 years and classified into three physical activity categories. Resting heart rate provided the basis for five categories: <60 bpm, 60-69 bpm, 70-79 bpm, 80-89 bpm, and >90 bpm. Lower resting heart rates were correlated with higher levels of physical activity, and with lower cancer mortality rates.

Steenland et al. (1995) reported an inverse association between pulse and cancer mortality in the general population. The data for this study came from the National Health and Nutrition Survey I Follow-Up conducted in the early 1970s and then repeated in 1987. The authors found a modest positive trend between heart rate (highest quartile compared to lowest quartile) and all cancers for men, but not for women. They observed no significant effect for nonrecreational physical activity. The authors caution that lack of participation in nonrecreational physical activity may be an artifact of an existing condition that limits physical activity.

Current research certainly does not justify claims that physical activity can affect all kinds of cancer mortality; however, the observed inverse correlation between low resting heart rates and cancer mortality could be an indicator of a general inverse association between physical fitness and cancer. We need more data.

Colon Cancer

Earlier studies examining the association between physical activity and cancer of the intestinal tract combined data for colon and rectal cancers. We know now that the effect of exercise on colon cancer may be different from that on rectal cancer (USDHHS 1996). The presence of adenomatous polyps in the colon and rectum are believed to be precursors of colorectal cancers. Sandler and colleagues (1995) reported that the risk of developing colorectal adenomatous polyps was inversely associated with physical activity.

Most of the research on physical activity and colon cancer has focused on occupational physical activity, with the majority of studies showing that this type of activity plays a protective role against developing colon cancer. Of the 18 studies described in the Surgeon General's Report in 1996 (USDHHS 1996), 14 reported a statistically significant inverse relationship between occupational physical activity and the risk of colon cancer. More recently Kiningham (1998) reviewed 36 studies of men and 21 studies of women, and concluded that physically active men appear to have about half the colon cancer risk of sedentary men. The relationship between women's physical activity and colon cancer was less clear than that observed in men. Many of the studies reviewed included few women with high or moderately high levels of physical activity, so the statistical power to distinguish a difference between activity groups was low. Nevertheless, the bulk of the data suggested a trend toward decreased risk with increased activity in both men and women.

Significant Studies

Some researchers have done more carefully designed assessments of leisure-time physical activity or total physical activity in longitudinal or retrospective studies. Most studies show inverse relationships between physical activity and colon cancer.

A case-control Swedish study of 163 men and 189 women, who had been diagnosed with colon cancer, along with 512 matched controls, obtained from a computerized registry of the population of Stockholm County, examined the relationships of occupational and leisure-time physical activity with incidence of colon cancer. Cases were obtained from various hospitals in Stockholm County and from the regional cancer registry. The researchers assessed dietary intake of fiber, fat, protein, browned meat surface, and total energy (Gerhardsson et al. 1990), and stratified participants by levels of leisure-time and occupational physical activity. After adjusting for age, body mass index, and diet, the authors observed a higher incidence of colon cancer in the lower than in the higher physical activity group. There was, in fact, a dose-response relationship between increased levels of physical activity and lower risk of colon cancer.

Giovannucci and colleagues (1995) evaluated data from 47,723 men aged 40-75 years, recording weekly participation in leisure-time physical activity and risk of cancer. The investigators used a recreational physical activity index to stratify individuals into quintiles, from least active to most active. This study was unique in that the investigators were able to control for history of endoscopic screening or any diagnosis of polyp, as well as dietary components. Not only did the most active quintile have the lowest incidence of colon cancer, but there was also an inverse dose-response relationship between physical activity and incidence of colon cancer.

Conclusions About Exercise and Colon Cancer

Substantial evidence shows that physical activity—after adjusting for family history; for dietary intake of fat, fiber and total energy; and in some instances for presence of polyps—is inversely related to colon cancer. It is impossible to determine the most beneficial kind of physical activity, since researchers did not design their projects for that purpose. Studies on occupational physical activity, in spite of their crudeness, do suggest that occupations with higher energy expenditure enjoy a protective benefit against the development of colon cancer.

In studies of leisure-time physical activity, the protective effect seems to occur among those engaged in higher levels of physical activity. Besides the direct effects that physical activity has on the immune system, the following mechanisms may partially explain the indirect benefits of exercise in preventing of colon cancer:

1. **Shortened intestinal transit time**—most likely because higher-intensity exercises increase peristaltic movement.

2. **Decreased body fat**—abdominal obesity and high-fat diets are risk factors for colon cancer.

3. **Secretion of F-series prostaglandins**—these have been associated with increased gut motility and decreased rates of colonic cell division.

4. **Reduced hyperinsulinemia**—insulin is a growth factor for colonic mucosal cells; and any factor that increases insulin levels may increase colon cancer risk (Kingham 1998).

Suggestions for Future Research

We need the ability to assess physical activity more precisely in order to determine the intensities, frequencies, and durations that more effectively prevent chronic diseases. Using job titles to estimate occupational physical activity is hardly satisfactory. Furthermore, given that cancer is a complex disease with multiple etiologic factors, we have yet to solve the problem of controlling for multiple factors—e.g., diet, environmental carcinogens, and socioeconomic status—that are important in evaluating the evidence of a protective effect of physical activity against colon cancer.

Longitudinal studies would benefit from multiple assessments of physical activity throughout individuals' lives. Additionally, the complexities in both the etiology and the development of colon cancer call for careful analyses of intakes of dietary fiber, alcohol, tobacco smoke, fat, and total energy—and also for controls relating to family histories of adenomatous polyps and colon cancer. Few, if any, studies to date have properly assessed all of these confounding factors.

Rectal Cancer

As previously explained, earlier studies of physical activity and cancer of the digestive tract usually combined data for colon and rectal cancer. Most recent studies on rectal cancer failed to report a consistent protective effect of physical activity. Although researchers have reported both positive and negative correlations between occupational physical activity and the risk of developing rectal cancer, most studies have observed no relationship one way or the other. Researchers with more precise measurements of leisure-time and total physical activity found inconclusive results (Giovannucci et al. 1995; Lee et al. 1991). It appears from current research that neither occupational nor leisure-time physical activity affect rectal cancer (USDHHS 1996).

Breast Cancer

More women are diagnosed with breast cancer every year than with any other cancer. It is true that effective treatment, early detection, and modification of risk factors have decreased mortality rates due to breast cancer in recent years—yet breast cancer is still the leading cancer killer after lung cancer. Epidemiological data have suggested that obesity, fat intake, nulliparity, and full-term pregnancy after age 35 years are possible risk factors.

Significant Studies

Frisch et al. (1985) described an independent and inverse correlation between physical activity and breast cancer. They contacted more than 5,300 alumnae from 10 colleges or universities who attended their respective institutions between the years of 1925 and 1981. About half of these women were former athletes, who were matched by a random sample of nonathletes from the same schools. Nonathletes were 86% more likely to develop breast cancer than their athlete counterparts, even after controlling for traditional risk factors.

Some research, however, has found a positive relationship between physical activity and breast cancer. Dorgan and colleagues (1994) found that women in the highest quartile of physical activity were more likely to develop breast cancer than women in the lowest quartile. The researchers followed more than 2,300 women in the Framingham Heart Study for approximately 30 years, finally observing that physically active women had 1.6 times the breast cancer risk of those in the least active quartile. This study had the advantage of periodic examinations and adjustments for several confounding factors. However, lack of additional assessments of physical activity after 1954 may not accurately describe secular trends in physical activity among women during these years.

More recently, Chen et al. (1997) found that leisure-time physical activity either during adolescence or in adulthood played no protective role against breast cancer. For this study the investigators selected 747 women aged 21-45 years from the Seattle-Puget Sound Surveillance, Epidemiology, and End Results registry who had developed breast cancer and matched them with 961 women from the same area who were free from cancer and otherwise healthy. Leisure-time physical activity was assessed for the two-year period immediately prior to the time of diagnosis, and for the period when the participants had been between the ages of 12 and 21 years. Breast cancer was associated with neither frequency of partici-pation in physical activity, nor hours per week engaged in physical activity, nor METs per week, whether before diagnosis or during adolescent years.

Other retrospective case-control studies have observed a protective role of exercise against breast cancer. Apter (1996) examined 537 women aged 50-64 years and matched them with 492 randomly selected women. This time Apter found that, compared to women who reported no exercise, there was a slightly decreased risk of breast cancer in women who exercised more than 1.5 hours per week in the two years before the diagnosis of breast cancer. There was no association between the risk of breast cancer and intensity of exercise at ages 12-21 years.

Bernstein et al. (1994) studied 545 women aged 40 years or younger who had been diagnosed with breast cancer, and compared them with a control group of 545 healthy women from the same neighborhood matched according to age, race, and parity history. The investigators recorded the hours per week each woman engaged in leisure-time physical activity after reaching menarche, and classified the women into five categories of physical activity. Women who spent 3.8 hours per week of leisure-time physical activity were less likely (OR = 0.42, 95% CI, 0.27-0.64) to develop cancer than women who engaged in no leisure-time physical activity (all other known risk factors being controlled). There was a dose-response relationship, with higher weekly amounts of physical activity related to lower risks of developing breast cancer. The authors concluded that participation in physical activity after menarche is protective against breast cancer.

Mezzetti et al. (1998) examined the effects of diet and physical exercise on breast cancer risks in 2,569 Italian women, aged 23-74 years. The experimenters stratified women by menopausal status (pre- and post-), age, education, body mass index, and alcohol intake. Physical exercise included self-reported intensity of activity at work and during leisure time. Women with low levels of physical exercise had 50% higher risk of developing breast cancer than women who were highly active. The protective effect of physical exercise was stronger among post- than among premenopausal women. In women less than 45 years old, Gammon and colleagues (1998) found that physical activity had no protective role against breast cancer. These women reported the intensity and frequency of physical activity during three different time periods that were relevant to two possible biological mechanisms. The authors did not observe a reduced risk of breast cancer among young women with increased recreational physical activity in adolescence, in young adulthood, or during the year prior to interviews.

Findings from longitudinal, case-control, and retrospective studies are inconclusive concerning the effect of physical activity in preventing breast cancer (Lee 1995; USDHHS 1996). Major problems in some of these epidemiologic studies include crude and incomplete measurements of physical activity and inadequate control for potential confounding factors (Friedenreich and Rohan 1995). Designs of these studies also failed to accurately account for the duration, frequency, and intensity of the physical activity, making it very difficult at present to suggest what type, duration, frequency, or intensity is more protective against breast cancer.

The existence of protective effects is certainly biologically plausible. Exercise can modify production and metabolism of estrogen and progesterone, which are known to affect the development of breast cancer. Other possible mechanisms could involve the effect of physical activity on menstrual cycle, body fat, and fat distribution.

Bernstein et al. (1987) studied the effects of moderate-intensity physical activity on the menstrual cycle, and found that adolescent girls who engaged in moderate physical activity had a threefold increase in the likelihood of an anovulatory menstrual cycle. Expenditure of more than 750 kcal of energy per week was associated with menstrual cycles that averaged 2.4 days shorter than those of less physically active girls (Bernstein et al. 1987). These results suggest that moderate physical activity during adolescence might also reduce breast cancer risk by delaying menarche, reducing the number of ovulatory cycles, and thereby reducing a woman's cumulative exposure to ovarian hormones (Kiningham 1998). The inverse relationship between physical activity and obesity in older women suggests the possibility that the protective role is associated with age at menopause (Friedenreich and Rohan 1995).

Conclusions About Exercise and Breast Cancer

More often than not, researchers have reported positive correlations between exercise and lower rates of breast cancer. Differences in methodological design may be responsible for the inconsistent results—some studies found the opposite. At present, there are inconclusive results to suggest that moderate-intensity confers better protection than vigorous-intensity physical activity. Exercise early and later in life may alter the ages of menarche and menopause, respectively—both of which may in turn affect breast cancer rates. Other

possible mechanisms of action include reductions in endogenous steroid exposure, alterations in menstrual cycle patterns, increased energy expenditure, reduction in body weight, changes in insulin-like and other growth factors, and enhancement of natural immune mechanisms (Hoffman-Goetz et al. 1998)

Prostate Cancer

Physicians diagnose approximately 165,000 new cases of prostate cancer each year, making it the most frequently diagnosed cancer among men. The prevalence of this cancer varies considerably from one racial group to another—blacks in the United States have one of the highest, if not the highest, rates of prostate cancer in the world. Treatment for this disease can be very disabling. As with breast cancer, the relationship between physical activity and prostate cancer is inconclusive.

Significant Studies

Of the 10 epidemiologic studies of cardiorespiratory fitness, leisure-time activity, or total physical activity reviewed in the Surgeon General's Report (USDHHS 1996), only five observed a benefit of physical activity for reducing risk of prostate cancer. Few studies have found a significant negative association, where increased physical activity increases the risk. Research examining the relationship between occupational physical activity and prostate cancer has found no significant association in either direction. Lee and colleagues (1992) reported on the incidence of prostate cancer in a longitudinal cohort of 17,719 men aged 30-79 years. They observed a protective effect for men whose age was 70 years or more and who expended 4,000 kcal or more per week, compared to men who expended less than 1,000 kcal per week. For younger men, however, there was no significant association between exercise level and the risk of prostate cancer.

Between 1971 and 1989 Oliveira et al. (1996) studied the association between cardiorespiratory fitness and prostate cancer in nearly 13,000 men from the the Aerobics Institute in Dallas. These men, aged 20-80 years, underwent a preventive medical examination that included an exercise treadmill test to estimate cardiorespiratory fitness, and at different intervals provided (via questionnaires) information on physical activity and prostate cancer. Stratifying the subjects by quartile of cardiorespiratory fitness and controlling for age, body mass index, and smoking habits, the investigators observed a protective effect of cardiorespiratory fitness among participants who were younger than 60 years. Participation in physical activity (self-reported via questionnaire) was also inversely associated with prostate cancer in all participants. Those who spent 3,000 kcal/week on exercise had lower risk (RR = 0.37, 95% CI, 0.14-0.98) of developing prostate cancer than those who spent less than 1,000 kcal/week.

Conclusions About Exercise and Prostate Cancer

Kiningham (1998) speculated that exercise could exert a suppressive effect on prostate cancer development by decreasing testosterone levels. Men with prostate cancer have higher levels of endogenous testosterone than men without the cancer, and aerobically trained men are reported to have lower testosterone levels than sedentary men (Kiningham 1998). However, the relationship between physical activity and sex hormone levels has not been studied as extensively in men as in women. It is also possible that exercise alters the metabolism of fat in a way that decreases its potential association with certain types of malignancies. We need more studies with better assessment of possible confounding factors such as smoking, sexual practices, alcohol consumption, measurements of circulating hormones, cardiorespiratory fitness, body composition, and improved physical activity.

Physical Activity and the Prevention of Osteoporosis and Falls

Osteoporosis is characterized by decreased bone mass and structural deterioration of the bone tissue, leading to bone fragility and increased susceptibility to fractures. It occurs most often among postmenopausal white women. Approximately 25 million Americans are currently afflicted with osteoporosis, with nearly 1.5 million fractures reported each year among people aged 45 years and older.

Risk factors for osteoporosis in the U.S. are many, the greatest being gender and age, i.e., being an older woman. More general risk factors are advanced age, early menopause, premenopausal removal of the ovaries, being Caucasian, being of Asian ethnicity, use of steroids, prolonged bed rest, menstrual irregularity,

anorexia nervosa, and family history. Decreased risk is found with heavy exercise, African American ethnicity, being overweight, use of estrogen, and dietary calcium intake. We need more research on the apparently deleterious effects of alcohol intake, cigarette smoking, use of thiazide diuretics, and excess caffeine intake, and the apparent benefits of fluoridated water and participation in moderate-intensity physical activity (USDHHS 1991).

Exercise and Osteoporosis

It is well established that bones adapt to the stresses imposed upon them through exercise training, heavy lifting, occupational work, or even housework. The effect of exercise in the primary *prevention* of osteoporosis is not as well documented as its effect in the *treatment* of osteoporosis, partially because it is difficult and costly to design studies for this purpose. Nevertheless, several investigators (Conroy et al. 1993; Grimston et al. 1993; Kirchner et al. 1996; Nichols et al. 1994; Rubin et al. 1993) have found that children who engaged in weightbearing or high-impact sports had greater bone density than children involved in swimming or low-impact sports. This observation has significance for public health, since achieving peak bone mass during physical maturity can affect development of osteoporosis later in life. It is troubling that children are more inactive now than they were in previous generations, and that girls engage in less physical activity than boys (Andersen et al. 1998; USDHHS 1996)—in fact, women of all ages are less physically active (especially in vigorous activity) than men (Crespo et al. 1996).

For exercise to produce long-term protection against age-related bone loss, it must be maintained for life. For example, Dalsky et al. (1988) had women exercise between 70% to 90% of their $\dot{V}O_2$max 3 times per week for 50-60 minutes. At the end of the study, lumbar bone mineral content increased 6%; yet after little more than a year of no exercise, the lumbar bone mineral content fell by 5%.

Lifetime physical activity is related to bone mineral density, but not to the incidence of osteoporotic fractures. In a long-term study, Greendale et al. (1995) measured bone mineral density of 1,014 women and 689 men. Exercise habits were calculated beginning in the teenage years, at around 30 years of age, again at around 50 years, and finally at approximately 73 years of age. Bone mineral density in the hip was greater in the current and lifelong recreational exercisers than in those who engaged in mild or no exercise. Yet the authors found no protective effect of exercise against osteoporotic fractures in older men and women.

Exercise and the Prevention of Falls

Physical activity may help prevent falls and fractures among older persons. One component of physical fitness is balance, which has a favorable impact on the prevention of falls (Province et al. 1995). Improved muscle strength certainly can reduce the risk of falls and fractures—and the decline in muscle strength in older persons is correlated with a loss of balance and subsequently with an increased rate of falls (Judge et al. 1994). It also appears that increased strength of the muscles that produce ankle dorsiflexion can protect against falls (Lord et al. 1991).

Both endurance exercise and strength training exercise have potential benefits in preventing osteoporosis, falls, and fractures. Strength training reduces muscle weakness associated with loss of balance and increased falls; moreover, weightbearing endurance training can help maintain bone mineral density and overall cardiorespiratory fitness.

Exercise in the Prevention of Arthritis

Arthritis is one of the most prevalent chronic diseases. Osteoarthritis, the most common form of arthritis, is characterized by degeneration of cartilage and new growth of bone around the joint. In older persons, arthritis is responsible for more days of limited activity than any other disease; and it is one of the most cited reasons for disability (see figure 9.6). More than 60% of women over the age of 75 report that they have arthritis (Collins 1997).

Running and other sports activities have not been associated with osteoarthritis in people who have not had joint injuries. The primary risk factors for osteoarthritis include joint trauma, obesity, and repetitive joint usage. Obesity can have a causal role in osteoarthritis of the knee. In longitudinal studies, obesity predicts the development of knee osteoarthritis in both men and women. Occupations that require excessive use of specific joints (e.g., bending the knees) are associated with knee osteoarthritis, while farming has been associated with hip osteoarthritis (Nieman 1996).

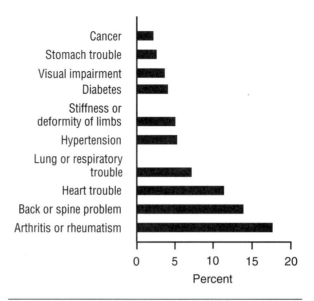

Figure 9.6 Percentage of persons aged 15+ years reporting selected conditions as the cause of their disability in the United States, 1991-1992.
Source: Centers for Disease Control and Prevention 1994.

Because joint trauma is one of the strongest predictors of osteoarthritis, it is difficult to determine whether contact sports or regular noncontact exercise is more effective in preventing osteoarthritis. Cross-sectional and cohort studies suggest that people involved in recreational running over long periods of time have no higher risk of developing osteoarthritis of the knee or the hip than people who engage in no leisure-time physical activity (Lane 1995; Panush et al. 1995) Competitive athletes who train at higher intensities, or compete in sports where specific joints are used excessively, carry the same risk of developing osteoarthritis as people whose occupations require repetitive use of certain joints. Lane et al. (1987) reported that long-distance runners aged 50-72 years had less physical disability and greater functional capacity than average members of the community. These runners sought medical services less often, weighed less, and experienced less musculoskeletal disability as they got older.

Some level of physical activity is necessary to preserve joint function. There is no conclusive evidence that physical activity either causes or prevents osteoarthritis. Injuries sustained in competitive or contact sports, however, can have a comparable effect to that of joint trauma, and thus increase the risk of osteoarthritis.) (Nieman 1996)

Exercise in the Prevention of Low Back Pain

Low back pain is one of the most prevalent conditions in the United States. Between 60% and 80% of U.S. adults have reported back pain at some time during their lives—and close to 50% reported having that pain within a given year (Lahad et al. 1994). Figure 9.6 shows that back or spine problems are among the most commonly cited reasons for disability among people aged 15 years or older in the United States, right after arthritis or rheumatism. Low back pain is usually temporary, however, and fewer than 10% of people suffering from low back pain become chronic sufferers (Collins 1997).

The most commonly cited prevention interventions in the literature are

- back flexion, back extension, and general fitness exercises;
- patient education on back mechanics and ergonomic techniques to prevent injury; and
- mechanical back supports (corsets).

Lahad et al. (1994) described three mechanisms by which exercise can prevent low back pain. First, exercise can strengthen the back muscles and increase trunk flexibility, preventing injury and decreasing its severity. Second, exercise can increase blood supply to the spine muscles and joints, and to intervertebral disks, minimizing the risk of injury and enhancing the body's natural healing and repair mechanisms. Third, exercise can improve mood and the perception of pain. Most of the studies reviewed by Lahad et al. reported that both exercise of trunk muscles and aerobic exercise were effective and mildly protective against future back pain. Exercise also helps prevent lower back pain by combating obesity, thereby reducing abdominal fat and its disproportionate strain in the lower back.

In summary, exercise—either in the form of aerobic exercise or strengthening of the trunk muscles—appears to be mildly protective against development of low back pain in asymptomatic individuals. Furthermore, exercise has been shown to improve psychological well-being and to reduce fatigue and stress.

Physical Activity and Primary Prevention of Obesity

Although there is plenty of literature about exercise in the *treatment* of obesity, only limited research has dealt with physical activity in the *primary prevention* of obesity. Americans are more overweight now than they have ever been (Kuczmarski et al. 1994). Whereas in 1976-1980 about 25% of Americans were overweight, by 1988-1994 the figure was approximately 33%. Using the new guidelines released by the National Obesity Education Initiative, almost half of the U.S. population is overweight (BMI ≥ 25) (NIH 1998). Currently about a quarter of the population does not engage in leisure-time physical activity—an estimate that has changed little since 1985 (Crespo et al. 1996). Reductions in other forms of physical activity can partially explain the increase in overweight. This section addresses physical activity in the *prevention* of excess weight, rather than in the treatment of obesity.

Both obese children and obese adults are less active than normal-weight people. Early studies had observed that obese children spent 40% less time engaging in physical activity than children who were not overweight. Furthermore, on average obese men walk about 3.7 miles per day (in the course of normal activities) compared to 6.0 miles for those of normal weight; and obese women walk approximately 2.0 miles per day compared to 4.9 miles for normal weight women (Bullen et al. 1964; Chirico and Stunkard 1960).

Ambiguity of the Evidence

In spite of the above-mentioned studies, few data exist to unequivocally suggest that physically active people are less likely to become obese than inactive people, i.e., that exercise *prevents* obesity. Cross-sectional studies reveal an inverse relationship (Andersen et al. 1998; Crespo and Wright 1995; DiPietro 1995)—physically active populations exhibit a lower prevalence of obesity than their physically inactive counterparts. Yet the evidence cannot accurately answer whether people are obese because they exercise less, or they exercise less because they are obese.

Ching et al. (1996) analyzed data from the Health Professionals Follow-Up Study, to examine if physical activity or watching TV has independent effects on becoming overweight. Between 1988 and 1990, close to 18,000 men between the ages of 40-75 had provided follow-up information. After adjusting for age and smoking status, the investigators found that more active men (highest quintile) were less likely to become overweight than men in the other four quintiles. Men in the higher third and fourth quintiles were also less likely to become overweight than those in the lowest (first) quintile of physical activity. Time spent watching TV was positively associated with overweight status. Thus, independent of TV watching, physical activity (either strenuous or moderate) conferred protective effects against becoming overweight in this sample of men, especially among those in the highest quintile of physical activity.

Children who spend more time in physical activity during physical education do not necessarily have less adipose tissue than children that engaged in less physical activity. Sallis and colleagues (1997) evaluated a health-related physical education program for fourth and fifth grade students, designed to increase the amount of physical activity in which children engage during their physical education period and also outside of school. In a quasi-experimental design, seven schools were randomly assigned to one of three conditions. The groups included (1) physical education classes led by an exercise specialist, (2) physical education led by a teacher, and (3) a control group that participated in the usual type of physical education for these seven schools. After two years of follow-up, the amount of time spent in physical activity increased significantly in the intervention groups compared to the control group—along with significant improvement in abdominal strength and endurance, and in cardiorespiratory endurance. Yet the intervention and control groups did not differ significantly in skinfold measurements or in participation in physical activities outside of school.

Even when physically active people continue to engage in high-intensity physical activity throughout their lives, exercise appears unable to prevent weight gain associated with aging. Dr. Paul T. Williams (1997) studied nearly 8,000 runners aged 18 years and older, monitoring them longitudinally and obtaining distance run per week through a questionnaire. This National Runners' Health Study classified the runners into five categories based on distance run in a given week: <16 km, 16-32 km, 32-48 km, 48-64 km, and >64 km. Williams observed that the rate of weight gain through middle age was the same in both shorter-distance and longer-distance runners, and concluded that physical activity guidelines either (1) should recommend substantial *increases* in activity over time, or (2) should use age-adjusted overweight standards. More to the point was the inability of a constant level of physical activity to prevent the age-related weight gain.

Suggestions for Further Research

We need more studies that can assess body weight, fat mass, sedentary activities, and physical activity prospectively in men and women, and in boys and

girls of different social classes. Obesity is a complex condition that responds to multiple cues from the environment and also has a genetic component that is not completely clear. The effect of culture, education, occupation, gender, marital status, and neighborhood safety are all key elements in the implementation of a physically active lifestyle.

Physical Activity and Psychological Well-Being

Some mental conditions are chronic, with complex etiologies. Itself a physical stressor, exercise raises blood pressure, perspiration, heart rate, blood sugars, body temperature, and oxygen supply, and stimulates the release of catecholamines. These changes in turn produce acute alterations in moods and mental states. Whether these acute physiological changes of physical activity are responsible for a preventive effect of exercise in maintaining good mental health over time is still unclear. Also, the type of physical activity people engage in seems to affect their moods differently. Recreational or leisure-time physical activities seem to exert a better mood profile, or sense of well-being, than occupational or household activities.

Significant Studies

Longitudinal studies have found a negative association between hours per week or calories per week engaged in physical activity and risk of being diagnosed with depression later in life. People who engaged in three or more hours of sports or play per week at baseline were nearly 25% less likely to be diagnosed with depression than those engaging in sports or play less than one hour a week. A similar level of protection occurred among those who reported spending 2,500 kcal per week in physical activity when compared to those who spent less than 1,000 kcal a week (Paffenbarger et al. 1994).

Camacho et al. (1991) found involvement in active sports, swimming or walking, daily exercise, and gardening to be negatively associated with depressive symptoms among men and women aged 20 years or more in a population study in Alameda County, California. The researchers collected baseline data in 1965 and data on depressive symptoms in 1974, and classified participants into three levels of physical activity: low, moderate, and high. Compared to those in the high-activity groups, low-activity men and women had higher risks of showing symptoms of depression. The moderately active groups did not differ significantly from the highly active groups of men and women. An interesting aspect of these studies (Camacho et al. 1991; Paffenbarger et al. 1994) was the negative dose-response relationship between physical activity and depression.

Weyerer (1992) published a rather short-term longitudinal study, with baseline assessments in 1975-1979 and follow-ups during 1980-1984. Based on one question that assessed frequency of physical activity, he classified individuals into regular, occasional, or no exercise groups. A psychiatric interview among participants, who were 16 years of age or older at baseline, provided the basis for the depression variable. Physical activity showed no statistically significant relationship with depression in men or women.

Gaps in Our Knowledge

At present we do not have enough evidence to suggest a threshold that must be crossed in the intensity, the frequency, or the duration of physical activity to prevent chronic mental disorders. We know of acute changes in physiological responses to exercise that may exert a protective benefit against acute mood changes. We also have evidence that in endurance athletes too much strenuous exercise in one bout leads to mood disturbances that may contribute to adverse mental health. Thus, for the general population, too strenuous a physical activity regimen may have a deleterious effect on mental health (USDHHS 1996). Anecdotal evidence abounds that, after a hard day of work and mental tension, one of the best remedies is a "time-out" 30-minute jog. We need more research to better understand the biological mechanisms that may link such episodic but regular bouts of exercise with improved mental health.

Summary

Physical activity and physical fitness appear to be effective in preventing many chronic diseases. More importantly, *the chronic diseases that produce the largest limitations in physical activity are also those most amenable to prevention through physical activity.*

Moderate-intensity physical activity can prevent or delay coronary heart disease. The risk of inactivity is more common among women and the oldest population than among men. Several chronic diseases are more prevalent among older individuals; and while the mechanisms by which physical activity can ame-

liorate these diseases are usually not clear, the existence of positive effects from exercise is often well established. Exercise can help prevent hypertension by improving insulin sensitivity and the sensitivity of baroreceptors—but we need more research to identify clear thresholds and types of physical activity for prevention of hypertension in special populations. The indirect effect of exercise on fibrinogens, body composition, and blood flow dynamics are also emerging issues of interest.

Exercise is clearly beneficial in the prevention of type 2 diabetes. Besides its effect on body weight, physical activity helps improve insulin sensitivity and reduce insulin resistance.

The causes of cancer are many and complex. The bulk of research has shown exercise to be protective against colon cancer, breast cancer, and prostate cancer (the leading cancer killers, along with lung cancer). Moreover, all cancer mortality appears inversely associated with lower heart rates, a physical fitness indicator (Lee 1995).

Research on the effect of exercise in preventing bone loss, osteoporosis, fractures, and falls shows that endurance and muscular strength exercises seem to be beneficial in protecting or improving bone health at any age. Participation in physical activity early in life diminishes the risk of osteoporosis later in life. Osteoarthritis, the most common form of arthritis, is not associated with increased participation in physical activity. Improved balance and muscular strength exercise (especially in the lower extremities) may provide additional protective benefit against falls among the elderly.

Although body weight strongly tends to increase with age, lifetime physical activity may help to prevent the excess weight gain observed with aging. Exercise is not a risk factor for low back pain, and may be more likely to help prevent low back pain than to cause it. Physically active persons appear less likely to suffer from depression and acute anxiety; we need more research to understand the effect of exercise on other psychological disorders.

In summary: to prevent the onset of many chronic diseases, people can benefit by participating in moderate-intensity physical activity for at least 30 minutes most days of the week, and also by regularly engaging in muscular strength, flexibility, and endurance exercise.

References

Abbot, R.D., B.L. Rodriguez, C.M. Burchfiel, and J.D. Curb. 1994. Physical activity in older middle-aged men and reduced risk of stroke: the Honolulu Heart Program. *Am J Epidemiol* 139:881-893.

American College of Sports Medicine. 1993. Position stand: physical activity, physical fitness, and hypertension. *Med Sci Sports Exerc* 25:i-x.

Andersen, L.B., and J. Haraldsdottir. 1995. Coronary heart disease risk factors, physical activity, and fitness in young Danes. *Med Sci Sports Exerc* 27:158-163.

Andersen, R.E., C.J. Crespo, S.J. Bartlett, L.J. Cheskin, and M. Pratt. 1998. Vigorous physical activity and television watching habits among U.S. children and their relation to body weight and level of fatness. *JAMA* 279:938-942.

Anderson, R.N., K.D. Kochanek, and S.L. Murphy 1997. *Report of final mortality statistics, 1995.* Monthly vital statistics report, 45(11) Supplement 2. Hyattsville, Maryland: National Center for Health Statistics.

Apter, D. 1996. Hormonal events during female puberty in relation to breast cancer risk. *Eur J Cancer Prev* 5:476-482.

Berlin J.A., and G.A. Colditz. 1990. A meta-analysis of physical activity in the prevention of coronary heart disease. *Am J Epidemiol* 132:612-628.

Bernstein L., B.E. Henderson, R. Hanisch, J. Sullivan-Halley, and R.K. Ross. 1994. Physical exercise and reduced risk of breast cancer in young women. *J Natl Cancer Inst* 86:1403-1408.

Bernstein, L., R.K. Ross, R.A. Lobo, R. Hanisch, M.D. Krailo, and B.E. Henderson. 1987. The effects of moderate physical activity on menstrual cycle patterns in adolescence: implications for breast cancer. *Br J Cancer* 55:681-685.

Bijnen, F.C.H., E.J.M. Feskens, C.J. Caspersen, S. Giampaoli, A.M. Nissinen, A. Menotti, W.L. Mosterd, and D. Kromhout. 1996. Physical activity and cardiovascular risk factors among elderly men in Finland, Italy, and The Netherlands. *Am J Epidemiol* 143:553-561.

Blair, S.N., N.N. Goodyear, L.W. Gibbons, and K.H. Cooper. 1984. Physical fitness and incidence of hypertension in healthy normotensive men and women. *JAMA* 252:487-490.

Blair, S.N., J.B. Kampert, H.W. Kohl III, C.E. Barlow, C.A. Macera, R.S. Paffenbarger Jr., and L.W. Gibbons. 1996. Influences of cardiorespiratory fitness and other precursors on cardiovascular disease and all-cause mortality in men and women. *JAMA* 276:205-210.

Blair, S.N., H.W. Kohl III, C.E. Barlow, R.S. Paffenbarger Jr., L.W. Gibbons, and C.A. Macera. 1995. Changes in physical fitness and all-cause mortality: a prospective study of healthy and unhealthy men. *JAMA* 273:1093-1098.

Bouchard, C. 1993. Heredity and health related fitness. *Physical Activity and Fitness Research Digest,* President's Council on Physical Fitness and Sports, November:1-8.

Bullen, B.A., R.B. Reed, and J. Mayer. 1964. Physical activity of obese and nonobese adolescent girls appraised by motion picture sampling. *Am J Clin Nutr* 14:211-213.

Camacho, T.C., R.E. Roberts, N.B. Lazarus, G.A. Kaplan, and R.D. Cohen. 1991. Physical activity and depression: evidence from the Alameda County Study. *Am J Epidemiol* 134:220-231.

Caspersen, C.J., K.E. Powell, and G.M. Christenson. 1985. Physical activity, exercise, and physical fitness: definitions and distinctions for health related research. *Public Health Rep* 100:126-131.

Centers for Disease Control and Prevention. 1994. Prevalence of disabilities and associated health conditions—United States, 1991-1992. *MMWR* 43:730-739.

Chen, C.L., E. White, K.E. Malone, and J.R. Daling. 1997. Leisure time physical activity in relation to breast cancer among young women (Washington, United States). *Cancer Causes Control* 8:77-84.

Ching, P.L.Y.H., W.C. Willett, E.B. Rimm, G.A. Colditz, S.L. Gortmaker, and M.J. Stampfer. 1996. Activity level and risk of overweight in male health professionals. *Am J Public Health* 86:25-30.

Chirico, A.M., and A.J. Stunkard. 1960. Physical activity and human obesity. *N Engl J Med* 263:935-940.

Chow, W., M. Dosemeni, W. Zheng, R. Vetter, J.K. McLaughlin, Y. Gao, and W.J. Blot. 1993. Physical activity and occupational risk of colon cancer in Shanghai, China. *Int J Epidemiol* 22:23-29.

Collins, J.G. 1997. Prevalence of selected chronic conditions: United States, 1990-1992. National Center for Health Statistics. *Vital Health Statistics* 10(194).

Conroy, B.P., W.J. Kraemer, C.M. Maresh, S.J. Fleck, M.H. Stone, and A.C. Fry. 1993. Bone mineral density in elite junior Olympic weightlifters. *Med Sci Sports Exerc* 26:1103-1109.

Crespo, C.J., S. Keteyian, G.W. Heath, and C.T. Sempos. 1996. Prevalence of leisure time physical activity among U.S. adults. Results from the National Health and Nutrition Examination Survey. *Arch Intern Med* 156:93-98.

Crespo, C.J., and E. Roccella. 1997. Increased hypertension among those who are less active in the United States. *Med Sci Sports Exerc* 29 (Suppl. 5):39.

Crespo, C.J., and J.D. Wright. 1995. Prevalence of overweight among active and inactive U.S. adults from the Third National Health and Nutrition Examination Survey (abstract). *Med Sci Sports Exerc* 27(Suppl. 5):409.

Cruz-Vidal, M., R. Costas Jr., M.R. Garcia-Palmieri, P.D. Sorlie, and E. Herzmark. 1979. Factors related to diabetes mellitus in Puerto Rican men. *Diabetologia* 28:300-307.

Dalsky, G.P., K.S. Stocke, and A.A. Ehsani. 1988. Weight bearing exercise training and lumbar bone mineral content in postmenopausal women. *Ann Intern Med* 108:824-828.

Daltroy, L.H., M.D. Iversen, M.G. Larson, R. Lew, E. Wright, J. Ryuan, C. Zwerling, A.H. Fossel, and M.H. Liang. 1997. A controlled trial of an educational program to prevent low back injuries. *N Engl J Med* 337:322-328.

Diabetes Data Group. 1995. *Diabetes in America.* 2d ed. NIH Publication 95-1468. Bethesda, MD: National Institutes of Health.

DiPietro, L. 1995. Physical activity, body weight, and adiposity: an epidemiologic perspective. *Exerc Sport Sci Rev* 23:275-303.

Dorgan, J.F., C. Brown, M. Barrett, G.L. Splasnky, B.E. Kreger, R.B. D'Agostino, D. Albanes, and A. Schatzkin. 1994. Physical activity and risk of breast cancer in the Framingham Heart Study. *Am J Epidemiol* 139:662-669.

Eaton, C.B., K.L. Lapane, C.E. Garber, A.R. Assaf, T.M. Lasater, and R.A. Carleton. 1995. Physical activity, physical fitness, and coronary heart disease risk factors. *Med Sci Sports Exerc* 27:340-346.

Erickson, P., R. Wilson, and I. Shannon. 1995. Years of healthy life. Statistical notes. Healthy People 2000. National Center for Health Statistics: Hyattsville, MD. 7:1-16.

Folsom, A.R., D.K. Arnett, R.G. Hutchingson, F. Liao, L.X. Clegg, and L.S. Cooper. 1997. Physical activity and incidence of coronary heart disease in middle-aged women and men. *Med Sci Sports Exerc* 29:901-909.

Folsom, A.R., R.J. Prineas, S.A. Kaye, and R.G. Munger. 1990. Incidence of hypertension and stroke in relation to body fat distribution and other risk factors in older women. *Stroke* 21:701-706.

Friedenreich, C.M., and T.E. Rohan. 1995. A review of physical activity and breast cancer. *Epidemiology* 6:311-317.

Frisch, R.E., G. Wyshak, N.L. Albright, T.E. Albright, I. Schiff, and K.P. Jones. 1985. Lower prevalence of breast cancer and cancers of the reproductive system among former college athletes compared to nonathletes. *Br J Cancer* 52:885-891.

Gammon, M.D., J.B. Schoenberg, J.A. Britton, J.L. Kelsey, R.J. Coates, D. Brogan, N. Potischman, C.A. Swanson, J.R. Daling, J.L. Stanford, and L.A. Brinton. 1998. Recreational physical activity and breast cancer risk among women under age 45 years. *Am J Epidemiol* 147:273-280.

Gerhardsson, M., G. Steineck, U. Hagman, A. Rieger, and S.E. Norell 1990. Physical activity and colon cancer: a case-referent study in Stockholm. *Int J Cancer* 46:985-989.

Giovannucci, E., A. Ascherio, E.B. Rimm, G.A. Colditz, M. Stampfer, and W.C. Willett. 1995. Physical activity, obesity, and risk of colon cancer and adenoma in men. *Ann Intern Med* 122:327-334.

Greendale, G.A., E. Barret-Connor, S. Edelstein, S. Ingles, and R. Haile. 1995. Lifetime leisure exercise and osteoporosis. The Rancho Bernardo Study. *Am J Epidemiol* 141:951-959.

Grimston, S.K., N.D. Willows, and D.A. Hanley. 1993. Mechanical loading regime and its relationship to bone mineral density in children. *Med Sci Sports Exerc* 25:1203-1210.

Hara, H., T. Kawase, M. Yamakido, and Y. Nishimoto. 1983. Comparative observation of micro- and macroangiopathies in Japanese diabetics in Japan and U.S.A. In *Diabetic microangiopathy*, ed. H. Abe and M. Hoshi. Basel: Karger.

Haskell, W.L. 1995. Physical activity in the prevention and management of coronary heart disease. *Physical Activity and Fitness Research Digest*, President's Council on Physical Fitness and Sports, March:1-8.

Heath, G.W., J. Gavin, J. Hinderlites, J. Hagberg, S. Bloomfield, and J. Holloszy. 1983. Effects of exercise and lack of exercise on glucose tolerance and insulin resistance. *J Appl Physiol* 55:512-517.

Helmrich, S.P., D.R. Ragland, and R.S. Paffenbarger Jr. 1994. Prevention of non-insulin-dependent diabetes mellitus with physical activity. *Med Sci Sports Exerc* 26:824-830.

Hoffman-Goetz, L., M.E. Reichman, A. McTiernan, M.I. Goran, W. Demark-Wahnefried, and D. Apter. 1998. Possible mechanism mediating an association between physical activity and breast cancer. *J Natl Cancer Inst* 83 (3 Suppl.):621-628.

Housley, E., G.C. Leng, P.T. Donnan, and F.G. Fowkes. 1993. Physical activity and risk of peripheral arterial disease in the general population: Edinburgh Artery Study. *J Epidemiol Community Health* 47:475-480.

Judge, J.O., R.H. Whipple, and L.I. Wolfson. 1994. Effects of resistive and balance exercises on isokinetic strength in older persons. *J Am Geriatr Soc* 42:937-946.

Kawate, R., M. Yamakido, Y. Nishimoto, P.H. Bennett, R.F. Hamman, and W.C. Knowler. 1979. Diabetes mellitus and its vascular complications in Japanese migrants on the island of Hawaii. *Diabetes Care* 2:161-170.

Kaye, S.A., A.R. Folsom, J.M. Sprafka, R.J. Prineas, and R.B. Wallace. 1991. Increased incidence of diabetes mellitus in relation to abdominal adiposity in older women. *J Clin Epidemiol* 44:329-334.

Kiely, D.K., P.A. Wolf, L.A. Cuppies, A.S. Beiser, and W.B. Kannel. 1994. Physical activity and stroke risk: The Framingham Study. *Am J Epidemiol* 140:608-620.

Kiningham, R.B. 1998. Physical activity and the primary prevention of cancer. *Oncology* 25:515-536.

Kirchner, E.M., R.D. Lewis, and P.J. O'Connor. 1996. Effect of past gymnastics participation on adult bone mass. *J Appl Physiol* 80:225-232.

Knapick, J., J. Zoltick, H.C. Rottner, J. Phillips, C. Bielenda, B. Jones, and F. Drews. 1993. Relationships between self-reported physical activity and physical fitness in active men. *Am J Prev Med* 9:203-208.

Kriska, A. 1997. Physical activity and the prevention of type II (non-insulin dependent) diabetes. *Research Digest*, President's Council on Physical Fitness and Sports, June:1-8.

Kuczmarski, R.J., K.M. Flegal, S.M. Campbell, and C.L. Johnson. 1994. Increasing prevalence of overweight among U.S. adults. The National Health and Nutrition Examination Surveys, 1960-1991. *JAMA* 272:205-211.

Kujala, U.M., S. Sarna, J. Kaprio, and M. Koskenvuo. 1996. Hospital care in later life among former world-class Finnish athletes. *JAMA* 276:216-220.

Lahad, A., A.D. Malter, A.O. Berg, and R.A. Deyo. 1994. The effectiveness of four interventions for the prevention of low back pain. *JAMA* 272:1286-1291.

Lakka, T.A., and J.T. Salonen. 1993. Moderate to high intensity conditioning leisure time physical activity and high cardiorespiratory fitness are associated with reduced plasma fibrinogen in eastern Finnish men. *J Clin Epidemiol* 46:1119-1127.

Lamaitre, R.N., S.R. Hechbert, B.M. Psaty, and D.S. Siscovick. 1995. Leisure time physical activity and the risk of nonfatal myocardial infarction in postmenopausal women. *Arch Intern Med* 155:2302-2308.

Lane, N.E. 1995. Exercise: a cause of osteoarthritis. *J Rheumatol* 22 (Suppl. 43):3-6.

Lane, N.E., D.A. Bloch, P.D. Wood, and J.F. Fried. 1987. Aging, long-distance running, and the development of musculoskeletal disability. *Am J Med* 82:772-780.

Laughlin, M.H. 1994. Effects of exercise training on coronary circulation: introduction. *Med Sci Sports Exerc* 26:1226-1229.

Lee, I.M. 1995. Physical activity and cancer. *Research Digest*, President's Council on Physical Fitness and Sports, June:1-8.

Lee, I.M., R.S. Paffenbarger Jr., and C. Hsieh. 1992. Physical activity and risk of prostatic cancer among college alumni. *Am J Epidemiol* 135:169-179.

Leon, A.S. 1991. Effects of exercise conditioning on physiologic precursors of coronary heart disease. *J Cardiopulm Rehabil* 11:46-57.

Leon, A.S., and J. Connet for the MRFIT Research Group. 1991. Physical activity and 10.5 year mortality in the multiple risk factor intervention trial (MRFIT). *Int J Epidemiol* 20:690-697.

Leon, A.S., and J. Norstrom. 1995. Evidence of the role of physical activity and cardiorespiratory fitness in the prevention of coronary heart disease. *Quest* 47:311-319.

Linsdted, K.D., S. Tonstad, and J.W. Kuzma. 1991. Self-report of physical activity and patterns of mortality in Seventh-Day Adventist men. *J Clin Epidemiol* 44:355-364.

Lord, S.R., R.D. Clark, and I.W. Webster. 1991. Physiological factors associated with falls in an elderly population. *J Am Geriatr Soc* 39:1194-1200.

Manson, J.E., D.M. Nathan, A.S. Krolewski, M.J. Stampfer, W.C. Willett, and C.H. Hennekens. 1992. A prospective study of exercise and incidence of diabetes among U.S. male physicians. *JAMA* 268:63-67.

Manson, J.E., E.B. Rimm, M.J. Stampfer, G.A. Colditz, W.C. Willett, and A.S. Krolewski. 1991. Physical activity and incidence of non-insulin-dependent diabetes mellitus in women. *Lancet* 338:774-778.

McBride, P., J. Einerson, P. Hanson, and K. Heindel. 1992. Exercise and the primary prevention of coronary heart disease. *Medicine, Exercise, Nutrition, and Health* 1:5-15.

Mezzetti, M., C.L. Vecchia, A. Decarli, P. Boyle, R. Talamini, and S. Franceschi. 1998. Population attributable risk for breast cancer: diet, nutrition, and physical exercise. *J Natl Cancer Inst* 90:389-394.

Morris, J.N. 1994. Exercise in the prevention of coronary heart disease: today's best buy in public health. *Med Sci Sports Exerc* 26: 817-814.

Morris, J.N., A. Kagan, D.C. Pattison, M.J. Gardness, and P.A.B. Raffle. 1966. Incidence and prediction of ischemic heart disease in London busmen. *Lancet* 2:553-559.

National High Blood Pressure Education Program. 1997. *Sixth report of the joint national committee on detection, evaluation, and treatment of high blood pressure.* NIH Publication No. 98-4080. Bethesda, MD: National Heart, Lung, and Blood Institute.

National Institutes of Health, Consensus Development Conference. 1996. Physical activity and cardiovascular health. *JAMA* 276:241-246.

National Obesity Education Initiative. 1998. Clinical guidelines on the identification, evaluation, and treatment of overweight and obesity in adults. The evidence report. National Institutes of Health; National Heart, Lung, and Blood Institute. Bethesda, Maryland.

Nichols, D.L., C.F. Sanborn, S.L. Bonnick, V. Ben-Ezra, B. Gench, and N.M. DiMarco. 1994. The effects of gymnastics training on bone mineral density. *Med Sci Sports Exerc* 26:1220-1225.

Niebauer, J., and J.P. Cooke. 1996. Cardiovascular effects of exercise: role of endothelial shear stress. *J Am Coll Cardiol* 28:1652-1660.

Nieman, D.C. 1996. *Fitness and sports medicine. A health related approach.* 3d ed. Palo Alto, CA: Bulls Publishing.

Nieman, D.C., V.D. Cook, D.A. Henson, J. Suttles, W.J. Rejeski, P.M. Ribist, O.R. Fagoaga, and S.L. Nehlsen-Cannarella. 1995. Moderate exercise training and natural killer cell cytotoxic activity in breast cancer patients. *Int J Sports Med* 16:334-337.

Nieman, D.C., and S.L. Nehlsen-Cannarella. 1992. Exercise and infection. In *Exercise and disease*, ed. R.R. Watson and M. Eisinger. Boca Raton, FL: CRC Press.

Oliveira, S.A., H.W. Kohl III, D. Trichopoulos, and S.N. Blair. 1996. The association between cardiorespiratory fitness and prostate cancer. *Med Sci Sports Exerc* 28:97-104.

Paffenbarger, R.S. Jr., I.M. Lee, and R. Leung. 1994. Physical activity and personal characteristics associated with depression and suicide in American college men. *Acta Psychiatr Scand Supp* 377:16-22.

Paffenbarger, R.S. Jr., A.L. Wing, R.T. Hyde, and D.L. Jung. 1983. Physical activity and incidence of hypertension in college alumni. *Am J Epidemiol* 117:245-257.

Panush, R.S., C.S. Hanson, J.R. Caldwell, S. Longley, J. Stork, and R. Thoburn. 1995. Is running associated with osteoarthritis? *J Clin Rheumatol* 1:35-39.

Pate, R.R., M. Pratt, S.N. Blair, W.L. Haskell, C.A. Macera, C. Bouchard, B. Buchner, W. Ettinger, G.W. Heath, A.C. King. A. Kriska, A.S. Leon, B.H. Marcus, J. Morris, R.S. Paffenbarger Jr., K. Patrick, M.L. Pollock, J.M. Rippe, J. Sallis, and J.H. Wilmore. 1995. Physical activity and public health. A recommendation from the Centers for Disease Control and Prevention and the American College of Sports Medicine. *JAMA* 273:402-407.

Peters, K.D., K.D. Kochanek, and S.L. Murphy. 1998. Deaths: final data for 1996. *National Vital Statistics Report* 47:1-100.

Powell, K.E., and S.N. Blair. 1994. The public health burdens of sedentary living habits: theoretical but realistic estimates. *Med Sci Sports Exerc* 26:851-856.

Province, M.A., E.C. Hadley, M.C. Hornbrook, L.A. Lipsitz, J.P. Miller, and C.D. Mulrow. 1995. The effects of exercise on falls in elderly patients: a preplanned meta-analysis of the FICSIT trials. *JAMA* 273:1341-1347.

Ravussin, E., P.H. Bennett, M.E. Valencia, L.O. Schulz, and J. Esparza. 1994. Effects of traditional lifestyle on obesity in Pima Indians. *Diabetes Care* 17:1067-1074.

Rockhill, B., G.A. Colditz, D. Spiegelman, S.E. Hankinson, J.E. Manson, D.J. Hunter, and W.C. Willett. Physical activity and breast cancer risk in a cohort of young women. 1998. *J Natl Cancer Inst* 90:1155-1160.

Rubin, K., V. Schirduan, P. Gendreau, M. Sarfarazi, R. Mendola, and G. Dalsky. 1993. Predictors of axial and peripheral bone mineral density in healthy children and adolescents, with special attention to the role of puberty. *J Pediatr* 123:863-870.

Sallis, J.F., T.L. McKenzie, J.E. Alcaraz, B. Kolody, N. Faucette, and M.F. Hovell. 1997. The effects of a 2-year physical education program (SPARK) on physical activity and fitness in elementary school students. *Am J Public Health* 87:1328-1334.

Sandler, R.S., M.L. Pritchard, and S.I. Bangdiwala. 1995. Physical activity and risk of colorectal adenomas. *Epidemiology* 6:602-606.

Sedgwick, A.W., D.W. Thomas, and M. Davies. 1993. Relationships between change in aerobic fitness and changes in blood pressure and plasma lipids in men and women: the "Adelaide 1000" 4-year follow up. *J Clin Epidemiol* 46:141-151.

Smutok, M., C. Reece, and P. Kokkinos. 1994. Effects of exercise training modality on glucose tolerance in men with abnormal glucose regulation. *Int J Sports Med* 15:283-289.

Steenland, K., S. Nowlin, and S. Palu. 1995. Cancer incidence in the National Health and Nutrition Survey I. Follow-up data: diabetes, cholesterol, pulse and physical activity. *Cancer Epidemiol Biomarkers Prev* 4:807-811.

Taylor, R.J., P.H. Bennett, G. LeGonidec, J. Lacoste, D. Combe, and M. Joffres. 1983. The prevalence of diabetes mellitus in a traditional-living Polynesian population: the Wallis Island survey. *Am J Public Health* 6:334-340.

U.S. Department of Health and Human Services. 1991. *Osteoporosis research, education, and health promotion.* NIH Publication No. 91-3216. Bethesda, MD: National Institute of Arthritis and Musculoskeletal and Skin Diseases.

U.S. Department of Health and Human Services, Centers for Disease Control and Prevention, National Center for Chronic Disease Prevention and Health Promotion. 1996. *Physical activity and health: A report of the Surgeon General.* Atlanta: Centers for Disease Control and Prevention.

Wannamethee, G., and A.G. Shaper. 1992. Physical activity and stroke in British middle aged men. *Br Med J* 304:597-601.

Wannamethee, G., A.G. Shaper, and P.W. Macfarlane. 1993. Heart rate, physical activity, and mortality from cancer and other noncardiovascular disease. *Am J Epidemiol* 137:735-748.

Weyerer, S. 1992. Physical inactivity and depression in the community: evidence from the Upper Bavarian Field Study. *Int J Sports Med* 13:492-496.

Williams, P.T. 1997. Evidence for the incompatibility of age-neutral overweight and age-neutral physical activity standards from runners. *Am J Clin Nutr* 65:1391-1396.

Part III

Exercise in the Rehabilitation of Specific Diseases and Conditions

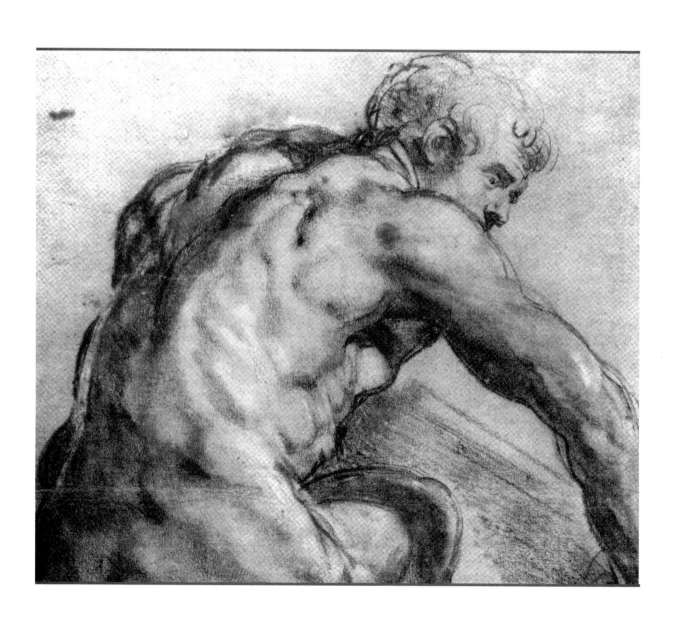

Chapter 10

Heart Diseases

Ruy S. Moraes, MD, MSc, and Jorge P. Ribeiro, MD, ScD

Case Study

A businessman had an uncomplicated inferior myocardial infarction in July 1988, at the age of 47. Before the myocardial infarction, he was sedentary and he smoked 30 cigarettes per day. His fasting plasma LDL-cholesterol level was 180 mg/dl, there was poorly controlled arterial hypertension, and his body mass index was 32 kg/m². An echocardiogram demonstrated left ventricular hypertrophy, with inferior akinesis and global ejection fraction of 63%. An exercise tolerance test limited by fatigue at 4 METs demonstrated 2 mm downsloping ST segment depression on the electrocardiogram, compatible with myocardial ischemia at a rate-pressure product of 24,000. He was discharged from the hospital on 100 mg daily of both atenolol and aspirin.

Two weeks after discharge from the hospital, the patient entered a comprehensive cardiac rehabilitation program that included a low-fat diet, smoking cessation, and exercise training five times per week. Over the 10 years that followed, the patient attended more than 80% of the scheduled exercise sessions. He was able to quit smoking, his plasma fasting LDL-cholesterol declined to 116 mg/dl, his blood pressure was adequately controlled on atenolol 50 mg daily, and his body mass index was reduced to 25 kg/m². A maximal exercise tolerance test performed in 1998 demonstrated a functional capacity of 12 METs limited by fatigue, with 1 mm ST segment depression at a rate-pressure product of 30,000. An echocardiogram demonstrated normal left ventricular wall thickness, inferior hypokinesis, and a global ejection fraction of 69%.

In the United States, cardiovascular disease causes half of all deaths as well as a great deal of suffering and disability. Coronary artery disease alone is responsible for 1.6 million myocardial infarctions per year, of which 500,000 result in death before hospitalization. Of those patients who are admitted to the hospital with myocardial infarction, 15% die during hospitalization and another 10% die within a year. The mortality rate from coronary artery disease has declined dramatically since 1965, mainly due to widespread efforts to reduce risk factors (Manson et al. 1992). Exercise training has played an important role in the primary prevention of cardiac diseases. Recently, new information has been available on the effects of exercise on risk factors, morbidity, and mortality of cardiac disease—including the role of exercise in secondary prevention (Smith et al. 1995).

The World Health Organization defines cardiac rehabilitation as the sum of activities required to ensure cardiac patients the best possible physical, mental, and social conditions so that they may, by their own efforts, regain a normal place in the community and lead an active, productive life (World Health Organization Expert Committee 1964). Thus, cardiac rehabilitation implies a multidisciplinary approach to cardiovascular disease that has exercise training as the cornerstone but also involves psychological, behavioral, and vocational support (Thompson et al. 1996). This chapter covers the rationale for and basic principles of physical exercise in cardiac rehabilitation.

Responses and Adaptations of Cardiac Patients to Exercise

Chapters 3, 4, and 5 described both the physiological responses to a single exercise session and the physiological adaptations to chronic exercise training for healthy individuals. The pathophysiology of exercise in heart disease, as well as the potential risks and benefits of exercise, may differ according to specific clinical conditions.

Coronary Artery Disease

Angina or left ventricular dysfunction may limit maximal functional capacity in patients with coronary artery disease. As is true in healthy individuals, exercise programs for these patients lead to improved exercise capacity as well as lower, submaximal heart rate, systolic blood pressure, and plasma catecholamines (Redwood et al. 1972). After a training pro-

gram, lower myocardial oxygen uptake occurs at a certain submaximal intensity, and these patients are able to tolerate higher exercise intensities before experiencing angina or manifestations of myocardial ischemia. Figure 10.1 compares the effects of exercise training to those of β-blockers or coronary revascularization in coronary patients with angina pectoris. For most patients with inducible ischemia, the main effect of exercise training is a reduction in oxygen demand by the heart. There is no evidence that exercise training induces collateral coronary formation in humans. However, as also shown in figure 10.1, long-term programs that include high training intensities or dietary interventions may improve myocardial blood flow (Froelicher et al. 1984; Hagberg 1991; Ribeiro et al. 1984; Schuler et al. 1988; Schuler et al. 1992), which may be related to regression of coronary artery disease (Hambrecht et al. 1993) or improved endothelial function (Franklin and Kahn 1996; Laughlin et al. 1996).

Arterial Hypertension

During incremental dynamic exercise, patients with established systemic hypertension present higher sys-

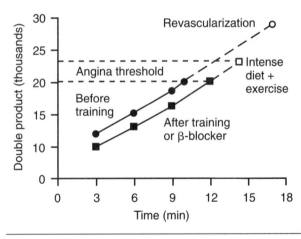

Figure 10.1 Response of the double product (heart rate × systolic blood pressure) to an exercise test, with increments in power every 3 minutes, in a patient with exercise-induced angina pectoris before (●) and after (■) interventions. After commonly used exercise conditioning or β-blockers (—■), the patient is able to tolerate a higher exercise intensity before angina appears. The onset of angina (angina threshold) occurs at the same double product compared to before intervention. After coronary revascularization with angioplasty or surgery (– –○), the patient is able to tolerate a higher exercise intensity without angina due to improvement in myocardial blood flow. After prolonged and intense physical training with dietary intervention (– –□), the patient is able to tolerate a higher exercise intensity due to both reduction in myocardial oxygen uptake and improvement in myocardial blood flow.

tolic and diastolic blood pressures for a given level of oxygen uptake as compared with normal individuals (Lund-Johansen 1967; Sannerstedt 1966). Although some have proposed exercise testing as a means of detecting individuals at risk of hypertension, there is little clinical evidence to support this concept (Liao et al. 1987). Blood pressure may be reduced for several hours after exercise. Some studies have suggested that exercise training programs may contribute to the reduction of blood pressure in patients with hypertension. However, Blumenthal et al. (1991) had difficulty isolating the effects of exercise training when they accounted for co-interventions (e.g., reduction in body weight) and recorded measurements from 24-hour ambulatory blood pressure devices. Important increments in both systolic and diastolic pressure occur during exercise with static components such as weight lifting. Although some have argued that hypertensive patients should avoid static exercise, the evidence indicates that patients using such training actually present the same blood pressure adaptations as those who engage in dynamic exercise (Blumenthal et al. 1991).

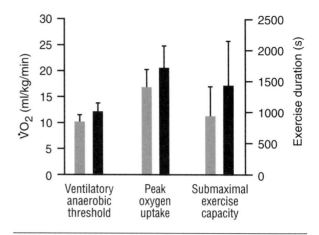

Figure 10.2 Mean ± standard deviation values for the ventilatory anaerobic threshold and peak oxygen uptake (both in ml/kg/min) during incremental tests, and exercise duration (in seconds) on submaximal, constant load protocols measured before (■) and after (■) 16 to 24 weeks of training in 12 patients with chronic heart failure. Maximal and submaximal exercise capacity increased significantly in these patients.
Adapted, by permission, from M.J. Sullivan, M.B. Higginbotham, and F.R. Cobb, 1989, "Exercise training in patients with chronic heart failure delays ventilatory anaerobic threshold and improves submaximal performance," *Circulation* 79:326-7.

Left Ventricular Dysfunction

Patients with congestive heart failure due to systolic dysfunction may present a marked limitation of exercise capacity. In symptomatic patients, functional capacity is usually less than 50% of normal for their ages, while in asymptomatic patients exercise capacity may be 60% to 70% of that predicted for their ages (Liang et al. 1992). Hemodynamic responses to exercise parallel this reduction in functional capacity, with inappropriate chronotropic (Colucci et al. 1989) and inotropic response (Weber et al. 1982), as well as reduced blood flow to exercising muscles (Arnold et al. 1990). The ventilatory response to exercise may also be abnormal, with increased ventilatory drive, increased respiratory dead space, and increased cost of breathing (Ribeiro et al. 1987; Sovijarvi et al. 1992). Skeletal muscle abnormalities in these patients include early lactate release, decreased mitochondrial size, reduced oxidative enzymes, type II fiber atrophy, and altered muscle metabolic responses (Drexler et al. 1992; Mancini et al. 1992; Minotti et al. 1991; Sullivan et al. 1990). In these patients, physical training improves submaximal as well as maximal exercise performance (figure 10.2) (Sullivan et al. 1989). The magnitude of the improvement in functional capacity is similar to and additional to that obtained by pharmacologic therapy (Ribeiro et al. 1985). However, some heart failure patients, particularly those with reduced cardiac output response to exercise, may

not improve functional capacity with exercise training (Wilson et al. 1996). Finally, physical training also induces partial reversal of autonomic as well as skeletal muscle abnormalities (Coats et al. 1992; Shephard 1996).

Valvular Heart Disease

Hemodynamic responses to exercise are quite different in patients with the most common presentations of valvular heart disease. In severe aortic stenosis, the reduction of peripheral vascular resistance during dynamic exercise may result in syncope (Atwood et al. 1988). Because diastolic duration and regurgitation volume decrease during exercise in patients with aortic regurgitation, these patients tolerate exercise well (Weber et al. 1986). In mitral stenosis, this same reduction in diastolic duration impairs left ventricular filling and may reduce cardiac output and increase pulmonary pressure. In mild to moderate mitral regurgitation, cardiac output is maintained during exercise. There is little information on the effects of exercise training in patients with valvular heart disease. Douard et al. (1997) demonstrated that patients with mitral stenosis treated with percutaneous commissurotomy improved their exercise capacity more with physical training than control patients who did not exercise. In general, patients with mild to moderate valvular heart disease and a near normal hemodynamic response to exercise may participate in training programs with the benefit of maintaining exercise capacity (Cheitlin et al. 1994). However, patients with severe valvular heart disease should exercise under close supervision.

Cardiac Arrhythmia

Activation of the sympathetic nervous system may contribute to development of ventricular arrhythmias during exercise, and cardiac patients have a higher risk for sudden death during vigorous exercise than healthy individuals. Chronic exercise training, however, can reduce resting and submaximal exercise plasma catecholamine concentrations, enhance heart rate variability, and improve baroreflex gain, reflecting increased vagal tone—thus chronic exercise may benefit patients with ventricular arrhythmias (Malfatto et al. 1996). Indeed, a study in dogs with experimentally induced myocardial infarction demonstrated that exercise conditioning increased the ventricular fibrillation threshold through an increase in vagal and a decrease in sympathetic tone (Billman et al. 1984). A retrospective clinical study also suggested that long-term cardiac rehabilitation could reduce the incidence

of ventricular arrhythmias by the effect of exercise training on the autonomic nervous system (Hertzeanu et al. 1993). Despite these favorable observations, patients with complex ventricular arrhythmias should exercise under close supervision.

Effect of Cardiovascular Drugs on Exercise Responses and Adaptations

In order to document inducible myocardial ischemia, exercise testing should be conducted without any drugs that interfere with the responses of heart rate and blood pressure to exercise. When evaluating patients before they start a formal training program, however, patients should be tested on their usual medications. Table 10.1 describes the effects of frequently used cardioactive drugs on cardiovascular responses and adaptations to exercise. To improve compliance, ask your patients before each exercise session if they have taken their appropriate medications.

Table 10.1   Effects of Commonly Used Drugs on the Responses and Adaptations to Exercise

Drug	Responses		Adaptations
	Heart rate	Blood pressure	Functional capacity
β-blockers	–	–	– + in angina
Arterial vasodilators	0/+	–	0
Calcium antagonists Dihydropiridines	0/+	–	0 + in angina
Diltiazem/verapamil	–	–	0 + in angina
Digitalis	–	0	+ in heart failure
Diuretics	0	–	0
Angiotensin converting inhibitors	0	–	+ in heart failure
Antiarrhythmic agents	0/–	0	0

0 = no significant effect; – = reduction; + = increase

Evaluation of Cardiac Patients

Although in the past most patients referred for cardiac rehabilitation were at low risk for cardiac events, today many high-risk patients participate in exercise programs. You need adequate risk stratification and objective measurement of exercise capacity in order to plan individualized programs.

Risk Stratification

Before starting any outpatient exercise program, perform an exercise tolerance test to establish the patient's limits of functional capacity, maximum heart rate, and maximum systolic blood pressure; to look for signs of ischemia or ventricular dysfunction; and to check for arrhythmias. This information permits you to stratify risk for complications during exercise (see "Risk Assessment in Cardiac Rehabilitation," page 180) and prescribe the optimum exercise intensity. While annual reevaluations are sufficient for low-risk patients, you probably should test moderate- to high-risk patients every six months. Reevaluate patients after any change in clinical status suggesting cardiovascular deterioration, or after any new intervention (e.g., a change in medication or the use of revascularization procedures), to determine if exercise is still safe. As appropriate, prescribe a new exercise intensity.

Evaluation of Exercise Capacity

Physicians traditionally have assessed exercise capacity in cardiac patients by subjectively evaluating symptoms resulting from ordinary physical activity. Such information permits use of a categorical scale such as one proposed by the Criteria Committee of the New York Heart Association (1964). Although useful in clinical practice because of its simplicity, this classification system has poor reproducibility, and does not reflect the entire continuum of exercise capacities (Goldman et al. 1981). One can improve the estimate of exercise capacity by questioning patients about their performance on daily activities with known metabolic costs (Lee et al. 1988), but still with significant misclassification. Estimation of exercise capacity from the total duration on a specific exercise protocol may correlate well with measured maximal oxygen uptake (Franciosa 1984); but oxygen uptake kinetics may differ in patients with heart disease,

making the estimation of the metabolic cost of exercise inaccurate (Roberts et al. 1984). Another inexpensive method for estimating submaximal exercise capacity is a self-paced walking protocol that measures the distance achieved by the patient in six minutes (Guyatt et al. 1985).

Cardiopulmonary exercise testing, with measurement of expired gases and determination of anaerobic threshold and peak oxygen uptake, allows objective evaluation of functional capacity and of the effect of medical interventions. It also helps define the prognosis in cardiac patients whose main limitations are not due to myocardial ischemia (Mancini et al. 1991; Ribeiro et al. 1985; Weber et al. 1982). Results from cardiopulmonary exercise testing may also reveal whether exertional dyspnea is secondary mainly to pulmonary or mainly to cardiac disease (Messner-Pellenc et al. 1994). For patients who are limited by myocardial ischemia, standard exercise testing is appropriate for the assessment of exercise capacity.

Indications for Cardiac Rehabilitation

Cardiac rehabilitation originally was developed for patients recovering from myocardial infarction. For many years, myocardial infarction was managed with several weeks of bed rest, in the belief that it was necessary for complete healing of the myocardium. Because prolonged bed rest may result in loss of muscular mass, bone reabsorption, anemia, thromboembolic events, pulmonary infections, cardiovascular deconditioning, postural hypotension, and tachycardia, survivors were so physically and emotionally limited that returning to normal life was a significant challenge. In recent decades, the concept of early ambulation after myocardial infarction has been well established. Furthermore, early coronary recanalization, risk stratification, and intervention for those at higher risk have gotten most patients out of bed on the second day of hospitalization, and discharged from the hospital after five to seven days. Higher-risk patients, however, may still endure prolonged bed rest and its consequences.

Traditionally, physicians recommended cardiac rehabilitation after myocardial infarction to restore patients' functional capacity and to allow them an active life. Today, the degree of functional impairment after myocardial infarction depends more on the degree of left ventricular dysfunction and the presence of residual ischemia than on the effects of prolonged bed rest. Although functional capacity on

Risk Assessment in Cardiac Rehabilitation

Low-risk patients

- New York Heart Association (NYHA) class I or II
- Exercise capacity > 6 METs
- Absence of heart failure
- Absence of signs of ischemia at rest or during an exercise test intensity < 6 METs
- Appropriate rise in systolic blood pressure during exercise
- Absence of sequential ecotopic ventricular contractions
- Capacity to self-monitor exercise intensity

Moderate- to high-risk patients

- Two or more myocardial infarctions
- NYHA class III or greater
- Exercise capacity < 6 METs
- ST depression ≥ 4 mm or angina during exercise
- Fall in systolic blood pressure during exercise
- Previous episode of primary cardiac arrest
- Ventricular tachycardia during exercise < 6 METs
- Unable to self-monitor exercise intensity
- Any life-threatening clinical problem

Adapted, by permission, from G. Fletcher et al., 1995, "Exercise standards. A statement for health professionals from the American Heart Association," *Circulation* 91: 602-3.

hospital discharge is normal in many cases, regular exercise training promotes important metabolic and cardiovascular adaptations that positively affect secondary prevention. Thus, cardiac rehabilitation is suitable for a great variety of clinical conditions, as listed on page 181 in "Indications for Cardiac Rehabilitation."

Contraindications for Cardiac Rehabilitation

Contraindications for starting or maintaining an exercise program are listed in the box on page 181. Before each exercise session, ask your patient about the

appearance of new symptoms and for any change in the presentation of their symptoms. Give close attention to changes in the pattern of angina for patients with coronary artery disease, and to weight gain in patients with left ventricular dysfunction. Always measure blood pressure and heart rate. Whenever there is doubt about the safety of performing an exercise session, notify the patient's clinician.

Exercise Prescription for the Cardiac Patient

Encourage cardiac patients to exercise during hospitalization and to maintain active lifestyles after dis-

Indications for Cardiac Rehabilitation

- Abnormal exercise test indicating ischemia
- Post-myocardial infarction patients
- Stable angina
- Coronary artery bypass surgery
- Post-percutaneous transluminal coronary angioplasty
- Compensated congestive heart failure
- Cardiomyopathy
- Post-heart transplantation
- After other cardiac surgery
- Patients with pacemaker or automatic implantable cardioverter defibrillator
- Peripheral vascular disease
- High-risk cardiovascular disease ineligible for surgical intervention
- Sudden cardiac death syndrome
- End-stage renal disease
- At risk for coronary artery disease

Adapted from American College of Sports Medicine 1995a.

Contraindications for Cardiac Rehabilitation

- Unstable angina
- Resting SPB > 200 mm Hg or DBP > 110 mm Hg
- Orthostatic blood pressure drop of > 20 mm Hg with symptoms
- Critical aortic stenosis
- Acute systemic illness or fever
- Uncontrolled arrhythmias
- Resting heart rate > 120 beats/min
- Uncompensated heart failure
- Third-degree AV block (without pacemaker)
- Active pericarditis or myocarditis
- Recent embolism
- Thrombophlebitis
- Resting ST segment displacement > 2 mm
- Uncontrolled diabetes
- Severe orthopedic problems
- Other metabolic problems

Adapted from American College of Sports Medicine 1995a.

charge. Inpatient and outpatient programs present different characteristics.

Inpatient Rehabilitation

For patients recovering from myocardial infarction, exercise during hospitalization helps prevent the deconditioning effects of bed rest and prepare the patients to face the demands of daily physical activities after discharge. For most patients, these daily tasks demand less than 4 METs (1 MET = 3.5 ml/kg/min = the average oxygen uptake while sitting). In uncomplicated cases, you can encourage patients during the first 48 hours of hospitalization to perform arm and leg range-of-motion movements, self-care activities, and low-resistance exercises (figure 10.3). The posture during these activities should progress from lying to sitting to standing, according to the patient's capacity. Supervision during this period is done by nurses, physical or occupational

therapists, or exercise physiologists—all with special training (Pashkow et al. 1988). On the third day after discharge from coronary care unit, patients should start walking for short periods of time, with close monitoring of heart rate, of blood pressure while standing, and, if necessary, of EKG. The exercise heart rate should not exceed 20 beats per minute above resting heart rate, and systolic blood pressure should not exceed 20 mm Hg above resting levels. In the beginning, total exercise duration should be around 20 minutes, twice a day, distributed in intermittent bouts lasting 3-5 minutes, with rest periods of 1-2 minutes between bouts. We recommend that you first increase exercise duration (10-15 minutes of continuous activity), and then raise intensity. During exercise, have the staff watch carefully for symptoms of myocardial ischemia, pulmonary congestion, or a drop in blood pressure. If any of these occurs, interrupt the session and reevaluate the patient before restarting exercise (ACSM 1995b).

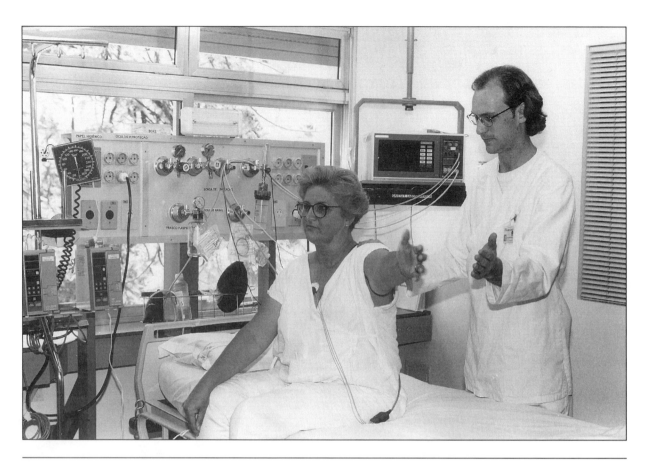

Figure 10.3   Post-myocardial infarction patient performing arm range-of-motion movements under supervision in the intensive care unit. Courtesy of COFIR – Hospital Moinhos de Vento.

Outpatient Programs

After you have stratified them according to risk, you can offer cardiac patients a variety of outpatient exercise programs.

Type of Exercise

Most exercise training in cardiovascular rehabilitation aims to enhance the response of a dysfunctional heart to all kinds of stress—i.e., to diminish the cardiovascular response for a given level of challenge. Aerobic exercise is more efficient in this matter than anaerobic, and is the first choice for cardiac rehabilitation. Most studies using aerobic exercise to control angina in coronary patients have found significant reductions of symptoms (Hagberg 1991; Redwood et al. 1972; Ribeiro et al. 1984).

It is important that predominantly aerobic exercises fulfill the following criteria: low-intensity start; smooth progression; low rate of musculoskeletal injury; and ease of performance and of monitoring. The most popular aerobic exercises are walking and stationary cycling, whose results differ little for most patients. But note that walking demands much more effort for overweight patients than for lean patients—it raises heart rate and blood pressure quickly and imposes a considerable amount of stress on the musculoskeletal system. Most overweight patients find cycling to be both safer and more enjoyable than walking as they start an exercise program.

Patients who use their arms in the workplace will require upper-body exercise before returning to work after a myocardial infarction. Although marked and fast elevations in blood pressure and heart rate occur during heavy weightlifting and isometric exercise, resistive exercise can be safe and useful with proper medical supervision and cardiovascular monitoring (Ghilarducci et al. 1989) (figure 10.4). Low-intensity resistive training may be performed as early as two to eight weeks after myocardial infarction or cardiac surgery (i.e., 0.5- to 4.0-kg hand weights, dumbbells, and elastics). More intense strength training should wait until the patient is aerobically well trained (Verrill 1998; Verrill et al. 1992).

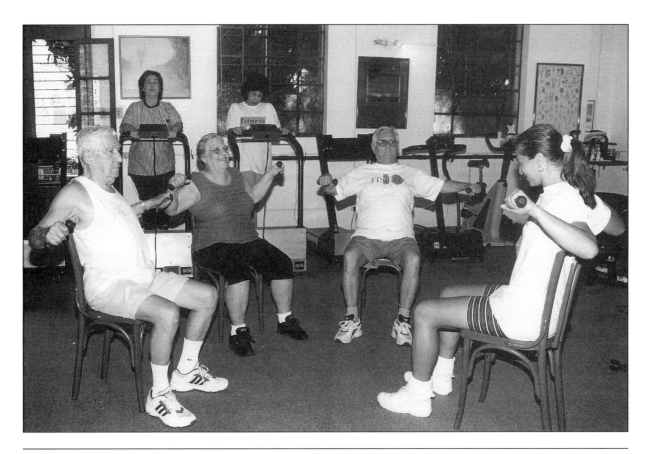

Figure 10.4   Low-intensity resistive training in an outpatient cardiac rehabilitation program.
Courtesy of FISICOR - Cardiac Rehabilitation Center.

Duration and Frequency

To increase aerobic capacity, exercise should last a minimum of 20 minutes, always beginning with a warm-up period and finishing with a cooldown, at least three times a week. The best results in terms of both weight loss and functional capacity occur with a caloric expenditure of about 800 to 1,000 calories/week, which implies 40- to 60-minute sessions three to five times a week. Some studies have demonstrated that burning 2,200 calories/week can induce plaque reduction. To reach this goal, patients must be highly motivated, exercising intensely for 60 minutes five to six times a week. Patients with very low functional capacity, who experience fatigue after a few minutes of exercise, will benefit from short periods of exercise many times a day (DeBusk et al. 1990).

Target Exercise Intensity

The safety of exercise training for cardiac patients depends mostly on the prescribed intensity. Based on

information obtained from an exercise tolerance test, you can calculate a safe exercise intensity range in several ways. "Range of Exercise Intensities for Cardiac Rehabilitation," on page 184, lists common methods for estimating target exercise intensity. The next-to-last item on that list, the "rating of perceived exertion," refers to the patient's perception of the difficulty of each level of exercise, according to the "Borg Scale" listed on page 184. To understand the scale and its administration it is necessary for all users to read *Borg's Perceived Exertion and Pain Scales* (Champaign, IL: Human Kinetics, 1998).

Researchers recently have explored the lower as well as the higher limits of exercise prescription. On one hand, studies have demonstrated that post-myocardial infarction patients may improve functional capacity after training programs that require less than 45% of maximal oxygen uptake (Blumenthal et al., 1988) or as low as 20 beats per minute above resting heart rate (Gobel et al. 1991). These low-intensity programs may result in higher compliance (Lee et al. 1996). On the other hand, selected patients who

Range of Exercise Intensities for Cardiac Rehabilitation

- Workload corresponding to 50% to 80% of $\dot{V}O_2max$

- 70% to 85% of maximal heart rate (HRmax)

- 50% to 75% of heart rate reserve plus heart rate at rest (HRrest)

  $([HRmax - HRrest] \times 50\%) + HRrest$

  $([HRmax - HRrest] \times 75\%) + HRrest$

- Rate of perceived exertion 12 to 16 on the Borg scale

- 10 bpm below the point that abnormal responses occur in the exercise test

Borg Scale for Rating Perceived Exertion (1998)

6	No exertion at all
7	Extremely light
8	
9	Very light
10	
11	Light
12	
13	Somewhat hard
14	
15	Hard (heavy)
16	
17	Very hard
18	
19	Extremely hard
20	Maximal exertion

Borg RPE scale
© Gunnar Borg, 1970, 1985, 1994, 1998

Reprinted, by permission, from G. Borg, 1998, *Borg's Perceived Exertion and Pain Scales* (Champaign, IL: Human Kinetics), 31.

participated in high-intensity exercise programs (70% to 90% of maximal oxygen uptake) for over a year improved left ventricular function and significantly reduced exercise-induced myocardial ischemia at higher myocardial oxygen uptake (Hagberg 1991). Take special care with patients recovering from large anterior Q-wave myocardial infarctions, with left ventricular dysfunction, as they may experience adverse ventricular remodeling over time with early mobilization and exercise training (Jugdutt et al. 1988). Although some studies have not confirmed this observation (Giannuzzi et al. 1992; Rowe et al. 1989), you probably should manage these patients more conservatively.

During the first training sessions, keep exercise intensity in the lower end of the calculated range of intensities. This will permit patients to feel comfortable and confident, and to be free of muscle pains after the sessions. As appropriate for a given patient's cardiovascular and muscular responses, you can gradually and safely increase workload and exercise intensity toward the higher end of the calculated range.

Pulse irregularity makes it difficult to use heart rate to prescribe exercise intensity for patients with atrial fibrillation; instead, use maximal exercise capacity and rate of perceived exertion in setting exercise intensity for these patients (Mertens and Kavanagh 1996). When the patient presents abnormal responses during exercise testing (see "Abnormal Exercise Responses During Stress Testing," page 185), heart rate during exercise training should be at least 10 beats below the heart rate related to the abnormalities.

During the first weeks after coronary artery bypass surgery, patients are still recovering from the surgical trauma, with pain from the thoracotomy and in the leg from which the saphenous vein was removed. For this reason, exercise training in this period usually is prescribed without a previous exercise test. During exercise sessions, keep heart rate around 20 beats per minute above resting heart rate and prescribe only low-level aerobic activity. Complete thoracotomy healing takes around 45-60 days, so upper body exercises in this period can include no resistance. Because of pain and fear, many patients avoid even moving their arms freely when they walk. It is very important that you respect their limitations in this period and provide whatever physical support is needed to prevent falls. After four to eight weeks, most patients can perform an exercise test for formal exercise prescription. Exercise training in this phase is exactly the same as it is for post-myocardial infarction patients. The preference is for aerobic exercises that rapidly increase maximal oxygen consumption. Strength training in these patients is useful to improve muscle strength, especially in the upper body,

Abnormal Exercise Responses During Stress Testing

- Progressive angina, dyspnea, paleness
- ST depression
- Drop in systolic blood pressure
- Systolic blood pressure > 240 mm Hg
- Diastolic blood pressure > 110 mm Hg
- Left ventricular dysfunction
- Complex ventricular arrhythmias
- EKG abnormalities

but has a smaller impact on maximal oxygen consumption (Wosornu et al. 1996).

Supervision

Outpatient exercise training programs for cardiac patients have different levels of supervision, depending on the time after the index event and the risk for developing cardiac complications during exercise (which is related to the severity of the underlying disease). This supervision can be as strict as continuous electrocardiographic monitoring during sessions, for those patients considered as high risk, right after hospital discharge; or no supervision at all for very low-risk patients 12 weeks following a myocardial infarction (see "Risk Assessment in Cardiac Rehabilitation," page 180).

Electrocardiographic monitoring may be appropriate during the first 6 to 12 sessions, gradually reduced to once a week, once a month, or only during symptoms, according to each patient's needs. Individuals at high risk for cardiac complications during exercise, or unable to self-regulate activity levels, may need longer periods of continuous electrocardiographic monitoring. After this intensely monitored phase, patients may enter a gymnasium- or community-based program that offers controlled exercise in an enjoyable environment (figure 10.5). This is the ideal setting to promote self-confidence and risk factor control. Patients have the opportunity to exchange experiences with each other, and group activities help them to increase exercise adherence. Gymnasium staff usually include registered nurses, physical therapists, exercise physiologists, and physical educators, all trained in current basic and advanced cardiac life support. Supervising physicians must be available for

emergency response and consultation, but need not be present in the gym (Vongvanich et al. 1996). Staff-to-patient ratio can be from 1-to-1 to 1-to-4 in continuously monitored programs during the first 12 weeks, and from 1-to-10 to 1-to-20 for group supervised programs (Haskell 1978). For low-risk patients, home exercise rehabilitation is an alternative to supervised group programs. Different monitoring and communication techniques—e.g., regular phone contacts, mail, fax, video recording, Internet, and transtelephonic electrocardiographic monitoring (Balas et al. 1997)—are safe, inexpensive, and convenient for some patients (DeBusk et al. 1985). Finally, exercise training without supervision is acceptable for low-risk patients who are able to prudently control their own exercise intensity.

Safety

Heart disease, vigorous exercise, and death have long been associated with each other in the popular mind. Since exercise increases myocardial oxygen consumption, it may be deleterious to a compromised heart. In recent years, scientists have extensively investigated the impact of exercise on the heart, learning that this potentially harmful activity actually can be effective in treating heart disease. According to the cardiac arrest rate reported in the United States for cardiac patients in exercise rehabilitation programs, the average risk is 1 cardiac arrest for 59,142 patient-hours of exercise training. Risk may increase when untrained patients perform intense levels of exercise, like jogging; it tends to decrease with activities like walking, cycling, or treadmill walking with continuous electrocardiographic monitoring (Fletcher et al. 1995). Probably because of close exercise supervision, the successful resuscitation rate for cardiac arrest in rehabilitation programs is around 85% (Haskell 1978; Van Camp and Peterson 1986).

Outcomes of Cardiac Rehabilitation Programs

Over the past decades, considerable amount of information has accumulated on the outcomes of cardiac rehabilitation programs.

Mortality

Many studies have been unable to detect any small, but clinically important, benefits of cardiac rehabilitation

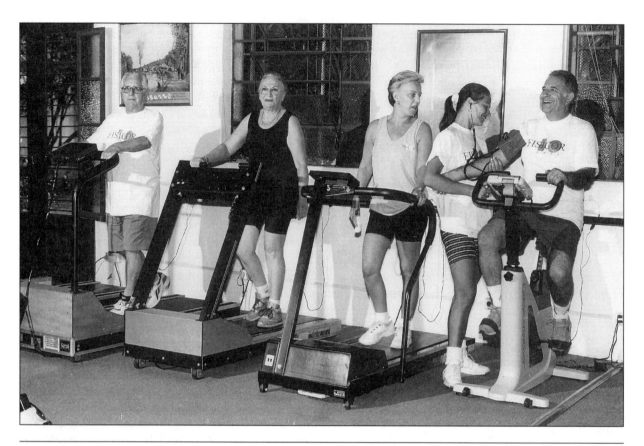

Figure 10.5 Community-based cardiac rehabilitation program that offers a controlled and enjoyable environment.
Courtesy of FISICOR - Cardiac Rehabilitation Center.

on mortality rates (Haskell, 1994). Two well-conducted meta-analyses (O'Connor et al. 1989; Oldridge et al. 1988), however, using prospective studies that compared patients enrolled in cardiac rehabilitation programs versus usual care, found that post-myocardial infarction patients in cardiac rehabilitation programs have lower rates both of overall mortality and of cardiovascular death, but no differences in the incidence of recurrent myocardial infarction. Patients enrolled in rehabilitation programs can expect a reduction of 20% to 25% in mortality rates—very similar to results obtained with use of β-blockers.

Functional Capacity

Patients enrolled in an exercise program for eight weeks may expect an increase in maximum oxygen consumption of about 30%, depending on their previous functional capacity. Patients with lower functional capacity benefit the most. After coronary artery bypass surgery, patients experience a spontaneous and gradual increase in functional capacity over 48 months (Weiner et al. 1981); exercise training significantly improves this response, allowing earlier return to work

(Fletcher et al. 1988). In a recent training study, the greatest improvement in functional capacity occurred in patients who recovered from myocardial infarction and subsequently had coronary artery bypass surgery; those with the lowest ejection fractions had the greatest increase in exercise capacity (Shiran et al. 1997).

Risk Factor Modifications

Secondary prevention of coronary artery disease—a well-established intervention based on risk factor modification—increases survival, improves quality of life, and reduces both the incidence of subsequent myocardial infarction and the need for interventional procedures. However, it is difficult to implement lifestyle changes for risk modification (Smith et al. 1995). Because of its multidisciplinary approach, cardiac rehabilitation is the ideal setting in which to promote the necessary behavior changes (Gordon and Haskell 1997). As a sole intervention, exercise conditioning can positively affect some of the most important known risk factors (Blair et al. 1993). Exercise increases high-density lipoproteins and decreases both low-density lipoproteins and triglycerides, with small changes in total cholesterol (Lavie and Milani 1996b; Tran and Weltman 1985). In obese patients, these benefits are even greater when associated to weight loss (Lavie and Milani 1996a). Obesity is a risk factor for coronary artery disease (Donahue et al. 1987) and adversely influences other risk factors. Exercise alone cannot always affect weight loss—dietary interventions are usually mandatory. Increases in the level of physical activity improve insulin sensitivity, sometimes preventing non-insulin-dependent diabetes mellitus (Helmrich et al. 1991). Intense endurance training in older people enhances fibrinolysis, possibly reducing the risk of acute thrombosis (Stratton et al. 1991). Although exercise is frequently recommended as a nonpharmacologic treatment for hypertension (Kelley and McClellan 1994), there is still controversy about its effectiveness in nonobese patients (Blumenthal et al. 1991); in obese patients exercise may promote weight loss, which is related to reductions in blood pressure (Schotte and Stunkard 1990). In sum: risk factor modification may be one of the main benefits of cardiac rehabilitation.

Vocational Status

Reemployment after an acute cardiac event depends on factors such as age, educational status, severity of the underlying disease, functional capacity, physician's advice, and the patient's perception of health. An exercise tolerance test after a myocardial infarction is one of the key steps in helping patients return to work. It provides information about the severity of the underlying disease and the functional capacity, and helps patients improve their perception of health. Three weeks after an uncomplicated myocardial infarction, patients may have a functional capacity of more than 7 METs, which meets the physical requirements of most white-collar jobs. For these patients, early return to work does not increase the incidence of recurrent cardiac events (Dennis et al. 1988). For high-risk patients with low functional capacity, exercise training seems to help them return to work faster (Hertzeanu et al. 1993). Manual laborers also may require lower and upper body conditioning before resuming their usual professional activities.

Psychosocial Benefits

Acute cardiovascular events strongly affect people's emotional lives. After a myocardial infarction, about 70% of patients report fatigue or lack of energy and are concerned about issues like physical health, re-turn to work, sex life, engaging in physical activities, and the possibility of living an enjoyable life in all aspects (Doerfler et al. 1997). Around 15% to 20% of patients develop signs of depression, which increases the risk of future cardiac events (Carney et al. 1987). Cardiac rehabilitation has been very successful in improving the psychosocial aspects of patients' lives after a major cardiac event. Patients who participate in cardiac rehabilitation programs report improvement in well-being, health, and functional abilities. They also consume fewer tranquilizers and are less depressed when compared to patients not enrolled in cardiac rehabilitation (Denollet and Brutsaert 1995; Lavie and Milani 1997; Milani et al. 1996). These positive effects are not yet fully explained. There is evidence that persons with a low level of activity are at increased risk of developing depression (Camacho et al. 1991), and that intense physical training can improve depression scores (Beniamini et al. 1997). Since cardiac rehabilitation improves fitness and provides an objective assessment of functional capacity, it may create more confidence in patients as they prepare for the usual challenge of daily activities (Dafoe and Huston 1997).

Cost Effectiveness

Since economic resources for health assistance are increasingly more scarce, economic evaluation of health services has become an important issue in modern medicine. To calculate the real cost of an intervention, one must consider health-related improvements in quality of life in addition to reductions in morbidity and mortality. Quality of life is a function not only of physical health, but of the complex interactions among the physical, psychological, and social domains of health (Pashkow et al. 1995; Testa and Simonson 1996). Patients with the same health status may perceive their realities in very distinct ways, having vastly different levels of satisfaction with their lives (Mayou and Bryant 1993).

Investigators have evaluated the costs of cardiac rehabilitation mainly as a secondary prevention measure after acute myocardial infarction. Together with an estimated reduction in mortality of 25% (O'Connor et al. 1989; Oldridge et al. 1988), cardiac rehabilitation reduces costs by lowering the incidence of rehospitalization and of emergency visits (Bondestam et al. 1995; Oldridge et al. 1993). Cardiac rehabilitation after acute myocardial infarction is estimated to cost only US$2,130 per year of life saved, using health care costs of 1985 (Ades et al. 1992); and US$4,950 per year of life saved using 1995 figures (Ades et al. 1997; NIH Consensus 1996). Compared to other interventions after acute myocardial infarction—such as coronary artery revascularization, thrombolytic reperfusion, β-adrenergic blocker therapy, angiotensin converting enzyme inhibitor therapy, lipid lowering therapy, and anti-platelet therapy—only smoking cessation programs are more cost-effective.

Summary

Cardiac rehabilitation is a safe, cost-effective intervention that increases functional capacity, usually improves psychosocial status, and may reduce working disability in a variety of cardiac diseases. Patients with lower functional capacity benefit the most. In post-myocardial infarction patients, exercise training may reduce mortality and improve risk factor profile. Finally, exercise programs for selected patients with coronary artery disease may reduce the progression and even improve the regression of coronary atherosclerosis.

References

Ades, P.A., D. Huang, and S.O. Weaver. 1992. Cardiac rehabilitation and participation predicts lower hospitalization costs. *Am Heart J* 123:916-921.

Ades, P.A., F.J. Pashkow, and J.R. Nestor. 1997. Cost-effectiveness of cardiac rehabilitation after myocardial infarction. *J Cardiopulm Rehab* 17:222-231.

American College of Sports Medicine. 1995a. *Guidelines for exercise testing and prescription.* 5th ed. Baltimore: Williams & Wilkins.

American College of Sports Medicine. 1995b. Position stand. Exercise for patients with coronary artery disease. *Med Sci Sports Exerc* 26:i-v.

Arnold, J.M.O., J.P. Ribeiro, and W.S. Colucci. 1990. Muscle blood flow during forearm exercise in patients with severe heart failure. *Circulation* 82:465-472.

Atwood, J.E., S. Kawanishi, J. Myers, and V.F. Froelicher. 1988. Exercise testing in patients with aortic stenosis. *Chest* 93:1083-1087.

Balas, E.A., F. Jaffrey, G.J. Kuprerman, S.A. Boren, G.D. Brown, F. Pinciroli, and J.A. Mitchell. 1997. Electronic communication with patients. Evaluation of distance medicine technology. *JAMA* 278:152-159.

Beniamini, Y., J.J. Rubenstein, L.D. Zaichkowsky, and M.C. Crim. 1997. Effects of high-intensity strength training on quality-of-life parameters in cardiac rehabilitation patients. *Am J Cardiol* 80:841-846.

Billman, G.E., P.J. Schwartz, and H.L. Stone. 1984. The effects of daily exercise on susceptibility to sudden cardiac death. *Circulation* 69:1182-1189.

Blair, S.N., K.E. Powell, T.L. Bazzarre, J.L. Early, L.H. Epstein, L.W. Green, S.S. Harris, W.L. Haskell, A.C. King, J. Koplan, B. Marcus, R.S. Paffenbarger, and K.K. Yeager. 1993. Physical inactivity. Workshop V. *Circulation* 88:1402-1405.

Bloch, A., J.P. Maeder, J.C. Haissly, J. Felix, and H. Blackburn. 1974. Early mobilization after myocardial infarction: a controlled study. *Am J Cardiol* 34:152-157.

Blumenthal, J.A., W.J. Rejeski, M. Walsh-Riddle, C.F. Emery, H. Miller, S. Roark, P.M. Ribisl, P.B Morris, P. Brubaker, and R.S. Williams. 1988. Comparison of high- and low-intensity exercise training after acute myocardial infarction. *Am J Cardiol* 61:26-30.

Blumenthal, J.A., W.C. Siegel, and M. Appelbaum. 1991. Failure of exercise to reduce blood pressure in patients with mild hypertension. Results of a randomized controlled trial. *JAMA* 266:2098-2104.

Bondestam, E., A. Breikss, and M. Hartford. 1995. Effects of early rehabilitation on consumption of medical care during the first year after acute myocardial infarction in patients ≥ 65 years of age. *Am J Cardiol* 75:767-771.

Borg, G. 1998. *Borg's perceived exertion and pain scales.* Champaign, IL: Human Kinetics.

Camacho, T.C., R.E. Roberts, N.B. Lazarus, G.A. Kaplan, and R.D. Cohen. 1991. Physical activity and depression: evidence from the Alameda County Study. *Am J Epidemiol* 134: 220-231.

Carney, R.M., M.W. Rich, A. Tevelde, J. Saini, K. Clark, and A.S. Jaffe. 1987. Major depressive disorder in coronary artery disease. *Am J Cardiol* 60:1273-1275.

Cheitlin, M.D., P.S. Douglas, and W.W. Parmley. 1994. 26th Bethesda Conference. Recommendations for determining eligibility for competition in athletes with cardiovascular abnormalities. Task Force 2. Valvular heart disease. *J Am Coll Cardiol* 24:874-880.

Coats, A.J.S., S. Adamopoulos, A. Radaelli, A. McCance, T.E. Meyer, L. Bernardi, P.L. Solda, P. Davey, O. Ormerod, C. Forfar, J. Conway, and P. Sleight. 1992. Controlled trial of physical training in chronic heart failure. *Circulation* 85:2119-2131.

Colucci, W.S., J.P. Ribeiro, M.B. Rocco, R.J. Quigg, M.A. Creager, J.D. Marsh, D.F. Gauthier, and L.H. Hartley. 1989. Impaired chronotropic response to exercise in patients with congestive heart failure. Role of postsynaptic β-adrenergic desensitization. *Circulation* 80:314-323.

Criteria Committee of the New York Heart Association. 1964. *Nomenclature and criteria for diagnosis of diseases of the heart and great vessels.* Boston: Little, Brown.

Dafoe, W., and P. Huston. 1997. Current trends in cardiac rehabilitation. *Can Med Assoc J* 156:527-532.

DeBusk, R.F., W.L. Haskell, N.H. Miller, K. Berra, and C.B. Taylor. 1985. Medically directed at-home rehabilitation soon after clinically uncomplicated myocardial infarction: a new model for patient care. *Am J Cardiol* 55:251-257.

DeBusk, R.F., U. Stenestrand, M. Sheehan, and W.L. Haskell. 1990. Training effects of long versus short bouts of exercise in healthy subjects. *Am J Cardiol* 65:1010-1013.

Dennis, C., N. Houston-Miller, R.G. Schwartz, D.K. Ahn, H.C. Kraemer, D. Gossard, M. Juneau, C.B. Taylor, and R.F. DeBusk. 1988. Early return to work after uncomplicated myocardial infarction. Results of a randomized trial. *JAMA* 260:214-220.

Denollet, J., and D.L. Brutsaert. 1995. Enhancing emotional well-being by comprehensive rehabilitation in patients with coronary heart disease. *Eur Heart J* 16: 1070-1078.

Doerfler, L.A., L. Pbert, and D. DeCosimo. 1997. Self-reported depression in patients with coronary artery disease. *J Cardiopulm Rehab* 17:163-170.

Donahue, R.P., R.D. Abbott, E. Bloom, D.M. Reed, and K. Yano. 1987. Central obesity and coronary heart disease in men. *Lancet* 1:821-824.

Douard, H., L. Chevalier, L. Labbe, A. Choussat, and J.P. Brouset. 1997. Physical training improves exercise capacity in patients with mitral stenosis after balloon valvuloplasty. *Eur Heart J* 18:464-469.

Drexler, H., U. Riede, T. Munzel, H. Konig, E. Funke, and H. Just. 1992. Alterations of skeletal muscle in chronic heart failure. *Circulation* 85:1751-1759.

Fletcher, B.J., A. Lloyd, and G.F. Fletcher. 1988. Outpatient rehabilitative training in patients with cardiovascular disease: emphasis on training method. *Heart Lung* 17:199-205.

Fletcher, G.F., G. Balady, S.N. Blair, J. Blumenthal, C. Caspersen, B. Chaitman, S. Epstein, E.S.S. Froelicher, V.F. Froelicher, I.L. Pina, and M.L. Pollock. 1996. Statement on exercise: benefits and recommendations for physical activity programs for all Americans. A statement for health professionals by the committee on exercise and cardiac rehabilitation of the Council on Clinical Cardiology, American Heart Association. *Circulation* 94:857-862.

Fletcher, G.F., G. Balady, V.F. Froelicher, L.H. Hartley, W.L. Haskell, and M.L. Pollock. 1995. Exercise standards. A statement for health professionals from the American Heart Association. *Circulation* 91:580-615.

Franciosa, J.A. 1984. Exercise testing in chronic congestive heart failure. *Am J Cardiol* 53:1447-1450.

Franklin, B.A, and J.K. Kahn. 1996. Delayed progression or regression of coronary atherosclerosis with intense risk factor modification. *Sports Med* 22:306-320.

Froelicher, V., D. Jensen, F. Genter, M. Sullivan, M.D. McKirman, K. Witztum, J. Scharf, M.L. Strong, and W. Ashburn. 1984. A randomized trial of exercise training in patients with coronary heart disease. *JAMA* 252:1291-1297.

Ghilarducci, L.E., R.G. Holly, and E.A. Amsterdam. 1989. Effects of high resistance training in coronary artery disease. *Am J Cardiol* 64: 866-870.

Giannuzzi, P., P.L. Temporelli, L. Tavassi, A. Corra, M. Gattone, A. Imparatto, A. Giordano, C. Schweiger, L. Sala, and C. Maliverni. 1992. EAMI—exercise in anterior myocardial infarction. An ongoing multicenter randomized study. Preliminary results on left ventricular function and remodeling. *Chest* 101 [Suppl.] 315S-321S.

Gobel, A.J., D.J. Hare, P.S. Macdonald, R.G. Oliver, M.A. Reid, and M.D. Worcester. 1991. Effects of early programmes of high and low intensity exercise on physical performance after transmural myocardial infarction. *Brit Heart J* 65:126-131.

Goldman, L., B. Hashimoto, E.F. Cook, and J.A. Loscalzo. 1981. Comparative reproducibility and validity of systems for assessing cardiovascular functional class: advantages of a new specific activity scale. *Circulation* 6:1227-1234.

Gordon, N.F., and W.L. Haskell. 1997. Comprehensive cardiovascular disease risk reduction in a cardiac rehabilitation setting. *Am J Cardiol* 80:69H-73H.

Guyatt, G.H., M.J. Sullivan, and P.J. Thompson. 1985. The 6 minute walk: a new measure of exercise capacity in patients with chronic heart failure. *Can Med Assoc J* 132:919-923.

Hagberg, J.M. 1991. Physiologic adaptations to prolonged high-intensity exercise training in patients with coronary artery disease. *Med Sci Sports Exerc* 23:661-667.

Hambrecht, R., J. Niebauer, C. Marburger, M. Grunze, B. Kalborer, K. Haner, G. Schlorf, W. Kubler, and G. Schulor. 1993. Various intensities of leisure time physical activity in patients with coronary artery disease. Effects on cardiorespiratory fitness and progression of coronary atherosclerotic lesions. *J Am Coll Cardiol* 22:468-477.

Haskell, W. L. 1978. Cardiovascular complications during exercise training of cardiac patients. *Circulation* 57:920-924.

Haskell, W.L. 1994. The efficacy and safety of exercise programs in cardiac rehabilitation. *Med Sci Sports Exerc* 26:815-823.

Helmrich, S.P., D.R. Ragland, R.W. Leung, and R.S. Paffenbarger. 1991. Physical activity and reduced occurrence of non-insulin-dependent diabetes mellitus. *New Engl J Med* 325:147-152.

Hertzeanu, H.L., J. Shemesh, L.A. Aron, A.L. Aron, E. Peleg, T. Rosenthal, M. Motro, and J.J. Kellermann. 1993. Ventricular arrhythmias in rehabilitated and nonrehabilitated post-myocardial infarction patients with left ventricular dysfunction. *Am J Cardiol* 71:24-27.

Jugdutt, B.I., B.L. Michorowski, and C.T. Kappagoda. 1988. Exercise training after anterior myocardial infarction. Importance of left ventricular function and topography. *J Am Coll Cardiol* 12:362-372.

Kelley, G., and P. McClellan. 1994. Antihypertensive effects of aerobic exercise. A brief meta-analytic review of randomized controlled trials. *Am J Hypertens* 7:115-119.

Laughlin, M.H., R.M. McAllister, J.L. Jasperse, D.A. Crader, and V.H. Huxley. 1996. Endothelium mediated control of the coronary circulation. Exercise training-induced vascular adaptations. *Sports Med* 22:228-250.

Lavie, C.J., and R.V. Milani. 1996a. Effects of cardiac rehabilitation and exercise training in obese patients with coronary artery disease. *Chest* 109:52-56.

Lavie, C.J., and R.V. Milani. 1996b. Effects of nonpharmacologic therapy with cardiac rehabilitation and exercise training in patients with low levels of high-density lipoprotein cholesterol. *Am J Cardiol* 78:1286-1289.

Lavie, C.J., and R.V. Milani. 1997. Effects of cardiac rehabilitation, exercise training, and weight reduction on exercise capacity, coronary risk factors, behavioral characteristics, and quality of life in obese coronary patients. *Am J Cardiol* 79:397-401.

Lee, J.Y., B.E. Jensen, A. Oberman, G.F. Fletcher, B.J. Fletcher, and J.M. Raczynski. 1996. Adherence in the training levels comparison trial. *Med Sci Sports Exercise* 28:47-52.

Lee, T.H., J.B. Shammash, J.P. Ribeiro, L.H. Hartley, J. Sherwood, and L. Goldman. 1988. Estimation of maximum oxygen uptake from clinical data: performance of the Specific Activity Scale. *Am Heart J* 115:203-204.

Liang, C., D.K. Stewart, T.H. LeJemtel, P.C. Kirlin, K.M. McIntyre, H.T. Robertson, R. Brown, A.W. Moore, K.L. Wellington, L. Cahill, M.N. Galvao, P.A. Woods, C. Garces, and P. Held. 1992. Characteristics of peak aerobic capacity in symptomatic and asymptomatic subjects with left ventricular dysfunction. *Am J Cardiol* 69:1207-1211.

Liao, Y., L.A. Emidy, F.C. Gosch, and J. Stamler. 1987. Cardiovascular responses to exercise of patients in a trial on the primary prevention of hypertension. *J Hypertens* 5:317-321.

Lund-Johansen, P. 1967. Hemodynamics in early essential hypertension. *Acta Med Scand* 183(Suppl. 482):1-105.

Malfatto, G., M. Facchini, R. Bragato, G. Branzi, L. Sala, and G. Leonetti. 1996. Short and long term effects of exercise training on the tonic autonomic modulation of heart rate variability after myocardial infarction. *Eur Heart J* 17:532-538.

Mancini, D.M., H. Eisen, W. Kussmaul, R. Mull, L.H. Edwards, and J.R. Wilson. 1991. Value of peak oxygen consumption for optimal timing of cardiac transplantation in ambulatory patients with heart failure. *Circulation* 83:778-786.

Mancini, D.M., G. Walter, N. Reichek, R. Lendkinski, K.K. McCully, J.L. Mullen, and J.R. Wilson. 1992. Contribution of skeletal muscle atrophy to exercise intolerance and altered muscle metabolism in heart failure. *Circulation* 85:1364-1373.

Manson, J.E., H. Tosteson, and P.M. Ridker. 1992. The primary prevention of myocardial infarction. *New Engl J Med* 326:1406-1416.

Mayou, R., and B. Bryant. 1993. Quality of life in cardiovascular disease. *Br Heart J* 69:460-466.

Mertens, D.J., and T. Kavanagh. 1996. Exercise training for patients with chronic atrial fibrillation. *J Cardiopulm Rehab* 16:193-196.

Messner-Pellenc, P., C. Ximenes, C.F. Brasileiro, J. Mercier, R. Grolleau, and C.G. Préfaut. 1994. Cardiopulmonary exercise testing. Determinants of dyspnea due to cardiac or pulmonary limitation. *Chest* 106:354-360.

Milani, R.V., C.J. Lavie, and M.M. Cassidy. 1996. Effects of cardiac rehabilitation and exercise training programs on depression in patients after major coronary events. *Am Heart J* 132:726-732.

Minotti, J.R., I. Christoph, R. Oka, M.W. Weiner, L. Wells, and B.M. Massie. 1991. Impaired skeletal muscle function in patients with congestive heart failure. *J Clin Invest* 88:2077-2082.

NIH consensus development panel on physical activity and cardiovascular health. 1996. Physical activity and cardiovascular health. *JAMA* 276:241-246.

Oldridge, N., W. Furlong, D. Feeny, G. Torrance, G. Guyatt, J. Crowe, and N. Jones. 1993. Economic evaluation of cardiac rehabilitation soon after acute myocardial infarction. *Am J Cardiol* 72:154-161.

Oldridge, N.B., G.H. Guyatt, M.E. Fischer, and A.A. Rimm. 1988. Cardiac rehabilitation after myocardial infarction. Combined experience of randomized clinical trials. *JAMA* 260:945-950.

O'Connor, G.T., J.E. Buring, S. Yusuf, S.Z. Goldhaber, E.M. Olmstead, R.S. Paffenbarger, and C.H. Hennekens. 1989. An overview of randomized trials of rehabilitation with exercise after myocardial infarction. *Circulation* 80:234-244.

Pashkow, F.J., P.S. Pashkow, and M.N. Schafer. 1988. *Successful cardiac rehabilitation: The complete guide for building cardiac rehab programs.* 1st ed. Loveland, CO: The HeartWatchers Press.

Pashkow, P., P.A. Ades, C.F. Emery, D.J. Frid, N.H. Miller, G. Peske, J.Z. Reardon, J.H. Schiffert, D. Southard, and R.L. ZuWallack. 1995. Outcome measurement in cardiac and pulmonary rehabilitation by the AACVPR Outcomes Committee. *J Cardiopulm Rehab* 15:394-405.

Redwood, D.R., D.R. Rosing, and S.E. Epstein. 1972. Circulatory and symptomatic effects of physical training in patients with coronary-artery disease and angina pectoris. *New Engl J Med* 286:959-965.

Ribeiro, J.P., L.H. Hartley, and W.S. Colucci. 1985. Effects of acute and chronic pharmacologic interventions on exercise and performance in patients with congestive heart failure. *Heart Failure* 1:102-111.

Ribeiro, J.P, L.H. Hartley, J. Sherwood, and A. Herd. 1984. The effectiveness of a low lipid diet and exercise in the management of coronary artery disease. *Am Heart J* 108:1182-1189.

Ribeiro, J.P., A. Knutzen, M.B. Rocco, L.H. Hartley, and W.S. Colucci. 1987. Periodic breathing during exercise in severe heart failure. *Chest* 92:555-556.

Roberts, J.M., M. Sullivan, V.F. Froelicher, F. Gender, and J. Myers. 1984. Predicting oxygen uptake from treadmill testing in normal subjects and coronary artery disease patients. *Am Heart J* 108:1454-1460.

Rowe, M.H., M.V. Jelinek, N. Liddell, and M. Hugens. 1989. Effect of rapid mobilization on ejection fractions and ventricular volumes after acute myocardial infarction. *Am J Cardiol* 63:1037-1041.

Sannerstedt, R. 1966. Hemodynamic response to exercise in patients with arterial hypertension. *Acta Med Scand* 180 (Suppl. 458):7-101.

Schotte, D.E., and A.J. Stunkard. 1990. The effects of weight reduction on blood pressure in 201 obese patients. *Arch Int Med* 150:1701-1704.

Schuler, G., R. Hambrecht, G. Schlierf, M. Grunze, S. Methfessel, K. Hanet, and W. Kubler. 1992. Myocardial perfusion and regression of coronary artery disease in patients on a regimen of intense physical exercise and low fat diet. *J Am Coll Cardiol* 19:34-42.

Schuler, G., G. Schlierf, A. Wirth, H.P. Mautner, H. Scheurlen, M. Thumm, H. Roth, F. Scharz, M. Kohlmeier, H.C. Mehmel, and W. Kubler. 1988. Low-fat diet and regular, supervised physical exercise in patients with symptomatic coronary artery disease. Reduction of stress-induced myocardial ischemia. *Circulation* 77:172-181.

Shephard, R.J. 1996. Exercise for patients with congestive heart failure. *Sports Med* 23:75-92.

Shiran, A., S. Kornfeld, S. Zur, A. Laor, Y. Karelitz, A. Militianu, A. Merdler, and B.S. Lewis. 1997. Determinants of improvement in exercise capacity in patients undergoing cardiac rehabilitation. *Cardiology* 88:207-213.

Smith, S.C., S.N. Blair, M.H. Criqui, G.F. Fletcher, V. Fuster, B.J. Gersh, A.M. Gotto, L. Gould, P. Greenland, S.M. Grundy, M.N. Hill, M.A. Hlatky, N. Houston-Miller, R.M. Krauss, J. LaRosa, I.S. Ockene, S. Oparil, T.A. Pearson, E. Rapaport, and R.D. Starke, for the Secondary Prevention Panel. 1995. Preventing heart attack and death in patients with coronary disease. *Circulation* 92:2-4.

Sovijarvi, A.R.A., H. Naveri, and H. Leinonen. 1992. Ineffective ventilation during exercise in patients with chronic congestive heart failure. *Clinical Physiology* 12:399-408.

Stratton, J.R., W.L. Chandler, R.S. Schwartz, M.D. Cerqueira, W.C. Levy, S.E. Kahn, V.G. Larson, K.C. Cain, J.C. Beard, and I.B. Abrass. 1991. Effects of physical conditioning on fibrinolytic variables and fibrinogen in young and old healthy adults. *Circulation* 83:1692-1697.

Sullivan, M.J., H.J. Green, and F.R. Cobb. 1990. Skeletal muscle biochemistry and histology in ambulatory patients with long-term heart failure. *Circulation* 81:518-527.

Sullivan, M.J., M.B. Higginbotham, and F.R. Cobb. 1989. Exercise training in patients with chronic heart failure delays ventilatory anaerobic threshold and improves submaximal performance. *Circulation* 79:324-329.

Testa, M.A., and D.C. Simonson. 1996. Assessment of quality-of-life outcomes. *New Engl J Med* 334:835-840.

Thompson, D.R., G.S. Bowman, A.L. Kitson, D.P. de Bono, and A. Hopkins. 1996. Cardiac rehabilitation in the United Kingdom. Guidelines and audit standards. *Heart* 75:89-93.

Tran, Z.V., and A. Weltman. 1985. Differential effects of exercise on serum lipid and lipoprotein levels seen with changes in body weight. A meta-analysis. *JAMA* 254:919-924.

Van Camp, S.P., and R.A. Peterson. 1986. Cardiovascular complications of cardiac rehabilitation programs. *JAMA* 256:1160-1163.

Verrill, D.E. 1998. Resistive exercise training in cardiac rehabilitation. In *Training techniques in cardiac rehabilitation*, ed. P.S. Fardy, B.A. Franklin, J.P. Porcari, and D.E. Verrill, 41-87. Champaign, IL: Human Kinetics.

Verrill, D.E., E. Shoup, G. McElveen, K. Witt, and D. Bergey. 1992. Resistive exercise training in cardiac patients. Recommendations. *Sports Med* 13:171-193.

Vongvanich, P., M.J. Paul-Labrador, and N.B. Merz. 1996. Safety of medically supervised exercise in a cardiac rehabilitation center. *Am J Cardiol* 77:1383-1385.

Weber, K., J.S. Janicki, and P.A. McElroy. 1986. Cardio-pulmonary exercise testing in the evaluation of mitral and aortic valve incompetence. *Herz* 11:88-96.

Weber, K., G. Kinasewitz, J. Janicki, and A. Fishman. 1982. Oxygen utilization and ventilation during exercise in patients with chronic heart failure. *Circulation* 65:1213-1223.

Weiner, D.A., C.H. McCabe, R.L. Roth, S.S. Cutler, R.L. Berger, and T.J. Ryan. 1981. Serial exercise testing after coronary artery bypass surgery. *Am J Cardiol* 101:149-154.

Wilson, J.R., J. Groves, and G. Rayos. 1996. Circulatory status and response to cardiac rehabilitation in patients with heart failure. *Circulation* 94:1567-1572.

World Health Organization Expert Committee. 1964. *Rehabilitation of patients with cardiovascular disease*. Technical Report Series #270. Geneva: World Health Organization.

Wosornu, D., D. Bedford, and D. Ballantyne. 1996. A comparison of the effects of strength and aerobic exercise training on exercise capacity and lipids after coronary artery bypass surgery. *Eur Heart J* 17:854-863.

Chapter 11

Respiratory Disease

Bartolome R. Celli, MD

Case Study

A 63-year-old woman, S.W., smoked one pack of cigarettes per day from age 17 to age 59. She had begun to experience dyspnea at age 57, and was diagnosed with chronic obstructive pulmonary disease (COPD) at age 59. Although she stopped smoking, her dyspnea continued to progress (at first appearing only with moderate efforts). Over the past year, however, she had become unable to walk up one flight of stairs, and the dyspnea occurred during activities of daily living (washing, bathing, and dressing). She began to limit her exercise, and used a nephew's wheelchair when she went out. She began to use low-flow oxygen at age 62.

A routine chest roentgenogram revealed a right upper lobe nodule measuring 2 centimeters, which had not appeared in an X ray two years earlier. Computerized tomography confirmed the nodule.

There were no mediastinal nodes. The same scan confirmed severe hyperinflation, and demonstrated the presence of inhomogeneous changes more prominent in the upper lobes.

Laboratory exams were within normal limits, including cardiac echocardiogram. Physiologic evaluation showed severe airflow obstruction, with a forced vital capacity of 2.05 L and a forced expiratory volume in one second (FEV1) of 0.52 L after bronchodilators. The residual volume determined by plethysmography showed severe air trapping with a value 260% of predicted. S.W.'s six-minute walking distance was 120 meters, and maximal oxygen uptake in a progressive cardiopulmonary exercise test was 11 ml/kg/min. The working diagnosis was that of neoplasm, very likely malignant, in the right upper lobe.

By conventional criteria S.W. was inoperable, because her FEV1 was very low (26% of predicted). Nevertheless, we explained to her that we could remove the nodule using recently developed lung volume reduction surgery. Even though she understood that poor functional capacity (as expressed by the six-minute walking test) generally predicts poor outcome with this procedure, she wanted to be aggressive and was willing to "do anything" to qualify for the procedure.

We began her on an intense pulmonary rehabilitation program that included lower-extremity exercise at 70% of the determined $\dot{V}O_2$max and upper-extremity unsupported exercise. To aid in the postoperative period, we instructed her in deep-breathing exercises and in assisted cough. S.W. began the program with daily sessions as an inpatient, completing it with three weeks of outpatient training for a total of 20 sessions. Retesting revealed less dyspnea with exercise, and she was able to walk 285 meters over six minutes. Her peak oxygen uptake had risen to 13 ml/kg/min.

S.W.'s lung volume reduction surgery, which included resection of the nodule, revealed adenocarcinoma of the lung. She recovered in the acute ward of St. Elizabeth's Medical Center for eight days, and was discharged to a rehabilitation facility to continue the program while a small persistent leak (drained with a Heimlich tube) closed. After the leak closed on the 16th day after surgery, S.W. went home. After eight months, the mass has not recurred.

S.W. is still dyspneic, but no longer uses the wheelchair. She has not required hospitalization, and her oxygen requirements have decreased 0.5 liter per minute. She walks daily, and her last six-minute walking distance was 268 meters.

Commentary: This case documents the extreme limitations characteristic of patients with severe COPD. It also shows the frequent association between COPD and lung cancer, as both share cigarette smoking as a common risk factor. More importantly, it shows how pulmonary rehabilitation that includes exercise training can significantly improve certain outcomes. S.W. was well-prepared and confident as she faced surgery. She was also able to walk longer and experience less dyspnea at a higher functional level. It is also possible that the educational components of her pulmonary rehabilitation (especially those that helped her control her breathing) helped improve her postoperative recovery.

Patients with chronic respiratory diseases decrease their overall physical activity, because any form of exercise often results in worsening dyspnea. The progressive deconditioning associated with inactivity initiates a vicious cycle in which dyspnea increases at ever lower physical demands. With time, the patients adopt a breathing pattern (usually fast and shallow) that is detrimental to overall gas exchange, thus worsening their symptoms. Physical reconditioning is a broad therapeutic concept that unfortunately has been equated with simple lower extremity exercise training. This chapter addresses the concept of respiratory muscle training and resting. It reviews current knowledge about reconditioning in broad terms, critically analyzing the effects and roles of leg and arm training, and giving practical recommendations. It also reviews the concept of breathing retraining in its broad definition.

The data on which our current knowledge of reconditioning is based have been obtained from patients with intrinsic lung disease—such as emphysema, bronchitis, bronchiectasis, cystic fibrosis, and acute respiratory failure. Very little is known about reconditioning in patients with pure "pump failure," such as those with degenerative neuromuscular diseases. There is every reason to believe that, in these patients, physical exercise may worsen rather than improve their overall function and sensation of well-being. On the other hand, pure breathing retraining, such as slow deep breathing, could have a more universal application as long as extra loads are not placed on already weakened and dysfunctional respiratory muscles. As will be reviewed in this chapter, patients with symptomatic "pump failure" may benefit more from ventilatory assistance and resting than from further training.

With these exceptions in mind, this chapter reviews the general principles of physical reconditioning and, specifically, lower and upper extremity training.

Physical Reconditioning

Physical reconditioning is the most important factor in rehabilitating patients with symptomatic respiratory disease. An understanding of the principles and components of exercise conditioning is necessary for anyone who wants to incorporate them in the treatment of such patients.

General Principles

The short- and long-term effects of systematic exercise conditioning have been the subject of extensive investigation. In normal individuals, participation in a well-designed exercise training program results in several objective changes:

- There is increased maximal oxygen uptake—primarily due to increases in blood volume, hemoglobin, and heart stroke volume—with improvement in peripheral utilization of oxygen.
- With specific training, there is increase in muscular strength and endurance—primarily resulting from enlargement of muscle fibers and improved blood and energy supply to the targeted muscle groups.
- Muscle coordination improves.
- Body composition changes, with increased muscle mass and loss of adipose tissue.
- The individual's sense of well-being improves.

In patients with obstructed airflow, participation in a similar program will result in different outcomes depending on the severity of the obstruction. Patients with mild to moderate disease usually respond similarly to healthy individuals; patients with severe obstruction will increase exercise endurance and improve their sensation of well-being with little if any increase in maximal oxygen uptake. Several recent studies have shown improvement in outcomes different from simple exercise performance. They include: improved muscle enzyme content, less dyspnea at a similar work level, and decreased production of lactic acid at isowork. Although an initial training effect has been shown, there has been no systematic investigation regarding the effect of maintenance programs on any of the outcomes, including exercise performance.

Chronic obstructive pulmonary disease decreases tolerance to exercise. The most important factors thought to contribute to this limitation of exercise are

- alterations in pulmonary mechanics,
- abnormal gas exchange,
- dysfunction of the respiratory muscles,
- alterations in cardiac performance,
- malnutrition, and
- development of dyspnea.

Although less well characterized, other factors deserve to be mentioned: smoking, abnormal peripheral muscle function, and polycythemia. While the most severely affected patients cannot reach exercise levels where training effects are thought to occur (above anaerobic threshold), a large body of evidence supports exercise training as a beneficial therapeutic tool in helping these patients achieve their full potential.

Physiologic Adaptation to Training

In order to prescribe exercise for patients with severe pulmonary problems, we must understand several principles of exercise training:

1. Specificity of training
2. Intensity, frequency, and duration of the exercise load, and
3. Detraining effect

1. **Specificity of training.** The training of muscles or muscle groups is beneficial only to the trained muscle.

High-resistance, low-repetition stimulus (e.g., weight lifting) increases muscle strength, whereas low-resistance, high-repetition training increases muscle endurance. Strength training increases myofibrils in certain muscle fibers, whereas endurance training increases the number of capillaries and mitochondrial content in the trained muscles.

The training is specific to the trained muscle. Clausen et al. (1973) trained subjects with their arms and legs and observed that the decreased heart rate observed for arm muscle training could not be transferred to the leg group and vice versa. Davis and Sargeant (1975) showed that if training was completed for one leg, the beneficial effect could not be transferred to exercise involving the untrained leg. More recently Belman and Kendregan (1981) tested eight COPD patients who for six weeks trained only their arms, and seven who trained only their legs. Improvements occurred only in the exercise for which the patients trained. Interestingly, biopsies taken before and after the training program revealed no changes in muscle enzyme content in the trained muscles.

2. **Intensity, frequency, and duration of the exercise load.** These factors profoundly affect the degree of the training effect. Although athletes usually train at maximal or near maximal levels in order to rapidly achieve the desired effects, middle-aged nonathletes may require less intense exercise. Siegel et al. (1970) showed that training sessions of 30 minutes about three times a week for 15 weeks significantly improved maximal oxygen uptake, *if* heart rate was raised over 80% of predicted maximal rate. In patients with chronic lung disease, research by several authors suggests that the greater the number of sessions and the more intense (as a function of maximal performance), the better the results.

Belman and Kendregan (1981) had patients with chronic lung disease exercise four times per week at 30% of their maximal capabilities, gradually increasing their loads as they could individually tolerate the increases. After six weeks, 9 of the 15 patients significantly improved their endurance times. The relatively low training level (30% of maximal) may help explain why six of the patients failed to increase their endurance times. Niederman et al. (1991), who started their subjects at 50% of maximal cycle ergometer level and increased intensity on a weekly basis, observed endurance improvement in most patients. Other authors have used higher starting exercise levels and have achieved higher endurance (Holle et al. 1988; Mohsenifar et al. 1983; Zack and Palange 1985; ZuWallack et al. 1991).

The most thorough study in this regard is that of Casaburi and colleagues. They studied 19 patients with moderate COPD (mean ± SD FEV1 [forced expiratory volume in 1 second] of 1.8 ± 0.53 L), who could achieve anaerobic threshold both before and after randomly assigned, low-intensity (50% of maximal) or high-intensity (80% of maximal) exercise. The high-intensity training program was more effective than the low; and after training there was a drop in ventilatory requirement for exercise that was proportional to the drop in lactate at a given work rate (Casaburi et al. 1991). It appears that a training effect occurs with an exercise intensity at least 50% of maximal, and that the intensity can be increased as tolerated. Yet any exercise is better than none, and good results have been shown even for patients with minimal exercise performance (ZuWallack et al. 1991).

The number of exercise sessions required to improve endurance is a matter of debate (Belman and Kendregan 1981; Make and Buckolz 1991). Table 11.1 shows that, in general, increases in observed endurance time are a function of the number of sessions. Since stopping the exercise results in loss of the training effect, the optimal plan should involve an intense training phase and a maintenance phase. Difficulty

in implementing the latter results in the frequently observed failure to maintain and preserve the beneficial effects of training—yet no study in any respiratory disease has addressed this important issue.

3. **Detraining effect.** The effect achieved by training is lost after the exercise is stopped. Saltin et al. (1968) showed that bed rest in normal subjects resulted in a significant decrease in maximal oxygen uptake within 21 days. When the subjects resumed their exercise programs, it took between 10 and 50 days for the values to return to those seen before resting. Keens et al. (1977) examined ventilatory muscle endurance after training in normal subjects who had undergone ventilatory muscle training. Within one month after they stopped training, the subjects had lost the training effect they had achieved. It seems important to continue to train, but the minimum practical and effective timing of maintenance training remains to be determined.

Patients in our program exercise at 70% of the maximal work achieved in a test day. The work is increased weekly, as tolerated by the patients. We aim to complete 24 sessions, typically in an outpatient setting with three weekly sessions. Hospitalized patients can complete the program more quickly, by performing them on a daily basis. Each session lasts 30 minutes if tolerated by the patient. If the patient cannot tolerate 30 minutes of exercise, the program is begun as tolerated by the patient and no further load is provided until the patient can complete the 30-minute session. When metabolic measurements are not possible, we determine a target work rate by using a Borg visual analog scale of the perception of dyspnea. Refer to Horowitz et al. (1997) for further description of this approach—it is helpful to use dyspnea and not heart rate to set performance targets for patients with lung disease, as breathlessness constitutes their most important complaint.

Table 11.1	Number of Exercise Sessions in Studies on Exercise Endurance		
Author	**Sessions**	**Endurance change**	
Belman	45	50%	
Epstein	19	30%	
Make	12	12%	

Lower Extremity Exercise

Several studies have shown that leg exercise benefits patients with lung disease (Beaumont et al. 1985; Christie 1968; Hughes and Davidson 1983; Moser et al. 1980; Paez et al. 1967).

Studies on Lower Extremity Exercise

Working with 39 dyspneic patients younger than 70 years and not on oxygen, Cockcroft et al. (1981) randomly assigned subjects to a treatment group that spent six weeks in a rehabilitation center where they underwent gradual endurance exercise training, and to a control group that received medical care but was given no special advice to exercise. After four months, the control group also was admitted to the rehabilitation center for six weeks. As was true for the treated patients, they were instructed to exercise at home afterward. Both groups were similar at baseline. After rehabilitation, only 2 of the 16 control patients manifested improvement in dyspnea and cough, whereas 16 of 18 patients in the treatment group improved. More importantly, the treated patients showed significant improvement in the 12-minute walk and in peak oxygen uptake when compared with the controls.

Sinclair and Ingram (1980) studied 33 patients with chronic bronchitis and dyspnea. The 17 patients randomly assigned to the treatment group climbed up and down on two 24-cm steps twice daily. The exercise time was increased to tolerance. The patients exercised at home and were evaluated by the treatment team weekly. The control group did not exercise. After six months, there were no changes in the degree of airflow obstruction in either group; nor was there improvement in strength of the quadriceps, the minute ventilation, and heart rate. Yet the trained patients significantly increased their performance in the 12-minute walk test.

More recently, O'Donnell et al. (1993) compared breathlessness, six-minute walking distance, and cycle ergometer work between two age-matched groups of patients with moderate COPD. The group trained in endurance exercise (n = 23) significantly reduced their dyspnea scores, and increased both distance walked and their cycle ergometry work, when compared to the control group (n = 13). This trial is important in that it not only documented increased endurance, but for the first time evaluated the patients'

perceptions of dyspnea—the most problematic symptom and the one leading to physical limitation.

Since those initial studies, several randomized trials have documented the beneficial effect of lower extremity exercise (Goldstein et al. 1994; Reardon et al. 1994; Ries et al. 1995; Wijkstra et al. 1994). Perhaps most important is the study by Ries et al. (1995), who assigned patients either to an education support group (n = 62) or to a similar educational program with the addition of three walking exercises per week for eight weeks (n = 57). After 2 months—and still at 4, 6, and 12 months—the exercise group showed increased exercise endurance, less dyspnea with exercise, less dyspnea with activity of daily living, and an increase (not statistically significant) in survival. This landmark study clearly establishes the benefit of exercise in pulmonary rehabilitation. Table 11.2 summarizes the results of several studies.

Physiologic Changes Resulting From Exercise

The mechanism by which exercise endurance is improved remains a matter of debate. Several studies, including those of Paez et al. (1967) and Mohsenifar et al. (1983), have demonstrated a drop in heart rate at similar work levels—a hallmark of a training effect for the specific exercise. This effect may be related to a decrease in exercise lactate level, as suggested by Woolf and Suero (1969). More recent evidence in support of a training effect is provided by the study of Casaburi and colleagues, whose COPD patients showed reduced exercise lactic acidosis and ventilation in response to training. The reduction was proportional to the intensity of training: there was a 12% decrease in the lactic acidosis rise in patients trained with the low work rate (50% of maximum), and a 32% decrease in those trained with the high work rate (80% of maximum). Both groups exhibited significant decreases in heart rate after training (Casaburi et al. 1991). Other studies have failed to document either increases in maximum O_2 uptake, or decreases in heart rate or lactate. The most important study in this group, by Belman and Kendregan (1981), failed to show a decrease in heart rate at the same workload as represented by the $\dot{V}O_2$. They also observed no change in oxidative enzyme content of muscle after training, as determined through analysis of biopsies. Interestingly, nine of the treated patients improved their exercise endurance. As stated previously, it is possible that this study used too low a

Table 11.2		Controlled Studies of Rehabilitation With Exercise in Patients With COPD		
Author	**No. patients**	**Duration**	**Course**	**Results**
Cockroft	18 T	Daily	16 weeks	↑12 MW ↑VO₂
	16 C	—	—	No change
Sinclair	17 T	Daily	40 weeks	↑FVC ↑12 MW
	16 C	—	—	No change
O'Donnell	23 T	Daily	8 weeks	↑FVC ↑12 MW ↓Dyspnea
	13 C	—	—	No change
Reardon	10 T	2 × week	6 weeks	↓Dyspnea
	10 C	—	—	No change
Ries	57 T	Daily	8 weeks	↑Exercise capacity ↓Dyspnea ↑Self-efficacy
	62 C	Daily education	8 weeks	No change
Wijkstra	28 T	Daily at home	12 weeks	↑Exercise capacity ↑Quality of life
	15 C	—	—	No change
Goldstein	45 T	Daily	24 weeks	↑6 MW VO₂ ↓Dyspnea ↓S.O.B.
	44 C	None	24 weeks	No change

T = treated; C = controls; MW = minute walk test; FVC = forced vital capacity; VO₂ = peak oxygen uptake; S.O.B. = shortness of breath

training effort, since training was started at 30% of the maximum achieved during their testing. This possibility is supported by two studies by Maltais and colleagues. First they showed that muscle biopsies from the legs of patients with COPD had decreased levels of mitochondrial oxidative enzymes (Maltais et al. 1995); subsequently, they observed significant increases in the mitochondrial enzymes after exercise training (Maltais et al. 1996), as well as delayed onset of the lactase threshold.

The evidence therefore indicates that patients with COPD can be trained to a level that produces physiologic changes consistent with improved muscle performance (figure 11.1).

Can Severely Affected Patients Benefit?

Two studies addressed the issue of whether patients with the most severe COPD can undergo exercise training. It is an important question: many patients with the most severe COPD do not exercise to the

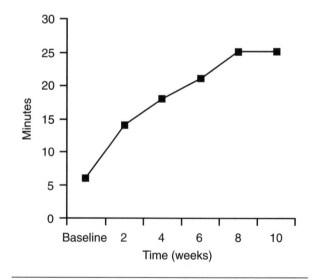

Figure 11.1 Average endurance time that 12 patients with COPD could sustain a submaximal workload targeted at 70% of maximal work measured in a cycle ergometer test. Patients were tested at baseline and at 2 weeks interval test, training 3 times weekly. Plateau was reached at 8 weeks (24 sessions) of training.

intensity required to reach their anaerobic threshold or to train the cardiovascular system.

Niederman et al. (1991) studied 33 patients with different degrees of COPD (FEV1 ranging from 0.33 L to 3.82 L). After training, there was no correlation between the degree of obstruction in these patients and their observed improvement—the patients with very low FEV1 were as likely to improve as the patients with high FEV1. Similarly, ZuWallack et al (1991) evaluated 50 patients with COPD (FEV1 range from 0.38 L to 3.24 L) before and after exercise training. They observed inverse relationships between the level of improvement and the baselines for 12-minute walking distance and for $\dot{V}O_2$. They concluded that patients with poor performance, on either the 12-minute walking distance or maximal exercise test, are not necessarily poor candidates for an exercise program. These data suggest that any patient capable of undergoing leg exercise endurance training will benefit from a program that includes leg exercise.

Type of Exercise and Testing

Different studies have used different training techniques. Most studies include walking both as a measurement of exercise tolerance and of the training program. The classic 6- or 12-minute walk (6 or 12 MWD—the distance walked over 6 or 12 minutes) is very good for patients with moderate to severe COPD but may not be taxing enough for patients with less airflow obstruction (McGavin et al. 1976). Performance on the 12 MWD actually predicted survival in one study. In our own studies of stair climbing, we found we could estimate the peak oxygen uptake from the number of steps climbed during a symptom-limited test (Pollock et al. 1993). Several researchers have used treadmills or steps for testing purposes, even when the training consisted of walking—oxygen uptake is higher for stair climbing or treadmill testing than for the more commonly used leg ergometry, presumably because the former uses more body muscles than leg cycling. Leg ergometry is a very popular testing device and has been the training apparatus for most recent studies. It is certainly smaller than the treadmill; and with relatively inexpensive units on the market, it is possible to place several together and train a number of patients simultaneously.

All the studies quoted relied on either inpatient or outpatient hospital training. Little information is available regarding implementation of such programs at home. In a unique report, O'Hara et al. (1984) enrolled 14 patients with moderate COPD (FEV1 = 1.17 ± 0.76 L) in a home exercise program. All pa-

tients walked daily while carrying a lightweight backpack (2.6 ± 0.5 kg). Half also did weightlifting and limb-strengthening exercises, including wrist curls, arms curls, partial leg squats, calf raises, and supine dumbbell press. The initial backpack load of 4.3 ± 0.9 kg was increased weekly by 1.2 ± 0.5 kg for six weeks, reaching 10.4 ± 2.6 kg by the last week. The weightlifters performed 10 repetitions three times—avoiding dyspnea, breath-holding, and fatigue—for a total time of 30 minutes daily. Patients documented their exercises in a diary. Health care personnel visited the patients weekly. After training, all weightlifters had reduced their minute ventilation during bicycle ergometry, when compared with controls. Furthermore, the weight-trained patients showed a 16% increase in exercise endurance. This study suggests that patients can engage in exercise training in the comfort of their homes, with relatively inexpensive programs and no hospital visits. More recent data confirm that supervised home exercise programs achieve the same outcomes as those in hospitals (Wijkstra et al. 1994).

In our pulmonary rehabilitation program we use an electrically braked ergometer for testing, and mechanically controlled ergometers for training, on either an outpatient or inpatient basis, depending on the patient's condition. See "Training Method for Leg Exercise" (below) for a practical discussion of how we train our patients. The program may be tailored to each individual and to the available training equipment.

Upper Extremity Exercise

It is unfortunate that most of our knowledge about rehabilitation exercise conditioning derives from programs emphasizing leg training. Performance of many everyday tasks requires not only the hands, but also

---

Training Method for Leg Exercise

1. Train at 60% of maximal work capacity (as determined by an exercise test, not necessarily by evaluating heart rate).

2. Increase work every 5th session as tolerated.

3. Monitor dyspnea and heart rate.

4. Increase work after 20-30 minutes of submaximal targeted work.

5. Aim for 24 sessions.

the concerted action of other muscle groups that control upper torso and arm positioning. Some muscles of the upper torso and shoulder girdle serve both respiratory and postural functions. Muscles such as the upper and lower trapezius, latissimus dorsi, serratus anterior, subclavius, and pectoralis minor and major possess both thoracic and extrathoracic anchoring points. They may help position the arms or shoulders; or, if given an extrathoracic fulcrum (such as fixing the arms in a supported position), they may exert a pulling force on the ribcage. In patients with chronic airflow obstruction, as severity worsens, the diaphragm loses its capacity to generate force, and the muscles of the rib cage become more important in generating inspiratory pressures (Martinez et al. 1990). When patients perform unsupported arm exercise, some of the shoulder girdle muscles decrease their participation in ventilation; tasks involving complex purposeful arm movements may affect the pattern of ventilation.

Studies on Upper Extremity Exercise

Tangri and Wolf (1973) used a pneumobelt to study breathing patterns in seven patients with COPD, while they performed simple activities of daily living such as tying their shoes and brushing their teeth. The patients developed an irregular and rapid pattern of breathing with the arm exercise. After the exercise, the patients breathed faster and deeper, which according to the authors was done to restore the blood gases to normal.

We have explored the ventilatory response to unsupported arm exercise and compared it with the response to leg exercise in patients with severe chronic lung disease (Celli et al. 1986). Arm exercise resulted in dyssynchronous thoracoabdominal excursion that was not due solely to diaphragmatic fatigue. The dyspnea reported by the patients was associated with a dyssynchronous breathing pattern. We concluded that unsupported arm exercise could shift work to the diaphragm and in some way lead to dyssynchrony. To test this hypothesis, we plotted pleural pressure (Ppl) versus gastric pressure (Pg) (measured with gastric and endoesophageal balloons), evaluating the changes as well as the ventilatory responses to unsupported arm exercise. We compared these results with those from leg cycle ergometry in normal subjects and in patients with airflow obstruction (Celli et al. 1988; Criner and Celli 1988), and found increased diaphragmatic pressure excursion with arm exercise. We also found alterations in the pattern of pressure generation, with more contribution by the diaphragm

and abdominal muscles of respiration and less contribution by the inspiratory muscles of the rib cage.

Our knowledge of ventilatory response to arm exercise was based on arm cycle ergometry. It is known that at a given work load in normal subjects, arm cranking is more demanding than leg cycling as shown by higher VO_2, VE, heart rate, blood pressure, and lactate production (Bobbert 1960; Davis et al. 1976; Steinberg et al. 1967). At maximal effort however, VO_2, VE, cardiac output, and lactate levels are lower during arm than during leg cycle ergometry (Martin et al. 1991; Reybrouck et al. 1975). Very little is known about the metabolic and ventilatory cost of simple arm elevation. Some recent reports underscore the importance of arm position in ventilation. Banzett et al. (1988) showed that arm bracing increases the capacity to sustain maximal ventilation, when compared to lifting the elbows from the braced position. Others have shown a decrease in the maximum attainable workload, and increases in both oxygen uptake and ventilation, at any given workload when normal subjects exercised with their arms elevated (Dolmage et al. 1993; Maestro et al. 1990). We evaluated the metabolic and respiratory consequence of simple arm elevation in patients with COPD (Martinez et al. 1990). Patients who held their arms in front of them, parallel to the floor, significantly increased both VO_2 and VCO_2, with concomitant increases in heart rate and VE. Evaluating ventilatory muscle recruitment patterns by continuous recording of Pg and Ppl, we observed increased contribution of diaphragmatic and abdominal muscle toward ventilation. The observations suggest that if we train the arms to perform more work, or if we decrease the ventilatory requirement for the same work, we should improve a patient's capacity to perform arm activity.

Results of Upper Extremity Exercise

Several studies using both arm and leg training have shown that the addition of arm training results in improved performance that is for the most part task-specific.

Belman and Kendregan (1981) observed a significant increase in arm exercise endurance after exercise training. Lake et al. (1990) had patients engage in arm exercise, leg exercise, or both. There were increases in exercise endurance for arm ergometry in the arm training group, for leg ergometry in the leg training group, and increases in both arm and leg ergometry in the combined group. In addition there was an improved sensation of well-being in the combined group. Ries et al. (1988) compared the effects of two forms of arm exercise—gravity resistance, and modified proprioceptive neuromuscular facilitation—with no arm exercise in a group of 45 patients with COPD who were involved in a comprehensive, multidisciplinary pulmonary rehabilitation program. Even though only 20 patients completed the program, they showed improved performance on tests that were specific for the training, and a decrease in fatigue in all the tests.

A group of cystic fibrosis patients studied by Keens et al. (1977) underwent upper extremity training consisting of swimming and canoeing for 1.5 hours daily. After six weeks, they exhibited increased upper extremity endurance; most importantly, their increase in maximal sustainable ventilatory capacity was similar to that obtained with ventilatory muscle training. This suggests that arm exercise training programs can train ventilatory muscles.

Because simple arm elevation results in significant increases in $\dot{V}O_E$, $\dot{V}O_2$, and VCO_2, we studied 14 patients with COPD before and after eight weeks of three-times-weekly, 20-minute sessions of unsupported arm and leg exercise. Our study was part of a comprehensive rehabilitation program to test whether arm training decreases ventilatory requirement for arm activity. There was a 35% decrease in the rise of $\dot{V}O_2$ and VCO_2 brought about by arm elevation, associated with a significant decrease in $\dot{V}O_E$ (Couser et al. 1993)(figure11.2). Because the patients also trained their legs, we could not conclude that the improvement was due to the arm exercise. To answer this question, we had patients with COPD undergo either unsupported arm training (n = 11) or resistance breathing training (n = 14). After 24 sessions, arm endurance increased only for the unsupported arm training group. Interestingly, maximal inspiratory pressure increased significantly for both groups, indicating that by training the arms, we may induce ventilatory muscle training for those rib cage muscles that hinge on the shoulder girdle (Epstein et al. 1991).

Upper Extremity Rehabilitation Programs

Based on the information available, we include arm exercise in our rehabilitation program. As seen in "Training Method for Supported (Ergometry) Arm Exercise" and "Training Method for Unsupported Arm Exercise" (below), the methods for supported and unsupported exercises vary in their implementation.

Training Method for Supported (Ergometry) Arm Exercise

1. Train at 60% of maximal work capacity (as determined by an exercise test, not necessarily by evaluating heart rate).

2. Increase work every 5th session as tolerated.

3. Monitor dyspnea and heart rate.

4. Train for as long as tolerated up to 30 minutes.

Training Method for Unsupported Arm Exercise

1. Dowel (weight = 750 grams).

2. Lift to shoulder level for 2 minutes, one repetition for each breath.

3. Rest for 2 minutes.

4. Repeat sequence as tolerated for up to 32 minutes.

5. Monitor dyspnea and heart rate.

6. Increase weight (250 grams) every 5th session as tolerated.

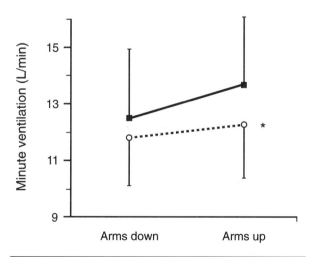

Figure 11.2 Minute ventilation measured with arms down and after two minutes of arm elevation before unsupported arm training (■). After 19 sessions of unsupported arm training, the patients manifested a significant decrease in minute ventilation during arm elevation (○). *p < .05 using paired t-test.

Reprinted, by permission, from J. Couser et al., 1993, "Pulmonary rehabilitation that include arm exercise, reduces metabolic and ventilatory requirements for simple arm elevation," *Chest* 103:37-38.

Our patients generally perform arm ergometry for 20 minutes per session, starting at 60% of the maximal work (measured in watts) achieved in the exercise test and increasing the work weekly as tolerated. We monitor dyspnea and heart rate. For patients whose limiting symptom is dyspnea at minimal work, we exercise them at 60% of the work that makes them stop. In the most severe patients, the heart rate is unreliable—they may be tachycardic even at rest, and may not show any significant increase with exercise. In these patients, dyspnea may be a more reliable index to follow.

In unsupported arm exercise training, patients lift a dowel (750 g) to shoulder level in the same rhythm as their breathing rate. For a total of 30 minutes, they exercise for two minutes then rest for two minutes. We monitor dyspnea and heart rate; and we increase the load by 250 grams each week, as tolerated. We aim to complete 24 sessions.

Martinez et al. (1993) compared unsupported arm training with arm ergometry training. Endurance time improved significantly for both groups, but un-supported arm training decreased oxygen uptake at the same workload when compared to arm cranking training. They concluded that arm exercise against gravity may be more effective in training patients for activities that resemble those of daily living.

Table 11.3 summarizes an increasing body of evidence that upper extremity exercise training results in improved performance for arm activities in general, and decreases ventilatory requirements for upper extremity activities similar to those in the exercise. The net result is an improvement in the capacity of patients to perform activities of daily living.

Respiratory Muscles and Breathing Training

Leith and Bradley (1976) first demonstrated that, like their skeletal counterparts, the respiratory muscles of normal individuals can be specifically trained to im-

Table 11.3		Controlled Studies of Arm Exercise in Patients With COPD			
Author	**No. patients**	**Duration**	**Course**	**Type**	**Results**
Keens	7 arms	1.5 hr/day	4 wk	Swimming/canoeing	↑VMT (56%)
	4 VMT	15 min/day	4 wk	VMT	↑VME (52%)
	4 control	—	—	VMT	↑VME (22%)
Belman	8 arms	20 min 4 ×/wk	6 wk	Arm ergometry	↑Arm cycle No ↑ PFT
	7 legs	20 min 4 ×/wk	6 wk	Cycle ergometry	↑Leg cycle No ↑ PFT
Lake	6 arms	1 hr 3 ×/wk	8 wk	Several types	No change in PImax or VME
	6 legs	1 hr 3 ×/wk	8 wk	Walking	No change in PImax or VME
	7 arms and legs	1 hr 3 ×/wk	8 wk	Combined	No change in PImax or VME
Ries	8 gravity resistance arms	15 min/day	6 wk	Low-resistance, high-repetition	↑Arm endurance ↓Dyspnea
	9 neuromuscular facilitation	15 min/day	6 wk	Weight lifts	↑Arm endurance ↓Dyspnea
	11 controls	—	6 wk	Walk	No change
Epstein	13 arms	30 min/day	8 wk	UAE	↓VO_2 and VE for arm elevation ↑PImax
	10 VMT	30 min/day	8 wk	VMT	↑PImax and VME

VMT = ventilatory muscle training; VME = ventilatory muscle endurance; PFT = pulmonary function tests; PImax = maximal inspiratory pressure; UAE = unsupported arm elevation

prove their strength or their endurance. Subsequent to that observation, a number of studies have shown that a training response will occur if there is sufficient stimulus. An increase in inspiratory muscle strength (and perhaps endurance) should result in improved respiratory muscle function by decreasing the ratio of the pressure required to breath (PI) and the maximal pressure that the respiratory system can generate (PImax). The PI/PImax ratio, which represents the effort required to complete each breath as a function of the force reserve, is the most important determinant of fatigue in loaded respiratory muscles (Roussos and Macklem 1982). Since patients with COPD have reduced inspiratory muscle strength, considerable efforts have been made to define the role of respiratory muscle training in these patients.

Ventilatory Muscle Strength and Endurance Training

In some cases, training ventilatory muscles is extremely effective. In others, it is of no use or even counterproductive. Every clinician should be well aware of when such training is or is not appropriate.

Strength Training

A high-intensity, low-frequency stimulus is needed to train respiratory muscles. Inspiratory muscles are trained by inspiratory maneuvers performed against a closed glottis or shutter.

Several studies have shown an increase in maximal inspiratory pressures when the respiratory muscles have been specifically trained for strength. Lecoq and colleagues studied nine patients (some of whom had COPD) who, after four weeks of training, showed a 50% increase in PImax (Lecoq et al. 1970). Reid and Warren (1984) observed a 53% increase in PImax in six COPD patients after five weeks of training. Both groups noticed a smaller but significant increase in expiratory muscle pressure. Decreasing PI/PImax through respiratory muscle strength training does not appear to be clinically important. Yet respiratory muscle strength often increases as a by-product of endurance training achieved with the use of resistive loads. It is possible that some of the benefits observed after endurance training may relate to the increased strength.

Endurance Training

Endurance is achieved through low-intensity, high-frequency training programs, of which there are three

types: flow resistive loading, threshold loading, and voluntary isocapneic hyperpnea.

Flow Resistive Loading and Threshold Loading

In flow resistive training, the load is created primarily by decreasing the inspiratory breathing hole size—provided that frequency, tidal volume, and inspiratory time are held constant. Although most studies in patients with COPD have shown an improvement in the time that a given respiratory load can be maintained (ventilatory muscle endurance), the results must be interpreted with caution since it has been shown that endurance can be influenced and actually increased with changes in the pattern of breathing. Threshold loading can result in some muscle training, by assuring that at least the inspired pressure is high enough to ensure training, independent of inspiratory flow rate. Although breathing pattern is important (inspiratory time or T_I and respiratory rate), it is not as critically important as inspired pressure.

Because many studies have not been controlled, it is difficult to attribute their results to the training. The controlled studies summarized in table 11.4 show an increase in the endurance time during which the ventilatory muscles could tolerate a known load; some show a significant increase in strength (Belman and Shadmehr 1988; Chen et al. 1985; Harver et al. 1989; Larson et al. 1988) and a decrease in dyspnea during the performance of inspiratory load and exercise (Epstein et al. 1991; Falk et al. 1985). In the studies that evaluated systemic exercise performance, there was a minimal increase in walking distance (Jones et al. 1985; Larson et al. 1988; Lisboa et al. 1994; Pardy et al. 1981; Weiner et al. 1992).

Weiner and colleagues assigned 36 COPD patients to one of three groups. Group 1 received specific ventilatory muscle threshold training (VMT) combined with general exercise reconditioning; group 2 received exercise training alone; group 3 received no training. VM training improved VM strength and endurance (as is already known), but patients treated with the combination of exercise and VMT manifested a significant increase in exercise tolerance when compared with those who only exercised (Weiner et al. 1992). In a companion article, the same group reported that asthmatic patients treated with VMT not only increased strength but also showed improvements in asthma symptoms, number of hospitalizations, number of emergency department visits, frequency of school or work absenteeism, and amount of medication consumption (Weiner et al. 1992). Lisboa et al. (1994) have shown that VMT at 30% of PImax seems

Table 11.4   Controlled Trials of Ventilatory Muscle Resistive Training in COPD

Author	No. patients	Type	Frequency	Duration	Results
Pardy	9	RB	2 ×/day	8 wk	↑ET ↑12 MW
	8	PT	3 ×/wk	8 wk	No change
Larson	10	RB	30 min/day 30% PImax	8 wk	↑PImax ↑ET ↑12 MW
	12	RB	Daily	8 wk	No ↑ PI, end time, or 12 MW
			15% PImax	30 min	
Harver	10	RB	15 min 2 ×/day	8 wk	↑PImax
	9	Sham	15 min 2 ×/day	8 wk	No change
Belman	8	RB	Daily	6 wk	↑ET (30 min) ↑PImax
	9	RB	Daily	6 wk	30 min
Chen	7	RB	Daily	4 wk	↑ET (30 min)
	6	Sham	Daily	4 wk	No change (30 min)
Bjerre	14	RB	45 min/day	6 wk	↑ET, no exercise
	14	Sham	45 min/day	6 wk	No change
Falk	12	RB	Daily	12 mo	↑ET (45 min), no exercise
	15	Sham	Daily	12 mo	No change
Noseda	12	RB	Daily	8 wk	↑ET (30 min)
	13	Breathing exercise	Daily	8 wk	No change
Jones	7	RB	Daily	10 wk	↑Exercise end (30 min)
	6	Sham	Daily	10 wk	↑Exercise end
	8	Exercise	Daily	10 wk	↑Exercise end
Weiner	12	RB and exercise	Daily	3 mo	↑↑Exercise ↑PImax
	12	Exercise	Daily	3 mo	↑Exercise
	12	Control	None	3 mo	No change
Lisboa	10	RB 12% PImax	Daily	5 wk	No change
	10	RB 30% PImax	Daily	5 wk	↑PImax ↑ET ↓Dyspnea

RB = resistive breathing; PT = physical therapy; ET = endurance time for loaded breathing; PImax = maximal inspiratory pressure; Exercise end = leg exercise endurance

not only to increase leg ergometry endurance; it also improves baseline dyspnea score and decreases breathlessness with exercise.

It is clear that VMT with resistive breathing results in improved VM strength and endurance. In COPD, however, it is not clear whether this effort results in decreased morbidity or mortality, or offers any clinical advantage that makes it worth the effort. In many studies, compliance has been low—with up to 50% of all pulmonary patients failing to complete the programs. On the other hand, if confirmed by others, the studies by Weiner and coworkers (1992) and Lisboa et al. (1994) suggest that this form of treatment for asthmatics should be further explored.

Ventilatory Isocapneic Hyperpnea

This is a training method by which patients maintain high levels of ventilation over time (15 minutes, two or three times daily). The oxygen and carbon dioxide are kept constant in the breathing circuit. In an uncontrolled study, patients with COPD not only increased their maximal sustained ventilatory capacity but also increased arm and leg exercise performance after six weeks of training (Harver et al. 1989). Two controlled studies (table 11.5) also reported increases in maximal sustainable ventilatory capacity (MSVC) in COPD in patients trained for six weeks, but their improvement in exercise endurance was no better than that of the control group (Belman and Mittman 1980; Ries and Moser 1986).

It seems that respiratory muscle training results in increased strength and capacity of the muscles to endure a respiratory load. There is debate as to whether it also results in improved exercise performance or improved performance in activities of daily living. Knowing the respiratory muscle factors that may contribute to ventilatory limitation in COPD, one might logically predict that increases in strength and endurance should help respiratory muscle function. But this is perhaps only important in the capacity of the patients to handle inspiratory loads, for example in acute exacerbations of their disease. It is less likely that ventilatory muscle training will greatly affect systemic exercise performance.

Ventilatory Muscle Training for Intensive Care Patients

Few data exist to justify training the ventilatory muscles of patients in intensive care. It is apparent that as soon as patients are left to breathe on their own (as during any form of weaning), their respiratory muscles are being retrained. We actually use this "training method" whenever we place patients on either T-piece or low synchronized intermittent mandatory ventilation (SIMV), although we don't generally analyze the results as we would for a formal training method. More often, we think of training in terms of additional, external loads in addition to spontaneous respiration.

Studies

Few researchers have studied patients recovering from ventilatory failure. Belman and colleagues reported improvement in two patients who had difficulty weaning from mechanical ventilation; after respiratory muscle threshold training, they were able to come off mechanical ventilation (Belman et al. 1981). In a larger but still uncontrolled study, Aldrich et al. (1989) recruited 30 patients who had suffered from stable chronic respiratory failure for at least three weeks, but who had failed repeated weaning attempts. Patients with active infections or unstable cardiovascular, renal, or endocrine problems were excluded, as were those with gross malnutrition (albumin < 2.5 g/dl) or neuromuscular disease. Training consisted of intermittently breathing through one inspiratory

| Table 11.5 | Controlled Trials of Ventilatory Isocapneic Hyperpnea in Patients With COPD |

Author	No. patients	Type	Frequency	Duration	Results
Ries	5	VIH	45 min	6 wk	↑MSVC ↑Exercise
	7	Walking	45 min	6 wk	↑Exercise
Levine	15	VIH	15 min	6 wk	↑MSVC ↑Exercise ↑ADLs
	17	IPPB	15 min	6 wk	↑ADLs ↑Exercise

VIH = ventilatory isocapneic; MSVC = maximal sustainable ventilatory capacity; ADLs = activities of daily living; IPPB = intermittent positive pressure breathing

resistor while either spontaneously breathing or being supported at two to eight breaths per minute with SIMV. The patients' PImax improved from 37 ± 15 to 46 ± 15 cm H_2O while vital capacity increased from 561 ± 325 to 901 ± 480 ml. Of the 30 patients, 12 were weaned after 10 to 46 days of training (40% success). Because the study was uncontrolled and used a selected group of patients, its findings may not apply to most patients recovering from respiratory failure; furthermore, the success rate is little different from those reported in weaning facilities that have not used VMT (Alrich et al. 1989). Before ventilatory muscle training can be recommended as a form of treatment for patients with respiratory failure, more rigorous research is needed.

Caution Is Necessary

It is important to understand that ventilatory muscle training, especially with resistive or threshold loading, may be deleterious. Breathing at high tension time index with either a PI/PImax or prolonged inspiratory time over the total duration of a respiratory cycle (T_I/T_{TOT}) may induce muscle fatigue (Bellemare and Grassino 1982). Because the muscles of ventilation cannot be rested, as is customary in the training of peripheral muscles in athletes, fatigue may precipitate ventilatory failure in COPD patients. Increased PI is an intrinsic part of VMT, hence it is possible that if an intense enough program is enforced, fatigue may actually be precipitated.

Breathing Retraining

There are other less conventional forms of training that are open to critical review, but that are conceptually solid and may offer new avenues of treatment. The ventilated patient has a high ventilatory drive—patients who failed a ventilator weaning trial manifest higher drive than those patients who successfully weaned.

Biofeedback

Holliday and Hyers studied 40 patients after at least seven days of mechanical ventilation, weaning them either with conventional methods or with electromyographic feedback training, using the frontalis signal to indicate tension and induce relaxation. They also used surface EMG of the intercostals and diaphragm as indicators of respiratory muscle activity. Compared with the control group, the biofeedback group had fewer mean ventilator days. Their tidal volume and mean inspiratory flow increased significantly when corrected by diaphragmatic EMG amplitude (which was interpreted as improved diaphragmatic efficiency). The authors concluded that breathing retraining resulted in a more efficient breathing pattern, which in turn decreased dyspnea and anxiety and allowed for quicker weaning time in the treated patients (Holliday and Hyers 1990).

To further study some of these factors, we measured the work of breathing (determined by the pressure time integral of the excursions of the continuously recorded Ppl) before and after rehabilitation in 16 patients with COPD. There were no changes in pulmonary functions, but there was a significant decrease in the pressure time index at the exercise isotime after rehabilitation (table 11.6). This drop was due mostly to a decrease in respiratory frequency (Benditt et al. 1990).

Finally, retraining in breathing techniques or pursed-lip breathing that decreases breathing fre-

Table 11.6	Work of Breathing, Exercise Endurance, and Maximal Transdiaphragmatic Pressure Before and After Pulmonary Rehabilitation		
	Endurance time (sec)	**∫ Pesdt (Cm H_2O · min)**	**Pdimax (Cm H_2O)**
Pre-rehab	434	288	48
Post-rehab	512*	219*	52

*$p < .05$

Pdimax = maximal transdiaphragmatic pressure; ∫ Pesdt = work of breathing as estimated by the pressure time index calculated from continuous recording of endoesophageal pressure

quency has resulted in increases in tidal volume oxygen saturation and decreases in dyspnea (Roa et al.).

In a previously cited work from our laboratory, analysis of the many factors that may have contributed to improved exercise endurance for upper extremity exercise after upper extremity training indicated that the most striking was a drop in mean inspiratory flow (VT/T_1) at exercise isotime (Epstein et al. 1997). We believe this may represent better coordination of the respiratory muscles.

Yoga

There are other ways to improve ventilatory patterns. Yoga teaches control of posture and voluntary control of breathing, the latter including rapid abdominal maneuvers and/or slow deep breaths with apnea at the end of inspiration and expiration. The breathing rate may be brought down to 6 breaths per minute.

Stanescu et al. (1981) compared breathing patterns of eight well-trained yoga practitioners with eight controls matched for gender, age, and height. The yoga group had a breathing pattern of ample tidal volume and slow frequency, and a lower ventilatory response to CO_2 rebreathing. The mechanisms of these effects are not clear, but they include habituation to chronic overstimulation of stretch receptors. Since ventilation is automatically controlled by structures in the upper medulla and brain stem, and is voluntarily controlled by the cortex, sustained slow deep breathing may become a "learned" reflex. Whatever the mechanisms, these responses may have practical applications. Tandon (1980) studied the effects of yoga breathing in patients with COPD. The yoga-trained patients controlled dyspnea and improved their exercise tolerance better than the controls.

Postural Changes

Habitual positioning may determine musculoskeletal tone and contraction. Over the last few years, increasing attention has been given to the voluntary inhibition of these musculoskeletal tone and contraction patterns. This focus has been particularly useful for singers. Austin and Pullin (1984) found that proprioceptive musculoskeletal education for better posture improved peak expiratory flow rate, maximal voluntary ventilation, and maximal inspiratory and expiratory pressures in normal subjects. These lessons have not been systematically evaluated in patients with lung disease, but breathing retraining (pursed-lip breathing and diaphragmatic breathing) is a form of therapy that resembles the above-mentioned techniques.

Pursed-Lip Breathing

Pursed-lip breathing (PLB) slows the breathing rate and increases tidal volume. It shifts the recruitment pattern of ventilatory muscles from one that is predominantly diaphragmatic to one that recruits more accessory muscles of the rib cage and abdominal muscles of exhalation (Roa et al. 1991). This shift may contribute to the relief of dyspnea reported by patients when they adopt PLB. Patients on ventilators cannot use pursed-lip breathing techniques. But administration of expiratory retardants or positive-end expiratory pressure improves oxygenation; it also decreases respiratory rate, augments ventilation, and improves the work of breathing in weaning patients. Since pursed-lip breathing (PLB) and positive end expiratory pressure (PEEP) may have similar physiologic effects, the former therapy is often indicated once the latter has been discontinued.

Summary

A critical review of the literature indicates that leg and arm exercise training improve exercise performance and seem to have physiological explanations different from simple dyspnea desensitization. Implementation of such elementary training programs is within the reach of virtually any facility, and will result in better quality of life for patients with respiratory disease.

There are more unresolved questions than known facts about training and respiratory muscle function. A wealth of information will be gained if systematic scientific analysis is applied to answer many of the questions we have addressed in this review. It is rewarding to see that widespread interest in applied respiratory physiology has begun to produce results that may benefit the large number of patients suffering from disabling respiratory diseases, and for whom there are no other viable therapeutic options.

References

Aldrich, T.K., J.P. Karpel, and R.M. Uhrlass. 1989. Weaning from mechanical ventilation: Adjunctive use of inspiratory muscle resistive training. *Crit Care* 17:143-7.

Austin, J., and G. Pullin. 1984. Improved respiratory function after lessons in the Alexander technique of musculoskeletal education. *Am Rev Respir Dis* 129:A275.

Banzett, R., G. Topulus, D. Leith, and C. Natios. 1988. Bracing arms increases the capacity for sustained hyperpnea. *Am Rev Respir Dis* 138:106-9.

Beaumont, A., A. Cockcroft, and A. Guz. 1985. A self-paced treadmill walking test for breathless patients. *Thorax* 40:459-64.

Bellemare, F., and A. Grassino. 1982. Evaluation of diaphragmatic fatigue. *J Appl Physiol* 53:1196-206.

Belman, M.J. 1981. Respiratory failure treated by ventilatory muscle training (VMT): a report of two cases. *Eur J Respir Dis* 62:391-3.

Belman, M.J., and B.A. Kendregan. 1981. Exercise training fails to increase skeletal muscle enzymes in patients with chronic obstructive pulmonary disease. *Am Rev Respir Dis* 123:256-61.

Belman, M.J., and C. Mittman. 1980. Ventilatory muscle training improves exercise capacity in chronic obstructive pulmonary disease patients. *Am Rev Respir Dis* 121:273-80.

Belman, M.J., and R. Shadmehr. 1988. Targeted resistive ventilatory muscle training in chronic obstructive pulmonary disease. *J Appl Physiol* 65:2726-35.

Benditt, J., M. Pollock, E. Breslin, and B. Celli. 1990. Comprehensive pulmonary rehabilitation decreases the work of breathing during leg cycle ergometry in patients with severe chronic airflow obstruction (CAO). *Am Rev Respir Dis* 141:A509.

Bjerre-Jempsen, K., N. Secher, and A. Kok-Jensen. 1981. Inspiratory resistance training in severe chronic obstructive pulmonary disease. *Eur J Respir Dis* 62:405-11.

Bobbert, A.C. 1960. Physiological comparison of three types of ergometry. *J Appl Physiol* 15:1007-14.

Casaburi, R., A. Patessio, F. Ioli, S. Zanabouri, C. Donner, and K. Wasserman. 1991. Reductions in exercise lactic acidosis and ventilation as a result of exercise training in patients with obstructive lung disease. *Am Rev Respir Dis* 143:9-18.

Celli, B., G. Criner, and J. Rassulo. 1988. Ventilatory muscle recruitment during unsupported arm exercise in normal subjects. *J Appl Physiol* 64:1936-41.

Celli, B., J. Rassulo, and B. Make. 1986. Dyssynchronous breathing associated with arm but not leg exercise in patients with COPD. *N Engl J Med* 314:1485-90.

Chen, H., R. Dukes, and B. Martin. 1985. Inspiratory muscle training in patients with chronic obstructive pulmonary disease. *Thorax* 131:251-5.

Christie, D. 1968. Physical training in chronic obstructive lung disease. *Br Med J* 2:150-1.

Clausen, J., K. Clausen, B. Rasmussen, and J. Trap-Jensen. 1973. Central and peripheral circulatory changes after training of the arms or legs. *Am J Physiol* 225:675-82.

Cockcroft, A., M. Saunders, G. Berry. 1981. Randomized controlled trial of rehabilitation in chronic respiratory disability. *Thorax* 36:200-3.

Couser, J., F. Martinez, and B. Celli. 1993. Pulmonary rehabilitation that include arm exercise, reduces metabolic and ventilatory requirements for simple arm elevation. *Chest* 103:37-38.

Criner, G., and B. Celli. 1988. Effect of unsupported arm exercise on ventilatory muscle recruitment in patients with severe chronic airflow obstruction. *Am Rev Respir Dis* 138:856-67.

Davis, C., and A. Sargeant. 1975. Effects of training on the physiological responses to one and two legged work. *J Appl Physiol* 38:377-81.

Davis, J., P. Vodak, J. Wilmore, J. Vodak, and P. Kwitz. 1976. Anaerobic threshold and maximal power for three modes of exercise. *J Appl Physiol* 41:549-50.

Dolmage, T., L. Maestro, M. Avendano, and R. Goldstein. 1993. The ventilatory response to arm elevation of patients with Chronic Obstructive Pulmonary Disease. *Chest* 104:1097-100.

Epstein, S., E. Breslin, J. Roa, and B. Celli. 1991. Impact of unsupported arm training (AT) and ventilatory muscle training (VMT) on the metabolic and ventilatory consequences of unsupported arm elevation (UAE) and exercise (UAEx) in patients with chronic airflow obstruction. *Am Rev Respir Dis* 143:81A.

Epstein, S., B. Celli, F. Martinez, J. Couser, J. Roa, M. Pollock, and J. Benditt. 1997. Arm training reduces the VO_2 and VE cost of unsupported arm exercise and elevation in chronic obstructive pulmonary disease. *J Cardpulm Rehabil* 17:171-177.

Falk, P., A. Eksen, K. Kolliker, and J.B. Andersen. 1985. Relieving dyspnea with an inexpensive and simple method in patients with severe chronic airflow limitation. *Eur J Respir Dis* 66:181-6.

Goldstein, R.S., E. Gort, D. Stubing, M.A. Avendano, and G.H. Guyatt. 1994. Randomized trial of respiratory rehabilitation. *Lancet* 344:1394-1398.

Harver, A., D. Mahler, and J. Daubenspeck. 1989. Targeted inspiratory muscle training improves respiratory muscle function and reduces dyspnea in patients with chronic obstructive pulmonary disease. *Ann Int Med* 111:117-24.

Holle, R., D. Williams, J. Vandree, G. Starks, and R. Schoene. 1988. Increased muscle efficiency and sustained benefits in an outpatient community hospital-based pulmonary rehabilitation program. *Chest* 94:1161-68.

Holliday, J., and T. Hyers. 1990. The reduction of weaning time from mechanical ventilation using tidal volume and relaxation biofeedback. *Am Rev Respir Dis* 141:1214-20.

Horowitz, M., B. Littenberg, and D. Mahler. 1997. Dyspnea ratings for prescribing exercise intensity in patients with COPD. *Chest* 109:1169-1175.

Hughes, R., and R. Davidson. 1983. Limitations of exercise reconditioning in COPD. *Chest* 83:241-9.

Jones, D., R. Thomson, and M. Sears. 1985. Physical exercise and resistive breathing training in severe chronic airways obstruction. Are they effective? *Eur J Respir Dis* 67:159-66.

Keens, T., I. Krastins, E. Wannamaker, H. Levinson, D. Crozier, and A. Bryan. 1977. Ventilatory muscle endurance training in normal subjects and patients with cystic fibrosis. *Am Rev Respir Dis* 116:853-60.

Lake, F., K. Hendersen, T. Briffa, J. Openshaw, and A.W. Musk. 1990. Upper limb and lower limb exercise training in patients with chronic airflow obstruction. *Chest* 97:1077-82.

Larson, J., M. Kim, and J. Sharp. 1988. Inspiratory muscle training with a pressure threshold breathing device in patients with chronic obstructive pulmonary disease. *Am Rev Respir Dis* 138:689-96.

Lecog, A., L. Delhez, and S. Janssens. 1970. Reentrainement de la fonction motrice ventilatoire chez des insuffisants respiratoire chroniques. *Acta Tuberc Pneumol Belg* 61:63-9.

Leith, D., and M. Bradley. 1976. Ventilatory muscle strength and endurance training. *J Appl Physiol* 4:508-16.

Levine, S., P. Weiser, and J. Guillen. 1986. Evaluation of a ventilatory muscle endurance training program in the rehabilitation of patients with chronic obstructive pulmonary disease. *Am Rev Respir Dis* 133:400-6.

Lisboa, C., V. Munoz, T. Beroiza, A. Leiva, and E. Cruz. 1994. Inspiratory muscle training in chronic airflow limitation: comparison of two different training loads with a threshold device. *Eur Respir J* 7:1266-1270.

Maestro, L., T. Dolmage, M. Avendano, and R. Goldstein. 1990. Influence of arm position in ventilation during incremental exercise in healthy individuals. *Chest* 98:113(S).

Make, B., and R. Buckolz. 1991. Exercise training in COPD patients improves cardiac function. *Am Rev Respir Dis* 143:80A.

Maltais, F., P. Leblanc, C. Simard, J. Jobin, C. Berube, J. Bruneau, L. Carrier, and R. Belleau. 1996. Skeletal muscle adapation to endurance training in patients with chronic obstructive pulmonary disease. *Am J Respir Crit Care Med* 154:442-447.

Maltais, F., A. Simard, J. Simard, J. Jobin, P. Desgagnes, and P. LeBlanc. 1995. Oxidative capacity of the skeletal muscle and lactic acid kinetics during exercise in normal subjects and in patients with COPD. *Am J Respir Crit Care Med* 153:288-293.

Martin, T., J. Zeballos, and I. Weisman. 1991. Gas exchange during maximal upper extremity exercise. *Chest* 99:420-5.

Martinez, F., J. Couser, and B. Celli. 1990. Factors influencing ventilatory muscle recruitment in patients with chronic airflow obstruction. *Am Rev Respir Dis* 142:276-82.

Martinez, F., P. Vogel, D. DuPont, I. Stanopoulos, A. Gray, and J.F. Beamis. 1993. Supported arm exercise vs. unsupported arm exercise in the rehabilitation of patients with chronic airflow obstruction. *Chest* 103:1397-2002.

McGavin, C., S. Gupta, and G. McHardy. 1976. Twelve minute walking test for assessing disability in chronic bronchitis. *Br Med J* 1:822-3.

Mohsenifar, Z., D. Horak, H. Brown, and S. Koerner. 1983. Sensitive indices of improvement in a pulmonary rehabilitation program. *Chest* 83:189-92.

Moser, K., G. Bokinsky, R. Savage, C. Archibald, and P. Hansen. 1980. Results of comprehensive rehabilitation programs. *Arch Int Med* 140:1596-601.

Niederman, M., P. Clemente, A. Fein, S. Feinsilver, D. Robinson, J. Ilowite, and M. Bernstein. 1991. Benefits of a multidisciplinary pulmonary rehabilitation program. Improvements are independent of lung function. *Chest* 99:798-804.

Noseda, A., J. Carpiaux, and N. Vandeput. 1987. Resistive inspiratory muscle training and exercise performance in COPD patients. A comparative study with conventional breathing retraining. *Bull Eur Physiopathol Respir* 23:457-63.

O'Donnell, D., K. Webb, and M. McGuire. 1993. Older patients with COPD: benefits of exercise training. *Geriatrics* 48:59-66.

O'Hara, W., B. Lasachuk, P. Matheson, M. Renahan. D. Schloter, and E. Lilker. 1984. Weight training and backpacking in Chronic Obstructive Pulmonary Disease. *Respir Care* 29:1202-10.

Paez, P., E. Phillipson, M. Mosangkay, and B. Sproule. 1967. The physiologic basis of training patients with emphysema. *Am Rev Respir Dis* 95:944-53.

Pardy, R., R. Livingston, and P. Despas. 1981. Inspiratory muscle training compared with physiotherapy in patients with chronic airflow limitation. *Am Rev Respir Dis* 123:421-5.

Pollock, M., J. Roa, J. Benditt, and B. Celli. 1993. Stair climbing (SC) predicts maximal oxygen uptake in patients with chronic airflow obstruction. *Chest* 104:1378-1383.

Reardon, J., E. Awad, E. Normandin, F. Vale, B. Clark, and R. ZuWallack. 1994. The effect of comprehensive outpatient pulmonary rehabilitation on dyspnea. *Chest* 105:1046-1048.

Reid, W., and C. Warren. 1984. Ventilatory muscle strength and endurance training in elderly subjects and patients with chronic airflow limitation: a pilot study. *Physio Canada* 36:305-11.

Reybrouck, T., G. Heigenhouser, and J. Faulkner. 1975. Limitations to maximum oxygen uptake in arm, leg and combined arm-leg ergometry. *J Appl Physiol* 38:774-9.

Ries, A., B. Ellis, and R. Hawkins. 1988. Upper extremity exercise training in chronic obstructive pulmonary disease. *Chest* 93:688-92.

Ries, A., R. Kaplan, T. Linberg, and L. Prewitt. 1995. Effects of pulmonary rehabiliation on physiologic and psychosocial outcomes in patients with chronic obstructive pulmonary disease. *Ann Int Med* 122:823-827.

Ries, A., and K. Moser. 1986. Comparison of isocapneic hyperventilation and walking exercise training at home in pulmonary rehabilitation. *Chest* 90:285-289.

Roa, J., S. Epstein, E. Breslin, T. Shannon, and B. Celli. 1991. Work of breathing and ventilatory muscle recruitment during pursed lip breathing. *Am Rev Respir Dis* 143:A77.

Roussos, C., and P. Macklem. 1982. The respiratory muscles. *N Engl J Med* 307:786-97.

Saltin, B., G. Blomquist, J. H. Mitchell, R. Johnson Jr., K. Wildenthal, and C. Chapman. 1968. Response to exercise after bed rest and training. *Circulation* 38(5 Suppl):VII1-78.

Scheinhorn, D., and C. Ho. 1991. Avoiding home mechanical ventilation; the regional weaning center. Proceeding International Conference on Pulmonary Rehabilitation and Home Mechanical Ventilation 3:A35.

Siegel, W., G. Blonquist, and J. Mitchell. 1970. Effects of a quantitated physical training program on middle-aged sedentary man. *Circulation* 41:19-29.

Sinclair, D., and C. Ingram. 1980. Controlled trial of supervised exercise training in chronic bronchitis. *Br Med J* 1:519-21.

Stanescu, D., B. Nemery, C. Veriter, and C. Marechal. 1981. Pattern of breathing and ventilatory response to CO_2 in subjects practicing hatha-yoga. *J Appl Physiol* 51:1625-29.

Steinberg, J., P. Astrand, B. Ekblom, J. Royce, and P. Sattin. 1967. Hemodynamic response to work with different muscle groups, sitting and supine. *J Appl Physiol* 22:61-70.

Tandon, M. 1980. Adjunct treatment with yoga in chronic severe airways obstruction. *Thorax* 33:514-517.

Tangri, S., and C. Woolf. 1973. The breathing pattern in chronic obstructive lung disease, during the performance of some common daily activities. *Chest* 63:126-7.

Weiner, P., Y. Azgad, and R. Ganam. 1992. Inspiratory muscle training, combined with general exercise reconditioning in patients with COPD. *Chest* 102:1351-6.

Weiner, P., Y. Azgad, R. Ganam, and M. Weiner. 1992. Inspiratory muscle training in asthma. *Chest* 102:1357-61.

Wijkstra, P., R. Van Altena, J. Kraan, V. Otten, D. Postma, and G. Koeter. 1994. Quality of life in patients with chronic obstructive pulmonary disease improves after rehabilitation in house. *Eur Respir J* 7:269-274.

Woolf, C., and J. Suero. 1969. Alterations in lung mechanics and gas exchange following training in chronic obstructive lung disease. *Chest* 55:37-44.

Zack, M., and A. Palange. 1985. Oxygen supplemented exercise of ventilatory and nonventilatory muscles in pulmonary rehabilitation. *Chest* 88:669-75.

ZuWallack, R., K. Patel, J. Reardon, B. Clark, and E. Normandin. 1991. Predictors of improvement in the 12-minute walking distance following a six-week outpatient pulmonary rehabilitation program. *Chest* 99:805-08.

Chapter 12

Diabetes Mellitus

Edward S. Horton, MD

Case Study

A 52-year-old accountant, J.P., was referred to us for evaluation and treatment of newly diagnosed type 2 diabetes mellitus. He stated that he has been overweight most of his adult life, which he attributes to his sedentary occupation. He has a history of hypertension and hyperlipidemia, which are being treated with a thiazide diuretic and an HMG Co-A reductase inhibitor respectively. He reluctantly admitted to some increasing fatigue, nocturia, and difficulty reading because of blurred vision. He also had noted polyuria, which he attributed to excessive coffee intake. He currently smokes one pack of cigarettes a day and has a 30-year history of smoking. His father had type 2 diabetes and died of a myocardial infarction at age 53.

On physical examination, J.P. was 5 feet 10 inches tall, weighed 235 pounds, and had a sitting blood pressure of 145/92 mmHg. He was obese, with, pre-

dominantly, an abdominal distribution of body fat, but otherwise appeared generally well. Fundoscopic examination revealed hard exudates, microaneurysms, and some blot hemorrhages, but no neovascularization. Cardiovascular examination was normal except for moderate hypertension, and carotid and peripheral pulses were normal without bruits. On neurological examination, the ankle jerks were absent and vibration sense was diminished, but touch sensation was normal when tested with a 10-g filament. Laboratory tests revealed a fasting plasma glucose of 260 mg/dl, hemoglobin A1C 9.2%, total cholesterol 220 mg/dl, LDL-cholesterol 105 mg/dl, HDL-cholesterol 32 mg/dl, and triglycerides 400 mg/dl. Urinalysis revealed glucosuria, but no albuminuria or ketone bodies.

We reconfirmed that J.P. does have type 2 diabetes mellitus, as well as inadequately treated hypertension, dsylipidemia, and obesity. In addition,

Case Study (cont.)

he has moderately severe background retinopathy and has early peripheral neuropathy.

Our treatment goal was to institute a lifestyle modification program to reduce his body weight by 7-10% through dietary modification and increased aerobic exercise, to reduce cardiovascular risk factors through smoking cessation, and to treat his hypertension and dyslipidemia more effectively. After an initial three-month trial of appropriate diet and exercise, glycemic control would be reassessed, and oral antidiabetic agents started, if necessary, to achieve control of his hyperglycemia.

To achieve these goals, the thiazide diuretic was replaced by an angiotensin converting enzyme inhibitor (ACEI), and the HMG Co-A reductase inhibitor was continued at the same dose. We referred J.P. to our diabetes management team for basic education and implementation of a calorically restricted diet that provided a daily negative energy balance of 500 to 1,000 kcal and followed the National Cholesterol Education Program Step 1 Guidelines. He was seen by the exercise physiologist who assessed his physical fitness and prescribed a program of moderate-intensity aerobic exercise for 30 to 45 minutes daily for at least five days per week. Because of the peripheral neuropathy, appropriate shoes were recommended, and exercises such as cycling, rowing, and swimming were prescribed rather than jogging or running. J.P. also undertook a smoking cessation program and decreased his coffee drinking as part of his lifestyle modification program.

After three months, J.P. lost 15 pounds and was successfully exercising five days a week. His blood pressure was 135/85, fasting glucose was 140 mg/dl, and hemoglobin A1C was 7.8%. Total cholesterol was 215 mg/dl, LDL-cholesterol 100 mg/dl, HDL-cholesterol 38 mg/dl, and triglycerides 300 mg/dl. His symptoms of fatigue, blurred vision, nocturia, and polyuria were much improved; and he had decreased his smoking to one or two cigarettes per day. Because of his substantial progress, we elected to continue the same program and did not start him on an oral antidiabetic agent at that time. This proved to be a good decision, since he continued to improve over the next three months with a further 10-pound weight loss and improvement in his glucose, blood pressure, and lipid levels.

This case illustrates several points about type 2 diabetes mellitus. First, as many as 50% of patients will have evidence of long-term complications when diabetes is first diagnosed. A thorough history and physical examination are required before starting a program of exercise and lifestyle modification. Second, patients with type 2 diabetes frequently have multiple risk factors for cardiovascular disease. In this case, hypertension, dyslipidemia, obesity, and cigarette smoking were all present and had to be addressed in the treatment plan. Third, a program of lifestyle modification to treat the diabetes and comorbidities requires a team approach involving diabetes education, nutrition, exercise physiology, and behavior modification, as well as appropriate medications. Finally, such an approach can be very successful in achieving the goals of treatment and should form the basis on which all other therapies are built. Over time, many patients with type 2 diabetes will require the addition of oral antidiabetic drugs or insulin, but a healthy lifestyle remains a fundamental pillar of the treatment program.

There are approximately 16 million people with diabetes in the United States and over 110 million worldwide. Over 90% have type 2 diabetes, and the incidence is increasing rapidly in many populations. Perhaps one-third to one-half of people with type 2 diabetes in the United States are receiving no treatment, because their disease is undiagnosed. In those who are diagnosed, treatment is frequently inadequate, leading to long-term complications that might be prevented. In the United States, diabetes is still the leading cause of new-onset blindness, of chronic renal failure requiring dialysis or kidney transplant, and of nontraumatic lower-extremity amputation. Approximately 60% of mortality in diabetes is due to coronary artery and other heart disease, while 15% results from cerebrovascular disease. The costs of treating diabetes and its complications may exceed 100 billion dollars per year in the United States—or nearly 15% of the total health care budget. Because of the increased mortality and morbidity associated with diabetes and the high costs of medical care for people with diabetes, it is imperative that physicians become more familiar with diabetes and its treatment. A healthy lifestyle, including increased physical activity and weight reduction, is essential both to prevent and to treat diabetes. This chapter reviews current information about diabetes—including the diagnosis, pathophysiology, and classification of its different forms—and discusses the role of physical (particularly aerobic) exercise as a key element in its treatment.

What Is Diabetes?

Diabetes mellitus is not a single disease but a group of metabolic disorders characterized by increased fasting and postprandial blood glucose concentrations that result from decreased insulin secretion, decreased insulin action, or both.

Although defects in the regulation of glucose metabolism are considered to be the primary abnormality in diabetes, alterations in lipid and protein metabolism also can occur—including hyperlipidemia and a protein catabolic state in inadequately treated patients. The most common symptoms of diabetes are related to chronic **hyperglycemia** and include fatigue, increased thirst and urination (**polydipsia** and **polyuria**), weight loss, increased hunger (**polyphagia**), blurred vision, poor wound healing, and increased susceptibility to infections. Prolonged, severe hyperglycemia may lead to dehydration, mental confusion, and loss of consciousness (**hyperosmolar nonketotic syndrome**)—or, when severe insulin deficiency is present, to **diabetic ketoacidosis** and death.

Hypoglycemia may occur in patients treated with insulin or drugs that stimulate insulin secretion. Symptoms of hypoglycemia include those associated with activation of the sympathetic nervous system such as tachycardia, palpitations, perspiration, and sensations of anxiety or hunger. With severe or prolonged hypoglycemia, neuroglucopenia may lead to mental confusion, loss of consciousness, or seizures. Symptoms usually respond rapidly to restoration of normal blood glucose concentrations; but prolonged, untreated hypoglycemia may lead to permanent brain damage.

The major morbidity and mortality of diabetes is related to long-term complications of chronic hyperglycemia. These include potential loss of vision; chronic renal failure; damage to peripheral nerves—leading to loss of sensation, foot ulcers, Charcot joints, and risk of amputation; and damage to the autonomic nervous system—causing gastrointestinal, genitourinary, and cardiovascular symptoms, as well as sexual dysfunction. Collectively these have been termed the **microvascular complications** of diabetes, and their development and progression are clearly linked to the degree and duration of hyperglycemia (DCCT 1993; Ohkubo et al. 1995; UKPDS 1998).

People with diabetes also have an increased incidence of **macrovascular diseases** including atherosclerotic cardiovascular, peripheral vascular, and cerebrovascular disease. The increased risk of atherosclerosis in diabetes is multifactorial and not well understood. Hyperglycemia may play a role, but diabetes is associated with increases in many of the recognized risk factors for atherosclerosis in nondiabetic individuals: hypertension, hyperlipidemia, obesity, insulin resistance, and alterations in the regulation of thrombosis and fibrinolysis. When adjustments are made for these risk factors, however, the incidence of coronary artery disease is still significantly greater in people with diabetes compared to those without the disease (Kannel 1990; Koskinen et al. 1992). Current research is directed toward understanding the relative roles and mechanisms by which hyperglycemia, hyperinsulinemia, and insulin resistance may contribute to the increased risk of macrovascular disease in diabetes.

Classification of Diabetes

Several pathogenic processes are involved in the development of diabetes—ranging from destruction of insulin-producing pancreatic beta cells by autoimmune, toxic, or other mechanisms, to defects in regulation of insulin secretion and action on its target tissues. Insulin deficiency may be "absolute," as in the case of pancreatic beta cell destruction; or "relative," when insulin secretion is present but inadequate to maintain blood glucose within the normal range.

In 1997, an expert committee of the American Diabetes Association revised the **diagnostic criteria** and classification of diabetes (ADA 1997). The new classification divides diabetes into four major diagnostic groups, based on etiology.

- In **type 1 diabetes,** destruction of beta cells leads to absolute insulin deficiency. The damage may be immune-mediated or idiopathic.
- **Type 2 diabetes,** the most common form of the disease, is characterized by relative insulin deficiency. Patients may range from predominantly insulin-resistant with relative insulin deficiency to a predominantly insulin-secretory defect with only mild to moderate insulin resistance.
- A large number of other specific, but generally uncommon, forms of diabetes have been defined—including diabetes associated with genetic

defects of beta cell function or insulin action, or with diseases of the endocrine pancreas; diabetes induced by various endocrinopathic drugs or chemicals; diabetes caused by various infections; uncommon forms of immune-mediated diabetes; and other genetic syndromes sometimes associated with diabetes.

- Finally, **gestational diabetes mellitus (GDM)** refers to diabetes that first appears during pregnancy, usually during the second or third trimester. In most cases, glucose tolerance returns to normal after delivery; but women with a history of GDM are at increased future risk of developing type 2 diabetes. Untreated GDM is frequently associated with fetal macrosomia, complicated delivery, and increased neonatal morbidity.

The ADA also modified the diagnostic criteria for diabetes from those previously used, and created a new category of **impaired fasting glucose**. Criteria for diagnosing **impaired glucose tolerance** remained unchanged, however, and are still based on the plasma glucose concentration two hours after a 75-gram oral glucose load. See "Criteria for the Diagnosis of Diabetes Mellitus, Impaired Glucose Tolerance, and Impaired Fasting Glucose."

Pathogenesis of Type 1 and Type 2 Diabetes

The most common cause of type 1 diabetes is autoimmune destruction of the pancreatic beta cells, which can occur rapidly or over many months or years. Markers of the immune process, which often appear before the onset of clinical diabetes, include islet cell autoantibodies, insulin autoantibodies, autoantibodies to glutamic acid decarboxylase, and autoantibodies to the tyrosine phosphatases IA-2 and IA-2B. There are also strong HLA (human leukocyte antigen) associations, with linkage to the *DQA* and *DQB* genes. Autoimmune destruction of the beta cells has multiple genetic modulators with both susceptibility and protective alleles, and is also related to environmental factors that are not well understood. Current research seeks to identify and modulate the autoimmune process in susceptible individuals, with the goal of preventing or delaying the onset of clinical diabetes and preserving residual beta cell function in those who have already developed diabetes. Once diabetes is established, treatment with insulin is required to maintain blood glucose concentration as close to normal as possible in order to relieve symp-

Criteria for the Diagnosis of Diabetes Mellitus, Impaired Glucose Tolerance, and Impaired Fasting Glucose

Diabetes Mellitus

- Symptoms of diabetes plus casual glucose concentration ≥ 200 mg/dl (11.1 mmol/L). Casual is defined as any time of day without regard to time since last meal. The classic symptoms of diabetes include polyuria, polydipsia, and unexplained weight loss.

  or

- Fasting plasma glucose ≥ 126 mg/dl (7.0 mmol/L). Fasting is defined as no caloric intake for at least 8 hours.

  or

- Plasma glucose ≥ 200 mg/dl (11.1 mmol/L) 2 hours after the oral ingestion of a glucose load equivalent to 75 g anhydrous glucose dissolved in water in a previously fasting subject (oral glucose tolerance test—OGTT).

In the absence of unequivocal hyperglycemia with acute metabolic decompensation, these criteria should be confirmed on a different day.

Impaired Glucose Tolerance

Plasma glucose ≥ 140 mg/dl (7.8 mmol/L) and <200 mg/dl (11.1 mmol/L) 2 hours after oral ingestion of a glucose load equivalent to 75 g anhydrous glucose dissolved in water in a previously fasting subject (OGTT).

Impaired Fasting Glucose

Fasting plasma glucose ≥ 110 mg/dl (6.1 mmol/L) and <126 mg/dl (7.0 mmol/L).

Source: American Diabetes Association 1997.

toms, restore metabolism, and prevent the development of acute and long-term complications of the disease.

Unlike type 1 diabetes, type 2 diabetes is associated not with beta cell destruction and absolute insulin deficiency, but rather with defects in the regulation of insulin secretion and action. Several factors contribute to development of type 2 diabetes. The disease is strongly familial and polygenic in character. As yet undetermined genetic factors contribute to both insulin resistance and impaired beta cell function.

A number of environmental factors contribute to insulin resistance. The most important of these are obesity (particularly intra-abdominal fat deposition), physical inactivity, and advancing age. Thus, as the population becomes older, fatter, and less physically active, insulin resistance increases and the incidence of type 2 diabetes also increases at a rapid rate. Figure 12.1 illustrates the sequence of events in the development of type 2 diabetes. Since insulin secretion adequately compensates for the insulin resistance before diabetes develops, the body is able to maintain normal fasting and postprandial plasma glucose concentrations. As insulin resistance increases, insulin secretion can no longer fully compensate, and impaired glucose tolerance develops. Genetic factors and the presence of increased glucose and/or free fatty acid concentrations may further impair beta cell function—leading in turn to further worsening of glucose tolerance and eventually to the development of overt diabetes.

Interventions that reduce insulin resistance, such as weight reduction and increased physical exercise, are the first steps in both the prevention and treatment of type 2 diabetes. A large number of cross-sectional and prospective studies show that regular physical exercise decreases the risk of developing type 2 diabetes (Helmrich et al. 1991; Kriska et al. 1991; Manson et al. 1991; Manson et al. 1992).

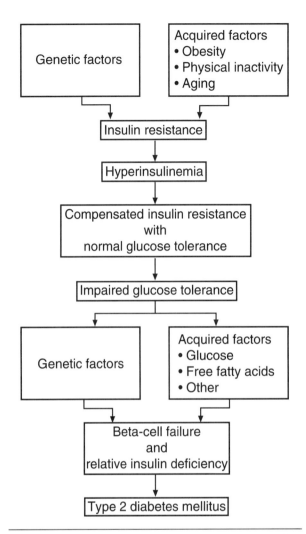

Figure 12.1   Steps in the development of type 2 diabetes mellitus. *Source:* Kruszynska and Olefsky 1996.

Exercise in Type 1 Diabetes

Before the discovery of insulin, diet and exercise were the principal therapies for diabetes. However, the ability to exercise was often severely limited in patients with type 1 diabetes, because of the associated metabolic abnormalities—including muscle wasting, dehydration, and ketosis. Survival was rarely longer than two to three years. With the advent of insulin therapy in 1921, vigorous exercise became possible for patients with type 1 diabetes, although difficult to manage. Successful therapy of type 1 diabetes depends on a carefully managed interaction among food intake, physical exercise, and insulin administration. Increased knowledge about metabolic regulation in response to acute exercise and physical training, along with development of newer insulin preparations and methods for self-monitoring of blood glucose, now make it possible for people with type 1 diabetes to participate in a wide variety of recreational and competitive sports. Many such individuals have become world-class athletes. However, the appropriate role of physical exercise in the treatment of type 1 diabetes is still somewhat controversial. Some health care professionals instruct all individuals with diabetes to exercise regularly as an integral part of their treatment plan; others merely evaluate and educate patients so they can participate in exercise and sports if they wish to do so. The latter approach has gained favor in recent years. Physicians are realizing that exercise can present both benefits and significant risks to patients with type 1 diabetes—and that appropriate advice requires careful evaluation of each patient with regard to his or her personal desires, the types of exercise to be performed, and the relative benefits and risks involved. Most diabetologists now seek to educate those with type 1 diabetes who want to participate in sports or other forms of physical exercise; but they do not recommend exercise for everyone. Educational programs should enable patients to maintain good metabolic control before, during, and after exercise, and to avoid or minimize the various complications of exercise (Horton 1988).

Potential Benefits

Regular physical exercise benefits the health of nearly everyone, including those with diabetes. See "Benefits of Exercise for Patients With Type 1 Diabetes." In addition to acutely lowering blood glucose (Berger et al. 1977; Kemmer et al. 1979) and increasing insulin sensitivity (Bjorntorp et al. 1970; Sato et al. 1984), regular exercise improves several of the recognized risk factors for cardiovascular disease. Serum cholesterol and triglyceride concentrations may decline with physical training, due to decreases in low-density and very low-density lipoproteins (Huttunen et al. 1979; Lipson et al. 1980), and increases in high-density lipoprotein cholesterol (Wood and Haskell 1979). Also, mild to moderate hypertension declines (Horton 1979), resting pulse rate and cardiac work decrease, and physical working capacity—usually measured as maximal aerobic capacity ($\dot{V}O_2$max)—increases with physical training. Since people with diabetes are at increased risk for developing cardiovascular disease, all of the above effects may provide the rationale for encouraging daily exercise. Psychological benefits of exercise—such as an increased sense of well-being, improved self-esteem, and an enhanced quality of life—are also important for people with diabetes, who must cope with the anxieties and limitations of living with a chronic disease.

Although exercise can acutely lower blood glucose and increase insulin sensitivity, some studies have failed to demonstrate a beneficial effect of regular exercise on long-term glycemic control in patients with type 1 diabetes (Wallberg-Henriksson et al. 1986; Zinman et al. 1977); others have shown that a program of regular exercise does result in improved glucose control (Marrero et al. 1988; Stratton et al. 1987). The negative results may be attributable to increased food intake that compensates for the increased energy expenditure of exercise, so that average blood glucose concentrations throughout a 24-hour period may not be altered (Zinman et al. 1977). One probably should not prescribe exercise programs for patients with type 1 diabetes for the sole purpose of

Benefits of Exercise for Patients With Type I Diabetes

1. Lower blood glucose concentrations during and after exercise
2. Improved insulin sensitivity and decreased insulin requirement
3. Improved lipid profile
   - Decreased triglycerides
   - Slightly decreased LDL-cholesterol
   - Increased HDL-cholesterol
4. Improvement in mild-to-moderate hypertension
5. Increased energy expenditure
   - Adjunct to diet for weight reduction
   - Increased fat loss
   - Preservation of lean body mass
6. Cardiovascular conditioning
7. Increased strength and flexibility
8. Improved sense of well-being and quality of life

improving long-term glycemic control. It is probably best to initiate an exercise program for such people only if they express strong desires to participate in sports or to obtain the general health benefits of an exercise program.

Risks

Exercise presents several risks for patients with type 1 diabetes (see "Risks of Exercise for Patients With Type 1 Diabetes"). Weigh these risks against the potential benefits when advising patients about participation in vigorous physical activity. Hypoglycemia may occur during or after exercise; and superimposing exercise on the insulin-deficient state may lead to rapid increases in blood glucose and the development of ketosis. Even in well-controlled individuals, brief periods of high-intensity exercise may cause hyperglycemia.

In adults, exercise may precipitate angina pectoris, myocardial infarction, cardiac arrhythmias, or

Risks of Exercise for Patients With Type 1 Diabetes

1. Hypoglycemia
   - Exercise-induced hypoglycemia
   - Late-onset postexercise hypoglycemia

2. Hyperglycemia after very strenuous exercise

3. Hyperglycemia and ketosis in insulin-deficient patients

4. Precipitation or exacerbation of cardiovascular disease
   - Angina pectoris
   - Myocardial infarction
   - Arrhythmias
   - Sudden death

5. Worsening of long-term complications of diabetes
   - Proliferative retinopathy
     a. Vitreous hemorrhage
     b. Retinal detachment
   - Nephropathy
     a. Increased proteinuria
   - Peripheral neuropathy
     a. Soft-tissue and joint injuries
   - Autonomic neuropathy
     a. Decreased cardiovascular response to exercise
     b. Decreased maximum aerobic capacity
     c. Impaired response to dehydration
     d. Postural hypotension
     e. Altered gastrointestinal function

sudden death if there is underlying coronary artery disease. Exercise may also worsen several of the long-term complications of diabetes. Physical activity does not appear to affect the development or progression of proliferative retinopathy in patients with type 1 diabetes (Cruickshanks et al. 1995), but individuals who have proliferative retinopathy are at increased risk for developing retinal or vitreous hemorrhages or retinal detachment. Although there is no firm evidence that these complications occur more frequently during or following exercise, it is usually recommended that individuals with proliferative retinopathy should avoid extremely vigorous exercise that increases blood pressure or causes jarring of the head. While vigorous exercise also increases proteinuria (Mogensen and Vittinghu 1975; Viberti et al. 1978), it is probably a transient hemodynamic response—exercise appears to have no deleterious effect on the progression of renal disease.

Injuries to soft tissues and joints may occur when patients with peripheral neuropathy engage in vigorous exercise. In those with autonomic neuropathy, physical working capacity may significantly decrease (Storstein and Jervell 1979), accompanied by increased resting pulse rate and reduced cardiovascular response to exercise (Hilsted et al. 1979; Kahn et al. 1986; Margonato et al. 1986), lower $\dot{V}O_2$max (Rubler 1981), and impaired response to dehydration. Gastroparesis, with altered rates of gastric emptying, may affect the absorption of food, fluid, and electrolytes.

Carefully screen adults for long-term complications of diabetes prior to prescribing an exercise program of moderate to vigorous intensity. In addition to a complete history and physical examination, complete a dilated retinal examination to identify proliferative retinopathy; renal function tests, including a screen for microalbuminuria; and a neurological examination for peripheral and autonomic neuropathy. For individuals age 35 or older, an exercise stress test can help screen for undiagnosed ischemic cardiac disease.

However, long-term epidemiological data for children with type 1 diabetes suggest that regular physical activity early in life is not associated with an adverse effect on health; in fact, it may be beneficial (LaPorte et al. 1986).

Management of exercise in patients with type 1 diabetes requires knowledge of the integrated cardiovascular, hormonal, and neural responses that ensure delivery of oxygen and fuel to muscles, to the central nervous system, and to other organ systems, and that remove potentially toxic metabolic end products. Chapters 3 and 4 describe these processes in detail. In brief, metabolic fuels are regulated by a complex system that involves both (1) breakdown of glycogen and triglyceride stores within muscle tissue, and (2) increased delivery of glucose and free fatty acids (FFAs) from the circulation. Blood glucose concentrations are maintained during exercise by increased hepatic glucose output, derived from hepatic glycogenolysis and gluconeogenesis, and from the digestion and absorption of ingested carbohydrates. Normally, hepatic glucose output is closely linked to glucose utilization; and blood glucose concentration is maintained within the normal range during exercise. Hypoglycemia is rare and occurs only with extreme, prolonged, and exhausting exercise.

During exercise, circulating FFA concentrations increase through release from adipose tissue triglycerides; exercising muscles and the liver then take up the FFAs and oxidize them for energy. Insulin plays a key role in regulating both glucose and FFA metabolism during exercise. It inhibits hepatic glucose production and stimulates peripheral glucose uptake, thus lowering the blood glucose concentration. It also inhibits lipolysis in adipose tissue, decreasing the release of FFAs—an important energy source for both the muscles and the liver. During exercise, activation of the sympathetic nervous system normally inhibits insulin secretion, decreasing plasma concentrations to a low physiological level and thereby increasing hepatic glucose production and adipose tissue lipolysis. Following the cessation of exercise, there is a transient increase in insulin secretion that reverses the increased rates of hepatic glucose production and lipolysis. Because patients with type 1 diabetes depend on exogenous insulin, they lack this finely tuned system—and regulation of metabolic fuel homeostasis during and after exercise is difficult to achieve. Too much insulin results in hypoglycemia, whereas too little leads to hyperglycemia and ketosis.

In the following sections we discuss common problems that patients with type 1 diabetes encounter in response to physical exercise, as well as the strategies used to prevent these problems.

Exercise-Induced Hypoglycemia

Whereas changes in blood glucose are very small in normal subjects during exercise, several factors may complicate glucose regulation during and following exercise in patients with type 1 diabetes. Since exercise potentiates the hypoglycemic effect of injected insulin, regular physical activity leads to decreased insulin requirements and increased risk of hypoglycemic reactions. Several studies have confirmed that physical training increases sensitivity to insulin (Horton 1986). Athletes have normal or increased tolerance to oral glucose, in conjunction with low basal and glucose-stimulated insulin responses (Lohmann et al. 1978), and physical inactivity rapidly results in decreased glucose tolerance (Lipman et al. 1972). Both normal subjects and patients with diabetes have a 30%-35% increase in insulin-stimulated glucose disposal after physical training, when studied by the hyperinsulinemic-euglycemic clamp technique (DeFronzo et al. 1983). This increase in insulin sensitivity correlates well with the training-induced increase in $\dot{V}O_2$max, and is due primarily to increased glucose uptake by muscle, associated with an increase in skeletal muscle GLUT 4 (glucose transporter isoform 4) content (Goodyear et al. 1992b).

Acute exercise in untrained subjects leads to increased insulin sensitivity and increased glucose metabolism—which persist for several hours following the exercise (Bogardus et al. 1983). These increases appear to stem from the need to replenish decreased muscle and liver glycogen stores and to increased glucose metabolism in muscle. Unless an individual adjusts the insulin dose, the increased sensitivity to insulin during and after exercise may result in hypoglycemia.

Another problem for people with type 1 diabetes is that plasma insulin concentrations do not respond to exercise in a normal manner, thus upsetting the balance between peripheral glucose utilization and hepatic glucose production. Plasma insulin concentrations do not decrease during exercise; they may even increase because of enhanced insulin absorption from the injection site. This effect of exercise on insulin absorption is most marked with short-acting insulin, and when the injection site is in an exercising part of the body (Koivisto and Felig 1978). At rest, soluble human insulin is absorbed more rapidly than is porcine insulin; but during exercise this difference disappears, both being absorbed more rapidly than in the resting condition. The increased absorption rate during exercise is not associated with increased cutaneous blood flow, but may be due to mechanical stimulation of the injection site (Fernqvist et al. 1986). It is preferable to choose an injection site in a nonexercising part of the body (e.g., the abdominal wall).

Enhanced insulin absorption during exercise is most likely to occur when the injection occurs shortly before the onset of exercise, due to increased absorption of insulin from the subcutaneous tissue. The longer the interval between injection and the onset of exercise, the less significant this effect will be and the less important it is to choose the site of injection to avoid an exercising area. The injection site (such as the thigh, abdomen, or arm) may affect the rate of insulin absorption more than the exercise itself. To avoid this problem, individuals should postpone vigorous exercise for at least 60-90 minutes after an insulin injection. Even with this precaution, however, plasma insulin concentrations do not decrease in a normal way during exercise in insulin-treated patients, possibly impairing glucose homeostasis.

The sustained insulin levels during exercise may enhance peripheral glucose uptake and stimulate glucose oxidation by exercising muscle. However, the major effect is an inhibition of hepatic glucose production (Zinman et al. 1977). The high insulin levels inhibit both glycogenolysis and gluconeogenesis. Even though counter-regulatory hormone responses may be normal or even enhanced, blood glucose concentration falls because the hepatic glucose production rate cannot match the rate of peripheral glucose utilization. During mild to moderate exercise of short duration, this decrease may be beneficial; but during more prolonged exercise, hypoglycemia may result.

It is now well recognized that one of the trade-offs for intensive metabolic control is an increased incidence of severe hypoglycemic reactions, many of which are associated with exercise. One possible mechanism for the increased incidence of exercise-induced hypoglycemia in patients on intensive insulin therapy is a subnormal response of epinephrine, growth hormone, and cortisol when blood glucose is lowered to 50 mg/dl (Simonson et al. 1985). Strict control of blood glucose by insulin pump therapy significantly decreases the threshold glucose concentration for epinephrine and growth hormone release, and increases the liver's sensitivity to insulin for inhibiting glucose production (Amiel et al. 1987). Thus, intensively treated patients achieve much lower blood glucose concentrations before counter-regulatory mechanisms are activated and hepatic glucose production increases.

Autonomic neuropathy may also contribute to exercise-induced hypoglycemia. Studying patients who experienced frequent hypoglycemic reactions during intensive insulin therapy, White et al. (1983) found that defective autonomic nervous system function was associated with decreased catecholamine responses and inadequate glucose counter-regulation to insulin-induced hypoglycemia. In addition, patients with autonomic neuropathy often do not develop the classic warning signs of hypoglycemia before developing severe neuroglucopenia—further compounding the problem of exercise-induced hypoglycemia.

Strategies to avoid hypoglycemia during prolonged, vigorous exercise include decreasing insulin dosage prior to exercise and eating supplemental carbohydrates before and during exercise. For example, individuals should inject insulin at least 60 minutes before exercise and decrease the dose by 25% to 50%. If blood glucose is less than 100 mg/dl, they should take supplemental carbohydrates prior to and during exercise.

In patients treated with an insulin pump, blood glucose responses following breakfast and in response to exercise are similar to those in normal control subjects; and there is an appropriate 30% decrease in insulin requirement during exercise. Infusing insulin at a constant rate—i.e., when it is not decreased during exercise—can cause symptomatic hypoglycemia, further demonstrating the interaction between insulin and exercise in lowering blood glucose concentration in insulin-treated subjects (Nelson et al. 1982).

Caron and colleagues (1982) studied metabolic responses, in type 1 diabetes and in normal subjects, to 45 minutes of moderate-intensity aerobic exercise performed 30 minutes after breakfast on one day and compared the results to the metabolic responses following breakfast without any exercise on another day. In the controls, exercise rapidly reversed the expected postprandial rise in blood glucose and insulin concentrations, and both returned to fasting levels within 45 minutes. When the normal subjects stopped exercising, there was a moderate rebound in glucose and insulin concentrations that did not exceed those occurring after breakfast alone. Thus, the postbreakfast exercise significantly but transiently lowered blood glucose concentrations in the normal individuals. In the diabetic subjects (treated with subcutaneous insulin), the responses were variable. Blood glucose concentrations improved for most of the subjects, remaining lower after breakfast and even through lunch. Some, however, showed improved glucose levels only during lunch. A few showed no significant improvement at all. Thus, the effect of postprandial exercise on blood glucose concentrations, and the appropriate adjustments in insulin dosage, may vary considerably from person to person. Individuals should experimentally determine their own responses in order to achieve improved glucose control and avoid symptomatic hypoglycemia.

Postexercise Hypoglycemia

Another major problem for people with type 1 diabetes is postexercise hypoglycemia. Many diabetics experience increased insulin sensitivity and have hypoglycemic reactions several hours following exercise, in some cases even the following day. In one study (MacDonald 1987), 16% of 300 young patients with type 1 diabetes who were followed prospectively for two years experienced postexercise, late-onset hypoglycemia—usually occurring at night 6 to 15 hours after the completion of unusually strenuous exercise or play. Although the mechanism of postexercise hypoglycemia is not well understood, it is most likely due to increased glucose uptake and glycogen synthesis in the previously exercised muscle groups, associated with increased insulin sensitivity and activation of glycogen synthase in skeletal muscle (Bogardus et al. 1983). Hepatic glycogen stores also recover following exercise, but at a slower rate than in muscle, so that increased requirements for dietary carbohydrate may persist for up to 24 hours following prolonged, glycogen-depleting exercise. Various strategies have been used to prevent postexercise hypoglycemia—including decreasing pre-exercise doses of intermediate- or short-acting insulin, and taking supplemental feedings after exercise—but no universal guidelines are totally effective. Treatment regimens must be individualized.

Exercise-Induced Hyperglycemia

In contrast to moderate-intensity, sustained exercise (during which blood glucose concentrations remain constant or decrease slightly), short-term, high-intensity exercise at $\geq$ 80% of $\dot{V}O_2$max is normally associated with a transient increase in blood glucose levels (Mitchell et al. 1988). In nondiabetic exercisers, blood glucose peaks 5 to 15 minutes after exercise ends, and then gradually returns to the pre-exercise level within 40 to 60 minutes. This glycemic response to intense exercise results from marked stimulation of hepatic glucose production, so that it exceeds the rate of glucose uptake in muscle. This stimulation is associated with activation of the sympathetic nervous system; with a sharp rise in glucose counter-regulatory hormones (particularly epinephrine); and with a suppression of insulin secretion. The energy for muscular contraction comes predominantly from glycolysis and from oxidation of glucose derived from breakdown of muscle glycogen—glucose uptake from the circulation increases only gradually. Hepatic glucose production, on the other hand, is stimulated rapidly by the decrease in portal vein insulin concentration, by an increase in the glucagon-to-insulin ratio, and by the rapid rise in plasma epinephrine. When exercise is stopped, there is a rapid, two- to threefold increase in plasma insulin, which has an inhibitory effect on hepatic glucose production and increases postexercise glucose uptake in muscle. As a result, the transiently elevated blood glucose concentration returns rapidly to normal (Calles et al. 1983).

Because this highly integrated response to brief, high-intensity exercise is abnormal in type 1 diabetes, sustained hyperglycemia may occur. Mitchell and associates (1988) studied the effects of exercise to exhaustion at 80% $\dot{V}O_2$max on glucose and hormone responses, both in diabetics treated with insulin pumps and in normal controls. Blood glucose rose to much higher levels during postexercise recovery in the diabetic subjects than in the normals, and remained elevated for the entire two-hour postexercise observation period. Pre-exercise glucose concentra-

tion affected the pattern of postexercise hyperglycemia, which was considerably greater when the pre-exercise level was elevated. The most likely mechanism of the sustained hyperglycemic response is intense autonomic nervous system stimulation of hepatic glucose production, and the absence of any increase in plasma insulin during postexercise recovery.

Since many sports and recreational activities require relatively short periods of very high-intensity exercise, the sustained hyperglycemic response to this type of exercise may present a problem for people with diabetes. At present there are no clear guidelines for prevention or management of this response, although it is possible that administration of small doses of insulin following exercise may shorten the period of hyperglycemia. Careful self-monitoring of blood glucose levels before, during, and following exercise of different intensities and duration may help individuals to develop strategies that minimize the risks of either hyper- or hypoglycemia.

Exercise-Induced Ketosis

When insulin-dependent individuals exercise in the presence of severe insulin deficiency, hyperglycemia and ketosis can develop. The onset of exercise increases peripheral glucose utilization, but also enhances lipolysis, and stimulates hepatic glucose production and ketogenesis. The already poor metabolic control rapidly becomes worse, and instead of lowering blood glucose, the exercise results in a rise in blood glucose and the development of ketosis (Berger et al. 1977). The mechanism for the rapid development of ketosis is not altogether clear. Recent studies suggest that there is a defect in peripheral clearance of ketones rather than a marked increase in ketogenesis during exercise in insulin-deprived individuals (Fery et al. 1987). Individuals with type 1 diabetes should check their blood glucose concentration and urine ketones prior to undertaking vigorous physical activity. If they note blood glucose greater than 250 mg/dl and ketones in their urine or blood, they should postpone the exercise and take supplemental insulin to reestablish good metabolic control.

Strategies for Management of Exercise in Type 1 Diabetes

"Suggested Strategies to Avoid Hypo- or Hyperglycemia During and After Exercise" is a helpful reference. Individuals anticipating exercise should plan to start it one to three hours after a meal, when the

Suggested Strategies to Avoid Hypo- or Hyperglycemia During and After Exercise

1. Adjustments to the insulin regimen

   • Take insulin at least one hour before exercise. If less than one hour before exercise, inject in a nonexercising part of the body.
   • Decrease the dose of both short- and intermediate-acting insulin before exercise.
   • Alter daily insulin schedule.

2. Meals and supplemental feedings

   • Eat a meal one to three hours before exercise and check to see that blood glucose is in a safe range (100 to 250 mg/dl) before starting exercise.
   • Take carbohydrate snacks or beverages during exercise—at least every 30 minutes if exercise is vigorous and of long duration. Monitor blood glucose during exercise, if necessary, to determine size and frequency of feedings needed to maintain safe glucose levels.
   • Increase food intake for up to 24 hours after exercise (depending on its intensity and duration) to avoid late-onset postexercise hypoglycemia.

3. Self-monitoring of blood glucose and urine ketones

   • Monitor blood glucose before, during, and after exercise to determine the need for and the effect of changes in insulin dosage and feeding schedule.
   • Delay exercise if blood glucose is <100 mg/dl or >250 mg/dl and ketones are present. Use supplemental feedings or insulin to correct glucose and metabolic control before starting exercise.

4. Determination of unique metabolic responses

   • Learn individual glucose responses to different types, intensities, and conditions of exercise.
   • Determine effects of exercise at different times of the day (e.g., morning, afternoon, or evening) and effects of physical training on blood glucose responses.

blood glucose is above 100 mg/dl. If exercise is prolonged and vigorous, they should have frequent carbohydrate snacks during exercise, and extra food following the exercise to avoid postexercise hypoglycemia. If exercise is intermittent, of high intensity and short duration, hyperglycemia may be a problem, and small supplemental doses of insulin may be needed during postexercise recovery.

No precise guidelines indicate how much carbohydrate one should eat during prolonged exercise to avoid hypoglycemia. However, one can make some estimate of energy requirements based on the intensity and duration of the physical exercise to be performed. In most situations, a snack containing 15-25 g of carbohydrate every 30 minutes during prolonged exercise will maintain normal blood glucose concentration.

Individuals who plan exercise in advance may alter their insulin dosages and schedules to decrease the likelihood of hypoglycemia during or following exercise. Those who take a single dose of intermediate-acting insulin may decrease the dose by 30%-35% on the morning prior to exercise. Or they may change to a split-dose regimen—taking 2/3 of the usual dose in the morning, and 1/3 before the evening meal if they need supplemental insulin following the exercise. Those who use a combination of intermediate- and short-acting insulin may decrease the short-acting dosage by 50%, or even omit it altogether prior to exercise. They may also decrease the intermediate-acting insulin before exercise and take supplemental doses of short-acting insulin after exercise if needed.

Those using multiple daily injections of short-acting insulin may decrease the dose before exercise by 30%-50%, adjusting postexercise doses based on glucose monitoring and their personal experience with postexercise hypoglycemia. If they use insulin pumps, they may decrease the basal infusion rate during exercise, and decrease or even omit premeal boluses. Although failure to make these adjustments may result in hypoglycemia during exercise (Schiffrin et al. 1984), this has not been a universal experience. In practice, individuals can adjust intra- and postexercise basal infusion rates as well as premeal boluses based on glucose monitoring and personal experience. In advising patients regarding these strategies, always stress the individual nature of the problem—including the need for careful glucose monitoring and for carefully recording their experiences. If their exercise patterns are relatively consistent with respect to the time of day and the intensity/duration of the exercise, your patients can often develop a routine program to avoid hypo- or hyperglycemia during or following exercise.

If their exercise is unusual or without a strong pattern, then frequent glucose monitoring will help them make adjustments in insulin dosage and in the frequency and size of supplemental snacks.

Exercise in Type 2 Diabetes

The role of exercise in the management of type 2 diabetes is quite different from that in type 1 diabetes. Approximately 80% of people with type 2 diabetes are obese and insulin-resistant, and only about 35% require insulin therapy. Exercise-induced hypoglycemia is uncommon, even in insulin-treated patients, and physicians often prescribe exercise—along with diet and oral antidiabetic agents—to achieve and maintain weight reduction and improve glycemic control. There is abundant evidence that regular physical exercise protects against the development of type 2 diabetes in high-risk populations. Along with the prevention and treatment of obesity by dietary restriction, increased physical activity is an important component of life-style modification for people with impaired glucose tolerance, with a family history of type 2 diabetes, or with other risk factors for its development.

As with type 1 diabetes, exercise presents specific risks and benefits for each patient. While exercise-induced hypoglycemia and acute regulation of blood glucose are less of a problem in type 2 than in type 1 diabetes, the risks of cardiovascular disease and musculoskeletal injuries are generally greater. People with type 2 diabetes develop the same long-term complications as those with type 1 diabetes—including retinopathy, nephropathy, neuropathy, and macrovascular disease—and must be screened for these before starting an exercise program. Proper selection of exercise type, intensity, and duration can avert most of the risks, although for some patients a program of physical exercise may be impractical or contraindicated.

Exercise and Insulin Sensitivity

Bjorntorp and colleagues (1973) first suggested the use of physical exercise to treat the insulin resistance associated with obesity and type 2 diabetes. They observed that physically active middle-aged men had significantly lower fasting insulin concentrations and lower insulin responses to oral glucose than untrained men of the same age and body weight (Bjorntorp et al. 1972). This finding suggested that regular physical activity is associated with increased insulin sensitivity, and led them to study the effects of physical training in obese patients with normal glucose tolerance but insulin resistance. After 12 weeks of moderate-intensity aerobic exercise (30-60 minutes, five days/week), there was no change in the subjects' blood glucose responses—but insulin levels were significantly lower, both fasting and following glucose administration (Bjorntorp et al. 1970). Subsequently, numerous investigators have used a variety of techniques to demonstrate increased insulin sensitivity and responsiveness in physically trained subjects (Horton 1986). For example, both normal subjects and patients with type 2 diabetes have a 30%-35% increase in insulin-stimulated glucose disposal after physical training, when studied by the hyperinsulinemic-euglycemic clamp technique (DeFronzo et al. 1983; Sato et al. 1984). This increased insulin sensitivity correlates closely with the training-induced increase in $\dot{V}O_2$max (Rosenthal et al. 1983; Yki-Jarvinen and Koivisto 1983); presumably it is due mainly to increased glucose uptake in skeletal muscle, since no changes have been observed in hepatic glucose production rates. Recently it has also been demonstrated that resistance training improves insulin sensitivity in people with type 2 diabetes without increasing $\dot{V}O_2$max (Ishii et al. 1998).

The increase in insulin sensitivity and responsiveness associated with physical conditioning rapidly disappears when exercise is discontinued. Burstein et al. (1985) found that much of the effect is gone within 60 hours; others have demonstrated that the effect is no longer present after 5-7 days without exercise. In a study by Bogardus and colleagues (1984) comparing the effects in type 2 diabetes of a very low-calorie diet with the same diet plus a physical (mainly aerobic) training program, the physically trained group had a significant increase in insulin-stimulated glucose disposal rates; the group treated by diet alone had no change after three months of treatment. The rise in insulin-stimulated glucose disposal in the diet-plus-exercise group was due entirely to increased nonoxidative glucose disposal, presumably reflecting increased glycogen synthesis. Since the glucose clamp procedures were done 5-7 days after the last exercise session in this study, these data presumably demonstrate a true effect of physical training rather than a carryover effect from the last bout of exercise.

In more recent studies, Mikines and associates (1988) observed that a single bout of aerobic exercise increased the sensitivity and responsiveness of insulin-stimulated glucose uptake in untrained individuals. The effect lasted at least two days, but was not observed after five days. In addition, physically trained subjects (as compared with untrained subjects) had increased insulin action 15 hours after their last training session. Five days after the last training session, insulin responsiveness remained elevated compared with that of untrained subjects, suggesting that training engenders a long-term adaptive increase in whole-body responsiveness to insulin (Mikines et al. 1989). Although the mechanism of this increase is not yet known, it may be related to increased capillary density in skeletal muscle, to enhanced oxidative capacity of skeletal muscle, or to other adaptations to training such as elevated skeletal muscle GLUT 4 content (Goodyear et al. 1992b).

Despite the increase in insulin-stimulated glucose uptake that can last 5-7 days following cessation of exercise in previously trained subjects, patients with type 2 diabetes generally do not have improved fasting blood glucose concentrations during this same period. Some researchers, however, have observed that physical training is associated with lower glycosylated hemoglobin levels (Schneider et al. 1984)—likely the cumulative result of decreased blood glucose concentrations during and after aerobic exercise rather than a specific effect of physical training. Since moderate-intensity aerobic exercise usually lowers blood glucose concentrations toward normal in hyperglycemic patients with type 2 diabetes, and since increased insulin-stimulated glucose disposal persists for many hours following a single bout of exercise (Devlin and Horton 1985), it is likely that regular exercise 4-7 days a week may decrease blood glucose and glycohemoglobin concentrations without a significant effect on fasting blood glucose or glucose response to meals. Thus, the net effect of exercise repeated on a regular basis would be to improve long-term blood glucose control in patients with type 2 diabetes.

Guidelines for Exercise in Type 2 Diabetes

Before starting an exercise program, all patients should have a complete history and physical examination—with particular attention to identifying any long-term complications of diabetes that may affect exercise safety or tolerance. Individuals over 35 years old should have a stress test if they intend to start a program of moderate or vigorous exercise (ACSM 1995). The test will help identify previously undiagnosed ischemic heart disease, and abnormal blood pressure responses to exercise. All individuals also should have a dilated retinal examination to identify proliferative

retinopathy, renal function tests (including screening for microalbuminuria), and a neurological examination to determine peripheral and/or autonomic neuropathy. To avoid significant risks or worsening complications, individuals with abnormalities should engage only in exercises of appropriate type and intensity. In general, an exercise program should consist of moderate-intensity aerobic exercises that can be sustained for 30 minutes or longer and that result in a sustained heart rate of 60%-70% of the individual's predetermined maximum heart rate. Patients with no proliferative retinopathy or significant hypertension may tolerate some resistance training or high-intensity exercises.

Each exercise session should begin with a warm-up of low-intensity aerobic exercise and stretching for 5-10 minutes to prevent musculoskeletal injuries. The moderate- to high-intensity exercise phase should last at least 30 minutes, with longer durations as tolerated by the level of physical conditioning. Patients should monitor their heart rates periodically during exercise, to ensure that they are in the target range. Each exercise session should conclude with a cooldown phase of 5-10 minutes to reduce the risk of postexercise cardiovascular and musculoskeletal complications. Activities such as walking, stretching, and slow, rhythmic exercises are appropriate.

To significantly increase cardiovascular fitness, to improve insulin sensitivity and glycemic control, and to lose or maintain reduced body weight, patients should exercise at least three days a week. Five to seven days a week is preferable. Individual or group activities are appropriate, and many patients find that variety sustains their interest. For individuals who are new to exercise or who have significant complications of diabetes, supervised exercise programs may be beneficial. Most patients, however, do not require formal supervision once they have completed an initial assessment and established an appropriate exercise program. Although blood glucose regulation during exercise in type 2 diabetes differs from normal in several ways, elevated blood glucose concentrations usually fall toward normal with moderate-intensity exercise. Exercise-induced hypoglycemia is rare. Exceptions may occur in patients taking insulin or sulfonylureas, but not metformin, thiazolidinediones, or α-glucosidase inhibitors. Patients treated by diet alone need not use supplemental feedings before, during, or after exercise, except when the exercise is exceptionally vigorous or of long duration. Individuals being treated with sulfonylureas or insulin may need supplemental feedings to prevent hypoglycemia; they may also decrease insulin doses to avoid hypoglycemia.

Summary

The role and management of physical exercise in patients with diabetes mellitus is complex, and is associated with both benefits and significant risks. In type 1 diabetes, the main goal should be to educate patients about regulation of blood glucose during and after exercise by glucose monitoring and appropriate adjustments in food intake and insulin administration. Individuals with type 2 diabetes should employ regular exercise and diet to achieve and maintain weight reduction (in obese patients), to reduce insulin resistance, to improve glycemic control, and to reduce cardiovascular risk factors including hypertension and hyperlipidemia. Those at risk of developing type 2 diabetes should engage in regular exercise as a preventive measure.

Before starting an exercise program, all patients with diabetes should undergo a careful medical evaluation to determine their general state of health, the presence and degree of long-term complications of diabetes, and any limitations or contraindications to exercise. Particular attention should be paid to the cardiovascular system, since people with diabetes have an increased risk of coronary artery disease (which may be asymptomatic). A dilated eye examination to detect proliferative retinopathy, an evaluation of renal function, and a neurological and musculoskeletal examination are important to detect diabetic complications that may be aggravated by exercise.

Exercise programs should be tailored to each individual's goals and medical condition. Patients must become proficient and faithful in self-monitoring—learning through careful experimentation the effects of specific types, intensities, and durations of exercise on their blood glucose. By following these guidelines, most diabetic patients can exercise effectively and safely.

References

American College of Sports Medicine. 1995. *Guidelines for exercise testing and prescription.* 5th ed., 3-26. Philadelphia: Lea & Febiger.

American Diabetes Association. 1997. Report of the expert committee on the diagnosis and classification of diabetes mellitus. *Diabetes Care* 20:1183-97.

Amiel, S.A., W.V. Tamborlane, D.C. Simonson, and R.S. Sherwin. 1987. Defective glucose counterregulation after strict control of insulin-dependent diabetes mellitus. *N Engl J Med* 316:1376-83.

Berger, M., P. Berchtold, H.-J. Cuppers, H. Drost, H.K. Kley, W.A. Muller, W. Wiegelmann, H. Zimmermann-Telschow, F.A. Gries, H.L. Kruskemper, and H. Zimmerman. 1977. Metabolic and hormonal effects of muscular exercise in juvenile type diabetics. *Diabetologia* 13:355-65.

Bjorntorp, P., K. de Jounge, L. Sjostrom, and L. Sullivan. 1970. The effect of physical training on insulin production in obesity. *Metabolism* 19:631-37.

Bjorntorp, P., K. de Jounge, L. Sjostrom, and L. Sullivan. 1973. Physical training in human obesity. II. Effects of plasma insulin in glucose intolerant subjects without marked hyperinsulinemia. *Scand J Clin Lab Invest* 32:42-45.

Bjorntorp, P., M. Fahlen, G. Grimby, A. Gustafson, J. Holm, P. Renstrom, and T. Schersten. 1972. Carbohydrate and lipid metabolism in middle aged physically well-trained men. *Metabolism* 21:1037-42.

Bogardus, C., E. Ravussin, D.C. Robbins, R.R. Wolfe, E.S. Horton, and E.A.H. Sims. 1984. Effects of physical training and diet therapy on carbohydrate metabolism in patients with glucose intolerance and non-insulin dependent diabetes mellitus. *Diabetes* 33:311-18.

Bogardus, C., P. Thuillez, E. Ravussin, B. Vasquez, M. Narimiga, and S. Azhar. 1983. Effect of muscle glycogen depletion on in vivo in insulin action in man. *J Clin Invest* 72:1605-10.

Burstein, R., C. Polychronakos, C.J. Toeus, J.D. MacDougall, H.J. Guyda, and B.I. Posner. 1985. Acute reversal of the enhanced insulin action in trained athletes. *Diabetes* 34:756-60.

Calles, J., J.J. Cunningham, L. Nelson, N. Brown, E. Nadel, R.S. Sherwin, and P. Felig. 1983. Glucose turnover during recovery from intensive exercise. *Diabetes* 32:734-38.

Caron, D., P. Poussier, E.B. Marliss, and B. Zinman. 1982. The effect of postprandial exercise on meal-related glucose intolerance in insulin-dependent diabetic individuals. *Diabetes Care* 5:364-69.

Cruickshanks, K.J., S.E. Moss, R. Klein, and B.E. Klein. 1995. Physical activity and the risk of progression of retinopathy or the development of proliferative retinopathy. *Ophthalmology* 102:1177-82.

DeFronzo, R.A., E. Ferranni, and V. Koivisto. 1983. New concepts in the pathogenesis and treatment of non-insulin dependent diabetes mellitus. *Am J Med* 74:52-81.

Devlin, J.T., and E.S. Horton. 1985. Effects of prior high-intensity exercise on glucose metabolism in normal and insulin-resistant men. *Diabetes* 34:973-79.

Diabetes Control and Complications Trial Research Group. 1993. The effect of intensive treatment of diabetes on the development and progression of long-term complications in insulin-dependent diabetes mellitus. *N Engl J Med* 329:977-86.

Fernqvist, E., B. Linde, J. Ostman, and R. Gunnarsson. 1986. Effects of physical exercise on insulin absorption in insulin-dependent diabetics. A comparison between human and porcine insulin. *Clin Physiol* 6:489-98.

Fery, F., V. deMaetalaer, and E.O. Balasse. 1987. Mechanism of the hyperketonemic effect of prolonged exercise in insulin-deprived type 1 (insulin-dependent) diabetic patients. *Diabetologia* 30:298-304.

Goodyear, L.J., M.F. Hirshman, E.D. Horton, and E.S. Horton. 1992a. Effect of exercise training and chronic glyburide treatment on glucose homeostasis in diabetic rats. *J Appl Physiol* 72:143-48.

Goodyear, L.J., M.F. Hirshman, P.M. Valyou, and E.S. Horton. 1992b. Glucose transporter number, function and subcellular distribution in rat skeletal muscle after exercise training. *Diabetes* 41:1091-99.

Helmrich, S.P., D.R. Ragland, R.W. Leung, and R.S. Paffenbarger. 1991. Physical activity and reduced occurrence of non-insulin-dependent diabetes mellitus. *N Engl J Med* 325:147-52.

Hilsted, J.J., H. Galbo, and N.J. Christensen. 1979. Impaired cardiovascular responses to graded exercise in diabetic autonomic neuropathy. *Diabetes* 28:313-19.

Horton, E.S. 1979. The role of exercise in the treatment of hypertension in obesity. *Int J Obes* 5(Suppl. 1):89-92.

Horton, E.S. 1986. Exercise and physical training: effects on insulin sensitivity and glucose metabolism. *Diabetes Metab Rev* 2:1-17.

Horton, E.S. 1988. Role and management of exercise in diabetes mellitus. *Diabetes Care* 11:201-11.

Huttunen, J.K., E. Lanisimies, E. Voutilainen, C. Ehnholm, F. Hietanen, I. Pantila, O. Siitonen, and R. Rauramua. 1979. Effect of moderate physical exercise on serum lipoprotein. *Circulation* 60:1220-29.

Ishii, T., T. Yamakita, T. Sato, S. Tanaka, and S. Fuji. 1998. Resistance training improves insulin sensitivity in NIDDM subjects without altering maximal oxygen uptake. *Diabetes Care* 21:1353-55.

Kahn, J.K., B. Zola, J.E. Juni, and A.I. Vinik. 1986. Decreased exercise heart rate and blood pressure response in diabetic subjects with cardiac autonomic neuropathy. *Diabetes Care* 9:389-94.

Kannel, W.B. 1990. Diabetes, fibrinogen, and risk of cardiovascular disease: the Framingham experience. *Am Heart J* 120:672-76.

Kemmer, F.W., P. Berchtold, M. Berger, A. Starke, H.-J. Cuppers, F.A. Gries, and H. Zimmerman. 1979. Exercise-induced fall of blood glucose in insulin-treated diabetics unrelated to alteration of insulin mobilization. *Diabetes* 28:1131-37.

Koivisto, V., and P. Felig. 1978. Effects of leg exercise on insulin absorption in diabetic patients. *N Engl J Med* 298:77-83.

Koskinen, P., M. Manttari, V. Manninen, J.K. Huttunen, O.P. Heinonen, and M.H. Frick. 1992. Coronary heart disease incidence in NIDDM patients in the Helsinki heart study. *Diabetes Care* 15:820-25.

Kriska, A.M., S.N. Blair, and M.A. Pereira. 1991. The potential role of physical activity in the prevention of non-insulin dependent diabetes mellitus: the epidemiological evidence. *Exerc Sports Sci Rev* 22:121-43.

Kruszynska, Y.T., and J.M. Olefsky. 1996. Cellular and molecular mechanisms of non-insulin dependent diabetes mellitus. *J Investig Med* 44:413-28.

LaPorte, R.E., J.S. Dorman, N. Tajima, K.J. Cruickshanks, T.J. Orchard, D.E. Cavender, D.J. Becker, and A.L. Drash. 1986.

Pittsburgh insulin-dependent diabetes mellitus morbidity and mortality study: physical activity and diabetic complications. *Pediatrics* 78:1027-33.

Lipman, R.L., P. Raskin, T. Love, J. Triebwasser, F.R. LeCocq, and J.J. Schnure. 1972. Glucose intolerance during decreased physical activity in man. *Diabetes* 21:101-07.

Lipson, L.C., R.W. Bonow, E. J. Schaefer, H. Brewer, and F.T. Lindren. 1980. Effect of exercise condition on plasma high-density lipoprotein and other lipoproteins. *Atherosclerosis* 37:529-38.

Lohmann, D., F. Liebold, W. Heilmann, H. Senger, and A. Pohl. 1978. Diminished insulin response in highly trained athletes. *Metabolism* 27:521-42.

MacDonald, M.J. 1987. Postexercise late-onset hypoglycemia in insulin-dependent diabetic patients. *Diabetes Care* 10:584-88.

Manson, J.E., D.M. Nathan, A.S. Krolewski, M.J. Stampfer, W.C. Willett, and C.H. Hennekens. 1992. A prospective study of exercise and incidence of diabetes among US male physicians. *JAMA* 268:63-67.

Manson, J.E., E.B. Rimm, M.J. Stampfer, G.A. Colditz, W.C. Willett, A.S. Krolewski, B. Rosner, C.H. Hennekens, and F.E. Speizer. 1991. Physical activity and incidence of non-insulin dependent diabetes mellitus in women. *Lancet* 338:774-78.

Margonato, A., P. Gerundini, G. Vicedomini, M.C. Gilardi, G. Pozza, and F. Fazio. 1986. Abnormal cardiovascular response to exercise in a young asymptomatic diabetic patient with retinopathy. *Am Heart J* 112:554-60.

Marrero, D.G., A.S. Fremion, and M.P. Golden. 1988. Improving compliance with exercise in adolescents with insulin-dependent diabetes mellitus: results of a self-motivated home exercise program. *Pediatrics* 81:519-25.

Mikines, K.J., B. Sonne, P.A. Farrell, B. Tronier, and H. Galbo. 1988. Effect of physical exercise on sensitivity and responsiveness to insulin in humans. *Am J Physiol* 254:E248-59.

Mikines, K.J., B. Sonne, B. Tronier, and H. Galbo. 1989. Effects of acute exercise and detraining on insulin action in trained men. *J Appl Physiol* 66:704-11.

Mitchell, T.H., G. Abraham, A. Shiffrin, L.A.Leiter, and E.B. Marliss. 1988. Hyperglycemia after intense exercise in IDDM subjects during continuous subcutaneous insulin infusion. *Diabetes Care* 11:311-17.

Mogensen, C.E., and E. Vittinghu. 1975. Urinary albumin excretion during exercise in juvenile diabetes. *Scan J Clin Lab Invest* 35:295-300.

Nelson, J.D., P. Poussier, E.B. Marliss, A.M. Albisser, and B. Zinman. 1982. Metabolic response of normal man and insulin-infused diabetics to postprandial exercise. *Am J Physiol* 242:E309-16.

Ohkubo, Y., H. Kishikawa, E. Araki, T. Miyata, S. Isami, S. Motoyoshi, Y. Kojima, N. Furuyoshi, and M. Shichiri. 1995. Intensive insulin therapy prevents the progression of diabetic microvascular complications in Japanese patients with non-insulin-dependent diabetes mellitus: a randomized prospective 6-year study. *Diabetes Res Clin Pract* 28:103-17.

Olefsky, J.M. 1989. Pathogenesis of non-insulin-dependent (type 2) diabetes. In *Endocrinology*. 3d ed., ed. L.J. DeGroot, 1369-88. Philadelphia: Saunders.

Rosenthal, M., W.L. Haskell, R. Solomon, A. Widstrom, and G.M. Reaven. 1983. Demonstration of a relationship between level of physical training and insulin-stimulated glucose utilization in normal humans. *Diabetes* 32:408-11.

Rubler, S. 1981. Asymptomatic diabetic female exercise testing. *NY State J Med* 81:1185-91.

Sato, Y., A. Iguchi, and N. Sakamoto. 1984. Biochemical determination of training effects using insulin clamp technique. *Horm Metab Res* 16:483-86.

Schiffrin, A., S. Parikh, E.B. Marliss, and M.M. Desrosier. 1984. Metabolic response to fasting exercise in adolescent insulin-dependent diabetic subjects treated with continuous subcutaneous insulin infusion and intensive conventional therapy. *Diabetes Care* 7:255-60.

Schneider, S.H., L.F. Amoroso, A.K. Khachadurian, and N.B. Ruderman. 1984. Studies on the mechanism of improved glucose control during exercise in type 2 (non-insulin-dependent) diabetes. *Diabetologist* 26:355-60.

Simonson, D.C., W.V. Tamborlane, R.A. DeFronzo, and R.S. Sherwin. 1985. Intensive insulin therapy reduces the counterregulatory hormone responses to hypoglycemia in patients with type 1 diabetes. *Ann Int Med* 103:184-90.

Storstein, L., and J. Jervell. 1979. Response to bicycle exercise testing of long standing juvenile diabetics. *Acta Med Scand* 205:227-30.

Stratton, R., D.P. Wilson, R.K. Endres, and D.E. Goldstein. 1987. Improved glycemic control after supervised 8 week exercise program in insulin-dependent diabetic adolescents. *Diabetes Care* 10:589-93.

United Kingdom Prospective Diabetes Study Group (UKPDS33). 1998. Intensive blood glucose control with sulfonylureas or insulin compared with conventional treatment and risk of complications in patients with type 2 diabetes. *Lancet* 352:837-53.

Viberti, G.C., R.J. Jarrett, M. McCartney, and H. Keen. 1978. Increased glomerular permeability to albumin induced by exercise in diabetic subjects. *Diabetologia* 14:293-300.

Wallberg-Henriksson, H., R. Gunnarsson, S. Rossner, and J. Wahren. 1986. Long-term physical training in female type 1 (insulin-dependent) diabetic patients: absence of significant effect on glycemic control and lipoprotein levels. *Diabetologia* 29:53-57.

White, N.H., D. Skor, P.E. Cryer, D.M. Bier, L. Levandoski, and J.V. Santiago. 1983. Identification of type 1 diabetic patients at increased risk for hyperglycemia during intensive therapy. *N Engl J Med* 308:485-91.

Wood, P.D., and W.L. Haskell. 1979. Effect of exercise on plasma high density lipoproteins. *Lipids* 14:417-27.

Yki-Jarvinen, H., and V.A. Koivisto. 1983. Effects of body composition on insulin sensitivity. *Diabetes* 32:965-69.

Zinman, B., F.T. Murray, M. Vranic, A.M. Albisser, B.S. Leibel, P.A. McClean, and E.B. Marliss. 1977. Glucoregulation during moderate exercise in insulin treated diabetics. *J Clin Endocrinol Metab* 45:641-52.

Chapter 13

Selected Arthritides

Rheumatoid Arthritis, Osteoarthritis, Spondylarthropathies, Systemic Lupus Erythematosus, Polymyositis/ Dermatomyositis, and Systemic Sclerosis

Maura Daly Iversen, SD, PT, MPH, Matthew H. Liang, MD, MPH, and Sang-Cheol Bae, MD, PhD, MPH

Case Study

A 35-year-old secretary, B.P., has classical seropositive erosive rheumatoid arthritis. Two years into her course on Plaquenil and NSAIDs, she has little or no functional limitations, though she increasingly has to arrange her day according to the physical demands of her activities. Her occupation requires mild lifting and a great deal of typing.

B.P.'s general physical examination and vital signs are normal, the physical findings limited only to her joints. She complains of neck pain, but has no objective findings, and has mild synovitis of her wrists and second through fourth metacarpophalangeal joints (MCPs) with mild ulnar deviation. Elbows are minimally involved, and she has a rheumatoid nodule on her left elbow. Her knees show small effusions and fine crepitus; the rest of her examination is normal.

What rehabilitation program would you advise? What restrictions to her activities would you recommend?

Rehabilitation program for B.P.: This patient presents with early, stable rheumatoid arthritis (RA). Her rehabilitation program therefore should include a combination of range-of-motion exercises for the involved joints, strength training (both static and dynamic), and aerobics to maximize her endurance and function. It should address static posture (particularly while typing), ergonomic factors, and adaptive equipment (wrist splints). The patient's education would include a thorough discussion of her disease and information on how to modify her exercise program based on her disease activity.

Arthritis and musculoskeletal disorders are among the most common chronic conditions, affecting approximately 37 million people in the United States (Lawrence et al. 1989) and resulting in severe activity limitations. The 100+ forms of these disorders—which spare neither age nor race—can cause joint pain, deformity, and disability. Some systemic rheumatic conditions can lead to death. Arthritis and musculoskeletal conditions are classified generally as systemic versus nonsystemic, and monoarticular versus polyarticular; polyarticular diseases may be subclassified as inflammatory, metabolic, or degenerative (Decker 1983). Table 13.1 lists selected rheumatic diseases, their pathology, and clinical presentation.

All joint diseases are associated with a series of events that compound one another—principally joint stiffness, pain and deformity, soft tissue contracture, muscle atrophy, general deconditioning, and diminished function. Patients with inflammatory or non-inflammatory joint disease can have decreased muscle strength and atrophy surrounding the involved joint. The reduced strength may result from inactivity, inflammation of muscles, or inhibition of muscle contraction due to joint inflammation. Agents used to treat these conditions (e.g., corticosteroids or hydroxychloroquine, which can cause myopathy) may compound the reduction in strength (Gerber 1990). It is even possible, in the case of osteoarthritis of the knee, that weakness is not the result of but a cause of the disease (Slemenda et al. 1997); we need more research in this area.

Restrictions in joint mobility and deformity are common in arthritis. Decreased joint range of motion and deformities may result from pain, soft tissue contractures, poor posture, improper positioning, joint capsule thickening, joint effusion, and subluxation of the joints (Semble et al. 1990). Collagen shortens when not periodically stretched, resulting in loss of

Table 13.1	Features of Rheumatic Diseases	
Disease	**Dominant pathology**	**Clinical presentation**
Rheumatoid arthritis (RA)	Synovitis	Symmetrical and bilateral joint involvement
		Joint pain, swelling, stiffness, contracture
		Muscle weakness and fatigue
Osteoarthritis (OA)	Cartilage degeneration	Weightbearing joints involved
		Joint pain
		Joint malalignment
		Muscle weakness
Spondylarthropathies	Enthesitis	Axial skeleton, hip, shoulder, knee
		Reduced spinal flexibility
		Pain
Systemic lupus erythematosus (SLE)	Systemic inflammation	Diverse and varied organ involvement
		Fatigue
Polymyositis/dermatomyositis (PM/DM)	Myositis	Proximal weakness
		Decreased ROM/contracture
Scleroderma	Fibrosis	Skin and visceral organs involved
		Contracture of soft tissue
		Respiratory involvement

articular structures such as articular cartilage (Gerber 1990). Systemic or local inflammatory disease may impair cardiopulmonary function or restrict activity, leading to contracture, muscle atrophy, diminished stamina and endurance, general deconditioning, and diminished function.

During the past 20 years, scientists have done a tremendous amount of research on the efficacy of strengthening and aerobic exercises in managing arthritis and musculoskeletal symptoms. Research data show clearly that exercise maximizes range of motion (Brighton et al. 1993), muscle strength (Ekdahl et al. 1990; Lyngberg et al. 1994), endurance (Ekblom et al. 1975; Harkcom et al. 1985; Minor et al. 1989), proper joint alignment, function (Stenstrom et al. 1996; Semble et al. 1990), and bone density (Aloia et al. 1978). Yet clinicians continue to prescribe suboptimal exercise levels, or they prescribe exercise only as an afterthought. The reasons in part stem from the belief that exercising patients with inflammatory arthritides could stress the joints and supporting tissues and cause more joint inflammation (Jensen and Lorish 1994). In a recent survey, about 80% of rheumatologists believed range-of-motion exercises were useful in managing the symptoms of rheumatoid arthritis, while only 42% believed aerobic exercises were useful (Iversen 1996).

This chapter reviews the major rheumatic conditions, their major symptoms, and the studies of exercise in the management of these physical symptoms.

Rheumatoid Arthritis

Rheumatoid arthritis (RA) is a chronic, systemic, inflammatory disorder of unknown etiology. The prevalence of rheumatoid arthritis—about 1% to 2% of the population (Lawrence et al. 1989)—increases with age. It affects women twice as often as men, tends to slightly shorten life expectancy (Harris 1990), and often causes a great deal of suffering.

Rheumatoid disease primarily affects the synovium of diarthrodial joints, resulting in synovitis. It is characterized by exacerbations and remissions. Joint involvement is generally symmetrical. If uncontrolled, rheumatoid synovitis results in progressive, disabling, joint destruction. Extra-articular manifestations of rheumatoid arthritis may involve the heart, lungs, blood vessels, skin, and nervous system (Harris 1990). Fatigue, which is common, probably results from production of cytokines, deconditioning, depression, and altered biomechanics from affected joints (which re-

quire greater energy expenditure for the same activities). All these factors significantly limit function and restrict independence of arthritic individuals.

The goals of rehabilitation in the management of rheumatoid arthritis are to maximize strength, flexibility, endurance, and mobility, and to promote the patient's independence. In designing an exercise program, consider the extent and stage of the joint impairments as well as factors which may affect the patient's motivation and compliance. Secondary psychosocial effects from this chronic illness are pervasive and include depression, reduced confidence in the ability to manage the disease, and disruption of personal relationships (Smedstad and Liang 1997; Stenstrom 1994). Depression and reduced self-confidence decrease motivation to perform exercises; social support for exercise increases the chance that the patient will participate in an exercise program, whether short-term or long-term. In fact, positive social support for exercise increases the likelihood by 300% that a patient will adhere to a program (Iversen 1996).

Joint Pain

Pain is common and disabling in rheumatoid arthritis. During acute flares, therapeutic cold helps to reduce inflammation and relieve pain; heat is avoided as it may exacerbate the inflammatory process. When the inflammation resolves, patients may apply either heat or cold to relieve pain and other joint symptoms, based on their preference, disease states, and treatment goals (Hayes 1996). Exercise also may help reduce joint pain. Ekdahl et al. (1990) found that circulating endorphin levels increase in proportion to the intensity and frequency of dynamic exercise. These endogenous opiates may be responsible for the decrease in pain experienced with exercise.

Joint Stiffness, Swelling, and Contractures

Rheumatoid arthritis can lead to tightening of the soft tissues, tendons, and joint capsules. Loss of bone and cartilage reduces joint space, structurally restricting joint motion. Because range-of-motion exercises may maximize joint function, patients with early disease should perform range-of-motion and flexibility exercises daily on affected joints. During acute flares, they should perform two to three repetitions of range-of-motion exercises once a day, either independently or with assistance (Swezey 1974). As inflammation subsides, passive stretching will increase joint range of motion. Patients may apply heat prior to stretching tissues into a more normal range, as it appears to increase the extensibility of collagen and maximize the stretching effect (Hicks 1994; Warren et al. 1976).

Research shows that range-of-motion exercises safely and efficiently maximize joint motion in patients with variable disease activity; they do not appear to increase joint damage, joint flares, or swelling over periods ranging from 6 weeks to 48 months (Brighton et al. 1993; Ekblom et al.1975; Lyngberg et al. 1988; Perlman et al. 1990; van den Ende et al. 1996). Table 13.2 illustrates the variety of exercise studies in rheumatoid arthritis.

Weakness

Strengthening programs enhance muscular strength and contractility, improving patients' ability to perform activities of daily living. Patients with RA are weaker than their healthy counterparts; those with severe disease have 33% to 55% less strength compared to healthy individuals (Nordesjo et al. 1983). In rheumatoid arthritis, muscle weakness may result from a variety of both direct and indirect manifestations of the disease process. For example, patients with RA exhibit type I and type II muscle fiber atrophy (Semble et al. 1990), which may be related to pathological changes within the tissue and/or to disuse. Because myositis can be subtle in rheumatoid arthritis, you should check muscle enzymes if you suspect its presence. If the myositis is not severe, patients may participate in exercise and achieve a training effect (Gerber 1990).

Strengthening programs may be static or dynamic, or a combination of the two. In **static exercises** (also known as isometric exercises), an individual generates muscle tension without changing muscle length or moving through the joint range. These exercises help prevent muscle atrophy; they also produce less inflammation and fewer changes in intra-articular pressure than do other forms of resistive exercise (Hicks 1994). Patients tolerate them well, even during periods of acute joint inflammation (Semble 1995). However, since sustained static exercises may place high demands on cardiac function, they are relatively contraindicated in the presence of ischemic heart disease or congestive heart failure. Patients with these conditions should consult the appropriate specialists.

Dynamic exercise is exercise in which muscle fibers lengthen or shorten, allowing the joint to move through a range of motion and generate a force. In general, the combination of low resistance and high repetitions enhances endurance; higher resistance and low repetitions produce muscle hypertrophy and increase strength. **Isokinetic exercise**, another form of dynamic exercise, is performed on machines that control the velocity of muscle contraction. Since the machines provide uniform resistance (which is proportional to muscle strength) at each point in the range, the machine speed controls the muscle torque.

Relevant Studies

Both static and dynamic strengthening programs lead to muscle fiber hypertrophy and improved strength and function in patients with rheumatoid arthritis. In a 7-week static exercise program in which patients with RA performed three maximal contractions of six seconds duration, three times a week (Machover and Sapecky 1966), patients increased their static quadriceps strength by 23%. Strength of the contralateral quadriceps increased 17%, perhaps as a result of muscle tension overflow—contraction of the exercising muscle produced tension in the matching nonexercising muscle, leading to a slight improvement in strength. Several subjects reported increased joint pain with the six-second maximal contraction.

To study the effects of isokinetic and isometric exercise on joint pain and swelling, Wessel and Quinney (1984) assigned 32 patients with stable disease either to a 7-week program of isokinetic or static exercises or to a control group. Both exercise groups trained on a Cybex II isokinetic dynamometer. The static group trained with the speed of the machine set at 0 degrees per second (allowing no range-of-motion through the joint) and were asked to extend their knees with maximal force against the input arm for three seconds at knee angles of 30, 60, and 90 degrees. A one-minute rest period was allowed between each contraction. The isokinetic group followed a similar procedure, except that patients performed contractions of the quadriceps through 90 degrees of motion at a speed of 180 degrees/second. One-minute rest periods followed three sets of six repetitions with each leg. Although clinicians have generally believed that static exercises create less stress on the joints than dynamic resistive exercises, the static exercise group reported significantly higher pain than the isokinetic group (24.8 vs. 18.1, $p < .05$). This unexpected finding may relate to the speed of the isokinetic contraction: the higher the velocity of the contraction, the less force was produced, resulting in less discomfort during exercise. Neither group noted measurable changes in joint swelling, although the

Table 13.2		Exercise in Rheumatoid Arthritis		
Author	**Subject (no.)**	**Study design**	**Intervention**	**Result**
Machover and Sapecky 1966	11 male patients, disease not classified; varying disease activity	Pre-post	7 wks of static quadriceps exercise, 3 maximal contractions of 6 sec duration, 3 ×/day, 5 days/wk	23% increase in quadriceps strength and a 17% increase in contralateral quadriceps strength; no joint flares noted
Ekblom et al. 1975	34 with non-active disease, Class II-III	RCT	6 wks general rehabilitation (1×/day) plus: ROM or strength training and aerobic bicycle ergometry, 5 days/wk, 20-40 min/day	The endurance training group decreased walk test time by 14%, increased VO$_2$ 20%, reported less pain; no change in articular indices in either group
Ekblom et al. 1975	30 with non-active disease, Class II, III	RCT	6 mo follow-up on patients enrolled in study described above	6 patients who exercised ≥ 4 ×/wk demonstrated sustained benefits
Wessel and Quinney 1984	32 with stable disease, Class II	RCT	7 wks of either static or isokinetic exercise, 3 ×/wk vs. control	No change in knee swelling detectable; exercise pain about 25% greater in isometric than isokinetic group
Harkcom et al. 1985	20 with non-active disease, Class II		12 wks of low intensity bicycle exercise 3 ×/wk at 70% max heart rate, 50 rpm; 4 groups: 15, 25, 35 minutes, and control group	17/20 completed; all exercisers improved aerobic capacity (VO$_2$max); exercise duration (mean increase 3.4 min), symptoms, and pain; only the 35-min group demonstrated statistically significant differences in aerobic capacity
Lyngberg et al. 1988	8 with moderate disease activity, Class I-III	Pre-post	8 wks of graded bicycle ergometer, 45-min, 2 ×/wk, static and ROM exercises	Aerobic capacity increased; patients reported fewer swollen joints and increased strength of the knee extensors and foot plantar flexors

(continued)

CRH = corticotropin-releasing hormone; PT = physical therapy; RCT = randomized clinical trial; ROM = range-of-motion exercises.

Author	Subject (no.)	Study design	Intervention	Result
Minor et al. 1989	40 with variable disease activity	RCT	12 wks aerobic walking; aerobic aquatic aerobic ROM, 3 ×/wk for 60 min	Improved endurance and aerobic capacity in walkers and aquatic groups; anxiety, depression, and physical activity AIMs improved; no difference in joint activity among groups
Perlman et al. 1990	53 with Class I-III, disease activity not reported	Pre-post	16 wks of aerobic dance, flexibility, strength exercises, and patient education; 2 ×/wk for 2 hrs/wk	43/53 completed; decrease in articular pain ($p = .033$) and swelling ($p < .004$); mean improvements in 50-ft walk 2 sec, and increased perception of general health; no effect on disease activity
Ekdahl et al. 1990	67 with low to moderate disease activity, Class II	RCT	6 wks of home exercises and supervised PT visits; 4 groups: dynamic plus 12 PT visits; dynamic plus 4 PT visits; static exercise plus 12 PT; static plus 4 PT visits; patients followed for 3 more mo	62/67 completed; significant increases in strength, endurance, and function; dynamic exercisers increased aerobic capacity by 30%; effects still seen at 3 mo; no significant change in static groups; no joint flares in any group
Brighton et al. 1993	44 with active disease, Class I	RCT	48 mo of hand exercises; reinforcement provided when necessary	Significant increases in grip strength and pincer grip strength in the exercise group
Baslund et al. 1993	18 with moderate disease activity	RCT	8 wks progressive bike training, 4-5 ×/wk for 35 min at 80% $\dot{V}O_2$max	Max VO_2 uptake increased 18% trained vs. 6% controls; heart rate at stage 2 and perceived exertion decreased; no change in immune response

Table 13.2   (continued)

Table 13.2   *(continued)*

Author	Subject (no.)	Study design	Intervention	Result
Hansen et al. 1993	75 with mixed disease activity, Class I-II	RCT	2-year study; 4 groups exercising 45 min total (15 min general, 30 min aerobic) 3 ×/wk: self-exercisers (SE); SE plus weekly group exercise; SE plus weekly group and PT exercises; and a group without instruction	65/75 completed; no significant differences between groups; strength increased in all groups; no change in aerobic fitness; no difference in X-ray progression of disease
Lyngberg et al. 1994	11 with mild to moderate disease activity, Class II or III	Pre-post	3 wks isokinetic exercise followed by 3 wks static exercise, 3 ×/wk at 50% max voluntary contraction	9/11 completed; 21% mean increase in knee extensor muscle strength; no joint flares or adverse effects
Hakkinen et al. 1994	43, disease activity not stated	RCT	10 mo progressive dynamic strength training (2-3 ×/wk at 40%-60% max) vs. regular activity (3-4 ×/wk)	39/43 completed; exercisers increased bilateral dynamic strength 32% and unilateral strength by 49%; ESR decreased and function increased; only slight changes in joints of subjects
Ekdahl et al. 1994	30 RA with low to moderate disease activity, Class II; & 20 healthy	RCT	6 wks of (1) high intensity (60 min 2 ×/wk); (2) low intensity dynamic exercise; (3) control	47/50 completed; initially RA and healthy subjects differed in CRH levels; RA exercisers increased CRH levels (3 pmo/L; $p < .05$) compared to others; significant difference in β-endorphin levels in RA and healthy exercisers
Hall et al. 1996	148 with Class I, II, III	RCT	4 wks; 30 min 2 ×/wk seated immersion, hydrotherapy; land exercise or relaxation	139/148 completed; all patients improved physically and emotionally; 27% decrease in joint tenderness; average knee ROM increased 6.6 degrees in women in hydrotherapy; at 3 mo hydrotherapy group maintained improvements

(continued)

Table 13.2   (continued)

Author	Subject (no.)	Study design	Intervention	Result
Stenstrom et al. 1996	54 with Class I, II disease	RCT	2 groups; dynamic exercise or relaxation training, 5 ×/wk for 30 min for 3 mo	48/54 completed; dynamic group improved walking speed (md diff = 0.7) and perceived exertion ($p < .05$); relaxation group improved on Nottingham Health Profile, joint tenderness, and lower extremity muscle function
Rall et al. 1996	30 RA patients with well-controlled disease	RCT	12 wk program with 4 groups: 8 healthy elders, 8 RA, and 8 young healthy; performed resistance exercises 2 ×/wk at 80% 1 rep max contraction; 6 elderly performed warm-up swimming exercises	Exercisers increased muscle strength compared to controls: RA 57%, young exercisers 44%, elderly exercisers 35%; no change in joint symptoms; RA patients reported improvements in pain and fatigue
Van den Ende et al. 1996	100 with stable disease	RCT	12 wk exercise with 12 wk follow-up; 4 groups: dynamic weightbearing exercises and bike, ROM and static exercises in group, supervised ROM and static exercises; or home ROM and static exercises	90/100 completed; 17% increase in aerobic capacity and muscle strength, 16% increase in joint mobility in high intensity group; gain lost after stopping; no damage to joints
Senstrom et al. 1997	54 with RA Class I and II disease & 6 PA	RCT	12 mo program; 2 groups: dynamic training or relaxation 5 ×/wk for 3 mo then 2-3 ×/wk for 9 mo	Improved physical impact (median 1.7 vs. 1.2, $p \le .05$) and work effects (AIMS2) in dynamic group; relaxation group less pain and emotional reaction

Adapted, by permission, from J.E. Hicks, 1994, "Exercise in rheumatoid arthritis," *Phys Med Rehabil Clin N Am* 5:708, 717.

crude measure of joint swelling (circumferential measurements) may not have been sensitive to change.

Lyngberg et al. (1994) saw improvements in muscle strength from a six-week strengthening program comprising three weeks of isokinetic exercise for the right knee extensors, followed by three weeks of static knee exercises for the left knee extensors. Using an isokinetic dynamometer, patients performed 48 repetitions of relatively low-intensity exercise (50% of maximal voluntary contraction) at four different angular velocities, three times per week for 15 minutes during the first three weeks of the trial. In the subsequent three weeks, the subjects trained their left knee extensors using static exercises at 50% of the maximal voluntary contraction at two joint angles, 60 and 90 degrees. They held each contraction for three seconds. Nine of the 11 patients with mild to moderate disease activity completed the study, with a mean increase in knee strength of 21% in the isokinetic program. The relatively large increase in strength with this modest exercise program may be attributed to the patients' low baseline level of conditioning. This static exercise program, however, led only to an insignificant increase in knee extensor strength. The subjects tolerated the static exercise training no better than the isokinetic program of similar intensity.

Ekdahl et al. (1990) randomized RA patients to a six-week program of either dynamic or static lower extremity exercises, in combination with physical therapy visits. The dynamic groups performed dynamic resistive weightbearing exercises and exercises to increase balance and coordination (figure 13.1). The static groups performed joint mobility exercises and static exercises at a submaximal level. All patients were also instructed in a home program. During the six-week period, patients in the dynamic training group demonstrated a 30% increase in aerobic capacity and greater improvements in both isometric and isokinetic strength and endurance tests compared to patients in the static exercise group. Although the dynamic groups exercised at a relatively high intensity, their joint symptoms did not worsen. Dynamic exercises appeared superior to static training in promoting lower extremity muscle function among patients with stable disease; with the addition of a home exercise program, these training effects were evident at the three-month follow-up.

To evaluate the impact of a high-intensity exercise program on muscle strength, Rall and colleagues (1996) enrolled 30 subjects: 8 healthy untrained subjects, 8 untrained subjects with RA, and 14 untrained healthy elderly subjects. The healthy elderly were randomized to either the dynamic resistance exercise or to the warm-up exercise in a swimming pool. Subjects in the high-intensity resistive exercise group trained all major muscle groups twice a week at 80% of their 1-repetition maximal contraction. After 12 weeks, the subjects with RA had a 57% increase in strength, the young healthy exercisers a 44% increase, and the healthy elderly subjects a 36% increase in strength. Subjects with RA also reported a 21% reduction in joint pain and a 38% decrease in fatigue. Although the sample was small, this study is unique in comparing (1) the effects of the exercise program on both young and old healthy individuals, with (2) its effects on RA patients.

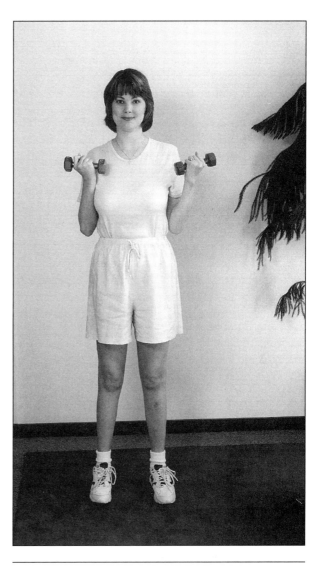

Figure 13.1 An RA patient can perform dynamic resistive weightbearing exercise as long as the exercised joint is not inflamed.

Conclusions About Strength Exercises and Rheumatoid Arthritis

In summary, static and dynamic exercises increase muscle strength in patients with rheumatoid arthritis over periods of 3 to 12 weeks. Static exercises produce less intra-articular force and place less shear force across joints (leading to less discomfort during exercise), and are appropriate during acute flares to prevent muscle atrophy. Patients with stable disease tolerate dynamic as well as static exercises; and the former lead to greater improvements in muscle strength and function. Isokinetic exercises performed at high speeds, such as a velocity of 180 degrees per second, appear to reduce the discomfort normally associated with dynamic exercise. As most studies of dynamic strengthening exercises in RA do not include patients with active or severe disease, one should not generalize the results of these studies to such populations—we recommend that individuals avoid dynamic strengthening exercises during acute flares. Other contraindications to dynamic exercises in RA include the presence of ligamentous laxity, which may increase the risk of ligament rupture during strengthening programs; and the presence of tense popliteal cysts, which could rupture during isokinetic testing (Hicks 1994).

Fatigue and Endurance

Aerobic exercise can improve immune responses, aerobic capacity, endurance, and function in healthy individuals (Åstrand and Rodahl 1986). Patients with RA have decreased aerobic capacity compared to healthy subjects; but with short-term conditioning programs they can improve both their cardiovascular fitness (by 20%, as measured by $\dot{V}O_2$max) and their physical function (Ekblom et al. 1975; van den Ende et al. 1996). Training regimens of 50% to 80% of $\dot{V}O_2$max appear to be best. Most maximal stress tests for RA patients use a modified Bruce protocol and employ bicycle ergometers to reduce stress on weightbearing joints. Bicycling, swimming or aquatic exercises, and walking are also appropriate aerobic activities for RA patients' joints (see figure 13.2). The buoyancy of water facilitates exercises that are difficult to perform on land. Warm water also relaxes muscle spasms and reduces pain. The recommended water temperature for patients with arthritis is 37 to 40 degrees Celsius (Gerber and Hicks 1990). There has been little research on aquatic programs for RA patients, although theoretically they are ideal for maximizing range of motion and endurance in such patients.

Relevant Studies

Baslund and colleagues (1993) evaluated the effects of an eight-week, moderate-intensity bicycle training program on the immune system of 18 patients with moderate RA disease activity. In this randomized trial, the researchers found a training effect, as measured by maximal O_2 uptake, but no changes in natural killer cell activity, blood mononuclear cells, plasma cytokines, or lymphocyte proliferative responses.

Harkcom et al. (1985) tested patients with RA at three levels of low-intensity aerobic conditioning for 35, 25, or 15 minutes, performed three times a week

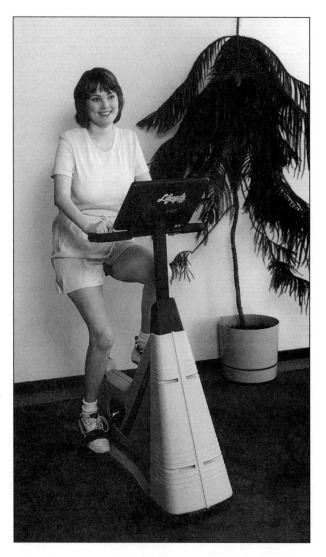

Figure 13.2 Bicycling is a safe and effective approach to exercise that patients can do at home.

over a 12-week period. The 35-minute, low-intensity conditioning program produced statistically significant improvements in aerobic capacity (6.9 ml/kg/minute on average). The 25- and 15-minute programs appeared to improve aerobic capacity, but the improvements were not statistically significant. A comparison of all three exercise groups to the control group showed an increase in mean aerobic capacity of 6.2 ml/kg/minute and a mean increase in endurance test time of 3.4 minutes. All exercisers reported significant decreases in joint pain and swelling compared to the nonexercising controls ($p < .01$). This study demonstrated that a low-intensity conditioning program of as little as 15 minutes' duration, performed three times per week over a three-month

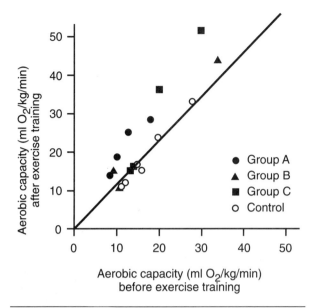

Figure 13.3 Aerobic capacity for each subject before and after exercise training. *P* < .05 for group A. Group A = 14 min final total duration exercise. Group B = 25 min final total duration exercise. Group C = 35 min final total duration exercise.
Adapted, by permission, from T.M. Harkcom et al., 1985, "Therapeutic value of graded aerobic exercise training in rheumatoid arthritis," *Arthritis Rheum* 28:35.

period, could improve aerobic capacity in patients with RA (see figure 13.3).

In a large randomized controlled trial, van den Ende et al. (1996) found improvements in aerobic capacity, muscle strength, and joint mobility with a 12-week program of high-intensity exercise. Patients were allocated to either

- a high-intensity dynamic program, including weightbearing exercises and bicycling, in which patients exercised at 70% to 85% of their age-predicted maximal heart rate;

- a low-intensity group exercise program, consisting of range-of-motion and static strengthening exercises for the trunk and lower extremity;

- a low-intensity individual range-of-motion and static exercise program, with instructions by a physical therapist; or

- a written home program of range-of-motion and static exercises.

The high-intensity exercise group met for one hour, three times per week; the low-intensity exercise group met for one hour, twice a week; the patients receiving individual instruction also performed their exercises twice a week. Patients in the home program were encouraged to exercise twice a week for at least 15 minutes. Following the 12-week program, the high-

intensity group demonstrated a 17% increase in aerobic capacity and knee muscle strength and a 15% increase in joint mobility; both low-intensity groups demonstrated a small increase (about 7%) in knee muscle strength. The home exercise participants did not differ significantly from baseline on any measure. Joint symptoms did not increase in any of the groups and actually decreased among the high-intensity exercisers. Twelve weeks after discontinuation of the program, the improvements in aerobic capacity and joint mobility were no longer present—although the gains in 50-foot walk time and muscle strength remained.

While earlier studies examined the benefits of bicycle ergometry (Ekblom et al. 1975; Harkcom et al. 1985), more recent research has focused on alternative forms of aerobic exercise for RA patients. Minor and colleagues (1989) tested how aerobic walking and aquatic programs could improve aerobic capacity in patients with RA. In addition to the improvements in aerobic capacity for both groups, patients reported improvements in mood. Perlman and colleagues (1990) studied the effects of a 16-week dance exercise program consisting of two-hour sessions, twice a week. Subjects reported significant decreases in articular pain, as measured by the Arthritis Impact Measurement Scale (mean difference = 7 points, $p <$ .05), and in swelling ($t = 3.05$, $p < .01$); they also improved their functional capacity, as measured by the 50-ft walk test ($t = 4.89$, $p < .001$). Again, the subjects reported no adverse effects, suggesting that patients with stable disease tolerate weightbearing aerobic exercise programs well.

Few studies have rigorously evaluated the efficacy of hydrotherapy on physical and psychological outcomes in patients with RA. Hall and colleagues (1996) randomly assigned patients to four weeks of hydrotherapy, seated immersion, land exercises, or relaxation training. Each session met twice a week for 30 minutes. All subjects improved both physically and emotionally. Subjects in the hydrotherapy group reported 27% less joint tenderness than patients in the other groups. Women in the hydrotherapy treatment increased their total combined knee range of motion by 6.6 degrees. At follow-up, hydrotherapy patients maintained their emotional and psychological improvements.

Conclusions About Aerobic Conditioning and Rheumatoid Arthritis

Studies of aerobic conditioning in RA have varied considerably in the frequency, duration, intensity, and mode of exercise tested, as well as the outcomes measured (physiologic versus self-report). While it is difficult to combine these results in a quantitative manner, the collective data support the notion that short-term aerobic exercise programs, in which patients exercise at least three times per week, can increase aerobic capacity by about 20% and can improve both endurance and mood. A significant problem with programs of short duration (6 to 12 weeks), however, is that the benefits are not maintained once the program has ended. Programs of longer duration and intensity produce the greatest aerobic effects. The conflicting results surrounding the impact of aerobic exercise on joint symptoms may reflect the variation in patient selection and sample size, and the use of differing measures of disease activity and joint symptoms. Aerobic exercise programs that incorporate weightbearing exercises, once believed to be harmful, have proven to be well tolerated by patients with stable disease. In our experience, it is very difficult for patients to adhere to these programs over the course of a chronic disease. Programs must be flexible, incorporating a variety of exercise modes that reduce boredom and enable patients to modify their programs based on their joint symptoms. Research is needed to assess the benefits of such programs for patients with varying levels of disease activity, and to determine the intensity required to maintain long-term aerobic effects.

General Recommendations

The degree of synovitis, amount of joint destruction and deformity, and the patient's pain tolerance set the parameters for the types and amounts of exercises prescribed. Patients in an acute flare should generally engage in static strengthening and gentle range-of-motion exercises, and should receive instruction in joint protection techniques to minimize trauma to inflamed joints. These patients should not do resistive exercises, since there is a possibility of tendon rupture. Static exercises, on the other hand, do not require joint movement—yet they generate maximal muscle contractions and improve muscle strength. Static exercises of six-second duration appear most effective for maximizing strength; individuals should perform them once a day on each muscle group during an acute flare. Table 13.3 summarizes the exercise recommendations.

RA patients should perform range-of-motion exercises daily to prevent loss of motion. This is important because joints generally feel more comfortable in flexion—which relieves pressure and discomfort

but may lead to flexion contractures. During a flare, two to three repetitions of active range-of-motion exercises help maximize joint mobility while placing minimal stress on the articular structures. Performing these exercises in the evening may reduce the early morning stiffness commonly experienced by patients with active disease (Byers 1985). As the inflammation subsides, the exercise program can expand to include 8 to 10 daily repetitions of these exercises for each involved joint.

During remissions or relatively inactive disease, patients with rheumatoid arthritis may undertake a more active exercise program that incorporates active range-of-motion exercises as well as strength and endurance training. Aerobic exercise sessions of as little as 15 minutes' duration, performed three times per week, increase aerobic capacity in patients with rheumatoid arthritis (Harkcom et al. 1985) without placing undue stress on joints.

Patients with RA should let their pain determine the intensity of the program. Acute pain during exercise indicates a need to modify the program; vague, diffuse pain that resolves in less than two hours does not indicate a need for program modification (Hayes 1996). Patients must recognize the warning signs of an acute flare—including redness, inflammation, pain, and stiffness—and learn how to modify their exercise program in accordance with their disease activity. Exercise instructions should include the intensity, frequency, and duration at which each exercise should be performed.

In summary, exercise is a proven method for improving function, endurance, and mood in patients with rheumatoid arthritis. Short-term programs of static and dynamic exercises have demonstrated improvements in muscle strength ranging from 27% to 57%, with little effect on joint effusion and pain. These exercises may even reduce joint synovitis. Short-term aerobic exercise, whether supervised or unsupervised, produces increases of up to 20% in aerobic capacity. However, there has been little research on the long-term effects of these exercises on joint integrity, and on the various stages of disease for which beneficial short-term effects obtain. Research is needed to describe the effects of long-term exercise training on joint structures and its impact on synovitis.

Osteoarthritis

Osteoarthritis (OA), also called osteoarthrosis and degenerative joint disease, is the most common form

Disease	Disease status	Recommendation
RA[#]	Acute flare "hot joint"	Active ROM exercises to involved joints: 2 repetitions/joint/day.
	Subacute	Active ROM exercises: 8-10 repetitions/joint/day.
		Static exercises: 4-6 contractions of 6 second duration.
		Isotonic exercises with light resistance; avoid if joints are unstable, or in presence of tense popliteal cysts or of internal joint derangement.
		Aerobic training (15-20 minutes, 3 × week). Cardiac evaluation for men over 35 and women over 45 is recommended. Establish heart rate parameters and use perceived rating of exertion scale (e.g., BORG).
	Stable or inactive	Active ROM and flexibility exercises.
		Static and dynamic strength training; avoid dynamic exercises if joints are unstable, or in presence of tense popliteal cyst(s).
		Aerobic training 15-20 minutes, 3 × week. Cardiac evaluation for men over 35 and women over 45 is recommended. Establish heart rate parameters and use perceived rating of exertion scale (e.g., BORG).
OA of hip and knee	Mild pain	Active ROM exercises (10 repetitions), 3-5 repetitions of flexibility and static exercises (8-10 repetitions of 6 second duration).
		Dynamic exercises especially to quadriceps and hamstrings (8-10 repetitions).
		Low-impact aerobic activities (pool, bicycling) 20 minutes, 3 × week.
		Static and dynamic exercises reduce to 5 repetitions, plus 3-5 repetitions of flexibility exercises to maintain muscular balance around joints.
	Moderate pain	Low-impact aerobic exercises (pool, biking) 20 min, 3 × week.
		Static and dynamic exercises (no resistance) 3-5 repetitions (contraindication: internal joint derangement).
	Severe pain	Low- to no-impact aerobic exercises (pool).
	Bone-on-bone	Same as severe, but few to no repetitions of dynamic exercises.
		Patient education very important.

(continued)

ROM = range-of-motion exercises

[#]Adapted, by permission, from J.E. Hicks, 1994, "Exercise in rheumatoid arthritis," *Phys Med Rehabil Clin N Am* 5:701-727. Remaining recommendations based on clinical practice and/or exercise literature.

Disease	Disease status	Recommendation
Spondylarthropathies		Stretching of pectorals, back extensors, hamstrings, psoas and active ROM exercises (8-10 × day).
		Breathing exercises (diaphragmatic & lateral costal expansion) frequently throughout day.
		Dynamic exercises especially for trunk and hip muscles 5-8 repetitions.
		Aerobic exercises (pool especially helpful in presence of hip involvement) 20 minutes, 3 × week.
SLE	Active but stable	Active ROM if synovitis present and endurance activities as tolerated.
	Inactive	Dynamic exercises, 8 to 10 repetitions.
		Aerobic exercises (bicycle, pool), 20 minutes, 3 × week.
PM/DM	Active but stable	Use RA guidelines for strengthening as a basis.
	Inactive	Active ROM & static exercises, 8-10 repetitions.
		Dynamic exercises, 8-10 repetitions (note: careful with eccentric exercises, use fewer repetitions).
		Aerobic exercises as tolerated (20 minutes, 3 × week).
Scleroderma		Active ROM exercises, heating of tissue prior to stretching helpful, or use prolonged stretch.
		Dynamic and static exercises 8-10 repetitions.
		Aerobic exercises 20 minutes, 3 × week.

Table 13.3   (continued)

of chronic arthritis. It increases with age and affects nearly 40 million individuals in the United States. Although its exact pathogenesis is unknown, genetic, environmental, and biological determinants are important. **Primary osteoarthritis**, the most common, includes a number of clinical syndromes of specific joints for which there is no etiologic basis. **Secondary osteoarthritis** is osteoarthritis due to underlying factors that accelerate age-related degeneration of cartilage. The factors include osteoarthritis from inflammatory arthritis (such as rheumatoid arthritis or spondylarthritis), osteoarthritis secondary to metabolic diseases (such as hemochromatosis, acromegaly, or diabetes), and osteoarthritis secondary to congenital abnormalities of the joint (which leave the joint surfaces incongruous, thereby accelerating damage of cartilage in specific areas).

Whether primary or secondary, the pathology of osteoarthritis is in the cartilage, which—over time, with variable amounts of inflammation and changes in loading across the joint surface—is destroyed. On X ray the classic appearance includes unequal joint space narrowing, eburnation of the subchondral bone, osteophytes, and subchondral cysts (see figure 13.4). These findings increase in frequency after the age of 50. One of the most impressive features of the epidemiology of OA is the lack of concordance between X-ray pictures and symptoms—roughly 2/3 of pa-

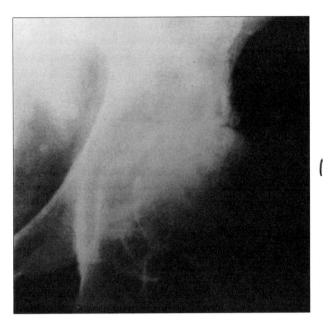

Figure 13.4 Moderately advanced osteoarthritic changes are present, with assymetric joint space narrowing and superior migration of the femoral head. Eburnation and cystic changes are seen in the subchondral region.
Reprinted, by permission, from W.N. Kelley et al., 1997, *Textbook of rheumatology*, 5th ed. (Philadelphia: W.B. Saunders), 665.

tients with radiographic features have few or no symptoms (Patients with early involvement experience joint stiffness with progressive cartilage destruction, and pain when loading the affected joint. Secondary contractures occur around the involved joint and contiguous joints. These contractures can be biomechanically disadvantageous and can increase energy requirements for the patient. Depending on the joints involved, discomfort may limit specific functional activities. The most commonly affected and symptomatic joints are the apophyseal joints of the spine, the distal and proximal interphalangeal joints, the carpometacarpal joint, the first metatarsal phalangeal joint, and the knee, hip, and patellofemoral joints. OA of the axial and of the large weightbearing joints has the greatest negative impact on patient mobility.

Finger Stiffness/Pain

Osteoarthritis of the fingers causes not only pain, aching, or stiffness, but also an unsightly appearance. With severe deformities, some patients may be unable to grip objects tightly or to make a tight fist. Very often with time the finger pain or stiffness diminishes, probably because the deformities prevent motion. There has been little study of range-of-motion

exercise regimens for osteoarthritis in the fingers. In one small trial, yoga and relaxation techniques over a ten-week period diminished pain and tenderness, and improved joint motion (Garfinkel et al. 1994).

Stiffness and Discomfort in Knees and Hips

Exercise prescriptions for hip and knee osteoarthritis aim to improve active and passive joint movement, to strengthen muscles, and to provide aerobic conditioning. The joint stiffness and post-weight loading discomfort of hip or knee osteoarthritis lead to functional deficits such as difficulties with transfers, prolonged standing, and walking. Studies of exercise regimens in osteoarthritis of the knee and hip have not been stratified for severity, nor is it clear how or whether such regimens affect the underlying pathology.

Muscle Weakness

It is generally believed that OA causes joint symptoms that reduce activity and contribute to disease-specific muscle atrophy and general deconditioning. However, a recent study suggests that muscle weakness may be more a cause than a result of knee osteoarthritis (Slemenda et al. 1997). Muscle weakness may alter the biomechanics of the joint and place unequal forces across the joint surface. Joint laxity from muscle inhibition and joint space narrowing distributes the forces across the cartilage surface unequally and can accelerate the process of cartilage degeneration. Patients with advanced radiographic structural changes have the worst deformity, range of motion, quadriceps weakness, and deconditioning (Philbin et al. 1995). Disuse atrophy probably results from ligament stretching, reflex inhibition from pain, capsular contraction, and joint irritation due to pain and effusion. Atrophy of the quadriceps muscle group due to reflex inhibition starts a vicious cycle, increasing force across the damaged cartilage and altering the mechanics of the patellofemoral joint. Malalignment of the patella and abnormal tracking may produce retropatellar pain and chondromalacia patellae. Because muscle weakness and deconditioning accompany OA of the hip and knee, improving both is a goal of rehabilitation. Since few investigators have studied the effectiveness of such rehabilitation programs, there are no data on their potential long-term adverse effects on cartilage, and few data on long-term compliance.

Relevant Studies

For individuals with mild to moderate osteoarthritis of the knee or hip, a 12-week aerobic exercise program (walking or in water) increased aerobic capacity by almost 20% without exacerbating joint symptoms; and it decreased pain by almost 10% and morning stiffness by 20 minutes. Minor and colleagues tested 80 patients with mild osteoarthritis of the hip, knee, or ankle for three months with three interventions:

1. A stretching and strengthening exercise program
2. The same program combined with aerobic pool activities
3. The same program combined with aerobic walking

All patients had supervised range-of-motion and isometric exercises three times a week for an hour. The two aerobic exercise groups also did up to 30 minutes of exercise to increase their heart rates to 60%-80% of baseline maximum. At three months, the researchers assessed 80% of the participants for maximum oxygen uptake as a measure of aerobic capacity, for flexibility, for exercise endurance on a treadmill, for their time to walk 50 feet, and for self-reported health status. The pool and walking programs increased aerobic capacity 20% and 19%, respectively, whereas the control group had no change. In no case was there exacerbation of joint symptoms in the two aerobic groups; on average, moreover, pain decreased by almost 10% and morning stiffness by 20 minutes. Physical activity, anxiety, and depression also improved in both aerobic groups significantly more than for the controls (Minor et al. 1989).

The best test of the aerobic exercise was done by Kovar and her colleagues, who randomly assigned 102 patients with primary knee osteoarthritis to either

• an eight-week program of lectures, group discussions, and supervised light stretching and strengthening followed by up to 30 minutes of walking; or
• routine care and telephone follow-up calls three times a week (control group).

The unblinded investigators evaluated 92% of the patients and 88% of the controls at baseline and at eight weeks. Intervention participants had an 18% increase in six-minute walking test time, compared with a 17% decrease in controls. The intervention group also improved more than controls on the self-reported measures of physical activities, arthritis pain, and use of medications (Kovar et al. 1992).

Ettinger and his colleagues randomized 439 community-dwelling subjects 60 years or older, with radiographic knee osteoarthritis, pain, and physical disability, to

• an aerobic exercise program,
• a resistance exercise program, or
• a health education program (Ettinger et al. 1997).

The researchers measured the following: self-rated disability and knee pain, performance (based on measures of physical function), X-ray score, aerobic capacity, and knee muscle strength. Overall, patients in the aerobic or resistance exercise groups had modest improvements in pain and disability, and better scores on performance measures and function, than those in the health education group. The effects were smaller than those observed in previous studies; the authors speculated that differences between the three raters might not be apparent since *all* interventions—even education alone—had previously been shown to be effective. Prior exercise behavior was the strongest predictor of exercise compliance in this population (Rejeski et al. 1997).

Conclusions About Exercise and Osteoarthritis in the Knees and Hips

Aerobic exercise improves endurance and reduces fatigue, but has modest effects on muscle strength. With structured exercise (three times/week over four months), individuals can improve strength and endurance—leading to decreased dependency and pain, and increased functional activity. Some of these benefits continue for up to eight months after an intense program (Fisher et al. 1991).

Despite the evidence that symptoms of osteoarthritis of the hip and knee can be improved with exercise, most patients do not have an exercise prescription. Even when physicians prescribed exercise, only a small percentage of patients exercised in a manner that can achieve a therapeutic effect (Dexter 1992). Certain patients with osteoarthritis of the hip can exercise at home as effectively as with outpatient hydrotherapy to improve joint mobility and increase muscle strength (Green et al. 1993).

In summary: patients with mild to moderate knee and hip osteoarthritis can safely train (at least short-term) the quadriceps muscles and engage in effective aerobic exercise without exacerbating joint symptoms. When patients are supervised and compliant, the results are good. In practice, however, where patients have to sustain the exercise program over a long period, the results may be less impressive; and no one has studied the long-term and possible adverse effects of such programs. Because of the practical barriers and the lack of supporting data, these modalities are not widely used or pursued aggressively in most patients.

Gait Problems in Osteoarthritis

Contracture of soft tissues and of tendons surrounding a joint, destruction of joint cartilage, persistent faulty posture, or an imbalance between agonist and antagonist muscle groups may lead to limited joint motion and abnormal gait. Although a flexed position minimizes intra-articular pressure and reduces pain, it leads to flexion contracture. Evaluations of regimens to correct or prevent contractures are almost nonexistent. In practice, heat followed by passive range-of-motion (ROM) exercises and joint mobilization often can help prevent or at least reduce contractures. Patients also should assume appropriate positions during extended inactivity or sleep, and engage in active ROM exercises to maximize functional range and strength. Patients with knee flexion contractures should not sleep with pillows under the knee. In difficult cases, serial casting or splinting can reduce contracture when followed by maintenance exercises.

Loss of joint motion at the hip has functional effects that some clinicians may not appreciate. A flexion contracture across the acetabulum toward the lateral margin (Hicks et al. 1993) increases valgus forces at the knee and ankle and causes inefficient gait patterns and increased energy expenditure; it also impairs both sitting and gait at the hip, and may affect personal hygiene and sexual function. Loss of hip range adversely affects the spine and other joints, including the knee and ankle. Preventive posturing, as in prone lying, is important. Repetitive sit-to-stand exercise maintains strength in hip and knee extensors and can be started with standing up from a seat whose level is progressively lowered as the maneuver becomes easier to complete. For patients unable to tolerate full-gravity exercise, the use of water allows exercise with reduced load.

Six patients with severe OA of the hip, who were waiting for total hip arthroplasty, increased hip adduction by 8.3 degrees, increased type I and II fiber cross-sectional area, and increased glycogen levels after passive muscle stretching perpendicular to the direction of the adductor muscle (without hip movement). The subjects stretched with a 20- to 30-kg

force applied manually for 30 seconds, rested for 10 seconds, and repeated; sessions lasted 25 minutes, five days a week for four weeks (Leivseth et al. 1989).

In summary, gait problems are common in patients with OA of any of the weightbearing joints and are a clue to underlying pathology of the soft tissues or the joints themselves. Left untreated, they can cause problems. Clinicians should be attentive to the diagnosis, and design treatments that maximize joint function.

Spondylarthropathies

Spondylarthropathies include a group of disorders: ankylosing spondylitis (AS), reactive arthritis (Reiter's disease), psoriatic arthritis, enteropathic arthritis, juvenile onset spondylarthropathy, and undifferentiated spondylarthropathy. The common finding of these diseases is spondylitis, sacroillitis, and enthesitis, an inflammation of the tendons at their insertion into bone; all result in low back stiffness/pain. Over years, spinal ankylosis may develop at a variable rate and pattern. In extreme cases of AS, the entire spine may fuse in a flexed position. Besides axial spine involvement, peripheral joints may be affected—especially hip, shoulder, or knee. Rehabilitation guidelines for RA are generally appropriate for patients with peripheral arthritis. Stiffness, pain, and restrictions in spinal mobility limit the functional abilities of most patients. The prototypic spondylarthropathy, AS, occurs in about 0.1% of the general Caucasian population—predominantly seen in males, although some studies suggest its prevalence ratio of men to women may be as high as 1:1 (Gran and Husby 1993). The possible reasons for the underestimation of AS among women include: the tradition of regarding AS as a disease of men; fear of exposing female pelvic organs to radiation; a more benign course; and peripheral arthritis in women, which suggests alternative diagnoses. Although researchers have focused most exercise therapy studies on AS rather than other spondylarthropathies, there is no reason to believe that the results of such research involving spinal symptoms would not apply to the other disorders. Table 13.4 summarizes these studies.

The goals of exercise prescription are to maximize range of motion, maintain and improve spinal mobility, and maintain a neutral posture. Exercises should include passive range-of-motion activity, and should aim to strengthen the extensors and stretch the flexors. These patients may have a rigid thorax and kyphosis due to bony ankylosis of the thoracic

Table 13.4		Studies of Exercise in AS		

Author	Subject (no.)	Study design	Intervention	Result
O'Driscoll et al. 1978	35	Pre-post	3 wk inpatient active neck mobilizing exercise	25/35 completed; significant improvement in flexion/extension, total lateral flexion and total rotation of neck
Bulstrode et al. 1987	39	Nonrandomized controlled trial	3 wk inpatient passive stretching exercise of hip	Significant increase in all ROM of hip except flexion
Viitanen et al. 1992	505	Retrospective	3-4 wk inpatient physiotherapy	7-37% increase in thoracolumbar flexibility, Schober test, occiput to wall distance, cervical rotation, chin to chest distance, finger to floor distance, chest expansion and vital capacity
Russel et al. 1993	57	Nonrandomized controlled trial, 2-6 mo follow-up study	Once per week for 1.5 hr physiotherapy	Increase in extension but no change in any other spinal movement; following over 2-6 mo, loss of flexion and lateral bend but no change in extension
Kraag et al. 1990	53	RCT	4 mo home physiotherapy	Intention to treat analysis: significant improvement in finger to floor distance, functional disability but no difference in pain, spinal alignment, Schober test
Kraag et al. 1994	46	8 mo follow-up study of Kraag et al. 1990	4 mo home physiotherapy	Initial improvement achieved was maintained in finger to floor distance

vertebrae, costovertebral, costotransverse, sternoclavicular, and sternomanubrial joints. Pulmonary function testing may show restrictive physiology, but with normal pulmonary compliance, diffusing capacity, and blood gases. Fisher et al. (1990) observed a weak association between chest expansion and vital capacity, and between vital capacity and exercise tolerance as measured by maximum oxygen capacity ($\dot{V}O_2$max). However, there was no association between chest expansion and exercise tolerance. The authors recommend placing a stronger emphasis on encouraging patients with AS to participate in regular aerobic exercise as well as exercises to maximize spinal mobility.

Limited Spinal Mobility

Several studies have shown improvements in spinal, hip, and neck movement from three- or four-week inpatient intensive physiotherapy, involving bending,

Table 13.4 (continued)

Author	Subject (no.)	Study design	Intervention	Result
Hidding et al. 1993	144	RCT	9 mo group physical therapy vs. home therapy	Intention to treat analysis: group physical therapy proved superior to home therapy in improving thoracolumbar mobility, fitness, and global assessment
Hidding et al. 1994	68	RCT continuation of Hidding et al. 1993	18 mo group physical therapy vs. home therapy	Intention to treat analysis: global health and functioning were sustained or even improved further if group physical therapy is continued; spinal mobility decreased slightly in both group and home therapy
Viitanen et al. 1995	141	Pre-post, 15 mo follow-up study	3-4 week inpatient physiotherapy	All 9 mobility measurements; vital capacity, fitness index improved after treatment; 15 mo later, all measurements except chest expansion and vital capacity were still better
Carbon et al. 1996	11	Pre-post self-controlled study	30-min cycle ergometry	Exercising unaffected body can elicit immediate short-term beneficial effect of affected body (improvement in spinal flexibility and a reduction in pain)

stretching, and/or strengthening exercises (Bulstrode et al. 1987; O'Driscoll et al. 1978; Viitanen et al. 1992). However, long-term follow-up studies after 2 to 15 months of short-term intensive physiotherapy, followed by unsupervised home exercise, showed mixed results in improving spine mobility (Hidding et al. 1993; Russell et al. 1993; Viitanen et al. 1995). If rehabilitation is started before a significant deformity occurs, it is effective; but short-term supervised physiotherapy might also be effective regardless of disease duration (Hidding et al. 1993, Viitanen et al. 1995). Russell and colleagues (1993) observed that vigorous exercise—including warm-up exercises fol-

lowed by high-powered aerobics sessions, hydrotherapy, and floor exercises for an average of one and one-half hours per week—had the immediate postexercise effect of improving the range of motion. Yet the general trend in the following six months was for the range of flexion and lateral bend to *decrease* slowly. The presence or absence of exercise did not appear to affect the rate at which loss of range of motion occurred. These contradictory results might be explained by the numbers studied, patient selection, retrospective study design, the lack of adequate control subjects, or the poor reproducibility of some spine motion measurements (Roberts et al. 1988).

A four-month home exercise program combined with patient education was effective in the treatment of patients with AS (Kraag et al. 1990). Including education about the disease process and its physical management, this program aimed to decrease local as well as generalized pain, increase spinal mobility and function, improve pulmonary vital capacity, increase muscle strength and endurance, improve exercise compliance, and enhance psychosocial adjustment. Patients in the treatment group showed significant improvements in finger-to-floor distance and functional ability ($p < .001$), but not with regard to pain (100 mm visual analog scale) or lumbar flexion (Schober test). The benefits from the treatment program remained after eight months (Kraag et al. 1994).

Hidding and colleagues (1993) showed that nine months of supervised group physical therapy was superior to individualized therapy in improving thoracolumbar mobility and fitness, and significantly improved general health as perceived by the patients. Group therapy consisted of one-hour physical training to improve mobility of the spine and peripheral joints and to strengthen muscles of the trunk and legs, followed by one hour of sporting activities such as volley or badminton and one hour of hydrotherapy. A follow-up study noted sustained or improved global health and function in the treatment group, but slightly decreased spinal mobility in both treatment and control groups over the longer term (Hidding et al. 1994). It's possible that the group therapy patients' higher compliance with home exercises strengthened the beneficial effects of group therapy (or vice versa).

Fatigue and Endurance

Carbon et al. (1996) reported that aerobic exercise of 30 minutes' duration using cycle ergometry produced immediate increases in spinal flexibility and bilateral cervical tilt, and a reduction in pain; but these improvements steadily waned, and all had disappeared by three to five hours. Although the mechanism responsible for increasing spinal mobility has yet to be elucidated, an exercise-induced rise in plasma cortisol (which has anti-inflammatory properties) and β-endorphins (which have analgesic effects) might play a role. So, exercising those regions of the body unaffected by disease can elicit short-term beneficial effects above systemically mediated mechanisms.

Summary

Few of the studies were properly controlled or randomized; most were short-term and had small sample numbers; no one has addressed side effects such as spinal fractures; and a variety of anthropometric techniques were used as outcome measurements, such as Schober's test, modified Schober's test, chest expansion, Smythe test, finger-to-floor test, occiput-to-wall test, or neck rotation test. It is clear that no single measurement is thoroughly reliable or even undeniably valid. For example, Roberts et al. (1988) demonstrated that warm-up improved performance for patients and normal subjects in measures of finger-to-floor distance and cervical rotation, but not in the Schober's test or chest expansion measures.

Nevertheless, the overall clinical impression is that some exercise is beneficial for at least the symptoms of stiffness. In practice, we must adjust exercise programs to the stage of the disease and the patients' problems. In patients with advanced ankylosed spine or ankylosed osteoporotic spine, vigorous spinal exercise may cause spinal fractures and is unlikely to improve mobility significantly. Since patient compliance is the key to long-term success, it is important to incorporate exercise into routine activities. To enhance and reinforce proper posture, for example, patients may want to read in the prone position or sleep on a hard bed with a low pillow height. Recreational exercises such as swimming, volleyball, or badminton provide carryover of the exercise program. Group exercise therapy can socially reinforce continuing exercise, and is less costly than individual programs (Bakker et al. 1994).

Systemic Lupus Erythematosus

Systemic lupus erythematosus (SLE) is a multisystem autoimmune disease, characterized by excessive autoantibody production and immunologically mediated tissue injury. It can affect any organ in the body—including cardiac, pulmonary, neuropsychiatric, gastrointestinal, hematological, renal, and musculoskeletal involvement. Estimated to afflict 40 or 50 per 100,000 population, lupus is more prevalent in women (particularly in their reproductive years) and in African Americans. Advances in managing lupus with corticosteroid and immunosuppressive agents have improved survival and reduced morbidity. Improved survival makes rehabilitation important, but there are few studies on the efficacy of rehabilitation in management.

You should individualize exercise strategies for your lupus patients. In those with predominant arthralgias or arthritis, we recommend the rehabilitation techniques used in rheumatoid arthritis. Avoid loading involved joints in patients with avascular necrosis, who can make use of programs (e.g., aquatic exercises) that combine range-of-motion and isometric exercises that do not stress affected joints. Manage patients with muscle weakness caused by myositis or steroid-induced myopathy with the strategy for polymyositis/dermatomyositis (discussed later, page 248).

Fatigue or decreased endurance is particularly marked and common in SLE and is problematic in both active and inactive disease. Its pathophysiology is uncertain. In some cases it may be due to actual myositis, low aerobic exercise capacity (Viitanen et al. 1995), cardiopulmonary involvement, or depression. It is important to determine whether fatigue is a manifestation of active disease or the result of some other treatable factors such as anemia, depression, or myositis.

Lupus patients often complain of fatigue without any specific reasons. For those patients, aerobic exercise might be helpful. Ten patients in a study by Robb-Nicholson et al. (1989) improved their aerobic capacity by 19% after an eight-week supervised aerobic program including walking, bicycling, and jogging; the 10 controls improved only 8%. The changes correlated with decreased fatigue. Exercise did not exacerbate disease. Since such an intensive supervised program might not be practical, Daltroy et al. (1995) tested a minimally supervised home aerobic training program, observing smaller but statistically nonsignificant improvements in fitness, depression, fatigue and helplessness. Even though there is limited evidence concerning its efficacy, you certainly can prescribe aerobic exercise with no concern for patients' safety (see table 13.5). Future research should address how to improve compliance with aerobic training.

Polymyositis/ Dermatomyositis

Polymyositis and dermatomyositis (PM/DM) are rare idiopathic inflammatory disorders of the muscles. Proximal limb muscle weakness is characteristic and sometimes associated with neck and respiratory muscle weakness. Although PM/DM are primarily diseases of skeletal muscles, the skin, heart, lungs, gastrointestinal tract, or joints may be involved.

The goal of exercise for most patients is to maximize muscle strength. When synovitis occurs, joints may lose range of motion; exercise can help prevent contractures or improve range of motion. With ex-

Table 13.5		Exercise in SLE and PM/DM		
Author	**Subject (no.)**	**Study design**	**Intervention**	**Result**
Robb-Nicholson et al. 1989	23 SLE	RCT	Supervised 8 wk anaerobic exercise	Anaerobic capacity ($\dot{V}O_2$max) increased by 19% in contrast to 8% in controls
Daltroy et al. 1995	34 SLE	Randomized controlled 2 stage trial	1st stage: moderately supervised 3 mo aerobic exercise; 2nd stage: minimally supervised 3 mo aerobic exercise	Better, but not significantly in exercise tolerance test, fatigue, depression, and helplessness at 3 mo; unsupervised home exercise program may benefit few patients only
Escalante et al. 1993	5 PM	Alternate treatment design	Resistive exercise	Muscle strength improved without rise in muscle enzyme
Hicks et al. 1993	1 PM	Case report	4 wk supervised isometric exercise	Muscle strength improved without rise in muscle enzyme

treme ectopic calcification (most commonly seen in children), maintaining a functional range may be very difficult. Preserving range of motion is particularly important in children and in markedly weakened adults, who can develop contractures rapidly. In the acute, active phase, it is common practice to avoid strengthening exercises for fear of aggravating muscle inflammation. However, Hicks et al. (1993) showed that static exercise significantly increased strength without a significant postexercise creatinine phosphate kinase (CPK) rise in one patient with active, stable polymyositis. Furthermore, resisted exercise increased muscle strength without clinically significant rises in serum levels of muscle enzyme in five patients with active, stable polymyositis (Escalante et al. 1993). Data on exercise in patients with active disease are limited, and more research is sorely needed.

It is difficult to make any definitive statement at this time. You can prescribe active exercises in patients with active, stable disease, but you should closely monitor these patients for elevation in muscle enzymes or increased muscle pain. Be cautious in prescribing eccentric exercises, which are required for functional activities—in healthy individuals, eccentric exercises are associated with greater postexercise discomfort. The mechanism for this increased pain is unknown, but it may be related to mechanical stress. Patients with PM/DM may be at even greater risk of postexercise discomfort because of the inflammatory nature of their disease; they should begin an exercise program with fewer repetitions of eccentric exercises per set, increasing their effort gradually, as tolerated. Although there are no empirical data regarding the benefits of breathing exercises, we recommend them to strengthen respiratory muscles.

Systemic Sclerosis

Systemic sclerosis is a rare connective tissue disease characterized by fibrosis of the skin and potential involvement of the visceral organs such heart, lung, kidney, and gastrointestinal tract. There are no data regarding exercise in patients with scleroderma, and, therefore, exercise guidelines rely on anecdotal observations.

Contractures of the fingers in limited disease or in other joints with more extensive skin and tendon involvement are traditionally treated with range-of-motion exercise; yet its efficacy is unstudied. The same is true with strengthening programs in cases of muscle involvement. Therapy is usually futile with severe,

advanced muscle involvement, although it is often done for psychological reasons. Restrictive lung disease, interstitial fibrosis, and pulmonary hypertension may occur; they may be relatively asymptomatic, or may present with marked pulmonary involvement. In one study, working capacity—measured by cardiac and pulmonary function, joint mobility, and muscle strength—averaged 51% of the predicted normal value, and ventilation at maximal workload was high despite normal arterial blood gases and normal physiologic dead space (Blom-Bulow et al. 1983). It is possible that impeded mobility of respiratory and locomotive organs increases muscle metabolism, thereby increasing demand on ventilation.

Although clinicians often recommend aerobic training for patients with systemic sclerosis, there is no evidence regarding its usefulness or even whether it is safe or tolerated. The latter needs special attention, since in the aforementioned study one-third of exercising patients developed arrhythmias—supraventricular and ventricular extrasystoles in bigeminy and/or trigeminy, or showers of extrasystoles of multifocal origin (Blom-Bulow et al. 1993). These arrhythmias might result from myocardial fibrosis. Ventricular tachycardia plays an important role in sudden death.

Improving Patient Adherence

Doctors' attitudes and beliefs influence the way in which they present options to their patients; they also modify the dynamics of the conversation, directly affecting even whether or not rehabilitation programs are prescribed (Iversen 1996).

Research in the field of persuasion (Cialdini et al. 1993) indicates that exposure to others' opinions and beliefs strongly influences attitude change—especially when the messages are personally relevant and when delivered by experts (doctors in the case of clinical encounters), either through reinforcing the use of exercise or by communicating misgivings. In the United States, physicians and nurses have many opportunities to promote exercise among their patients. The greatest barrier to the success of such promotion is the providers' lack of confidence in their ability to promote change (Iverson et al. 1985).

Few studies have focused on arthritis patients' adherence to exercise prescriptions, but the impression is that compliance rates are fairly low, in the range of 35% to 60% (Bradley 1989; Deyo 1982; Stenstrom et al. 1997). In specific subgroups the compliance rates may be even lower. Factors associated with nonadherence in arthritis treatment include education, gender, and age; features of the disease (such as disease activity or severity); characteristics of the treatment source (hospital or clinic); and the quality of the doctor-patient interaction (Hicks 1985). For example, the more severe the patients' disease, the more likely they are to comply with the treatment regimen. However, more complex treatment regimens are associated with lower compliance rates. Demographic factors and characteristics of the treatment source (hospital-based versus clinic) explain only a small proportion of differences in compliance rates. Beliefs and attitudes, including patients' confidence in their ability to manage the disease, explain a fair amount of the differences seen in compliance with treatments (Gecht et al. 1996). For example, Stenstrom et al. (1997) have shown that high self-confidence and previous participation in exercise strongly predict exercise compliance at one year among patients with inflammatory rheumatic diseases.

Patient compliance strongly mediates functional outcomes. Carefully consider each patient's physical and psychosocial characteristics, as well as his or her own beliefs regarding the effectiveness of exercise, when designing a rehabilitation program (Iversen 1996). Iversen (1996) and Jensen and Lorish (1994) have demonstrated how patients' and providers' attitudes about the effectiveness of exercise in managing arthritis symptoms can affect the patients' intention to exercise as well as their subsequent exercise behavior. Godin (1987) has shown that the pleasantness or unpleasantness associated with exercise is a stronger determinant of intention to exercise than patients' perceptions of the effectiveness of the exercise. Always describe the positive attributes of your prescribed exercise program (e.g., warm-water exercises are soothing and relaxing), along with the benefits of exercise (e.g., enhanced mood, improved appearance, and increased functional mobility), in order to enhance adherence to it.

In chronic arthritides, exercise prescriptions are "exercises for life." Patients who are successful in adhering to an exercise regimen are those who have learned to modify their program to accommodate the specific features of their disease. In order to instruct patients properly, you must understand the role of the various types of exercise (dynamic versus static strength training; aerobic exercise; range-of-motion exercises), and when to prescribe each exercise. Then you must convey this information clearly and concisely to your patients in terms they can understand. A skillful communicator elicits patients' expectations of exercise, their perceived barriers to adhering to the prescription, and their confidence in performing the exercises appropriately. Using this information as a framework, you can collaborate with patients in setting goals.

The next step is to incorporate exercises into activities of daily living. For example, patients can perform postural exercises in front of the mirror either before or after a shower and range-of-motion exercises at the edge of the bed before going to sleep, to reduce early morning stiffness and discomfort.

Feedback enhances adherence to exercise programs. Providing target heart rates based on age-adjusted predicted heart rate values (ACSM 1995), or targeting particular levels of perceived exertion (Borg 1982), can be especially useful to ensure that patients achieve aerobic benefits from their exercise programs. Similarly, they can use a log of these results to track progress and exercise-induced symptoms. By encouraging patients to participate in recreational activities and linking them with community resources, you can increase their physical activity while also enhancing their psychological well-being. The National Arthritis Foundation has designed exercise programs specifically for patients with arthritis. These programs, such as PACE (People with Arthritis Can Exercise) are taught by certified instructors educated in the principles of exercise as they pertain to individuals with arthritis. Exercise videos are also available through the Arthritis Foundation as an adjunct or alternative to home exercises. For a summary of suggestions for helping patients stick with their exercise programs, see "Tips for Enhancing Patient Adherence to Exercise" (on next page).

The final step in enhancing compliance is to help patients identify significant others who will support their participation in exercise. Educating the partners along with the patients will reinforce patient learning and increase adherence to the program. This multifaceted approach in the design and implementation of an exercise regimen will enhance patient carryover and safety.

Summary

This chapter discusses the role of exercise therapy in several arthritic conditions, the pathology of each condition, the evidence supporting the use of various exercise modalities, and the strengths and limitations of these studies. Future research areas are suggested. We highlight the importance of prescribing the correct frequency, duration, intensity, and type

Tips for Enhancing Patient Adherence to Exercise

1. Elicit patient's beliefs and attitudes regarding the benefits of exercise and past experience with exercise.

2. Discuss patient's expectations of exercise.

3. Establish realistic goals. Small, incremental, attainable goals will encourage and promote long-term adherence.

4. Help patient identify and reduce barriers to exercise.

5. Promote the positive attributes of exercise.

6. Provide written instructions and have patient demonstrate exercises.

7. Provide intensity, frequency, and duration of each form of exercise, whether aerobic or strength training.

8. Teach patient to take a radial pulse and give patient an exercise range heart rate (e.g., 60% to 80% age-predicted heart rate).

9. Encourage use of an exercise diary or log.

10. Link patient to community resources (such as the Arthritis Foundation).

11. Incorporate recreational activities.

12. Identify a significant other to support patient's participation in exercise.

of exercise, and present techniques to enhance patient adherence to exercise regimens and to help health care providers develop goals of exercise therapy with their patients, based on the patients' disease, status, goals for rehabilitation, and preferences for treatment.

References

Aloia, J.F., S.H. Cohn, J.A. Ostuni, R. Cane, and K. Ellis. 1978. Prevention of involutional bone loss by exercise. *Ann Int Med* 89:356-358.

American College of Sports Medicine. 1995. *Guidelines for exercise testing and prescription*. Philadelphia: Lea & Febiger.

Åstrand, P.O., and K. Rodahl. 1986. *Textbook of work physiology: Physiological bases of exercises*. New York: McGraw-Hill.

Bakker, C., A. Hidding, S. van der Linden, and E. van Doorslaer. 1994. Cost effectiveness of group physical therapy compared to individualized therapy for ankylosing spondylitis. A randomized controlled trial. *J Rheumatol* 21:264-268.

Baslund, B., K. Lyngberg, V. Andersen, J. Halkjaer Kristensen, M. Hansen, M. Klokker, and B.K. Pedersen. 1993. Effect of 8 weeks of bicycle training on the immune system of patients with rheumatoid arthritis. *J Appl Physiol* 75:1691-1695.

Blom-Bulow, B., B. Jonson, and K. Bauer. 1983. Factors limiting exercise performance in progressive systemic sclerosis. *Semin Arthritis Rheum* 13:174-181.

Borg, G.A. 1982. Psychophysical bases of perceived exertion. *Med Sci Sports Exer* 14:377-381.

Bradley, L.A. 1989. Adherence with treatment regimens among adult rheumatoid arthritis patients: current status and future directions. *Arthritis Care Res* 2:S33-9.

Brighton, S.W., J.E. Lubbe, and C.A. van der Merwe. 1993. The effect of a long-term exercise programme on the rheumatoid hand. *Br J Rheumatol* 32:392-395.

Bulstrode, S.J., J. Barefoot, R.A. Harrison, and A.K. Clarke. 1987. The role of passive stretching in the treatment of ankylosing spondylitis. *Br J Rheumatol* 26:40-42.

Byers, P.H. 1985. Effect of exercise on morning stiffness and mobility in patients with rheumatoid arthritis. *Res Nurs Health* 8:275-281.

Carbon, R.J., M.G. Macey, D.A. McCarthy, F.P. Pereira, J.D. Perry, and A.J. Wade. 1996. The effect of 30 minute cycle ergometry on ankylosing spondylitis. *Br J Rheumatol* 35:167-177.

Cialdini, R.B. 1993. *Influence: The psychology of persuasion*, rev. ed. New York: Quill/Morrow.

Daltroy, L.H., C. Robb-Nicholson, M.D. Iversen, E.A. Wright, and M.H. Liang. 1995. Effectiveness of minimally supervised home aerobic training in patients with systemic rheumatic disease. *Br J Rheumatol* 34:1064-1069.

Decker, J.L. 1983. American Rheumatism Association nomenclature and classification of arthritis and rheumatism. *Arthritis Rheum* 26:1029-1032.

Dexter, P.A. 1992. Joint exercises in elderly persons with symptomatic osteoarthritis of the hip or knee. Performance patterns, medical support patterns, and the relationship between exercising and medical care. *Arthritis Care Res* 5:36-41.

Deyo, R.A. 1982. Compliance with therapeutic regimens in arthritis: issues, current status, and a future agenda. *Semin Arthritis Rheum* 12:233-244.

Ekblom, B., O. Lovgren, M. Alderin, M. Fridstrom, and G. Satterstrom. 1975. Effect of short-term physical training on patients with rheumatoid arthritis. A six-month follow-up study. *Scand J Rheumatol* 4:87-91.

Ekblom, B., O. Lovgren, M. Alderin, M. Fridstrom, and G. Satterstrom. 1975. Effect of short-term physical training on patients with rheumatoid arthritis I. *Scand J Rheumatol* 4:80-86.

Ekdahl, C., S.I. Andersson, U. Moritz, and B. Svensson. 1990. Dynamic versus static training in patients with rheumatoid arthritis. *Scand J Rheumatol* 19:17-26.

Ekdahl, C., R. Ekman, I. Petersson, and B. Svensson. 1994. Dynamic training and circulating neuropeptides in patients with rheumatoid arthritis: a comparative study with healthy subjects. *Int J Clin Pharmacol Res* 14:65-74.

Escalante, A., L. Miller, and T.D. Beardmore. 1993. Resistive exercise in the rehabilitation of polymyositis/dermatomyositis. *J Rheumatol* 20:1340-1344.

Ettinger, W.H. Jr., R. Burns, S.P. Messier, W. Applegate, W.J. Rejeski, T. Morgan, S. Shumaker, M.J. Berry, M. O'Toole, J. Monu, and T. Craven. 1997. A randomized trial comparing aerobic exercise and resistance exercise with a health education program in older adults with knee osteoarthritis. The Fitness Arthritis and Seniors Trial (FAST). *JAMA* 277:25-31.

Fisher, L.R., M.I. Cawley, and S.T. Holgate. 1990. Relation between chest expansion, pulmonary function, and exercise tolerance in patients with ankylosing spondylitis. *Ann Rheum Dis* 49:921-925.

+Fisher, N.M., D.R. Pendergast, G.E. Gresham, and E. Calkins. 1991. Muscle rehabilitation: its effect on muscular and functional performance of patients with knee osteoarthritis. *Arch Phys Med Rehabil* 72:367-374.

Garfinkel, M.S., H.R. Schumacher Jr., A. Husain, M. Levy, and R.A. Reshetar. 1994. Evaluation of a yoga based regimen for treatment of osteoarthritis of the hands. *J Rheumatol* 21:2341-2343.

Gecht, M.R., K.J. Connell, J.M. Sinacore, and T.R. Prochaska. 1996. A survey of exercise beliefs and exercise habits among people with arthritis. *Arthritis Care Res* 9:82-88.

Gerber, L.H. 1990. Exercise and arthritis. *Bull Rheum Dis* 39:1-9.

Gerber, L.H., and J.E. Hicks. 1990. Exercise in rheumatic disease. In *Therapeutic exercise,* ed. J.V. Basmajian and S.L. Wolf. Baltimore: Williams & Wilkins.

Godin, G. 1987. Importance of the emotional aspect of attitude to predict intention. *Psychol Reports* 61:719-723.

Gran, J.T., and G. Husby. 1990. Ankylosing Spondylitis in women. *Semin Arthritis Rheum* 19:303-312.

Gran, J.T., and G. Husby. 1993. The epidemiology of ankylosing spondylitis. *Semin Arthritis Rheum* 22:319-334.

+ Green, J., F. McKenna, E.J. Redfern, and M.A. Chamberlain. 1993. Home exercises are as effective as outpatient hydrotherapy for osteoarthritis of the hip. *Br J Rheumatol* 32:812-815.

Hakkinen, A., K. Hakkinen, and P. Hannonen. 1994. Effects of strength training on neuromuscular function and disease activity in patients with recent-onset inflammatory arthritis. *Scand J Rheumatol* 23:237-242.

Hall, J., S.M. Skevington, P.J. Maddison, and K. Chapman. 1996. A randomized and controlled trial of hydrotherapy in rheumatoid arthritis. *Arthritis Care Res* 9:206-215.

Hansen, T.M., G. Hansen, A.M. Langgaard, and J.O. Rasmussen. 1993. Long-term physical training in rheumatoid arthritis.

A randomized trial with different training programs and blinded observers. *Scand J Rheumatol* 22:107-112.

Harkcom, T.M., R.M. Lampman, B.F. Banwell, and C.W. Castor. 1985. Therapeutic value of graded aerobic exercise training in rheumatoid arthritis. *Arthritis Rheum* 28:32-39.

Harris, E.D. Jr. 1990. Rheumatoid arthritis. Pathophysiology and implications for therapy [published erratum appears in *New Engl J Med* 1990 Oct 4; 323(14):996]. *New Engl J Med* 322:1277-1289.

Hayes, K.W. 1996. Heat and cold in the management of rheumatoid arthritis. In *Rehabilitation of persons with rheumatoid arthritis,* ed. R.W. Chang. Gaithersburg, Maryland: Aspen Publishers.

Hicks, J.E. 1985. Compliance: a major factor in the successful treatment of rheumatic disease. *Compr Ther* 11:31-37.

Hicks, J.E. 1994. Exercise in rheumatoid arthritis. *Phys Med Rehabil Clin of N Am* 5:701-727.

Hicks, J.E., F. Miller, P. Plotz, T.H. Chen, and L. Gerber. 1993. Isometric exercise increases strength and does not produce sustained creatinine phosphokinase increases in a patient with polymyositis. *J Rheumatol* 20:1399-1401.

Hidding, A., and S. van der Linden. 1995. Factors related to change in global health after group physical therapy in ankylosing spondylitis. *Clin Rheumatol* 14:347-351.

Hidding, A., S. van der Linden, M. Boers, X. Gielen, L. de Witte, A. Kester, B. Dijkmans, and D. Moolenburgh. 1993. Is group physical therapy superior to individualized therapy in ankylosing spondylitis? A randomized controlled trial. *Arthritis Care Res* 6:117-125.

Hidding, A., S. van der Linden, and L. de Witte. 1993. Therapeutic effects of individual physical therapy in ankylosing spondylitis related to duration of disease. *Clin Rheumatol* 12:334-340.

Hidding, A., S. van der Linden, X. Gielen, L. de Witte, B. Dijkmans, and D. Moolenburgh. 1994. Continuation of group physical therapy is necessary in ankylosing spondylitis: results of a randomized controlled trial. *Arthritis Care Res* 7:90-96.

Iversen, M.D. 1996. The influence of expectations and attitudes on doctor-patient communication and health outcomes in arthritis. PhD diss., Harvard School of Public Health.

Iverson, D.C., J.E. Fielding, R.S. Crow, and G.M. Christenson. 1985. The promotion of physical activity in the United States population: the status of programs in medical, worksite, community, and school settings. *Public Health Rep* 100:212-224.

Jensen, G.M., and C.D. Lorish. 1994. Promoting patient cooperation with exercise programs: linking research, theory, and practice. *Arthritis Care Res* 7:181-189.

Kovar, P.A., J.P. Allegrante, C.R. MacKenzie, M.G. Peterson, B. Gutin, and M.E. Charlson. 1992. Supervised fitness walking in patients with osteoarthritis of the knee. A randomized, controlled trial. *Ann Int Med* 116:529-534.

Kraag, G., B. Stokes, J. Groh, A. Helewa, and C. Goldsmith. 1990. The effects of comprehensive home physiotherapy and supervision on patients with ankylosing spondylitis—a randomized controlled trial. *J Rheumatol* 17:228-233.

Kraag, G., B. Stokes, J. Groh, A. Helewa, and C. Goldsmith. 1994. The effects of comprehensive home physiotherapy and supervision on patients with ankylosing spondylitis—an 8-month follow-up. *J Rheumatol* 21:261-263.

Lawrence, R.C., M.C. Hochberg, J.L. Kelsey, F.C. McDuffie, T.A. Medsger Jr., W.R. Felts, and L.E. Shulman. 1989. Estimates of the prevalence of selected arthritic and musculoskeletal diseases in the United States. *J Rheumatol* 16:427-441.

Leivseth, G., J. Torstensson, and O. Reikeras. 1989. Effect of passive muscle stretching in osteoarthritis of the hip. *Clin Sci* 76:113-117.

Lyngberg, K., B. Danneskiold-Samsoe, and O. Halskov. 1988. The effect of physical training on patients with rheumatoid arthritis: changes in disease activity, muscle strength and aerobic capacity. A clinically controlled minimized cross-over study. *Clin Exp Rheumatol* 6:253-260.

Lyngberg, K.K., B.U. Ramsing, A. Nawrocki, M. Harreby, and B. Danneskiold-Samsoe. 1994. Safe and effective isokinetic knee extension training in rheumatoid arthritis. *Arthritis Rheum* 37:623-628.

Machover, S., and A.J. Sapecky. 1966. Effect of isometric exercise on the quadriceps muscle in patients with rheumatoid arthritis. *Arch Phys Med Rehabil* 47:737-741.

Minor, M.A., J.E. Hewett, R.R. Webel, S.K. Anderson, and D.R. Kay. 1989. Efficacy of physical conditioning exercise in patients with rheumatoid arthritis and osteoarthritis. *Arthritis Rheum* 32:1396-1405.

Nordesjo, L., B. Nordgren, and A. Wigirew. 1983. Isometric strength and endurance in patients with severe rheumatoid arthritis or osteoarthritis in the knee joints. *Scand J Rheumatol* 12:152-156.

O'Driscoll, S.L., M.I. Jayson, and H. Baddeley. 1978. Neck movements in ankylosing spondylitis and their responses to physiotherapy. *Ann Rheum Dis* 37:64-66.

Perlman, S.G., K.J. Connell, A. Clark, M.S. Robinson, P. Conlon, M. Gecht, P. Caldron, and J.M. Sinacore. 1990. Dance-based aerobic exercise for rheumatoid arthritis. *Arthritis Care Res* 3:29-35.

Philbin, E.F., G.D. Groff, M.D. Ries, and T.E. Miller. 1995. Cardiovascular fitness and health in patients with end-stage osteoarthritis. *Arthritis Rheum* 38:799-805.

Rall, L.C., S.N. Meydani, J.J. Kehayias, B. Dawson-Hughes, and R. Roubenoff. 1996. The effect of progressive resistance training in rheumatoid arthritis. Increased strength without changes in energy balance or body composition. *Arthritis Rheum* 39:415-426.

Rejeski, W.J., L.R. Brawley, W. Ettinger, T. Morgan, and C. Thompson. 1997. Compliance to exercise therapy in older participants with knee osteoarthritis: implications for treating disability. *Med Sci Sports Exer* 29:977-985.

Robb-Nicholson, C., L.H. Daltroy, H. Eaton, V. Gall, E. Wright, L.H. Hartley, P.H. Schur, and M.H. Liang. 1989. Effects of aerobic conditioning in lupus fatigue: a pilot study. *Br J Rheumatol* 28:500-505.

Roberts, W.N., M.H. Liang, L.M. Pallozzi, and L.H. Daltroy. 1988. Effects of warming up on reliability of anthropometric techniques in ankylosing spondylitis. *Arthritis Rheum* 31:549-552.

Russell, P., A. Unsworth, and I. Haslock. 1993. The effect of exercise on ankylosing spondylitis—a preliminary study. *Br J Rheumatol* 32:498-506.

Semble, E.L. 1995. Rheumatoid arthritis: new approaches for its evaluation and management. *Arch Phys Med Rehabil* 76:190-201.

Semble, E.L., R.F. Loeser, and C.M. Wise. 1990. Therapeutic exercise for rheumatoid arthritis and osteoarthritis. *Semin Arthritis Rheum* 20:32-40.

Slemenda, C., K.D. Brandt, D.K. Heilman, S. Mazzuca, E.M. Braunstein, B.P. Katz, and F.D. Wolinsky. 1997. Quadriceps weakness and osteoarthritis of the knee. *Ann Int Med* 127:97-104.

Smedstad, L.V., and M.H. Liang. 1997. Psychosocial management of rheumatic diseases. In *Textbook of rheumatology*, ed. W.N. Kelley, T. Harris, S. Ruddy, and C.B. Sledge. Philadelphia: W.B. Saunders.

Stenstrom, C.H. 1994. Therapeutic exercise in rheumatoid arthritis. *Arthritis Care Res* 7:190-197.

Stenstrom, C.H., B. Arge, and A. Sundbom. 1996. Dynamic training versus relaxation training as home exercise for patients with inflammatory rheumatic diseases. A randomized controlled study. *Scand J Rheumatol* 25:28-33.

Stenstrom, C.H., B. Arge, and A. Sundbom. 1997. Home exercise and compliance in inflammatory rheumatic diseases—a prospective clinical trial. *J Rheumatol* 24:470-476.

Swezey, R.L. 1974. Essentials of physical management and rehabilitation in arthritis. *Semin Arthritis Rheum* 3:349-368.

van den Ende, C.H., J.M. Hazes, S. le Cessie, W.J. Mulder, D.G. Belfor, F.C. Breedveld, and B.A. Dijkmans. 1996. Comparison of high and low intensity training in well controlled rheumatoid arthritis. Results of a randomised clinical trial. *Ann Rheum Dis* 55:798-805.

Viitanen, J.V., K. Lehtinen, J. Suni, and H. Kautiainen. 1995. Fifteen months' follow-up of intensive inpatient physiotherapy and exercise in ankylosing spondylitis. *Clin Rheumatol* 14:413-419.

Viitanen, J.V., J. Suni, H. Kautiainen, M. Liimatainen, and H. Takala. 1992. Effect of physiotherapy on spinal mobility in ankylosing spondylitis. *Scand J Rheumatol* 21:38-41.

Warren, C.G., J.F. Lehmann, and J.N. Koblanski. 1976. Heat and stretch procedures: an evaluation using rat tail tendon. *Arch Phys Med Rehabil* 57:122-126.

Wessel, J., and H.A. Quinney. 1984. Pain experienced by persons with rheumatoid arthritis during isometric and isokinetic exercise. *Physiotherapy Canada* 36:131-134.

Chapter 14

Neuromuscular Disease

David D. Kilmer, MD, and Susan Aitkens, MS

Case Study

A 44-year-old woman with hereditary motor and sensory neuropathy, type I (HMSN), came to us for rehabilitation. She was independent functionally in self-care, but reported difficulty with fine motor tasks. Distal weakness in the lower extremities led her to use ankle-foot orthoses in community ambulation, but she noted increasing fatigue as she walked longer distances. Although she used to enjoy walking and gardening, she now spent most of her day sedentary at home.

We carefully assessed her interests and motivations, and her reasons for not exercising, and formulated realistic goals for an exercise prescription. She probably had a component of disuse weakness due to lack of activity, and worked at a higher percentage of her maximal capacity during routine physical activities. An exercise program to build her muscular endurance was the primary focus—so we initially prescribed a 15-minute walking program three days a week, at an intensity requiring fairly hard breathing but maintaining the ability to carry on a conversation. We also encouraged her to garden or perform other enjoyable recreational activity on alternate days, working toward a goal of some physical exertion each day; but we cautioned her to stop exercising if she noted any increased muscle weakness or pain. Initially testing her lower extremity strength with a hand-held dynamometer in the clinic, we scheduled subsequent tests at one-month intervals to reassure both the patient and ourselves of her progress and to motivate her to continue the program.

At the three month follow-up, the patient reported that she was able to walk 45 minutes without stopping, and had increased energy to enjoy her garden. She still had to be careful not to perform continuous physical activity for more than one hour, lest she endure excessive soreness and fatigue the following day. Objective strength testing using hand-held dynamometry showed no significant improvement or decrement of isometric force.

Despite advancing knowledge regarding the beneficial effects of habitual physical exercise in the able-bodied population over the last several decades, the role of exercise in the rehabilitation of diseases of the peripheral nervous system remains unclear. The term **neuromuscular diseases (NMDs)** encompasses disorders of the anterior horn cell, peripheral nerve, neuromuscular junction, and skeletal muscle. Each specific disease may respond differently to exercise. However, researchers commonly group NMDs together due to their relative rarity and common clinical issues: progressive muscular weakness, fatigability, and disability. Until recently, clinicians have understood few of the specific structural or biochemical abnormalities distinguishing many conditions, with diseases diagnosed primarily by common clinical characteristics.

This situation is changing. There is now a high level of scientific interest in the molecular basis for a number of diseases of the peripheral nervous system. The ultimate goal is to determine the genes and gene products responsible for normal and abnormal functioning of the motor unit. However, it will be clear from this chapter that we still know little about how diseased muscle responds to physical activity. The basic principles of an adaptive response to muscle overload may not be valid in neuromuscular conditions, and in fact certain types of exercise could be detrimental. This chapter reviews current understanding of the effects of exercise in neuromuscular disease, discusses etiologies for the decline in neuromuscular function in these disorders, and makes reasonable exercise recommendations based upon the limited scientific research available.

Physiologic and Functional Consequences of Neuromuscular Diseases

This discussion highlights diseases at each anatomic level of the peripheral nervous system leading to progressive impairment, disability, and compromised exercise performance. The primary focus is on hereditary diseases, since few exercise studies exist in acquired diseases such as polymyositis and Guillain-Barré syndrome. It should be evident that motor weakness is the common thread linking each disorder.

Anterior Horn Cell

Amyotrophic lateral sclerosis (ALS) results in degeneration of bulbar and spinal motor neurons, causing progressive, usually rapid, loss of strength both in the limbs and bulbar musculature. It is known to affect maximal oxygen uptake and work capacity early in the disease, possibly due to functional skeletal muscle loss as well as deconditioning (Sanjak et al. 1987). ALS subjects may also have a higher oxygen cost for a given level of submaximal work (Sanjak et al. 1987). Spasticity and other causes of biomechanical inefficiency are important contributing factors.

Recent work suggests abnormal muscle fatigability in ALS patients, possibly due to an abnormality distal to the muscle membrane (Sharma et al. 1995; Sharma and Miller 1996). The implications of these findings for exercise performance and rehabilitation are not known.

Other causes of anterior horn cell dysfunction include primarily autosomal recessive **spinal muscular atrophies (SMA)** of childhood and adult onset, resulting in gradual loss of lower motor neuron function. In general, an earlier onset of weakness implies more severe disability, with a higher likelihood of contractures, progressive scoliosis, and restrictive lung disease (Carter et al. 1995a). An exercise program may be appropriate for persons with the later onset forms.

Peripheral Nerve

The most common hereditary neuropathy leading to disability is **hereditary motor and sensory neuropathy, type I (HMSN, or Charcot-Marie-Tooth Disease)**. The majority of cases are associated with duplication of a gene locus on chromosome 17 involved in peripheral nerve myelination (Murakami et al. 1996). The primary pathology of this autosomal dominant disorder is uniform demyelination of peripheral nerve progressing to axonal degeneration, manifested by weakness and sensory loss primarily in the feet and hands. However, systematic studies demonstrate significant deficits in proximal muscle strength as well, even in mildly affected subjects (Carter et al. 1995b; Lindeman et al. 1994). These deficits correspond with a reduction in functional abilities (Lindeman et al. 1994). It is unclear whether the proximal weakness is a direct result of the neuropathy, or is related to disuse.

A closely related hereditary disease of the peripheral nerve, termed **hereditary motor and sensory neuropathy, type II**, involves axonal degeneration as the primary pathology rather than demyelination as in type I. There seems to be less proximal muscular involvement with this disease, with less overall disability. It is not known if exercise responses differ between the forms of hereditary neuropathy.

Neuromuscular Junction

The most common neuromuscular junction disorder is **myasthenia gravis (MG)**, caused by antibodies directed against acetylcholine receptors. Characteristic symptoms include fluctuating weakness exacerbated by physical exertion. Unlike other NMDs considered here, MG may be treatable with anticholinesterase and cytotoxic medications, although in generalized MG there may be persistent muscle weakness. Aerobic and strength characterization studies have not been performed in MG.

Muscle

The muscular dystrophies comprise a heterogeneous group of hereditary diseases exhibiting progressive loss of muscle fibers, resulting in weakness first usually noted in proximal musculature. The most common dystrophy is **Duchenne muscular dystrophy (DMD)**, an X-linked, recessive, rapidly progressive disease of boys causing gait difficulty during childhood, wheelchair dependence in late childhood or early adolescence, and death by the early third decade. **Becker's muscular dystrophy (BMD)** follows a similar pattern of weakness and shares X-linked inheritance, but typically has a later onset and a much slower rate of progression.

The protein **dystrophin**, which is deficient in DMD, is closely associated with the cell membrane (Bonilla et al. 1988; Hoffman et al. 1987). Although its exact function is not known, dystrophin is probably important in maintaining the cytoskeletal framework of the muscle cell during active muscle contraction (Ervasti and Campbell 1993). When dystrophin is absent (as in DMD), or decreased or altered (as in BMD), the muscle fiber may be predisposed to damage with normal activities. More recently, the dystrophin-associated glycoproteins or other membrane constituents have been found to be abnormal or absent in subtypes of **limb-girdle muscular dystrophy syndromes (LGS)**, possibly causing disorders of skeletal muscle similar to but less severe than those seen in DMD (Brown 1997). Whether other muscular dystrophies or neuropathic disorders have structural muscle cell membrane defects is not yet known. Although the genetic defect in **myotonic muscular dystrophy (MMD)** is known to involve the presence of CTG codon repeating sequences on chromosome 19, the ramifications of this abnormality at the muscle cellular level are not yet clear (Brook et al. 1992). Table 14.1 lists the major muscular dystrophies and current knowledge about the deficient or abnormal proteins.

With knowledge of muscle cell membrane abnormalities in at least some dystrophies, it seems plausible that activities stressing the muscle fiber, such as physical exertion, might be detrimental for persons with these disorders. Indeed, intense physical exercise results in marked release of creatine kinase in a number of myopathies, implying muscle membrane damage. The lack of dystrophin may weaken the sarcolemma, making muscles more susceptible to injury (Moens et al. 1993; Petrof et al. 1993; Weller et al. 1990). As we gain further knowledge about the function of these cellular proteins, researchers may be able to design scientifically based protocols, using different types of exercise interventions, to determine beneficial and detrimental effects of physical activity on the muscle fiber.

Subjects with DMD and other dystrophies have reduced maximal oxygen uptake during exercise, probably due to loss of functional muscle mass rather than a defect in muscle energy metabolism (Haller et al. 1983; Haller and Lewis 1984; Sockolov et al. 1977). In fact, there is some evidence for an inverse relationship between leg weakness and maximal oxygen uptake (Carroll et al. 1979). However, since muscle strength and endurance may affect daily physical abilities more than cardiorespiratory limitations in NMD, improving maximal oxygen uptake is of limited value (Bar-Or 1996). Progressive loss of muscle fibers with motor weakness is the hallmark of the dystrophies. The primary goals of intervention should be to maintain or reverse loss of strength and function.

Causes of Reduced Neuromuscular Function in NMD

Progressive muscle weakness from the disease is only one cause of the disability resulting from disorders of the peripheral nervous system. In fact, disability may be out of proportion to the severity of muscle involvement. Other factors often play an important role in defining the extent of one's disability, and these components may be primarily amenable to an exercise program.

Muscle Disuse

Disuse of muscle fibers results in reduced myofibril size, decreased fiber cross-sectional area, lower force production, and reduced muscle endurance

Table 14.1   Classification of the Major Muscular Dystrophies

Dystrophies with exercise-training investigations

Dystrophy	Inheritance	Responsible chromosome	Altered gene product
Duchenne (DMD)	Sex-linked recessive	X	Dystrophin (absent)
Becker's (BMD)	Sex-linked recessive	X	Dystrophin (partial/abnormal)
Myotonic (MMD)	Autosomal dominant	19	Myotonin protein kinase
Facioscapulohumeral (FSH)	Autosomal dominant	4	–
Limb-girdle 1A/1C (LGS)	Autosomal dominant	5 (1A), 1 (1B), 3 (1C)	–
Limb-girdle 2A/2G (LGS)	Autosomal recessive	Various	Various sarcoglycans

Selected dystrophies without exercise-training investigations

Dystrophy	Inheritance	Responsible chromosome	Altered gene product
Emery-Dreifuss	Sex-linked recessive	X	Emerin
Classic merosin-positive congenital muscular dystrophy (CMD)	Autosomal recessive	–	–
Classic merosin-negative CMD	Autosomal recessive	6	Merosin
Fukuyama CMD	Autosomal recessive	9	–
Walker-Warburg Syndrome CMD	Autosomal recessive	9	–
Scapuloperoneal	Autosomal dominant	14	–
Autosomal dominant distal myopathy	Autosomal dominant	12	–
Autosomal recessive distal myopathy	Autosomal recessive	2	–
Oculopharyngeal	Autosomal dominant	14	–

(Appel 1990). Although there is no direct evidence linking muscle disuse with disability in persons with NMD, clinical experience as well as limited studies examining aerobic fitness suggest that persons with neuromuscular disorders are sedentary and poorly conditioned (McCrory et al. 1998; Wright et al. 1996). Likely explanations include poor physical fit-

ness skills learned during childhood and adolescence, social isolation, concern from health care professionals and physical educators about the potential harm from exercise, and lack of available adapted programs (Kilmer and McDonald 1995). Further evidence comes from the frequent clinical observation that short periods of bed rest, particularly in rapidly progressive disorders such as DMD, result in significant loss of strength and function that may not be reversible (Vignos 1983).

It seems clear that muscle disuse usually contributes to the muscular weakness, easy fatigability, and poor endurance seen with NMD. In the nonmetabolic myopathies and neuropathic syndromes, there appear to be no primary defects in muscle oxidative transport or phosphorylation. However, muscle adapts to imposed stresses, likely resulting in low concentrations of important enzymes in these pathways. Diseased muscle may therefore respond in a similar fashion as intact muscle to progressive overload during aerobic training.

The biomechanical disadvantage in persons with NMD, due to weakness and/or sensory loss, leads to inefficient performance of physical tasks. For example, weakness in the prime movers of a joint forces the musculature to work at a higher percentage of maximal capacity, leading to fatigue (Dolmage and Cafarelli 1991). Recruitment of secondary, less efficient muscles further increases the energy expended to perform a task, fatiguing muscle more rapidly (figure 14.1). It is not surprising that patients complain of poor work capacity, fatigue, and muscle soreness when they attempt physical tasks. This phenomenon is noted in the post-polio population with residual muscle weakness (Borg et al. 1988; Perry et al. 1988). These people often adopt sedentary, inactive lifestyles, increasing the spiral of disability. A key question for researchers and clinicians is the relative contribution of disuse in an individual patient's disability, and potential for reversal without damaging the muscle.

Muscle Overuse and Eccentric Contractions

NMD patients often say they "pay the price" for physical exertion, reporting residual muscle soreness and fatigue for several days following exercise. Clinicians have long been concerned about potential damaging effects of vigorous exercise (commonly called **overwork weakness**) in NMD patients. This concern is pervasive, despite lack of evidence from systematic studies in NMD subjects showing deleterious effects of exercise. Evidence for overwork weakness is only anecdotal, known from a series of case reports.

An influential case series in the 1950s reported signs of overwork weakness in poliomyelitis patients during both supervised submaximal resistance exercise and unsupervised community activities (Bennett and Knowlton 1958). In a pathologic study of a person with DMD, the greatest degeneration occurred

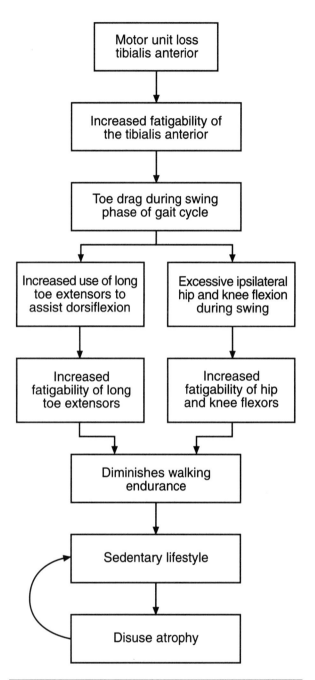

Figure 14.1 An example of the cascade of dysfunction that may occur with weakness in the prime mover of a joint, in this case the tibialis anterior.
Adapted, by permission, from D.D. Kilmer, 1996, Functional anatomy of skeletal muscle. In *Physical Medicine and Rehabilitation and State of the Art Reviews* 10:3, edited by K. Shankar (Philadelphia: Hanley & Belfus), 413-426.

in muscles undergoing sustained physical activity, suggesting the possibility of overwork weakness (Bonsett 1963). Additional circumstantial evidence exists in a report of persons with **facioscapulohumeral dystrophy (FSH)**, demonstrating greater weakness in the dominant limb subjected to heavy loads during work or involved in unsupervised weight lifting (Johnson and Braddom 1971). However, a natural history profile reports frequent asymmetric upper extremity weakness in FSH (Kilmer et al. 1995).

Recent work involving experimental models of muscle overuse in able-bodied subjects may have relevance for the NMD population. It is well established that a bout of maximal **eccentric (lengthening) contractions** causes damage to muscle fibers and results in transient muscle weakness over a period of weeks (Clarkson et al. 1992; Friden and Lieber 1992). This weakness is associated with delayed muscle soreness, changes in resting joint angle, and elevations of creatine kinase. There appears to be high strain on individual fibers rather than equal transmittal of load through the entire muscle, possibly disrupting the cytoskeletal framework with myofibrillar damage (Friden and Lieber 1992; Lieber and Friden 1993; Lieber et al. 1996). The actual muscle fiber damage may result from calcium influx through the disrupted sarcolemma, stimulating protease and phospholipase activity within the muscle cell (Armstrong et al. 1991). However, an adaptive response seems to occur, and a repeated bout within several months causes less damage (Clarkson et al. 1992). It is not known if this adaptive response occurs in diseased skeletal muscle or whether damage is cumulative.

In the primary animal model of DMD, the mdx mouse, there is a similar lack of dystrophin but with a milder phenotypic expression of weakness and muscle necrosis (Cooper 1989). Several studies demonstrate that muscles from mdx mice sustain greater injury than those from control mice after eccentric exercise, resulting in higher levels of intracellular calcium and potential muscle necrosis (Franco and Lansman 1990; Stedman et al. 1991; Turner et al. 1991). Jacobs and colleagues (1996) mechanically induced muscle damage in prednisone-treated mice, which sustained less damage than controls. The authors suggest that prednisone protects against mechanically induced damage, possibly by stabilizing the muscle cell membrane. Prednisone is known to help slow the rate of progression in human DMD (Fenichel et al. 1991).

There may be similarities between models of muscle overuse from eccentric muscle contractions and weakness in diseases of the muscle fiber cytoskeletal framework. Indeed, Edwards et al. (1984) proposed that submaximal eccentric contractions, so important in postural muscles during routine activities, may damage diseased muscle over time. This hypothesis is attractive in light of recent findings that, in a number of dystrophies, abnormalities in sar-

colemmal structural proteins may increase susceptibility to mechanical damage from routine eccentric contractions. Myopathic patients complaining of soreness and weakness on the day after unusual exertion may be manifesting the untoward effects of eccentric muscle contractions. Dystrophic muscle may not repair itself sufficiently to return strength to a baseline level.

The only way to avoid eccentric contractions in daily life would be to live in a gravity-free environment. However, there is now at least a theoretical rationale to design exercise programs minimizing this type of muscular contraction, made particularly feasible by use of isokinetic dynamometers. In a study of patients with post-polio muscular atrophy, a training technique involving primarily concentric contractions showed beneficial strengthening results with no serological or histological evidence of muscular damage (Spector et al. 1996).

Cardiopulmonary Involvement

When it directly affects the cardiopulmonary system, NMD compromises exercise performance—as certainly occurs in some neuromuscular disorders, particularly DMD (McDonald et al. 1995b), BMD (McDonald et al. 1995a), and MMD (Johnson et al. 1995). In DMD, cardiomyopathy becomes a clinical concern during the adolescent years, along with restrictive lung disease from weakness of the respiratory musculature. At this stage, however, profound extremity and truncal weakness already severely limit exercise capacity. Even during earlier stages of the disease, Sockolov et al. (1977) observed reduced maximal work rate and endurance along with reductions in stroke volume, cardiac output, and peripheral oxygen utilization.

In the slowly progressive disorders, BMD may exhibit disproportionately severe cardiomyopathy as compared with skeletal myopathy (McDonald et al. 1995a), and MMD presents well-described cardiac conduction defects (Johnson et al. 1995)—but the extent to which either problem limits exercise performance is not known.

In most other NMDs, deconditioning likely plays a more prominent role in reduced stroke volume and cardiac output than intrinsic cardiac malfunction. While Carroll et al. (1979) demonstrated a wide range of exercise capacities among subjects with various NMDs, there were generally reductions in maximal oxygen uptake. Haller et al. (1983) noted similar ratios between NMD subjects and controls for cardiac output and systemic O_2 difference from rest to maximal exercise, implying normal cardiac function.

Body Weight

That many persons with NMD are overweight, with increased adiposity compared to similar-aged controls (McCrory et al. 1998), probably results from a sedentary lifestyle, poor nutritional choices, and reduced income. Important ramifications of this problem include

- increased muscular demand for movement, causing the muscle to work at a higher percentage of its maximal capacity;
- accentuated biomechanical inefficiencies due to altered body habitus; and
- increased atherosclerotic risk factors for ischemic cardiac disease.

Reversing this tendency to become overweight may lead to improved function.

Contractures

A comprehensive review of hereditary NMDs found that, with the exception of DMD, joint contractures were not a significant functional problem until people were forced to rely on wheelchairs (McDonald et al. 1995b). This is not surprising, since contractures are generally a consequence of muscle imbalances, chronic postural adjustments to maintain the ability to stand and take steps, and habitual wheelchair use, leading to more significant weakness and limited exercise capacity (Vignos 1983). In DMD, progression of contractures in the heelcords, hip flexors, and iliotibial bands may allow continued upright standing at the cost of reduced muscle endurance and increased work during ambulation. In other NMDs, contractures do not limit exercise performance until late in the disease.

Effects of Resistance (Strengthening) Exercise in NMD

The first controlled study of strengthening exercise used a high-resistance regimen in 24 rapidly and slowly progressive NMD patients over a one-year period, reporting strength improvement throughout the first four months of exercise with a subsequent plateau in strength (Vignos and Watkins 1966). The authors determined that, since the degree of improvement was related to the initial strength of the exercised muscle, exercise programs should begin early in the course of disease (see table 14.2).

Milner-Brown and Miller (1988) had 16 patients with gradually progressive NMD (6 FSH, 4 MMD, 3 SMA, 1 BMD, 1 LGS, and 1 idiopathic polyneuropathy) perform elbow curls using dumbbells, and knee extensions using ankle weights. They initially used weights that could be lifted a maximum of 12-15 times, and completed one set on alternate days—gradually increasing the number of sets, training days, and weight over time to model a high-resistance weight training program. While most patients demonstrated strength gains, those with severely weak muscles (<10% normal strength) generally did not improve. The authors concluded that NMD patients should initiate weight training at the onset of muscle weakness, as the training provides no benefit once muscles have become severely weak.

McCartney et al. (1988) trained 5 subjects with NMD (3 spinal muscular atrophy, 1 LGS, 1 FSH) over a nine-week period, three times per week. The progressive weight training program was based on initial one-repetition maximums (1 RM) for single arm curl and double leg press; the contralateral limb served as control for the arm exercise. By the end of the study, the strength of the trained arms had increased between 19% and 34%, while the strength of the untrained arms had changed between −14% and +25%, demonstrating cross-training effects in some cases. Leg strength increased from 11% to 50%. Muscular endurance also improved considerably. By the end of the training period, the pretraining 1 RM could be lifted from 3 to 48 times in the trained limbs, and from 1 to 13 times in the untrained limbs. The authors concluded that strength training may be useful in managing selected NMDs.

Aitkens and colleagues (1993) studied moderate resistance exercise in 14 control and 27 slowly progressive NMD subjects over a 12-week period, three days per week. They prescribed submaximal exercise, using ankle and wrist weights and a handgrip exerciser (table 14.3). Both groups demonstrated significant increases in most strength measures. Since the strength gains did not significantly differ between the exercised and nonexercised limbs in either group, a cross-training effect was apparent.

Table 14.2   Summary of Strength Training Studies in NMD

Author	Study population and sample size	Duration of training	Training modality	Training protocol	Response(s)
Vignos and Watkins 1966	Various NMD (24)	12 months	Weight training (multiple muscle groups)	Unspecified, but based on 10-repetition maximum (RM)	Strength increased; % increase correlated with initial strength
Milner-Brown and Miller 1988	Various NMD (12)	>12 months (variable)	Weight training (elbow flexion and knee extension)	Initially 1 set of 10 reps based on 15 RM performed on alternate days; gradually increased to a maximum of 5 sets 4 days per wk; protocol individualized	Strength increased significantly when the initial degree of strength loss was not severe (<10%)
McCartney et al. 1988	Various NMD (5)	9 wks	Weight training (arm curl and leg press)	3 days per wk; initially 2 sets of 10-12 reps at 40% max; gradually progressed to 3 sets of 10-12 reps (1 set at 50%, 60%, and 70% max); contralateral arm control	Strength and muscular endurance increased; considerable inter-subject variability Cross-training effect in nonexercised limb
Aitkens et al. 1993	Slowly progressive NMD (27) and able-bodied controls (14)	12 wks	Weight training (elbow flexion, knee extension, grip)	See table 14.3	Significant improvement in most strength measures (not grip) in both groups; cross-training effect
Kilmer et al. 1994	Slowly progressive NMD (10) and able-bodied controls (6)	12 wks	Weight training (elbow flexion, knee extension)	See table 14.4	Results mixed; some increase in leg strength coupled with decrease in arm strength in NMD
Lindeman et al. 1995	MMD (33) and HMSN (29); non-exercise control group	24 wks	Weight training (knee extension and flexion, hip extension and flexion)	3 days per week; initially 3 sets of 25 reps at 60% of 1 RM; progressed to 3 sets of 10 reps at 80% of 1 RM	In MMD group, no change in strength In HMSN group, increased strength of knee extensors

The same research group modified the moderate-resistance protocol described above into a high-resistance program with 10 slowly progressive NMD and 6 control subjects, again using elbow flexion and knee extension exercise (Kilmer et al. 1994) (table 14.4). The results of this regimen were less consistent in the NMD group than those of the moderate-resistance study. While most strength parameters showed improvement over the 12-week period, a few indices declined in the NMD group. Finding no benefit of high- vs. moderate-resistance protocol, the researchers suggested caution with high-resistance exercise.

The only randomized, controlled trial of strength training in NMD examined 33 subjects with MMD and 29 subjects with HMSN (Lindeman et al. 1995), exercising three times per week over 24 weeks. Initially subjects completed three sets of 25 repetitions

| Table 14.3 | | | | Moderate-Resistance Exercise Training Schedule Over 12 Weeks | | | | | | |

	Knee extension			Elbow flexion			Hand grip		
Week	Sets	Reps	% max*	Sets	Reps	% max*	Sets	Reps	% max*
1	3	4	30	3	4	10	3	4	100
2	3	6	30	3	6	10	3	4	100
3	3	8	30	3	8	10	3	4	100
4	3	8	30	3	8	10	3	4	100
5	3	4	35	3	4	15	3	4	100
6	3	6	35	3	6	15	3	4	100
7	3	8	35	3	8	15	3	4	100
8	3	8	35	3	8	15	3	4	100
9	3	4	40	3	4	20	3	4	100
10	3	6	40	3	6	20	3	4	100
11	3	8	40	3	8	20	3	4	100
12	3	8	40	3	8	20	3	4	100

*Exercise performed 3 days per week based on one-repetition maximum weight.
Adapted, by permission, from S.A. Aitkens, M.A. McCrory, D.D. Kilmer, and E.M. Bernauer, 1993, "Moderate resistance exercise program: Its effect is slowly progressive neuromuscular disease," *Arch Phys Med Rehabil* 74:711-715.

at 60% of 1 RM, increasing to three sets of 10 reps at 80% of 1 RM as the study progressed. In the MMD group, investigators found no deleterious or beneficial effect on strength. In the HMSN group, there was a significant increase in the strength (14%) of the knee extensors, and a nonsignificant increase of 13% for knee flexors. Neither group experienced a change in muscle endurance—but because the endurance test was a timed maximal *isometric* contraction sustained at 80% of maximal voluntary contraction, and the training was *dynamic*, this finding is not surprising. The authors also noted that most participants enjoyed the training and intended to continue exercising.

No one has examined the relative contribution of neural factors versus actual muscle fiber hypertrophy in NMD strengthening studies. However, during brief 8- to 12-week protocols, improved recruitment of motor units and efficiency of contraction (neural factors) are probably the primary causes for increases in strength. The cross-training effects described above to the nonexercised limb are consistent with this conclusion.

In summary, it appears there are significant benefits to appropriate strength training in persons with slowly progressive NMD, particularly if they start training before significant weakness has evolved. Limited research suggests that high-resistance is no more beneficial than moderate-resistance exercise. Importantly, there have been no signs of overwork weakness in these systematic investigations.

Effects of Aerobic (Endurance) Exercise in NMD

Because the hallmark of NMD is motor weakness, more investigators have dealt with muscle strengthening than with aerobic capacity. This discussion demonstrates the challenges of aerobic testing in this population and reviews the few studies performed.

Week	Exercise days per week	Sets	Repetitions per set*
Table 14.4	High-Resistance Exercise Training Schedule Over 12 Weeks for Knee and Elbow Exercise		
1	3	1	10
2	3	2	10
3	3	3	10
4	3	4	10
5	4	4	10
6	4	4	10
7	4	4	10
8	4	4	10
9	4	5	10
10	4	5	10
11	4	5	10
12	4	5	10

*Based on maximum weight lifted 12 times.

Adapted, by permission, from D.D. Kilmer, M.A. McCrory, N.C. Wright, S.A. Aitkens, and E.M. Bernauer, 1994, "The effect of a high resistance exercise program in slowly progressive neuromuscular disease," *Arch Phys Med Rehabil* 75: 560-563.

Testing Approaches

Since NMD subjects may have difficulty with stability and ambulation, measuring aerobic capacity with graded bicycle ergometry offers significant advantages (i.e., it is stationary and provides support) over treadmill exercise. Additionally, it is possible to start at a very low work rate (e.g., 0 to 200 kilopond-meters/min) and increase the exercise intensity in small increments. It is often a challenge to find the "right" protocol for a given subject population: if the protocol is too rapid or aggressive, a weaker subject cannot keep pace; if it is excessively slow-paced, local muscular fatigue (legs) can cause premature termination of the test.

An additional challenge in testing the aerobic capacity of NMD subjects is determining the end point. One end point is a clearly defined $\dot{V}O_2$max, i.e., the point at which oxygen uptake plateaus in response to an increase in work. Even in motivated, healthy individuals, achieving this objectively definable end point is an arduous task. It is often be-

yond the physical capacity of NMD subjects. Another end point is "volitional fatigue," the theoretical limit beyond which a subject no longer can continue the prescribed protocol. This end point is highly dependent on the motivation of the subject, the influence of the person administering the protocol (e.g., verbal encouragement), and established discontinuation criteria. For example, if a given pace is established and a subject starts to slow down, the point of test termination becomes arbitrary and unclear.

Typical aerobic testing protocols are continuous, with an increase in workload every 1-2 minutes. Most exercise protocols involving NMD subjects do not achieve steady-state oxygen consumption at each progressive workload. In general, poorly conditioned individuals require longer to reach steady state at any given workload—yet it is desirable to achieve steady state if the oxygen cost of a given submaximal exercise level is of interest. This generally requires that each step be longer in duration, e.g., 3-5 minutes.

Response to Training

After earlier studies demonstrated reduced aerobic capacity in persons with NMD, several investigators examined the response of individuals with NMD to aerobic exercise training. Florence et al. (1984) tested four control and eight NMD subjects (various slowly progressive or nonprogressive disorders) in a 12-week aerobic training program, three days per week. The subjects performed six five-minute bouts on a bicycle ergometer, with a two-minute rest period between each bout, at 70% of each individual's previously determined $\dot{V}O_2$max. The $\dot{V}O_2$max increased significantly in both groups, the majority of the increase occurring in the first six weeks. After 12 weeks of training, the NMD subjects increased $\dot{V}O_2$max from 24.2 ± 3.2 to 29.6 ± 3.4 ml/min/kg, and the control subjects increased from 29.9 ± 1.4 to 35.5 ± 2.0 ml/min/kg. The two groups responded similarly to the training program when expressed as a percentage of the initial value. Interestingly, the increase in $\dot{V}O_2$max in the NMD subjects brought their values up to the initial level of the healthy control subjects. The authors concluded that persons with a variety of neuromuscular disorders can develop relatively normal adaptations to training, although they cautioned that there may be disease-specific differences.

Wright et al. (1996) studied the effects of a 12-week, home-based aerobic walking program on eight NMD subjects (five MMD, two HMSN, one LGS). Subjects exercised at training heart rates (HR) corresponding to resting heart rate plus 50%-60% of heart rate reserve (Reserve HR = Max HR − Resting HR). They began with 15-minute exercise periods and increased to 30 minutes 3-4 days per week. Graded exercise testing to volitional fatigue using a semirecumbent cycle ergometer found significant decreases in submaximal heart rate and systolic blood pressure for a given work load following the training period; increases in $\dot{V}O_2$max were not significant. Although both studies demonstrated modest improvements in function without untoward effects, it is not yet possible to draw firm conclusions about the role of endurance exercise training in diseases of the peripheral nervous system.

Exercise Recommendations in Neuromuscular Disorders

Before prescribing exercise for persons with NMD, be sure to differentiate between **physical activity** and exercise, terms often used interchangeably. Casperson (1989) defines **exercise** as a subcategory of physical activity, involving planning, structure, and repetition leading to improved fitness. With NMD, it may be beneficial to prescribe physical activities not clearly defined as exercise. For example, gardening does not meet the strict definition of exercise, but as a physical activity may be a successful method to slowly improve endurance in a person with limited motivation and resources, and easy fatigability. Indeed, low levels of activity such as walking and gardening, although not improving maximal oxygen uptake, may reduce the risk of coronary artery disease in the general population; a condition certainly important in the NMD population as well (Leon and Connett 1991). Unstructured activities are more feasible in this disabled group because of their low levels of employment (Fowler et al. 1997). There are often limited financial resources to join health clubs, purchase equipment, and travel to events.

Based on our understanding of available research, our general recommendations for strengthening programs include focusing on muscles with greater than

Exercise Prescription Recommendations

- To improve compliance, consider both a formal exercise program and enjoyable physical activities.

- Include activities with opportunities for social development and personal accomplishment.

- Strengthening programs should emphasize concentric rather than eccentric muscle contractions.

- High-resistance strengthening programs probably have no benefit over moderate-resistance programs.

- Muscles with less than antigravity strength have little capacity to improve: the program should focus on stronger muscles.

- Periodically monitor muscle strength to assess for possible overwork weakness, particularly in unsupervised programs.

- Activity modification should include periods of physical activity alternating with rest.

antigravity strength, emphasizing concentric rather than eccentric muscle contractions, and encouraging moderate- rather than high-resistance weight training.

When feasible, structured and supervised exercise programs for NMD patients are highly desirable. You can define and ensure the exercise mode, intensity, frequency, and rest periods. In fact, some advocate that NMD patients use only therapist-supervised programs, although others have found beneficial improvements in both strength and endurance measures using home-based programs (Aitkens et al. 1993; Kilmer et al. 1994; Vignos 1983; Wright et al. 1996). If a therapist-supervised program is not available or not practical, and the patient is motivated to perform a home program, it is prudent to follow the patient closely for the first several months using quantitative strength measures to reassure yourself and the patient. The hand-held dynamometer is a quick, inexpensive, and reliable device to measure strength in this population (Kilmer et al. 1997).

Adequate rest is an important component of exercise prescriptions in NMD. Extrapolating from the post-polio population, there is evidence that alternating periods of activity and rest forestall the development of fatigue (Agre and Rodriguez 1991). These same principles should benefit patients with other diseases of the peripheral nervous system.

Do not overlook the potential psychological benefits of exercise. Being involved in a sport, even at a low level, can have tremendous effects on self-esteem. Participating in an exercise program improves energy, reduces weight, and often brings a new sense of independence.

Summary

This chapter highlights the consequences of peripheral nervous system pathology for exercise performance, including the specific neuromuscular defects associated with compromised physical abilities. Disability in NMD is a complex phenomenon, however, and many other factors play an important role, including muscle disuse, cardiopulmonary involvement, excess body weight, and contractures. Muscle overuse is a particular concern in NMD; although no one has conclusively demonstrated the association experimentally, overuse may be related to habitual or sporadic eccentric muscular contractions.

Overcoming the psychological and social barriers that make the NMD population sedentary is a challenge to clinicians working with these patients. Unfortunately, review of the scientific literature does not yet allow us to confidently assure safety and effec-

tiveness for all types of exercise. A prudent and thoughtful exercise prescription takes into account the person's goals, motivations, abilities, limitations, and concerns. A personalized, well-devised physical activity program may currently be the most effective prescription we can give to people with NMD to improve their quality of life, enhance self-image, and provide greater energy for both work and play.

Acknowledgments

This work was supported by Research and Training Grant H133B0026-96 from the National Institute on Disability and Rehabilitation Research (NIDRR), United States Department of Education.

References

Agre, J.C., and A.A. Rodriquez. 1991. Intermittent isometric activity: its effect on muscle fatigue in postpolio subjects. *Arch Phys Med Rehabil* 72:971-975.

Aitkens, S.G., M.A. McCrory, D.D. Kilmer, and E.M. Bernauer. 1993. Moderate resistance exercise program: its effect in slowly progressive neuromuscular disease. *Arch Phys Med Rehabil* 74:711-715.

Appell, H.J. 1990. Muscular atrophy following immobilisation. *Sports Med* 10:42-58.

Armstrong, R.B., G.L. Warren, and J.A. Warren. 1991. Mechanisms of exercise-induced muscle fibre injury. *Sports Med* 12:184-207.

Bar-Or, O. 1996. Role of exercise in the assessment and management of neuromuscular disease in children. *Med Sci Sports Exerc* 28:421-427.

Bennett, R.L., and G.C. Knowlton. 1958. Overwork weakness in partially denervated skeletal muscle. *Clin Orthop* 12:22-29.

Bonilla, E., C.E. Samitt, A.F. Miranda, A.P. Hays, G. Salviati, S. DiMauro, L.M. Kunkel, E.P. Hoffman, and L.P. Rowland. 1988. Duchenne muscular dystrophy: deficiency of dystrophin at the muscle cell surface. *Cell* 54:447-452.

Bonsett, C.A. 1963. Pseudohypertrophic muscular dystrophy: distribution of degenerative features as revealed by anatomic study. *Neurology* 13:728-738.

Borg, K., J. Borg, L. Edstrom, and L. Grimby. 1988. Effects of excessive use of remaining muscle fibers in prior polio and LV lesion. *Muscle Nerve* 11:1219-1230.

Brook, J.D., M.E. McCurrach, H.G. Harley, A.J. Buckler, D. Church, H. Aburatani, K. Hunter, V.P. Stanton, J.P. Thirion, and T. Hudson. 1992. Molecular basis of myotonic dystrophy expansion of a trinucleotide (CTG) repeat at the 3' end of a transcript encoding a protein kinase family member. *Cell* 68:799-808.

Brown, R.H. 1997. Dystrophin-associated proteins and the muscular dystrophies. *Ann Rev Med* 48:457-466.

Carroll, J.E., J.M. Hagberg, M.H. Brooke, and J.B. Shumate. 1979. Bicycle ergometry and gas exchange measurements in neuromuscular diseases. *Arch Neurol* 36:457-461.

Carter, G.T., R.T. Abresch, W.M. Fowler Jr., E.R. Johnson, D.D. Kilmer, and C.M. McDonald. 1995a. Profiles of neuromuscular diseases: spinal muscular atrophy. *Am J Phys Med Rehabil* 74:S150-159.

Carter, G.T., R.T. Abresch, W.M. Fowler Jr., E.R. Johnson, D.D. Kilmer, and C.M. McDonald. 1995b. Profiles of neuromuscular diseases: hereditary motor and sensory neuropathy, types I and II. *Am J Phys Med Rehabil* 74:S140-S149.

Casperson, C.J. 1989. Physical activity epidemiology: concepts, methods, and applications to exercise science. In *Exercise and sport sciences reviews*. Vol. 17, ed. K. Pandolf, 423-473. Baltimore: Williams & Wilkins.

Clarkson, P.M., K. Nosaka, and B. Braun. 1992. Muscle function after exercise-induced muscle damage and rapid adaptation. *Med Sci Sports Exerc* 24:512-520.

Cooper, B.J. 1989. Animal models of Duchenne and Becker muscular dystrophy. *Br Med Bull* 45:703-718.

Dolmage, T., and E. Cafarelli. 1991. Rate of fatigue during repeated submaximal contractions of human quadriceps muscle. *Can J Physiol Pharmacol* 69:1410-1415.

Edwards, R.H.T., D.A. Jones, D.J. Newham, and S.J. Chapman. 1984. Role of mechanical damage in pathogenesis of proximal myopathy in man. *Lancet* 8376:548-551.

Ervasti, J.M., and K.P. Campbell. 1993. A role for the dystrophin-glycoprotein complex as a transmembrane linker between laminin and actin. *J Cell Biol* 122:809-823.

Fenichel, G.M., J.M. Florence, A. Pestronk, J.R. Mendell, R.T. Moxley 3d, R.C. Griggs, M.H. Brooke, J.P. Miller, J. Robison, W. King, L. Signore, S. Pandya, J. Schierbecker, and B. Wilson. 1991. Long-term benefit from prednisone therapy in Duchenne muscular dystrophy. *Neurology* 41:1874-1877.

Florence, J.M., M.H. Brooke, J.M. Hagberg, and J.E. Carroll. 1984. Endurance exercise in neuromuscular disease. In *Neuromuscular diseases*, ed. G. Serratrice, 577-581. New York: Raven Press.

Fowler, W.M. Jr., R.T. Abresch, T.R. Koch, M.L. Brewer, R.K. Bowden, and R.L. Wanlass. 1997. Employment profiles in neuromuscular diseases. *Am J Phys Med Rehabil* 76:26-37.

Franco, A. Jr., and J.B. Lansman. 1990. Calcium entry through stretch-inactivated ion channels in mdx myotubes. *Nature* 344:670-673.

Friden, J., and R.L. Lieber. 1992. Structural and mechanical basis of exercise-induced muscle injury. *Med Sci Sports Exerc* 24:521-530.

Haller, R.G., and S.F. Lewis. 1984. Pathophysiology of exercise performance in muscle disease. *Med Sci Sports Exerc* 16:456-459.

Haller, R.G., S.F. Lewis, J.D. Cook, and C.G. Blomqvist. 1983. Hyperkinetic circulation during exercise in neuromuscular disease. *Neurology* 33:1283-1287.

Hoffman, E.P., R.H. Brown Jr., and L.M. Kunkel. 1987. Dystrophin: the protein product of the Duchenne muscular dystrophy locus. *Cell* 51:919-928.

Jacobs, S.C., A.L. Bootsma, P.W. Willems, P.R. Bar, and J.H. Wokke. 1996. Prednisone can protect against exercise-induced muscle damage. *J Neurol* 243:410-416.

Johnson, E.R., R.T. Abresch, G.T. Carter, D.D. Kilmer, W.M. Fowler Jr., B.J. Sigford, and R.L. Wanlass. 1995. Profiles of neuromuscular diseases: myotonic dystrophy. *Am J Phys Med Rehabil* 74:S104-S116.

Johnson, E.W., and R. Braddom. 1971. Over-work weakness in facioscapulohumeral dystrophy. *Arch Phys Med Rehabil* 52:333-336.

Kilmer, D.D. 1996. Functional anatomy of skeletal muscle. In *Physical Medicine Rehabilitation State of the Art Reviews* 10:3, ed. K. Shankar, 413-426. Philadelphia: Hanley & Belfus.

Kilmer, D.D., R.T. Abresch, M.A. McCrory, G.T. Carter, W.M. Fowler Jr., E.R. Johnson, and C.M. McDonald. 1995. Profiles of neuromuscular diseases: facioscapulohumeral muscular dystrophy. *Am J Phys Med Rehabil* 74:S131-S139.

Kilmer, D.D., M.A. McCrory, N.C. Wright, S.A. Aitkens, and E.M. Bernauer. 1994. The effect of a high resistance exercise program in slowly progressive neuromuscular disease. *Arch Phys Med Rehabil* 75:560-563.

Kilmer, D.D., M.A. McCrory, N.C. Wright, R.A. Rosko, H.R. Kim, and S.A. Aitkens. 1997. Reliability of hand-held dynamometry in persons with neuropathic weakness. *Arch Phys Med Rehabil* 78:1364-1368.

Kilmer, D.D., and C.M. McDonald. 1995. Childhood progressive neuromuscular disease. In *Sports and exercise for children with chronic health conditions*, ed. B. Goldberg, 109-121. Champaign, IL: Human Kinetics.

Leon, A.S., and J. Connett. 1991. Physical activity and 10.5 year mortality in the Multiple Risk Factor Intervention Trial (MRFIT). *Int J Epidemiology* 20:690-697.

Lieber, R.L., and J. Friden. 1993. Muscle damage is not a function of muscle force but active muscle strain. *J Appl Physiol* 74:520-526.

Lieber, R.L., L.E. Thornell, and J. Friden. 1996. Muscle cytoskeletal disruption occurs within the first 15 min of cyclic eccentric contraction. *J Appl Physiol* 80:278-284.

Lindeman, E., P. Leffers, J. Reulen, F. Spaans, and J. Drukker. 1994. Reduction of knee torques and leg-related functional abilities in hereditary motor and sensory neuropathy. *Arch Phys Med Rehabil* 75:1201-1205.

Lindeman, E., P. Leffers, F. Spaans, J. Drukker, J. Reulen, M. Kerckhoffs, and A. Koke. 1995. Strength training in patients with myotonic dystrophy and hereditary motor and sensory neuropathy: a randomized clinical trial. *Arch Phys Med Rehabil* 76:612-20.

McCartney, N., D. Moroz, S.H. Garner, and A.J. McComas. 1988. The effects of strength training in patients with selected neuromuscular disorders. *Med Sci Sports Exerc* 20:362-368.

McCrory, M.A., H.R. Kim, N.C. Wright, C.A. Lovelady, S. Aitkens, and D.D. Kilmer. 1998. Energy expenditure, physical activity and body composition of ambulatory adults with hereditary neuromuscular disease. *Am J Clin Nutr* 67:1162-1169.

McDonald, C.M., R.T. Abresch, G.T. Carter, W.M. Fowler Jr., E.R. Johnson, and D.D. Kilmer. 1995a. Profiles of neuromuscular diseases: Becker's muscular dystrophy. *Am J Phys Med Rehabil* 74:S93-S103.

McDonald, C.M., R.T. Abresch, G.T. Carter, W.M. Fowler Jr., E.R. Johnson, D.D. Kilmer, and B.J. Sigford. 1995b. Profiles of neuromuscular diseases: Duchenne muscular dystrophy. *Am J Phys Med Rehabil* 74:S70-S92.

Milner-Brown, H.S., and R.G. Miller. 1988. Muscle strengthening through high-resistance weight training in patients with neuromuscular disorders. *Arch Phys Med Rehabil* 69:14-19.

Moens, P., P.H. Baatsen, and G. Marechal. 1993. Increased susceptibility of EDL muscles from mdx mice to damage induced by contractions with stretch. *J Muscle Res Cell Motil* 14:446-451.

Murakami, T., C.A. Garcia, L.T. Reiter, and J.R. Lupski. 1996. Charcot-Marie-Tooth disease and related inherited neuropathies. *Medicine* 75:233-250.

Perry, J., G. Barnes, and J.K. Gronley. 1988. The postpolio syndrome: an overuse phenomenon. *Clin Orthop* 233:145-162.

Petrof, B., J.B. Shrager, H.H. Stedman, A.M. Kelly, and H.L. Sweeney. 1993. Dystrophin protects the sarcolemma from stresses developed during muscle contraction. *Proc Natl Acad Sci* 90:3710-3714.

Sanjak, M., D. Paulson, R. Sufit, W. Reddan, D. Beaulieu, L. Erickson, A. Shug, and B.R. Brooks. 1987. Physiologic and metabolic response to progressive and prolonged exercise in amyotrophic lateral sclerosis. *Neurology* 37:1217-1220.

Sharma, K.R., J.A. Kent-Braun, S. Majumdar, Y. Huang, M. Mynhier, M.W. Weiner, and R.G. Miller. 1995. Physiology of fatigue in amyotrophic lateral sclerosis. *Neurology* 45:733-740.

Sharma, K.R., and R.G. Miller. 1996. Electrical and mechanical properties of skeletal muscle underlying increased fatigue in patients with amyotrophic lateral sclerosis. *Muscle Nerve* 19:1391-1400.

Sockolov, R., B. Irwin, R.H. Dressendorfer, and E.M. Bernauer. 1977. Exercise performance in 6-to-11-year-old boys with Duchenne muscular dystrophy. *Arch Phys Med Rehabil* 58:195-201.

Spector, S.A., P.L. Gordon, I.M. Feuerstein, K. Sivakumar, B.F. Hurley, and M.C. Dalakas. 1996. Strength gains without muscle injury after strength training in patients with postpolio muscular atrophy. *Muscle Nerve* 19:1282-1290.

Stedman, H.H., H.L. Sweeney, J.B. Shrager, H.C. Maguire, R.A. Panettieri, B. Petrof, M. Narusawa, J.M. Leferovich, J.T. Sladky, and A.M. Kelly. 1991. The mdx mouse diaphragm reproduces the degenerative changes of Duchenne muscular dystrophy. *Nature* 352:536-539.

Turner, P.R., P.Y. Fong, W.F. Denetclaw, and R.A. Steinhardt. 1991. Increased calcium influx in dystrophic muscle. *J Cell Biol* 115:1701-1712.

Vignos, P.J. Jr. 1983. Physical models of rehabilitation in neuromuscular disease. *Muscle Nerve* 6:323-338.

Vignos, P.J. Jr., and M.P. Watkins. 1966. Effect of exercise in muscular dystrophy. *JAMA* 197:843-848.

Weller, B., G. Karpati, and S. Carpenter. 1990. Dystrophin-deficient mdx muscle fibers are preferentially vulnerable to necrosis induced by experimental lengthening contractions. *J Neurol Sci* 100:9-13.

Wright, N.C., D.D. Kilmer, M.A. McCrory, S.A. Aitkens, B.J. Holcomb, and E.M. Bernauer. 1996. Aerobic walking in slowly progressive neuromuscular disease: effect of a 12-week program. *Arch Phys Med Rehabil* 77:64-69.

Chapter 15

Spinal Cord Injury

Michael G. Lacourse, PhD, Kristen E. Lawrence, MS, Michael J. Cohen, PhD, and Robert R. Young, MD

Case Study

Steve, a moderately physically fit 32-year-old accountant, sustained a complete spinal cord injury at the T-5 level while on a white-water rafting vacation. Upon evaluating him soon after the accident, Steve's kinesiotherapist advised him to improve his range of motion, upper body strength, and endurance so that he could complete activities of daily life, including transfers and wheelchair mobility. Steve's plan of care included progressive resistance exercises, range-of-motion activities, therapeutic standing, manual wheelchair mobility, balance training, and other activities of daily living. After three months of physical training for one hour a day, three days a week, Steve became 100% independent in his transfers to and from bed, a car, the commode, the bathtub, and a chair or sofa. His muscular endurance and strength also increased, allowing him to operate a wheelchair for long distances, including ascending and descending ramps and curbs. He was able to participate in therapeutic standing in a portable standing frame or in parallel bars with long leg braces, and has completed driver training. Through a program of exercises and activities, Steve has achieved a good deal of independence in his daily life and was motivated to continue his training outside of the hospital with a wheelchair sports organization.

Spinal cord injury (SCI) produces a number of neuromuscular, skeletal, hormonal, metabolic, and psychological changes in the injured individual. Potential benefits of exercise and physical activity are, of course, drastically altered. Recent data indicate a marked change in the activity pattern of the central nervous system in response to spinal cord injury: massive deafferentation leads to reorganization of the cerebral cortex, and probably of subcortical connections as well. These facts should influence our thinking about using physical activity to improve motor performance and muscle strength in individuals who have spinal cord injury.

In this chapter we first review the available data regarding skeletal and muscular changes after spinal cord injury. Electrical stimulation may partially prevent morphologic and metabolic changes in muscle after injury. We also review the cardiorespiratory adaptations and hormonal changes in people with SCI.

Next, we review the somatosensory and motor cortical reorganization in individuals with SCI, and the data derived from PET scans and transcranial magnetic stimulation. These studies suggest that an alternate form of motor rehabilitation might be appropriate for people with SCI, and we will discuss motor imagery as one possibility for improving muscle strength and function. See "Summary of Benefits That Individuals With SCI Derive From Exercise" (page 269).

Effects of Chronic Inactivity on Individuals With SCI

The importance of regular exercise and sports participation for the rehabilitation of individuals with spinal cord injuries has been recognized since World War II. Despite this awareness, there remains little understanding of how exercise may influence the quality of life for individuals with SCI (Noreau and Shephard 1992). Spinal cord injury generally reduces an individual's ability to participate in the vigorous daily activities needed to maintain a healthy lifestyle; it thereby increases the prevalence of secondary impairments such as cardiovascular disease and non-insulin-dependent diabetes mellitus.

Chronic inactivity is well known to have debilitating effects on lifestyle, and may increase morbidity and mortality even for able-bodied individuals. According to a 1995 consensus report from the National Institutes of Health, the absence of frequent vigorous physical activity is a major risk factor for

cardiovascular disease (NIH 1995). The problem is more acute for individuals with SCI—their mortality rate from cardiovascular disease is 228% higher than in the general population (Kocina 1997). Regular participation in a structured exercise program may reduce the risk of cardiovascular disease as well as improve autonomy for the performance of activities of daily living.

Physical inactivity may also lead to bone demineralization, atrophy of both skeletal and cardiac muscle, decreased lean body mass, reduced body water content and blood volume, and increased body fat (Figoni 1993). Physically inactive men with SCI have levels of body fat that put them at high risk for diseases associated with obesity, while physically active men with SCI have lower but still above-average levels of body fat (Kocina 1997). Since bone mineral content decreases approximately 25%-50% in paralyzed limbs (the degree of loss dependent on the level, completeness, and duration of the injury), 100% of people with SCI have osteoporosis of a paralyzed limb (Kocina 1997). Skeletal muscle atrophy leads to a 30% reduction in body protein and a 15% reduction in the ratio of total body water to body weight.

The more rostral the level of spinal cord trauma, the greater and more severe the loss of somatic and autonomic nervous system function (Davis 1993). Lesions in the thoraco-lumbar regions cause varying loss of function, depending on the level and completeness of the injury—including impaired sensorimotor function of the lower limbs, poor bowel and bladder control, and some loss of sexual ability. Injuries above the first thoracic vertebra (causing quadriplegia) lead to additional loss of function, depending on the level and completeness of the injury—including loss of sensorimotor function of the upper limbs, diaphragmatic inspiratory control, respiratory/thoracic muscle pump, intrinsic control of arterial and venous blood vessels, cardiovascular reflexes, and local metabolic processes in active muscles (Figoni 1993). Moreover, a spinal cord injury may disrupt autonomic reflexes required for normal physical activity.

While a spinal cord injury usually precludes full participation in many physical activities available to able-bodied persons, various exercise modalities and sports have been successfully modified for such individuals. Wheelchair ergometry, arm-crank ergometry, functional neuromuscular stimulation, functional magnetic stimulation, and hybrid exercise protocols that combine arm-crank ergometry and functional electrical stimulation can improve muscle strength and increase capacity for aerobic activity. Some strength training devices have been adapted for use by the disabled; and increasingly popular wheelchair

Summary of Benefits That Individuals With SCI Derive From Exercise

Musculoskeletal

1. Decreased rate (or possible cessation) of bone density loss
2. Increased strength and endurance

Cardiovascular

3. Increased stroke volume and decreased total peripheral resistance
4. Reduced resting and submaximal heart rate
5. Reduced blood pressure during exercise
6. Increased exercise capacity
7. Increased HDL- ("good") cholesterol; decreased total cholesterol and LDL- ("bad") cholesterol
8. Decreased risk for cardiovascular disease

Neural

9. Reduced spasticity
10. Accelerated peripheral nerve regeneration

Hormonal

11. Enhanced insulin sensitivity

General/Other

12. Accelerated wound healing
13. Weight loss, fat loss
14. Increased employability
15. Increased independence: ability to complete activities of daily life without assistance

Selected citations

1. Hangartner et al. 1994; Leeds et al. 1990; Kaplan et al. 1978
2. Bremner et al. 1992; Pollack et al. 1989; Davis et al. 1986; Davis and Shephard 1990

3. Faghri et al. 1992; Hooker et al. 1992a; Hooker et al. 1992b; Davis et al. 1990
4. Davis and Shephard 1988

5. Kim et al. 1993; Ragnarsson 1988; Faghri et al. 1992
6. Hoffman 1986
7. Brenes et al. 1986; Hooker and Wells 1989

8. NIH 1995; Figoni 1993

9. Daly et al. 1996
10. Daly et al. 1996

11. Burstein et al. 1996

12. Daly et al. 1996
13. Kocina 1997
14. Noreau and Shephard 1992
15. Noreau and Shephard 1992

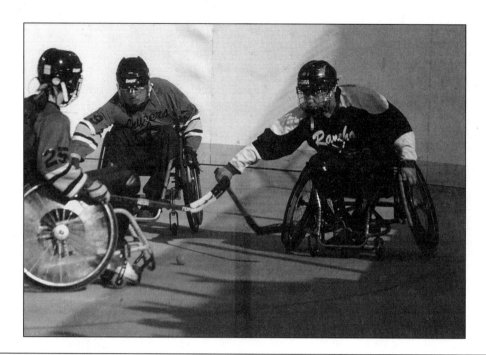

Figure 15.1   Diego Rodriguez of the Rancho Kings wheelchair hockey team.
Courtesy of the Rancho Los Amigos Medical Center.

sports such as basketball, track and field, and hockey are available to individuals with different injury levels (see figure 15.1). Exercise not only improves muscle strength and endurance, cardiorespiratory function, and range of motion; it may increase the probability of obtaining gainful employment for individuals with SCI (Noreau and Shephard 1992).

Musculoskeletal Adaptations to Physical Activity in Individuals With SCI

Spinal cord injury leads to partial or complete loss of volitional control of muscles innervated below the level of injury, loss of muscle strength and endurance, and demineralization of bone. The loss of muscle strength and endurance also inhibits cardiorespiratory response to exercise, since local fatigue prevents muscles from maintaining prescribed workloads. Regular exercise through either voluntary activity or electrical stimulation of paralyzed muscles can increase strength and endurance of persons with SCI (Bremner et al. 1992; Pollack et al. 1989) and decrease the rate of bone demineralization (Abramson and Delagi 1961; Garland et al. 1992; Hangartner et al. 1994; Kaplan et al. 1978; Kaplan et al. 1981; Lew

1987). In maintaining the viability of muscle tissue, exercise also can speed rehabilitation and increase the chance for partial recovery when and if spinal motor neurons are reconnected with descending motor axons (Mira 1982).

Muscle

Disuse atrophy (denervation of muscles paralyzed by a spinal cord injury) presents special problems for the rehabilitation of individuals with SCI. Damage to spinal motoneurons or ventral root axons produces denervation of muscles in the dermatomes supplied by the portion of the spinal cord involved in the injury zone. To a limited extent, some denervated muscle fibers may become reinnervated by sprouts from axons of motoneurons that are still connected to higher motor centers. This accounts for spontaneously increased strength in some of the more rostral paralyzed muscles. Without reinnervation, or without transplantation of functioning nerves into these denervated muscles, they undergo irreversible denervation atrophy and cannot be activated by ordinary electrical stimuli with pulse widths of a millisecond or less.

Muscle Property Changes Following SCI

Most musculoskeletal deconditioning occurs during the initial six months postinjury (Sloan et al. 1994), when morphological and metabolic changes in muscles render them unsuitable for prolonged periods of contraction (Riley and Allin 1973). Martin and colleagues (1992) examined the tibialis anterior of five motor-complete (C6-T4) spinal cord injured patients 2-11 years postinjury. Compared with five normal controls subjects, individuals with SCI had a substantially lower proportion of type I fibers, smaller cross-sectional area (no difference in area between fiber types), 40% reduction in absolute enzymatic activity of type I and II fibers, significantly lower capillary-to-fiber ratio, and lower succinate dehydrogenase (SDH) activity for both type I and II fibers (type II fibers seemed more affected than type I). Furthermore, Grimby et al. (1976) found significantly lower SDH and phosphofructokinase activities in lower extremity muscles of individuals with SCI (low cervical or thoracic level lesions) than in the deltoid muscles. Overall, spinal cord injuries appear to effect a shift from slow oxidative fibers to fast glycolytic fibers.

Effects of Physical Activity on Muscle Strength and Endurance

SCI patients may engage in muscle strength and endurance training either volitionally or through electrical stimulation (ES) techniques. The injury level determines the type of training. Although some modified strength training equipment is available for individuals with quadriplegia, such people usually must use ES to train muscles. People with paraplegia have more options for upper extremity training, and may use electrical stimulation techniques to condition lower extremity muscles.

Upper Extremity Strength Training

Upper extremity muscle strength and endurance are important for wheelchair propulsion and for performing daily activities such as lifting oneself in and out of a car. Individuals with paraplegia can use several exercise modalities to condition upper extremity muscles, including wheelchair and arm crank ergometry, standard and modified static exercises, isokinetic and isotonic exercise equipment, and active participation in wheelchair sports. A common perception is that, because ergometry and wheelchair sports are primarily aerobic, they may not provide sufficient stimulus to promote muscle hypertrophy and increased strength. Yet there is substantial evidence that these exercise modalities can increase both muscle strength and endurance.

Davis et al. (1986) found that wheelchair athletes have 10%-57% greater arm power than inactive individuals with paraplegia; Grimby (1980) observed 20%-100% increases in shoulder abduction torque with wheelchair training and swimming. Wheelchair basketball players have hypertrophied type II muscle fibers (Tesch and Karlsson 1983)(see figure 15.2). Despite the differences between active and inactive individuals with paraplegia, well-trained wheelchair athletes have low to average concentrations of both aerobic and anaerobic enzymes per unit mass of muscles above the injury zone, as compared with normal, untrained individuals (Grimby 1980).

Davis and Shephard (1990) assessed changes in isokinetic strength following 16 weeks of forearm ergometer training. Despite the aerobic nature of the exercise, the researchers found increased muscle power in the two muscle groups controlling the exercise (i.e., shoulder extension and elbow flexion). The exercise group also demonstrated some gains of muscle

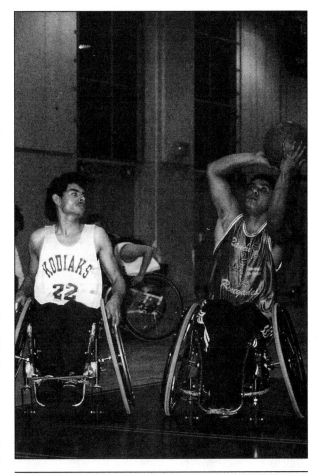

Figure 15.2 Ramon Cervantes of the Rancho Renegades wheelchair basketball team.
Courtesy of the Rancho Los Amigos Medical Center.

function (both peak and average muscle power), especially at higher velocities of contraction. Nilsson et al. (1975) found that, after seven weeks of triceps strength training, individuals with paraplegia increased overall muscle strength by 19% and overall muscular endurance by 80%.

Electrical Stimulation

Electrical stimulation (ES) is an alternative form of therapy that may substitute for volitional exercise to increase muscle strength and improve functional motor performance. As is true with disuse atrophy in nonparalyzed individuals, paralyzed but innervated muscles weaken after spinal cord injury because they lose intracellular contractile proteins—they behave like muscles composed primarily of fast, type II (anaerobic, fatigable) fibers when first stimulated electrically (Gibson et al. 1989). With chronic electrical stimulation, such muscles develop increased protein synthesis and become typical slow muscles composed of type I (aerobic, nonfatigable) fibers (Martin et al. 1992).

With **functional neuromuscular stimulation (FNS)**, also called **functional electrical stimulation (FES)**, lower motor neurons are electrically excited via surface, percutaneous, or implanted electrodes that produce muscle contraction either during a functional motor task or against some external load (Yarkony et al. 1992). The benefits of functional neuromuscular stimulation include reversal of muscle atrophy and alteration of muscle characteristics (Pette and Vrbova 1985), modification of spasticity and rigidity (Stefanovska et al. 1991), accelerated wound healing (Vodovnik and Karba 1992), and accelerated peripheral nerve regeneration (Nix and Hopf 1983). FNS alters tissue characteristics such as skeletal muscle blood flow, and alleviates abnormal behavior such as spasticity. The most well-documented FNS effect on tissue function and structure is a change in fundamental characteristics of skeletal muscle: skeletal muscle exposed to prolonged functional demands responds first with metabolic changes, then with structural adaptations (Borgens et al. 1981; Brown et al. 1976; Pette and Vrbova 1985; Pette et al. 1973; Salmons and Henriksson 1981). Several recent reviews describe FNS/FES techniques (Glaser 1994; Kralj et al. 1993; Yarkony et al. 1992).

Electrical stimulation of surviving motor axons can activate muscles innervated by spinal segments caudal to the injury zone. These muscles have undergone disuse atrophy but are not denervated. They contract even when they are first stimulated, although with a force markedly reduced from normal, and they

fatigue rapidly. Such muscles cannot perform useful functions with electrical stimulation; they require exercise and training to increase their force output and reduce their fatigability. In their pioneering studies of individuals with quadriplegia, Peckham and colleagues demonstrated that chronic, low-frequency (10-15 Hz) electrical stimulation of the motor nerves innervating these muscles for a few seconds, followed by a few seconds of rest, for an hour or two a day over a span of a month or two, results in forces at least quadruple those seen initially, with much less fatigability. Such muscles are then suitable for functional electrical stimulation (Peckham et al. 1976).

Martin et al. (1992) examined the effects of electrical stimulation on changes in morphology and metabolic properties of muscle. Five SCI patients (motor-complete, C6-T4) self-administered a 24-week progressive program of electrical stimulation of the tibialis anterior. They experienced a significant increase in the proportion of type I fibers, a 29% increase in the ratio of capillaries to fibers (not significant), a significant increase in SDH activity for both fiber types (with the greatest increase in type II fibers), and an overall increase in muscle endurance. Stimulation did not influence the distribution of fiber sizes in the patients with SCI, and did not increase the activity of myofibrillar ATPase in either fiber type. Electrical stimulation generally enhanced the oxidative capacity and endurance properties of the paralyzed muscles, but had no effect on fiber size and strength.

Bone

There is substantial bone remodeling in people with SCI, with bone resorption occurring at a faster rate than bone formation (Chantraine et al. 1986; Miniare et al. 1974). The degree of remodeling depends on the degree of spasticity, amount of physical activity, diet, and lifestyle (Hangartner et al. 1994).

Changes in Bone Density Following SCI

Physical inactivity leads to bone demineralization and a higher incidence of osteoporosis (Hangartner et al. 1994; Kaplan et al. 1978; Leeds et al. 1990). Immediately following a spinal cord injury, an increase in calcium and hydroxyproline excretion creates a negative calcium balance and eventually leads to demineralization and a decline in bone density (Chantraine et al. 1986; Hangartner et al. 1994; Leeds et al. 1990) that may continue for several years. In one study

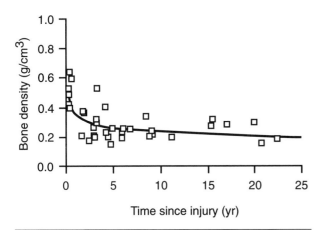

Figure 15.3 Subcortical bone density at the distal end of the tibia in a group of 37 SCI patients measured before the start of the FES exercise training. The regression line of bone density vs. time post injury is of the form y = ax^b.

Reprinted, by permission, from T.N. Hangartner et al., "Tibial bone density loss in SCI patients: effects of FES exercise," *J Rehabil Res Dev* 31(1): 55.

involving nine individuals with SCI, equilibrium between bone resorption and synthesis did not occur until approximately two years postinjury (Sloan et al. 1994). In another study, Hangartner et al. (1994) measured bone density in 37 SCI patients with various postinjury durations. Regression analysis showed the loss in bone density during the first two years postinjury to be 51.5% for trabecular, 44.2% for subcortical, and 32.7% for cortical bone (figure 15.3 shows the subcortical data). Overall, the loss of trabecular bone density is about 70% by seven years postinjury, with little loss thereafter. Significant osteoporotic changes have been observed as soon as four weeks postinjury in iliac crest bone biopsies (Claus-Walker et al. 1972; Naftchi et al. 1980).

Effects of Physical Activity on Bone Density

Clinicians use various modes of exercise—such as standing, ambulation, and FES—to reduce bone demineralization. Although reversals of osteopenia have been reported in able-bodied individuals following ambulation training, there are inconsistent findings concerning the effects of ambulation on bone density of individuals with SCI (Abramson and Delagi 1961; Claus-Walker et al. 1972; Claus-Walker et al. 1977; Donaldson et al. 1970; Kaplan et al. 1981; Guttmann 1976). Kaplan et al. (1978) provided ambulation training for eight SCI patients (T4-L5) and measured fecal calcium before and after training. Ambulation training significantly decreased hypercalciuria and positively altered calcium balance in patients with SCI who were less than three months

postinjury, with smaller changes in those who were more than six months postinjury. Unfortunately, the researchers provided no details on the nature of the training program.

Leeds et al. (1990) trained six individuals with quadriplegia three days each week for three months using FES-cycle ergometry, and found no significant changes in bone mineral density in the femoral neck, Ward's triangle, or trochanter. A follow-up study of three additional men demonstrated that even after three years of FES-cycle ergometry, there were no changes in bone mineral content.

In the aforementioned study by Hangartner and colleagues (1994), 37 SCI patients with varying postinjury durations performed a 12-week (36-session) FES program of knee extension or leg cycling. The reduction in bone loss averaged between 0.2% and 3.3% per year for all bone parameters at the distal end of the tibia, and for trabecular bone density at the proximal end of the tibia. FES did not increase bone density during the exercise period.

Sloan et al. (1994) examined the effects of a three-month exercise program of FES-induced cycling on 12 individuals with incomplete SCI. The researchers measured bone mineral density before and after the exercise program in two of the subjects—one less than a year postinjury, and one greater than four years postinjury. There was some increase of bone mineral density in the more recently injured subject, but no change in the long-term patient. FES appears to have little or no effect on bone mineral density of subjects who are several years postinjury and a small effect on bone mineral density of subjects who have recent injuries.

Hangartner and colleagues (1994) recommend caution when loading the legs through standing, walking, or other forms of physical rehabilitation. Instead of attempting to reverse the osteoporosis that occurs post-SCI, it may be more realistic to prevent bone mineral density loss with FES or other weightbearing or resistive exercises introduced early in the rehabilitation process.

Cardiorespiratory Adaptations to Physical Activity in Individuals With SCI

Spinal cord injury prevents the use of large leg muscles during volitional exercise. Without the contribution of these powerful muscles, it is difficult to derive central cardiovascular benefits from physical training. The smaller muscles of the upper body, such as those used during arm crank ergometry, are generally not strong enough to allow exercise of sufficient intensity or duration to improve cardiovascular fitness. Cardiovascular function is influenced by several physiological factors, including cardiac output (CO), heart rate (HR), stroke volume (SV), oxygen uptake ($\dot{V}O_2$max), blood pressure (BP), and temperature regulation. We will discuss the effects of spinal cord injury and physical activity on each of these factors.

Cardiac Output, Heart Rate, and Stroke Volume

According to McArdle and colleagues (1994), **cardiac output** is the primary indicator of the circulatory system's functional capacity to meet the demands of physical activity. It is computed as the product of heart rate and stroke volume ($CO = HR \times SV$). With inactivity due to paralysis, the heart, like skeletal muscle, becomes less efficient; and because it ejects less blood with each contraction, it must contract more frequently to meet even resting circulatory requirements.

In addition to reduced cardiac efficiency, individuals with SCI experience a decrease in sympathetic activity and venous return. When compared with able-bodied persons, people with SCI exhibit **circulatory hypokinesis**, which is a reduced CO for any exercise intensity. On average, individuals with paraplegia have 25% less CO than controls at rest, and 68% less CO than controls during maximal exercise (percentages vary based on lesion level) (Hoffman 1986). Reduced sympathetic nerve outflow limits cardiovascular adaptation to exercise in SCI individuals, whose heart rate response to activity increases in comparison to able-bodied persons (Davis 1993). Sedentary individuals with quadriplegia have an even lower heart rate response to exercise than persons with paraplegia, and therefore a greatly reduced CO relative to able-bodied controls.

Lower extremity skeletal muscles assist with venous return during exercise and recovery. Because individuals with SCI are incapable of voluntarily contracting lower extremity muscles, the pumping activity necessary for sufficient venous return during exercise does not occur. Spasticity in paralyzed muscles can assist, but there is an overall decrease in CO and, consequently, an inadequate distribution of blood to exercising muscles (VanLoan et al. 1987). In order to compensate for the decreased CO, individuals with a

spinal cord injury must become more efficient at cellular oxygen extraction. Figoni et al. (1988) observed that men with quadriplegia deliver blood and O_2 at a slower rate from the heart to the periphery, but extract O_2 from the capillaries at a faster rate than able-bodied men.

Cardiovascular training can increase CO by improving the efficiency of the circulatory system. In a study involving 36 sessions of FES-leg cycle ergometry training, submaximal exercise CO increased significantly in persons with paraplegia, while stroke volume increased significantly and heart rate decreased significantly for individuals with both paraplegia and quadriplegia (see figure 15.4) (Faghri et al. 1992). These adaptations to exercise are similar to those observed in able-bodied persons.

The increased active muscle mass and enhanced vasodilation that result from hybrid training protocols have led to declines in both resting and exercise total peripheral resistance in the blood vessels (Davis et al. 1990; Hooker et al. 1992a; Hooker et al. 1992b; Shenberger et al. 1990). In a study comparing active and inactive individuals with paraplegia, Davis and Shephard (1988) found that submaximal heart rate was lower for the active group than for the inactive, and that stroke volume and CO were higher for the active group. In a review, Shephard (1988) cites studies suggesting that increased posttraining stroke

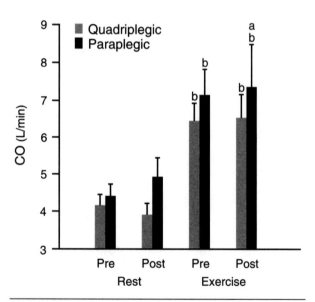

Figure 15.4 Cardiac output (CO) response of people with spinal cord injury at rest and during submaximal exercise pre- and post-FES-leg cycle ergometry training. Values are means ± SE. a, Significant changes pretraining to posttraining at rest and/or exercise; b, significant changes rest to exercise.
Reprinted, by permission, from P.D Faghri, R.M. Glaser, and S.F. Figoni, 1992, "Functional electrical stimulation leg cycle," *Archives of Physical Medicine and Rehabilitation* 73:1089.

volume results from decreased end-systolic volume—the latter due to decreased afterload associated with increased upper body muscle strength. In individuals with quadriplegia, the higher lesion level and ensuing abolishment of cerebral control of the sympathetic nervous system cause a smaller exercise response and thus a reduced capacity for cardiovascular function improvement. Faghri et al. (1992) suggest that long-term training may be necessary to increase benefits for individuals with quadriplegia.

Blood Volume and Hemoglobin Content

Individuals with spinal cord injuries tend to exhibit reduced blood volume and blood hemoglobin content, especially immediately postinjury. Figoni et al. (1988) explained the blood volume decrease by venous pooling in the lower body combined with the extrusion of plasma from lower-body capillaries into the tissues. Knutsson and colleagues (1973) observed that the average man with SCI has a blood volume of 5.15 ± 0.82 L, vs. 6.05 ± 0.82 L for the average able-bodied man. For women, the average values are 3.68 L (range = 3.0-4.2, standard deviation not reported) versus 4.3 ± 0.61 L. Hemoglobin content follows a similar trend. For men with SCI, the average hemoglobin content was 9.46 ± 1.63 g/kg vs. 10.23 ± 1.18 g/kg for the able-bodied; for women, the values were 7.57 ± 1.47 g/kg (SCI) and 8.07 ± 0.86 g/kg (able-bodied). The difference was statistically significant in the male subjects.

According to Lipetz and associates (1997), the condition of **anemia** is defined as blood hemoglobin values <13 g/dl. They observed anemia in 65% of 46 individuals with acute spinal cord injuries—most commonly in those with complete quadriplegic injuries. One year later, only three (6.8%) were still anemic, suggesting that anemia in acutely injured people may be transitory, resulting from blood loss, pain medication, stress, and/or erythropoietin resistance secondary to acute injury. Individuals with chronic spinal cord injuries who exhibit low blood hemoglobin content should be examined for factors such as chronic inflammatory lesions, blood loss, post-traumatic stress, and high usage of aspirin or NSAIDs that could contribute to anemia.

Unfortunately, exercise has little or no direct effect on blood volume or hemoglobin content (Gass and Camp 1979; Knutsson et al. 1973). To some extent, the posttraining increase in CO can compensate for these deficits by increasing overall circulation.

Oxygen Uptake

Oxygen uptake is defined as the usage of oxygen by the cells. During exercise, need for oxygen in active cells throughout the body increases due to its role in energy (ATP) synthesis. **Maximum oxygen uptake** ($\dot{V}O_2$max), the point at which oxygen uptake either plateaus or increases only slightly even if the workload increases (McArdle et al. 1994), is an important indicator of cardiovascular function. In fact, an increase in maximum oxygen uptake is considered to be the most significant change in cardiovascular function with aerobic exercise (McArdle et al. 1994). In addition to the numerous factors that may affect $\dot{V}O_2$max in able-bodied persons (age, sex, training state) (Åstrand and Rodahl 1977), there are impairments specific to a spinal cord injury. For example, lesion level may explain 46% of the variability in $\dot{V}O_2$max (Burkett et al. 1990). Higher lesions (quadriplegia) lead to poorer cardiovascular performance than thoracic or lumbar lesions (Burkett et al. 1990; VanLoan et al. 1987).

In many studies involving individuals with SCI, the term $\dot{V}O_2$peak is used instead of $\dot{V}O_2$max, to indicate a limit on the ability to reach a true maximal value. It is still possible, however, for exercise to have an effect on oxygen uptake in the spinal cord injured, as reported in a review of 13 cardiorespiratory training studies (Hoffman 1986). Hoffman reported that in all but one study, exercise capacity increased, as demonstrated by either increased $\dot{V}O_2$max, increased work performance, and/or decreased submaximal exercise measures ($\dot{V}O_2$, heart rate) following physical training using various modes, intensities, and session durations. After 4 to 20 weeks of training, average improvement in $\dot{V}O_2$max was 20% (range 0%-61%).

Blood Pressure

Adaptations in both systolic blood pressure (SBP) and diastolic blood pressure (DBP) suggest improved cardiovascular function in individuals with SCI after participation in an exercise program. Following at least five weeks of training, researchers have seen reductions in peak SBP (Faghri et al. 1992; Kim et al. 1993; Ragnarsson 1988) and in peak DBP (Faghri et al. 1992; Pollack et al. 1989; Ragnarsson 1988) during exercise. Fewer adaptations to training occur in resting BP values, but Faghri et al. (1992) did find an increase in resting SBP in individuals with quadriplegia. Subjects with higher-level lesions also demonstrated lower mean exercise SBP and DBP, and an abnormal SBP exercise response as compared to persons with paraplegia and controls (Drory et al. 1990): monitoring BP of this group during exercise may be important for safety reasons. Persons with paraplegia tend to exhibit training responses in SBP and DBP similar to those of controls, both at rest and during exercise (Drory et al. 1990).

Autonomic dysreflexia is a condition peculiar to the spinal cord injured that can lead to high blood pressure during exercise. It is usually limited to persons with injuries above the major splanchnic outflow (often at or above T6), with both complete and incomplete injuries. Painful or noxious stimuli below the level of injury trigger pathological reflexes via somatic or autonomic nerve pathways (Comarr and Eltorai 1995). Electrical stimulation exercises (such as FES) often induce autonomic dysreflexia because, according to able-bodied persons, the stimulation is painful (Ashley et al. 1993). Symptoms include, but are not limited to, sweating, headache, elevated blood pressure (as high as 300/220), goose pimples, nausea, flushing in face and neck, and convulsions. Although some athletes with spinal cord injuries induce autonomic dysreflexia as a way to improve performance, it is potentially a very dangerous condition, and can lead to cerebral hemorrhage and cardiac arrhythmia (Ashley et al. 1993). It is therefore important to monitor blood pressure carefully during FES.

Temperature Regulation

SCI patients are limited to upper-body exercises, which may cause more thermal stress than lower-body exercises. Increased thermal stress results from the decrease in venous return that occurs with lower extremity inactivity, and from the ensuing decrease in blood distribution (Sawka et al. 1989). In addition, since the SCI population tends to demonstrate very little, if any, sweating below the lesion level, there is decreased blood flow to the skin and reduced heat loss via evaporation (Hopman et al. 1993). In order to maintain CO while allowing for heat loss through evaporation (which decreases blood volume), able-bodied persons exhibit a "cardiovascular drift," i.e., an increase in heart rate with a steady pace of activity. Individuals with lesions above T6 do not appear able to make this compensation, and thus exhibit a decrease in CO over time with continuous exercise and a decrease in their ability to regulate body temperature (Hopman et al. 1993).

Hormonal and Metabolic Adaptations to Physical Activity in Individuals With SCI

Individuals with SCI tend to have insufficient hormonal and metabolic responses to exercise (Kjaer et al. 1996). Normal responses require a functional motor center, afferent nerves from working muscles, and an intact central nervous system. Individuals with SCI exhibit only humoral feedback and spinal or simple autonomic nervous reflex mechanisms, which are insufficient for an adequate exercise response (Kjaer et al. 1996). Table 15.1 summarizes hormonal and metabolic responses in people with SCI.

Blood Glucose/Insulin Response

Kjaer and colleagues found that, in exercising control subjects, both glucose production and utilization increased, and plasma glucose decreased slightly. During FES in SCI patients training at the same $\dot{V}O_2$ as the controls, glucose utilization increased, glucose production did not change, and plasma glucose decreased. Plasma insulin increased in SCI subjects during FES, while controls exercising at the same $\dot{V}O_2$ exhibited only a small response (Kjaer et al. 1996). Burstein et al. (1996) found no apparent disruption in glucose homeostasis in a moderately active spinal cord injured (paraplegia) group, as compared with controls. This was in contrast to the belief that, with muscular atrophy, SCI impairs glucose uptake. The daily activities and moderate exercise of these subjects may have increased upper-body musculature, compensating metabolically for lower-body muscular atrophy. In another study (Dearwater et al. 1986), both active and inactive SCI subjects exhibited significantly lower fasting serum glucose levels, but similar insulin values—suggesting increased insulin sensitivity—as compared with controls. The response appears to be a function of neuronal control of glucose metabolism rather than of physical activity. In summary, injury seems to decrease both resting and exercise blood glucose levels, and to increase insulin levels during exercise. Moderate physical activity may improve glucose homeostasis through an increase in muscle mass, thereby enhancing insulin sensitivity.

Table 15.1	Summary of Hormonal and Metabolic Characteristics of Individuals With Spinal Cord Injury as Compared With Able-Bodied Individuals		
	SCI vs. able-bodied at rest	**Able-bodied during exercise**	**SCI during exercise**
Plasma glucose	SCI lower	Little or no change	Decrease
Plasma insulin	Little or no difference	Decrease during some activities, or no change	Increase during some activities, or no change
Lactic acid	Little or no difference	Increase	Larger response than able-bodied
Somatotropin	SCI higher	Increase	Larger response than able-bodied
ACTH	Little or no difference	Increase	Increase during some activities, or no change
β-endorphins	Little or no difference	Increase	Increase during some activities, or no change
Testosterone	SCI returns to baseline after stabilization following initial trauma-induced suppression	Increase	Increase
Catecholamines	SCI lower	NE: increase E: no change	NE: increase during some activities (still lower than resting able-bodied), or no change E: no change
Renin	Little or no difference	Progressive increase during exercise, then decline at termination	Increase that continues throughout recovery
Cholesterol	SCI higher	Decrease with chronic exercise	Decrease with chronic exercise
Metabolism	SCI lower	Increase	Increase

NE = norepinephrine; E = epinephrine

Lactic Acid Response

Individuals with spinal cord injuries show an increased lactic acid response to FES exercise when compared with able-bodied controls performing a voluntary activity (Kjaer et al. 1996). SCI individuals attain a larger activation of glycolysis than normal for power output and $\dot{V}O_2$ levels (Hooker et al. 1990). Pollack and colleagues (1989) suggest that lactic acid accumulation may occur more promptly in SCI persons who participate in upper-body exercise, due to more rapid depletion of energy resources than occurs during lower-body exercise at the same intensity. Hooker et al. (1990) suggest that the high blood lactate accumulation seen in individuals with SCI may be due to: (1) the deconditioned state of paralyzed leg muscle, (2) the preferential recruitment of type II (fast, glycolytic) muscle fibers during FES exercise, (3) a diminished circulatory response to exercise due to sympathetic dysfunction, or (4) a decreased capacity for blood lactate clearance. Lactic acid levels may significantly limit exercise duration and/or intensity for the spinal cord injured. In comparing adaptations to wheelchair ergometry training at low and moderate intensities in SCI subjects, Hooker and Wells (1989) found that the latter more effectively lowered lactic acid response during submaximal exercise.

Hormonal Responses

The endocrine system produces, stores, and releases hormones. As the chemical messengers of the body, hormones play an important role in almost all aspects of human function and help maintain internal homeostasis in many situations. Exercise is a physical stressor that activates numerous paths in the endocrine system (McArdle et al. 1994).

Somatotropin

The growth hormone **somatotropin** promotes cell division and cellular proliferation throughout the body, facilitates protein synthesis, decreases carbohydrate utilization, and increases use of lipids for energy. Secretion is directly related to exercise intensity (McArdle et al. 1994). Individuals with spinal cord injuries have higher resting levels of somatotropin than able-bodied persons. In one study, these levels increased dramatically during arm crank ergometry and voluntary exercise (with no change during FES)—suggesting that motor center activity stimulates somatotropin response (Kjaer et al. 1996).

Adrenocorticotropic Hormone and β-Endorphins

Adrenocorticotropic hormone (ACTH) regulates hormonal output from the adrenal cortex, directly enhances lipid metabolism, increases rates of gluconeogenesis, and stimulates protein catabolism. β-endorphins (BE) increase pain tolerance, improve appetite control, and reduce anxiety, tension, anger, and confusion. BE is what triggers the "exercise high." Both ACTH and BE increase in response to exercise (McArdle et al. 1994); trained SCI people have higher levels of BE at rest than their sedentary counterparts (Kjaer et al. 1996). For individuals with spinal cord injuries, plasma ACTH and BE increase during FES, while only ACTH increases during arm crank ergometry. The latter response, however, is not seen in able-bodied controls. The increase in ACTH and BE in SCI persons during most forms of exercise suggests that humoral feedback or autonomic nervous reflex mechanisms compensate somehow for the

lack of central command and nervous feedback (Kjaer et al. 1996).

Testosterone

Testosterone augments release of somatotropin and is responsible for increases in muscle mass and decreases in body fat (McArdle et al. 1994). In the able-bodied, serum total and free testosterone increase during short-term strenuous exercise and decrease during and after prolonged exercise (Wheeler et al. 1996). With chronic endurance training, there is a reduction in total testosterone and in the available portion in circulation (Wheeler et al. 1994). Trained and untrained individuals with chronic SCI show testosterone responses to exercise similar to those of able-bodied people (Wheeler et al. 1994; Wheeler et al. 1996). Thus, humoral responses seem to be involved in the testosterone response and its abolition (Wheeler et al. 1994).

Catecholamines

The adrenal medulla secretes the catecholamines **norepinephrine (NE)** and **epinephrine (E)**, increasing their release in response to increased intensity and duration of exercise. NE and E affect the heart, blood vessels, and glands in the same way as direct stimulation by the sympathetic nervous system (McArdle et al. 1994). Kjaer and colleagues found lower resting plasma levels of NE and E in SCI individuals than in controls. NE rose during FES, but was still lower than in resting controls and did not rise during arm crank ergometry. E never rose in the spinal cord injured. That there generally was less increase in catecholamines during FES for SCI individuals than during exercise for able-bodied individuals suggests that central command and somatic afferent feedback from muscles are important in their regulation (Kjaer et al. 1996). In another study, Wheeler and colleagues (1996) found that NE significantly increased with exercise in the able-bodied and spinal cord injured, although the individuals with SCI started and remained at lower levels. E levels were unchanged for both groups.

Renin

Renin, released in response to restricted blood flow to the kidneys, stimulates production of angiotensin and release of aldosterone from the adrenal cortex. **Aldosterone**, in turn, regulates sodium reabsorption, increases blood volume, and increases CO and BP. In the able-bodied, renin release increases progressively during exercise (McArdle et al. 1994). In SCI individuals, plasma renin increases during exercise (more during FES than during arm-crank ergometry) and continues to increase throughout recovery, while able-bodied controls exhibit a decline in renin levels after the termination of exercise. Trained SCI individuals have lower renin levels at rest than sedentary SCI individuals, suggesting that compensatory mechanisms can increase sympathetic nervous activity and thus increase plasma renin, which maintains blood pressure in individuals with SCI (Kjaer et al. 1996).

Cholesterol

In able-bodied persons, a direct relationship exists between **low-density lipoprotein** cholesterol (**LDL**) and coronary heart disease (CHD) (Galbo 1983), and an inverse relationship exists between **high-density lipoprotein** (**HDL**) and CHD (Kjaer, Perko, et al. 1994). Based on HDL levels, individuals with paraplegia are at 90% greater risk for CHD than controls and 350% greater risk than runners (Hardison et al. 1987). HDL increases as time since injury increases; even at its highest levels, however, SCI patients have some of the lowest HDL concentrations of any population (Brenes et al. 1986). Moderate upper-body conditioning may positively alter the lipid-lipoprotein profile of individuals with SCI (Hooker and Wells 1989); and in active individuals with paraplegia, overall profiles are within the normal range despite high levels of body fat. $\dot{V}O_2$max varies inversely with LDL levels and directly with HDL levels (Bostom et al. 1991). Male SCI athletes have higher total HDL and lower total cholesterol than sedentary SCI men, with HDL levels slightly below the mean for sedentary male controls (Brenes et al. 1986). Moderate activity can lead to decreases in total cholesterol and LDL, combined with increases in HDL, that can lower CHD risk more than 20% (Hooker and Wells 1989). As with able-bodied persons, aerobic fitness is clearly an important tool for CHD prevention in individuals with spinal cord injuries (see figure 15.5).

Metabolic Response

Individuals with spinal cord injuries often experience an initial drop in weight, followed by weight gain and decreases in energy expenditure and caloric requirements that are related to the level of injury and amount of deactivated muscle. In the early phases of rehabilitation, individuals with SCI need up to 54%

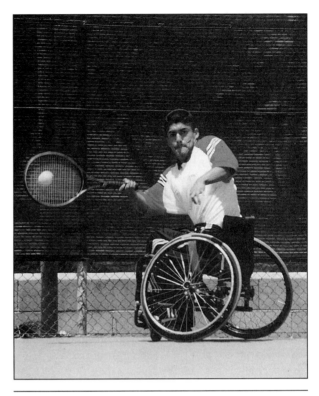

Figure 15.5 Ramon Cervantes of the Rancho Smashers wheelchair tennis team.
Courtesy of the Rancho Los Amigos Medical Center.

fewer calories than predicted by formulas for able-bodied persons (Cox et al. 1985). Energy expenditure in sedentary persons is largely determined by resting metabolic rate, which is an important factor in weight management. Exercise that increases muscle size and strength also increases activity of muscle fibers even at rest—thereby increasing resting metabolic rate and lean body mass. This higher metabolic rate increases energy expenditure and may help to decrease or prevent the weight and body fat gains often seen in individuals with SCI.

Cortical Adaptations to Physical Activity in Individuals With SCI

Depending on its level and severity, SCI results in moderate to profound loss of sensory, kinesthetic, and proprioceptive input to the brain and an equally profound loss of controlled motor activity. A growing body of research has demonstrated plasticity of the somatosensory cortex following deafferentation from peripheral injury (Cusick et al. 1990; Garraghty and Kaas 1991; Sanes et al. 1990), experimental or adventitious amputation (Kelahan and Doetsch 1984; Merzenich et al. 1984), or experimental or traumatic SCI (Casanova et al. 1991; Chau and McKinley 1991; Cohen et al. 1991). Brain reorganization also occurs following sustained peripheral stimulation (Jenkins et al. 1990; Recanzone et al. 1990) and learning (Recanzone et al. 1992; Recanzone et al. 1993). Merzenich and others (1984) found that after amputation of one or two digits in monkeys, adjacent cortical somatropic fields expanded over a period of months to years (Pons et al. 1991), filling in the deafferented areas. Similar findings have been reported in raccoons (Kelahan and Doetsch 1984) and in cats subsequent to experimental SCI (Casanova et al. 1991; Chau and McKinley 1991). Recent reports of chronic (up to 12 years) experimental deafferentation found that cortical reorganization is substantially more extensive than previously surmised and may indicate that reorganization occurs at subcortical levels (Pons et al. 1991; Ramachandran 1993; Ramachandran et al. 1992).

Transcranial magnetic stimulation and magnetoencephalography have provided corroborating evidence in amputees (Sica et al. 1984; Topka et al. 1991; Yang 1994) and in individuals with quadriplegia (Levy et al. 1990). Recently, magnetic field tomography revealed reorganization of somatosensory receptive fields to a more "normal" pattern following surgical separation of congenitally webbed fingers (Mogliner et al. 1993). Transcranial magnetic stimulation was used to map the motor cortex of four acute C5-6 individuals with SCI (6-17 days postinjury). Expanded cortical maps of the preserved contralateral biceps muscle were reported as early as six days postinjury (Streletz et al. 1995), indicating early motor reorganization. In contrast, focal transcranial magnetic stimulation was used to map motor cortical representations of the biceps brachii, deltoid, and triceps muscles in 12 control subjects, 5 subjects with complete cervical SCI, and 5 with incomplete cervical SCI. The authors tested both relaxed and gently contracted muscles, but did not find evidence for expanded motor cortical representations in the groups with spinal cord injuries (Brouwer and Hopkins-Rosseel 1997).

Perceptual and Cognitive Functioning

Though the accumulated data convincingly demonstrate that somatosensory cortical reorganization occurs following central deafferentation such as in SCI, and motor reorganization probably also occurs, we do not know if the reorganization alters processing of somatosensory or motor information. A few studies have measured electrophysiological correlates of arousal, perception, or cognition in SCI groups. Although inconclusive and methodologically questionable, relatively old studies of electroencephalographic (EEG) activity generally indicated a slowing of overall brain activity in SCI (Adey et al. 1968; Kaplan and Stearns 1949; Merlis and Watson 1949). Because EEG data were similar to those from sensory deprivation experiments, investigators concluded that individuals with SCI have decreased arousal (Zubek 1969). In an attempt to manipulate arousal level by altering incentive levels, Hester (1971) tested functionally complete individuals with SCI on a verbal serial coding task and a reaction time task. Although the SCI and control groups had similar error rates for any task/incentive combination, the SCI subjects had significantly slower performance speed. Because no measures of arousal were taken, it is unknown if the manipulation altered arousal.

More recent studies have attempted to directly assess perceptual and cognitive functioning in SCI. Using EEG measures, Richards and colleagues (1982) studied individuals with paraplegia and quadriplegia using an auditory vigilance task. EEG arousal states, measured during the vigilance task, were similar for controls and both experimental groups. Healthy persons with quadriplegia due to older injuries had superior vigilance performance and the sharpest auditory acuity. A follow-up study assessed auditory perception in outpatients with quadriplegia using a dichotic listening task while recording auditory evoked potentials and auditory thresholds. SCI subjects did not differ from controls on measures of auditory threshold or evoked potentials, but the SCI group was consistently more accurate than controls in aspects of the dichotic listening task. Because the SCI subjects were, in a sense, stimulus-starved (low brain arousal level), and thus more attentive to external stimuli, the investigators argued that the data reflected attention-motivational differences between able-bodied and SCI individuals (Richards et al. 1986).

Cohen and colleagues (1992) assessed attention-arousal mechanisms in persons with paraplegia and quadriplegia by manipulating intensity of auditory and visual stimuli while measuring the event-related potential (ERP) at the C3 and C4 cortical recording sites (primary sensorimotor areas). Overall, SCI groups had attenuated ERP amplitudes compared to a control group. Though the paraplegia and quadriplegia groups did not significantly differ from each other, the group with quadriplegia had a flatter ERP. The difference among groups was most evident in the P200 component, which is believed to reflect processing of stimulus intensity. Though SCI groups' ERPs were flatter, their P200s did differentiate stimulus intensities. To assure that the electrophysiological changes were due to processing and not transmission of the stimulus, the researchers studied brain auditory evoked response (BAER) in a group with paraplegia, a group with quadriplegia, and a control group. As predicted, no differences appeared in these near-field waves (Ament et al. 1995).

To replicate and extend the finding of attenuated ERPs and to assess the effect of SCI on selective attention, Cohen and colleagues (1996) used a tactile "oddball" paradigm to examine the P300 component of the ERP. All groups successfully maintained target counts and produced significantly larger P300 amplitudes with longer latencies to target versus nontarget trials. However, for all stimulus conditions, SCI groups had significantly attenuated P300s compared to the control group. In fact, in the group with quadriplegia, the response was virtually absent to nontarget stimuli—but even though the SCI groups had smaller P300 amplitudes, the amplitudes and latencies varied predictably with changes in stimulus qualities.

To summarize: signal transmission and recognition, as measured by BAER, are normal in SCI. Resting EEG appears to be lower in SCI than in control groups; but when measured during cognitive tasks, there are no group amplitude differences. Those with quadriplegia tend to perform better than controls on some tasks with higher cognitive demands. ERP data from various paradigms show a general reduction in several components, yet the ERP continues to differentiate task-related aspects of the experiments. The attenuation is related to level of injury, but not to the probability of a concomitant head injury or the concurrent use of CNS-active drugs.

Brain Metabolism

Recent positron emission tomography (PET) studies of motor and somatosensory reorganization further support the brain mapping and ERP studies. When moving a joystick with the affected arm, patients with acquired hemidystonia had significantly increased regional cerebral blood flow (rCBF) in the contralateral prefrontal premotor cortex, rostral supplementary motor area, bilateral sensorimotor cortex, insula, mesial parietal cortex, and ipsilateral cerebellum (Ceballos-Bauman et al. 1995). In a study of people with upper limb amputations—either adventitious (with prominent phantom limb symptoms) or congenital—Kew and colleagues (1994) reported that rCBF increased over a wider area in the trau-

matic amputee group. Following restitution of hand function in patients with hemiplegic subcortical strokes due to ischemic infarction of the basal ganglia or thalamus, rCBF showed larger activation areas for the motor and the sensory hand areas contralateral to the affected hand (Weder et al. 1994).

Though the degree of central deafferentation and loss of motor control are much greater in SCI than in virtually any other deafferentating injury or disease, only one recent PET study (Roelcke et al. 1997) has used modern brain imaging methodology to investigate the subject. Four individuals with complete quadriplegia, seven with complete paraplegia, and twelve control subjects had glucose metabolic PET scans following a period of rest. Global glucose metabolic activity was lower in the SCI subjects. Statistical parametric mapping (SPM) determined that SCI subjects had relatively increased metabolic activity in the supplemental motor area, putamen, and anterior cingulate, compared to the rest of the brain; and relatively decreased activity in the midbrain, cerebellar hemispheres, and temporal cortex. The authors concluded that the lower overall metabolic activity represented cerebral deafferentation due to the SCI, while the relative increases in secondary motor areas might be related to secondary disinhibition in these regions.

Cohen et al. (submitted for review) conducted two PET experiments to determine regional cerebral glucose metabolism of chronic SCI subjects. Experiment I tested individuals with paraplegia during a finger-tapping task, while Experiment II measured those with quadriplegia during a continuous performance task. Images were analyzed with statistical parametric mapping (SPM 96). Compared to the controls, the group with paraplegia had relatively increased metabolism in the spinocerebellum and in the superior parietal lobes, but decreased relative metabolism in the frontal lobes and in the somatosensory and sensorimotor motor cortex in the area controlling the hand, fingers, wrist, and head.

Results from Experiment II revealed that the group with quadriplegia, compared to its control group, had higher relative metabolism in visual association areas and in cortices subserving sensation and motor control of the body areas disconnected from the brain. Areas of decreased relative activity included cortices controlling language, cognitive, and somatomotor functions in areas that could be sensed and controlled. These results may stem from alterations of normal feed-forward and feedback control of neural mechanisms; or they may reflect motor systems executing overlearned, overused movements.

Several recent experiments with finger tapping by able-bodied individuals, with either PET or functional magnetic resonance imaging (fMRI) dependent variables, reported high metabolic activity in the contralateral primary sensorimotor cortex in the vicinity representing the hand (Blinkenberg et al. 1996; Boecker et al. 1994; VanGelderen et al. 1995; Yang et al. 1994). Lower metabolic activity in the relevant contralateral primary motor cortex, along with some increased activity in the spinocerebellum, is indicative of brain activity seen with overpracticed motor responses or with recovery of motor function following a CNS injury. Ghez and Fahn (1981) stated that the cerebellum appears to be involved in compensating for injury to the motor system and in learning new motor programs. Evarts (1980) suggested that motor reorganization following brain injury probably depends on adaptive modification of input-output relationships in the cerebellum. It might also be argued that subjects with paraplegia and quadriplegia "overlearn" responses from their sentient motor areas. For example, those with paraplegia use hands and arms for functions usually performed by legs and feet; and those with quadriplegia use head and neck movement for writing, control of wheelchairs, and other activities of daily living. These "overlearned" motor behaviors require less cortical control and more guidance by the cerebellum.

Another interesting finding in SCI was increased metabolic activity in the superior parietal lobe, an area involved in body image and body orientation in space. There are anecdotal reports that persons with SCI may have a distorted body image, though the psychological meaning of this increased activity is unclear.

Using Motor Imagery Techniques to Improve Muscle Strength and Motor Performance in Individuals With SCI

There are many well-documented alterations in the musculoskeletal and cortical sensorimotor systems following spinal cord injury. Structured physical activity appears to mitigate some of those alterations, so that an individual with SCI may regain some motor function, increase physical fitness, and decrease risk for secondary impairments such as cardiovascular disease. Structured physical activity is often impossible immediately following an injury, however, because of pain, skeletal instability, or muscular dysfunction.

There is a growing belief that alternative forms of motor rehabilitation used immediately postinjury can prevent loss of muscle strength and function. Decety and Ingvar (1990) suggest that motor imagery may facilitate the recovery of functional motor activity when physical practice is difficult, painful, or cannot be carried out during motor rehabilitation.

Neurological Adaptations to Strength Training

Although the objective of rehabilitation in individuals with incomplete injuries is to partially restore the strength of muscles below the injury zone, there are also immediate and profound decreases in EMG activity and muscle fiber cross-sectional area that occur in functioning limbs that are immobilized during bed rest (Fournier et al. 1983). The rapid reduction in muscle strength results in a loss of functional capacity and may extend the duration of recovery from injury. Such individuals should initiate resistance training as soon as possible after injury to minimize the loss of muscle strength and to begin functional rehabilitation.

Normal improvements in muscle strength from resistance training arise from interaction of several factors—neural (e.g., motor unit recruitment, discharge rate, intermuscular coordination), mechanical (e.g., moment-arm), and muscular (e.g., muscle length and cross-sectional area) (Enoka 1994). Neural adaptations effect initial improvements in muscle strength, while changes in muscle mass bring about later increases (Sale 1988). While a complete description of the neural adaptations responsible for the initial increase in muscle strength is not yet available, some of the potential mechanisms include

- improved intermuscular coordination (Rutherford and Jones 1986),
- decreased coactivation of agonist/antagonist muscles (Carolan and Cafarelli 1992), and
- increased synchronization of single motor units (Milner-Brown et al. 1973).

Muscular adaptations include muscle hypertrophy, hyperplasia, and an increase in specific tension (i.e., force that a muscle can produce per cross-sectional area). Hormonal, metabolic, and mechanical factors mediate these changes. Perhaps the most revealing evidence that initial increases in muscle strength are primarily neural is from Yue and Cole (1992), who found that imagined muscle contractions alone increased maximum muscle strength 22% over a four-week period. Contrast this gain with a 30% increase among subjects who performed actual muscle contractions, and

3% in controls who did not train. Based on this evidence, we can speculate that individuals with SCI who have incomplete injuries may increase or maintain muscle strength by performing imagined muscle contractions during physical rehabilitation.

Motor Imagery

Psychologists and sport coaches use **motor imagery** techniques in training athletes to perform highly skilled movements (Suinn 1984); therapists rarely use them for physical rehabilitation following SCI (Decety and Boisson 1990). Motor imagery refers to the systematic and repeated inner rehearsal of a movement without any associated muscular activity. A large number of studies support the effectiveness of mental imagery for improving motor performance (Feltz and Landers 1983; Kohl and Roenker 1980). Although it's possible that the beneficial effects of imagery arise from motivational factors that increase the overall arousal of the performer (Paivio 1986), they are more likely due to adaptations of the neural mechanisms involved in movement (Finke 1979; Johnson 1982). Recent theories of action attribute a central role to imagery during the initiation and direction of higher order action plans, which in turn control motor activity (Gopher 1984; Kelso and Wallace 1978).

The neural basis for the effects of imagery on motor performance remains hypothetical. One possibility is that efferent discharges produced during imagery prime descending motor pathways (Jeannerod 1994). There is some evidence that imagery activates muscle at a low level (Jeannerod and Mouret 1962; Shaw 1938; Shaw 1940); other research, however, failed to observe any muscle activity during imagery (Decety et al. 1993; Yue and Cole 1992). Mellah et al. (1990) found that a small proportion of low-threshold biceps motor units in monkeys are active during the preparation period for arm flexion, but stop firing just prior to movement. The motor units apparently increase the stiffness of the muscle prior to the movement command. It is possible that motor imagery activates these low-threshold motor units, which are difficult to detect using surface electrodes.

Decety and colleagues (1994) used PET to examine brain activation in subjects imagining the performance of a grasping task. They observed activation at the cortical level in the inferior part of the frontal gyrus, the prefrontal areas (areas 9, 8, and 46), and the anterior cingulate cortex; and at the subcortical level in the basal ganglia and cerebellum. Each of these areas is normally associated with motor behavior. These data support previous research, which shows that motor learning during mental practice

involves rehearsal of neural pathways related to the cognitive stages of motor control (Decety et al. 1991; Yue and Cole 1992). Despite the well-known effects of motor imagery on motor performance, no one has yet studied motor imagery in SCI patients or as a general technique for rehabilitation (Decety and Boisson 1990).

Cortical areas activated during visual imagery are similar to those activated during visual perception (Goldenberg, Podreka, Steiner et al. 1989; Goldenberg, Podreka, Uhl et al. 1989; Roland and Friberg 1985). It is possible that motor imagery activates cortical areas normally associated with motor preparation (Jeannerod 1994). Using PET, fMRI, and measurements of rCBF, researchers have observed cortical activation during movement preparation in the supplementary motor area (SMA) (Colebatch et al. 1991; Evarts 1984; Fox and Hitchcock 1987; Roland 1984; Roland et al. 1980), primary motor cortex (Kim et al. 1993; Grafton et al. 1991), Rolandic region (Roland et al. 1980), contralateral sensorimotor areas, ipsilateral sensorimotor areas, medial frontal cortex (Hallett et al. 1994), cerebellum (Decety et al. 1990), and basal ganglia (Roland et al. 1982); while imagery activates the SMA (Roland 1984; Roland et al. 1980; Fox and Hitchcock 1987), premotor cortex, and posterior inferior premotor area (Fox and Hitchcock 1987). Rao et al. (1993) used fMRI to examine activation during the performance and imagination of simple and complex finger movements. They found that both conditions activated the SMA and the premotor cortex. Eccles (1982) suggested that the SMA may act as an interface between concept formation and motor execution.

It appears that cortical activation during motor imagery is related to task constraints, with no-choice and multiple-choice conditions activating different regions (Deiber et al. 1991), simple and sequential movements producing different levels of activation (Shibasaki 1993), and larger muscles being activated more than smaller muscles (Colebatch et al. 1991). The differences are likely due to the amount of motor preparation required to perform tasks of varying complexity and effort.

Together, these findings suggest that motor imagery and motor preparation share common neural substrates and may be functionally equivalent (Jeannerod 1994). Consequently, motor imagery may be effective for organizing neural activity to produce skilled movements. If so, rehabilitation of SCI patients should combine motor imagery with physical practice to re-activate cortical motor circuits following injury.

Motor imagery produces changes in heart and respiratory rates as well as in cortical activation. Decety et al. (1991) and Wang and Morgan (1992) observed increases in heart and respiratory rates compared with resting levels in able-bodied subjects performing motor imagery tasks such as running on a treadmill or pedaling a bicycle ergometer. No muscle activity accompanied these changes. Autonomic responses such as increased heart and respiratory rate in the absence of muscular work can only be attributed to a central influence similar to that observed during motor preparation (Jeannerod 1994).

Although stimulation of the brain stem of paralyzed animals induces fictive locomotion that leads to increased heart rate (Eldridge et al. 1985), no one has yet verified changes in heart and respiratory rates accompanying motor preparation in SCI (Jeannerod 1994). The correlation of autonomic responses with both motor imagery and motor preparation suggests that these responses, in addition to changes in cortical activation detected with EEG, may be used as indicators of motor imagery performance in individuals with SCI.

Imagined Strength Training for Individuals With SCI

In addition to activating various cortical and subcortical regions, motor imagery appears to modulate spinal excitability and may lead to increases in maximum strength. Kiers et al. (1997) observed mild increases in H-reflex amplitude in subjects who were mentally simulating the performance of a hand movement; Bonnet et al. (1997) found large increases in H-reflex amplitude during imagined performance of a foot press. The amplitude of the H-reflex in each of these studies is greater than at rest, but not as great as during actual movement. There is other evidence, however, that the amplitude of the H-reflex remains unchanged during mental simulation of movement relative to rest (Kasai et al. 1997; Yahagi et al. 1996). While the question of spinal excitability during imagery remains equivocal, there is some reason to believe that mental simulation of movement activates spinal circuits in addition to various cortical and subcortical regions.

Perhaps the most compelling evidence for the use of motor imagery to increase muscle strength comes from a study by Yue and Cole (1992). Subjects trained their hypothenar muscles five days per week for four weeks by repeatedly performing maximal static muscle contractions. One group actually performed the maximal static contractions, while a second group only imagined performing the contractions. A third group served as a control and did not exercise the hypothenar muscle. No groups exhibited changes in

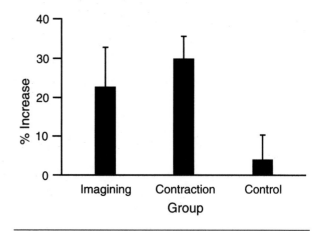

Figure 15.6 Mean and standard deviation of percentage increases of left 5th finger abduction force of each group.
Reprinted, by permission, from G. Yue and K.J. Cole, 1992, "Strength increases from the motor program: comparison of training with maximal voluntary and imagined muscle contractions," *Journal of Neurophysiology* 67:1117.

the electrically evoked abduction twitch force of the hypothenar muscle, indicating an absence of muscle hypertrophy. Mean abduction force, however, increased 30% for the contraction group, 22% for the imagined contraction group, and 3% for the control group (see figure 15.6). Yue and Cole believe the increase in abduction force without a concomitant increase in twitch force can be explained by changes in central motor programming/planning. This finding is consistent with existing literature that attributes initial gains in strength during a strength training program to various neural adaptations.

We recently asked subjects to perform a series of submaximal static muscle contractions using a hand dynamometer (Romero et al. 1998). We factorially combined two levels of peak force (PF) (PF > 60% MVC, and PF < 10% MVC) with two levels of TPF, or time to peak force (TPF > 500 msec, and TPF < 200 msec), to yield four unique force-time profiles. Subjects repeatedly performed or imagined performing muscle contractions with each of the profiles, and we used the results to determine whether cortical activation was similar during actual and imagined muscle contractions. We measured cortical activation by recording event-related potentials from the primary and supplementary motor areas, and measured muscle activation using integrated EMG from the flexor digitorum longus. The cross-correlation of the average ERP during rapid high force movements and imagined high force movements was 0.78 at the FCz recording site (primarily supplementary motor area). The cross-correlations between the actual and imagined movements ranged from 0.95 to 0.98 for the remaining force-time profiles. The cross-correlation

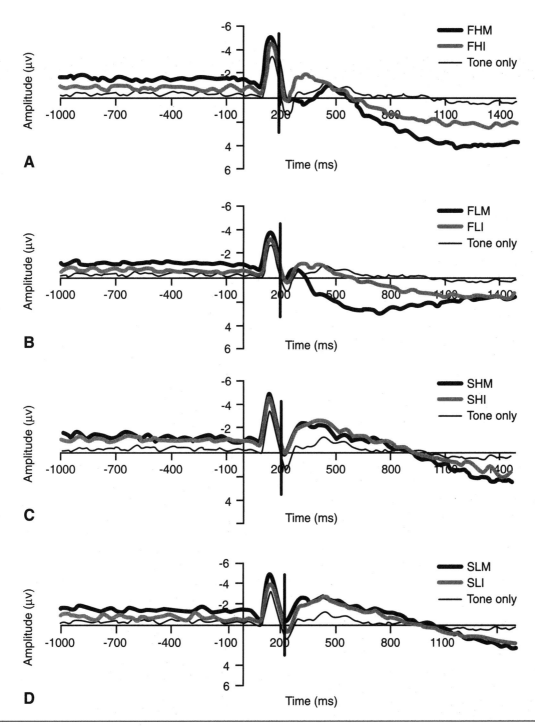

Figure 15.7   ERPs averaged across subjects for all experimental conditions vs. tone only: (A) fast-high condition; (B) fast-low condition; (C) slow-high condition; (D) slow-low condition. Abbreviations: F = fast; S = slow; H = high force; L = low force; M = movement; I = imagery. Reprinted, by permission, from D. Romero et al., 1998, "Event-related potentials during executed and imagined sub-maximal isometric muscle contractions," *Journal of Sport and Exercise Psychology* 20 (Supplement):539.

between all imagery conditions and a tone-only control condition ranged from 0.72 to 0.82. In general, the ERP profiles recorded from the supplementary motor area during the performance of actual and imagined movements were nearly indistinguishable (see figure 15.7).

Although the data are limited, it appears that an imagined static muscle contraction activates the supplementary motor area in a manner similar to when movements are actually performed, and that imagined muscle contractions can lead to increased muscle strength over a four-week training period. These findings are significant for the rehabilitation of nonparalyzed muscles in patients with SCI who are unable to physically practice because of pain or dysfunction. It is possible that a training program consisting only of imagined muscle contractions could successfully maintain muscle strength when limbs are temporarily paralyzed or immobilized (Decety and Ingvar 1990).

Summary

This chapter provides an overview of the many neuromusculoskeletal, cardiovascular, hormonal, and metabolic changes that result from SCI, as well as the potential benefits of physical activity for mitigating some of these changes. While active exercise is likely to provide the most profound improvements in function, individuals with SCI must take several precautions when exercising (see "Precautions Specific to Exercise and Individuals With SCI," below). Other modalities (e.g., electrical stimulation) and training techniques (e.g., motor imagery) are likely to become effective adjuncts to active exercise, particularly during the acute phase of rehabilitation. Future rehabilitation strategies for individuals with SCI will probably involve a combination of physical exercise, electrical stimulation, and mental rehearsal of movement, along with various pharmacological agents.

Acknowledgments

The authors recognize the contributions of Dr. Barry Lavay, California State University, Long Beach, for reviewing earlier drafts of the manuscript; the Kinesiotherapy Department at the Veterans Affairs Medical Center, Long Beach, for providing information about their rehabilitation program and protocols; and Lisa Hilborn and the Rancho Los Amigos Wheelchair Sports Program of Downey, CA, for providing photographs of athletes in wheelchairs. This project was partially funded by a Department of Veterans Affairs medical research grant to Dr. Michael Cohen and Dr. Michael Lacourse.

Precautions Specific to Exercise and Individuals With SCI

1. Temperature regulation problems may occur due to high thermal stress of upper-body exercises, lack of sweat response below lesion level, and lack of heart rate compensation during steady-state activity.

2. The restricted ability to exercise at moderate- to high-intensity levels (due to reliance on smaller muscle groups of the upper body) may be further inhibited by local muscle fatigue.

3. Decreased cardiac output (because of reduced cardiac efficiency and decreased venous return) reduces the amount of oxygen available to active muscles and may limit duration and intensity of exercise.

4. Because of their decreased sympathetic nervous system response, limited cardiovascular adaptation to exercise prevents most active individuals with SCI from achieving fitness levels beyond those of sedentary able-bodied persons.

5. Exercise may cause an abnormal decrease in systolic blood pressure in individuals with quadriplegia.

6. Autonomic dysreflexia may occur during electrical stimulation exercises.

7. Individuals with SCI do not exhibit the necessary cardiovascular and respiratory changes just prior to and at the onset of exercise that allow prompt removal of lactic acid. Therefore lactic acid buildup may limit duration and intensity of activity.

8. Clinicians administering FES should be especially careful while preparing SCI patients—because these individuals cannot feel pain or discomfort from incorrect electrode application, they are more easily wounded in regions below the lesion level.

In general, exercise programs for individuals with SCI should be similar to those of severely deconditioned able-bodied people—activity should begin at a very low intensity and progress by small increments.

References

Abramson, A.S., and E.F. Delagi. 1961. Influence of weight-bearing and muscle contraction on disuse osteoporosis. *Arch Phys Med Rehab* 42:147-51.

Adey, W.R., E. Bors, and R.W. Porter. 1968. EEG sleep patterns after high cervical lesions in man. *Arch Neurol* 19:337-83.

Ament, P.A., M.J. Cohen, S.L. Schandler, M. Sowa, and M. Vulpe. 1995. Auditory P3 event related potentials (ERP) and brainstem auditory evoked responses (BAER) after spinal cord injury in humans. *J Spinal Cord Med* 18:208-15.

Ashley, E.A., J.J. Laskin, L.M. Olenik, R. Burnham, R.D. Steadward, D.C. Cumming, and G.D. Wheeler. 1993. Evidence of autonomic dysreflexia during FES in individuals with SCI. *Paraplegia* 31:593-605.

Åstrand, P.O., and K. Rodahl. 1977. *Textbook of work physiology: Physiological bases of exercise.* 2d ed. New York: McGraw-Hill.

Blinkenberg, M., C. Bonde, S. Holm, C. Svarer, J. Anderssen, O.B. Paulson, and I. Law. 1996. Rate dependence of regional cerebral activation during performance of a repetitive motor task: a PET study. *J Cereb Blood Flow Metab* 16:794-803.

Boecker, H., A. Kleinschmidt, M. Requardt, W. Hanicke, K.D. Merboldt, and J. Frahm. 1994. Functional cooperativity of human cortical motor areas during self-paced simple finger movements. A high resolution MRI study. *Brain* 117:1231-9.

Bonnet, M., J. Decety, M. Jeannerod, and J. Requin. 1997. Mental simulation of action modulates the excitability of spinal reflex pathways in man. *Brain Res Cogn Brain Res* 5:221-8.

Borgens, R.B., E. Reoderer, and M.J. Cohen. 1981. Enhanced spinal cord regeneration in lamprey by applied electric fields. *Science* 213:611-7.

Bostom, A.G., M.M. Toner, W.D. McArdle, T. Montelione, C.D. Brown, and R.A. Stein. 1991. Lipid and lipoprotein profiles relate to peak aerobic power in SCI men. *Med Sci Sports Exerc* 23:49-54.

Bremner, L.A., K.E. Sloan, R.E. Day, E.R. Scull, and T. Ackland. 1992. A clinical exercise system for paraplegics using FES. *Paraplegia* 30:647-55.

Brenes, G., S. Dearwater, R. Shapera, R.E. LaPorte, and E. Collins. 1986. High density lipoprotein cholesterol concentrations in physically active and sedentary SCI persons. *Arch Phys Med Rehab* 67:445-50.

Brouwer, B., and D.H. Hopkins-Rosseel. 1997. Motor cortical mapping of proximal upper extremity muscles following spinal cord injury. *Spinal Cord* 35:205-12.

Brown, M.D., M.E. Cotter, H.W. Standte, and G. Vrbova. 1976. The effects of different patterns of muscle activity on capillary density, mechanical properties and structure of slow and fast rabbit muscles. *Pflugers Arch* 361:241-50.

Burkett, L.N., J. Chisum, W. Stone, and B. Fernhall. 1990. Exercise capacity of untrained SCI individuals and the relationship of peak oxygen uptake to level of injury. *Paraplegia* 28:512-21.

Burstein, R., G. Zeilig, M. Royburt, Y. Epstein, and A. Ohry. 1996. Insulin resistance in paraplegics—effect of one bout of acute exercise. *Int J Sports Med* 17:272-6.

Carolan, B., and E. Cafarelli. 1992. Adaptations in coactivation after isometric resistance training. *J Appl Physiol* 73:911-7.

Casanova, C., P.A. McKinley, and S. Molotchnikoff. 1991. Responsiveness of reorganized primary somatosensory (SI) cortex in chronic spinal cats. *Somatosens Mot Res* 8:65-76.

Ceballos-Bauman, A.O., R.E. Passingham, C.D. Marsden, and D.J. Brook. 1995. Motor reorganization in acquired hemidystonia. *Ann Neurol* 37:746-57.

Chantraine, A., B. Nusgens, and C.M. Lapiere. 1986. Bone remodeling during the development of osteoporosis in paraplegia. *Calcif Tissue Int* 38:323-7.

Chau, C.W., and P.A. McKinley. 1991. Chronological observations of primary somatosensory cortical maps in kittens following low thoracic (T12) spinal cord transection at 2 weeks of age. *Somatosens Mot Res* 8:355-76.

Claus-Walker, J., R.J. Campos, R.E. Carter, C. Vallbona, and H.S. Lipscomb. 1972. Calcium excretion in quadriplegia. *Arch Phys Med Rehab* 53:14-20, 37.

Claus-Walker, J., J. Singh, C.S. Leach, D.V. Hatton, C.W. Hubert, and N. DiFerrante. 1977. The urinary excretion of collagen degradation products by quadriplegic patients and during weightlessness. *J Bone Joint Surg* 59:209-12.

Cohen, L.G., H. Topka, R.A. Cole, and M. Hallett. 1991. Leg paresthesias induced by magnetic brain stimulation in patients with thoracic spinal cord injury. *Neurology* 41:1283-8.

Cohen, M.J., P.A. Ament, S.L. Schandler, and M. Vulpe. 1996. Changes in the P300 component of the tactile event related potential due to spinal cord injury. *Paraplegia* 34:107-12.

Cohen, M.J., R.J. Haier, M.G. Lacourse, R.R. Young, and J.H. Fallon. Submitted for review. Regional cerebral glucose metabolic activity in spinal cord injured humans during motor and cognitive tasks. *Somatosens Mot Res*.

Cohen, M.J., S.L. Schandler, and M. Vulpe. 1992. Event-related potentials during orienting to auditory and visual stimulation in spinal cord injured humans. *Paraplegia* 30:864-71.

Colebatch, J.G., M.P. Deiber, R.E. Passingham, K.J. Friston, and R.S. Frackowiak. 1991. Regional cerebral blood flow during voluntary arm and hand movements in human subjects. *J Neurophysiol* 65:1392-1401.

Comarr, A.E., and I. Eltorai. 1995. Autonomic dysreflexia/hyperreflexia. *J Spinal Cord Med* 20:345-52.

Cox, S.A.R., S.M. Weiss, E.A. Posuniak, P. Worthington, M. Prioleau, and G. Heffley. 1985. Energy expenditure after SCI: an evaluation of stable rehabilitating patients. *J Trauma* 25:419-23.

Cusick, C.G., J.T. Wall, J.H. Whiting Jr., and R.G. Wiley. 1990. Temporal progression of cortical reorganization following nerve injury. *Brain Res* 537:355-8.

Daly, J.J., B. Marsolais, L.M. Mendell, W.Z. Rymer, A. Stefanovska, J.R. Wolpaw, and C. Kantor. 1996. Therapeutic neural effects of electrical stimulation. *IEEE Trans Rehab Eng* 4:218-30.

Davis, G.M. 1993. Exercise capacity of individuals with paraplegia. *Med Sci Sports Exerc* 25:423-432.

Davis, G.M., P.R. Kofsky, J.C. Kelsey, and R.J. Shepard. 1981. Cardiorespiratory fitness and muscular strength of wheelchair users. *Can Med Assoc J* 125:1313-23.

Davis, G.M., F.J. Servedio, R.M. Glaser, S.C. Gupta, and A.G. Suryaprasad. 1990. Cardiovascular responses to arm cranking and FNS-induced leg exercise in paraplegics. *J Appl Physiol* 69:671-7.

Davis, G.M., and R.J. Shephard. 1988. Cardiorespiratory fitness in highly active versus inactive paraplegics. *Med Sci Sports Exerc* 20:463-8.

Davis, G.M., and R.J. Shephard. 1990. Strength training for wheelchair users. *Br J Sports Med* 24:25-30.

Davis, G.M., S. Tupling, and R.J. Shephard. 1986. Dynamic strength and physical activity in wheelchair users. In *Sports and disabled athletes*, ed. C. Sherrill. Champaign, IL: Human Kinetics.

Dearwater, S.R., R.E. LaPorte, R.J. Robertson, G. Brenes, L.L. Adams, and D. Becker. 1986. Activity in the SCI patient: an epidemiologic analysis of metabolic parameters. *Med Sci Sports Exerc* 18:541-4.

Decety, J., and D. Boisson. 1990. Effect of brain and spinal cord injuries on motor imagery. *Eur Arch Psychiatry Neurol Sci* 240:39-43.

Decety, J., and D.H. Ingvar. 1990. Brain structures participating in mental stimulation of motor behavior: a neuropsychological interpretation. *Acta Psychol* 73:13-34.

Decety, J., M. Jeannerod, D. Durozard, and G. Baverel. 1993. Central activation of autonomic effectors during mental simulation of motor actions in man. *J Physiol* 461:549-63.

Decety, J., M. Jeannerod, M. Germain, and J. Pastene. 1991. Vegetative response during imagined movement is proportional to mental effort. *Behav Brain Res* 42:1-5.

Decety, J., D. Perani, M. Jeannerod, V. Bettinardi, B. Tadary, R. Woods, J.C. Mazziotta, and F. Fazio. 1994. Mapping motor representations with positron emission tomography. *Nature* 371:600-2.

Decety, J., H. Sjoholm, E. Ryding, G. Stenberg, and D.H. Ingvar. 1990. The cerebellum participates in mental activity: tomographic measurements of regional cerebral blood flow. *Brain Res* 535:313-7.

Deiber, M.P., R.E. Passingham, J.G. Colebatch, K.J. Friston, P.D. Nixon, and R.S. Frackowiak. 1991. Cortical areas and the selection of movement: a study with positron emission tomography. *Exp Brain Res* 84:393-402.

Donaldson, C.L., S.B. Hulley, J.M. Vogel, R.S. Hattner, J.H. Bayers, and D.E. McMillan. 1970. Effect of prolonged bed rest on bone mineral. *Metabolism* 19:1071-84.

Drory, Y., A. Ohry, M.E. Brooks, D. Dolphin, and J.J. Kellermann. 1990. Arm crank ergometry in chronic SCI patients. *Arch Phys Med Rehab* 71:389-92.

Eccles, J.C. 1982. The initiation of voluntary movements by the supplementary motor area. *Arch Psychiatr Neurol Sci* 231:423-41.

Eldridge, F.L., D.E. Millhorn, J.P. Kiley, and T.G. Waldrop. 1985. Stimulation by central command of locomotion, respiration, and circulation during exercise. *Respir Physiol* 59:313-37.

Enoka, R.M. 1994. *Neuromechanical basis of kinesiology.* Champaign, IL: Human Kinetics.

Evarts, E.V. 1980. Brain control of movement: possible mechanisms of function. In *Recovery of function: Theoretical considerations for brain injury rehabilitation*, ed. P. Bach-y-Rita. Bern, Switzerland: Hans Huber.

Evarts, E.V. 1984. Hierarchies and emergent features in motor control. In *Dynamic aspects of neocortical function*, ed. G.M. Edelman, W.E. Gall, and W.M. Cowan. New York: Wiley.

Faghri, P.D., R.M. Glaser, and S.F. Figoni. 1992. FES leg cycle ergometer exercise: training effects on cardiorespiratory responses of SCI subjects at rest and during submaximal exercise. *Arch Phys Med Rehab* 73:1085-93.

Feltz, D.L., and D.M. Landers. 1983. The effects of mental practice on motor skill learning and performance: a meta-analysis. *J Sport Psychol* 5:25-57.

Figoni, S.F. 1993. Exercise responses and quadriplegia. *Med Sci Sports Exerc* 25:433-41.

Figoni, S.F., R.A. Boileau, B.H. Massey, and J.R. Larsen. 1988. Physiological responses of quadriplegic and able-bodied men during exercise at the same VO_2. *Adapt Phys Act Q* 5:130-9.

Finke, R.A. 1979. The functional equivalence of mental images and errors of movement. *Cognit Psychol* 11:235-64.

Fournier, M., R.R. Roy, H. Perham, C.P. Simard, and V.R. Edgerton. 1983. Is limb immobilization a model of muscle disuse? *Exp Neurol* 80:147-56.

Fox, J.E., and E.R. Hitchcock. 1987. F wave size as a monitor of motor neuron excitability: the effect of deafferentation. *J Neurol Neurosurg Psychiatry* 50:453-9.

Galbo, H. 1983. *Hormonal and metabolic adaptation to exercise.* New York: Thieme-Stratton.

Garland, D.E., C.A. Stewart, R.H. Adkins, S.S. Hu, C. Rosen, F.J. Liotta, and D.A. Weinstein. 1992. Osteoporosis after spinal cord injury. *J Orthop Res* 10:371-80.

Garraghty, P.E., and J.H. Kaas. 1991. Large-scale functional reorganization in adult monkey cortex after peripheral injury. *Proc Natl Acad Sci* 88:6976-80.

Gass, G.C., and E.M. Camp. 1979. Physiological characteristics of trained paraplegic and tetraplegic subjects. *Med Sci Sports* 11:256-65.

Ghez, C., and S. Fahn. 1981. The cerebellum. In *Principles of neural sciences*, ed. E.R. Kandel and J.H. Schwartz. New York: Elsevier/North-Holland.

Gibson, J.N.A., W.L. Morrison, C.M. Serimgeour, K. Smith, P.J. Stoward, and M.J. Rennie. 1989. Effects of therapeutic percutaneous electrical stimulation of atrophic human quadriceps on muscle composition, protein synthesis and contractile properties. *Eur J Clin Invest* 19:206-12.

Glaser, R.M. 1994. Functional neuromuscular stimulation. Exercise conditioning of SCI patients. *Int J Sports Med* 15:142-8.

Goldenberg, G., I. Podreka, M. Steiner, K. Willmes, E. Suess, and L. Deecke. 1989. Regional cerebral blood flow patterns in visual imagery. *Neuropsychologia* 27:641-64.

Goldenberg, G., I. Podreka, F. Uhl, M. Steiner, K. Willmes, and L. Deeke. 1989. Cerebral correlates of imagining colours, faces and a map—I. SPECT of regional cerebral blood flow. *Neuropsychologia* 27:1315-28.

Gopher, D. 1984. The contribution of vision-based imagery to the acquisition and operation of a transcription skill. In *Handbook of physiology: The nervous system,* ed. V.B. Brooks and M.D. Bethesda. Berlin: Springer-Verlag.

Grafton, S.T., R.P. Woods, J.C. Mazziotta, and M.E. Phelps. 1991. Somatotopic mapping of the primary motor cortex in humans: activation studies with cerebral blood flow and positron emission tomography. *J Neurophysiol* 66:735-43.

Grimby, G. 1980. Aerobic capacity, muscle strength, and fiber composition in young paraplegics. In *First international medical congress on sports for the disabled,* ed. H. Natvig. Oslo: Royal Ministry for Church and Education.

Grimby, G., C. Broberg, I. Krotiewska, and M. Krotiewski. 1976. Muscle fiber composition in patients with traumatic cord lesion. *Scand J Rehabil Med* 8:37-42.

Guttmann, L. 1976. *Spinal cord injuries: Comprehensive management and research.* 2d ed. London: Blackwell Scientific.

Hallett, M., R.M. Dubinsky, T. Zeffiro, and S.M. Bierner. 1994. Comparison of glucose metabolism and cerebral blood flow during cortical motor activation. *J Neuroimaging* 4:1-5.

Hangartner, T.N., M.M. Rodgers, R.M. Glaser, and P.S. Barre. 1994. Tibial bone density loss in SCI patients: effects of FES exercise. *J Rehabil Res Dev* 31:50-61.

Hardison, G.R. Jr., R.G. Israel, and G.W. Somes. 1987. Physiological responses to different cranking rates during submaximal arm ergometry in paraplegic males. *Adapt Phys Act Q* 4:95-105.

Hester, G.A. 1971. Effects of functional transection of spinal cord on task performance under varied emotional conditions. *Psychophysiology* 8:451-61.

Hoffman, M.D. 1986. Cardiorespiratory fitness and training in quadriplegics and paraplegics. *Sports Med* 3:312-30.

Hooker, S.P., S.F. Figoni, R.M. Glaser, M.M. Rodgers, B.N. Ezenwa, and P.D. Faghri. 1990. Physiologic responses to prolonged electrically stimulated leg-cycle exercise in the SCI. *Arch Phys Med Rehab* 71:863-9.

Hooker, S.P., S.F. Figoni, M.M. Rodgers, R.M. Glaser, T. Mathews, A.G. Suryaprasad, and S.C. Gupta. 1992a. Metabolic and hemodynamic responses to concurrent voluntary arm crank and electrical stimulation leg cycle exercise in quadriplegics. *J Rehabil Res Dev* 29:1-11.

Hooker, S.P., S.F. Figoni, M.M. Rodgers, R.M. Glaser, T. Mathews, A.G. Suryaprasad, and S.C. Gupta. 1992b. Physiologic effects of electrical stimulation leg cycle exercise training in SCI persons. *Arch Phys Med Rehab* 73:470-6.

Hooker, S.P., and C.L. Wells. 1989. Effects of low- and moderate-intensity training in spinal cord-injured persons. *Med Sci Sports Exerc* 21:18-22.

Hopman, M.T.E., B. Oeseburg, and R.A. Binkhorst. 1993. Cardiovascular responses in persons with paraplegia to prolonged arm exercise and thermal stress. *Med Sci Sports Exerc* 25:577-83.

Jeannerod, M. 1994. The representing brain: neural correlates of motor intention and imagery. *Behav Brain Sci* 17:187-245.

Jeannerod, M., and J. Mouret. 1962. Etude des mouvements oculaires observés chez l'homme au cours de la veille et du sommeil. *Comptes Rendus de la Société de Biologie* 156:1407-10.

Jenkins, W.M., M.M. Merzenich, M.T. Ochs, T. Allard, and E. Guic-Robles. 1990. Functional reorganization of primary somatosensory cortex in adult owl monkeys after behaviorally controlled tactile stimulation. *J Neurophysiol* 63:82-104.

Johnson, P. 1982. The functional equivalence of imagery and movement. *Q J Exp Psychol* 34:349-65.

Kaplan, L.I., and E. Stearns. 1949. Electroencephalographic studies in spinal cord disease. *Arch Neurol Psychiatr* 62:293-303.

Kaplan, P.E., B. Gandhavadi, L. Richards, and J. Goldschmidt. 1978. Calcium balance in paraplegic patients: influence of injury duration and ambulation. *Arch Phys Med Rehab* 59:447-50.

Kaplan, P.E., W. Roden, E. Gilbert, L. Richards, and J.W. Goldschmidt. 1981. Reduction of hypercalciuria in tetraplegia after weight-bearing and strengthening exercises. *Paraplegia* 19:289-93.

Kasai, T., S. Kawai, M. Kawanishi, and S. Yahagi. 1997. Evidence for facilitation of motor evoked potentials (MEPs) induced by motor imagery. *Brain Res* 744:147-50.

Kelahan, A.M., and G.S. Doetsch. 1984. Time-dependent changes in functional organization of somatosensory cerebral cortex following digit amputation in adult raccoons. *Somatosens Res* 2:49-81.

Kelso, J.A.S., and S.A. Wallace. 1978. Conscious mechanisms in movement. In *Information processing in motor control and learning,* ed. G. Stelmach. New York: Academic Press.

Kew, J.J., M.C. Ridding, J.C. Rothwell, R.E. Passingham, P.N. Leigh, S. Sooriakumaran, R.S. Frackowiak, and D.J. Brooks. 1994. Reorganization of cortical blood flow and transcranial magnetic stimulation maps in human subjects after upper limb amputation. *J Neurophysiol* 72:2517-24.

Kiers, L., B. Fernando, and D. Tomkins. 1997. Facilitatory effect of thinking about movement on magnetic motor-evoked potentials. *Electroencephalogr Clin Neurophysiol* 105:262-8.

Kim, S.Y., K.J. Cho, C.I. Park, T.S. Yoon, D.Y. Han, S.K. Kim, and H.L. Lee. 1993. Effect of wheelchair ergometer training on SCI paraplegics. *Yonsei Med J* 34:278-86.

Kjaer, M., G. Perko, N.H. Secher, R. Boushel, N. Beyer, S. Pollack, A. Horn, A. Fernandes, T. Mohr, S.F. Lewis, and H. Galbo. 1994. Cardiovascular and ventilatory responses to electrically induced cycling with complete epidural anaesthesia in humans. *Acta Physiol Scand* 151:199-207.

Kjaer, M., S.F. Pollack, T. Mohr, H. Weiss, G.W. Gleim, F.W. Bach, T. Nicolaisen, H. Galbo, and K.T. Ragnarsson. 1996. Regulation of glucose turnover and hormonal responses during electrical cycling in tetraplegic humans. *Am J Physiol* 271:R191-9.

Knuttson, E., E. Lewenhaupt-Olsson, and M. Thorsen. 1973. Physical work capacity and physical conditioning in paraplegic patients. *Paraplegia* 11:205-16.

Kocina, P. 1997. Body composition of spinal cord injured adults. *Sports Med* 23:48-60.

Kohl, R.M., and D.L. Roenker. 1980. Mechanism involvement during skill imagery. *J Mot Beh* 15:179-90.

Kralj, A.R., T. Bajd, M. Munih, and R. Turk. 1993. FES gait restoration and balance control in SCI patients. *Prog Brain Res* 97:387-96.

Leeds, E., J. Klose, W. Ganz, A. Serafini, and B.A. Green. 1990. Bone mineral density after bicycle ergometry training. *Arch Phys Med Rehab* 71:207-9.

Levy, W.J., V.E. Amassian, M. Traad, and J. Cadwell. 1990. Focal magnetic coil stimulation reveals motor cortical system reorganization in humans after traumatic quadriplegia. *Brain Res* 10:130-4.

Lew, R.D. 1987. The effects of FNS on disuse osteoporosis. Paper presented at the 10th Annual RESNA Conference, San Jose, CA.

Lipetz, J.S., S.C. Kirshblum, K.C. O'Connor, S.J. Voorman, and M.V. Johnston. 1997. Anemia and serum protein deficiencies in patients with traumatic spinal cord injury. *J Spinal Cord Med* 20:335-40.

Martin, T.P., R.B. Stein, P.H. Hoeppner, and D.C. Reid. 1992. Influence of electrical stimulation on the morphological and metabolic properties of paralyzed muscle. *J Appl Physiol* 72:1401-6.

McArdle, W.D., F.I. Katch, and V.L. Katch. 1994. *Essentials of exercise physiology.* Philadelphia: Lea & Febiger.

Mellah, S., L. Rispal-Padel, and G. Riviere. 1990. Changes in excitability of motor units during preparation for movement. *Exp Brain Res* 82:178-86.

Merlis, J.K., and C.W. Watson. 1949. Electroencephalogram after injury to spinal cord in man. *Arch Neurol Psychiatry* 61:695-8.

Merzenich, M.M., R.J. Nelson, M.P. Stryker, M.S. Cyander, A. Schoppmann, and Z.M. Zook. 1984. Somatosensory cortical map changes following digit amputation in adult monkeys. *J Comp Neurol* 224:591-605.

Milner-Brown, H.S., R.B. Stein, and R. Yemm. 1973. The contractile properties of human motor units during voluntary isometric contractions. *J Physiol* 228:285-306.

Miniare, P., P. Meunier, C. Edouard, J. Bernard, P. Courpron, and J. Bourret. 1994. Quantitative histological data on disuse osteoporosis: comparison with biological data. *Calcif Tissue Res* 17:57-73.

Mira, J.C. 1982. Degenerescence et regeneration des nerfs periferiques: observations ultrastructurales et electrophysiologique, aspects quantitatifs et consequences musculaires. In *Aspects biologiques de la regeneration du nerf periferique.* Paris: Edition Volal.

Mogliner, A., J.A. Grossman, U. Ribary, M. Joliot, J. Volkman, D. Rapaport, R.W. Beasley, and R.R. Llinas. 1993. Somatosensory cortical plasticity in adult humans revealed by magnetoencephalography. *Proc Natl Acad Sci* 90:593-7.

Naftchi, N.E., A.T. Viau, G.H. Sell, and E.W. Lowman. 1980. Mineral metabolism in spinal cord injury. *Arch Phys Med Rehab* 61:139-42.

National Institutes of Health. 1995. *Physical Activity and Cardiovascular Health Consensus Statement Online.* http://text.nlm.nih.gov/nih/cdc/www/101txt.html.

Nilsson, S., P. Staff, and E. Pruett. 1975. Physical work capacity and the effect of training on subjects with long standing paraplegia. *Scand J Rehabil Med* 7:51-6.

Nix, W.A., and H.C. Hopf. 1983. Electrical stimulation of regenerating nerve and its effect on motor recovery. *Brain Res* 416:308-14.

Noreau, L., and R.J. Shephard. 1992. Return to work after SCI: the potential contribution of physical fitness. *Paraplegia* 30:563-72.

Paivio, A. 1986. *Mental representations: A dual coding approach.* Oxford: Clarendon Press.

Peckham, P.H., J.T. Mortimer, and E.B. Marsolais. 1976. Alteration in the force and fatigability of skeletal muscle in quadriplegic humans following exercise induced by chronic electrical stimulation. *Clin Orthop* 114:326-34.

Pette, D., M.E. Smith, H.W. Staudle, and G. Vrbova. 1073. Effects of long-term electrical stimulation on some contractile and metabolic characteristics of fast rabbit muscles. *Pflugers Arch* 338:257-72.

Pette, D., and G. Vrbova. 1985. Neural control of phenotypic expression in mammalian muscle fibers. *Muscle Nerve* 8:676-89.

Pollack, S.F., K. Axen, N. Spielholz, N. Levin, F. Haas, and K.T. Ragnarsson. 1989. Aerobic training effects of electrically induced lower extremity exercises in SCI people. *Arch Phys Med Rehab* 70:214-9.

Pons, T.P., P.E. Garraghty, A.K. Ommaya, J.H. Kaas, E. Taub, and M. Mishkin. 1991. Massive cortical reorganization after sensory deafferentation in adult macaques. *Science* 252:1860-75.

Ragnarsson, K.T. 1988. Physiologic effects of FES-induced exercises in SCI individuals. *Clin Orthop* Aug:53-63.

Ramachandran, V.S. 1993. Behavioral and magnetoencephalographic correlates of plasticity in the adult human brain. *Proc Natl Acad Sci* 90:10413-20.

Ramachandran, V.S., M. Stewart, and D.C. Rogers-Ramachandran. 1992. Perceptual correlates of massive cortical reorganization. *Neuroreport* 3:583-6.

Rao, S.M., J.R. Binder, P.A. Bandettini, T.A. Hammeke, F.Z. Yetkin, A. Jesmanowicz, L.M. Lisk, G.L. Morris, W.M. Mueller, L.D. Estkowski, E.C. Wong, V.M. Haughton, and J.S. Hyde. 1993. Functional magnetic resonance imaging of complex human movements. *Neurology* 43:2311-8.

Recanzone, G.H., T.T. Allard, W.M. Jenkins, and M.M. Merzenich. 1990. Receptive-field changes induced by peripheral nerve stimulation of SI in adult cats. *J Neurophysiol* 63:1213-25.

Recanzone, G.H., M.M. Merzenich, W.M. Jenkins, K.A. Grajski, and H.R. Dinse. 1992. Topographic reorganization of the hand representation in cortical area owl monkeys trained in a frequency-discrimination task. *J Neurophysiol* 67:1031-56.

Recanzone, G.H., C.E. Schreiner, and M.M. Merzenich. 1993. Plasticity in the frequency representation of primary auditory cortex following discrimination training in adult owl monkeys. *J Neurosci* 13:87-103.

Richards, J.S., M. Hirt, and L. Melamed. 1982. Spinal cord injury: sensory restriction perspective. *Arch Phys Med Rehabil* 63:195-9.

Richards, J.S., M.R. Seitz, and W.A. Eisele. 1986. Auditory processing in spinal cord injury: a preliminary investigation from a sensory deprivation perspective. *Arch Phys Med Rehabil* 67:115-7.

Riley, D.A., and E.F. Allin. 1973. The effects of inactivity, programmed stimulation and denervation on the histochemistry of skeletal fibre type. *Exp Neurol* 40:391-413.

Rodgers, M.M., R.M. Glaser, S.F. Figoni, S.P. Hooker, B.N. Ezenwa, S.R. Collins, T. Mathews, A.G. Suryaprasad, and S.C. Gupta. 1991. Musculoskeletal responses of SCI individuals to functional neuromuscular stimulation-induced knee extension exercise training. *J Rehabil Res Dev* 28:19-26.

Roelcke, U., A. Curt, A. Otte, J. Missimer, R.P. Maguire, V. Dietz, and K.L. Leenders. 1997. Influence of spinal cord injury on cerebral sensorimotor systems: a PET study. *J Neurol Neurosurg Psychiatry* 62:61-5.

Roland, P.E. 1984. Organization of motor control by the normal human brain. *Hum Neurobiol* 2:205-16.

Roland, P.E., and L. Friberg. 1985. Localization of cortical areas activated by thinking. *J Neurophysiol* 53:1219-43.

Roland, P.E., B. Larsen, N.A. Lassen, and E. Skinhoj. 1980. Supplementary motor area and other cortical areas of organization of voluntary movements in man. *J Neurophysiol* 43:118-36.

Roland, P.E., E. Meyer, T. Shibasaki, Y.L. Yamamoto, and C.J. Thompson. 1982. Regional cerebral blood flow changes in cortex and basal ganglia during voluntary movements in normal human volunteers. *J Neurophysiol* 48:467-80.

Romero, D.H., M.G. Lacourse, M.J. Cohen, and K.E. Lawrence. 1998. Event-related potentials during executed and imagined sub-maximal isometric muscle contractions. *J Sport Exerc Psychol* 20 (Suppl.):S29.

Rutherford, O.M., and D.A. Jones. 1986. The role of learning and coordination in strength training. *Eur J Appl Physiol* 55:100-5.

Sale, D.G. 1988. Neural adaptation to resistance training. *Med Sci Sport Exerc* 20:S135-45.

Salmons, S., and J. Henriksson. 1981. The adaptive response of skeletal muscle to increased use. *Muscle Nerve* 4:94-105.

Sanes, J.N., S. Suner, and J.P. Donoghue. 1990. Dynamic organization of primary motor cortex to target muscles in adult rats I. Long-term patterns of reorganization following motor or mixed peripheral lesions. *Exp Brain Res* 79:479-91.

Sawka, M.N., W.A. Latzka, and K.B. Pandolf. 1989. Temperature regulation during upper body exercise: able-bodied and SCI. *Med Sci Sports Exerc* 21:S132-40.

Shaw, W.A. 1938. The distribution of muscular action potentials during imaging. *Psychol Rec* 2:195-216.

Shaw, W.A. 1940. The relation of muscular action potentials to imagined weight lifting. *Arch Psychol* 35:5-50.

Shenberger, J.S., G.J. Leaman, M.M. Neumyer, T.I. Musch, and L.I. Sinoway. 1990. Physiologic and structural indices of vascular function in paraplegics. *Med Sci Sports Exerc* 22:96-101.

Shepard, R.J. 1988. Sports medicine and the wheelchair athlete. *Sports Med* 4:226-47.

Shibasaki, H. 1993. Recent advances in non-invasive studies of higher brain functions. *Brain Dev* 15:423-7.

Sica, R.E.P., O.P. Sanz, L.P. Cohen, J.D. Freyre, and M. Panizza. 1984. Changes in the N1-P1 component of the somatosensory cortical evoked response in patients with partial limb amputation. *Electroencephalogr Clin Neurol* 24:415-27.

Sloan, K.E., L.A. Bremner, J. Byrne, R.E. Day, and E.R. Scull. 1994. Musculoskeletal effects of an electrical stimulation induced cycling programme in the spinal injured. *Paraplegia* 32:407-15.

Stefanovska, A., S. Rebersek, R. Bajd, and L. Vodovnik. 1991. Effects of electrical stimulation on spasticity. *CRC Phys Rehab Med* 3:59-99.

Streletz, L.J., J.K. Belevich, S.M. Jones, A. Bhushan, S.H. Shah, and G.J. Herbison. 1995. Transcranial magnetic stimulation: cortical motor maps in acute spinal cord injury. *Brain Topogr* 7:245-50.

Suinn, R.N. 1984. Imagery and sports. In *Cognitive sport psychology*, ed. W.F. Straub and J.M. Williams. Lansing, N.Y.: Sport Science Associates.

Tesch, P.A., and J. Karlsson. 1983. Muscle fiber type characteristics of M. deltoideius in wheelchair athletes. Comparisons with other trained athletes. *Am J Physiol Med* 62:239-43.

Topka, H., L.G. Cohen, R.A. Cole, and M. Hallett. 1991. Reorganization of corticospinal pathways following spinal cord injury. *Neurology* 41:1276-83.

VanGelderen, P., N.F. Ramsey, G. Liu, J.H. Duyn, J.A. Frank, D.R. Weinberger, and C.T. Moonen. 1995. Three-dimensional functional magnetic resonance imaging of human brain on a clinical 1.5-T scanner. *Proc Natl Acad Sci* 92:6906-10.

VanLoan, M.D., S. McCluer, M. Loftin, and R.A. Boileau. 1987. Comparison of physiological responses to maximal arm exercise among able-bodied, paraplegics and quadriplegics. *Paraplegia* 25:397-405.

Vodovnik, L., and R. Karba. 1992. Treatment of chronic wounds by means of electric and electromagnetic fields, part 2: literature review. *Med Biol Eng Comput* 30:257-66.

Wang, Y., and W.P. Morgan. 1992. The effect of imagery perspectives on the psychophysiological responses to imagined exercise. *Behav Brain Res* 52:167-74.

Weder, B., U. Knorr, H. Herzog, B. Nebeling, A. Kleinschmidt, Y. Huang, H. Steinmetz, H.J. Freund, and R.J. Seitz. 1994. Tactile exploration of shape after subcortical ischaemic infarction studied with PET. *Brain* 117:593-605.

Wheeler, G.D., E.A. Ashley, V. Harber, J.J. Laskin, L.M. Olenik, D. Sloley, R. Burnham, R.D. Steadward, and D.C. Cumming. 1996. Hormonal responses to graded-resistance, FES-assisted strength training in SCI. *Spinal Cord* 34:264-7.

Wheeler, G.D., D.C. Cumming, R. Burnham, I. Maclean, B.D. Sloley, Y. Bhambhani, and R.D. Steadward. 1994. Testosterone, cortisol, and catecholamine responses to exercise stress and autonomic dysreflexia in elite quadriplegic athletes. *Paraplegia* 32:292-9.

Yahagi, S., K. Shimura, and T. Kasai. 1996. An increase in cortical excitability with no change in spinal excitability during motor imagery. *Percept Mot Skills* 83:88-290.

Yang, T.T., C.C. Gallen, V.S. Ramachandran, S. Cobb, B.J. Schwartz, and F.E. Bloom. 1994. Noninvasive detection of cerebral plasticity in adult somatosensory cortex. *Neuroreport* 5:701-4.

Yarkony, G.M., E.J. Roth, G. Cybulski, and R.J. Jaeger. 1992. Neuromuscular stimulation in SCI: I: Restoration of functional movements of the extremities. *Arch Phys Med Rehab* 73:78-86.

Yue, G., and K.J. Cole. 1992. Strength increases from the motor program: comparison of training with maximal voluntary and imagined muscle contractions. *J Neurophysiol* 67:1114-23.

Zubek, J.P. 1969. *Sensory deprivation: 15 years of research.* New York: Appleton-Century-Crofts.

Chapter 16

Stroke

Joel Stein, MD

Case Study

A 73-year-old man came to the hospital after sudden onset of right-sided weakness and dysarthria. Charles had a history of hypertension, and admitted to noncompliance with his medication. Finding a left internal capsule lacunar infarct, his neurologist started him on aspirin for prevention of recurrent stroke and transferred him to a rehabilitation facility. There he enrolled in a multidisciplinary program of rehabilitation, with extensive physical, occupational, and speech therapy. His dysarthria resolved, but he continued to experience a persistent hemiparesis. Because of his inadequate ankle dorsiflexion, we fitted Charles with a plastic ankle foot orthosis (AFO). His exercise program was primarily functionally oriented, and he made steady gains in both his activities of daily living (ADLs) and his mobility. Three weeks after his initial stroke, we discharged him to his home. He could walk independently with a straight cane and his AFO, and could perform most of his ADLs independently. He currently uses homemaker services to assist with shopping and cleaning, and receives additional physical and occupational therapy. Despite this therapy, he remains unable to use his upper right extremity except as a gross assist to stabilize objects, and continues to require the use of his cane and AFO. Despite his persistent deficits, Charles reports satisfaction with his recovery, and has resumed an active lifestyle, including working as a volunteer in a hospital.

Charles's case illustrates both the successes and challenges of stroke rehabilitation. Many individuals achieve considerable functional improvement after stroke, yet both the mechanisms of this improvement and the most effective treatment programs remain poorly understood. Improvement after stroke frequently falls substantially short of premorbid function, leaving considerable impairments in function. This chapter reviews current knowledge of the mechanisms of stroke recovery, and the role that exercise can play in facilitating this recovery.

Scope of the Problem

Stroke remains a major cause of morbidity and mortality in the United States, with approximately 600,000 new strokes occurring in the United States each year and 4,000,000 survivors alive today (AHA 1998). Exercise in asymptomatic individuals at risk for cerebrovascular disease is an important public health issue, as exercise favorably affects risk factors for stroke such as hypertension, plasma lipids, obesity, and reduced insulin sensitivity (Bronner et al. 1995). Studies by Gillum and colleagues (1996), Kiely and colleagues (1994), and Shinton (1997) have found an association between physical inactivity and the risk of stroke. Indeed, Shinton (1997) estimates that 79% of strokes could be averted through regular exercise and avoidance of both smoking and obesity. Yet other studies have found no clear protective benefit from exercise (Menotti et al. 1990), and the Surgeon General's report (USDHSS 1996) recently concluded that "The existing data do not unequivocally support an association between physical activity and the risk of stroke."

For individuals who sustain a stroke, therapeutic exercise forms a large part of the rehabilitation program, despite limited data on its efficacy and uncertainty about how best to design exercise programs for the stroke survivor. In this chapter, I summarize current knowledge regarding the efficacy of various forms of exercise and related therapies for recovering function poststroke, and make recommendations for designing such exercise programs.

How Much Exercise?

With the growth of managed care and increasing emphasis on containing costs, the issue of what constitutes the optimal amount of therapeutic exercise and overall rehabilitation poststroke has become a much

discussed, if not well-studied, issue. Most research in this area has examined the amount of rehabilitation provided, and the setting in which it is provided. The intensity of the overall rehabilitation program affects outcome (Kwakkel et al. 1997; Seitz et al. 1987; Sivenius et al. 1985), with intensive, hospital-based rehabilitation programs showing better functional outcomes than less intensive nursing home programs (Keith et al. 1995; Kramer et al. 1997). Despite these data, there has been a tendency of managed care programs to direct individuals to less intensive, nursing home-based rehabilitation programs (Retchin et al. 1997). There are also multiple reports (Indredavik et al. 1997; Kalra and Eade 1995; Kaste et al. 1995; Stevens et al. 1984; Strand et al. 1985), as well as a meta-analysis based largely on European studies (Stroke Unit Trialists' 1997), indicating that structured stroke units have better outcomes than general medical units (see figures 16.1 and 16.2). Although some research suggests that the benefits of structured stroke units apply to individuals with both intermediate and severe disability (Kalra et al. 1993; Kalra and Eade 1995), these European studies have limited applicability to the United States because they generally do not distinguish between acute and rehabilitative phases of treatment. Comparing rehabilitation care to conventional medical care, another meta-analysis confirmed improved rates of discharge home, but not other long-term benefits (Evans et al. 1995). While these studies help to validate the benefits of rehabilitation, they do not attempt to determine the optimum quantity and duration of exercise for individuals poststroke. In the absence of such data, physicians must base stroke rehabilitation exercise programs on clinical judgment—and, increasingly, on insurance coverage.

Recovery Versus Compensation

Individuals who sustain a stroke are, as a rule, more interested in recovery of neurologic function than in learning compensatory strategies. Rehabilitation exercise programs, however, tend to combine these two goals to varying degrees, in part because recovery of neurologic function is often unsatisfactory. It remains unclear to what extent exercise or other rehabilitation interventions can influence ultimate recovery. In competing for scarce rehabilitation resources, clinicians designing poststroke exercise programs must balance the goals of recovery versus compensation. For example, they can train an individual who has partially lost ankle dorsiflexion to try to recruit the tibialis anterior through cueing or biofeedback; or they

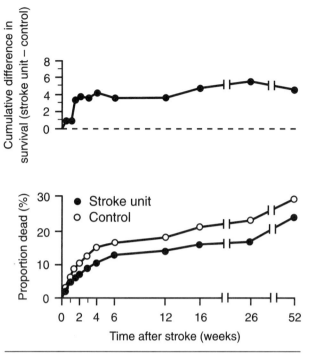

Figure 16.1 Proportion of patients known to have died after a stroke, with the cumulative difference between those treated on stroke units and on control (general medical) units.

This figure was first published in the BMJ (Stroke Unit Trialists' Collaboration, 1997, "Collaborative systematic review of the randomized trials of organized inpatient (stroke unit) care after stroke," *BMJ* 314:1151-59) and is reproduced by permission of the BMJ.

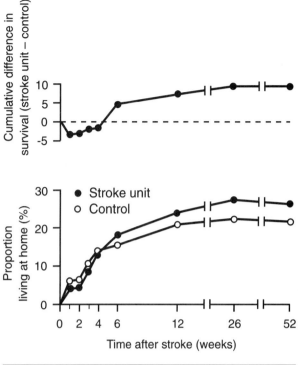

Figure 16.2 Proportion of patients living at home after a stroke, with the cumulative difference between those treated on stroke units and on control (general medical) units.

This figure was first published in the BMJ (Stroke Unit Trialists' Collaboration, 1997, "Collaborative systematic review of the randomized trials of organized inpatient (stroke unit) care after stroke," *BMJ* 314:1151-59) and is reproduced by permission of the BMJ.

can train the person to compensate by using a brace. The compensatory strategy of bracing may achieve more rapidly the functional goal of independent ambulation; but the cost may be less effort devoted to correcting the underlying motor deficit. Despite the centrality of this issue in the design of rehabilitation exercise programs, financial pressures—rather than scientific data—are determining the balance between these two approaches. The strong impetus to achieve independent functioning as quickly as possible has led to increased emphasis on compensatory approaches, rather than on attempts to facilitate recovery. While it may be argued that society should choose the least expensive approach (compensatory training) in the absence of evidence supporting a more expensive approach (facilitating recovery), I cannot overstate the importance of continuing to examine this issue.

Physicians prescribe therapeutic exercise for a variety of impairments that result from stroke. This chapter focuses on the use of exercise to improve motor control, strength, gait, balance, ataxia, sensation, and endurance. The use of exercise to learn compensatory strategies, per se, will not be discussed, though in practice this is intermingled with all of the above exercise programs.

Effects of Stroke on Neuromuscular Function

The effects of hemiparesis secondary to stroke on neuromuscular function are intertwined with the effects of deconditioning of the affected limb. Landin et al. (1977) found paretic leg muscles to have a reduction in blood flow, increased lactate production, and higher glycogen consumption than nonparetic leg muscles. Some of these effects may be due to changes in the proportion of fiber types (Potempa et al. 1996), though cause and effect are not clear even if the correlations are valid.

Motor neuron firing patterns are a major determinant of muscle fiber myosin isoform composition (Lomo 1989; Pette and Vrbova 1992; Salmons and Sreter 1976). Motor neuron firing rates and recruitment are reduced in hemiparetic individuals (Gemperline et al. 1995), perhaps explaining the observed changes in muscle fiber type composition.

Studies of fiber type proportions have yielded apparently conflicting results. Most have observed selective atrophy of type II muscle fibers (Brooke and Engel 1969; Dattola et al. 1993; Dietz et al. 1986; Scelsi et al. 1984; Slager et al. 1985). A few studies, however, revealed an increased prevalence of type IIa fibers in paretic muscles (Frontera et al. 1997; Jakobsson et al. 1991). While biopsy studies have mostly revealed atrophy, at least one researcher has reported some focal hypertrophy (Slager et al. 1985). Some of the observed variability in muscle histochemistry and morphometry may result from factors that experimenters did not control—specifically the severity of the weakness, the presence or absence of spasticity, patterns of compensation, and which specific muscle was studied. There is little information on the fiber composition of muscles of the nonparetic side poststroke, though one report found an increased proportion of type I fibers (Frontera et al. 1997). We do not know the effects of exercise on the fiber type proportions in muscle poststroke, and a trial of resistive and/or endurance exercises would be interesting.

Mechanisms of Motor Recovery Poststroke

The natural history of stroke usually includes a significant degree of recovery, including recovery of motor function. Animal models (Johansson et al. 1996; Ohlsson and Johansson 1995) suggest that environment plays a significant role in the recovery of motor function, though we do not fully understand the mechanism(s) and optimal timing of such environmental stimulation. A major, largely unrealized, goal of stroke treatment is to use a combination of medical, surgical, and exercise treatments to enhance this natural recovery of function poststroke.

Learning Versus Recovery

Assessing the effectiveness of exercise therapy for recovery is complicated by the simultaneous motor learning that undoubtedly occurs. There are no data to contradict the supposition that individuals poststroke can "learn" new motor skills in their involved limbs in a fashion similar (though attenuated) to that of healthy individuals. The ability to learn new motor skills appears to represent a continuum based on the severity of neurologic deficits—it is likely better preserved in those with less severe neurologic deficits, and may be absent in the densely plegic. Several

studies have shown that individuals with chronic, stable motor deficits due to strokes can improve their motor functioning after specialized intensive training (Lehmann et al. 1975; Tangeman et al. 1990; Taub and Wolf 1993; Werner and Kessler 1996; Wolf et al. 1989). The amount of recovery correlates with the intensity of rehabilitation (Langhorne et al. 1996; Nugent et al. 1994; Smith et al. 1981). Does this represent late recovery, or is it learning? Can the two phenomena truly be distinguished?

Cortical mapping has shown that, in both the intact (Nudo, Milliken et al. 1996; Pascual-Leone et al. 1994) and the injured (Nudo, Wise et al. 1996) brain, learning motor tasks leads to changes in the organization of the cerebral cortex. Advances in functional imaging techniques may eventually enable us to separate the phenomena of learning and recovery. It is possible that the conceptual distinction between motor recovery and motor learning reflects an artificial dichotomy, with both phenomena occurring through similar patterns of reorganization of the cerebral cortex.

Mechanisms of Motor Recovery

The mechanisms of stroke recovery are incompletely understood. One mechanism involves assumption of lost function by adjacent areas of undamaged brain tissue. Detailed topographic maps of the primary motor cortex have provided considerable information about the elements forming the well-known motor homunculus. The reorganization of cortical maps after cortical injury occurs in the motor system (Asanuma 1991; Jacobs and Donoghue 1991; Nudo, Wise et al. 1996) as well as in the sensory (Pons et al. 1988), visual (Kaas et al. 1990), and auditory systems (King and Moore 1991). This remapping of adjacent cortical tissue is influenced by retraining (i.e., rehabilitation) of the animal through practice of previously acquired motor tasks (see figure 16.3), and may not appear without this activity (Nudo, Wise et al. 1996). Indeed, there is evidence that the undamaged adjacent cerebral cortex may experience a shrinkage of the cortical map for the affected limb in the absence of any rehabilitative efforts (Nudo and Milliken 1996).

In another mechanism of functional recovery, homologous regions of the unaffected contralateral cerebral hemisphere substitute for the infarcted brain tissue (Fisher 1992; Glees 1980; Sabatini et al. 1994). The unaffected ipsilateral hemisphere may control motor function through uncrossed pyramidal fibers, which may constitute as many as 25% of the pyramidal tracts (Nyberg-Hansen and Rinvik 1963). Func-

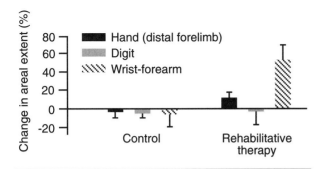

Figure 16.3 Changes in the cortical area size for the upper extremities in squirrel monkeys recovering from experimental cortical lesions. Comparison of rehabilitative therapy with control animals. Reprinted, by permission, from R.J. Nudo, B.M. Wise, F. SiFuentes, and G.W. Milliken. 1996. Neural substrates for the effects of rehabilitative training on motor recovery after ischemic infarct. *Science* 272:1791-94. Copyright 1996 American Association for the Advancement of Science.

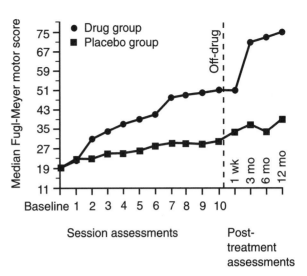

Figure 16.4 Median Fugl-Meyr motor scale scores over the course of combined amphetamine and exercise therapy sessions, with follow-up at 1 week after drug cessation and at 3, 6, and 12 months after stroke onset. Reprinted, by permission, from D. Walker-Batson, P. Smith, S. Curtis, H. Unwin, and R. Greenlee, 1995, "Amphetamine paired with physical therapy accelerates motor recovery after stroke. Further evidence," *Stroke* 26:22549.

tional MRI studies have found increased cortical activity in homologous areas contralateral to the stroke, as well as in undamaged regions adjacent to those affected by the stroke, suggesting that both mechanisms may play a role in recovery of motor function poststroke (Cramer et al. 1997).

Medical Interventions to Enhance Recovery

Medical interventions to influence motor recovery fall into two major categories.

• **Medications to limit damage during acute stroke.** Citicoline (CDP-choline) is a precursor of phosphatidylcholine, a key component of cell membranes. It has been suggested that citicoline limits damage from free radicals, and one study found that it reduces functional deficits poststroke (Clark et al. 1997) when started in the acute period.

• **Medications to enhance motor recovery in the postacute phase.** Amphetamines and related drugs are among the most promising of these agents, with both animal (Feeney et al. 1982; Hovda and Feeney 1984) and limited human data (Crisostomo et al. 1988; Walker-Batson et al. 1995) suggesting that they may enhance recovery. Interestingly, the human studies have combined exercise therapy with the administration of amphetamine, following the lead of animal studies that showed the effectiveness of combination therapies in stimulating motor recovery (Feeney et al. 1982; Hovda and Feeney 1984) (see figure 16.4). Growth factors also enhance recovery in animal models of acute stroke (Bethel et al. 1997; Kawamata et al. 1997), and appear affective even when administered several days after the stroke.

Animal data (Feeney et al. 1982) and limited human data (Goldstein 1995) suggest that some commonly used medications—including clonidine, prazosin, phenobarbital, phenytoin, dopamine receptor antagonists, and benzodiazepines—may hinder recovery from stroke.

Environmental and Behavioral Interventions to Enhance Motor Recovery

Environmental and behavioral interventions, with particular emphasis on therapeutic exercise, are the primary rehabilitative techniques for enhancing recovery poststroke. Several factors have limited direct study of the impact of rehabilitation interventions for enhancing motor recovery. These include

• the normal tendency for spontaneous recovery for several months poststroke,

• the difficulty in distinguishing clinically between recovery and motor learning,

• limitations in noninvasive assessment of subtle neurologic changes in living humans poststroke,

• difficulty in standardizing treatment, and

• difficulty conducting well-controlled studies during the early phase of recovery, where using an untreated control group (i.e., no rehabilitation) is considered unethical.

Animals provided with an enriched environment poststroke have better recovery of motor function (Johansson 1996; Ohlsson and Johansson 1995). Increased use of a paretic limb after experimental cortical injury can lead to a more normal pattern of dendritic arborization of pyramidal neurons (Jones and Schallert 1994).

Some limited animal data suggest, however, that *excessive* use of a paretic limb after experimental cortical injury can actually impede recovery, possibly due to the toxic effect of neurotransmitter release in the peri-infarct area. The researchers in this experiment created "excessive use" by immobilizing the nonparetic forelimb of a rat immediately after the cortical injury, and maintaining the forced use of the paretic limb for a 15-day period (Kozlowski et al. 1996). While extrapolating these data to humans is difficult, they suggest that extreme efforts to increase use of paretic limbs in the early poststroke period may be hazardous (Schallert et al. 1997).

Some researchers have studied sensory stimulation as a possible mediator of recovery in poststroke patients. Several studies found acupuncture to be helpful (Johansson et al. 1993; Magnusson et al. 1994; Naeser et al. 1992). Functional electrical stimulation (discussed on pages 299 and 302-303) may also exert its effects through increased sensory stimulation. The mechanisms by which acupuncture or other sensory stimulation modalities might influence stroke recovery remain speculative.

Exercise for Motor Control

The history of poststroke exercise for motor control is notable for the widespread clinical application of unproven treatment approaches. Multiple attempts to demonstrate the benefits of a particular therapeutic approach over a "standard" functionally oriented approach have failed to demonstrate any benefit. Dickstein et al. (1986) compared a functionally oriented program, proprioceptive neuromuscular facilitation (PNF) techniques, and the Bobath (neurodevelopmental or NDT) approach in 131 stroke patients. They found no differences among the three groups in functional ability, ambulation status, muscle tone, or isolated motor control. Hesse, Jahnke et al. (1994) found little benefit from an intensive four-week program of NDT-based exercise; and Butefisch and colleagues (1995) observed the NDT approach to be less effective in restoring motor control than a program of resisted flexion and extension exercises. Several trials have similarly failed to demonstrate any benefit of PNF techniques over conventional functionally oriented therapy (Logigian et al. 1983; Lord and Hall 1986; Stern et al. 1970). One comparison of NDT versus PNF showed no significant benefits of one treatment approach over the other (Wagenaar et al. 1990). Variations of these techniques, such as sensorimotor integrative treatment, apparently are no more effective than functionally oriented therapy programs (Jongbloed et al. 1989). Researchers continue to examine other techniques, such as ballistic movements, resisted agonist, and resisted antagonist movements (Trombly et al. 1986), but so far have found them to have no advantage over generally accepted techniques.

The Standard Approach

Despite its widespread application, there is no universally accepted definition of the "standard" functional approach: essentially, it involves providing physical assistance and encouragement for the stroke patient during functional or prefunctional tasks, and then gradually withdrawing this support as the individual's ability to perform desired activities improves. The therapeutic program typically incorporates instruction in compensatory techniques to improve functional abilities. Problems in defining this approach include the highly individualized nature of the treatment program, with variable emphasis on the "quality" of movement, and variable ratios of retraining paretic muscle groups versus encouraging compensation by unaffected muscle groups. Clinicians often fail to document the amount of time spent performing actual exercises, thus complicating efforts to determine a "dose-response" relationship between the amount of exercise and recovery.

Part of the decreased function after stroke may be due to "learned disuse," in which initial weakness of the paretic limb leads to failure to complete functional tasks with that limb. This failure leads in turn to a cessation of attempts to use the paretic limb, even as some neurologic improvement occurs. Thus continued failure to use the paretic limb is in part a learned behavior. Taub et al. (1993) and Wolf et al. (1989) examined restraint of uninvolved upper extremities in individuals with chronic stable hemiparesis. They coupled use of upper extremity restraints with intense training programs consisting of six hours per day of various functional activities using the affected upper extremity (eating, writing, card games, etc.). The paretic limbs significantly improved in motor function after intensive two-week training periods, and maintained the gains throughout a two-year follow-up (see figure 16.5). Preliminary data by

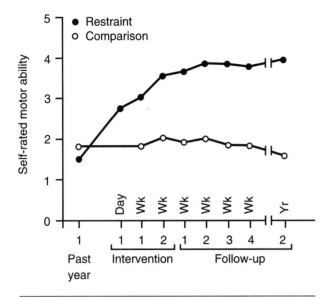

Figure 16.5 Self-rated motor ability based on activity logs for chronic stable poststroke subjects after paretic upper extremity training. Comparison of subjects who had training with restraint of the unaffected arm versus control group.

Reprinted, by permission, from E. Taub, N.E. Miller, T.A. Novack, E.W. Cook, W.C. Fleming, C.S. Nepomuceno, J.S. Connell, J.E. Crago,1993, "Technique to improve chronic motor deficit after stroke," *Arch Phys Med Rehabil* 74:347-54.

Taub and Wolf (1997) suggest that similar results may obtain through intensive physical training of the paretic limb without use of constraints in the normal upper extremity. Although demonstrated only in small groups of carefully selected subsets of hemiparetic individuals, these results are particularly intriguing, given that the historical outcomes of therapeutic exercise for upper extremity function have been quite disappointing. Only 5% of individuals who receive intensive therapy for upper extremity weakness poststroke regain functional use of the upper extremity during rehabilitation (Gowland 1982). Extrapolation of the work of Taub and Wolf to larger patient populations is premature—we need larger controlled clinical trials to validate these preliminary results.

Other studies have demonstrated that intensive therapeutic exercise programs can improve functional ability in patients with chronic stable deficits poststroke (Rodriquez et al. 1996; Tangeman et al. 1990), although some have found that the benefits are temporary and are not maintained after cessation of treatment (Wade et al. 1992). While it is possible that these improvements are due to motor learning rather than neurologic recovery, there are no data to reveal the mechanism of this improvement in function. Regression to prior functioning after cessation of the formal exercise program in some studies may indicate that the intervention was not effective in individuals with chronic deficits poststroke; or it may simply point to the need for some form of maintenance therapy.

Meaningful exercise appears more effective than meaningless exercise. In a supination task, Nelson et al. (1996) found that use of a simple dice game provided significantly more rotation than a rote, meaningless task. While the mechanism by which this effect takes place is not established, it is reasonable to hypothesize that increased motivation for a meaningful task leads to greater effort and a greater degree of muscle activation. Moreover, the specificity of exercise training applies to poststroke as well as to healthy individuals. In designing therapeutic exercise programs, be sure to incorporate functional type tasks instead of routine "mat" exercises whenever possible.

The optimal intensity of physical and occupational therapy remains undetermined. Interventions directed at increasing the intensity of gait training early after stroke (Richards et al. 1993) have shown only transient benefits. Others have found a dose-response effect in therapy for ambulation, with greater amounts of weightbearing exercise correlated with better ambulation status (Nugent et al. 1994). Sunderland and colleagues (1994) found that an "enhanced" physical therapy program (consisting of increased therapy time and efforts to increase functional use of the upper extremity) in the acute phase poststroke improved function at six months poststroke; after one year, however, there was no significant difference between the conventional and enhanced therapy groups.

Biofeedback and Functional Electrical Stimulation

Multiple approaches have been used to enhance the efficacy of therapeutic exercise poststroke. Providing enhanced feedback via monitoring of EMG or other activity has had particular appeal. Many researchers have examined the utility of biofeedback (BFB) to facilitate improved neuromuscular control (see table 16.1), and there have been three meta-analyses of data on this subject. Schleenbaker and Mainous (1993) reviewed eight controlled trials of biofeedback for hemiplegia, totaling 192 subjects, and found a significant benefit to EMG-BFB compared with conventional treatment or no treatment ($p < .00001$). Another meta-analysis on the same subject failed to demonstrate significant benefit of biofeedback (Moreland and Thomson 1993). A third and more recent meta-analysis (Glanz et al. 1995) also failed to demonstrate benefit using the outcome measure of improved range of motion. The limitations in study

Table 16.1   Biofeedback Trials

Author	Trial design	Treatment focus	Intervention	Duration of treatment	Length of follow-up	Results
Basmajian et al. (1975)*#	RCT n = 20 >3 months poststroke	Ankle dorsi-flexion	EMG-BFB + conventional PT vs. conventional PT	3 ×/wk × 5 wks	Variable	No benefit
Mroczek et al. (1978)	Nonrandomized crossover design n = 9 >1 year poststroke	Wrist extension, elbow flexion	EMG-BFB vs. conventional PT	3 ×/wk × 4 wks	None	Both beneficial in restoring AROM, no difference between treatments
Shiavi et al. (1979)	RCT n = 22 <1 month poststroke	Lower extremity	EMG-BFB + conventional PT vs. conventional PT	Varied	Variable	Improved muscle control; no functional assessment performed
Hurd et al. (1980)#	RCT n = 24 Mean 76 days post-stroke	Deltoid or tibialis anterior (each 1/2 of subjects)	EMG-BFB vs. sham BFB vs. un-treated control muscles; all continued usual therapy program	5 ×/wk × 2 wks	None	EMG-BFB and sham BFB equivalent, and both superior to control
Prevo et al. (1982)	Nonrandomized n = 18 >1 year poststroke	Upper extremity	EMG-BFB vs. conventional PT	28 sessions over 10 wks	None	No benefit on agonist function, though decreased abnormal co-contraction
Basmajian et al. (1982)*	RCT n = 37 25 months poststroke	Upper extremity	EMG-BFB vs. conventional therapy	3 ×/wk × 5 wks	None	No benefit
Burnside et al. (1982)*	RCT n = 22 0.512 years poststroke	Ankle dor-siflexion	EMG-BFB vs. conventional PT	2 ×/wk × 6 wks	6 wks	Increased strength in BFB group; no change in gait or range

*Included in meta-analysis by Schleenbaker and Mainous 1993

#Included in meta-analysis by Glanz et al. 1995

AROM = active range of motion; BFB = biofeedback; EMG = electromyography; LE = lower extremity; PT = physical therapy; RCT = randomized clinical trial; UE = upper extremity

Table 16.1   (continued)

Author	Trial design	Treatment focus	Intervention	Duration of treatment	Length of follow-up	Results
Wolf and Binder-Macleod (1983a)*	Controlled, nonran-domized n = 31 >1 year poststroke	Upper extremity	EMG-BFB of UE vs. no treatment	23 ×/wk × 26 wks	None	No functional benefit
Wolf and Binder-Macleod (1983b)*	Controlled, nonran-domized n = 36 >1 year poststroke	Lower extremity	EMG-BFB of LE vs. no treatment vs. EMG-BFB to UE only vs. relaxation training	5 ×/wk × 12 wks	None	Improved AROM; de-creased ambulatory aids; no change in walking speed
Inglis et al. (1984)*	RCT with crossover of control group n = 30 >6 months poststroke	Upper extremity	EMG-BFB vs. conven-tional PT	3 ×/wk × 7 wks	None	Improved AROM and muscle strength
John (1986)#	Crossover n = 12 12-280 (mean 75.5) days post-stroke	Lower extremity	EMG-BFB + conven-tional PT vs. conven-tional PT	Daily × 3 wks for 20 min	None	No benefit
Mulder et al. (1986)#	RCT n = 12 duration poststroke not given	Ankle dorsiflexion	EMG-BFB vs. neuro-developmen-tal treatment	3 ×/wk × 5 wks	None	No benefit
Basmajian et al. (1987)	RCT n = 29 112 months poststroke	Upper extremity	EMG-BFB + behaviorally oriented PT vs. conven-tional PT	3 ×/wk × 5 wks	9 months	No benefit
Cozean et al. (1988)*	RCT n = 36 mixed duration poststroke	Gait	EMG-BFB vs. FES vs. EMG-BFB + FES vs. conventional treatment	3 ×/wk × 6 wks	None	Improved gait velocity in EMG-BFB + FES group compared with control

(continued)

Table 16.1	(continued)					
Author	**Trial design**	**Treatment focus**	**Intervention**	**Duration of treatment**	**Length of follow-up**	**Results**
Crow et al. (1989)*	RCT n = 40 28 weeks poststroke	Upper extremity	EMG-BFB for UE vs. conventional therapy	6 wks	6 wks	No benefit
Mandel et al. (1990)#	RCT n = 37 >6 months poststroke	Gait	EMG-BFB vs. positional BFB vs. no-treatment control	2 ×/wk × 6 wks	3 months	Positional BFB improved walking speed compared with EMG-BFB and nontreated control
Colborne et al. (1993)	Crossover n = 8 >7 months poststroke	Gait	EMB-BFB vs. positional BFB vs. conventional PT	2 ×/wk × 4 wks	1 month	Some improvement in certain parameters of gait, but walking speed improved equally with all treatments
Intiso et al. (1994)	RCT n = 16 mean 9.8 months poststroke	Gait	EMG-BFB + conventional PT vs. conventional PT	15 sessions	None	Improved gait parameters, but no change in velocity

design and comparability and variations in biofeedback training techniques of the studies included in these meta-analyses raise the possibility of a type II error (inadequate sample size) (Glanz et al. 1995). The correlation between results of meta-analyses and those from large randomized clinical trials is only fair (LeLorier et al. 1997), and the conflicting results of these meta-analyses suggest the need for a large randomized clinical trial for biofeedback poststroke.

Most trials of biofeedback have focused on "standard" EMG biofeedback, in which a surface electrode is placed over the agonist muscle (and in some cases the antagonist muscle), and the patient receives visual and/or auditory feedback when EMG activity is produced in the agonist muscle. Other forms of biofeedback have been examined as well, though not as extensively. Biofeedback of joint position obtained via an electrogoniometer has been used in several studies involving the upper extremity (Greenberg 1980) and the lower extremity (Colborne et al. 1993; Mandel et al. 1990; Morris et al. 1992). These studies have consistently reported some improved control of movement as reflected by joint position when compared to control groups. The limited data comparing positional biofeedback to EMG biofeedback suggest that the former is superior (Mandel et al. 1990). Neither Morris and colleagues (1992) nor Colborne and colleagues (1993), however, have demonstrated improved gait velocity from biofeedback when comparing it with conventional physical therapy.

Another form of biofeedback has utilized force feedback using force plates, in an effort to more equally distribute weight over the paretic leg (Engardt 1994; Engardt et al. 1993). While this approach does allow for better force distribution and better performance on a sit-to-stand task, it has not shown an overall impact on functional status.

Functional electrical stimulation (FES) has also been studied using a variety of techniques, including low-level stimulation below the motor threshold and higher degrees of stimulation intended to induce a muscular contraction. Table 16.2 lists many of the published FES trials. A recent meta-analysis (Glanz et al. 1996) found evidence that FES appears to promote recovery of muscle strength poststroke.

An interesting combination of FES and biofeedback is EMG-triggered FES. In this technique, the target muscle surface EMG signal is monitored, and when it exceeds a preset threshold, an electrical volley is generated that causes completion of the desired movement. This technique shares features of both FES and biofeedback, and appeared to produce some benefit in an uncontrolled case series (Fields 1987) and in one small controlled study (Kraft et al. 1992). No research has demonstrated any benefit of this approach over standard FES techniques. A small pilot trial demonstrated efficacy of this technique over control treatment in acute stroke patients (Francisco et al. 1998). A similar technique of triggered FES has been used with positional rather than EMG feedback (Bowman et al. 1979; Winchester et al. 1983).

An interesting but as yet untested extension of this technique has been proposed (J. Chae, personal communication), in which the patient's activation of the agonist muscle is monitored using the EMG signal. As in EMG-triggered FES, an electrical stimulus is provided to the agonist muscle based on the presence of an EMG signal above a certain threshold. This technique differs from standard EMG-triggered FES in that FES continues as long as the individual continues to voluntarily activate the muscle, and ceases when the patient relaxes the muscle. This EMG-controlled FES system may prove to be a significant advance in combining the techniques of biofeedback and FES.

Although scientists have studied biofeedback for twenty years, its overall utility and most appropriate application remain unclear. Combining the technologies of EMG, FES, kinesiologic information, and force generation information may ultimately provide the best results with these techniques. At present, the available data on these techniques are inconclusive.

Balance Training

Although standing balance appears to correlate strongly with several measures of gait (Bohannon 1995), there is no conclusive evidence that exercise to improve balance leads to improved functional

ambulation. Platform training for balance impairments in hemiplegic stroke patients can help increase the magnitude of postural deviations tolerated on a perturbed platform (Hocherman et al. 1984), and can reduce lateral sway (Shumway-Cook et al. 1988) and standing symmetry (Winstein et al. 1989). The improvement in static standing balance does not appear to lead to improved gait symmetry or speed, however (Winstein et al. 1989).

Sitting balance is important both functionally and prognostically (Feigin et al. 1996). One study found that devices providing feedback regarding sitting angle can be useful (Dursun et al. 1996). Training programs involving seated reaching tasks appear to help improve sitting balance, but without any carryover into ambulatory ability (Dean and Shepherd 1997). In general, balance training appears useful to the extent that it is task-specific for a functional activity (e.g., sitting balance training to improve sitting balance). There is no evidence that balance training carries over from one activity to another, such as from standing balance to ambulation.

Other Techniques

To restore ambulatory ability in nonambulatory hemiparetic patients, several experiments have tested treadmill training with partial support of the patient's body (Dobkin et al. 1991; Hesse et al. 1994; Hesse et al. 1995). In their study of subacute stroke patients (mean duration poststroke 176.8 days), Hesse et al. (1995) found treadmill training with harness support to be significantly more effective in improving gait independence than standard physical therapy training. While intriguing, these studies need to be confirmed by larger and better controlled trials.

Use of robots to facilitate motor recovery has to date focused only on the proximal upper extremity—with robot-assisted movement of the arm, and visual and auditory feedback to enhance accuracy of movement. As the patient begins to perform functional patterns of movement, the support of the robot is gradually withdrawn (Aisen et al. 1997). While initial results are encouraging, we need to assess this treatment with larger studies—including long-term follow-up—before wider adoption.

Strengthening Exercises

Impairments of strength are a key issue in many individuals who have sustained a stroke, but are

Table 16.2			Functional Electrical Stimulation Trials			
Author	**Design**	**Treatment focus**	**Intervention**	**Duration of treatment**	**Length of follow-up**	**Results**
Merletti et al. (1978)*	RCT n = 49 0.5-15 months poststroke	Ankle dorsi-flexion	FES + conventional PT vs. conventional PT	1 month	3 months	Improved strength in FES group; no functional outcomes documented
Bowman et al. (1979)*	RCT n = 30 3-16 wks poststroke	Wrist extension	Electrogoniometer-triggered FES + conventional PT vs. conventional PT	2 ×/day × 4 wks	None	Increased wrist extensor torque and active ROM
Winchester et al. (1983)*	RCT n = 40 <6 month poststroke	Knee extension	Electrogoniometer-triggered FES + conventional PT vs. conventional PT	4 wks	None	Increased knee extensor torque, but no change in isolated knee extension control
Kraft et al. (1992)	Nonrandomized controlled trial n = 18 >6 months poststroke	Upper extremity	EMG-triggered FES vs. low-intensity continuous FES vs. proprioceptive neuromuscular facilitation vs. no treatment	3 months	9 months	3 treatment groups all had improved motor function compared with control; no difference among treatment modalities
Levin and Hui-Chan (1992)*	RCT, with crossover of some "placebo" subjects n = 13 >8 months poststroke	LE spasticity and ankle dorsiflexion	TENS to common peroneal nerve vs. low-intensity TENS	5 ×/wk × 3 wks	None	Decreased spasticity and increased dorsiflexion strength in treatment group

*Included in meta-analysis by Glanz et al. 1996

ECR = extensor carpi radialis; EMG = electromyography; FCR = flexor carpi radialis; FES = functional electrical stimulation; LE = lower extremity; PT = physical therapy; RCT = randomized clinical trial; ROM = range of motion; TENS = transcutaneous electrical stimulation

Table 16.2   (continued)

Author	Design	Treatment focus	Intervention	Duration of treatment	Length of follow-up	Results
Faghri et al. (1994)	RCT n = 26 11-21 days poststroke	Shoulder subluxation, pain, and function	FES + conventional PT vs. conventional PT	7 days/wk × 6 wks	6 wks	Reduced pain and subluxation; improved motor function
Bogataj et al. (1995)	Crossover n = 20 19 months poststroke	Gait	FES + conventional PT vs. conventional PT	3 wks	None	Improved gait parameters, but poor correlation with motor function
Hummelsheim et al. (1997)	Prospective case series n = 12 34 months poststroke	Wrist flexion and extension	FES to ECR and FCR + therapy	2 ×/day × 2 wks	None	No benefit from FES, but therapy improved function

notoriously difficult to separate from impairments of motor control. As would be expected, the best predictor of motor strength at the completion of rehabilitation is the motor strength at admission (Bohannon and Smith 1987). While some studies have demonstrated a correlation between muscle strength and functional ability (Bohannon and Andrews 1990; Hamrin et al. 1982; Sunderland et al. 1989), strength per se does not appear to be an independent predictor of gait performance after stroke (Bohannon 1995). A stroke survivor's ability to generate isokinetic torque at high velocities correlates better with his/her ambulatory function than does his/her ability to generate isometric torque (Nakamura et al. 1985), possibly reflecting the relationship between motor control and speed of movement in individuals after stroke.

Most trials of therapeutic exercise have concentrated on restoration of motor control rather than motor strength, and few have incorporated resistive exercises. Historically, some physicians have argued that resistive exercises might interfere with developing improved motor control (Bobath 1990), though no published evidence exists to support this conten-

tion. One experiment found that resistive finger extension exercises provided no significant benefit for restoring control of finger extension (Trombly and Quintana 1983; Trombly et al. 1986). Limited data suggest that resistive exercises may accelerate the *rate* of functional improvement when compared with a standard functionally oriented program, but not the ultimate functional *outcome* (Inaba et al. 1973).

In studying the relative benefits of concentric versus eccentric strengthening, Engardt et al. (1995) found both techniques equally effective for increasing muscle strength in the hemiparetic limb. Conflicting results have been found for the value of isokinetic strength training of the lower extremity poststroke: one study (Glasser 1986) observed no additional functional benefit to combining isokinetic training with standard physical therapy; another (Sharp and Brouwer 1997) reported that isokinetic strengthening of knee flexors and extensors in chronic stable poststroke individuals can increase both muscle strength and gait velocity, without adverse effects. The discrepancy between these two studies may be due in part to differences in study populations—Sharp and Brouwer tested chronic stable poststroke patients, while Glasser studied more recently affected individuals.

Some investigators have noted a modest correlation between spasticity and motor strength in the same muscle in hemiplegic stroke patients (Bohannon et al. 1987), but others have not seen the correlation (Nakamura et al. 1985). Spasticity does not correlate well with gait speed (Bohannon and Andrews 1990). Strengthening of hemiparetic muscles does not affect spasticity in those muscles (Sharp and Brouwer 1997), and the importance of spasticity in designing exercise programs poststroke appears limited.

Exercise for Ataxia

A small but significant number of individuals develop ataxia poststroke, most commonly after cerebellar injury. There is a paucity of scientific literature on the use of therapeutic exercise for rehabilitation of cerebellar ataxia. While physicians have advocated Frenkel's exercises for many years to treat ataxia (Urbsheit and Oremland 1990), there are few objective data to support their use. Limb weights appear to provide some benefit for both upper extremity functional tasks and for ambulation (Morgan 1975)(see figure 16.6). The optimal amount of weighting is patient-specific, with lighter or heavier weights reducing benefits. Case reports suggest that exercise training during both outpatient physical therapy (Gill-Body et al. 1997) and during comprehensive inpatient rehabilitation (Sliwa et al. 1994) provides some benefit for cerebellar ataxia. A small case series (Balliet et al. 1987) suggests that individuals with chronic stable ataxia may benefit from an exercise program that reduces the amount of weightbearing through the upper extremities. There

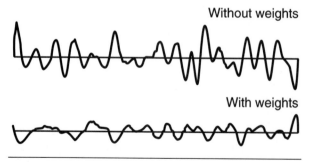

Without weights

With weights

Figure 16.6 Accelerometer traces recording hand movement towards a target in an ataxic individual, with and without wrist weights. Reprinted, by permission, from M.H. Morgan, 1975, "Ataxia and weights," *Physiotherapy* 61:332-34.

are case reports of the utility of EMG biofeedback for ataxia (Davis and Lee 1980; Guercio et al. 1997), but no controlled trials.

Exercise for Aerobic Conditioning

Deconditioning is highly prevalent poststroke, due in many cases to neurologic impairments that interfere with the ability to participate in aerobic conditioning exercise. Monga et al. (1988) found that stroke patients were unable to achieve the same workload as age-matched control subjects during lower extremity ergometry. Well-designed exercise programs for this population can reduce this deconditioning. Using an adapted bicycle ergometer, Potempa et al. (1995) found that a 10-week training period with gradually increasing workload resulted in significant improvements in maximal O_2 consumption, workload, and exercise duration in experimental subjects as compared with controls. Subjects also showed a significant reduction in systolic blood pressure at submaximal workloads.

The safety of aerobic and other physiologically stressful exercise has been a concern in stroke patients. Coronary artery disease (CAD) shares many of the risk factors for stroke, and the two conditions frequently coexist. In one angiographic series, 35% of individuals with transient ischemic attack (TIA), stroke, or asymptomatic carotid bruit had evidence of severe CAD (>70% stenosis of one or more coronary arteries), with only 7% having normal coronary arteries (Hertzer et al. 1985). Roth (1993) estimated that approximately 75% of individuals who have sustained a stroke have heart disease. The fact that cardiac disease is the most common cause of death in long-term poststroke survivors (Matsumoto et al. 1973) argues for both the importance of aerobic exercise in this population, as well as some caution in implementing such a program.

Because of the high prevalence of cardiac disease in the stroke population, exercise stress testing is necessary to assess the presence and severity of coronary artery disease in poststroke patients. While conventional treadmill or bicycle ergometry testing is often impractical due to neurologic deficits, a variety of adapted exercise testing techniques offer suitable substitutes. These include arm, leg, or combined arm and leg ergometry, supine bicycle ergometry (Moldover et al. 1984), wheelchair ergometry, and low-velocity treadmill testing (Macko et al. 1997). Others (Roth

1993) have used cardiac monitoring during physical therapy to check for possible ischemia or arrhythmia. Finally, Dipyridamole thallium^{201} testing or Dobutamine echocardiography can identify ischemia without exercise. Despite the availability of these techniques, however, no large-scale studies have demonstrated improved outcomes as a result of routine cardiac testing in individuals poststroke.

Other Benefits of Exercise

Stroke with resulting hemiplegia decreases bone mass on the hemiplegic side (Hamdy et al. 1993; Hamdy et al. 1995), with resulting increased risk of osteoporotic fractures. Although no published reports have examined the effects of increased exercise on bone mineral density in the hemiplegic leg, it is reasonable to hypothesize that it may be of some benefit in this population. See chapter 17 for a more detailed discussion of the role of exercise in the rehabilitation of osteoporosis.

Summary

Thirty years ago, a review of stroke treatment in the *New England Journal of Medicine* concluded, "It has not yet been demonstrated that patients receiving formal physical therapy after strokes recover more quickly or more completely than those who receive no therapy" (Browne and Poskanzer 1969). While this statement is no longer considered true, there remains much in the use of therapeutic exercise poststroke that is not scientifically based. Given the high human costs of stroke and the financial pressures to reduce unproven or unnecessary care, the need for definitive studies of rehabilitation interventions in stroke has never been more acute. The community of rehabilitation professionals needs to establish recommendations—based on *evidence*—that provide the most effective and efficient programs of therapeutic exercise for stroke survivors. Documentation of functional outcomes will be essential to convince third-party payers to continue coverage of the current array of rehabilitation programs.

References

Aisen, F.L., H.I. Krebs, N. Hogan, F. McDowell, and B.T. Volpe. 1997. The effect of robot-assisted therapy and rehabilitative training on motor recovery following stroke. *Arch Neurol* 54:443-46.

American Heart Association. 1998. *Heart and Stroke Statistical Update.* Dallas, TX: The Association.

Asanuma, C. 1991. Mapping movements within a moving motor map. *Trends Neuroscience* 14:217-18.

Balliet, R, K.B. Harbst, D. Kim, and R.V. Stewart. 1987. Retraining of functional gait through the reduction of upper extremity weightbearing in chronic cerebellar ataxia. *Int Rehabil Med* 8:149-53.

Basmajian, J.V., C. Gowland, M.E. Brandstater, L. Swanson, and J. Trotter. 1982. EMG feedback treatment of upper limb in hemiplegic stroke patients: a pilot study. *Arch Phys Med Rehabil* 63: 613-16.

Basmajian, J.V., C.A. Gowland, M.A. Finlayson, A.L. Hall, L.R. Swanson, P.W. Stratford, J.E. Trotter, and M.E. Brandstater. 1987. Stroke treatment: comparison of integrated behavioral-physical therapy vs traditional physical therapy programs. *Arch Phys Med Rehabil* 68:267-72.

Basmajian, J.V., C.G. Kukulka, M.G. Narayan, and K. Takebe. 1975. Biofeedback treatment of foot-drop after stroke compared with standard rehabilitation technique: effects on voluntary control and strength. *Arch Phys Med Rehabil* 56:231-36.

Bethel, A., J.R. Kirsch, R.C. Koehler, S.P. Finklestein, and R.J. Traystman. 1997. Intravenous basic fibroblast growth factor decreased brain injury resulting from focal ischemia in cats. *Stroke* 28:609-15.

Bobath, B. 1990. *Adult hemiplegia: Evaluation and treatment.* 3d ed., 60-61. Oxford, England: Butterworth Heinemann.

Bogataj, U., N. Gros, M. Kljajic, R. Acimovic, and M. Malezic. 1995. The rehabilitation of gait in patients with hemiplegia: a comparison between conventional therapy and multichannel functional electrical stimulation therapy. *Phys Ther* 75:490-502.

Bohannon, R.W. 1995. Standing balance, lower extremity muscle strength, and walking performance of patients referred for physical therapy. *Percept Mot Skills* 80:379-85.

Bohannon, R.W., and A.W. Andrews. 1990. Correlation of knee extensor muscle torque and spasticity with gait speed in patients with stroke. *Arch Phys Med Rehabil* 71:330-33.

Bohannon, R.W., P.A. Larkin, M.B. Smith, and M.G. Horton. 1987. Relationship between static muscle strength deficits and spasticity in stroke patients with hemiparesis. *Phys Ther* 67:1068-71.

Bohannon, R.W., and M.B. Smith. 1987. Upper extremity strength deficits in hemiplegic stroke patients: relationship between admission and discharge assessment and time since onset. *Arch Phys Med Rehabil* 68:155-57.

Bowman, B.R., L.L. Baker, and R.L. Waters. 1979. Positional feedback and electrical stimulation: an automated treatment for the hemiplegic wrist. *Arch Phys Med Rehabil* 60:492-502.

Bronner, L.L., D.S. Kanter, and J.E. Manson. 1995. Primary prevention of stroke. *New Engl J Med* 333:1392-1400.

Brooke, M.H., and W.K. Engel. 1969. The histographic analysis of human muscle biopsies with regard to fiber types. Part 2. Diseases of the upper and lower motor neuron. *Neurology* 19:378-93.

Browne, T.R. 3d, and D.C. Poskanzer. 1969. Treatment of strokes. *New Engl J Med* 281:594-602.

Burnside, I.G., S. Tobias, and D. Bursill. 1982. Electromyographic feedback in the remobilization of stroke patients: a controlled trial. *Arch Phys Med Rehabil* 63:217-22.

Butefisch, C., H. Hummelsheim, P. Densler, and K. Mauritz. 1995. Repetitive training of isolated movements improves the outcome of motor rehabilitation of the centrally paretic hand. *J Neurol Sci* 130:59-68.

Clark, W.M., S.J. Warach, and L.C. Pettigrew, R.E. Gammans, L.A. Sabounjian. 1997. A randomized dose-response trial of citicoline in acute ischemic stroke patients. *Neurology* 49:671-78.

Colborne, G.R., S.J. Olney, and M.P. Griffin. 1993. Feedback of ankle joint angle and soleus electromyography in the rehabilitation of hemiplegic gait. *Arch Phys Med Rehabil* 74:1100-6.

Cozean, C.D., W.S. Pease, and S.I. Hubbell. 1988. Biofeedback and functional electric stimulation in stroke rehabilitation. *Arch Phys Med Rehabil* 69:401-05.

Cramer, S.C., G. Nelles, R.R. Benson, J.D. Kaplan, R.A. Parker, K.K. Kwong, D.N. Kennedy, S.P. Finklestein, and B.R. Rosen. 1997. A functional MRI study of subjects recovered from hemiparetic stroke. *Stroke* 28:2518-27.

Crisostomo, E.A., P.W. Duncan, M. Propst, D.V. Dawson, and J.N. Davis. 1988. Evidence that amphetamine with physical therapy promotes recovery of motor function in stroke patients. *Ann Neurol* 23:94-97.

Crow, J.L., N.B. Lincoln, F.M. Nouri, and W. DeWeerdt. 1989. The effectiveness of EMG biofeedback in the treatment of arm function after stroke. *Int Disabil Studies* 11:155-60.

Dattola, R., P. Girlanda, G. Vita, M. Santoro, M.L. Roberto, A. Toscano, C. Venuto, A. Baradello, and C. Messina. 1993. Muscle rearrangement in patients with hemiparesis after stroke: an electrophysiological and morphological study. *European Neurology* 33:109-14.

Davis, A.E., and R.G. Lee. 1980. EMG biofeedback in patients with motor disorders: an aid for coordinating activity in antagonist muscle groups. *Can J Neurolog Sci* 7:199-206.

Dean, C.M., and R.B. Shepherd. 1997. Task-related training improves performance of seated reaching tasks after stroke. A randomized controlled trial. *Stroke* 28:722-28.

Dickstein, R., S. Hocherman, T. Pillar, and R. Shaham. 1986. Stroke rehabilitation. Three exercise therapy approaches. *Phys Ther* 66:1233-38.

Dietz, V., U. Ketelsen, W. Berger, and J. Quintern. 1986. Motor unit involvement in spastic paresis. *J Neurol Sci* 75:89-103.

Dobkin, B., E. Fowler, and R. Gregor. 1991. A strategy to train locomotion in patients with chronic hemiplegic stroke. *Ann Neurol* 30:278.

Dursun, E., N. Hamamci, S. Donmez, O. Tuzunalp, and A. Cakci. 1996. Angular biofeedback device for sitting balance of stroke patients. *Stroke* 27:1354-57.

Engardt, M. 1994. Rising and sitting down in stroke patients. Auditory feedback and dynamic strength training to enhance symmetrical body weight distribution. *Scand J Rehabil Med* (Suppl.) 31:1-57.

Engardt, M., E. Knutsson, M. Jonsson, and M. Sternhag. 1995. Dynamic muscle strength training in stroke patients: effects on knee extension torque, electromyographic activity, and motor function. *Arch Phys Med Rehabil* 76:419-25.

Engardt, M., T. Ribbe, and E. Olsson, 1993. Vertical ground reaction force feedback to enhance stroke patients' symmetrical bodyweight distribution while rising/sitting down. *Scand J Rehabil Med* 25:41-48.

Evans, R.L., R.T. Connis, R.D. Hendricks, and J.K. Haselkorn. 1995. Multidisciplinary rehabilitation versus medical care: a metaanalysis. *Soc Sci Med* 40:1699-706.

Faghri, P.D., M.M. Rodgers, R.M. Glaser, J.G. Bors, C. Ho, and P. Akuthota. 1994. The effects of functional electrical stimulation on shoulder subluxation, arm function recovery, and shoulder pain in hemiplegic stroke patients. *Arch Phys Med Rehabil* 75:73-79.

Feeney, D.M., A. Gonzales, and W. Law. 1982. Amphetamine, haloperidol and experience interact to affect rate of recovery after motor cortex injury. *Science* 217:855-57.

Feigin, L., B. Sharon, B. Czaczkes, and A.J. Rosin. 1996. Sitting equilibrium 2 weeks after a stroke can predict the walking ability after 6 months. *Gerontology* 42:348-53.

Fields, R.W. 1987. Electromyographically triggered electrical muscle stimulation for chronic hemiplegia. *Arch Phys Med Rehabil* 68:407-14.

Fisher, C.M. 1992. Concerning the mechanism of recovery in stroke hemiplegia. *Can J Neurol Sci* 19:57-63.

Francisco G., J. Chae, H. Chawla, S. Kirshblum, R. Zorowitz, G. Lewis, and S. Pang. 1998. Electromyogram-triggered neuromuscular stimulation for improving the arm function of acute stroke survivors: a randomized pilot study. *Arch Phys Med Rehabil* 79:570-5.

Frontera, W.R., L. Grimby, and L. Larsson. 1997. Firing rate of the lower motoneuron and contractile properties of its muscle fibers after upper motoneuron lesion in man. *Muscle Nerve* 20:938-47.

Gemperline, J.J., S. Allen, D. Walk, and W.Z. Rymer. 1995. Characteristics of motor unit discharge in subjects with hemiparesis. *Muscle Nerve* 18:1101-14.

Gill-Body, K.M., R.A. Popat, S.W. Parker, and D.E. Krebs. 1997. Rehabilitation of balance in two patients with cerebellar dysfunction. *Phys Ther* 77:534-552.

Gillum, R.F., M.E. Mussolino, and D.D. Ingram. 1996. Physical activity and stroke incidence in women and men: the NHANES I epidemiologic follow-up study. *Am J Epidemiol* 143:860-869.

Glanz, M., S. Klawansky, W. Stason, C. Berkey, and T.C. Chalmers. 1996. Functional electrostimulation in poststroke rehabilitation: a meta-analysis of the randomized controlled trials. *Arch Phys Med Rehabil* 77:549-553.

Glanz, M., S. Klawansky, W. Stason, C. Berkey, H. Phan, and N. Shah. 1995. Biofeedback therapy in poststroke rehabilitation: a meta-analysis of the randomized controlled trials. *Arch Phys Med Rehabil* 76:508-15.

Glasser, L. 1986. Effects of isokinetic training on the rate of movement during ambulation in hemiparetic patients. *Phys Ther* 66:673-76.

Glees, P. 1980. Functional reorganization following hemispherectomy in man and after small experimental lesions in primates. In *Recovery of function: Theoretical considerations for brain injury rehabilitation,* ed. P. Bach-y-Rita. Baltimore: University Park Press.

Goldstein, L.B., and the Sygen in Acute Stroke Study Investigators. 1995. Common drugs may influence motor recovery after stroke. *Neurology* 45:865-71.

Gowland, C. 1982. Recovery of motor function following stroke: profile and predictors. *Physiotherapy* 34:77-84.

Greenberg, S., and R.S. Fowler Jr. 1980. Kinesthetic biofeedback: a treatment modality for elbow range of motion in hemiplegia. *Am J Occup Ther* 34:738-43.

Guercio, J., R. Chittum, and M. McMorrow. 1997. Self-management in the treatment of ataxia: a case study in reducing ataxic tremor through relaxation and biofeedback. *Brain Injury* 11:353-62.

Hamdy, R.C., G. Krishnaswamy, V. Cancellaro, K. Whalen, and L. Harvill. 1993. Changes in bone mineral content and density after stroke. *Am J Phys Med Rehabil* 72:188-91.

Hamdy, R.C., S.W. Moore, V.A. Cancellaro, and L.M. Harvill. 1995. Long-term effects of strokes on bone mass. *Am J Phys Med Rehabil* 74:351-56.

Hamrin, E., G. Eklund, A.K. Hillgren, O. Borges, J. Hall, and O. Hellstrom. 1982. Muscle strength and balance in poststroke patients. *Upsala J Med Sci* 87:11-26.

Hertzer, N.R., J.R. Young, E.G. Beven, R.A. Graor, P.J. O'Hara, W.F. Ruschhaupt, V.G. de Wolfe, and L.C. Maljovec. 1985. Coronary angiography in 506 patients with extracranial cerebrovascular disease. *Arch Intern Med.* 145:849-52.

Hesse, S., C. Bertelt, M.T. Jahnke, A. Schaffrin, P. Baake, M. Malezic, and K.H. Mauritz. 1995. Treadmill training with partial body weight support compared with physiotherapy in nonambulatory hemiparetic patients. *Stroke* 26:976-81.

Hesse, S., C. Bertelt, A. Schaffrin, M. Malezic, and K.H. Mauritz. 1994. Restoration of gait in nonambulatory hemiparetic patients by treadmill training with partial bodyweight support. *Arch Phys Med Rehabil* 75:1087-93.

Hesse, S.A., M.T. Jahnke, C.M. Bertelt, C. Schreiner, D. Lucke, and K.H. Mauritz. 1994. Gait outcome in ambulatory hemiparetic patients after a 4-week comprehensive rehabilitation program and prognostic factors. *Stroke* 25:1999-2004.

Hocherman, S., R. Dickstein, and T. Pillar. 1984. Platform training and postural stability in hemiplegia. *Arch Phys Med Rehabil* 65:588-92.

Hovda, D.A., and D.M. Feeney. 1984. Amphetamine and experience promote recovery of locomotor function after unilateral frontal cortex injury in the cat. *Brain Res* 298:358-61.

Hummelsheim, H., M.L. Maier-Loth, and C. Eickhof. 1997. The functional value of electrical muscle stimulation for the rehabilitation of the hand in stroke patients. *Scand J Rehabil Med* 29:3-10.

Hurd, W.W., V. Pegram, and C. Nepomuceno. 1980. Comparison of actual and simulated EMG biofeedback in the treatment of hemiplegic patients. *Am J Phys Med* 59:73-82.

Inaba, M., E. Edberg, J. Montgomery, and M.K. Gillis. 1973. Effectiveness of functional training, active exercise, and resistive exercise for patients with hemiplegia. *Phys Ther* 53:28-35.

Indredavik, B., S.A. Slordahl, F. Bakke, R. Rokseth, and L.L. Haheim. 1997. Stroke unit treatment: longterm effects. *Stroke* 28:1861-66.

Inglis, J., M.W. Donald, T.N. Monga, M. Sproule, and M.J. Young. 1984. Electromyographic biofeedback and physical therapy of the hemiplegic upper limb. *Arch Phys Med Rehabil* 65:755-59.

Intiso, D., V. Santilli, M.G. Grasso, R. Rossi, and I. Caruso. 1994. Rehabilitation of walking with electromyographic biofeedback in footdrop after stroke. *Stroke* 25:1189-92.

Jacobs, K.M., and J.P. Donoghue. 1991. Reshaping the cortical motor map by unmasking latent intracortical connections. *Science* 251:944-47.

Jakobsson, F., L. Edstrom, L. Grimby, and L.E. Thornell. 1991. Disuse of anterior tibial muscle during locomotion and increased proportion of type II fibers in hemiplegia. *J Neurol Sci* 105:49-56.

Johansson, B.B. 1996. Functional outcome in rats transferred to an enriched environment 15 days after focal brain ischemia. *Stroke* 27:324-26.

Johansson, K., I. Lindgren, H. Widner, I. Wiklund, and B.B. Johansson. 1993. Can sensory stimulation improve the functional outcome in stroke patients? *Neurology* 43:2189-92.

John, J. 1986. Failure of electrical myofeedback to augment the effects of physiotherapy in stroke. *Int J Rehabil Res* 9:35-45.

Jones, T.A., and T. Schallert. 1994. Use-dependent growth of pyramidal neurons after neocortical damage. *J Neurosci* 14:2140-52.

Jongbloed, L., S. Stacey, and C. Brighton. 1989. Stroke rehabilitation: sensorimotor integrative treatment versus functional treatment. *Am J Occup Ther* 43:391-97.

Kaas, J.H., L.A. Krubitzer, and Y.M. Chino, A.L. Langston, E.H. Polley, and N. Blair. 1990. Reorganization of retinotopic cortical maps in adult mammals after lesions of the retina. *Science* 248:229-31.

Kalra, L., P. Dale, and P. Crome. 1993. Improving stroke rehabilitation: a controlled study. *Stroke* 24:1462-67.

Kalra, L., and J. Eade. 1995. Role of stroke rehabilitation units in managing severe disability after stroke. *Stroke* 26:2031-34.

Kaste, M., H. Palomaki, and S. Sarna. 1995. Where and how should elderly stroke patients be treated? A randomized trial. *Stroke* 26:249-53.

Kawamata, T., E.K. Speliotes, and S.P. Finklestein. 1997. The role of polypeptide growth factors in recovery from stroke. *Adv Neurol* 73:377-82.

Keith, R.A., D.B. Wilson, and P. Gutierrez. 1995. Acute and subacute rehabilitation for stroke: a comparison. *Arch Phys Med Rehabil* 76:495-500.

Kiely, D.K., P.A. Wolf, L.A. Cupples, A.S. Beiser, and W.B. Kannel. 1994. Physical activity and stroke risk: The Framingham Study. *Am J Epidemiol* 140:608-20.

King, A.J., and D.R. Moore. 1991. Plasticity of auditory maps in the brain. *Trends Neurosci* 14:21-27.

Kozlowski, D.A., C.D. James, and T. Schallert. 1996. Use-dependent exaggeration of neuronal injury after unilateral sensorimotor cortex lesions. *J Neurosci* 16:4776-86.

Kraft, G.H., S.S. Fitts, and M.C. Hammond. 1992. Techniques to improve function of the arm and hand in chronic hemiplegia. *Arch Phys Med Rehabil* 73:220-27.

Kramer, A.M., J.F. Steiner, R.E. Schlenker, T.B. Eilertsen, C.A. Hrincevich, D.A. Tropea, L.A. Ahmad, and E.G. Eckhoff. 1997. Outcomes and costs after hip fracture and stroke: a comparison of rehabilitation settings. *JAMA* 277:396-404.

Kwakkel, G., R.C. Wagenaar, T.W. Koelman, G.J. Lankhorst, and J.C. Koetsier. 1997. Effects of intensity of rehabilitation after stroke. A research synthesis. *Stroke* 28:1550-6.

Landin, S., L. Hagenfeldt, B. Saltin, and J. Wahren. 1977. Muscle metabolism during exercise in hemiparetic patients. *Clin Sci Mol Med.* 53:257-69.

Langhorne, P., R. Wagenaar, and C. Partridge. 1996. Physiotherapy after stroke: more is better? *Physiother Res Int* 1:75-88

Lehmann, J.F., B.J. Delatuer, and R.S. Fowler Jr., C.G. Warren, R. Arnhold, G. Schertzer, R. Hurka, J.J. Whitmore, A.J. Masock, and K.H. Chambers. 1975. Stroke: does rehabilitation affect outcome? *Arch Phys Med Rehabil* 56:375-82.

LeLorier, J., G. Gregoire, A. Benhaddad, J. Lapierre, and F. Derderian. 1997. Discrepancies between meta-analyses and subsequent large randomized controlled trials. *New Engl J Med* 337:536-42.

Levin, M.F., and C.W.Y. Hui-Chan. 1992. Relief of hemiparetic spasticity by TENS is associated with improvement in reflex and voluntary motor functions. *Electroencephelogr Clin Neurophysiol* 85:131-42.

Logigian, M.K., M.A. Samuels, and J.F. Falconer. 1983. Clinical exercise trial for stroke patients. *Arch Phys Med Rehabil* 64:364-67.

Lomo, T. 1989. Long term effects of altered activity on skeletal muscle. *Biomed Biochim Acta* 48:S432-44.

Lord, J.P., and K. Hall. 1986. Neuromuscular reeducation versus traditional programs for stroke rehabilitation. *Arch Phys Med Rehabil* 67:88-91.

Macko, R.F., L.I. Katzel, A. Yataco, L.D. Tretter, C.A. DeSouza, D.R. Dengel, G.V. Smith, and K.H. Silver. 1997. Low velocity graded treadmill stress testing in hemiparetic stroke patients. *Stroke* 28:988-92.

Magnusson, M., K. Johansson, and B.B. Johansson. 1994. Sensory stimulation promotes normalization of postural control after stroke. *Stroke* 25:1176-80.

Mandel, A.R., N.J. Nymark, S.J. Balmer, D.M. Grinnell, and M.D. O'Riain. 1990. Electromyographic versus rhythmic positional biofeedback in computerized gait retraining with stroke patients. *Arch Phys Med Rehabil* 71:649-54.

Matsumoto, N., J.P. Whisnant, L.T. Kurland, and H. Okazaki. 1973. Natural history of stroke in Rochester, Minnesota, 1955 through 1969: an extension of a previous study, 1945 through 1954. *Stroke* 4:20-29.

Menotti, A., A. Keys, H. Blackburn, C. Aravanis, A. Dontas, F. Fidanza, S. Giampaoli, M. Karvonen, D. Kromhout, and S. Nedeljkovic. 1990. Twenty-year stroke mortality and prediction in twelve cohorts of the Seven Countries Study. *Int J Epidemiol* 19:309-15.

Merletti, R., F. Zelaschi, D. Latella, M. Galli, S. Angeli, and M.B. Sessa. 1978. A control study of muscle force recovery in hemiparetic patients during treatment with functional electrical stimulation. *Scand J Rehabil Med* 10:147-54.

Moldover, J.R., M.C. Daum, and J.A. Downey. 1984. Cardiac stress testing of hemiparetic patients with a supine bicycle ergometer: preliminary study. *Arch Phys Med Rehabil* 65:470-76.

Monga, T.N., D.A. Deforge, J. Williams, and L.A. Wolfe. 1988. Cardiovascular responses to acute exercise in patients with cerebrovascular accidents. *Arch Phys Med Rehabil* 69:937-940.

Moreland, J., and M.A. Thomson. 1994. Efficacy of electromyographic biofeedback compared with conventional physical therapy for upper extremity function in patients following stroke: a research overview and metaanalysis. *Phys Ther* 74:534-43.

Morgan, M.H. 1975. Ataxia and weights. *Physiotherapy* 61:332-34.

Morris, M.E., T.A. Matyas, T.M. Bach, and P.A. Goldie. 1992. Electrogoniometric feedback: its effect on genu recurvatum in stroke. *Arch Phys Med Rehabil* 73:1147-54.

Mroczek, N., D. Halpern, and R. McHugh. 1978. Electromyographic feedback and physical therapy for neuromuscular retraining in hemiplegia. *Arch Phys Med Rehabil* 59:258-67.

Mulder, T., W. Hulstijn, and J. Van der Meer. 1986. EMG feedback and the restoration of motor control. A controlled group study of 12 hemiparetic patients. *Am J Phys Med* 65:173-88.

Naeser, M.A., M.P. Alexander, D. Stiassny-Eder, V. Galler, J. Hobbs, and D. Bachman. 1992. Real versus sham acupuncture in the treatment of paralysis in acute stroke patients: a CT scan lesion site study. *J Neuro Rehab* 6:163-73.

Nakamura, R., T. Hosokawa, and I. Tsuji. 1985. Relationship of muscle strength for knee extension to walking capacity in patients with spastic hemiparesis. *Tohoku J Experimental Med* 145:335-40.

Nelson, D.L., K. Konosky, K. Fleharty, R. Webb, K. Newer, V.P. Hazboun, C. Fontane, and B.C. Licht. 1996. The effects of an occupationally embedded exercise on bilaterally assisted supination in persons with hemiplegia. *Am J Occup Ther* 50:639-46.

Nudo, R.J., and G.W. Milliken. 1996. Reorganization of movement representations in primary motor cortex following focal ischemic infarcts in adult squirrel monkeys. *J Neurophysiol* 75:2144-49.

Nudo, R.J., G.W. Milliken, W.M. Jenkins, and M.M. Merzenich. 1996. Use-dependent alterations of movement representations in primary motor cortex of adult squirrel monkeys. *J Neurosci* 16:785-807.

Nudo, R.J., B.M. Wise, F. SiFuentes, and G.W. Milliken. 1996. Neural substrates for the effects of rehabilitative training on motor recovery after ischemic infarct. *Science* 272:1791-94.

Nugent, J.A., K.A. Schurr, and R.D. Adams. 1994. A dose-response relationship between amount of weightbearing exercise and walking outcome following cerebrovascular accident. *Arch Phys Med Rehabil* 75:399-402.

Nyberg-Hansen, R., and E. Rinvik. 1963. Some comments on the pyramidal tract, with special reference to its individual variations in man. *Acta Neurol Scand* 39:1-30.

Ohlsson, AL., and B.B. Johansson. 1995. The environment influences functional outcome of cerebral infarction in rats. *Stroke* 26:644-49.

Pascual-Leone, A., J. Grafman, and M. Hallett. 1994. Modulation of cortical motor output maps during development of implicit and explicit knowledge. *Science* 263:1287-89.

Pette, D., and G. Vrbova. 1992. Adaptation of mammalian skeletal muscle fibers to chronic electrical stimulation. *Rev Physiol Biochem Pharmacol* 120:115-202.

Pons, T.P., P.E. Garraghty, and M. Mishkin. 1988. Lesion-induced plasticity in the second somatosensory cortex of adult macaques. *Proc Natl Acad Sci* 85:5279-81.

Potempa, K., L.T. Braun, T. Tinknell, and J. Popovich. 1996. Benefits of aerobic exercise after stroke. *Sports Med* 21:337-46.

Potempa, K., M. Lopez, L.T. Braun, J.P. Szidon, L. Fogg, and T. Tincknell. 1995. Physiological outcomes of aerobic exercise training in hemiparetic stroke patients. *Stroke* 26:101-105.

Prevo, A.J., S.L. Visser, and T.W. Vogelaar. 1982. Effect of EMG feedback on paretic muscles and abnormal cocontraction in the hemiplegic arm, compared with conventional physical therapy. *Scand J Rehabil Med* 14:121-31.

Retchin, S.M., R.S. Brown, S-C.J. Yeh, D. Chu, and L. Moreno. 1997. Outcomes for stroke patients in Medicare fee for service and managed care. *JAMA* 278:119-24.

Richards, C.L., F. Malouin, S. Wood-Dauphinee, J.I. Williams, J.P. Bouchard, and D. Brunet. 1993. Task-specific physical therapy for optimization of gait recovery in acute stroke patients. *Arch Phys Med Rehab* 74:612-20.

Rodriquez, A.A., P.O. Black, K.A. Kile, J. Sherman, B. Stellberg, J. McCormick, J. Roszkowski, and E. Swiggum. 1996. Gait training efficacy using a home-based practice model in chronic hemiplegia. *Arch Phys Med Rehabil* 77:801-05.

Roth, E.J. 1993. Heart disease in patients with stroke: incidence, impact, and implications for rehabilitation. Part 1: Classification and prevalence. *Arch Phys Med Rehabil* 74:752-60.

Sabatini, U., D. Toni, P. Pantano, G. Brughitta, A. Padovani, L. Bozzao, and G.L. Lenzi. 1994. Motor recovery after early brain damage. *Stroke* 25:514-17.

Salmons, S., and F.A. Sreter. 1976. Significance of impulse activity in the transformation of skeletal muscle type. *Nature* 263:30-34.

Scelsi, R., S. Lotta, G. Lommi, P. Poggi, and C. Marchetti. 1984. Hemiplegic atrophy. *Acta Neuropathol* 62:324-31.

Schallert, T., D.A. Kozlowski, J.S. Humm, and R.R. Cocke. 1997. Use-dependent structural events in recovery of function. *Adv Neurol* 73:229-38.

Schleenbaker, R.E., and A.G. Mainous. 1993. Electromyographic biofeedback for neuromuscular reeducation in the hemiplegic stroke patient: a meta-analysis. *Arch Phys Med Rehabil* 74:1301-04.

Seitz, R.H., K.E. Allred, M.E. Backus, and J.A. Hoffman. 1987. Functional changes during acute rehabilitation in patients with stroke. *Phys Ther* 67:1685-90.

Sharp, S.A., and B.J. Brouwer. 1997. Isokinetic strength training of the hemiparetic knee: effects on function and spasticity. *Arch Phys Med Rehabil* 78:1231-36.

Shiavi, R.G., S.A. Champion, F.R. Freeman, and H.J. Bugel. 1979. Efficacy of myofeedback therapy in regaining control of lower extremity musculature following stroke. *Am J Phys Med* 58:185-94.

Shinton, R. 1997. Lifelong exposures and the potential for stroke prevention: the contribution of cigarette smoking, exercise, and body fat. *J Epidemiol Community Health* 51:138-43.

Shumway-Cook, A., D. Anson, and S. Haller. 1988. Postural sway biofeedback: its effect on reestablishing stance stability in hemiplegic patients. *Arch Phys Med Rehabil* 69:395-400.

Sivenius, J., K. Pyorala, O.P. Heinonen, J.T. Salonen, and P. Riekkinen. 1985. The significance of intensity of rehabilitation of stroke: a controlled trial. *Stroke* 16:928-31.

Slager, U.T., J.D. Hsu, and C. Jordan. 1985. Histochemical and morphometric changes in muscles of stroke patients. *Clin Orthop* 199:159-68.

Sliwa, J.A., S. Thatcher, and J. Jet. 1994. Paraneoplastic subacute cerebellar degeneration: functional improvement and the role of rehabilitation. *Arch Phys Med Rehabil* 75:355-57.

Smith, D.S., E. Goldenberg, A. Ashburn, G. Kinsella, K. Sheikh, P.J. Brennan, T.W. Meade, D.W. Zutshi, J.D. Perry, and J.S. Reebacket. 1981. Remedial therapy after stroke: a randomized controlled trial. *BMJ* 282:517-20.

Stern, P.H., F. McDowell, J.M. Miller, and M. Robinson. 1970. Effects of facilitation exercise techniques in stroke rehabilitation. *Arch Phys Med Rehabil* 51:526-31.

Stevens, R.S., N.R. Ambler, and M.D. Warren. 1984. A randomised controlled trial of a stroke rehabilitation ward. *Age Ageing* 13:65-75.

Strand, T., K. Asplund, S. Eriksson, E. Hagg, F. Lithner, and P.O. Wester. 1985. A non-intensive stroke unit reduced functional disability and the need for long-term hospitalisation. *Stroke* 16:29-34.

Stroke Unit Trialists' Collaboration. 1997. Collaborative systematic review of the randomized trials of organized inpatient (stroke unit) care after stroke. *BMJ* 314:1151-59.

Sunderland, A., D. Fletcher, L. Bradley, D. Tinson, R.L. Hewer, and T.D. Wade. 1994. Enhanced physical therapy for arm function after stroke: a one year follow up study. *J Neurol Neurosurg Psych* 57:856-58.

Sunderland, A., D. Tinson, L. Bradley, and R.L. Hewer. 1989. Arm function after stroke. An evaluation of grip strength as a measure of recovery and a prognostic indicator. *J Neurolog Neurosurg Psych* 52:1267-72.

Tangeman, P.T., D.A. Banaitis, and A.K. Williams. 1990. Rehabilitation of chronic stroke patients: changes in functional performance. *Arch Phys Med Rehabil* 71:876-80.

Taub, E., N.E. Miller, T.A. Novack, E.W. Cook, W.C. Fleming, C.S. Nepomuceno, J.S. Connell, and J.E. Crago. 1993. Technique to improve chronic motor deficit after stroke. *Arch Phys Med Rehabil* 74:347-54.

Taub, E., and S.L. Wolf. 1997. Constraint induced movement techniques to facilitate upper extremity use in stroke patients. *Top Stroke Rehabil* 3:38-61.

Trombly, C.A., and L.A. Quintana. 1983. The effects of exercise on finger extension of CVA patients. *Am J Occup Ther* 37:195-202.

Trombly, C.A., L. Thayer-Nason, G. Bliss, C.A. Girard, L.A. Lyrist, and A. Brexa-Hooson. 1986. The effectiveness of therapy in improving finger extension in stroke patients. *Am J Occup Ther* 40:612-17.

U.S. Department of Health and Human Services. 1996. *Physical activity and health: A report of the Surgeon General*, 102-7. Atlanta: U.S. Department of Health and Human Services, Centers for Disease Control and Prevention, National Center for Chronic Disease Prevention and Health Promotion.

Urbsheit, N.L., and B.S. Oremland. 1990. Cerebellar dysfunction. In *Neurological rehabilitation*. 2d ed., ed. D.A. Umphred, 597-618. St. Louis: Mosby.

Wade, D.T., F.M. Collen, G.F. Robb, and C.P. Warlow. 1992. Physiotherapy intervention late after stroke and mobility. *BMJ* 304:609-13.

Wagenaar, R.C., O.G. Meijer, P.C. van Wieringen, D.J. Kuik, G.J. Hazenberg, J. Lindeboom, F. Wichers, and H. Rijswijk. 1990. The functional recovery of stroke: a comparison between neurodevelopmental treatment and the Brunnstrom method. *Scand J Rehab Med* 22:1-8.

Walker-Batson, D., P. Smith, S. Curtis, H. Unwin, and R. Greenlee. 1995. Amphetamine paired with physical therapy accelerates motor recovery after stroke. Further evidence. *Stroke* 26:2254-9.

Werner, R.A., and S. Kessler. 1996. Effectiveness of an intensive outpatient rehabilitation program for postacute stroke patients. *Am J Phys Med Rehabil* 75:114-20.

Winchester, P., J. Montgomery, B. Bowman, and H. Hislop. 1983. Effects of feedback stimulation training and cyclical electrical stimulation on knee extension in hemiparetic patients. *Phys Ther* 63:1096-1103.

Winstein, C.J., E.R. Gardner, D.R. McNeal, P.S. Barto, and D.E. Nicholson. 1989. Standing balance training: effect on balance and locomotion in hemiparetic adults. *Arch Phys Med Rehabil* 70:755-62.

Wolf, S.L., and S.A. Binder-Macleod. 1983a. Electromyographic biofeedback applications to the hemiplegic patient: changes in upper extremity neuromuscular and functional status. *Phys Ther* 63:1393-1403.

Wolf, S.L., and S.A. Binder-Macleod. 1983b. Electromyographic biofeedback applications to the hemiplegic patient: changes in lower extremity neuromuscular and functional status. *Phys Ther* 63:1404-13.

Wolf, S.L., D.E. LeCraw, L.A. Barton, and B.B. Jann. 1989. Forced use of hemiplegic upper extremities to reverse the effect of learned nonuse among chronic stroke and head-injured patients. *Exp Neurol* 104:125-32.

Chapter 17

Osteoporosis

David M. Slovik, MD

Case Study

A 73-year-old woman, R.D., came to us with acute back pain after lifting a heavy object. She was independent, in good health, and participated in many outside activities.

She had a normal menarche at age 13 and had two children. She had no history of eating disorders or chronic illnesses. She considered herself nonathletic and rarely had participated in sport activities. Her nutritional status was "average" when growing up, although she liked milk and dairy products.

She had a natural menopause at age 50, but refused hormone replacement therapy. She occasionally took calcium supplements, and walked at the local mall one-half hour several times each week.

R.D.'s height was 61 inches (usual height 64 inches) and she weighed 105 pounds. She had a dorsal kyphosis and tenderness over several lumbar vertebrae and in the lumbar paravertebral area. Lumbosacral X rays showed end-plate compression of L1 and L3 vertebral bodies. Thoracic spine X rays also showed anterior wedge deformities of T10 and T12 vertebrae.

A femoral neck bone density by dual X-ray absorptiometry (DXA) showed a *t* score (compared to young female adult mean) of −3.2 standard deviations and a *z* score (compared to age-matched females) of −0.8 standard deviations. Additional workup revealed no secondary causes of osteoporosis.

We initially treated R.D. with analgesics and bed rest, progressing to activity as tolerated in subsequent weeks. We placed her on calcium supplementation, a multivitamin containing vitamin D, and antiresorptive therapy to slow bone loss. We also referred her to a physical therapist to begin a program of gentle abdominal and back-strengthening exercises and to learn how to care for her back and avoid future falls. After three months she had occasional low back discomfort late in the day, but was back to her independent state and able to participate in prior activities. A follow-up bone density measurement one year later was similar to the first reading, indicating no further bone loss.

Osteoporosis is a major public health problem because it leads to fractures—with resultant morbidity, loss of independence, chronic suffering, and increased mortality. Osteoporosis affects more than 25 million people in the United States, and predisposes to more than 1.3 million fractures annually—including over 500,000 vertebral, 250,000 hip, and 240,000 wrist fractures (Consensus Development Conference 1993; Riggs and Melton 1986). The lifetime risk of fracture is 40% for white women and 13% for white men from age 50; among those who live to be 90 years old, 33% of women and 17% of men suffer a hip fracture (Melton et al. 1992). Perhaps 90% of all hip and spine fractures among elderly white women are attributed to osteoporosis (Melton et al. 1997). The annual cost of caring for osteoporosis-related fractures in the United States in 1995 was $13.8 billion (Ray et al. 1997). As the elderly population grows, the incidence of fractures will increase. Any means of increasing bone mass, slowing bone loss, and lessening the likelihood of falling will have major long-term health benefits.

Osteoporosis has been defined as a systemic skeletal disease characterized by low bone mass and microarchitectural deterioration of bone tissue, with consequent increase in bone fragility and susceptibility to fracture (Consensus Development Conference 1993). The World Health Organization proposed that an individual with bone mineral density (BMD) or bone mineral content (BMC) more than 2.5 standard deviations below the young adult mean value has osteoporosis (Kanis et al. 1994).

Bone strength and health are related to many factors including genetics, nutrition, hormones, environmental influences, and physical activity. All of these factors are important to

- achieve the maximal amount of bone at the time of skeletal maturity (peak bone mass),
- maintain bone mass in adulthood, and
- slow the rate of bone loss in postmenopausal women.

Physical activity may be especially important, because it is something that most individuals can control. The prevention and treatment of osteoporosis involves nonpharmacologic and pharmacologic approaches. The former includes calcium and vitamin D supplementation, nutrition, lifestyle changes, and exercise. The latter includes hormone replacement, bisphosphonates, calcitonin, and selective estrogen receptor modulators (SERMs). A beneficial program often combines both.

Bone adapts to physical and mechanical loads by altering its mass and strength. Although the physiological mechanisms are unknown, the bones appear to change either as a result of direct impact from the weightbearing activity, or of the action of the muscles attached to bone. High levels of physical activity and loading can increase bone mass, while low levels may lead to less bone. This chapter explores the effects that physical activity and exercise have on the skeleton at various stages of life and in various populations.

Mechanical Properties of Bone: Effects of Exercise

The primary function of the skeleton is to provide structural support; a secondary role, however, is to act as a source of minerals. In serving these functions, bone responds to many factors, including mechanical loading; sufficient force can lead to increased bone density.

In normal individuals, bone architecture (mass, shape, and internal arrangement) is primarily determined by the individual's genetic inheritance and the response to functional load bearing (Lanyon 1996). Lanyon also states that when a load is applied to a structure, it deforms until the intermolecular forces within the structure prevent further deformation. These intermolecular forces are the stresses, which approximately equal the applied load divided by the load-carrying area (stress = force per unit area). The deformation produced by the applied load can be resolved into strains, with each strain defined as the ratio of change in the relevant dimension to the original dimension. Very high repetitive strains can lead to damage and fractures.

Studies in animals have demonstrated that the osteogenic response to dynamic compressive forces is related to the magnitude of the load (Rubin and Lanyon 1985) and the rate of loading (O'Connor et al. 1982).

Although the mechanisms are unclear, it appears that mechanical loads stimulate bone cells (osteoblasts and osteocytes) in the loaded bones to change calcium fluxes to increase production of prostacyclin, prostaglandin E2, nitric oxide, glucose-6-phosphate dehydrogenase (G6PD), and to increase RNA synthesis, with subsequent release of growth factors (American College of Sports Medicine 1995; Lanyon 1996).

Schwarz et al. (1996) reported that brief low- and high-intensity exercise by ten males (mean age 28 years) led to a significant increase in circulating insulin-like growth factors. The response was greater in the high-intensity group.

Disuse, Weightlessness, and Immobilization

The most dramatic example of the effect of physical activity on bone is the rapid, dramatic, and extensive loss of bone seen with any type of immobilization. Krolner and Toft (1983) reported that BMC of the spine decreased 0.9% per week in 34 patients aged 18-60 years who were hospitalized with low back pain due to protrusion of a lumbar intervertebral disk. Reambulation resulted in a gain in BMC, with restoration to nearly normal levels after four months. Goemaere et al. (1994) studied 53 patients with complete traumatic paraplegia of at least one year's duration. Compared to controls, the BMD of paraplegic patients was preserved in the lumbar spine but was markedly decreased in the proximal femur (−33%) and femoral shaft (−25%). In those performing passive weightbearing standing with the aid of a standing device, BMD of the femur was significantly higher than in those not performing these activities. Del Puente and colleagues (1996) found significant bone loss in the femoral neck in the paralyzed limbs of 48 hemiplegic subjects, the degree of bone loss directly correlated with the length of immobilization. Early studies with astronauts during space flight showed a significant increase in urinary calcium excretion and a decrease in BMC at the os calcis (Rambaut and Goode 1985). The mechanism of bone loss and immobilization is not understood. Immobilization can lead to rapid increases in osteoclastic bone resorption, urinary calcium excretion, and bone loss.

Physical Activity and Bone Mass

The effects of physical activity and exercise have been studied in many populations, at various ages, with different exercise regimens (some with confounding variables) and in cross-sectional and longitudinal studies. It is thus very difficult to answer the question, "Does exercise prevent bone loss, promote bone gain, or have any role in bone physiology?" without considering the specific population studied, the age and menopausal status of women included, and the type and intensity of the exercise program.

Athletes

Athletic training programs often include intense mechanical loading of specific bones or skeletal regions. The response to loading differs according to the magnitude of the load, the type of physical activity, and the level of exertion within the activity. Table 17.1, pages 328-336, summarizes many studies of intense exercise training in different athletic groups.

BMD is higher in the dominant playing forearm compared to the nondominant forearm of lifetime tennis players. In 35 active male tennis players aged 70-84 years, Huddleston et al. (1980) found that the bone mass of the radius midshaft ranged from 4%-33% greater in the playing arms compared with the nonplaying arms.

In a study of 51 professional tennis players, Jones and colleagues (1977) reported higher cortical bone density in the humerus of the playing arm. Haapasalo et al. (1996) found similar results in both young and older tennis players. A recent study by this same group (Haapasalo et al. 1998) found BMD also greater in the playing arm of female junior tennis players, with the benefit of unilateral activity becoming evident at the time of the adolescent growth spurt.

Kannus et al. (1995) reported that, in a group of tennis and squash players, BMD was significantly greater in the playing vs. the nonplaying arm compared to controls. The difference was 2-4 times greater in female players who started playing before or at menarche, than in those who started more than 15 years after menarche. Thus, high levels of activity before and during puberty have a larger impact on bone mass than activity started later.

Smith and Rutherford (1993) reported that male rowers have higher BMD of the lumbar spine and whole body compared with triathletes and sedentary controls. Each of the exercise groups devoted similar total hours to exercise each week, but the regimens differed: rowers used weights; the triathletes ran, swam, and cycled. Weightlifting appears to have a major influence on BMD.

Karlsson and coworkers (1993b) reported significantly higher BMD in hip, spine, and total body in weightlifters compared to controls. Similarly Conroy et al. (1993), using DXA to measure BMD in 25 elite junior Olympic weightlifters (mean age 17 years), found significantly greater BMD for the lumbar spine and proximal femur in the athletes compared with their age-matched controls, and also compared with an adult reference range (age 20-39 years). BMD correlated with strength in this study, as it did in a report by Virvidakis et al. (1990), who observed higher BMC of the forearm in junior competitive male weightlifters than in age-matched controls. Hamdy and colleagues (1994) reported higher BMD in weightlifters' upper limbs, but not in axial areas—resulting perhaps from a less intensive weightlifting program, or from less axial loading compared to that of Olympic lifters.

Female weightlifters exhibit a similar response—significantly higher BMD (compared to controls) at the lumbar spine, distal radius, and several lower extremity sites (Heinonen et al. 1993). BMC in young female body builders performing weightlifting resistance exercises was significantly higher than in nonexercising controls or in swimmers or runners who followed nonresistance exercise programs (Heinrich et al. 1990).

Resistance exercise comes in many forms. Slemenda and Johnston (1993) reported that 22 young female competitive skaters (aged 10-23), despite being thinner and having more oligomenorrhea or amenorrhea, had significantly greater skeletal densities compared to nonskaters in the lower part of the skeleton (pelvis and legs) and had similar densities at upper body sites. Karlsson et al. (1993a) measured BMD in 42 professional ballet dancers (17 men and 25 women), 28 of whom were still actively performing. After correcting for differences in body mass index, they found a significantly higher BMD in the lower extremities of female dancers and in the femoral neck of male dancers. In those dancers with a history of more than one year of amenorrhea, however, BMD of the spine was 7% lower than in the menstruating dancers.

Significant bone loss, along with menstrual irregularities and hypogonadism, often accompanies intense training programs or anorexia nervosa (AN) in young women. Young et al. (1994) studied the interrelationships of exercise, hypogonadism, and body weight in 44 female ballet dancers (mean age 17 years), 23 girls of comparable age with regular menstrual cycles (the controls), and 18 sedentary amenorrheic girls with AN. The total bone density in the dancers was similar to the controls and higher than that in girls with AN. At weightbearing sites (proximal femoral), dancers had bone density higher than girls with AN ($p <$ .01), and similar to controls, yet higher values compared to controls after adjustment for body weight. At nonweightbearing sites (ribs, arms, and skull), on the other hand, dancers had BMD similar to the girls with AN and lower than the controls. After correction for age and weight, BMD did not differ from normal at nonweightbearing sites in the dancers, or in the girls with anorexia nervosa. The authors suggest that weightbearing exercise may offset the effects of hypogonadism at predominantly cortical weightbearing sites such as the proximal femur. While nonweightbearing sites and weightbearing sites containing substantial trabecular bone may benefit little from weightbearing exercise, they still benefit significantly by maintenance of body weight (figure 17.1).

BMD in 101 retired elite female ballet dancers (mean age 51 years, mean time since retirement 25.6 years) was lower than that of controls at nonweightbearing sites (ultradistal and mid-third radius) but no different from that of controls at weightbearing sites (hip and spine) in a study by Khan et al. (1996); the latter finding is particularly interesting, since in their youth the dancers had multiple risk factors for osteoporosis—including greater prevalence of menstrual disturbances, greater lifetime alcohol intake, more smoking, and a lower calcium intake in adolescence. The retired dancers currently performed twice as much exercise as the controls. Note, however, that dancers who had experienced significant menstrual disturbance during their dancing years had 8% lower BMD of the lumbar spine, and 10% lower BMD of the ultradistal radius ($p <$ .05), than their eumenorrheic matched controls.

Gymnasts can achieve ground reaction forces as much as 18 times body weight (Taaffe et al. 1995). Robinson and colleagues (1995) studied bone mass and oligomenorrhea and amenorrhea in two groups of competitive female athletes with different skeletal loading patterns. They reported that, despite a similar prevalence of oligo- and amenorrhea, gymnasts had higher BMD than runners at the lumbar spine, proximal femur, and whole body, and higher BMD than controls at the femoral neck. Thus, high-impact exercises to the extent seen in female gymnasts may protect against bone loss associated with menstrual abnormalities.

Many young female athletes fit the "female athlete triad" characterized by disordered eating, menstrual dysfunction, and osteoporosis. Drinkwater and coworkers (1984) observed that young amenorrheic athletes had decreased vertebral (but not radial) BMD compared to that of athletes with regular cycles. A follow-up study (Drinkwater et al. 1986) reported that six of the seven original amenorrheic athletes who resumed menses had a marked increase of vertebral

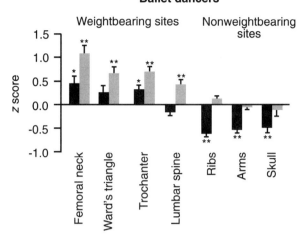

Ballet dancers

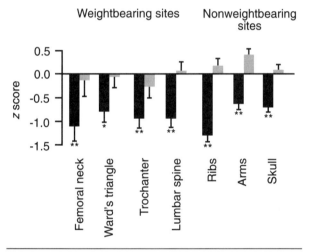

Girls with anorexia nervosa

Figure 17.1 Bone density (mean ± SEM) expressed as a z score adjusted for age alone ■ and for both age and weight ■ in ballet dancers and girls with anorexia nervosa. In dancers, the z scores were normal or increased at weightbearing sites and were reduced at nonweightbearing sites before, but not after, adjustment for body weight. The z scores were negative at all sites in girls with anorexia nervosa before, but not after, adjustment for body weight. * p < .05, ** p < .01 (compared to zero).

Reprinted, by permission, from N. Young et al., 1994, "Bone density at weightbearing and nonweightbearing sites in ballet dancers: the effects of exercise, hypogonadism, and body weight," *Journal of Clinical Endocrinology and Metabolism* 78:449-454, © The Endocrine Society.

BMD in 14.4 months. Fisher et al. (1986) reported that BMC of the lumbar spine was lower in amenorrheic runners, but positively correlated with estradiol levels in all women. Marcus et al. (1985) studied 11 elite women distance runners, mean age 20 years, with secondary amenorrhea. They found BMD of the lumbar spine in this group to be lower than that in similar runners with normal menstrual cycles and in

age-matched nonathlete controls, but higher than in runners with secondary amenorrhea and less physical activity. Thus, although intense exercise may reduce the impact of amenorrhea on bone mass, these runners are still at high risk for exercise-related fractures. In a recent study of 49 female athletes (primarily runners), Rencken and colleagues (1996) compared bone loss at multiple skeletal sites in 49 women runners with either amenorrhea or normal menstrual cycles. Amenorrheic athletes had significantly lower BMD at the lumbar spine and at multiple areas of the proximal femur, the femoral shaft, and tibia—including those sites that were subjected to impact loading during exercise. Myburgh et al. (1993) also reported significantly lower BMD in axial and appendicular sites in amenorrheic runners.

Several researchers have studied different loading exercises and training programs in collegiate female athletes. Fehling and colleagues (1995) compared BMD of collegiate female athletes who competed in impact-loading sports (volleyball and gymnastics) with that of athletes who participated in an active loading sport (swimmers), and also with nonathlete controls. The impact-loading group had significantly greater BMD at the lumbar spine, femoral neck, Ward's triangle, and total body compared to the active loading and control groups. Furthermore, oligomenorrhea and amenorrhea in the gymnastic group did not negatively affect BMD, supporting evidence that high magnitudes of mechanical loading may offset the detrimental effect of hormone deficiency. This is another example of the importance of site specificity in exercise programs. Taaffe et al. (1997) found comparable results. After either 8 or 12 months of training, the gymnasts (high-impact loading) in two separate studies had significant increases in BMD at the lumbar spine and femoral neck, compared to runners, swimmers, and controls. Again, these increases were independent of reproductive hormone status (figure 17.2).

Heinonen et al. (1995) examined 59 Finnish female athletes representing three sports with different skeletal loading (aerobic dancers, squash players, speed skaters). The highest BMD values were in sites receiving the highest impact, supporting the concept that high strain rates and high peak stresses are more effective in enhancing bone formation than low-force repetitions.

Intensive training and exercise programs may also lead to skeletal problems. As noted previously, female athletes who have menstrual abnormalities may have low bone density. Moreover, Myburgh and coworkers (1990) showed that in athletes (mainly runners) with similar training habits, those with stress fractures are

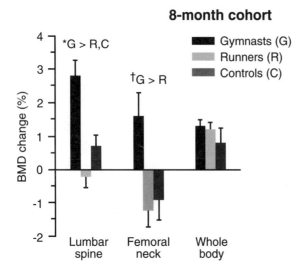

8-month cohort

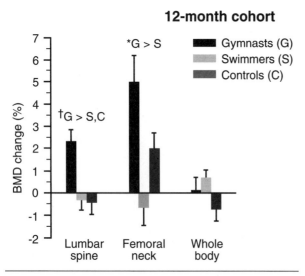

12-month cohort

Figure 17.2 Percent change in lumbar spine, femoral neck, and whole-body BMD for 8-month and 12-month cohorts. *$p < .001$, †$p < .01$. Values are mean ± SEM.
Reprinted, by permission of the American Society for Bone and Mineral Research, from D. Taaffe et al., 1995, "High-impact exercise promotes bone gain in well-trained female athletes," *Journal of Bone and Mineral Research* 12:255-260.

more likely to have lower bone density, lower dietary calcium intake, current menstrual irregularity, and lower contraceptive use.

The impact of intensive exercise and training programs has also been studied in male athletes. Investigating the impact of running on bone mass in 120 healthy physically active men (age 19-56 years) who ran 0-160 km/week, Hetland et al. (1993) found that long distance runners had a lower bone mass at the spine, femur, and forearm, and higher bone turnover, than nonrunning controls. There was no evidence of gonadal failure in this group. In fact, lumbar BMC— which was negatively correlated with the distance run

weekly—was 19% lower in the elite runners than in the healthy, active, but nonrunning controls. While Bilanin et al. (1989) observed a similar phenomenon—in this case, that vertebral BMD was 9.7% lower in 13 male long distance runners than in controls—other data are contradictory: Aloia and colleagues (1978) found no difference in BMC of the radius in marathon runners; Williams et al. (1984) reported that BMC of the os calcis increased during a 9-month marathon training program; and MacDougall et al. (1992) found no BMD differences at multiple sites between male runners (5-75 miles/ week) and controls, although the lower leg bone density was higher in the 15-20 mile/wk group.

A report by Klesges and coworkers (1996) illustrates how complicated this question is. These investigators measured BMC and calcium intake/losses in 11 members of a college Division I-A male basketball team. From preseason to late summer (approximately 11 months), total BMC decreased 6.1% and BMC of the legs decreased 10.5%, with dermal calcium losses of 422 mg per training session. Calcium supplementation was associated with increases in BMC. The authors concluded that bone loss is related to calcium intake, and that exercise is positively related to BMC—but only if calcium intake is sufficient to offset dermal loss. Although this study was very small, its implications are significant, demonstrating the need for more extensive investigation into the changes occurring within intensive training programs.

Childhood and Adolescence

Although osteoporosis is considered a disease of the elderly, predisposition for it begins in childhood and adolescence. It is extremely important to attain the maximal amount of bone at skeletal maturity (peak bone mass), which typically occurs by the end of late adolescence (Bonjour et al. 1991; Matkovic et al. 1994) although slight increases in bone mass may occur after this. The major determinant of peak bone mass is genetic, contributing up to 70%-80% of the variability. Environmental factors, including nutrition and exercise, are important for the remaining 20%-30% (Recker et al. 1992; Slemenda et al. 1991).

In a prospective study of 59 pairs of white monozygotic twins (age 5-14 years), Slemenda and coworkers (1991) investigated the influence of physical activity on BMD in children by using questionnaires filled out separately by the children and their mothers. Total time spent in weightbearing activity was significantly related to BMD in the radius and hip, independently of age or gender. A weaker, yet still positive correlation was present for the lumbar spine. Increases in peak skeletal mass may carry through into adulthood and ultimately lessen the incidence of osteoporotic fractures. A recent cross-sectional study by Bass and colleagues (1998) supports this theory. They measured BMD in 45 active prepubertal female gymnasts (mean age 10 years), 36 retired female gymnasts (mean age 25 years), and controls for each group. BMD in the active prepubertal gymnasts was 0.7-1.9 SD higher at the weightbearing sites than in controls, and increased as the duration of training increased. During 12 months, the increases in BMD of the total body, spine, and legs in the active prepubertal gymnasts was 30%-85% greater than in prepubertal controls. In the retired gymnasts, the BMD was 0.5-1.5 SD higher than in controls at weightbearing sites (figure 17.3). There was no diminution of BMD during the 20 years since retirement (mean 8 years), despite lower frequency and intensity of exercise. Thus, increases in bone density in the prepubertal years may have long-term effects into adulthood.

In 101 women age 20-35 years, McCulloch et al. (1990) reported that the mean bone density of the os calcis was significantly higher for those who participated in any kind of organized sport or fitness programs as children. Following 84 males and 98 females longitudinally from age 13 until age 28, however, Welten et al. (1994) found that only weightbearing activity and body weight contributed significantly to lumbar BMD at age 27. Weightbearing activity was the best predictor of BMD in males, and body weight was the best predictor in females. Greendale and co-workers (1995) investigated the association between BMD and lifetime physical activity in 1,703 adults (mean age 73); she found that, although current and lifetime exercise (including during the teen years) was positively associated with BMD of the hip, it did not protect against fractures.

Cooper et al. (1995) reported that growth and physical activity in childhood were important determinants of peak bone mass in 21-year-old women (n = 153), suggesting that growth may primarily determine the size of the skeletal envelope, while activity modulates the mineral density within the skeletal envelope. Slemenda and colleagues (1994), following 90 children (ages 6-14 years) for three years, also described physical activity as a significant predictor of BMD at all skeletal sites in the prepubertal group. Prepubertal children in the highest activity quartile had 4%-7% greater rates of mineralization than those in the lowest activity group. In contrast, Kroger et al. (1993) observed increases in BMD during adolescence, but no significant relationship between physical activity and the increment rate of bone density. These studies generally underline the importance of physical activity in childhood and adolescence, in achieving the highest peak bone mass.

Young Adult and Premenopausal Women

Although most bone mass accumulates by age 17-18, additional small increases in bone mass may occur in young adults after linear bone growth has stopped. Rodin et al. (1990) reported a 5% increase in spinal bone density in premenopausal women between the age groups 18-22 and 33-37 ($p < .03$).

After following 156 healthy young adult women (age 18-26 years) for up to five years, Recker et al. (1992) observed that the median gain in bone mass for the third decade of life was 4.8% for the forearm, 6.8% for lumbar BMD, and 12.5% for total body bone mineral. The rate of gain in spinal bone density was negatively correlated with age, but positively correlated with levels of physical activity as well as calcium intake. The authors suggest that lifestyle changes among college-aged women—involving relatively modest increases in physical activity and calcium intake—could effect a significant long-term reduction in the later risk of osteoporosis.

There are at present too many confounding factors in published research—heterogeneity of populations, varying levels of exercise (both in intensity

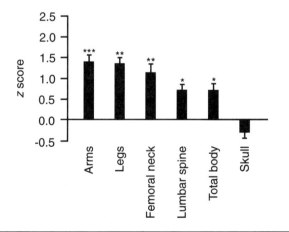

Figure 17.3 Cross-sectional data showing regional areal bone density expressed as a z score in retired female gymnasts. The z scores were higher than the predicted mean value in controls (represented by zero) at each site except the skull. * $p < .05$, ** $p < .01$, *** $p < .001$ compared to zero.
Reproduced from *J Bone Miner Res* 1998; 13:500-507, Figure 4 with permission of the American Society for Bone and Mineral Research.

and loading stresses to specific bones), variability in methods for measuring bone density, and variability in the designs of research projects—to permit an unambiguous claim that physical activity and exercise increase bone mass in young adult women. Despite the difficulties in interpreting these studies, however, several general principles are emerging. In particular: (1) there appears to be a positive correlation between activity level and BMD; and (2) activities that deliver high loads to specific bones appear most beneficial.

The effect of physical activity and exercise may vary with the groups studied. The previous sections discussed the effects of activity and exercise on the growing skeleton in childhood and adolescence. Another group to look at is young adult and premenopausal women.

Cross-Sectional Studies

Perhaps the best way to look at the data is to divide the studies into cross-sectional and interventional (Bouxsein and Marcus 1994; Gutin and Kasper 1992; Marcus et al. 1992; Snow et al. 1996).

As discussed on pages 315-318, unilateral exercise programs have shown that tennis and racquetball players have higher bone mass in their dominant compared with nondominant arms. In addition, elite athletes and long-term exercisers have greater bone mass than nonexercisers, particularly at sites undergoing the greatest mechanical loading. In gymnasts, in fact, high-impact loads at the hip from tumbling and dismounting may override the potential deleterious effects on bone of low gonadal function (Robinson et al. 1995).

Less clear, however, is the effect of less intense recreational sports activities and regular physical activity on bone mass. Aloia et al. (1988) measured physical activity in 24 healthy premenopausal women (mean age 39) using a motion sensor worn at the waist. Total physical activity levels were significantly correlated with BMD of the spine and with total body calcium, but not with BMD of the radius. In 161 healthy Asian women (aged 19-25 years), Hirota and colleagues (1992) found that those with the longest prior history of physical activity had the highest radial BMD. Lifetime physical activity correlated with BMD at the radius for 181 premenopausal women (aged 20-50 years) surveyed by Halioua and Anderson (1989). Davee et al. (1990) studied 27 premenopausal women (aged 20-30 years) with different long-term exercise programs. Those who supplemented aerobic exercise with muscle-building activities for more than one hour per week had higher spine densities than those who were sedentary or who participated in aerobic

exercises only. In addition, IGF-1 (insulin-like growth factor) levels were greatest in that group and correlated with hours of muscle building per week. In 38 premenopausal women (ages 24-28 years), Metz and colleagues (1993) found that 90 minutes of moderate physical activity weekly, correlated positively with radial BMD.

Others have not found similar results. Kirk and colleagues (1989) studied 10 premenopausal female recreational runners who ran more than 20 miles per week for at least two years. The generally higher vertebral bone density in younger runners vs. sedentary controls was not statistically significant, although there was a significant positive correlation between vertebral bone density and physical fitness as assessed by $\dot{V}O_2$max. Jacobson and colleagues (1984) reported that a group of athletic women aged 20-40 years had higher BMD than controls at the radius and lumbar spine. Picard et al. (1988) found no differences in BMC between a low-exercise and high-exercise group of women, aged 40-50 years, who followed their usual exercise pattern. For two years, Mazess and Barden (1991) followed 300 premenopausal women (aged 20-39 years), assessing activity with pedometer and accelerometer measurements over 48-hour periods. They find no relationship between current physical activity and bone density at several sites.

In summary: based on cross-sectional studies, there appears to be no clear-cut relationship between current activity status and bone status in moderately active people.

Intervention Studies

Prospective and (especially) randomized studies provide the clearest way to determine the effects of any intervention.

Nonrandomized Studies

The intensity and specificity of exercises may be most important. In a nonrandomized controlled 12-month study, Gleeson and coworkers (1990) compared 34 premenopausal women (mean age 33) who followed a modified Nautilus weightlifting program lasting 30 minutes three times per week with 34 matched controls. The weightlifting group had a nonsignificant increase in mean lumbar BMD; but when matched to the controls, who showed a small decrease, the difference between the groups was significant ($p < .05$). There was no difference in BMD of the os calcis. A more dramatic effect of weightlifting may not have occurred because (1) in contrast to the young elite weightlifters, these subjects' skeletons had stopped growing; or perhaps (2) the resistance exercises were not sufficiently strenuous. Smith et al. (1989) conducted a four-year nonrandomized aerobic and upper-body strength program in 142 (62 control and 80 exercise) pre- and postmenopausal women (mean age 50 years). Regardless of menopausal status, the exercise group—who participated in 45 minutes of physical activity three days per week—lost significantly less bone than controls in the radius, ulna, and humerus.

In contrast to the previous positive studies, Rockwell et al. (1990) compared 10 premenopausal women (mean age 36 years) in a weightlifting program with seven sedentary women (mean age 40 years). After nine months of weight training aimed at loading the axial skeleton and strengthening large muscle groups, the exercise group had a 4% decrease in lumbar BMD while the control group did not lose bone. No significant change in femoral density occurred in either group.

Randomized Studies

Several researchers have conducted randomized intervention exercise studies in young women.

In an eight-month intervention trial, Snow-Harter and colleagues (1992) randomly assigned 52 healthy college-aged women (mean age 19.9 years) to a control group, to a group that jogged three times weekly, or to a weightlifting group. Lumbar spine BMD showed small but significant increases of 1.2% in the weight training and 1.3% in the jogging groups. Proximal femur BMD did not change in any group. More prolonged loading of the hip may be needed for increases in BMD to occur.

Bassey and Ramsdale (1994) reported that after six months, 14 young women in a high-impact exercise program (mean age 32) had a significant increase of 3.4% in trochanteric BMD compared with 13 women in a low-impact control group (mean age 30). In the second six months, the control group crossed over to the high-impact exercise—and subsequently showed a significant increase of 4.1% in trochanteric BMD. Spinal BMD did not change. Heinonen et al. (1996) studied 98 premenopausal women (mean age 39) in a randomized 18-month trial of a high-impact exercise program. BMD at the femoral neck increased significantly more in the training group compared to controls (p = .006). Lohman et al. (1995) found similar results, wherein lumbar spine and femur trochanter BMD increased significantly for a group of premenopausal women (mean age 34) in a resistance exercise program. In a two-year randomized trial of 63 premenopausal women, Friedlander and coworkers (1995) found that an exercise program combin-

ing aerobics and weight training produced significant positive differences in BMD between the exercise and control groups at the spine, proximal femur, and calcaneus.

Contrary to the above studies, one randomized three-year study in 67 premenopausal women (mean age 36) reported that back extension and shoulder girdle weightlifting had no significant effect on BMD at the spine, hip, or radius (Sinaki et al. 1996).

These studies generally support a positive effect of physical activity on bone in premenopausal women, with high-impact programs having the most benefit. However, making any definitive statement is premature because of the wide differences among exercise programs, skeletal sites tested (e.g., spine, hip, forearm), and populations studied.

Postmenopausal Women

With advancing age after menopause, the most significant clinical consequence of bone loss is the occurrence of fractures. Low bone mass and falling are the two major risk factors for osteoporotic fractures later in life. A primary goal of exercise in postmenopausal women is to slow down and reverse bone loss, if possible, and to improve balance and motor strength in order to lessen the likelihood of falling and sustaining a fracture.

Determining the effects of exercise in postmenopausal women has not been simple. Results are often contradictory and difficult to compare because of many confounding variables including the ages of the subjects, their health and comorbid conditions, and their nutritional status—as well as differences in exercise regimens and methods, and sites of bone mass measurements. Table 17.2, pages 337-343, summarizes many randomized studies on bone mineral density in postmenopausal women.

Cross-Sectional Studies

The data from these studies in postmenopausal women are quite variable. Nelson et al. (1988) studied 18 sedentary and 15 endurance-trained postmenopausal women (mean age 62 years) who had run an average of 22.6 miles per week since menopause. The active women had significantly lower body weight, body fat, and estrone levels than the sedentary group; yet BMD of the spine, proximal femur, and radius did not differ between the two groups. When normalized for body weight, moreover, BMDs of the spine and radius were higher in the endurance-trained group.

Other studies of long-distance runners have also reported higher lumbar spine density. In 41 long-distance runners aged 50-72, Lane et al. (1986) observed that BMD of the lumbar spine was 40% higher than for matched controls. Michel and coworkers (1989) in a cross-sectional study found a strong correlation between lumbar BMD and moderate weightbearing exercise (up to 300 min/wk) in 23 postmenopausal women (mean age 57). Five women who exercised even more than the five hours/week, however, had lower BMD than the other exercisers. In a two-year longitudinal study of 40 female and male subjects over age 50, Michel and colleagues (1991) again found a high positive correlation between changes in exercise and changes in bone density in a moderate exercise group. In a subset of "overexercisers" (>300 minutes/week in females and >200 minutes/week in males) a negative correlation between exercise levels and BMD was found. On the other hand, Kirk et al. (1989) reported no differences in vertebral bone density between controls and nine postmenopausal long-distance runners.

Greendale et al. (1995) evaluated the relationship between use of leisure time, BMD, and osteoporotic fracture in community-dwelling adults (1,014 women and 689 men) with a mean age of 73. The researchers found positive associations between current exercise and BMD at the total hip, greater trochanter, intertrochanter, and femoral neck. Lifetime exercise was similarly associated, demonstrating as well a barely significant association with spinal BMD. These data suggested a protective effect of current and life-long exercise on hip BMD, but not on osteoporotic fracture, in older men and women. In a study of 100 postmenopausal women (age 50-68 years) by Ballard et al. (1990), those in a high-physical activity group had significantly greater BMD of the radial shaft, but not distal radius, than women in the low-activity group.

Clinicians and researchers usually have assessed aerobic fitness by measuring maximal oxygen consumption ($\dot{V}O_2$max). Evaluating 84 normal women, Pocock and coworkers (1986) found that aerobic fitness was the only significant predictor of femoral neck BMD in the 46 who were postmenopausal. Weight and fitness predicted lumbar BMD (figure 17.4).

Chow and colleagues (1986) studied 31 postmenopausal women (ages 50-59 years) and found a significant correlation between physical fitness and bone mass of the trunk and proximal femur; using neutron activation analysis (NAA), they expressed their data as a calcium bone index. Bevier et al. (1989) reported that, in 55 women aged 61-84 years, there was no relationship between aerobic capacity ($\dot{V}O_2$max) and

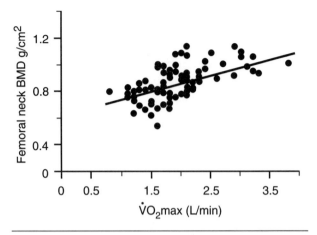

Figure 17.4 Plot of femoral neck BMD against physical fitness ($\dot{V}O_2$max) in 82 normal women. Equation for regression: femoral neck BMD = 0.61 + 0.13 ($\dot{V}O_2$max).
Reproduced from the *Journal of Clinical Investigation*, 1986, 78:618-621 by copyright permission of The American Society for Clinical Investigation.

BMD of the spine or forearm. However, in 36 men aged 63-80 years there was a significant correlation between $\dot{V}O_2$max and BMD of the lumbar spine. In a cross-sectional study of 55 postmenopausal women (mean age 73.5 years), Vico and colleagues (1995) reported that $\dot{V}O_2$max was the strongest predictor of proximal femur BMD, accounting for 10.8%-18.3% of the BMD variability. In addition, at the vertebral level, psoas surfaces constituted the best predictor of lumbar BMD. The anatomic connections between psoas muscles and vertebrae can explain such a relationship. Jacobson et al. (1984) reported significantly higher BMD in the radius in a group of women aged 55-70 years who regularly exercised, as compared to age-matched controls.

In addition to physical fitness, body composition and muscular strength appear positively correlated with BMD. Reid, Plank, and Evans (1992) found that, in premenopausal women, and Reid et al. (1992) found that, in postmenopausal women, total body fat mass was positively correlated to BMD throughout the skeleton. Bevier and colleagues (1989) found a significant correlation between fat mass and lean mass with each other and to spine BMD but not radius BMD in postmenopausal women aged 61-84 years. Grip strength correlated significantly with forearm density and spine density, yet the researchers found no correlation between back strength and lumbar BMD. This contrasts to the report by Sinaki et al. (1986), who found a significant correlation between lumbar spine BMD and back extensor strength in a younger postmenopausal group, aged 49-65 years. In this group, they also reported a positive correlation between lumbar spine BMD and the level of physical activity (Sinaki and Offord 1988). Sinaki et al. (1974) also found a significant correlation between midradius BMC and grip strength.

Snow-Harter and colleagues (1990) found muscle strength to be an independent predictor of BMD in 59 women aged 18-31 years; they theorized that muscle groups with attachments distant from the spine and hip may strongly affect BMD at these sites. In a group of 181 men and women aged 45-77 years, Hughes et al. (1995) observed significant associations between elbow extensor strength and radial BMD in both men and women; and between knee flexor muscle strength and lumbar BMD in women. Madsen et al. (1993) reported highly significant correlations between quadriceps strength and BMD of the proximal tibia in 66 healthy women, aged 21-78 years, including 24 women aged 60-78 years.

Interventional Studies

The best way to avoid the biases in cross-sectional studies is to use a prospective randomized intervention trial. This avoids the possibility that people predisposed to a type of exercise will self-select for participation in that exercise.

Nonrandomized Studies

In a group of nine postmenopausal women (mean age 53) who followed an exercise program using the guidelines of the President's Council on Physical Fitness three times a week for one year, Aloia et al. (1978) found an increase in total body calcium compared to a decrease in the control group. Cavanaugh and Cann (1988) reported that a moderately brisk walking program of one year's duration by 17 postmenopausal women (ages 49-64 years) did not prevent the loss of spinal bone density. Nelson and colleagues (1991) studied the effect of a one-year supervised walking program and increased calcium intake in 36 postmenopausal women (mean age 60 years). Subjects wore leaded belts (3.1 kg) around their waists and walked for 50 minutes four times a week. Trabecular BMD of the lumbar spine, as measured by computed tomography, increased 0.5% in the exercising women and decreased 7.0% in sedentary women. There was no significant change in femoral neck or radius BMD. The lack of response at some sites in these studies may be due to inadequate mechanical forces being applied.

In a study by Krolner and colleagues (1983), 16 postmenopausal women (mean age 61) participated for eight months (one hour twice weekly) in a moderate program of walking, running, and sitting/standing exercises. Lumbar spine BMC increased 3.5% in the training group and declined 2.7% in the controls ($p < .005$ between groups). There was no difference between the groups in forearm BMC. Dalsky et al. (1988) studied 35 postmenopausal women, aged 55-70 years, 17 of whom were in a weightbearing exercise training program consisting primarily of walking, jogging, and stair climbing. BMC of the lumbar spine significantly increased 5.2% in the exercise group after 9 months and 6.1% after 22 months. In those who stopped exercising, lumbar BMC fell to baseline, suggesting that exercise must be maintained to retain its benefit. Pruitt et al. (1992) studied 17 postmenopausal women (mean age 54) in a weight-training program using Universal Gym equipment, free weights, and ankle weights, three days per week for nine months. Lumbar BMD increased 1.6% and was significantly different from that of the control group, who lost 3.6%. There were no differences at the femoral neck or distal wrist.

A nine-month strength-training program prevented the loss of calcaneal bone in older women (mean age 72) in a study by Rundgren and colleagues (1984). Ayalon et al. (1987) studied 14 osteoporotic women (mean age 63) in a five-month program that specifically loaded the distal forearm. During the year prior to the study, BMD of the distal forearm significantly decreased in both the exercise and control group; but during the exercise period, it increased in the exercise group (+3.8%) while significantly decreasing in the control group (−1.9%). In 54 women (aged 36-67 years), Peterson and coworkers (1991) compared the effects of an endurance dance program, a program that combined endurance dance and resistance weight training, and a control sedentary program. Although muscle strength increased with weight training, there were no significant changes in BMD of the lumbar spine, hip region, or appendicular skeleton with either training program.

Kohrt and colleagues (1997) assigned 39 older, sedentary women (ages 60-74 years) to one of three groups:

- Exercises providing stress to the skeleton through ground-reaction forces (GRF)—i.e., walking, jogging, stair climbing
- Exercises through joint-reaction forces (JRF)—i.e., weight lifting, rowing
- Sedentary control group

Both the GRF and JRF exercise programs resulted in significant and similar increases in BMD of the whole body, lumbar spine, and Ward's triangle region of the proximal femur. The GRF program also produced a

3.5% increase in BMD of the femoral neck ($p < .01$). Although the JRF program did not increase BMD of the femoral neck, it increased lean body mass ($p < .01$) and strength ($p < .01$) and thus may still be important in reducing the risk for falls.

Randomized Studies

Chow and coworkers (1987) used NAA to measure bone mass in 48 postmenopausal women (ages 50-62 years), randomly assigning subjects to an aerobic exercise program, to a program of aerobic exercise plus strength training, or to a control group. At the end of one year the exercise groups did not differ significantly from each other, but both had greater bone mass than controls ($p < .05$).

Grove and Londeree (1992) randomly assigned 15 early postmenopausal women (ages 49-65 years) to a control group, a low-impact exercise group, or a high-impact group. Each exercise group had 20 minutes of supervised exercise three times a week. After one year, the control group had a significant decrease in lumbar BMD (−6.08%). Both exercise groups maintained BMD, and this was significantly different from the controls. Hatori and colleagues (1993) reported a significantly higher lumbar spine BMD in a high-intensity exercise group relative to control subjects after a seven-month program, while those in a moderate-intensity group did not differ significantly from controls. The high-intensity group walked three times per week for seven months with heart rates at about 110% of anaerobic threshold. Martin and Notelovitz (1993) reported that in 18 postmenopausal women within six years after the onset of menopause, those assigned to treadmill walking for one year had reduced spinal BMD loss compared with non-exercising similar women ($p < .05$).

In a study of 39 postmenopausal women (ages 50-70 years), Nelson and coworkers (1994) randomly assigned 20 women to a high-intensity strength-training program of workouts two days per week for one year, using five different exercises. The other 19 women were sedentary controls. Muscle mass, muscle strength, and dynamic balance significantly increased in the strength-trained women and decreased in the controls. Femoral neck BMD and lumbar spine BMD increased by 0.9% and 1.0%, respectively, in the strength-trained women, and decreased by 2.5% and 1.8%, respectively, in the controls ($p = .02$ and .04). Not only did the exercise program strengthen bone, but by improving muscle function and balance it probably lessened the likelihood of falling and sustaining a fracture as well (figure 17.5).

Notelovitz and colleagues (1991) randomly assigned 20 surgically menopausal women to receive

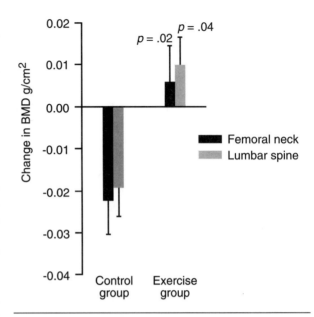

Figure 17.5 Changes in bone after the interventions (either no exercise, or high-intensity strength training). The values are means ± SE for individual changes in bone adjusted for age, smoking, and baseline bone mineral density, using analysis of covariance. BMD = bone mineral density.
Reprinted, by permission, from M.E. Nelson et al., 1994, "Effects of high-intensity strength training on multiple risk factors for osteoporotic fractures: a randomized controlled trial," *JAMA* 272:1909-1914. Copyrighted 1994, American Medical Association.

either estrogen (mean age 46 years) or estrogen plus a variable-resistance weight-training program involving Nautilus muscle strengthening/endurance equipment (mean age 43 years). After one year, lumbar spine BMD increased 8.3% in the exercise group, total body BMD increased 2.1%, and midshaft radial BMD increased 4.1%, compared to nonsignificant changes in the nonexercising group. Thus, variable-resistance training in estrogen-replete women added bone to both the axial and appendicular skeleton. Perhaps the difference between the beneficial results from resistance training in this study compared to other studies is that the patients in the Notelovitz study were younger and able to train at an intensity needed to maximally stress the muscle.

In a study of 120 postmenopausal women (mean age 56) who had low forearm bone density, Prince and colleagues (1991) randomly assigned them to an exercise program, to exercise plus calcium (1 gram daily), or exercise plus estrogen. Exercise alone did not prevent bone loss at the forearm. When combined with calcium, exercise slowed bone loss; but when combined with estrogen, exercise significantly increased BMD (figure 17.6).

Pruitt et al. (1995) compared the effects of 12-month high-intensity and low-intensity resistance training programs in 26 older postmenopausal

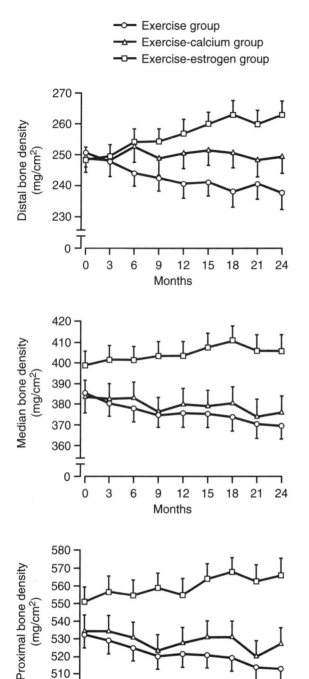

- ─○─ Exercise group
- ─△─ Exercise-calcium group
- ─□─ Exercise-estrogen group

Figure 17.6   Effects of three interventions on bone density at distal, median, and proximal forearm sites during a two-year study period. Values are means ± SE for all women remaining in each group at the time indicated. After two years there were 35 women remaining in the exercise group, 36 in the exercise-calcium group, and 32 in the exercise-estrogen group.

women aged 65-79 years. Despite an effective muscle strengthening program, resistance training did not produce significant changes in spine or proximal femur BMD in either the high- or low-intensity groups. The women in this study possessed good BMD on entrance, and the majority had taken hormone replacement therapy for at least one year prior to participation. The authors suggest that the resistance training in this study may not have differed sufficiently from activities (particularly of the lower limb) normally carried out by older, active women, thus being insufficient to produce increases in bone density. Yet such training may still confer benefits by improving strength and possibly balance, lessening the likelihood of falling or sustaining fractures.

Revel and coworkers (1993) evaluated 78 postmenopausal women—half in a psoas muscle training program, half in a deltoid training program (the control group). The psoas muscle attaches to the lumbar vertebrae. Losses in lumbar spine BMD were comparable in both groups after one year. However, in the subgroup of women who performed the psoas exercises assiduously for one year, there was a significantly smaller loss than in the controls. Sandler and colleagues (1987) studied 229 postmenopausal women—half were sedentary controls, and half walked more than seven miles a week for three years. Bone loss in the radius was similar in both groups, but changes in the cross-sectional area of the radius were significantly greater in the walkers with high grip strength than in controls with comparable high grip strength. The significance of this finding is not clear, but may indicate that some local muscular loading was involved. Sinaki et al. (1989) studied the effect of back-strengthening exercises on spinal BMD in 34 postmenopausal women, mean age 56. Despite an increase in back extensor muscle strength in the exercise group, there was no difference in the rate of bone loss between the exercise and control group. Perhaps the load generated on the back extensors was insufficient to adequately load the skeleton. Finally, Smidt et al. (1992) investigated the effect of a progressive resistance training program for trunk muscles in 22 early postmenopausal women (mean age 57). They found no significant differences in BMD between the exercise and control groups at the lumbar spine and proximal femur at the end of one year.

In summary, these prospective studies offer modest but variable evidence that increased activity—either through dynamic exercises or high-intensity weight training—may improve bone mass, muscle strength, and/or balance, possibly translating into fewer falls and fractures. The data are often contradictory, and we need to learn much more about specific exercises (both in type and intensity) in specific populations. Kelley (1998) recently used meta-analysis to examine the effects of exercise on regional BMD in postmenopausal women, analyzing 11 randomized trials yielding 40 outcome measures in a total of 719 subjects (370 exercise, 349 nonexercise). Kelley concluded that exercise may slow the rate of bone loss in postmenopausal women, but that it is premature to form strong conclusions regarding the effects of exercise on regional BMD. We need additional, well-designed studies.

Physical Activity, Fall Prevention, and Fractures

In 1990, there were an estimated 1.7 million hip fractures worldwide, most resulting from falls (Melton 1993). In a community of 336 elderly persons at least 75 years of age in New Haven, Connecticut, 32% fell during one year, 24% had serious injuries, and 6% had fractures (Tinetti et al. 1988). One out of every six white women in the United States will have a hip fracture during her lifetime (Cummings et al. 1989); among Americans aged 65 years or older, falls are the leading cause of death from injury (Sattin 1992). The incidence of hip fracture increases exponentially after age 65, and the rate of hip fracture among white women is twice that of white men (Sattin 1992). Those who survive often suffer long-term disability.

Low bone density is a major risk factor for hip fracture during a fall. Important risk factors for falling include lower- and upper-extremity weakness, low physical activity, gait abnormalities, poor balance, poor transfer skills, visual impairment, sedatives and other prescription medications, cognitive impairment, neurologic disorders, anxiety, and depression (Cummings et al. 1995; Greenspan et al. 1994; Grisso et al. 1991; Johnell et al. 1995; Rubenstein et al. 1994; Sudarsky 1990; Tinetti et al. 1988).

Changes in any of these risk factors may have important long-term clinical implications. The most significant benefit of exercise may be to modify some of these factors, improve neuromuscular function, and reduce the likelihood of falling. Johnell et al. (1995) felt that 50% of hip fractures result from potentially reversible risk factors. For older individuals, Greenspan et al. (1994) emphasized that the characteristics of falls—including the direction—are at least

as important as BMD in determining hip fracture risk. They suggest that reducing the odds of falling directly on a hip, or enhancing the hip's ability to withstand such an impact, could decrease the severity of falls and the risks of fractures. Interventions for these purposes include exercises to improve quadriceps strength, neuromuscular function, and gait.

Province and coworkers (1995) did a meta-analysis of the seven FICSIT studies (Frailty and Injuries: Cooperative Studies of Intervention Techniques). These are independent, randomized, controlled clinical trials assessing intervention efficacy in reducing falls and frailty in elderly patients. All included an exercise component for 10-36 weeks, with follow-ups for falls and injuries continuing for the two to four years of the study. A total of 2,328 subjects participated, including residents of two nursing homes and five community-dwelling sites. Although the minimum ages differed at the study sites, the youngest was 60 years. Female participation in the seven centers ranged from 42% to 81%. While the exercise component varied across the studies, all subjects trained in one or more areas of endurance, flexibility, balance platform, tai chi (dynamic balance), and resistance. Those subjects assigned to the interventions that included exercise or balance training had significantly fewer falls. Thus, exercise by elderly adults can reduce the risk of falls.

Fiatarone et al. (1994) conducted a randomized placebo-controlled trial comparing progressive resistance exercise training, multinutrient supplementation, both interventions, and neither in 100 frail nursing home residents (mean age 87.1 years) over a 10-month period. In the subjects who underwent exercise training, muscle strength increased by 113%, gait velocity by 11.8%, stair-climbing power by 28.4%, and thigh muscle areas by 2.7%. Levels of spontaneous activity also increased. Nutritional supplement had no effect on any primary outcome measure. Thus, even in a frail elderly population, high-intensity exercise training is a feasible and effective way to counter muscle weakness and physical frailty.

Using a multiple risk factor intervention that included an exercise program in 301 subjects over age 70, Tinetti et al. (1994) found a significant reduction in the risk of falling. In a one-year randomized controlled trial, Lord and coworkers (1996) studied 179 postmenopausal women (ages 60-85 years) who engaged in twice-weekly structured general aerobic exercise. The exercise group showed significant improvements in quadriceps strength and postural sway, but not BMD, when compared with the control group. Indices of fracture risk also decreased significantly in the exercise group, despite lack of improvement in BMD, implying that it is possible to lower fracture risk without improving bone density.

Elderly subjects appear to tolerate exercise well (even mild high-impact programs) when the activity is appropriate—particularly when health professionals take into consideration the participants' other medical conditions, and properly supervise the programs. Thus, lifestyle changes and exercise should significantly reduce falls and fractures.

Summary

The studies described in this chapter show that an exercise program can be established for nearly anyone, and that such programs may be helpful in building and maintaining bone mass, strengthening muscle, improving balance, and preventing falls and fractures. It is not yet clear precisely how to individually tailor exercise programs according to specific individuals' needs, or how long such programs should last. Yet it is important to individualize exercise programs—which should begin (when appropriate) only after medical clearance and under the supervision of a physician and a physical therapist.

Although there is much that we need to learn about the effect of exercise on bone health and os-teoporosis, at this time we can make several general statements:

1. Many studies support the beneficial effects of exercise.
2. Bone adapts to alterations in mechanical loading.
3. The skeleton responds in a site-specific manner to mechanical loading.
4. If the load is high enough, bone will respond.
5. To see an increase in BMD in specific areas, it is important to load the specific bones.
6. Physical activity may increase peak bone mass in childhood and adolescence, maintain bone mass in young adulthood, and slow bone loss in older subjects.
7. Young bones respond more favorably to mechanical loading than older bones.
8. Exercise may improve balance, strength, mobility, and gait, and lessen the likelihood of falling and sustaining a fracture.
9. Older postmenopausal women and even the frail elderly can tolerate appropriately designed strength training and resistance exercise programs, potentially improving both muscle strength and BMD.

Acknowledgments

I wish to thank Christine Carr for her typing of this manuscript.

Table 17.1   Effects of Intense Training Programs on Bone Mineral Density in Athletes

Author	Type of exercise program	Sex	Age mean (years)	Number of subjects	Bone measurement	Results
Jones et al. (1977)	Tennis (professional)	M	27	48	X rays of humerus	Cortical thickness on playing arm was greater by 35% in men and 28% in women compared with control site.
		F	24	30		
Huddleston (1980)	Tennis (lifetime)	M	70-84 (range)	35	BMC of forearm by SPA	Mean BMC 13% higher in playing than nonplaying arm.
Haapasalo et al. (1996)	Tennis (competitive)	M	25	17	BMD of humerus by DXA	Young men and women: significantly greater values in BMD, BMC, and cortical wall thickness in playing vs. nonplaying arm in tennis players and compared to controls.
		F	19	30		
		F	43	20		
	Control	M	25	16		Older women: significant difference but smaller than young.
		F	21	25		
		F	39	16		
Haapasalo et al. (1998)	Tennis	F	9.4-15.5 (different Tanner Stage)	91	BMD of lumbar spine, humerus, and radius by DXA	Tennis players: 1. In tennis players BMD difference were significantly greater in the playing vs. nonplaying arm at all Tanner Stages (mean difference 1.6-15.7%).
	Control	F	9.4-15.4 (different Tanner Stage)	58		2. In controls: mean difference −0.2 to 4.6% but significant at some humerus sites. 3. Players vs. control: difference (arms) significant at growth spurt (Tanner Stage III). Difference in lumbar spine significant at Tanner Stage IV. 4. Nonloaded, nondominant distal radius: no difference between players and controls at any Tanner Stage.

BMC = bone mineral content; BMD = bone mineral density; CT = computerized tomography; DPA = dual photon absorptiometry; DXA = dual X-ray absorptiometry; SPA = single photon absorptiometry

Table 17.1   (continued)

Author	Type of exercise program	Sex	Age mean (years)	Number of subjects	Bone measurement	Results
Kannus et al. (1995)	Tennis and squash	F	28	105	BMC of radius, humerus, and calcaneus	Compared to controls, the players had significantly larger side-to-side differences at all measured sites.
	Controls	F	27	50		
Heinonen et al. (1993)	Weightlifters	F	25	18	BMD of lumbar spine, femur, patella, tibia, calcaneus, distal radius by DXA	Weightlifters had significantly higher BMD than controls at all sites except femoral neck and calcaneus.
	Orienteers	F	23	30		
	Cross-country skiers	F	21	28		
	Cyclists	F	24	29		Orienteers had higher BMD than controls at distal femur and proximal tibia.
	Controls	F	23	25		
						Compared with other athlete groups, the weightlifters had higher BMD in lumbar spine, distal femur, patella, and distal radius.
Heinrich et al. (1990)	Swimmers	F	22	13	BMC of lumbar spine and femur by DPA; forearm by SPA	BMC of body builders significantly greater than swimmers, collegiate and recreational runners and controls.
	Collegiate runners	F	20	5		
	Recreational runners	F	30	11		
	Body builders (weightlifting)	F	26	11		
	Controls	F	25	18		
Nilsson and Westlin (1971)	Athletes: Weightlifters	M	21	11	BMD in distal end of femur by photon-absorption method	Athletes had significantly denser femurs than non-athletes.
	Throwers	M	24	4		BMD decreased with decreasing load. No difference between swimmers and controls.
	Runners	M	22	25		
	Soccer players	M	25	15		
	Swimmers	M	18	9		
	Controls: Exercising	M	23	24		In controls, exercise group had significantly higher BMD than nonexercisers.
	Nonexercising	M	23	15		
Gleeson et al. (1990)	Weightlifting (modified Nautilus weightlifting program)	F	33	34	BMD of lumbar spine by DPA; and os calcis by SPA	BMD lumbar spine: weightlifters +0.8% controls −0.5% $p < .05$
	Controls	F	33	38		No difference in os calcis.

(continued)

329

Table 17.1   (continued)

Author	Type of exercise program	Sex	Age mean (years)	Number of subjects	Bone measurement	Results
Slemenda and Johnston (1993)	Figure skaters	F	18	22	Total body bone mineral by DXA	Skaters had significantly higher BMD in legs and pelvis.
	Controls	F	16	22		BMD similar at upper-body sites.
Karlsson et al. (1993a)	Professional ballet dancers	M	40	17	Total body and regional BMD by DXA, and BMD of forearm by SPA	Male dancers had higher BMD in femoral neck ($p < .05$).
		F	36	25		
	Controls	M	age and sex matched to dancers	17		Female dancers had higher BMD in all hip measurements and in the legs ($p < .05$).
		F		25		
Young et al. (1994)	Ballet dancers	F	17	44	Total body and regional BMD by DXA	Total body BMD and proximal femur sites in dancers similar to girls with regular menses and higher than girls with anorexia nervosa ($p < .05$).
	Controls:					
	Regular menses	F	17	23		
	Amenorrhea/ anorexia nervosa	F	18	18		Lumbar spine and non-weightbearing sites: BMD in dancers similar to anorexia nervosa.
						When corrected for weight, BMD at weightbearing sites was higher in the dancers than girls with normal menses ($p < .01$).
Conroy et al. (1993)	Elite junior Olympic weightlifters	M	17	25	BMD of lumbar spine and proximal femur by DXA	BMD significantly higher in weightlifters at all sites compared to age-matched controls and adult reference range.
	Controls (no weightlifting)	M	17	11		
Virvidakis et al. (1990)	Junior competitive weightlifters	M	15-20 (range)	59	BMC of forearm by SPA	BMC of distal and proximal forearm significantly greater in weightlifters.

(continued)

Table 17.1   (continued)

Author	Type of exercise program	Sex	Age mean (years)	Number of subjects	Bone measurement	Results
Virvidakis (cont.)	Controls (normal physical activity)	M	age-matched	91		
Hamdy et al. (1994)	Weightlifting	M	27	11	BMC and BMD of lumbar spine and proximal femur by DPA	Upper limb BMD significantly greater in weightlifters compared to runners and recreational exercisers: similar to cross-trained athletes. No differences in spine or proximal femur.
	Running/ jogging	M	29	12		
	Cross-training (weightlifting and aerobic exercise)	M	31	8		
	Recreational exercise	M	28	9		
Smith and Rutherford (1993)	Rowing	M	21	12	BMD of lumbar spine and total body by DXA	Rowers: higher BMD of spine ($p < .01$) and total body ($p < .05$) compared to triathletes and controls.
	Triathletes	M	29	8		No difference in spine and total body BMD between triathletes and controls.
	Sedentary controls	M	22	13		Rowers: higher BMD of arms compared to controls ($p < .01$) but not triathletes.
Khan et al. (1996)	Ballet dancers (retired)	F	51	101	BMD of lumbar spine, wrist, proximal femur, and total body by DXA	Dancers vs. controls: no difference in BMD at spine or hip.
	Controls	F	52	101		Lower BMD at ultra-distal and mid-third radius in dancers ($p < .05$).
						No difference in the proportion of dancers and controls with osteopenia or osteoporosis (World Health Organization criteria).

(continued)

Table 17.1   *(continued)*

Author	Type of exercise program	Sex	Age mean (years)	Number of subjects	Bone measurement	Results
Robinson et al. (1995)	Gymnasts	F	20	21	BMD of lumbar spine, femoral neck, total body by DXA	Oligo- and amenorrhea: gymnasts 47% runners 30% controls 0%
	Runners	F	22	20		BMD lumbar spine: gymnasts > runners ($p = .0001$) controls > runners ($p < .01$)
	Controls (exercise <3 hr/wk)	F	19	19		BMD femoral neck: gymnasts > runners > controls ($p = .0001$) controls > runners ($p < .01$)
						BMD total body: gymnasts > runners ($p = .0001$)
						Bone mineral apparent density (adjusted for body size).
						Lumbar spine: gymnasts > controls and runners ($p = .0001$) controls > runners ($p < .01$)
						Femoral neck: gymnasts > controls and runners ($p = .0001$)
Drinkwater et al. (1984)	Athletes: runners and crew (amenorrheic)	F	25	14	BMD of lumbar spine by DPA; and radius by SPA	BMD of lumbar spine lower in amenorrheic athletes ($p < .01$). No difference in 2 radius sites.
	Athletes: runners and crew (eumenorrheic)	F	26	14		
Drinkwater et al. (1986)	Athletes: runners and crew (amenorrheic who regained menses)	F	28	7	BMD of lumbar spine by DPA; and radius by SPA	Regained menses group had an increase in BMD of spine of 6.2% ($p < .01$). Eumenorrheic group: no change.
	Athletes: runners and crew (eumenorrheic)	F	28	7		Amenorrheic group (n = 2) lost bone (−3.4%). No significant difference in radius.

(continued)

Table 17.1   (continued)

Author	Type of exercise program	Sex	Age mean (years)	Number of subjects	Bone measurement	Results
Drinkwater et al. (1986) (cont.)	Athletes: runners and crew (amenor-rheic)	F	±28	2		
Fisher et al. (1986)	Runners: amenorrheic	F	25	11	BMC of lumbar spine by DPA; and radius by SPA	BMD of spine: eumenorrheic > amenor-rheic ($p = .02$).
	eumenorrheic	F	30	24		BMD of radius: no differ-ence.
Marcus et al. (1985)	Elite distance runners: cyclic menses	F	24	6	BMD of lumbar spine by CT; and radius by SPA	BMD of spine: cyclic > amenorrhea ($p < .02$) controls > amenorrhea ($p < .05$)
	amenorrhea	F	20	11		
	Controls (non-athletes)	F	similar to above			BMD of forearm: no dif-ference.
Rencken et al. (1996)	Runners: amenorrheic	F	26	29	BMD of lumbar spine, proximal and shaft of fe-mur, tibia, and fibula by DXA	BMD was lower in amen-orrheic group at the lum-bar spine, proximal femur sites, femoral shaft, and tibia ($p < .01$).
	eumenorrheic	F	26	20		No difference at fibula.
Myburgh et al. (1993)	Runners: amenorrheic	F	29	12	BMD of lumbar spine, proximal fe-mur, total body by DXA; and radius by SPA	BMD was lower in the amenorrheic group at the lumbar spine, whole body, proximal femur sites, fe-moral shaft ($p < .05$ – $p < .005$).
	eumenorrheic	F	28	9		No difference at mid-radius and tibial shaft.
Fehling et al. (1995)	High impact: volleyball	F	20	8	BMD of lumbar spine, proximal fe-mur, and total body by DXA	Impact group (volleyball and gymnasts) had greater BMD at lumbar spine, fe-moral neck. Ward's triangle, total body, legs, pelvis com-pared to active loading (swimming) and controls ($p < .05$).
	gymnasts	F	20	13		
	Active loading: swimmers	F	20	7		
	Controls (exer-cise <1 hr/wk)	F	21	17		Gymnasts had greater BMD compared to all groups at right and left arm sites.

(continued)

Table 17.1   (continued)

Author	Type of exercise program	Sex	Age mean (years)	Number of subjects	Bone measurement	Results
Fehling et al. (1995) *(cont.)*						No difference at any site between swimmers and controls.
Taaffe et al. (1997)	Cohort I (8 months)				BMD of lumbar spine, femoral neck, and total body by DXA	Gymnasts from both cohorts had significant increases in BMD of the lumbar spine and femoral neck.
	gymnasts	F	20	26		
	runners	F	21	36		
	controls (exercise <3 hr/wk)	F	20	14		Gymnasts from both cohorts had significantly greater increases in BMD than the other athletes or controls at the spine ($p <$ .01); and compared to the other athletes at the femoral neck ($p <$ .05).
	Cohort II (12 months)					
	gymnasts	F	19	8		
	swimmers	F	20	11		
	controls (exercise <3 hr/wk)	F	19	11		No difference among groups for change in whole body BMD.
Heinonen et al. (1995)	Aerobic dancers	F	28	27	BMD lumbar spine, femur, patella, calcaneus, distal radius by DXA	Squash players had highest weight-adjusted BMD at all sites.
	Squash players	F	25	18		Compared with sedentary controls:
	Speed skates	F	21	14		• squash players had significantly higher BMD at lumbar spine (13.8%), femoral neck (16.8%), proximal tibia (12.6%), calcaneus (18.5%).
	Controls (physically active)	F	23	25		
	Controls (sedentary)	F	24	25		• aerobic dancers had significantly higher BMD at femoral neck (8.5%), proximal tibia (5.5%), calcaneus (13.6%), but significantly lower BMD in distal radius (−7.8%).
						• speed skaters had significantly higher BMD at distal femur (7.2%).
						• no difference between physically active and sedentary controls in BMD at any site.

(continued)

Table 17.1 (continued)

Author	Type of exercise program	Sex	Age mean (years)	Number of subjects	Bone measurement	Results
Hetland et al. (1993)	Long-distance runners (>100 km/wk)	M	32	22	BMC and BMD of lumbar spine, proximal femur, total body by DXA; and forearm by SPA	Long-distance runners had a significantly lower BMC in the lumbar spine, proximal femur, distal forearm, and total body than nonrunners.
	Controls (≤ 5 km/wk)	M	31	12		BMC of lumbar spine correlated negatively with weekly distance runners ($p < .0001$) and 19% lower than nonrunners.
	All subjects (0-160 km/wk)	M	32	120		A similar relationship at other sites except femoral neck.
MacDougall et al. (1992)	Runners: 5-10 mi/wk	M	28	5	BMD of whole body and regions by DPA	BMD in lower legs was significantly higher ($p < .05$) in the 15-20 mi/wk group than in 5-10 mi/wk group or control.
	15-20 mi/wk	M	29	11		
	25-30 mi/wk	M	28	12		
	40-55 mi/wk	M	30	9		Cross-sectional area of tibia and fibula normalized to body weight tended to be larger with increasing mileage; 40-50 mi/wk significantly greater than control.
	60-75 mi/wk	M	36	16		
	Controls (non-active)	M	33	22		No other differences in BMD.
Bilanin et al. (1989)	Long-distance runners (>64 km/wk)	M	29	13	BMD of lumbar spine and mid-tibia by DPA; and mid-radius by SPA	BMD of spine significantly lower in runners than nonrunners ($p < .05$).
	Controls (non-runners)	M	27	11		No difference between groups in tibia or radial BMD.
Aloia et al. (1978)	Marathon runners	M	42	30	BMC of radius by SPA	No difference between groups.
	Controls	M	45	16		
Williams et al. (1984)	Long-distance runners (9 month study):				BMC of os calcis by SPA	"Consistent" runners but not "inconsistent" runners showed significant increase in BMC over controls
	Consistent runners (mean 141 km/month)	M	48	7		

(continued)

Table 17.1   *(continued)*

Author	Type of exercise program	Sex	Age mean (years)	Number of subjects	Bone measurement	Results
Williams et. al (1984) *(cont.)*	Inconsistent runners (mean 65 km/month)	M	50	13		
	Controls (non-runners)	M	47	10		
Klesges et al. (1986)	Basketball	M	20	11	BMC of total body and regions by DXA	From preseason to late summer, overall decrease of 6.1% in total BMC and 10.5% decrease in BMC of the legs.

Table 17.2   Effects of Exercise on Bone Mineral Density in Postmenopausal Women in Randomized Studies

Author	Type of exercise program	Duration of study (months)	Age (years)	Number of subjects	Bone measurement	Results
Bassey and Ramsdale (1995)	High-impact exercise: 50 heel drops daily	12	54	20	BMD of lumbar spine, proximal femur, and radius by DXA	No significant increases in BMD at any site in either group.
	Control: flexibility and low-impact exercise		55	24		BMD at ultradistal radius site decreased in exercise group ($p < .001$).
Chow et al. (1987)	Aerobic exercise: 30 minutes of walking, jogging, dance 3 d/wk	12	57	17	Calcium bone index by neutron activation analysis	Bone mass significantly higher in both exercise groups compared to controls.
	Aerobics/strength training. Additional 10-15 minutes low-intensity strength training (free weights attached to wrists and ankles: 10 repetitions for each muscle group at 10 repetitions maximum 3 d/wk)		56	16		No difference between the exercise groups.
	Control (maintain current activity level)		56	15		
Grove and Londeree (1992)	High-impact group: supervised exercise ≥ 2 times their body weight, 20 min, 3 d/wk	12	57	5	BMD of lumbar spine by DPA	Control: -6.08% ($p = .002$). Both exercise groups: no change over time but both significantly different from conrol ($p < .05$).
	Low-impact group: supervised exercise ≤ 1.5 times their body weight, 20 min, 3 d/wk		54	5		No difference between low- and high-impact group

BMC = bone mineral content; BMD = bone mineral density; CT = computerized tomography; DPA = dual photon absorptiometry; DXA = dual energy X-ray absorptiometry; RM = repetition maximum; SPA = single photon absorptiometry

Table 17.2 (continued)

Author	Type of exercise program	Duration of study (months)	Age (years)	Number of subjects	Bone measurement	Results
Grove and Londeree (1992) (cont.)	Control (non-exercise)		56	5		
Hatori et al. (1993)	High-intensity: work intensity above anaerobic threshold (110% heart rate) walking 3 d/wk	7	56	12	BMD of lumbar spine by DXA	Control: decrease of 1.7%; high-intensity: increase of 1.1%; moderate-intensity: decrease of 1.0%
	Moderate-intensity: work intensity below anaerobic threshold (90% heart rate) walking 3 d/wk		58	9		High-intensity versus control: significant difference ($p < .05$); moderate-intensity versus control: no significant difference
	Control		58	12		
Heinonen et al. (1998)	Calisthenics: 3 sets of 16 repetitions of 8 different exercises to load muscles of lower extremities; additional wrist and ankle weight bands (1-2 kg) 4 d/wk	18	53	35	BMD of lumbar spine, femoral neck calcaneus, and radius by DXA	Linear trend of maintaining BMD of femoral neck in endurance group compared to control ($p < .05$); calisthenics group: non-significant
	Endurance: walking, jogging, ergometry, cycling, stair climbing, treadmill at 55-75% $\dot{V}O_2$max 4 d/wk		53	32		BMD other sites: no training effect in either group, except distal radius BMD of endurance group showed significant negative trend ($p = .006$)
	Controls stretching once per week		53	34		

Table 17.2   *(continued)*

Author	Type of exercise program	Duration of study (months)	Age (years)	Number of subjects	Bone measurement	Results
Lau et al. (1992)	Stepping up and down a block (9 in. in height) 100 times and then exercised (moving upper trunk while standing) 4 d/wk	10			BMD of lumbar spine and hip by DXA	Exercise did not have any significant effect on rate of bone loss at any site. Two-way analysis of variance showed significant interaction of calcium supplements and exercise at femoral neck ($p < .01$), but not at other sites.
	Placebo		75	12		
	Calcium (800 mg/d)		75	12		
	Exercise plus placebo		79	11		
	Exercise plus calcium (800 mg/d)		76	15		
Martin and Notelovitz (1993)	Treadmill exercise to 70-85% of maximal heart rate 3 sessions/wk	12			BMD of lumbar spine by DXA and forearm by SPA	No increase in BMD; but training attenuated loss of lumbar BMD in women who were ≤ 6 years after the onset of menopause.
	1. 30-min session		60	20		
	2. 45-min session		58	16		
	3. Control (maintain normal daily activities)		57	19		
Nelson et al. (1994)	High-intensity strength training (dynamic exercise including concentric and eccentric contractions): hip extension, knee extension, lateral pull-down, back extension, abdominal flexions (using pneumatic resistance machines); 3 sets of 8 reps at 80% of 1 RM during 45-min session 2 d/wk	12	61	20	BMD of lumbar spine, femoral neck, and total body by DXA	Femoral neck: exercise: +0.9% control: -2.5% $p = .02$ Lumbar spine: exercise: +1.0% control: -1.8% $p = .04$ Total body bone mineral: exercise: +0.0% control: -1.2% (NS)
	Control (maintain current physical activity level)		57	19		

(continued)

Table 17.2   *(continued)*

Author	Type of exercise program	Duration of study (months)	Age (years)	Number of subjects	Bone measurement	Results
Notelovitz et al. (1991)	Resistance circuit weight-training program using Nautilus equipment; 8 reps maxmum for each exercise; 15-20 min sessions 3 d/wk	12			BMD of lumbar spine, total body by DPA; and midshaft radius by SPA	Spine: exercise plus estrogen +8.3% p = .002; estrogen +1.5% p = NS
						Total body: exercise plus estrogen +2.1% p = .003; estrogen +0.6% p = NS
	Estrogen		46	11		
	Exercise plus estrogen		43	9		Midshaft radius: exercise plus estrogen +4.1% p = .01; estrogen −0.3% p = NS
Prince et al. (1991)	Supervised low-impact aerobic exercise for 1 hr/wk	24			BMD of three forearm sites by densiometer	Exercise: distal −2.6%; median −2.4%; proximal −2.0%
	Two brisk 30-min walks/wk					Exercise + calcium: distal −0.5%; median −1.3%; proximal −1.5%
	Exercise		57	41		
	Exercise plus calcium		57	39		Exercise + estrogen: distal +2.7%; median +0.8%; proximal +0.7%
	Exercise plus estrogen		55	40		
	Controls (normal bone density)		56	42		Controls: distal −2.7%; median −1.9%; proximal −1.5%
						Bone loss similar in controls and exercise group.
						Bone loss significantly lower in exercise-calcium group at distal and median site.
						Increase in BMD in exercise-estrogen group at all sites and significant from changes in all other groups.

(continued)

Table 17.2   (continued)

Author	Type of exercise program	Duration of study (months)	Age (years)	Number of subjects	Bone measurement	Results
Prince et al. (1995)	Exercise 4 hrs/wk: 2 hrs supervised weight-bearing class; 2 hrs walking; subjects asked to exercise at a rate to increase their heart rate to 60% of peak for age	24			BMD of lumbar spine, hip, and ultra-distal ankle by DXA	Femoral neck: exercise plus calcium: +0.28% ($p < .05$); calcium (both groups): −0.18%
	Placebo		63	42		No significant bone loss at the spine in any group.
	Exercise plus 1 gram calcium (tablets)		63	42		Significant reduction in rate of bone loss at ultradistal site of tibia for all groups compared to placebo, but no difference between exercise plus calcium group and calcium group.
	Calcium 1 gram (powder)		63	42		
	Calcium 1 gram (tablets)		62	42		
Pruitt et al. (1995)	High-intensity resistance training: 1 set of 14 repetitions at 40% 1 RM as warm-up followed by 2 sets of 7 repetitions at 80% 1 RM 3 d/wk	12	67	8	BMD of lumbar spine hip by DXA	Spine: high-intensity +0.7% low-intensity +0.5% controls −0.1%
	Low-intensity resistance training: 3 sets of 14 repetitions at 40% 1 RM; Nautilus and universal gym equipment used (10 exercises) 3 d/wk		68	7		Total hip: high-intensity +0.8% low-intensity +1.0% controls −0.9%
						Femoral neck: high-intensity −0.2% low-intensity +1.8% controls −0.9%
	Control (maintain current activity)		70	11		No significant change in BMD of spine or proximal femur (despite effective muscle-strengthening program).

(continued)

Table 17.2 *(continued)*

Author	Type of exercise program	Duration of study (months)	Age (years)	Number of subjects	Bone measurement	Results
Revel et al. (1993)	Psoas training: in sitting position, with 5-kg sandbag on knee, 60 flexions of each hip daily	12	57	39	BMD of lumbar spine by CT	No significant change in either group. In subgroup of "assiduous" exercisers, BMD loss significantly greater in the control group.
	Deltoid training (control): in sitting position, 1-kg sandbag on each hand, 60 abductions of both arms daily		56	39		
Sandler et al. (1987)	Walking: goal to achieve minimum walking of seven miles per week (at least 3 miles per session) 2 d/wk	36			Bone density of midshaft radius using CT	No difference in change in bone tissue density. Walking group had a significantly greater increase in cross-sectional area of the radius than the control group, but only for those in a high-grip strength group ($p < .05$).
	Exercise		58	114		
	Control		57	115		
Sinaki et al. (1989)	Back-strengthening exercises: backpack with weights equivalent to 30% of maximal isometric back muscle strength; in prone position, subject lifted backpack 10 times 5 d/wk	24			BMD of lumbar spine by DPA	Exercise: -1.4% $p < .001$ Control: -1.2% $p = .006$ NS difference between groups (back extensor strength increased more in exercise group than controls $p = .002$).
	Exercise		56	34		
	Control (no back exercises)		57	31		

(continued)

Table 17.2   (continued)

Author	Type of exercise program	Duration of study (months)	Age (years)	Number of subjects	Bone measurement	Results
Smidt et al. (1992)	Progressive resistive program for the trunk muscles: at 70% maximal strength, 3 sets of 10 repetitions of 3 exercises (sit-up, double leg raise, prone trunk extension) 3-4 d/wk	12			BMD of lumbar spine and hip by DPA	No significant differences between the exercise and control groups.
	Exercise		57	22		
	Control (maintain current lifestyle)		55	27		

References

Aloia, J.F., S.H. Cohn, T. Babu, C. Abesamis, N. Kalici, and K. Ellis. 1978. Skeletal mass and body composition in marathon runners. *Metabolism* 27:1793-1796.

Aloia, J.F., S.H. Cohn, J.A. Ostuni, R. Cane, and K. Ellis. 1978. Prevention of involutional bone loss by exercise. *Ann Intern Med* 89:356-358.

Aloia, J.F., A. Vaswani, J. Yeh, and S. Cohn. 1988. Premenopausal bone mass is related to physical activity. *Arch Intern Med* 148:121-123.

American College of Sports Medicine. 1995. Position stand on osteoporosis and exercise. *Med Sci Sports Exerc* 27:1-7.

Ayalon, J., A. Simkin, I. Leichter, and S. Raifmann. 1987. Dynamic bone loading exercises for postmenopausal women: effect on the density of the distal radius. *Arch Phys Med Rehabil* 68:280-283.

Ballard, J.E., B.C. McKeown, H.M. Graham, and S.A. Zinkgraf. 1990. The effect of high level physical activity (8.5 METs or greater) and estrogen replacement therapy upon bone mass in postmenopausal females, aged 50-68 years. *Int J Sports Med* 11:208-214.

Bass, S., G. Pearce, M. Bradney, E. Hendrich, P.D. Delmas, A. Harding, and E. Seeman. 1998. Exercise before puberty may confer residual benefits in bone density in adulthood: studies in active prepubertal and retired female gymnasts. *J Bone Miner Res* 13:500-507.

Bassey, E.J., and S.J. Ramsdale. 1994. Increase in femoral bone density in young women following high-impact exercise. *Osteoporos Int* 4:72-75.

Bassey, E.J., and S.J. Ramsdale. 1995. Weightbearing exercise and ground reaction forces: a 12-month randomized controlled trial of effects on bone mineral density in healthy postmenopausal women. *Bone* 16:469-476.

Bevier, W.C., R.A. Wiswell, G. Pyka, K.C. Kozak, K.M. Newhall, and R. Marcus. 1989. Relationship of body composition, muscle strength, and aerobic capacity to bone mineral density in older men and women. *J Bone Miner Res* 4:421-432.

Bilanin, J.E., M.S. Blanchard, and E. Russek-Cohen. 1989. Lower vertebral bone density in male long distance runners. *Med Sci Sports Exerc* 21:66-70.

Bonjour, J.P., G. Theintz, B. Buchs, D. Slosman, and R. Rizzoli. 1991. Critical years and stages of puberty for spinal and femoral bone mass accumulation during adolescence. *J Clin Endocrinol Metab* 73:555-563.

Bouxsein, M.L., and R. Marcus. 1994. Overview of exercise and bone mass. *Rheum Dis Clin North Am* 20:787-802.

Cavanaugh, D.J., and C.E. Cann. 1988. Brisk walking does not stop bone loss in postmenopausal women. *Bone* 9:201-204.

Chow, R., J.E. Harrison, C.F. Brown, and V. Hajek. 1986. Physical fitness effect on bone mass in postmenopausal women. *Arch Phys Med Rehabil* 67:231-234.

Chow, R., J.E. Harrison, and C. Notarius. 1987. Effect of two randomized exercise programmes on bone mass of healthy postmenopausal women. *Br Med J* 295:1441-1444.

Conroy, B.P., W.J. Kraemer, C.M. Maresh, S. Fleck, M.H. Stone, A.C. Fry, P.D. Miller, and G.P. Dalsky. 1993. Bone mineral density in elite junior Olympic weightlifters. *Med Sci Sports Exerc* 25:1103-1109.

Consensus Development Conference. 1993. Diagnosis, prophylaxis, and treatment of osteoporosis. *Am J Med* 94:646-650.

Cooper, C., M. Cawley, A. Bhalla, P. Egger, F. Ring, L. Morton, and D. Barker. 1995. Childhood growth, physical activity, and peak bone mass in women. *J Bone Miner Res* 10:940-947.

Cummings, S.R., D.M. Black, and S.M. Rubin. 1989. Lifetime risks of hip, Colles' or vertebral fracture and coronary heart disease among white postmenopausal women. *Arch Intern Med* 149:2445-2448.

Cummings, S.R., M.C. Nevitt, W.S. Browner, K. Stone, K.M. Fox, K.E. Engrud, J. Cauley, D. Black, and T.M. Vogt for the Study of Osteoporotic Fractures Research Group. 1995. Risk factors for hip fracture in white women. *N Engl J Med* 332:767-773.

Dalsky, G.P., K.S. Stocke, A.A. Ehsani, E. Slatopolsky, W.C. Lee, and S.J. Birge Jr. 1988. Weightbearing exercise training and lumbar bone mineral content in postmenopausal women. *Ann Intern Med* 108:824-828.

Davee, A.M., C.J. Rosen, and R.A. Adler. 1990. Exercise patterns and trabecular bone density in college women. *J Bone Miner Res* 5:245-250.

del Puente, A., N. Pappone, M.G. Mandes, D. Mantova, R. Scarpa, and P. Oriente. 1996. Determinants of bone mineral density in immobilization: a study on hemiplegic patients. *Osteoporos Int* 6:50-54.

Drinkwater, B.L., K. Nilson, C.H. Chesnut III, W. Bremner, S. Shainholtz, and M.B. Southworth. 1984. Bone mineral content of amenorrheic and eumenorrheic athletes. *N Engl J Med* 311:277-281.

Drinkwater, B.L., K. Nilson, S. Ott, and C.H. Chesnut III. 1986. Bone mineral density after resumption of menses in amenorrheic athletes. *JAMA* 256:380-282.

Fehling, P.C., L. Alekel, J. Clasey, A. Rector, and R.J. Stillman. 1995. A comparison of bone mineral densities among female athletes in impact loading and active loading sports. *Bone* 17:205-210.

Fiatarone, M.A., E.F. O'Neill, N.D. Ryan, K. Clements, G.R. Solares, M.E. Nelson, S.B. Roberts, J.J. Kehayias, L.A. Lipsitz, and W.J. Evans. 1994. Exercise training and nutritional supplementation for physical frailty in very elderly people. *N Engl J Med* 330:1769-1775.

Fisher, E.C., M.E. Nelson, W.R. Frontera, R.N. Turksoy, and W.J. Evans. 1986. Bone mineral content and levels of gonadotropins and estrogens in amenorrheic running women. *J Clin Endocrinol Metab* 62:1232-1236.

Friedlander, A.L., H.K. Genant, S. Sadowsky, N.N. Byl, and C.C. Gluer. 1995. A two-year program of aerobics and weight training enhances bone mineral density of young women. *J Bone Miner Res* 10:574-585.

Gleeson, P.B., E.J. Protas, A.D. LeBlanc, V.S. Schneider, and H.J. Evans. 1990. Effects of weight lifting on bone mineral density in premenopausal women. *J Bone Miner Res* 5:153-158.

Goemaere, S., M. Van Laere, P. DeNeve, and J.M. Kaufman. 1994. Bone mineral status in paraplegic patients who do or do not perform standing. *Osteoporos Int* 4:138-143.

Greendale, G.A., E. Barrett-Connor, S. Edelstein, S. Ingles, and R. Haile. 1995. Lifetime leisure exercise and osteoporosis. The Rancho Bernardo study. *Am J Epidemiol* 141:951-959.

Greenspan, S.L., E.R. Myers, L.A. Maitland, N.M. Resnick, and W.C. Hayes. 1994. Fall severity and bone mineral density as risk factors for hip fracture in ambulatory elderly. *JAMA* 271:128-133.

Grisso, J.A., J.L. Kelsey, B.L. Strom, G.Y. Chiu, G. Maislin, L.A. O'Brien, S. Hoffman, F. Kaplan, and the Northeast Hip Fracture Study Group. 1991. Risk factors for falls as a cause of hip fracture in women. *N. Engl J Med* 324:1326-1331.

Grove, K.A., and B.R. Londeree. 1992. Bone density in postmenopausal women: high impact vs. low impact exercise. *Med Sci Sports Exerc* 24:1190-1194.

Gutin, B., and M.J. Kasper. 1992. Can vigorous exercise play a role in osteoporosis prevention? A review. *Osteoporos Int* 2:55-69.

Haapasalo, H., P. Kannus, H. Sievänen, M. Pasanen, K. Uusi-Rasi, A. Heinonen, P. Oja, and I. Vuori. 1998. Effect of long-term unilateral activity on bone mineral density of female junior tennis players. *J Bone Miner Res* 13:310-319.

Haapasalo, H., H. Sievänen, P. Kannus, A. Heinonen, P. Oja, and I. Vuori. 1996. Dimensions and estimated mechanical characteristics of the humerus after long-term tennis loading. *J Bone Miner Res* 11:864-872.

Halioua, L., and J.J.B. Anderson. 1989. Lifetime calcium intake and physical activity habits: independent and combined effects on the radial bone of healthy premenopausal women. *Am J Clin Nutr* 49:534-41.

Hamdy, R.C., J.S. Anderson, K.E. Whalen, and L.M. Harvill. 1994. Regional differences in bone density in young men involved in different exercises. *Med Sci Sports Exerc* 26:884-888.

Hatori, M., A. Hasegawa, H. Adachi, A. Shinozaki, R. Hayashi, H. Okamo, H. Mizunuma, and K. Murata. 1993. The effects of walking at the anaerobic threshold level on vertebral bone loss in postmenopausal women. *Calcif Tissue Int* 52:411-414.

Heinonen, A., P. Kannus, H. Sievänen, P. Oja, M. Pasanen, M. Rinne, K. Uusi-Rasi, and I. Vuori. 1996. Randomized controlled trial of effect of high-impact exercise on selected risk factors for osteoporotic fractures. *Lancet* 348:1343-1347.

Heinonen, A., P. Oja, P. Kannus, H. Sievänen, H. Haapasalo, A. Mänttäri, and I. Vuori. 1995. Bone mineral density in female athletes representing sports with different loading characteristics of the skeleton. *Bone* 17:197-203.

Heinonen, A., P. Oja, P. Kannus, H. Sievänen, A. Mänttäri, and I. Vuori. 1993. Bone mineral density of female athletes in different sports. *Bone Miner* 23:1-14.

Heinonen, A., P. Oja, H. Sievänen, M. Pasanen, and I. Vuori. 1998. Effect of two training regimens on bone mineral den-

sity in healthy perimenopausal women: a randomized controlled trial. *J Bone Miner Res* 13:483-490.

Heinrich, C.H., S.B. Going, R.W. Pamenter, C.D. Perry, T.W. Boynden, and T.G. Lohman. 1990. Bone mineral content of cyclically menstruating female resistance and endurance trained athletes. *Med Sci Sports Exerc* 22:558-563.

Hetland, M.L., J. Haarbo, and C. Christiansen. 1993. Low bone mass and high bone turnover in male long distance runners. *J Clin Endocrinol Metab* 77:770-775.

Hirota, T., M. Nara, M. Ohguri, E. Manago, and K. Hirota. 1992. Effect of diet and lifestyle on bone mass in Asian young women. *Am J Clin Nutr* 55:1168-1173.

Huddleston, A.L., D. Rockwell, D. Kulund, and R.B. Harrison. 1980. Bone mass in lifetime tennis athletes. *JAMA* 244:1107-1109.

Hughes, V.A., W.R. Frontera, G.E. Dallal, K.J. Lutz, E.C. Fisher, and W.J. Evans. 1995. Muscle strength and body composition: associations with bone density in older subjects. *Med Sci Sports Exer* 27:967-974.

Jacobson, P.C., W. Beaver, S.A. Grubb, T.N. Taft, and R.V. Talmage. 1984. Bone density in women: college athletes and older athletic women. *J Orthop Res* 2:328-332.

Johnell, O., B. Gullberg, J.A. Kanis, E. Allander, L. Elffors, J. Dequcker, G. Dilsen, C. Gennari, A.L. Vaz, G. Lyritis, G. Mazzuoli, L. Miravet, M. Passeri, R.P. Cano, A. Rapado, and C. Ribot. 1995. Risk factors for hip fracture in European women: the MEDOS study. *J Bone Miner Res* 10:1802-1815.

Jones, H.H., J.D. Priest, W.C. Hayes, C.C. Tichenor, and D.A. Nagel. 1977. Humeral hypertrophy in response to exercise. *J Bone Joint Surg* 59A:204-208.

Kanis, J.A., L.J. Melton III, C. Christiansen, C.C. Johnston, and N. Khaltaev. 1994. The diagnosis of osteoporosis. *J Bone Miner Res* 9:1137-1141.

Kannus, P., H. Haapasalo, M. Sankelo, H. Sievanen, M. Paganen, A. Heinonen, P. Oja, and I. Vuori. 1995. Effect of starting age of physical activity on bone mass in the dominant arm of tennis and squash players. *Ann Intern Med* 123:27-31.

Karlsson, M.K., O. Johnell, and K.J. Obrant. 1993a. Bone mineral density in professional ballet dancers. *Bone Miner* 21:163-169.

Karlsson, M.K., O. Johnell, and K.J. Obrant. 1993b. Bone mineral density in weight lifters. *Calcif Tissue Int* 52:212-215.

Kelley, G.A. 1998. Exercise and regional bone mineral density in postmenopausal women: a meta-analytic review of randomized trials. *Am J Phys Med Rehabil* 77:76-87.

Khan, K.M., R.M. Green, A. Saul, K.L. Bennell, K.J. Crichton, J.L. Hopper, and J.D. Wark. 1996. Retired elite female ballet dancers and nonathletic controls have similar bone mineral density at weightbearing sites. *J Bone Miner Res* 11:1566-1574.

Kirk, S., C.F. Sharp, N. Elbaum, D.B. Enders, S.M. Simons, J.G. Mohler, and R.K. Rude. 1989. Effect of long distance running on bone mass in women. *J Bone Miner Res* 4:515-522.

Klesges, R.C., K.D. Ward, M.L. Shelton, W.B. Applegate, E.D. Cantler, G.M.A. Palmieri, K. Harmon, and J. Davis. 1996. Changes in bone mineral content in male athletes: mechanism of action and intervention effects. *JAMA* 276:226-230.

Kohrt, W.M., A.A. Ehsani, and S.J. Birge Jr. 1997. Effects of exercise involving predominantly either joint-reaction or ground-reaction forces on bone mineral density in older women. *J Bone Miner Res* 12:1253-1261.

Kroger, H., A. Kotaniemi, L. Kroger, and E. Alhava. 1993. Development of bone mass and bone density of the spine and femoral neck—a prospective study of 65 children and adolescents. *Bone Miner* 23:171-182.

Krolner, B., and B. Toft. 1983. Vertebral bone loss: an unheeded side effect of therapeutic bedrest. *Clin Sci* 64:537-540.

Krolner B., B. Toft, S.P. Nielsen, and T. Tondevold. 1983. Physical activity as prophylaxis against involutional vertebral bone loss: a controlled trial. *Clin Sci* 64:541-546.

Lane, N.E., D.A. Bloch, H.H. Jones, W.H. Marshall Jr., P.D. Wood, and J.F. Fries. 1986. Long distance running, bone density and osteoarthritis. *JAMA* 255:1147-1151.

Lanyon, L.E. 1996. Using functional loading to influence bone mass and architecture: objectives, mechanisms, and relationship with estrogen of the mechanically adaptive process in bone. *Bone* 18(Suppl.):37-43.

Lau, E.M.C., J. Woo, P.C. Leung, R. Swaminathan, and D. Leung. 1992. The effects of calcium supplementation and exercise on bone density in elderly Chinese women. *Osteoporos Int* 2:168-173.

Lohman, T., S. Going, R. Pamenter, M. Hall, T. Boyden, L. Houtkooper, C. Ritenbaugh, L. Bare, A. Hill, and M. Aickin. 1995. Effects of resistance training on regional and total bone mineral density in premenopausal women: a randomized prospective study. *J Bone Miner Res* 10:1015-1024.

Lord, S.R., J.A. Ward, and P. Williams. 1996. Exercise effect on dynamics stability in older women: a randomized controlled trial. *Arch Phys Med Rehabil* 77:232-236.

MacDougall, J.D., C.E. Webber, J. Martin, S. Ormerod, A. Chesley, E.V. Younglai, C.L. Gordon, and C.J.R. Blimkie. 1992. Relationship among running mileage, bone density, and serum testosterone in male runners. *J Appl Physiol* 73:1165-1170.

Madsen, O.R., O. Schaadt, H. Bliddal, C. Egsmose, and J. Sylvest. 1993. Relationship between quadriceps strength and bone mineral density of the proximal tibia and distal forearm in women. *J Bone Miner Res* 12:1439-1444.

Marcus, R., C. Cann, P. Madvig, J. Minkoff, M. Goddard, M. Bayer, M. Martin, L. Gaudiani, W. Haskel, and H. Genant. 1985. Menstrual function and bone mass in elite women distance runners: endocrine and metabolic features. *Ann Intern Med* 102:158-163.

Marcus, R., B. Drinkwater, G. Dalsky, J. Dufek, D. Rabb, C. Slemenda, and C. Snow-Harter. 1992. Osteoporosis and exercise in women. *Med Sci Sports Exerc* 24(Suppl.):301-307.

Martin, D., and M. Notelovitz. 1993. Effect of aerobic training on bone mineral density of postmenopausal women. *J Bone Miner Res* 8:931-936.

Matkovic, V., T. Jelic, G.M. Wardlaw, J.Z. Ilich, P.K. Goel, J.K. Wright, M.B. Andon, K.T. Smith, and R.P. Heaney. 1994. Timing of peak bone mass in caucasian females and its implication for the prevention of osteoporosis. Inference from a cross-sectional model. *J Clin Invest* 93:799-808.

Mazess, R.B., and H.S. Barden. 1991. Bone density in premenopausal women: effects of age, dietary intake, physical activity, smoking, and birth-control pills. *Am J Clin Nutr* 53:132-142.

McCulloch, R.G, D.A. Bailey, C.S. Houston, and B.L. Dodd. 1990. Effects of physical activity, dietary calcium intake and selected lifestyle factors on bone density in young women. *Can Med Assoc J* 142:221-227.

Melton, L.J. III, 1993. Hip fractures. A worldwide problem today and tomorrow. *Bone* 14(Suppl.):1-8.

Melton, L.J. III, E.A. Chrischilles, C. Cooper, A.W. Lane, and B.L. Riggs. 1992. How many women have osteoporosis? *J Bone Miner Res* 9:1005-1010.

Melton, L.J. III, M. Thamer, N.F. Ray, J.K. Chan, C.H. Chestnut III, T.A. Einhorn, C.C. Johnston, L.G. Raise, S.L. Silverman, and E.S. Siris. 1997. Factors attributable to osteoporosis: report from the National Osteoporosis Foundation. *J Bone Miner Res* 12:16-23.

Metz, J.A., J.J.B. Anderson, and P.N. Gallagher Jr. 1993. Intakes of calcium, phosphorus, and protein, and physical-activity level are related to radial bone mass in young adult women. *Am J Clin Nutr* 58:537-542.

Michel, B.A., D.A. Bloch, and J.F. Fries. 1989. Weightbearing exercise, overexercise, and lumbar bone density over age 50 years. *Arch Intern Med* 149:2325-2329.

Michel, B.A., N.E. Lane, D.A. Bloch, H.H. Jones, and J.F. Fries. 1991. Effect of changes in weightbearing exercise on lumbar bone mass after age fifty. *Ann Med* 23:397-401.

Myburgh, K.H., L.K. Bachrach, B. Lewis, K. Kent, and R. Marcus. 1993. Low bone mineral density at axial and appendicular sites in amenorrheic athletes. *Med Sci Sports Exerc* 25:1197-1202.

Myburgh, K.H., J. Hutchins, A.B. Fataar, S.F. Hough, and T.D. Noakes. 1990. Low bone density is an etiologic factor for stress fractures in athletes. *Ann Intern Med* 113:754-759.

Nelson, M.E., M.A. Fiatarone, C.M. Morganti, I. Trice, R.A. Greenberg, and W.J. Evans. 1994. Effects of high-intensity strength training on multiple risk factors for osteoporotic fractures: a randomized controlled trial. *JAMA* 272:1909-1914.

Nelson, M.E., E.C. Fisher, F.A. Dilmanian, G.E. Dallal, and W.J. Evans. 1991. A 1-year walking program and increased dietary calcium in postmenopausal women: effects on bone. *Am J Clin Nutr* 53:1304-1311.

Nelson, M.E., C.N. Meredith, B. Dawson-Hughes, and W.J. Evans. 1988. Hormone and bone mineral status in endurance-trained and sedentary postmenopausal women. *J Clin Endocrinol Metab* 66:927-933.

Nilsson, B.E., and N.E. Westlin. 1971. Bone density in athletes. *Clin Orthop* 77:179-182.

Notelovitz, M., D. Martin, R. Tesar, F.Y. Khan, C. Probart, C. Fields, and L. McKenzie. 1991. Estrogen therapy and variable-resistance weight training increase bone mineral in surgically menopausal women. *J Bone Miner Res* 6:583-590.

O'Connor, J.A., L.E. Lanyon, and H. MacFie. 1982. The influence of strain rate on adaptive bone remodeling. *J Biomech* 15:767-781.

Peterson, S.E., M.D. Peterson, G. Raymond, C. Gilligan, M.M. Checovich, and E.L. Smith. 1991. Muscular strength and bone density with weight training in middle-aged women. *Med Sci Sports Exerc* 23:499-504.

Picard, D., L.G. Ste-Marie, D. Coutu, L. Carrieri, R. Chartrand, R. Lepage, P. Fugere, and P.D. Armour. 1988. Premenopausal bone mineral content relates to height, weight and calcium intake during early adulthood. *Bone Miner* 4:299-309.

Pocock, N.A., J.A. Eisman, M.G. Yeates, P.N. Sambrook, and S. Eberl. 1986. Physical fitness is a major determinant of femoral neck and lumbar spine bone mineral density. *J Clin Invest* 78:618-621.

Prince, R., A. Devine, I. Dick, A. Criddle, D. Kerr, N. Kent, R. Price, and A. Randell. 1995. The effects of calcium supplementation (milk powder or tablets) and exercise on bone density in postmenopausal women. *J Bone Miner Res* 10:1068-1075.

Prince, R.L., M. Smith, I. Dick, R.I. Price, P.G. Webb, N.K. Henderson, and M.M. Harris. 1991. Prevention of postmenopausal osteoporosis: a comparative study of exercise, calcium supplementation, and hormone replacement therapy. *N Engl J Med* 325:1189-1195.

Province, M.A., E.C. Hadley, M.C. Hornbrook, L.A. Lipsitz, J.P. Miller, C.D. Mulrow, M.G. Ory, R.W. Sattin, M.E. Tinetti, and S.L. Wolf for the FICSIT Group. 1995. The effects of exercise on falls in elderly patients: a preplanned meta-analysis of the FICSIT trials. *JAMA* 273:1341-1347.

Pruitt, L.A., R.D. Jackson, R.L. Bartels, and H.J. Lehnhard. 1992. Weight-training effects on bone mineral density in early postmenopausal women. *J Bone Miner Res* 7:179-185.

Pruitt, L.A., D.R. Taaffe, and R. Marcus. 1995. Effects of a one-year high-intensity versus low-intensity resistance training program on bone mineral density in older women. *J Bone Miner Res* 10:1788-1795.

Rambaut, P.C., and A.W. Goode. 1985. Skeletal changes during space flight. *Lancet* 2:1050-1052.

Ray, N.F., J.K. Chan, M. Thaemer, and L.J. Melton III. 1997. Medical expenditures for the treatment of osteoporotic fractures in the United States in 1995: report from the National Osteoporosis Foundation. *J Bone Miner Res* 12:24-35.

Recker, R.R., K.M. Davies, S.M. Hinders, R.P. Heaney, M.R. Stegman, and D.B. Kimmel. 1992. Bone gain in young adult women. *JAMA* 268:2403-2408.

Reid, I.R., R. Ames, M.C. Evans, G. Sharpe, G. Gamble, J.T. France, T.M.T. Lim, and T.F. Cundy. 1992. Determinants of total body and regional bone mineral density in normal postmenopausal women—a key role for fat mass. *J Clin Endocrinol Metab* 75:45-51.

Reid, I.R., L.D. Plank, and M.C. Evans. 1992. Fat mass is an important determinant of whole body bone density in pre-

menopausal women but not in men. *J Clin Endocrinol Metab* 75:779-782.

Rencken, M.L., C.H. Chestnut III, and B.L. Drinkwater. 1996. Bone density at multiple skeletal sites in amenorrheic athletes. *JAMA* 276:238-240.

Revel, M., M.A. Mayoux-Benhamou, J.P. Rabourdin, F. Bagheri, and C. Roux. 1993. One-year psoas training can prevent lumbar bone loss in postmenopausal women: a randomized controlled trial. *Calcif Tissue Int* 53:307-311.

Riggs, B.L., and L.J. Melton III. 1986. Involutional osteoporosis. *N Engl J Med* 314:1676-1686.

Robinson, T.L., C. Snow-Harter, D.R. Taaffe, D. Gillis, J. Shaw, and R. Marcus. 1995. Gymnasts exhibit higher bone mass than runners despite similar prevalence of amenorrhea and oligomenorrhea. *J Bone Miner Res* 10:26-35.

Rockwell, J.C., A.M. Sorensen, S. Baker, D. Leahey, J.L. Stock, J. Michaels, and D.T. Baran. 1990. Weight training decreases vertebral bone density in premenopausal women: a prospective study. *J Clin Endocrinol Metab* 71:988-993.

Rodin, A., B. Murby, M.A. Smith, M. Caleffi, I. Fentiman, M.G. Chapman, and I. Fogelman. 1990. Premenopausal bone loss in the lumbar spine and neck of femur: a study of 225 Caucasian women. *Bone* 11:1-5.

Rubenstein, L.Z., K.R. Josephson, and A.S. Robbins. 1994. Falls in the nursing home. *Ann Intern Med* 121:442-451.

Rubin, C.T., and L.E. Lanyon. 1985. Regulation of bone mass by mechanical strain magnitude. *Calcif Tissue Int* 37:411-417.

Rundgren, A., A. Aniansson, P. Ljungberg, and H. Wetterqvist. 1984. Effects of a training programme for elderly people on mineral content of the heel bone. *Arch Gerontol Geriatr* 3:243-248.

Sandler, R.B., J.A. Cauley, D.L. Hom, D. Sashin, and A.M. Kriska. 1987. The effects of walking on the cross-sectional dimensions of the radius in postmenopausal women. *Calcif Tissue Int* 41:65-69.

Sattin, R.W. 1992. Falls among older persons: a public health perspective. *Annu Rev Public Health* 13:489-508.

Schwarz, A.J., J.A. Brasel, R.L. Hintz, S. Mohan, and D.M. Cooper. 1996. Acute effect of brief low- and high-intensity exercise on circulating insulin-like growth factor (IGF) I, II and IGF-binding protein-3 and its proteolysis in young healthy men. *J Clin Endocrinol Metab* 81:3492-3497.

Sinaki, M., M.C. McPhee, S.F. Hodgson, J.M. Merritt, and K.P. Offord. 1986. Relationship between bone mineral density of spine and strength of back extensors in healthy postmenopausal women. *Mayo Clin Proc* 61:116-122.

Sinaki, M., and K.P. Offord. 1988. Physical activity in postmenopausal women. Effect on back muscle strength and bone mineral density of the spine. *Arch Phys Med Rehabil* 69:277-280.

Sinaki, M., J.L. Opitz, and H.W. Wahner. 1974. Bone mineral content: relationship to muscle strength in normal subjects. *Arch Phys Med Rehabil* 55:508-512.

Sinaki, M., H.W. Wahner, E.J. Bergstrall, S.F. Hodgson, K.P. Offord, R.W. Squires, R.G. Swee, and P.C. Kao. 1996. Three-year controlled randomized trial of the effect of dose-specified loading and strengthening exercises on bone mineral density of spine and femur in nonathletic, physically active women. *Bone* 19:233-244.

Sinaki, M., H.W. Wahner, K.P. Offord, and S.F. Hodgson. 1989. Efficiency of nonloading exercises in prevention of vertebral bone loss in postmenopausal women: a controlled trial. *Mayo Clin Proc* 64:762-769.

Slemenda, C.W., J.Z. Miller, S.L. Hui, T.K. Reister, and C.C. Johnston Jr. 1991. Role of physical activity in the development of skeletal mass in children. *J Bone Miner Res* 6:1227-1233.

Slemenda, C.W., and C.C. Johnston. 1993. High intensity activities in young women: site specific bone mass effects among female figure skaters. *Bone Miner* 20:125-132.

Slemenda, C.W., T.K. Reister, S.L. Hui, J.Z. Miller, J.C. Christian, and C.C. Johnston Jr. 1994. Influences on skeletal mineralization in children and adolescents: evidence for varying effects of sexual maturation and physical activity. *J Pediatr* 125:201-207.

Smidt, G.L, S-Y. Lin, K.D. O'Dwyer, and P.R. Blanpied. 1992. The effect of high-intensity trunk exercise on bone mineral density of postmenopausal women. *Spine* 17:280-285.

Smith, E.L., C. Gilligan, M. McAdam, C. Ensign, and P. Smith. 1989. Deterring bone loss by exercise intervention in premenopausal and postmenopausal women. *Calcif Tissue Int* 44:312-321.

Smith, R., and O.M. Rutherford. 1993. Spine and total body bone mineral density and serum testosterone levels in male athletes. *Eur J Appl Physiol* 67:330-334.

Snow, C.M., J.M. Shaw, and C.C. Matkin. 1996. Physical activity and risk for osteoporosis. In *Osteoporosis*, ed. R. Marcus, D. Feldman, and J. Kelsey. San Diego: Academic Press.

Snow-Harter, C., M.L. Bouxsein, B.T. Lewis, D.R. Carter, and R. Marcus. 1992. Effects of resistance and endurance exercise on bone mineral status of young women: a randomized exercise intervention trial. *J Bone Miner Res* 7:761-769.

Snow-Harter, C., M.L. Bouxsein, B.T. Lewis, S. Charette, P. Weinstein, and R. Marcus. 1990. Muscle strength as a predictor of bone mineral density in young women. *J Bone Miner Res* 5:589-595.

Sudarsky, L. 1990. Gait disturbances in the elderly. *N Engl J Med* 322:1441-1446.

Taaffe, D.R., T.L. Robinson, C.M. Snow, and R. Marcus. 1997. High-impact exercise promotes bone gain in well-trained female athletes. *J Bone Miner Res* 12:255-260.

Taaffe, D.R., C. Snow-Harter, D.A. Connolly, T.L. Robinson, M.D. Brown, and R. Marcus. 1995. Differential effects of swimming versus weightbearing activity on bone mineral status of eumenorrheic athletes. *J Bone Miner Res* 10:586-593.

Tinetti, M.E., D.I. Baker, G. McAvay, E.B. Claus, P. Garrett, M. Gottschalk, M.L. Koch, K. Trainor, and R.I. Horwitz. 1994. A multifactorial intervention to reduce the risk of falling among elderly people living in the community. *N Engl J Med* 331:821-827.

Tinetti, M.E., M. Speechley, and S.F. Ginter. 1988. Risk factors for falls among elderly persons living in the community. *N Engl J Med* 319:1701-1707.

Torgerson, D.J., M.K. Campbell, and D.M. Reid. 1995. Lifestyle, environmental and medical factors influencing peak bone mass in women. *Br J Rheumatol* 34:620-624.

Vico, L., J.F. Pouget, P. Calmels, J.C. Chatard, M. Rehailia, P. Minaire, A. Geyssant, and C. Alexandre. 1995. The relations between physical ability and bone mass in women aged over 65 years. *J Bone Miner Res* 10:374-383.

Virvidakis, K., E. Georgiou, A. Korkotsidis, K.N. Talles, and C. Provkakis. 1990. Bone mineral content of junior competitive weightlifters. *Int J Sports Med* 11:244-246.

Welten, D.C., H.C.G. Kemper, G.B. Post, W. Van Mechelen, J. Twisk, P. Lips, and G.J. Teule. 1994. Weightbearing activity during youth is a more important factor for peak bone mass than calcium intake. *J Bone Miner Res* 9:1089-1096.

Williams, J.A., J. Wagner, R. Wasnick, and L. Heilbrun. 1984. The effect of long-distance running upon appendicular bone mineral content. *Med Sci Sports Exerc* 16:223-227.

Young, N., C. Formica, G. Szmukler, and E. Seeman. 1994. Bone density at weightbearing and nonweightbearing sites in ballet dancers: the effects of exercise, hypogonadism, and body weight. *J Clin Endocrinol Metab* 78:449-454.

Chapter 18

Mental Health

Richard C. Kaiser, MD

Case Study

A 32-year-old construction worker, J.C., lost his status in life after a workplace injury. He reported panic attacks each time he spoke to his ex-wife or his insurance company. He did not want to try any medications, but found instead that treadmill exercise twice a day significantly reduced these attacks. He began to use his treadmill to "walk off his anger or fear" on a daily basis.

S.B., a 45-year-old with chronic headaches, back pain, and depression from a motor vehicle accident, had responded modestly to antidepressant treatment. Yet she reported that walking her dog substantially improved her mood, en-ergy, and pain level, and that she could not miss a day.

P.K., 72 years old, developed major depression during his long rehabilitation from major cardiopulmonary illness. Antidepressants helped him regain his will to live. Once he began strength training and walked again with assistance, moreover, his spirits brightened and he noted his accomplishments with pride.

E.M., a 35-year-old physician, was under intense stress in a fast-paced field. She reported that jogging "cleared her mind" so that she could sleep well and start with a "clean emotional slate" the next day.

An Overview

The benefits of regular exercise to one's physical and mental health seem obvious. Improvements in mood, anxiety, and quality of life are common. Yet few clinicians prescribe exercise to treat disorders of mental health. And even when it is prescribed, depressed people often fail to adhere to their programs. In this chapter, I will explore the scientific evidence for the linkage of anxiety, mood, and motor function, and theorize how we may harness this linkage for the benefit of our patients.

Historical Background

The linkage between motor activity and mental illness has been known for centuries. Plato noted that one should "avoid exercising either mind or body without the other and thus preserve an equal and healthy balance between them." Centuries later, Burton's "Anatomy of Melancholy" (circa 17th century) linked depression and slowness of movement (see Jacobs 1994).

Epidemiological studies in recent decades have documented a consistent link between inactivity and mental illness in the general population (Paffenbarger et al. 1994). Stephens (1988) and others asserted that higher levels of physical activity are associated with general well-being, positive mood, and lower levels of anxiety and depression in the general population. Currently, the widespread public belief is that regular exercise ameliorates the effects of stress.

Defining "Exercise" and "Mental Health"

For the purposes of our discussion, I will often refer to "aerobic exercise" simply as exercise. Most researchers believe that aerobic exercise creates beneficial changes in the brain and the psyche. Most human studies of exercise, mood, and anxiety have subjects exercise at levels greater than 60% of their maximum oxygen uptake (VO_2max) for twenty minutes or more. This creates cardiac conditioning and activates the hypothalamic-pituitary-adrenal (HPA) response to stress. The resulting increase of neurochemicals (catecholamines and endorphins) in the bloodstream is often taken as evidence of similar effects within the brain—yet despite vigorous research efforts on the biochemical changes associated with exercise, the proper type, dosage, and duration of exercise required to enhance mental health remain

largely unknown. I will also mention several studies that have shown some mental health benefits from resistance weight training and relaxation exercises.

It is somewhat difficult to define mental health. *Stedman's Medical Dictionary* (26th ed., 1995) defines mental health as "a state of psychological well being in which the individual has achieved a satisfactory integration of his or her instinctual drives acceptable to both himself and his social milieu; or an appropriate balance of love, work, and leisure pursuits." Others define it as a lack of any diagnosable syndrome from the *Diagnostic and Statistical Manual of Mental Disorders IV* (American Psychiatric Association 1994), the more common of which are listed in "Common Psychiatric Disorders Studied in Exercise Rehabilitation" (pages 351-352). It is important to differentiate transient mood disorders from chronic pervasive syndromes that affect mental health.

Epidemiology

The syndromes most often considered *potentially* amenable to treatment with exercise include nonpsychotic depressive and anxiety disorders. In some epidemiologic studies, nearly three of ten persons aged 15-54 years report having a mental disorder (most commonly anxiety or depression) during the previous year (USDHHS 1996). Because typically only one in five of these affected individuals seeks professional treatment, the need for alternative treatments is great.

Mood disorders have a lifetime prevalence of about eight percent in the population, with depression and dysthymia accounting for the majority of cases (Regier et al. 1988). More severe forms of depressive mood disorders reveal common physiological symptoms termed "vegetative signs of depression": general slowing of the organism characterized by weight loss, abnormal menses, decreased libido, fatigue, and psychomotor retardation. Dysregulation of the HPA response to stress has been implicated in the development of the more severe symptoms (Gold et al. 1988).

Researchers have developed a number of theories to explain the etiology of depressive disorders and to help in designing treatments. Development of a depressive disorder in response to stress appears to result from a combination of genetics, temperament, and environmental factors. Loss, family dynamics, and conflicts often play pivotal roles in the onset, course, and recurrence of episodes of mood disorders (Gabbard 1994). Some individuals respond to stress by increasing activity through work, exercise, and enhanced efforts in spiritual or social ties; others

Common Psychiatric Disorders Studied in Exercise Rehabilitation

A: Depressive Mood Disorders

- **Major depressive episode** is characterized by two weeks of either *pervasively depressed mood* or *loss of interest*, combined with four or more of the following symptoms:

  1. Significant weight loss/gain
  2. A change in appetite
  3. Insomnia or hypersomnia
  4. Psychomotor agitation or retardation
  5. Fatigue
  6. Feelings of guilt or worthlessness
  7. Decreased concentration
  8. Recurrent thoughts of death

  Qualifiers to the above include the following: The symptoms are not part of a mixed (manic) episode; they must cause clinically significant distress or impairment in function; they are not due to the direct effects of a substance (e.g., alcohol) or medical condition (e.g., hypothyroidism), or recent bereavement of a loved one, all of which can cause symptoms similar to those of major depression.

  The mean age of onset is about age 40, with 50% having onset between ages 20 and 50. The lifetime prevalence of major depressive disorder is about 6% for men, 10% for women (Kaplan et al. 1994).

B: Other Depressive Mood Syndromes

- **Dysthymic disorder** is characterized by a two-year persistence of depressed mood, accompanied by at least two of the depressive symptoms listed above, without suicidal feelings.

- **Minor depressive disorder** is similar to a major depressive episode, but with only two to five of the depressive symptoms listed above.

- **Adjustment disorder** is diagnosed when a person has experienced identifiable stressors and develops emotional or behavioral symptoms within three months of the events. The symptoms may include depressed mood and anxiety, but not to the degree of a major mood disorder. Adjustment disorders are most common during young adulthood, but may occur at any age when faced with a serious life stressor.

- **Bipolar mood disorders** have cycles of elevated mood and activity alternating with periods of depression, and may exhibit loss of judgment, as well as psychosis.

C: Anxiety Disorders

- **Acute stress disorder.** The person has experienced, witnessed, or been confronted with an event involving actual or threatened death or serious injury to self or others. The person's response involves intense fear, helplessness, or horror. Symptoms include numbing, dissociation, avoidance of stimuli, nightmares, flashbacks, and hyperarousal.

(continued)

351

- **Post-traumatic stress disorder.** The symptoms of acute stress disorder persist for more than one month after the stressor.

- **Panic disorder.** Recurrent unexpected panic attacks, consisting of a period of intense fear or discomfort in which four or more of the following symptoms develop abruptly, reaching a peak within 10 minutes: palpitations, sweating, trembling, dyspnea, choking sensations, chest pain or discomfort, nausea/GI distress, dizziness, derealization, depersonalization, fear of losing control or of dying, paresthesias, chills/hot flushes. Often associated with social limitations and a fear of unexpected panic attacks in public places (agoraphobia).

- **Generalized anxiety disorder.** For at least six months, excessive anxiety and worry occurring frequently about a number of events and activities. Three of the following six symptoms prevailed over the previous six months: restlessness, easy fatigability, difficulty concentrating, irritability, muscle tension, sleep disturbance.

- **Adjustment disorder with anxiety.** Anxiety symptoms appear in the presence of an identifiable life stressor that occurred within the past three months.

D: Other Syndromes in Rehabilitation

Virtually any psychological disorder may appear in the rehabilitation setting. The trend to increase medical acuity in rehabilitation facilities has increased the prevalence of medically related psychiatric conditions. Patients with changes in mental status may appear to mimic anxiety or show depressive symptoms. The mental status may change due to medications, medical illness, hypoxia, alcohol or drug withdrawal, seizures, ongoing infections, psychosis, or a chronic dementing illness. Patients with chronic dementias or acute confusional states may appear depressed or anxious. Any deficits in cognitive or mental status should be investigated by a trained examiner. Prompt treatment with medications, behavioral measures, and cognitive cueing can improve rehabilitation potential. These illnesses are far too severe to be treated with exercise alone.

Major depressive episode diagnostic criteria, and definitions of mood disorders and anxiety disorders reprinted with permission from the *Diagnostic and Statistical Manual of Mental Disorders*, Fourth Edition. Copyright 1994 American Psychiatric Association.

respond negatively by succumbing to addictive substances or emotional disorders. Fortunately, most cases of major depression improve in 6-12 months even without specific treatment. If treated, the condition generally remits within 12 weeks. Depression is often a chronic relapsing illness, however, with an average of five to six episodes occurring over a 20-year period (Kaplan et al. 1994).

For moderate to severe depressive disorders, psychotherapy and antidepressant medications have proven more effective than placebo treatment (Elkin et al. 1989). However, mild depressive symptoms may show an equal response to many treatments, including placebos. Anxiety disorders have a lifetime prevalence of almost 15 percent in the general population, with phobias being the most common (Regier et al. 1988). Effective treatments include a variety of cog-

nitive, behavioral, and supportive psychotherapies, as well as placebos (Gabbard 1994). Medications such as benzodiazepines and antidepressants can lessen the severity and frequency of panic disorder. To gauge the effectiveness of differing treatment regimens, it is essential to stratify anxiety and depressive syndromes based on severity, and to compare treatments with placebos. Failure to test the placebo effect has been a confounding factor in many early studies of exercise and mental health.

Our Paleolithic Legacy

The link between inactivity and medical illness is well documented (Blair et al. 1995). Eaton, in his inspiring book, *The Paleolithic Prescription*, credits this link to the evolutionary mismatch between modern industrial society and our physiologic heritage. Early humans were hunter-gatherers, who engaged in regular daily aerobic walking or running. Their stresses were often acute, and they depended on their "fight-or-flight" stress response systems to survive. With the conversion to agricultural societies approximately 10,000 years ago, about 500 generations of humans adapted to a physically labor-intensive but less acutely unpredictable lifestyle. With the advent of the modern industrial age more than 200 years ago, the need for individuals to engage in aerobic exercise abruptly declined, while stresses continued to evoke primitive physiologic responses. Our animalistic stress response system stores tension, raises blood pressure, elevates heart rate and anxiety, and seeks release when confronted with a perceived danger. A modern manifestation of this response occurs in phobic reactions or panic attacks. Stress responses also play a role in cardiovascular illnesses (Blair et al. 1995). Despite development of a large cerebral cortex that acts as an emotional buffer system, human evolution has not kept pace with the lifestyle changes induced by modern industrial society. Increased use of computers is leading a growing segment of the population to become sedentary. Failure to place exercise back into our daily schedules—with a priority as great as eating our daily meals—will surely increase the incidence of stress-related illnesses.

Physical Rehabilitation and Mental Health

A large body of literature documents the broad beneficial effects of physical rehabilitation on psychological well-being. Investigators have also started to assess the psychological benefits of aerobic and resistance exercise for a variety of specific conditions, as is shown in table 18.1.

The Psychological Benefits of Physical Rehabilitation

Encouraging results of physical medicine and rehabilitation studies have led physicians and members of the lay public to conclude that physical exercise can improve one's mental health. Yet we must distinguish improvement in the quality of life of medically ill, mildly depressed individuals from that of chroni-

cally impaired psychiatric inpatients. There are many reasons behind the psychological benefits of physical rehabilitation programs: emotional gains may be due to increased attention and coaching by staff, patient expectancy for improvement, the overcoming of passivity and helplessness during the rehabilitation process (increased self-efficacy and mastery), or some combination of these factors.

The Usefulness of Modern Psychiatric Treatments in Physical Rehabilitation

Patients undergoing physical rehabilitation often experience moderate to severe psychiatric disorders (see table 18.2) that can interfere with the patients' desire and ability to exercise, prompting health care givers to deem them "resistant to physical rehabilitation." In such cases, the caregivers should ask a rehabilitation psychiatrist or psychologist to perform a thorough diagnostic interview and neuropsychiatric workup, and to recommend treatment with psychotherapy and medication as needed (Pet 1996). Judicious use of antidepressants, psychostimulants, pain medications, benzodiazepines, and other agents is often crucial to the recovery process (APA 1993, 1998). Psychotherapy, cognitive behavioral therapy (CBT), and relaxation techniques may significantly improve mood and anxiety disorders stemming from illness or disability (Cassem 1991; Pet 1996; Trexler and Fordyce 1996). These disorders also benefit from a variety of individual and group psychotherapies. It is especially appropriate that patients in a medical setting address issues of loss, isolation, injury to self-concept, and superstitious and fatalistic beliefs about illness (Cassem 1991). Bereavement for permanent loss of function and acceptance of new limitations is important in the long-term adaptation to serious disability (Trexler and Fordyce 1996).

Clinical Studies: The Effects of Exercise on Mental Health

Although the associations between physical activity, exercise, and mental health have been observed for centuries, scientifically proving the direct benefits of exercise on mental health has been difficult. A formidable group of researchers has held the literature to close scientific scrutiny and provided guidance on this subject.

Table 18.1   Recent Survey of Psychological Benefits of Exercise Rehabilitation Programs

Disorder	Author	Variables	Exercise program results
Asthma	Emtner et al. 1996	Anxiety/dyspnea	Improved anxiety and breathlessness
Cardiac	Kugler et al. 1994	Anxiety/depressive scores	Meta-analysis: a positive effect size for 13-15 studies
COPD	Carrieri-Kohlman et al. 1996	Anxiety/dyspnea	Exercise training improved symptoms independent of coaching
Elderly	McMurdo and Burnett 1992	Mood	Aerobics group improved in life satisfaction, perceived health
Elderly	Netz and Jacob 1994	Cognition	Aerobic exercise acutely improved cognition in hospitalized patients
Elderly	Okumiya et al. 1996	Neurobehavior	Aerobics improved behavior in community-dwelling elderly
Fibromyalgia	Wigers et al. 1996	Various symptoms over 4 yrs	Aerobic exercise superior or equal to stress management program
Geriatrics	Blumenthal et al. 1991	Mood/anxiety/quality-of-life measures	Improved with aerobics or yoga
Hemodialysis	Carney et al. 1987	Mood	Improved more with exercise vs. support groups
HIV	LaPerriere et al. 1994	Depression	Group aerobics improved affect and depression scores
Mitral valve prolapse	Scordo 1991	Anxiety	Aerobics decreased anxiety and chest pain frequency
Multiple sclerosis	Petajan 1996	Depression, quality-of-life measures	Aerobics improved significantly vs. controls
Pain	Anshel and Russel 1994	Pain tolerance/mood	Aerobics improved symptoms more than strength training or controls
PMS	Choi and Salmon 1995	Mood	Moderate exercise protected mood from depression
Rheumatoid arthritis	Noreau et al. 1995	Depression/anxiety/fatigue	Modified dance program improved symptoms
Smoking	Marcus et al. 1995	Nicotine dependency	Thrice weekly exercise aided smoking cessation

Discovering the Links Between Physical Fitness and Mental Health

William P. Morgan was one of the first to review the biochemical and clinical evidence linking physical fitness and mental health. Despite methodological limitations, his studies of the severely mentally ill found that psychopathology and physical fitness were inversely correlated: the greater the disorganization and severity of the illness, the less fit the patient. Cognitive and motivational deficits in the severely ill may have accounted for some of these results—depressed

Table 18.2	Rates of Major Depression in Rehabilitation Diagnostic Groups	
Diagnostic group	**Rate of depression (%)**	**Author**
Amputation	35-58	Gerhardt et al. 1984; Rybarczyk et al. 1992; Shukla et al. 1982
Chronic pain	28-87	Large 1986; Lindsay and Wyckoff 1981
Mulitple sclerosis	6-27	Lishman 1987
Oncology	6-25	Holland 1987; Massie and Holland 1990
Rheumatoid arthritis	19-50	Beckham et al. 1992
Spinal cord injury	2-30	Fullerton et al. 1981; MacDonald et al. 1987
Stroke	25-30	Tiller 1992
Traumatic brain injury	25	Federoff et al. 1992

Reprinted, by permission, from D.S. Bishop and L.R. Pet; Physical medicine and rehabilitation, In *Textbook of Consultation-Liaison Psychiatry*, edited by J.R. Rundell and M.G. Wise (Washington, DC: American Psychiatric Press), 1996, 755-80.

patients exhibited consistently low physical working capacity (a measure of fitness). Interestingly, greater initial physical fitness predicted rapid recovery from depression (Morgan 1994). It is difficult to get a physically healthy but severely psychologically depressed/anxious individual to exercise regularly and aerobically. Yet exercise appears to significantly reduce chronic anxiety: Martinson et al. (1989) found reductions in anxiety scores after eight weeks of either aerobics or weight training/relaxation in hospitalized psychiatric patients, and later found that involvement in exercise and sport reduced the likelihood of relapse among nonpsychotic adult psychiatric patients (Martinson 1994).

In a meta-analysis that examined 124 exercise and mental health studies for various interactions, Petruzzello and colleagues (1991) found that aerobic exercise was associated with significant reductions in chronic (trait) anxiety. The effects on acute (state) anxiety were less pronounced—equivalent to the effects of relaxation and meditation. The authors noted that significant changes in trait anxiety occurred chiefly in training programs that exceeded 10 weeks and whose sessions included at least 20 minutes of exercise.

Exercise Benefits in Normal Subjects

While there is evidence that physical activity and good mental health are associated in the general population (Stephens 1988), it has been difficult in clinical trials to demonstrate that exercise significantly affects mood in subjects who were not initially depressed (Lennox et al. 1990; Moses et al. 1989). When Goldwater and Collins (1985) randomly assigned healthy college students to cardiovascular conditioning or to low-intensity exercise five times per week, they noted greater mental health improvements in the aerobic group. Blumenthal et al. (1991) found that both aerobics and yoga led to improvements in depressive scores of normal older adults, as compared to controls. Despite few improvements on standard psychometric scales, subjects often reported that they were less anxious, less depressed, and had more energy; they also expressed greater life satisfaction.

Over the past thirty years, literally thousands of published studies have demonstrated an improvement in depression and anxiety with regular aerobic exercise—yet formal exercise therapy is not incorporated into most modern psychiatric rehabilitation protocols. Scientific scrutiny of the research data typically reveals methodological problems: the setting, dosage, and frequency of exercise have varied among studies; some researchers have incorrectly suggested that temporary improvement of a depressed or anxious affect implies long-term benefits for more severe mental health disorders; researchers often have examined subjects before and after eight or more weeks of treatment, but with no intermittent evaluations; and many studies have lacked adequate control groups; finally, authors frequently have failed to stratify subjects according to severity of illness, in order to discount the healing effects of group settings for exercise, and to exclude spontaneous remissions.

Critically reviewing the literature for scientific validity, Hughes (1984) found that only 12 of 1,100 published articles met scientific criteria for randomization and for placebo controls. Among the most common methodological flaws noted in the literature were small sample size, nonrandomization, inadequate psychological measures, and experimenter and subject biases. The paucity of well-designed research projects perhaps explains why most psychiatric rehabilitation includes no formal exercise therapy.

The Placebo Effect

The equivocally positive results of various exercise and relaxation regimens on chronic mood and anxiety states may in part be artifactual. Mild depression and anxiety can spontaneously subside in twelve weeks with little or no treatment. Depressed and anxious individuals may respond well to any added intervention through the power of belief. This effect is commonly known as the **placebo effect**, or as Benson (1996) has termed it, "remembered wellness."

To test this hypothesis, Desharnais and coworkers (1993) had 48 healthy normal young adults engage in a "health and fitness project" for 10 weeks. Both groups exercised aerobically to similar group regimens. The experimental subjects were told and frequently reminded that the program would help aerobic capacity and psychological well-being, while the control group received no such encouragement. Although both groups physically improved after 10 weeks of training, the "hyped" group had significantly higher self-esteem on psychological scales. Benson (1996) and others have advocated that we harness this power of belief for medical treatments, because of its widespread medical and psychological benefits. Medical science has generally scoffed at this notion. The placebo effect has been viewed as a unfounding factor in ascertaining the efficacy of medical treatments.

Randomized, Controlled Studies of Exercise and Mental Health

The power of belief can confound results of nearly any study of exercise and mood or anxiety—it is quite difficult to design a true placebo control group for exercise studies. Several researchers have published guidelines for increasing the scientific validity of research in this field (McDonald and Hodgdon 1991; Morgan 1994). Petruzello and colleagues (1991) offered several suggestions for further study in their meta-analysis of the literature on exercise and anxiety.

Martinson (1994) and others tried to establish strict scientific criteria to explore the effectiveness of exercise in treating psychiatric disorders. He recently noted several acceptable randomized controlled studies on clinically depressed subjects (see table 18.3). Controlled trials for aerobic exercise studies have included psychotherapy, meditation, and resistance weight training as comparative therapies. Most studies have used exercise as an adjunct to standard psychiatric treatments.

Our best scientific studies reveal that aerobic exercise is as good or better than meditation, psychotherapy, or weight training—and better than no treatment—in reducing depression in psychiatric patients (see table 18.3). However, information on the timing, dosage, setting, and expectancy factors of the subjects has often varied. Many studies have had trainers orient individuals or groups to the regimen. Especially when such trainers are respected clinicians (imparting a belief system and sense of enthusiasm), results of the exercise are confounded with the expectancy effect. Varied individual and group settings add social forces that may be therapeutic in themselves (Yalom 1985). Greist and coworkers (1979) taught exercisers to ignore depressive thoughts and to focus on bodily sensations and rhythms while running. These instructions added a relaxation and meditative component to the program, which was not considered in the analysis. Klein et al. (1985) and McCann and Holmes (1984) found that aerobic exercise was equivalent to or slightly better than muscle relaxation or yoga. Most of the remaining studies found that improvements with aerobic exercise were similar to those from weight training or resistance exercises in the reduction of depression scores.

Despite subtle differences, most studies showed a clear benefit from the use of various exercise programs as adjuncts to mental health care. Sexton et al. (1989) followed outpatient depressive neurotic patients assigned to a walking or jogging program for a year, and found improvements in depression and global symptoms. This effect was independent from aerobic fitness, although anxiety levels were lower in the fit group over time. This is one of the few studies showing that exercise may be an effective long-term treatment for mood and anxiety disorders.

Acute Versus Long-Term Effects

It is unclear whether the mood-altering and anxiety-reducing effects of exercise are due to single sessions, to long-term training effects, or to both. Most intensities of aerobic exercise appear to diminish acute

Table 18.3   Randomized Controlled Studies of Aerobic Exercise as Therapy
                    for Clinical Disorders of Mental Health

Author	(n)	Disorders	Group(s) vs. controls	Exercise regimen	Results
Greist et al. 1979	28	Minor depression	Aerobic vs. psychotherapy	<1 hr 3 ×/wk × 10 wk/ I, C	Both improved
Klein et al. 1985	74	Mixed depression	Aerobic vs. meditation/ relaxation vs. group psychotherapy	<1 hr 2 ×/wk × 12 wk; I, C	Improved equally
McCann and Holmes 1984	41	Major depression	Aerobic vs. meditation/ relaxation vs. controls	1 hr 3 ×/wk × 10 wk; I, G, C	Aerobic > relaxation > controls
Freemont and Craighead 1987	49	Major depression	Aerobic vs. cognitive psychotherapy vs. both	3 ×/wk × 10 wk	Improved equally
Martinson et al. 1985	49	Major depression	Aerobic vs. controls, inpatient psychotherapy	1 hr 3×/wk × 9 wk; I, G, C	Aerobic showed significant improvement vs. controls
Mutrie 1988	24	Major depression	Aerobic vs. weights vs. controls	1 hr 3 ×/wk × 4 wk	Aerobic > weights > controls
Doyne et al. 1987	40	Mixed depression	Aerobic vs. weights vs. controls	<1 hr 3×/wk × 8 wk; I	Aerobic = weights > controls
Sexton et al. 1989	25	Major depression	Aerobic walk vs. aerobic run	30 min 3×/wk × 8+ wk; G, I	Improved equally
Martinson et al. 1985	49	Major depression	Aerobic vs. controls, inpatient psychotherapy	1 hr 3×/wk × 8 wk; G, C	Improved equally
Veale et al. 1992	67	Depression	Aerobic vs. low-intensity exercise	3×/wk × 12 wks; G, C	Improved
Palmer et al. 1995	45	Substance abuse	Aerobics vs. weights, no control	45 min 3×/wk; I, G, C	Weights > aerobic
Broocks et al. 1998	46	Panic disorder	Aerobics vs. medical vs. control	1 hr 3×/wk; I, G, C	Medical ≥ aerobic > control

I = individual sessions; C = coach/trainer present; G = group sessions

or "state" anxiety. Higher intensities sometimes have shown delayed onset of anxiolysis, possibly due to the intensity of the temporary stress response (Raglin and Wilson 1996). However, Tate and Petruzello (1995) have shown "energetic arousal/positive affect" and state anxiety to improve more with higher-intensity ($\geq$70% $\dot{V}O_2$max) than with lower-intensity regimens.

Roth (1989) used a controlled, between-subjects design to document the immediate benefits of exercise on mood and anxiety among college students.

Noting that mental stress and the controlled scientific environment of testing might have interfered with the development of psychological changes, the author and his colleagues recommended that controlled studies use imagery and cognitive enhancements during exercise (Roth et al. 1990). Harte and Eifert (1995) recently documented that exercise setting, attention, and cognitive appraisal alters the emotional experience associated with exercise by altering levels of catecholamine and endocrine release.

After a meta-analysis of the clinical literature, North and associates (1990) concluded that exercise was as effective in decreasing chronic depression as was psychotherapy, and (surprisingly) that anaerobic and aerobic exercise were equally effective. The longer the study and more frequent the sessions, the more powerful the antidepressant effects. Exercise reduced state anxiety (acute anxiety) consistently, with an effect size of 1/4 standard deviation. Chronic exercise appears to reduce chronic anxiety traits by 1/3 standard deviation overall.

Petruzello and colleagues (1991), in their meta-analysis, found widespread support for the anxiolytic effect of acute aerobic exercise despite differing study methodologies. They observed that anxiolytic effects begin almost immediately after an aerobic exercise session and continue for at least two hours. Resistance weight training, in contrast, did not alter acute state anxiety, although it increased body awareness and blood pressure (Koltyn et al. 1995). Meta-analyses of the literature are useful in assessing trends toward significance, but are inherently limited by the methodology of the studies in their review.

Broocks and coworkers (1998) recently found that exercise is quite effective in treating panic disorder. They randomly assigned 42 patients with moderate to severe panic disorder either to 10 weeks of outdoor running (four miles, three times a week), to psychiatric medication (clomipramine), or to a placebo pill. Both exercise and medication led to a significant decrease in symptoms by all main efficacy measures, compared to the placebo. The authors concluded that aerobic exercise alone is associated with significant improvements in panic disorder, although it is less effective than psychiatric medication. Although critics may argue that outdoor running is a cognitive-behavioral approach to desensitize a patient to feared stimuli, this was not the intent of treatment. Studies such as this one will secure a place for exercise as a modern and effective psychiatric treatment for panic disorder.

Conclusions

Randomized and controlled clinical trials show that exercise is a useful and effective adjunct for treating major depressive and anxiety syndromes. To date, no studies have shown consistent advantages of aerobic exercise over other stress reduction therapies—possibly due to variations among individual responsiveness, to the strong placebo effect seen in any intervention with depression or anxiety, or to other unknown factors.

The widespread application of scientific standards of efficacy has shaped psychiatric care into a powerful treatment tool for the 21st century (Hyman 1998).

The scientific comparison of various meditative/stress-reducing and exercise regimens, while using controls with similar settings and expectations of benefit, will best validate future results. Use of standardized psychological diagnostic and measurement scales and the comparison of results to other modern psychiatric treatments will help convince the scientific community of the value of exercise as a treatment option for mild mental illnesses.

Changes in Brain Function Linked to Exercise and Mental Health

Since mood and anxiety disorders are linked to common neurochemical changes in the brain, understanding the neurochemistry of mental disorders will lay the foundation for further research into exercise and mental health. Aerobic exercise in particular may have the potential to create a healing effect on the brain through its action on several important neurotransmitter systems.

Neurobiology of Mood Disorders

In the past 40 years, scientists have gained revolutionary insight into the neurobiology and treatment of mood and anxiety disorders. Combined evidence from animal and human studies has implicated dysregulations of norepinephrine-, serotonin-, and dopamine-related pathways in depressive mood disorders (Hyman and Nestler 1993). Neuroendocrine dysregulations in depressive disorders often involve changes in the hypothalamic-pituitary-adrenal axis or the thyroid. Abnormal sleep cycles, appetitive, libidinal, and psychomotor changes may occur in depression (Kaplan et al. 1994). Anxiety disorders have been linked to norepinephrine, serotonin, and gamma amino butyric acid (GABA) neurotransmitter systems (Kaplan et al. 1994).

Mood disorders appear to involve the limbic system (figure 18.1)—a set of related brain structures involved with motivation, attention, emotion, and memory (Murray 1992). In 1937, Papez proposed that a circuit involving the hypothalamus, the mammilothalamic tract, the anterior thalamic nuclei, the cingulate gyrus, the hippocampus, the fornix, and again the hypothalamus represented the neuroanatomic substrate for emotional experience. The crucial role of the prefrontal cortex and amygdala in

Parietal region

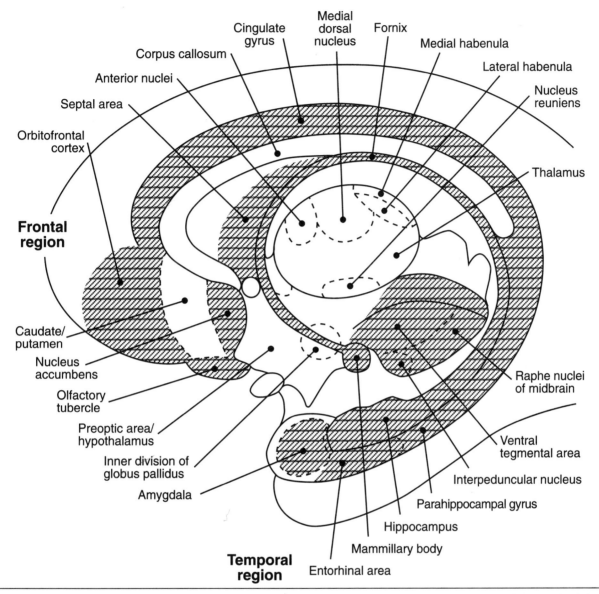

Figure 18.1 Sagittal schematic of the limbic system, showing locations of the major limbic structures and their relations to the thalamus, hypothalamus, and midbrain tegmentum.
Principles of Neuroanatomy by J.B. Angevine Jr. and C.W. Cotman, eds., © 1981 by Oxford University Press, Inc. Reprinted by permission.

modulating emotional experience was later added (Neylan 1995). Studies of various brain injuries and stroke syndromes linked depression with hypoactivity in frontal and parietal lobes of the cerebral cortex (Caplan and Ahmed 1992).

Dopamine: The Link Between Mood and Motor Function

Extensive animal research has revealed some of the pathways linking mood and motor function (Mogenson

et al. 1993). A small dopaminergic structure called the **nucleus accumbens** is thought to be the crossroads for turning motivation into action. Sometimes labeled the "pleasure center," the nucleus accumbens appears to be the locus of addictive behaviors in the brain. In this area, dopamine is often co-localized with brain opiates (Hyman and Nestler 1993).

Dopaminergic changes may play a role in the acute stimulant-like, mood-altering effects of exercise. In humans, psychostimulants such as amphetamines acutely release brain dopamine and norepinephrine to improve alertness and attention, and to elevate

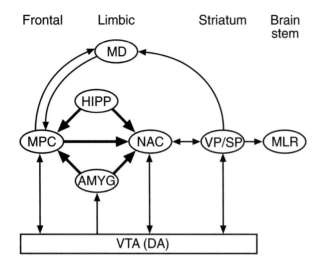

Frontal   Limbic   Striatum   Brain
stem

Figure 18.2 Simplified schematic diagram depicting the major circuity implicate in limbic-motor integration. Reciprocal connections exist in most sites. Dopaminergic neurons in the ventral tegmental area (VTA) modulate several sites and are under feedback control. The nucleus accumbens (NAC) contains endogenous opiate receptors. Abbreviations: MPC = medial prefrontal cortex; AMYG = amygdala; HIPP = hippocampus; NAC= nucleus accumbens; VP/SP = ventral and sub-pallidum (basal ganglia); MLR = mesencephalic locomotor region; MD = mediodorsal thalamic nucleus.
Adapted, with permission, from G.J. Mogenson et al., 1993. In *Limbic motor circuits and neuropsychiatry*, edited by P. Kalivas and C. Barnes (Boca Raton, FL: CRC Press), 193-236.

mood, while causing stereotypic locomotor activation symptoms (Mogenson et al. 1993). Actions designed to affect the meso-cortico-limbic "mood and motivation" tract typically affect the dopaminergic motor tract, and vice versa. Figure 18.2 shows a model of the limbic motor circuits. Deficits in dopaminergic tone have been implicated in depressive disorders, attention deficit disorders, fatigue syndromes, and addictive disorders (Kaplan et al. 1994). Our growing understanding of the intimate neurophysiologic linkage of motor activity and mood in the brain is a cornerstone to our insight into the relationship between physical activity and mental health.

Serotonin: Mood, Anxiety, and Motor Activities

Because of the successes and safety of serotonergic antidepressant agents, the neurotransmitter serotonin has gained much publicity as a modulator of mood. Not all clinicians know that the brain actually uses serotonin as a primary modulator of motor function. In rodent models, treadmill exercise regularly causes acute changes in central serotonergic transmission (Chaouloff 1997).

Jacobs and Fornal (1993) showed that, during tonic repetitive movements in mammals (such as treadmill

exercise), the serotonergic brain nuclei are increasingly activated to fire and to release serotonin. In their model, the forebrain initiates movement, sending signals to serotonergic neurons, to central pattern generators, and to motor neurons. Serotonergic neurons may orchestrate many functions—including modulation of motor activity and inhibition of sensor processing—that increase the animal's focus (Jacobs 1994). These researchers have suggested that the obsessive cleaning and repetitive activities seen in some nervous disorders might be an attempt to rectify acute deficits in brain serotonin. Others have wondered whether regular aerobic exercise may ameliorate depressive and anxiety disorders by preventing catecholamine depletion during stress (Ransford 1982).

Neurobiology of Anxiety Disorders

As with all mental disorders, theories about the causes of anxiety invoke both biological and psychological factors. Cognitive-behavioral therapies and medication have proven quite effective in reducing symptoms of panic and anxiety disorders (APA 1998). Combined evidence from animal and human studies of the neurobiology of anxiety disorders has led to an elegant and complex model involving the stress response system. Researchers have outlined pathways in the brain whereby the cerebral cortex or peripheral senses, upon discerning real or imagined danger, relay a message to the limbic system's amygdala (Goddard and Charney 1997). Chronic repetitive triggering of the fight-or-flight response through psychological anxiety is thought to be a cause of depressive and stress-related illnesses (Gold et al. 1988).

Brain Centers That Affect Anxiety Disorders

Upon receiving sensory information, the amygdala interprets the significance of a threat and sends information to the brain stem to increase arousal and alertness. It may also influence the basal ganglia to tense skeletal muscles and to cause locomotion as part of the fight-or-flight response. This may all occur beneath our conscious awareness. The paraventricular nucleus of the hypothalamus may be stimulated to provide the hormonal aspect of the stress response, simultaneously releasing ACTH and β-endorphins.

The cerebral cortex, which harbors our intellect, has input to this system and can activate or deactivate components through various pathways. For example, dental research has shown that certain words spoken to a patient can elicit a panic-like stress response. Individuals can decrease this anticipatory anxiety through exercise and meditation (Morse

1994). Some researchers suggest that individuals who develop chronic anxiety and panic disorders may have reinforced these fear pathways with overuse. Medication or active behavioral intervention is required to break the trigger points and response cycles (APA 1998).

Norepinephrine: Mood, Anxiety, and Cognitive Activities

The changes in central norepinephrine levels commonly noted in animal studies after aerobic exercise may account for the improved cognitive and motor acuities seen in human exercise research (Dustman et al. 1990). The noradrenergic (norepinephrine) system is involved in the orienting response to danger, and in overall alertness and arousal (Goddard and Charney 1997). For years, psychiatrists have treated depressive disorders, panic disorder, and anxiety with noradrenergic antidepressant agents. In rodent models, experimentally produced, continuously stressed lifestyles create docile animals that mimic human depression in physiology and behavior. This "learned helplessness" or "behavioral despair" results in norepinephrine neurotransmitter depletion in important brain regions. The depressant effect can even be reversed with the administration of noradrenergic antidepressant agents. Dishman (1997) has demonstrated that voluntary aerobic exercise can have antidepressant-like effects in this animal model.

Exercise-Induced Changes in Neurochemistry

Our direct evidence for changes in human brain biochemistry following exercise is limited by current technology. Physiologists have shown that aerobic exercise acutely affects many neurotransmitters—including dopamine, epinephrine, norepinephrine, serotonin, and endogenous opiates—that affect mood. In humans, however, changes in neurotransmitter levels have mostly been noted in the peripheral blood (Dimsdale and Moss 1980; Carr et al. 1981); and these changes—resulting from activation of the adrenal glands and the stress response system—are not necessarily associated with changes in brain chemistry. The blood-brain barrier prevents many blood-borne substances from affecting the brain. Obtaining cerebrospinal fluid samples for study is much more acceptable in animals than in humans.

Nevertheless, one National Institute of Mental Health (NIMH) study of depressed psychiatric inpatients did find evidence that physical activity can acutely alter brain biochemistry. Human participants served as their own controls, undergoing a lumbar puncture before and after a period of planned physical and/or emotional hyperactivity. Levels of serotonin, dopamine, and norepinephrine metabolites were significantly higher in the cerebrospinal fluid following prolonged psychomotor hyperactivity (Post et al. 1973).

Functional brain imaging during exercise may further our understanding of this process. Still in its infancy, this field has begun to document preferential increases in cerebral perfusion during various exercises (Madsen 1993). Electroencephalographic activation of the left frontal area of the brain occurs following acute exercise (Landers and Petruzello 1994). Some researchers have reported increased alpha waves (indicative of relaxation) following exercise, but larger samples are needed to validate these phenomena (Dustman et al. 1990).

While a review of animal research over the past 30 years is well beyond the scope of this chapter, I should note that researchers have demonstrated exercise-induced changes in brain neurotransmitter production and turnover in several animal species (Brown et al. 1979; Jacobs 1994). Recently Dishman's group (1997) has made progress by compensating for the inherent limitations of the rodent models of stress, depression, anxiety, and exercise. These researchers have shown that long-term voluntary exercise in rodents does increase catecholamine production and turnover in the brain stem, hippocampal, and frontal regions, and alters GABA receptor densities linked to anxiety. The effects appear to protect the animals against the catecholamine depletion caused in animal models of stress and depression.

The Stress Response and Endogenous Opiates

The stress response, or fight-or-flight, system is common to all mammals and helps protect the organism in acute danger. In modern humans, however, it is often activated by psychological stressors for which immediate physical activity is not the appropriate solution (Goddard and Charney 1997). An individual's appraisal of and sensitivity to life stressors may influence the onset and course of several mental and physical illnesses through the detrimental effects of accumulated stress responses (Gold et al. 1988; Post 1992).

Moderate aerobic exercise may help discharge the stress response system by simulating the flight response. Exercise-induced discharge of the stress response system is accompanied by a number of physiological changes—including the release of ACTH and cortisol (Luger et al. 1987), and release of endogenous opiates into the peripheral circulation (Carr et al. 1981).

The endogenous opiates of the brain are endorphins, enkephalins, and dynorphins. The β-endorphins are located in the arcuate nucleus of the hypothalamus, in the brain stem, and in the anterior pituitary. Enkephalin and dynorphin receptors are distributed widely throughout the central nervous system.

Beta-endorphins from the pituitary gland are released simultaneously with ACTH during the stress response. These neurochemicals have been touted as major contributors toward the beneficial effects of exercise on mood and anxiety states (Mondin 1996).

A number of studies have confirmed that plasma β-endorphin levels increase during intense aerobic physical activity (Goldfarb and Jamurtas 1997). Required intensity levels are often greater than 60% $\dot{V}O_2$max, and endorphins increase with increasing intensity and duration of exercise. Typically, β-endorphins peak 15 minutes after exercise ends and return to normal within an hour (Hoffmann et al. 1996). This acute biochemical change correlates with the clinical anxiety-reducing effects of exercise said to last one to four hours (Petruzello et al. 1991).

Some researchers have estimated that the level of opioid analgesia after an intense marathon run is the equivalent of up to 10 mg of morphine (Janal et al. 1984). In other circumstances, the amount of pituitary β-endorphin released to the blood may be much less than that required to elicit analgesia by peripheral injection, and may not cross the blood-brain barrier (Snyder 1978). Animal studies have revealed central opioid effects. Rodents given a running wheel and the opportunity to exercise had significantly higher cerebrospinal fluid β-endorphins after five weeks than those without a running wheel (Hoffmann et al. 1996). The effect persisted up to 48 hours after exercise—after which they became hyperaggressive, possibly due to opioid withdrawal. This increase in irritability following abrupt "exercise withdrawal" has been duplicated in human habitual exercisers (Mondin et al. 1996).

Researchers have not yet been able to demonstrate changes in brain enkephalins in response to human treadmill exercise (Farrell et al. 1987). However, in the peripheral nervous system, skeletal muscle ac-tivity may release dynorphin opioids during exercise. Muscle physiology studies have shown that exercise-fatigued muscles release dynorphin opioids to provide local analgesia (Hoffmann et al. 1996). Similar mechanisms may mediate the effects of acupuncture and the calming, pain-relieving effects of exercise.

During the period acutely following aerobic exercise, pain sensitivity decreases, pain thresholds rise, and blood pressure falls (Koltyn et al. 1995). Pretreatment with the partial opiate antagonist naloxone has abolished both postexercise hypogesia and hypotension (Janal 1996; Janal et al. 1984). The immediate calm and anxiolytic effect are not as easily reversible. However, when Daniel et al. (1992) pretreated aerobics class participants with naltrexone or placebo in a double-blind crossover study, they found that the opioid antagonist blocked the positive mood shifts noted following the exercise.

Although dopamine, norepinephrine, and serotonin are also involved in pain pathways, it is unclear what effects exercise-induced changes in these neurotransmitters have on pain perception. Aerobic exercise has been reported to raise pain thresholds (Anshel and Russel 1994). Use of aerobic exercise in pain management programs could potentially reduce the high comorbidity of mood, anxiety, and substance abuse disorders in this population.

Neuromuscular Explanations

Aerobically fit individuals have lower heart rates and higher thresholds to endure stress prior to exhaustion. This "physiologic toughening" or decreased "stress reactivity" may provide a protective effect against psychological reactions to stress (Aldana et al. 1996). However, excessive physical training to exhaustion can actually induce the detrimental effects of a chronically stressed state (Morgan 1994). Exercise-induced body warming is thought to relax skeletal muscle, similar to the effect of heat, massage, or bathing. This relaxed muscular state may trigger a **relaxation response**, similar to the muscular relaxation exercises used in meditative techniques. Thus periods of exertion lead to activation of homeostatic mechanisms that help return the body to physiological set points; relaxation may be the natural consequence (Bahrke and Morgan 1978).

Exercise and Neurochemistry: Conclusions

Current research is rapidly advancing our understanding of the neurochemistry of emotional changes as they are affected by aerobic exercise. However, other stimulatory and inhibitory neurotransmitters abound in the complex biochemical networks of the brain, and our current understanding of their interactions is simplistic at best (Hyman and Nestler 1993). Evidence for the direct acute effect of aerobic exercise on significant brain neurochemicals continues to accumulate. Stimulation of the motor system may affect mood and anxiety through a number of significant neurotransmitter systems in the brain. Discharge of the stress response system through exercise appears to activate endogenous opiate systems as well, imparting pain relief and relaxation effects from aerobic exercise. We need further research to understand how exercise can "discharge" stress, or bodily tension, through its many actions on the mind and body.

The Psychological Effects

While neurochemical explanations for the effects of exercise on the mind and body appear diverse, one needs only to look at the psychological explanations proposed in order to appreciate the scope of this subject. These include theories of exercise-induced self-hypnosis, meditation and relaxation effects, and improved sleep. Cognitive-behavioral and group psychologists have proposed mechanisms of improvement as well.

Self-Hypnosis and the Runner's High

Several investigators have attempted to quantify the experience that long distance runners term the **runner's high**—described as a period of euphoria with a lifting of spirits, increased creativity, increased insight, and a sense of well-being (Callen 1983; Sachs 1984). In Callen's survey, two-thirds of 30-mile runners in a group of 424 admitted to these sensations. Callen wrote, "About half the time the average runner will experience a period of elevated mood, a sense of well-being, and possibly a feeling of lightness during the second half of the run. In addition, he or she will occasionally notice somewhat unusual psychological experiences such as trance-like states, sensations of floating, various visual images, and dissociative periods." In order to achieve these experiences Sachs (1984) states that one needs to let go and have "a quiet mind, total involvement in the movement, letting play be aesthetic, and entering into the experience." Although many have theorized that these experiences result from release of endogenous opiates in the brain, no one has scientifically proven a biochemical mechanism.

Several researchers have theorized that running is a means of inducing self-hypnosis, distraction, and meditation. Eliciting the mind-body relaxation response can lower blood pressure, heart rate, and muscle tension (Benson 1975). One can elicit this response by simple maneuvers: repeating a word, sound, prayer, phrase, or a muscular activity, and passively disregarding everyday thoughts that come to mind, returning to the repetition.

Benson's group studied the use of exercise to elicit the relaxation response while walking, running, and partaking in tai chi classes (Brown 1995). They claimed that these meditative techniques could hasten the onset of the runners' high. Noting that athletes have described similar hypnotic experiences during their peak performances, sports psychologists have used visual imagery, relaxation, and meditation to improve athletic performance (Whelan et al. 1991).

Improved Sleep

Sleep deprivation leads to increased irritability, concentration problems, and cognitive deficits the following day. King et al. (1997) found significant sleep improvement in adults who exercised in a "healthy lifestyle" study. In this randomized, controlled trial, a moderate level of daily aerobics resulted in significant improvement in sleep quality, latency, and duration. Singh and coworkers (1997) found that a supervised nonaerobic weight training program three times per week improved sleep and depression measures by approximately twice that of controls. In polysomnographic sleep studies on 12 aerobically fit men and sedentary controls, Edinger et al. (1993) found that fit subjects had shorter sleep latencies, fewer awakenings, higher sleep efficiency, and more total slow waves than their sedentary counterparts. Daytime exercise was preferred over late evening sessions to avoid sleep fragmentation due to increased body heat and arousal. The potential to improve insomnia without the risks of medication is a significant development, and an important rationale for prescribing exercise as part of a treatment program.

Mastery and Self-Efficacy

In contemporary Western society, the tasks individuals perform have become increasingly cerebral, and stresses are often chronic and inescapable. Psychoanalysts were among the first to recognize our need to safely "work through" the animalistic fears, desires, jealousies, rages, and frustrations that occur in everyday life (Gabbard 1994). Physical activity provides a way to sublimate aggressive urges into a healthy, productive outlet. Performance of exercise routines provides a tangible way to accomplish and master a task with both immediate and long-term benefits. Feelings of "mastery" and "self-efficacy" improve greatly with exercise training, and improve self-esteem and outlook in the process (McAuley et al. 1995). **Self-efficacy** expectations are beliefs in one's capabilities to execute necessary courses of action to satisfy situational demands. These beliefs presumably influence the activities one chooses, the effort one expends, and the degree of persistence against adversity (Bandura 1977). Cognitive theorists have suggested that, in depression, a negative set of thoughts leads to a downward spiral of thought and affect. By changing behavior, exercise may catalyze a transformation of this cognitive set (North et al. 1990). Thus, exercise may allow one to combat feelings of loss and degradation. Aerobic training commonly results in improved body image ("body image cathexis") (Morgan 1994). McAuley and coworkers (1995) recommended that exercise regimens maximize feelings of mastery in order to enhance participation and compliance. Research has identified both intrinsic and extrinsic motivators for exercise participation (Frederick et al. 1996). Individuals who are more intrinsically motivated are more content than those who are concerned with ideal standards and goals.

Group Effects

It is widely known that physical activity improves health (Blair et al. 1995; Shephard 1997). Group exercise adds the many psychological benefits of a group experience, and may enhance compliance and emotional response to exercise. Yalom (1985) has identified several healing factors inherent in all group processes: instillation of hope, universality, imparting of information, altruism, socializing techniques, imitative behavior, catharsis, corrective experience, existential factors, cohesiveness, and interpersonal learning. Varied use of both individual and group settings in exercise research has both enhanced and confounded our understanding. We need more research that is designed to understand and maximize the benefits of these phenomena.

Discussion and Cautionary Notes

Generalizations are nearly impossible in this field of study. Exercise may relieve stress, but perhaps only short-term. The more one exercises, the greater the positive effects on mood, unless one exercises too much—in which case the more one exercises, the more deleterious

the effects. Frequent aerobic exercise may cause substantial positive changes in brain chemistry—yet it can also lead to withdrawal symptoms that are highly negative. We are just beginning to understand a few simple parts of several highly complex phenomena.

Theoretical Challenges

1. While the biochemical hypotheses for the acute effects of exercise are attractive, they do not fully mesh with our current theories of depression and anxiety. In mood and anxiety disorders, chronic changes in brain biochemistry are neither quickly nor permanently altered by the acute administration of catecholamine-enhancing psychostimulant or antidepressant agents. Rather, four or more weeks of treatment are required to create chronic changes in receptor densities in the brain. Evidence from psychostimulant and opiate research suggests that repeated acute effects can bring about chronic changes—but the changes can also lead to increased dependency on these substances (Hyman and Nestler 1993). Therefore, although exercise may cause acute fluctuations in neurotransmitters in certain brain regions, it may not follow that it is an adequate long-term antidepressant. Psychiatric medications, on the other hand, have undergone rigorous comparison and placebo studies to prove effectiveness. They offer fast, effective, reliable results and require little effort by participants. Rehabilitation medicine specialists recognize the difficulties in motivating the depressed or anxious patient to exercise effectively. We need long-term follow-up studies of the effects of daily exercise on mood and anxiety before we can justify its use as a sole therapeutic agent.

2. Common experience suggests that, despite any acute effects of exercise on brain chemistry, our ability to experience emotional changes during exercise depends on many factors. Compare the exhilaration of scoring a goal in a game of soccer with the feelings generated by running for a train. The exercise value may be equivalent in both activities, but the emotional value and euphoria differ dramatically. Despite advances in neuropsychiatry, the gateway between mood and motor function remains poorly understood. Humans have some intellectual control over their primitive impulses, and processing the meaning of events is a complex operation. We are beginning to see that the setting of physical activity has much to do with the onset of beneficial emotional effects (Harte and Eifert 1995; Stephens 1988). Further research is needed in this area.

3. Discharge of the stress response system through exercise may acutely reduce stress, but it provides only

symptomatic relief. In order to reduce their general tendency to react to stress with increased tension and anxiety, individuals must alter their cognitive and affective appraisal of stressors—possibly through counseling that encourages emotional growth and maturity. Exercise is best utilized as an adjunct to such treatments.

Individual Effects May Vary

Individuals respond differently to various psychiatric therapies and medications. Differences in temperament may be one cause of varying responsiveness to treatment.

Recent studies note varying HPA stress responsiveness in different subgroups of men (Petrides et al. 1997). The reasons for these differences are not wholly understood, but Cloninger (1987) has outlined a theoretical framework of personality types based on differences in the predominance of the various neurotransmitter systems. Individual families and cultures place differing values on physical activity, ranging from encouraging it to negating its importance. Such factors may influence individual motivation, self-esteem, and clinical outcome. Some individuals may become more fatigued or disinhibited after exercise. Aerobic exercise has occasionally been shown to trigger panic attacks, migraine headaches, asthma, and other conditions in some susceptible individuals. Although some panic disorder sufferers may become more anxious following acute exercise, those who become accustomed to the physiological changes of exercise may improve their symptoms (Broocks et al. 1998; Rief and Hermanutz 1996). Bipolar manic patients and anorexics should avoid excessive activity without close supervision from their physicians. Meditation and massage may also alter physiologic tone and reduce stress and anxiety, with results equivalent to those of most exercise studies (Bahrke and Morgan 1978). A number of relaxation techniques and psychotherapies are effective in stress reduction (Cotton 1990). Stressed individuals should be encouraged to explore options and seek resolution of their conflicts through various support systems and mechanisms (Cotton 1990). As with any treatment, some individuals may use exercise excessively and for detrimental purposes.

Exercise Addiction, Overtraining, and Anorexia

Several investigators have linked personality characteristics with those who exercise excessively (Yates et al. 1983). **Exercise dependence syndrome** is a disorder in which an athlete is unwilling to alter or discontinue training regimens despite medical contraindications. Psychological studies have found significantly higher exercise dependence in both marathoners and ultra-marathoners than in less frequent runners (Pierce 1994).

Several investigators have documented an **exercise withdrawal syndrome** in habitual daily exercisers. Three days of voluntary abstention from exercise often results in increased total mood disturbance, state anxiety, tension, depression, confusion, and vigor 24-48 hours later (Mondin et al. 1996). This may be due to a biochemical withdrawal syndrome, possibly related to declines in endogenous opioids.

Excessive exercise may be strongly related to preoccupation with weight. Male exercisers may have more obsessive-compulsive traits (Davis et al. 1993). A controlled study of psychiatrically hospitalized eating disorder patients showed that 78% engaged in excessive exercise. At least 60% were competitive athletes prior to their eating disorders, and sport or exercise predated their dieting. Davis and colleagues (1993) concluded that sport and exercise are an integral part of the pathogenesis and disease progression for a number of anorexic patients.

Overtraining occurs when healthy, nondepressed individuals exhibit signs of depression as a result of excessively high training loads. Mood disturbance increases in a dose-dependent manner with overtrained swimmers (Morgan 1994). This syndrome, often referred to as **staleness**, is characterized by decreased performance, inability to train at usual levels, chronic fatigue, muscle soreness, hypertension, and a sense of increased effort. Vegetative signs of this pseudo-depression include hypercortisolism, hormonal and hypothalamic dysregulation, insomnia, loss of appetite, and/or disturbed mood. It is believed that overtraining, far from being a method of stress reduction, rather creates a state of chronic stress. Prevention and management of overtraining syndromes has become a major field in sport psychology.

Guidelines

The following are suggestions for the safe and effective use of exercise as an adjunct to the treatment of psychological disorders.

1987 NIMH Findings

The conclusions of a 1987 NIMH consensus panel (Morgan and Goldston 1987) still hold true today:

1. Physical fitness is positively associated with mental health and well being.
2. Exercise is associated with the reduction of stress emotions.
3. Anxiety and depression are common symptoms of failure to cope with mental stress, and exercise has been associated with a decreased level of mild to moderate depression and anxiety.
4. Severe depression usually requires professional treatment, which may include medication, electroshock treatment, or psychotherapy, with exercise as an adjunct.
5. Physically healthy people who require psychotropic medication may safely exercise when exercise and medication are titrated under close medical supervision.

Use Exercise as an Adjunct to Modern Treatments

Evidence strongly predicts favorable results when exercise is combined with modern mental health treatments. The ideal frequencies and intensities of exercise remain unclear—most exercise and mental health studies have found that aerobic conditioning occurs only with regimens of 20 minutes or more, three times per week, at greater than 60% $\dot{V}O_2$max (Martinson 1994). The risks of excessive aerobic exercise include stress injuries and cardiovascular disorders. A full medical workup and cardiology examination should be precede any treatment regimen. Certain drugs (including tricyclic compounds) may raise or lower blood pressure, alter cardiac conduction times, lower seizure thresholds, show altered metabolism, or cause sedation or diplopia. Although many patients taking various psychiatric medications have safely engaged in exercise programs (Martinson 1994), few researchers have studied exercise as a combined pharmacologic augmentation strategy. Proper warm-up and cooldown periods and a moderation of activity level have always been the guidelines for safety.

The acute anxiolytic effects following aerobic exercise last one to four hours (Petruzello et al. 1991). A program that aspires to use exercise as a mood-enhancing, anxiolytic intervention might consider frequent performance of the treatment regimen. The use of several brief (20-minute) sessions of moderate aerobic exercise per day has not been well investigated. We need research on the benefits of frequent daily exercise.

Greist et al. (1979) found that exercise frequency should be at least three to five times per week. Unlike when they are training for aerobic conditioning, individuals exercising for psychological benefits should run comfortably and slow to a walk when appropriate. Fitness walking can decrease acute anxiety and affect mood (Rippe et al. 1988). Using a coach or "running therapist" may help motivate reluctant exercisers. The secret to success, according to Greist, is to "try to run each day in such a way that you would want to run again" (Greist et al. 1979).

Enhance Exercise With Inspiring Contexts

Reduced motor activity and motivation are the hallmarks of several mood and anxiety syndromes. Affected individuals may require psychotropic medication to achieve enough motivation to participate in exercise regimens. Setting *achievable* short-term goals during training is important to develop the mastery and self-efficacy that improve mental health.

Mental imagery strategies may enhance motivation and harness acute biochemical and psychological changes. Several authors have published reviews of the expanding literature documenting the effects of psychogenic factors on running efficiency and mood state (Crews 1992; Morgan 1985). Runners most likely to experience calm and the runner's high have been able to induce a tranquil meditative state during exercise (Callen 1983).

Evidence is growing for the effectiveness of combining exercise and meditation. Several authors have shown that various forms of mind-enhanced exercise affect mood elevation and anxiolysis, including meditation and tai chi (Brown et al. 1995; Jin 1992), yoga (Berger and Owen 1992), and various dance classes (Noreau 1995). These activities combine exercise with spirituality, meditation, music, coaching, and group social activity. Individuals who can become emotionally connected with their exercise routines will gain the greatest emotional benefit from them.

We very much need research trials that use exercise as an adjunct to psychiatric medical therapies (Moore and Blumenthal 1998). Individuals may benefit from exercise as a psychotherapeutic interlude. We need researchers to develop cognitive strategies that will enhance the meditative-relaxation effects of exercise. Once aware of the sources of stress, patients may begin to join therapists in formulating appropriate solutions to complex problems.

Aerobic exercise, resistance weight training, and meditation may simultaneously treat different symptoms. Randomized controlled research exploring the adjunctive treatment of mood and anxiety disorders with various combinations of exercise and meditation may help identify the specific anxiety and affective states best responsive to each type of regimen.

Summary

Epidemiological studies confirm that moderately physically active people are less likely to succumb to mental disorders than sedentary individuals. Physical medicine and rehabilitation programs are effective in improving the mental health of many of their participants. Individuals resistant to rehabilitation are often helped by modern psychiatric therapies and medication.

Scientific research provides encouraging support for the theory that aerobic exercise affects the major neurotransmitters involved in mood and anxiety. It may act as a mild psychostimulant, antidepressant, or opiate in humans. There is a gating mechanism between mood, anxiety, and motor function, which includes structures within the limbic system. The human stress response system may require regular exercise or relaxation techniques to return it to baseline. Repetitive perceived stressors exacerbate chronic ailments of modern society, and play a role in the course of mental health disorders. Individuals may alter their perception of stressors through various psychotherapies and personal growth experiences.

Clinical evidence suggests that moderate aerobic exercise at least three times per week for twenty minutes or more can provide an effective adjunct to treatments of mood and anxiety disorders. Psychological and physical barriers towards exercise need to be conquered for it to become useful for the majority of psychiatric clients. As Morgan (1994) has noted, while there is compelling evidence to support an *association* between exercise and mental health, there is as yet an absence of *causal evidence*. Physical conditioning may not be necessary to achieve mental health benefits from exercise. Nonaerobic weight training and relaxation exercises have also shown the potential to improve mental health, although they may act by different mechanisms. In most studies, the acute and chronic benefits of exercise regimens are readily observed among the initially depressed or anxious subjects.

Further research is needed to determine the optimal type, dosage, and setting of exercise in the adjunctive treatment of various psychological illnesses. Careful study designs must stratify subjects based on level of illness, and must control for the strong placebo effects of exercise.

Several positive psychological factors influence the antidepressant and anxiolytic effects of exercise. These include mastery, self-efficacy, sublimation, cognitive-behavioral change, group effects, self-hypnosis, physical relaxation, and improved sleep quality. Ideally, exercise should be part of a comprehensive stress management program that includes relaxation techniques, healthy diet and lifestyle changes, and the use of proven psychiatric treatments. Psychiatric medication and psychotherapy help offset the substantial tendency toward inactivity found in many mental illnesses. The context in which exercise occurs is a significant yet often neglected variable in the manifestation of psychological change. Research in exercise and mental health should explore various cognitive enhancements to exercise programs in order to attempt to generate more robust psychological benefits. Structured motivational programs may be required for enhanced participation.

The relationship between movement and mood has been noted for centuries. By combining neuropsychiatric, psychological, and physical rehabilitation research efforts, we may better understand and utilize those connections for the benefit of all.

Acknowledgments

This chapter benefited from editing by Walter Frontera MD, PhD, and Theodore A. Stern, MD. Research began at the Massachusetts General Hospital and Boston Medical Center Psychiatric training programs. Thanks to Edwin H. Cassem, MD, George B. Murray, MD, Clifford Askinazi, MD, and Ronald Calvanio, PhD, for their insights. A special thanks to my wife, Elizabeth Peters Kaiser, MD, for her support.

References

Aldana, S.G., L.D. Sutton, B.H. Jacobson, and M.G. Quirk. 1996. Relationships between physical activity and perceived stress. *Percept Mot Skills* 82:315-21.

American Psychiatric Association. 1993. Practice guideline for major depressive disorder in adults. *Am J Psychiatry* 150(Suppl.):1-26.

American Psychiatric Association. 1994. *Diagnostic and statistical manual of mental disorders.* 4th ed. Washington, DC: American Psychiatric Press.

American Psychiatric Association. 1998. Practice guideline for the treatment of patients with panic disorder. *Am J Psychiatry* 155(Suppl.):1-34.

Angevine, J.B. Jr., and C.W. Cotman, eds. 1981. *Principles of neuroanatomy*, 253-83. New York: Oxford University Press.

Anshel, M.H., and K.G. Russel. 1994. Effect of aerobic and strength training on pain tolerance, pain appraisal, and mood of unfit males as a function of pain location. *J Sport Sci* 12:535-47.

Bahrke, M.S., and W.P. Morgan. 1978. Anxiety reduction following exercise and meditation. *Cognitive Therapy and Research* 2:323-33.

Bandura, A. 1977. Self-efficacy theory: toward a unifying theory of behavioral change. *Psychol Review* 84:191-215.

Beckham J.C., C.J. D'Amico, J.R. Rice, J.S. Jordan, G.W. Divine, and W.B. Brook. 1992. Depression and level of functioning in patients with rheumatoid arthritis. *Can J Psychiatry* 37:538-43.

Benson, H. 1975. *The relaxation response*. New York: William Morrow.

Benson, H. 1996. *Timeless healing: The power and biology of belief*. New York: Simon & Schuster.

Berger, B.G., and D.R. Owen. 1992. Mood alteration with yoga and swimming: aerobic exercise may not be necessary. *Percept Mot Skills* 75(3 pt. 2):1331-43.

Blair, S.N., H.W. Kohl, C.E. Barlow, R.S. Paffenbarger, L.W. Gibbons, and C.A. Macera. 1995. Changes in physical fitness and all-cause mortality. *JAMA* 273:1093-98.

Blumenthal, J.A., C.F. Emery, D.J. Madden, S. Schniebolk, M. Walsh-Riddle, L.K. George, D.C. McKee, M.B. Higginbotham, F.R. Cobb, and R.E. Coleman. 1991. Long-term effects of exercise on psychological functioning in older men and women. *J Gerontol* 46:352-61.

Broocks, A., B. Bandelow, G. Pekrun, A. George, T. Meyer, U. Bartmann, U. Hillmer-Vogel, and E. Ruther. 1998. Comparison of exercise, clomipramine, and placebo in the treatment of panic disorder. *Am J Psychiatry* 155:603-09.

Brown, B.S., T. Payne, C. Kim, G. Moore, P. Krebs, and W. Martin. 1979. Chronic response of rat brain norepinephrine and serotonin levels to endurance training. *J Appl Physiol* 46:19-23.

Brown, D.R., Y. Wang, A. Ward, C.B. Ebbeling, L. Fortlage, E. Puleo, H. Benson, and J.M. Rippe. 1995. Chronic psychological effects of exercise and exercise plus cognitive strategies. *Med Sci Sports Exerc* 27:765-75.

Callen, K.E. 1983. Mental and emotional aspects of long-distance running. *Psychosomatics* 24:133-51.

Caplan, L.R., and I. Ahmed. 1992. Depression and neurological disease: their distinction and association. *Gen Hosp Psychiatry* 14:177.

Carney, R.M., B. Templeton, B.A. Hong, H.R. Harter, J.M. Hagberg, K.B. Schechtman, and A.P. Goldberg. 1987. Exercise training reduces depression and increases the performance of pleasant activities in hemodialysis patients. *Nephron* 47:194-98.

Carr, D.B., B.A. Bullen, G.S. Skrinar, M.A. Arnold, M. Rosenblatt, I.Z. Beitins, J.B. Martin, and J.W. McArthur. 1981. Physical conditioning facilitates the exercise induced secretion of beta endorphin and beta lipotropin in women. *N Engl J Med* 305:560.

Carrieri-Kohlman, V., J.M. Gormley, M.K. Douglas, S.M. Paul, and M.S. Stulbarg. 1996. Exercise training reduces dyspnea and the anxiety associated with it. Monitoring alone may be as effective as coaching. *Chest* 110:1526-35.

Cassem, N.H. 1991. Depression. In *Massachusetts General Hospital handbook of general hospital psychiatry*. 3d ed., ed. N.H. Cassem, 237-68. St. Louis: Mosby Year Book.

Chaouloff, F. 1997. Effects of acute physical exercise on central serotonergic systems. *Med Sci Sports Exerc* 29:58-62.

Choi, P.Y., and P. Salmon. 1995. Symptom changes across the menstrual cycle in competitive sportswomen, exercisers, and sedentary women. *Br J Clin Psychol* 34:447-60.

Cloninger, C.R. 1987. A systematic method for clinical description and classification of personality variants. *Arch Gen Psychiatry* 44:573-88.

Cotton, D.H.G. 1990. *Stress management: An integrated approach to therapy*. New York: Brunner/Mazel.

Crews, D.J. 1992. Psychological state and running economy. *Med Sci Sports Exerc* 24:475-82.

Daniel, M., A.D. Martin, and J. Carter. 1992. Opiate receptor blockade by naltrexone and mood state after acute physical activity. *Br J Sports Med* 26:111-15.

Davis, C., S.H. Kennedy, E. Ravelski, and M. Dionne. 1993. The role of physical activity in the development and maintenance of eating disorders. *Psychol Med* 24:957-67.

DeGeus, E.J., L.J. Van Doornen, and J.F. Orlebeke. 1993. Regular exercise and aerobic fitness in relation to psychological make-up and physiological stress-reactivity. *Psychosom Med* 55:347-63.

Desharnais, R., J. Jobin, C. Cote, L. Levesque, and G. Godin. 1993. Aerobic exercise and the placebo effect: a controlled study. *Psychosom Med* 55:149-54.

Dimsdale, J., and J. Moss 1980. Plasma catecholamines in stress and exercise. *JAMA* 243:340-42.

Dishman, R.K. 1997. Brain monoamines, exercise, and behavioral stress: animal models. *Med Sci Sports Exerc* 29:63-74.

Doyne, E.J., D.J Ossip-Klein, E.D. Bowman, K.M. Osborn, I.B. McDougall-Wilson, and R.A. Neimeyer. 1987. Running versus weight lifting in the treatment of depression. *J Consult Clin Psychol* 55:748-54.

Dustman, R.E., R.Y. Emmerson, R.O. Ruhling, D.E. Shearer, L.A. Steinhaus, S.C. Johnson, H.W. Bonekat, and J.W. Shigeoka. 1990. Age and fitness effects on EEG, ERPs, visual sensitivity and cognition. *Neurobiol Aging* 11:193-200.

Edinger, J.D., M.C. Morey, R.J. Sullivan, M.B. Higginbotham, G.R. Marsh, D.S. Dailey, and W.V. McCall. 1993. Aerobic fitness, acute exercise and sleep in older men. *Sleep* 16:351-59.

Eaton, S.B., M. Shostak, and M. Connor. 1988. *The paleolithic prescription*. New York: Harper & Row.

Elkin, I., T. Shea, J. Watkins, S.D. Imbert, S.M. Sotsky, J.F. Collins, D.R. Glass, P.A. Pilkonis, W.R. Leber, and J.P. Docherty. 1989. NIMH treatment of depression collaborative research program: general effectiveness of treatments. *Arch Gen Psychiatry* 46:971-82.

Emtner, M., M. Herala, and G. Stalenheim. 1996. High intensity physical training in adults with asthma. A 10 week rehabilitation program. *Chest* 109:323-30.

Etnier, J.L., and D.M. Landers. 1995. Brain function and exercise: current perspectives. *Sports Med* 19:81-85.

Farrell, P.A., A.B. Gustafson, W.P. Morgan, and C.B. Pert. 1987. Enkephalins, catecholamines, and psychological mood alterations: effects of prolonged exercise. *Med Sci Sports Exerc* 19:347-53.

Federoff, J.P., S.E. Starkstein, and A.W. Forrester. 1992. Depression in patients with acute traumatic brain injury. *Am J Psychiatry* 149:918-23.

Frederick, C.M., C. Morrison, and T. Manning. 1996. Motivation to participate, exercise affect, and outcome behaviors toward physical activity. *Percept Mot Skills* 82:691-701.

Freemont J., and L.W. Craighead. 1987. Aerobic exercise and cognitive therapy in the treatment of dysphoric moods. *Cognitive Therapy and Research* 2:241-251.

Fullerton, D.T., R.F. Harvey, M.H. Klein, and T. Howell. 1981. Psychiatric disorders in patients with spinal cord injuries. *Arch Gen Psychiatry* 38:1369-71.

Gabbard, G.O. 1994. *Psychodynamic psychiatry in clinical practice: The DSM IV edition*. Washington, DC: American Psychiatric Press.

Gerhardt, F., I. Florin, and T. Knapp. 1984. The impact of medical, reeducational, and psychological variables on rehabilitation outcome in amputees. *Int J Rehabil Res* 7:379-88.

Goddard, A.W., and D.S. Charney. 1997. Toward an integrated neurobiology of panic disorder. *J Clin Psychiatry* 58(Suppl. 2):4-11.

Gold, P.W., F.K. Goodwin, and G.P. Chrousos. 1988. Clinical and biochemical manifestations of depression: relation to the neurobiology of stress, part II. *N Engl J Med* 319:413-20.

Goldfarb, A.H., and A.Z. Jamurtas. 1997. β-Endorphin response to exercise: an update. *Sports Med* 24:8-16.

Goldwater, B.C., and M.L. Collins. 1985. Psychologic effects of cardiovascular conditioning: a controlled experiment. *Psychosom Med* 47:174-81.

Greist, J.R., M.H. Klein, R.R. Eischens, J. Faris, A.S. Gurman, and W.P. Morgan. 1979. Running as treatment for depression. *Compr Psychiatry* 20:41-54.

Gurevich, M., P.M. Kohn, and C. Davis. 1994. Exercise induced analgesia and the role of reactivity in pain sensitivity. *J Sports Sci* 12:549-59.

Harte, J.L., and G.H. Eifert. 1995. The effects of running, environment, and attentional focus on athletes' catecholamine and cortisol levels and mood. *Psychophysiology* 32:49-54.

Hoffmann, P., I.H. Jonsdottir, and P. Thoren. 1996. Activation of different opioid systems by muscle activity and exercise. *News Physiological Sciences* 11:223-28.

Holland, J.C. 1987. Managing depression in the patient with cancer. *CA Cancer J Clin* 37:366-71.

Hughes, J.R. 1984. Psychological effects of habitual aerobic exercise: a critical review. *Prev Med* 13:66-78.

Hyman, S.E. 1998. The now and future of NIMH. *Am J Psychiatry* 155(Suppl.):36-40.

Hyman, S.E., and E.J. Nestler. 1993. *The molecular foundations of psychiatry*. Washington, DC: American Psychiatric Press.

Jacobs, B.L. 1994. Serotonin, motor activity, and depression related disorders. *American Scientist* 82:456-63.

Jacobs, B.L., and C.A. Fornal. 1993. 5-HT and motor control: a hypothesis. *Trends Neurosci* 16:346-52.

Janal, M.N. 1996. Pain sensitivity, exercise and stoicism. *J R Soc Med* 89:376-81.

Janal, M.N., E.W.D. Colt, W.C. Clark, and M. Glusman. 1984. Pain sensitivity, mood and plasma endocrine levels in man following long-distance running: effects of naloxone. *Pain* 19:13-25.

Jin, P. 1992. The efficacy of Tai Chi, brisk walking, meditation, and reading in reducing mental and emotional stress. *J Psychosom Res* 36:361-70.

Judd, L.L. 1998. Historical highlights of the NIMH from 1946 to the present. *Am J Psychiatry* 155(Suppl.):3-7.

Kaplan, H.I., B.J. Sadock, and J.A. Grebb, eds. 1994. *Kaplan and Sadock's synopsis of psychiatry: Behavioral sciences, clinical psychiatry*. 7th ed. Baltimore: Williams & Wilkins.

Keller, M.B., P.W. Cavori, T.I. Mueller, W. Coryell, R.M. Hirschfeld, and T. Shea. 1992. Time to recovery, chronicity, and levels of psychopathology in major depression. *Arch Gen Psychiatry* 49:809.

King, A.C., R.F. Oman, G.S. Brassington, D.L. Bliwise, and W.L. Haskell. 1997. Moderate intensity exercise and self-rated quality of sleep in older adults: a randomized controlled trial. *JAMA* 277:32-37.

King, A.C., C.B. Taylor, and W.L. Haskell. 1993. Effects of differing intensities and formats of 12 months of exercise training on psychological outcomes in older adults. *Health Psychol* 12:292-300.

Klein, M.H., J.H. Greist, A.S. Gurman et al. 1985. A comparative outcome study of group psychotherapy vs. exercise treatments for depression. *International Journal of Mental Health* 13:148-77.

Koltyn, K.F., J.S. Raglin, P.J. O'Connor, and W.P. Morgan. 1995. Influence of weight training on state anxiety, body awareness, and blood pressure. *Int J Sports Med* 16:266-69.

Kugler, J., H. Seelbach, and G.M. Kruskemper. 1994. Effects of rehabilitation exercise programmes on anxiety and depression in coronary patients: a meta-analysis. *Br J Clin Psychol* 33:401-10.

Landers, D.M., and S.J. Petruzello. 1994. Physical activity, fitness, and anxiety. In *Physical activity, fitness and health*, ed. C. Bouchard, R.J. Shephard, and T. Stephens, 868-79. Champaign, IL: Human Kinetics.

LaPerriere, A, G. Ironson, M.H. Antoni, N. Schneiderman, N. Klimas, and M.A. Fletcher. 1994. Exercise and psychoneuroimmunology. *Med Sci Sports Exerc* 26:182-90.

Large, R.G. 1986. DSM III diagnoses in chronic pain: confusion or clarity? *J Nerv Ment Dis* 174:295-303.

Lennox, S.S., J.R. Bedell, and A.A. Stone. 1990. The effect of exercise on normal mood. *J Psychosom Res* 34:629-36.

Lindsay, P.G., and M. Wyckoff. 1981. The depression-pain syndrome and its response to antidepressants. *Psychosomatics* 22:571-77.

Lishman, W.A. 1987. Other disorders affecting the central nervous system. In *Organic psychiatry: The psychological consequences of cerebral disorder.* 2d ed., 588-650. Boston: Blackwell Scientific.

Luger, A., P.A. Deuster, S.B. Kyle, W.T. Gallucci, L.C. Montgomery, P.W. Gold, D.L. Loriaux, and G.P. Chrousos. 1987. Acute hypothalamic-pituitary-adrenal responses to the stress of treadmill exercise. *N Engl J Med* 316:1309-15.

MacDonald, M.R., W.R. Nielson, and M.G.P. Cameron. 1987. Depression and activity patterns of spinal cord injured persons living in the community. *Arch Phys Med Rehabil* 68:339-43.

Madsen, P.L. 1993. Blood flow and oxygen uptake in the human brain during various states of sleep and wakefulness. *Acta Neurol Scand* 88(Suppl. 148):5-25.

Marcus, B.H., A.E. Albrecht, R.S. Niaura, E.R. Taylor, L.R. Simkin, S.I. Feder, D.B. Abrams, and P.D. Thompson. 1995. Exercise enhances the maintenance of smoking cessation in women. *Addict Behav* 20:87-92.

Martinson, E.W. 1994. Physical activity and depression: clinical experience. *Acta Psychiatr Scand Suppl* 377:23-27.

Martinson, E.W., A. Hoffart, and O. Solberg. 1989. Comparing aerobic and non-aerobic forms of exercise in the treatment of clinical depression: a randomized trial. *Compr Psychiatry* 30:324-31.

Martinson, E.W., A. Medhus, and L. Sandvik. 1985. Effects of aerobic exercise on depression: a controlled study. *Br Med J* 291:109.

Massie, M., and J. Holland. 1990. Depression and the cancer patient. *J Clin Psychiatry* 51(Suppl. 7):12-17.

McAuley, E.S., M. Bane, and S.L. Mihalko. 1995. Exercise in middle aged adults: self efficacy and self presentational outcomes. *Prev Med* 24:319-28.

McCann, L., and D.S. Holmes. 1984. Influence of aerobic exercise on depression. *J Pers Soc Psychol* 46:1142-47.

McDonald, D.G., and J.A. Hodgdon. 1991. *The psychological effects of aerobic fitness training: Research and theory.* New York: Springer-Verlag.

McMurdo, M.E., and L. Burnett. 1992. Randomized controlled trial of exercise in the elderly. *Gerontology* 38:292-98.

Milani, R.V., C.J. Lavie, and M.M. Cassidy. 1996. Effects of cardiac rehabilitation and exercise training programs on depression in patients after major coronary events. *Am Heart J* 132:726-732.

Mogenson, G.J., S.M. Brudzynski, M. Wu et al. 1993. From motivation to action: a review of dopaminergic regulation of limbic, nucleus accumbens, ventral pallidum, pedunculopontine nucleus circuitries involved in limbic-motor integration. In *Limbic motor circuits and neuropsychiatry*, ed. P. Kalivas and C. Barnes, 193-236. Boca Raton, FL: CRC Press.

Mogenson, G.J., D.L. Jones, and C.Y. Yim. 1980. From motivation to action: functional interface between the limbic system and the motor system. *Prog Neurobiol* 14:69-97.

Mondin, G.W., W.P. Morgan, P.N. Piering, A.J. Stegner, C.L. Stotesbery, M.R. Trine, and M.Y. Wu. 1996. Psychological consequences of exercise deprivation in habitual exercisers. *Med Sci Sports Exerc* 28:1199-1203.

Moore, K.A., and J.A. Blumenthal. 1998. Exercise training as an alternative treatment for depression among older adults. *Alternative Therapies in Health and Medicine* 4:48-56.

Morgan, W.P. 1985. Psychogenic factors and exercise metabolism: a review. *Med Sci Sports Exerc* 17:309-16.

Morgan, W.P. 1994. Physical activity, fitness and depression. In *Physical activity, fitness, and health*, ed. C. Bouchard, R.J. Shephard, and T. Stephens, 851-67. Champaign IL: Human Kinetics.

Morgan, W.P. and S.E. Goldston, eds. 1987. *Exercise and mental health.* Washington, DC: Hemisphere.

Morse, D.R. 1994. Relaxed exercise. *Int J Psychosom* 41:17-22.

Moses, J., A. Steptoe, A. Mathews, and S. Edwards. 1989. The effects of exercise training on mental well being in the normal population: a controlled trial. *J Psychosom Res* 33:47-61.

Murray, G.B. 1992. Limbic music. *Psychosomatics* 33:16-23.

Mutrie, N. 1988. Exercise as a treatment for moderate depression in the UK health service. Presented at the Sport, Health Psychology and Exercise Symposium, Buckinghamshire, UK.

Neylan, T.C. 1995. Classic articles in neuropsychiatry: introduction to the series. *J Neuropsychiatry* 7:102-03.

Netz, Y., and T. Jacob. 1994. Exercise and the psychological state of institutionalized elderly: a review. *Percept Mot Skills* 79:1107-18.

Noreau, L., H. Martineau, L. Roy, and M. Belzile. 1995. Effects of a modified dance based exercise on cardiorespiratory fitness, psychological state, and health status of persons with rheumatoid arthritis. *Am J Phys Med Rehabil* 74:19-27.

North, T.C., P. McCullagh, and Z.V. Tran. 1990. Effect of exercise on depression. *Exerc Sport Sci Rev* 18:379-415.

Okumiya, K., K. Matsubayashi, T. Wada, S. Kimura, Y. Doi, and T. Ozawa. 1996. Effects of exercise on neurobehavioral function in community dwelling older people more than 75 years of age. *J Am Geriatr Soc* 44:569-72.

Paffenbarger, R.S. Jr., I.M. Lee, and R. Leung. 1994. Physical activity and personal characteristics associated with depression and suicide in American college men. *Acta Psychiatr Scand* (Suppl. 377):16-22.

Palmer, J.A., L.K. Palmer, K. Michels, and B. Thigpen. 1995. Effects of type of exercise on depression in recovering substance abusers. *Percept Mot Skills* 80:523-30.

Papez, J.W. 1937. A proposed mechanism of emotion. Reprinted in: *Journal of Neuropsychiatry*, 1995, 1:104-12.

Pet, L.R. 1996. Physical medicine and rehabilitation. In *Textbook of consultation-liaison psychiatry*, ed. J.R. Rundell and M.G. Wise, 755-80. Washington, DC: American Psychiatric Press.

Petajan, J.H. 1996. Impact of aerobic training on fitness and quality of life in multiple sclerosis. *Ann Neurol* 39:432-41.

Petrides, J.S., P.W. Gold, G.P. Mueller, A. Singh, C. Stratakis, G.P. Chrousos, and P.A. Deuster. 1997. Marked differences in functioning of the hypothalamic pituitary adrenal axis between groups of men. *J Appl Physiol* 82:1979-88.

Petruzzello, S.J., D.M. Landers, and B.D. Hatfield. 1991. A meta analysis on the anxiety reducing effects of acute and chronic exercise: outcomes and mechanisms. *Sports Med* 11:143-82.

Petruzzello, S.J., D.M. Landers, and W. Salazar. 1991. Exercise and anxiety reduction: examination of the thermogenic hypothesis. *Med Sci Sports Exerc* 23(Suppl.):S41.

Pierce, E.F. 1994. Exercise dependence syndrome in runners. *Sports Med* 18:149-55.

Post, R.M. 1992. Transduction of psychosocial stress into the neurobiology of affective disorders. *Am J Psychiatry* 149:999.

Post, R.M., J. Kotin, F.K. Goodwin, and E.K. Gordon. 1973. Psychomotor activity and cerebrospinal fluid amine metabolites in affective illness. *Am J Psychiatry* 130:67-72.

Raglin, J.S., and M. Wilson. 1996. State anxiety following 20 minutes of bicycle ergometer exercise at selected intensities. *Int J Sports Med* 17:467-71.

Ransford, C.P. 1982. A role for amines in the anti-depressant effect of exercise: a review. *Med Sci Sports Exerc* 14:1-10.

Regier, D.A., J.H. Boyd, J.D. Burke, D.S. Rae, J.K. Myers, M. Kramer, L.N. Robins, L.K. George, M. Karno, and B.Z. Locke. 1988. One month prevalence of mental disorders in the United States. *Arch Gen Psychiatry* 45:981.

Rief, W., and M. Hermanutz. 1996. Responses to activation and rest in patients with panic disorder and major depression. *Br J Clin Psychol* 35:605-16.

Rippe, J.M., A. Ward, J.P. Porcari, and P.S. Freedson. 1988. Walking for health and fitness. *JAMA* 259:2720-24.

Roth, D.L. 1989. Acute emotional and psychophysiological effects of aerobic exercise. *Psychophysiology* 26:593-602.

Roth, D.L., S.D. Bachtier, and R.B. Fillingim. 1990. Acute emotional and cardiovascular effects of stressful mental work during aerobic exercise. *Psychophysiology* 27:694-701.

Roth, D.L., and D.S. Holmes. 1985. Influence of physical fitness in determining the impact of stressful life events on physical and psychological health. *Psychosom Med* 47:164-73.

Rybarczyk, B.D., D.L. Nyenhuis, J.J. Nicholas, R. Schulz, R.J. Alioto, and C. Blair. 1992. Social discomfort and depression in a sample of adults with leg amputations. *Arch Phys Med Rehabil* 73:1169-73.

Sachs, M.J. 1984. The runners high. In *Running as therapy: An integrated approach*, ed. M.L. Sachs and G.W. Buffone, 273-87. Lincoln, NE: University of Nebraska Press.

Schildkraut, J.J. 1965. The catecholamine hypothesis of affective disorders: a review of supporting evidence. *Am J Psychiatry* 112:509-22.

Scordo, K.A. 1991. Effects of aerobic exercise training on symptomatic women with mitral valve prolapse. *Am J Cardiol* 67:863-68.

Sexton, H., A. Maere, and N.H. Dahl. 1989. Exercise intensity and reduction of neurotic symptoms: a controlled follow-up study. *Acta Psychiatr Scand* 80:231-35.

Shephard, R.J. 1997. Exercise and relaxation in health promotion. *Sports Med* 23:211-17.

Shukla, G.D., S.C. Sahu, and R.P. Tripathi. 1982. A psychiatric study of amputees. *Br J Psychiatry* 141:50-53.

Singh, N.A., K.M. Clements, and M.A. Fiatarone. 1997. A randomized controlled trial of the effect of exercise on sleep. *Sleep* 20:95-101.

Snyder, S.H. 1978. The opiate receptor and morphine like peptides in the brain. *Am J Psychiatry* 135:645-51.

Sonstrom, R.J., and W.P. Morgan. 1989. Exercise and self esteem: rationale and model. *Med Sci Sports Exerc* 21:329-37.

Stedman's Medical Dictionary. 26th ed. 1995. Baltimore: Williams & Wilkins.

Stephens, T. 1988. Physical activity and mental health in the United States and Canada: evidence from four population surveys. *Prev Med* 17:35-47.

Sutton, J.R., P.A Farrell, and V.J. Haber. 1988. Hormonal adaptation to physical activity. In *Exercise, fitness and health*, ed. C. Bouchard, R.J. Shephard, and T. Stephens, 217-50. Champaign, IL: Human Kinetics.

Tate, A.K., and S.J. Petruzzello. 1995. Varying the intensity of acute exercise: implications for changes in affect. *J Sports Med Phys Fitness* 35:295-302.

Tiller, J. 1992. Post-stroke depression. *Psychopharmacology* 106(Suppl.):S130-133.

Trexler, L.E., and D.J. Fordyce. 1996. Psychological perspectives on rehabilitation: contemporary assessment and intervention strategies. In *Physical medicine and rehabilitation*. 1st ed., ed. R.L. Braddom, 66-81. Philadelphia: W.B. Saunders.

Umphred, D.A. 1995. Limbic complex: influence over motor control and learning. In *Neurological rehabilitation*. 3d ed., ed. D.A. Umphred, 93-117. St. Louis: Mosby.

U.S. Department of Health and Human Services. 1996. *Physical activity and health: A report of the Surgeon General*. Atlanta: U.S. Department of Health and Human Services, Centers for Disease Control and Prevention, National Center for Chronic Disease Prevention and Health Promotion.

Veale, D., K. LeFevre, C. Pantelis, V. de Souza, A. Mann, and A. Sargeant. 1992. Aerobic exercise in the adjunctive treatment of depression: a randomized controlled trial. *J R Soc Med* 85:541-44.

Whelan, J.P., M.J. Mahoney, and A.W. Meyers. 1991. Performance enhancement in sport: a cognitive behavioral domain. *Behavior Therapy* 22:307-27.

Wigers, S.H., T.C. Stiles, and P.A. Vogel. 1996. Effects of aerobic exercise versus stress management treatment in fibromyalgia. A 4.5 year prospective study. *Scand J Rheumatol* 25:77-86.

Woods, S.W., G.E. Tesar, G.B.Murray, and N.H. Cassem. 1986. Psychostimulant treatment of depressive disorder secondary to medical illness. *J Clin Psychiatry* 47:12-15.

Yalom, I.D. 1985. *The theory and practice of group psychotherapy*. 3d ed. New York: Basic Books.

Yates, A., K. Leehey, and C.M. Shisslak. 1983. Running—an analogue of anorexia? *N Engl J Med* 308:251-55.

Chapter 19

Obesity

Edward Saltzman, MD, and Ronenn Roubenoff, MD, MHS

Case Study

Charles Larson, a 48-year-old white insurance agent, weighs 258 lbs (122 kg), and is 5'9" (175 cm) tall. When he played football in high school, he weighed 205 lbs (93 kg), then reduced to 190 lbs (86 kg) by age 24. At age 30 he again weighed 205 lbs (93 kg), and by age 40 he was 230 lbs (105 kg). He says he "watches what he eats," and is surprised to hear his current weight. Mr. L. becomes short of breath walking down the hall from the waiting room to the examining room. He says that he gets up to urinate once or twice per night. He denies smoking, but drinks "a couple of beers" each night. Blood pressure is 150/96 mm Hg (with a large cuff), and his heart rate is 88 bpm. A repeat blood pressure after sitting quietly is 148/96 mm Hg. General examination is unremarkable. Waist circumference is 46 inches, and hip circumference is 42 inches. Initial laboratory evaluation shows that his CBC and electrolytes are normal, his random glucose is 167 mg/dl, and urinalysis is unremarkable. He returns for further tests, including a fasting glucose of 128 mg/dl, and glucose two hours after an oral glucose load is 192 mg/dl.

Twenty-five mg daily of hydrochlorothiazide is prescribed for hypertension, and Mr. L. is sent to the dietitian for diet therapy of his metabolic disorders and obesity. The dietitian determines that Mr. L.'s usual dietary intake is 2,500 calories per day. His diet contains 42% of calories from fat. He is instructed in a diet that reduces his energy intake to 2,000 kcal, with 30% of calories from fat, and 2 grams of sodium.

At one-month follow-up, blood pressure has improved to 132/84, and weight to 254 lbs (115 kg). Mr. L.'s rate of weight loss (1 lb/week) is good, but exercise is added to insure continued loss and ability to stabilize at a satisfactory level. He is counseled to begin a walking program, taught how to take his pulse, and asked to walk 1 mile per day 3 times a week for 4 weeks, increasing to 2 miles per day 3-5 times per week. The pace should be brisk enough to reach a target heart rate of about 140 beats per minute ([220-age] × 0.85). He is encouraged to do this outdoors or indoors, and to consider joining a health club where he can use treadmills, bicycles, and other machines, swim, or do aerobics.

One year later, his weight is 217 lbs, his fasting glucose is 108 mg/dl, and his blood pressure is 130/80. He states he feels much better and did not realize before that he had been suffering from low energy and fatigue until these symptoms had resolved.

The prevalence of obesity is increasing rapidly in the United States and other developed countries, as well as in some developing countries. In June 1998, the National Institutes of Health (NIH) and National Heart, Lung, and Blood Institute (NHLBI) adopted a new scheme—which now aligns the U.S. with the World Health Organization—for classifying overweight and obesity (NHLBI 1998). Overweight is defined as a body mass index (BMI) of 25.0-29.9 kg/m², and obesity is defined as a BMI ≥ 30.0 kg/m². According to the most recent National Health and Nutrition Examination Survey (NHANES III), 39.4% of adult American men and 24.7% of adult American women are overweight, while 19.9% of men and 24.9% of women are obese (see "Definitions of Overweight"). Since these surveys were begun in 1960, the prevalence of overweight (utilizing the new criteria) has remained relatively stable, while the prevalence of obesity has increased substantially (table 19.1). These increases in the prevalence of obesity have occurred during a time when dietary intake of fat *as a percent of energy intake* in the United States has been stable or falling slightly, and dietary intake of fruits and vegetables has increased; however, the *total intake of energy* (and thus total fat intake) may have increased despite the compositional changes of the diet. However, there has been a progressive decline in physical activity in the United States, which coincides with the increase in obesity, suggesting that inadequate physical activity may play an important role in developing and maintaining obesity. If correct, this hypothesis provides an important rationale for aggressively prescribing exercise to prevent and treat obesity.

Definitions of Overweight

	BMI (kg/m²)
• Overweight	25-29.9
• Obese	30-39.9
• Extreme obesity	40+

Health Implications of Obesity

Obesity is a major public health problem in the developed world, and there is evidence that it is rapidly becoming a problem in the developing world. Obesity is a risk factor for diabetes, coronary artery disease, hypertension, gallstones, gout, and osteoarthritis, as well as cancer of the breast, colon, and prostate (Colditz et al. 1995; Hubert et al. 1983). These comorbidities increase the risk of premature mortality; they also increase risks of longer hospital stays and of more difficult recovery from various acute medical problems and from surgery. Even small reductions in weight can reduce the risks of developing these comorbidities, or at least reduce their severity. It is not necessary to reduce weight to the level of ideal body weight in order to see clinically signifi-

Table 19.1   Trends in the Prevalence of Overweight and Obesity in the United States 1960-1994

Survey	BMI (kg/m²)			
	25-29	30-34	35-39	40+
NHES I (1960-62)	30.5%	9.6%	2.4%	0.8%
NHANES I (1971-74)	32.0%	10.1%	2.8%	1.3%
NHANES II (1976-80)	31.5%	10.1%	3.1%	1.3%
NHANES III (1988-94)	32.0%	14.4%	5.2%	2.9%

Data shown are the proportion of the U.S. Population in each BMI category.

cant improvements in blood pressure or glycemic control. Moreover, it is unlikely that most obese individuals can achieve and maintain a loss of more than 10%-15% of starting weight with nonsurgical treatment. Thus, it is neither necessary nor realistic for most obese adults to slim down to published or perceived definitions of "ideal weight." People also are more likely to maintain a gradual weight loss, avoiding the wide swings in weight that occur with more restrictive diets, known popularly as "yo-yo" dieting. Increased physical activity is important to maintain reduced weight after an initial reduction phase.

Body Composition Through the Life Cycle

Of a healthy newborn child's total weight, 10%-15% is fat and approximately 25% is muscle. In contrast, a healthy young adult has 15%-25% fat and 40% muscle. With age, the ratio of fat to muscle increases even in healthy adults who maintain their weight throughout their lives. By the eighth decade, it is not unusual to see adults with 40% body fat even though their weights are within 20% of ideal. Most adults in the developed world gain weight between their twenties and their sixties, after which there is a slow decline in weight. During this time period, a gain of only one pound per year would lead to a 40-pound weight gain, of which 30 pounds are expected to be fat.

Comparing Weights—The Body Mass Index

The simplest way to assess obesity is to weigh a person. Because weight alone can be misleading, however— 150 pounds is low for a 6-foot tall man, but excessive for a 5'2" woman—researchers developed ways to compare weight for height, usually using one of several **body mass indices (BMIs)**. The most common such measure is the Quetelet index (weight in kg divided by the square of the height in meters), to which the simple term **BMI** typically refers. Because the BMI is designed to compare weights of people of different heights, it has a greater correlation with body weight than with height (Micossi and Harris 1990). Although useful, the BMI exhibits important age and gender biases—a BMI of 25 kg/m² does not represent the same body composition in men as in women,

or in young persons as in old persons. Clinicians have often used BMI to indicate body fatness: weight gain in adults is mostly fat, and BMI correlates reasonably well ($r \sim 0.5$-0.7) with fat mass (Micossi and Harris 1990; Roubenoff et al. 1995). However, it correlates equally well with lean mass. Calculation of BMI allows clinicians to assign initial classification of weight for height, but only after they consider mitigating factors. For example, there are obviously great differences between a 200-pound linebacker, who may be heavy but has a low percentage body fat and is very physically fit, and a 200-pound sedentary man with a protuberant abdomen and poor physical conditioning. Yet each may have the same BMI. Fortunately, such dramatic differences in body composition are usually apparent even to untrained observers.

BMI has been useful as an indicator of increased mortality risk. Risk of death increases with age; and when this risk is plotted against BMI, it is clear that a BMI greater than about 27 kg/m² is associated with an increased risk of death (Metropolitan Life Insurance Company 1980; Roberts 1989). This increased risk is attributed to the excess body fat of people with high BMIs, and their attendant reduced physical activity. Thus the **ideal body weight** is the range of weights (or BMIs) associated with the lowest risk of mortality in the population. Although some believe there is also increased risk of death at low BMIs (below 20 kg/m²) due to insufficient lean mass, such a discussion is beyond the scope of this chapter (see Forbes 1987). In reality, BMI is only a fair measure of body fatness—to use it as a surrogate for fatness may be necessary in a busy clinical practice and in large-scale epidemiologic studies, but it should not be encouraged or accepted uncritically. The best use of BMI lies in assessing individuals' weights, not their fatness.

Measuring Body Composition— Other Considerations

Over the past five decades, researchers have devised many methods to measure body composition. At the most basic level, the composition of the human body can be divided into two "compartments": fat and lean. **Lean body mass** comprises the body cell mass (muscle, viscera, and the immune system) and the intercellular connective tissue (bones, ligaments, tendons, extracellular water, and loose connective tissue), while fat mass includes the subcutaneous and visceral adipose cells and their fat (Roubenoff and Kehayias 1991). The muscle component of lean mass increases in response to exercise, especially weightbearing and resistance exercise. Fat mass increases in response to a positive energy balance. In adults, about 60%-80% of weight gain is fat, with the remainder lean mass (Forbes 1987). Methods that use the two-compartment approach include (in order of increasing precision) anthropometry (skinfolds and limb circumferences), bioelectrical impedance, and underwater weighing.

There are two major limitations of the two-compartment model: (1) It assumes that the compositions of the two compartments are fixed and known. (2) Since generally only one compartment is measured, and then subtracted from total weight to estimate the remaining compartment, errors in measuring the first compartment propagate to measurement of the second (Roubenoff and Kehayias 1991). The assumption that lean mass and fat mass are of uniform composition is demonstrably incorrect for critically ill patients or patients with edema—in whom extracellular fluids can increase while body cell mass decreases—and in the elderly, in whom intramuscular fat replaces contractile tissue so that lean mass is less lean than in young people (Roubenoff and Kehayias 1991; Van Pelt et al. 1998). As for error propagation, consider a 70-kg woman with 30% body fat—i.e., 21 kg of fat and 49 kg of lean mass. Measuring her lean mass (e.g., by bioimpedance) might introduce an absolute error of ± 2.45 kg, or ± 5%. Estimating fat mass by subtracting lean mass from total mass requires carrying the entire error over to the fat mass—but the ± 2.45 kg error for a mere 21 kg of fat becomes an error of ± 2.45 kg/21kg, or ± 11.1% (Roubenoff and Kehayias 1991)!

Although more complex ways to assess body composition are available for research purposes, they are not generally available in field or clinical settings. These include measurements of several body compartments—using total body potassium to measure body cell mass; neutron activation to measure body fat, calcium, nitrogen, and water; and isotope dilution using deuterium or tritium plus bromide given orally or intravenously to measure total body water and extracellular water. One technique that is becoming more available for body composition measurements is dual energy X-ray absorptiometry (DXA). This method entered routine clinical practice for measurement of bone density in the diagnosis and treatment of osteoporosis—but in order to assess bone density, DXA instruments must estimate the overlying lean and fat tissue in order to remove the effects of this overlying tissue on the calculation of bone density. Whole-body DXA scans can provide reasonably precise and accurate measure of body fatness and leanness. However, clinicians should be aware that, unlike the regional DXA scans of the spine and hip used for osteoporosis, whole-body

scans are considered a research technique and are not currently reimbursed by third-party payers. Table 19.2 compares the precision of techniques used in body composition analysis.

Etiology of Obesity

Development of obesity is a multifactorial process involving genetic, metabolic, and environmental factors. Genetic factors confer the potential for obesity, but it is the interaction between genetic and environmental factors—such as diet and level of physical activity—that result in weight gain. Gains in body weight by definition represent an imbalance between energy intake and energy expenditure—to maintain body weight, an individual must match intake and expenditure. To illustrate just how precise this regulation is, consider a small energy imbalance of +2% (or +50 kcal/day for an individual with total maintenance needs of 2500 kcal/day), an imbalance that can easily occur. That small imbalance, if persisting over one year, would result in a gain in body weight of approximately five pounds. In epidemiologic studies, the average weight gain in adults is between 0.5 and 2.0 pounds/year (Jeffrey and French 1997; Williamson 1993; Williamson et al. 1993), suggesting that most persons chronically maintain energy balance to greater than 99% tolerance. Discussion of the role of energy intake in obesity is well beyond the scope of this chapter; Roberts and colleagues (1996) have recently reviewed the contribution of energy intake and dietary factors to energy balance.

Total energy expenditure (TEE) comprises resting energy expenditure, the thermic effect of food, and energy expended on physical activity. **Resting energy expenditure (REE)** accounts for approximately 60%-75% of TEE, and represents the energy cost of essential biological functions such as respiration, cardiac function, and maintaining membrane potentials and ion gradients. The viscera and the brain contribute disproportionately to REE. While skeletal muscle at rest expends less energy per unit mass than many other tissues, the large total mass of muscle translates to a significant contribution to REE. The thermic effect of food (TEF) usually provides about 10% of TEE, reflecting the energy required to digest and assimilate ingested food. Energy expenditure for activity (EEA) is the most variable part of TEE, and can range from approximately 15% of TEE in sedentary persons to over 50% in active persons or athletes. The ratio of TEE:REE can be considered an index of physical activity (termed

Table 19.2   Precision of Techniques Used in Compartmental and Elemental Analysis of Body Composition

Technique	Target tissue	Precision (cv) (%)	Accuracy (subjective)
Anthropometry	Fat mass, LBM	5-10	Depends on observer
Underwater weighing	Fat mass	3	Excellent in healthy subjects
Bioelectrical impedance	LBM	<5	Depends on equations
TOBEC	LBM	<5	Depends on equations
^{40}K-counting	BCM, LBM	3	Excellent
Na_e/K_e	BCM, LBM	6	Good
^{3}H or D_2O dilution	TBW	3	Good
DXA	Bone	1-3	Excellent
Neutron capture	Protein (nitrogen)	5-10	Good
Neutron scattering	Fat (carbon)	2-3	Excellent
Neutron activation	Calcium (total body)	1	Excellent

TOBEC = total body electrical conductivity; Na_e/K_e = exchangeable sodium/potassium, based on radioactive sodium or potassium injection; cv = coefficient of variation; BCM = body cell mass; LBM = lean body mass; TBW = total body water.
Source: *Nutrition Reviews,* Volume 49, Number 6, page 166. Used with permission. All rights reserved. © 1991 International Life Sciences Institute, Washington, DC, USA.

physical activity level, or **PAL**). Since both TEE and REE can be elevated in obesity (see below), using absolute values of these measures may be confusing; it is therefore important to normalize levels of activity to REE.

In addition to being the most variable component of energy expenditure, energy spent on physical activity is the most difficult to measure accurately. Techniques employed include questionnaires and inventories, heart-rate monitoring, accelerometers worn on the belt or at other body sites, indirect calorimetry performed in a metabolic chamber over 24 hours, and the doubly labeled water method (DLW). Because subjects are restricted to a metabolic chamber environment during calorimetry testing, and therefore may not follow habitual levels of activity, this approach may underestimate TEE. DLW measures CO_2 production in free-living persons by administering stable isotopes of hydrogen and oxygen and following the disappearance of these isotopes in urine, blood, or sputum (Roberts 1989). While DLW is the most accurate way to determine TEE, it is also by far the most expensive and technically challenging, requiring expertise in administration and laboratory analysis of isotopes. As will be discussed below, measuring TEE by DLW while measuring REE by indirect calorimetry permits calculation of nonresting energy expenditure (or TEE minus REE), which includes energy expenditure associated with daily activities as well as with exercise.

Energy Expenditure: Relationship to Obesity

Two questions logically arise when one considers the relationship between obesity and energy expenditure: (1) Do obese persons expend less energy than their lean counterparts, thus allowing maintenance of the obese state? (2) Does a deficit in energy expenditure or any of its components promote obesity?

Cross-sectional studies reveal that, in absolute value, both total and resting energy expenditure are increased in the obese in comparison to lean counterparts. As measured by DLW, TEE is positively correlated with body weight (Rising et al. 1994; Schulz and Schoeller 1994). REE increases with weight gain, although in some regression models other factors (such as fat mass and genetics) account for additional variability of REE. While REE rises absolutely in the obese, its value per unit of lean mass is not appreciably different from that of leaner people.

Despite the absolute increase in TEE observed in obesity, the amount of energy expended on physical activity when normalized to the REE is actually lower in obese persons than in lean persons. Using DLW in combination with REE measured by indirect calorimetry, Roberts et al. (1995) observed an inverse relationship between percent of weight as body fat (%BF) and TEE/REE (figure 19.1). Other investigators using DLW have also found inverse relationships between fatness and energy spent on physical activity normalized for REE (Rising et al. 1994; Schulz and Schoeller 1994). Cross-sectional comparison of PAL from different studies does not consistently show a lower PAL for the obese; but within individual studies, the inverse relationship between obesity and PAL appears more consistently. This apparent discrepancy is possibly due to methodological differences between labs in using DLW to measure TEE. Using questionnaires to measure energy spent on leisure time activities, Gardner and Poehlman (1994) found that energy spent on leisure time activity (again normalized to REE) decreases as body fat increases. TEF is also measured as part of TEE; and although TEF appears to be lower in the obese, the actual significance of this deficit in relation to body weight remains unclear. It is likely that the overall small contribution of TEF to TEE, and the small magnitude of the differences observed with obesity,

make TEF a relatively minor factor in energy balance in comparison to REE and EEA.

Thus, although absolute levels of TEE and REE are increased in obese persons, nonresting energy expenditure is likely to be depressed relative to REE. Theoretically, the increased expenditure needed to support movement of excess weight (especially in weightbearing exercise) will partially offset this deficit. The cause of this low nonresting energy expenditure in obesity remains speculative; but in extreme obesity, deconditioning, dyspnea, and joint pain are likely contributors. In terms of overall energy balance, low nonresting energy expenditure is likely to contribute to maintenance of the obese state.

Energy Expenditure: Development of Obesity

The mere association between obesity and decreased PAL or EEA (relative to REE) provides no information about cause and effect. To evaluate if obesity *results* from low energy expenditure, some researchers have conducted prospective studies or studies in individuals who are no longer obese. Large epidemiologic studies attempting to prospectively link levels of physical activity to weight gain have rendered mixed results. In the NHANES I Epidemiologic Follow-Up Study, Williamson and coworkers (1993) evaluated recreational physical activity and body weight at baseline as well as changes in these parameters after ten years. As expected, baseline activity was inversely related to baseline weight, but baseline activity did not predict changes in weight at follow-up. Levels of activity at follow-up were inversely related to weight gain over ten years, and a decrease in activity or maintenance of a low level of activity over ten years was also associated with risk of weight gain. Similarly, in the Healthy Women Study, Owens et al. (1992) observed an inverse relationship between baseline physical activity and weight gain over three years. In the Health Professionals Follow-Up Study (Coakley et al. 1998), the men most likely to gain weight over four years were those who maintained a low level of activity or decreased activity, or who increased time spent watching television. As reviewed by Williamson (1996), a number of methodological and other issues (including the difficulty of accurately measuring physical activity) may hamper the ability of these observational studies to reach a consensus regarding predictive factors for weight gain.

Prospective trials utilizing 24-hour calorimetry or DLW may better estimate TEE (and hence activity, if REE is also measured), but such trials have been

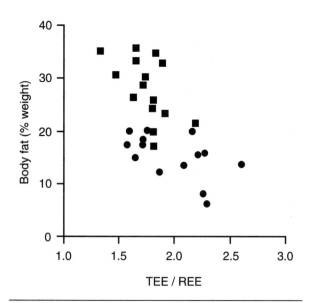

Figure 19.1   Relationship between body fat and the ratio of total energy expenditure to resting energy expenditure (TEE/REE) in young (●) and elderly (■) men.
Source: Katzel et al. 1995.

rare to date. Ravussin and colleagues (1988) examined 24-hour energy expenditure using a room calorimeter (respiratory chamber) in 95 Southwestern American Indians, and then followed the subjects' weight gain for up to two years. There was a significant inverse correlation between TEE at baseline and subsequent weight gain ($r = -0.33$, $p < .001$). Fifteen of the 95 subjects gained at least 7.5 kg during the follow-up period. Subjects who expended 200 kcal/day less than the group mean at the initial examination had a fourfold higher probability ($p < .02$) of gaining at least 7.5 kg over the next two years. To emphasize the previous discussion about the small difference between positive and negative energy balances, note that the mean difference in 24-hour energy expenditure between subjects who gained at least 7.5 kg and those who did not was only 87 kcal/day (2262 ± 194 kcal/day, vs. 2349 ± 133; $p = .12$).

Using the DLW method, Roberts and coworkers (1988) measured TEE in infants at three months of age and then assessed weight gain over the next nine months. At 12 months of age, infants who exceeded the 90th percentile of weight for height were considered overweight. At three months, the weight of infants who subsequently became overweight did not differ significantly from that of infants who did not become overweight (5.97 kg vs. 5.56 kg); but infants who eventually became overweight had a lower TEE than the other infants (61 kcal/kg vs. 80 kcal/kg, $p < .05$). These studies, along with the few others that measured TEE (Davies et al. 1991; Griffiths and Payne 1976; Griffiths et al. 1990) suggest that deficits in TEE may contribute to subsequent gains in weight.

Regular exercise seems to attenuate the increase in fat mass with age. Van Pelt et al. (1998) found that postmenopausal female runners (mean age 56 years; average 28 miles/week) averaged 23.4% body fat, compared to 15% body fat in premenopausal female runners (mean age 30 years; average 38 miles/week). Although this observation suggests that fat mass increases substantially with age even among highly active runners, note how these results compare with those of sedentary women studied at the same time: the postmenopausal sedentary women (mean age 61 years) had 40% body fat while the premenopausal sedentary women (mean age 29 years) had 27% body fat. Thus, the athletes had an age-related difference in their body fatness of 8.4%, while the sedentary women had a difference of 13.0%. These data suggest that habitual exercise reduced the age-related increase in body fatness by about 35% (13.0 − 8.4 divided by 13.0). In addition, the habitual exercisers were also significantly more fit than the sedentary

women at any age ($\dot{V}O_2$max 55 ± 0.9 vs. 42 ± 1.5 ml/kg/min). Although some caution is appropriate in interpreting cross-sectional rather than longitudinal data, these observations suggest that high levels of physical activity can prevent obesity.

While a large portion of TEE is determined by REE (and hence by lean mass), energy spent on physical activity remains an effective way to increase total expenditure. Since (as is often pointed out) a couple of cookies can overcome the caloric expenditure of an hour of exercise, it is relatively difficult to create a negative energy balance by physical activity alone. It is true that exercising an extra 100 or 200 calories per day amounts to only about 10% of the day's energy intake. Nevertheless, as discussed previously, the difference between positive and negative energy balance in most individuals is relatively small, so that even a small increase in physical activity can influence whether that day's balance is positive or negative. As table 19.3 shows, even moderate physical activity can lead to important caloric expenditures, especially in more obese people who require more energy to perform work on their body mass (i.e., to move).

Effect of Exercise on Dietary Intake

In contrast to evidence that a sedentary lifestyle predisposes humans to gain weight, physical activity level does not seem to affect food intake appreciably, either in terms of quantity or quality. In general, exercise does not appear to consistently influence the amount or the macronutrient composition (energy, protein, and fat) of ad libitum diets (King et al. 1997). It has been hypothesized, but not proven, that a more physically active lifestyle could entrain other healthy lifestyle choices—e.g., smoking cessation, reduced intake of dietary fat, and increased intake of fruits and vegetables. Because they expend more energy than sedentary people, athletes also tend to consume more energy and protein. In a study of nonobese women, increased energy intake compensated for increasing energy expenditure from exercise (Pi-Sunyer and Wood 1985). In several trials with obese persons, exercise without dietary restriction resulted in small losses of weight, but the energy imbalance was attributable to the additional energy expended on physical activity and not due to decreases in energy intake (Pi-Sunyer and Wood 1985). However, responses differed in other trials. Nieman and Onasch (1990) examined the effect of moderate exercise training (45 minutes, or about 5 km, of brisk walking five days a week for 15 weeks) on dietary quality in 36 sedentary, mildly obese women who were randomly

Table 19.3		Energy Costs of Moderate Physical Activity	
		Cost (kcal) of 1 hour of activity for a	
	METs	**70-kg woman**	**100-kg man**
Walking @ 3 mph	3.5	245	350
Running @ 6 mph	10	700	1000
Raking lawn	4	280	400
Pushing power mower	4.5	315	450
Slow freestyle swim	8	560	800
Doubles tennis	6	420	600
Volleyball	3	210	300
Golf/pulling clubs	5	350	500

A MET is equal to a multiple of resting energy expenditure (REE). Assigned MET value $\times$ body weight (kg) $\times$ (duration of activity/60 minutes) = kcal.

assigned to attend supervised exercise sessions or remain sedentary. All the women were encouraged to eat ad libitum. The women in the exercise group did not change their weights, while the control subjects gained about 1.1 kg ($p < .002$). The women in the exercise group tended to reduce their total energy intake, largely due to lower carbohydrate intake, while there was a mild increase in the control subjects ($p < .09$). Goran and Poehlman (1992) reported similar data for six young, healthy obese men (mean age 25, mean BMI 38 kg/m^2) who walked vigorously for 90 minutes per day five days a week to burn an average of 1,100 kcal per session. No attempt was made to alter their diet. The men initially increased their dietary energy intake in the first four weeks by about 300 calories per day, but over the next 12 weeks they progressively reduced their intake. By the end of the study, they were eating about 100 kcal/day less than they had at the beginning, while expending about 800 kcal/day more because of the exercise. As a result, they lost an average of 5.9 kg of body fat without a significant change in lean body mass. These data suggest that energy intake and expenditure may not be as tightly linked in obese adults as in normal-weight adults. We advise caution in interpreting these data, however: most of the food intake data in the above trials were collected by subjects' self-reports, which tend to reflect underreporting in the obese.

It has been postulated that exercise and energy intake in the obese (but not in normal-weight adults) may be dissociated because the large fat mass, with its corresponding large energy store and leptin production, acts as a buffer to prevent exercise from triggering hyperphagia. Another mechanism by which exercise may contribute to diminished energy intake is by increasing compliance with a hypocaloric diet. Racette et al. (1995) evaluated the effect of inclusion of aerobic exercise on weight loss over 12 weeks in subjects instructed to consume energy at a level of 75% of basal metabolic rate. Exercising subjects were instructed to consume additional energy to compensate for the cost of exercise. Subjects who exercised lost 10 $\pm$ 3.2 kg, while the nonexercising group lost 8.1 $\pm$ 2.3 kg ($p < .05$). Exercising subjects consumed energy (determined by DLW) at a level closer to the prescribed amount. Dietary compliance was inversely correlated with anxiety and depression ($r = -0.5$, $p = .05$), both of which frequently accompany dieting. This study suggests that inclusion of exercise may facilitate compliance with, and psychological tolerance of, a hypocaloric diet.

Effect of Exercise on Energy Expenditure

Resting energy expenditure increases with body size, and the increased absolute REE in obese people reflects that 25% of their excess weight is lean mass (Forbes 1987). When REE is expressed per kilogram of lean mass (or normalized to lean mass by other statistical means), there is no consistently observed difference between obese and leaner persons—suggesting that total quantity of cell mass, rather than the proportions or metabolic state of different types of cells, is the major determinant of REE in the obese (Ravussin et al. 1988). However, there are probably other small but important effects on REE, such as from genetic factors and fat mass. Ravussin et al. (1988) observed that people with low REE were more prone to develop obesity than people with higher REE; this difference withstood adjustment for lean body mass. People in the lowest tertile of REE gained an average of 2.75 kg/year, while those in the middle and upper tertiles had no significant gain per year ($p < .01$). The difference in total 24-hour energy expenditure between the low REE group and the other groups was only about 90 kcal/day.

Because of the large role of REE in determining daily energy requirements, there has been a great deal of interest in interventions that could increase REE and thus favor negative energy balance. In the 1960s, some physicians used thyroid hormone for this purpose; but attendant cardiac toxicity and ill effects on lean mass and bone mass make this a poor choice for bolstering thermogenesis. Other pharmacologic approaches to raising REE are under investigation. Ephedrine, taken orally, has been associated with increases in REE greater than 10% (Astrup et al. 1995); while this drug may hold promise for weight control, safety issues and long-term weight loss efficacy are not yet proven. Methylxanthines such as theophylline (Dash et al. 1994) and other common over-the-counter drugs such as aspirin are associated with small increases in energy expenditure. To date, however, no thermogenic drug has been approved in the U.S. for clinical use in treatment or prevention of obesity. Conversely, commonly prescribed drugs such as beta-adrenergic blockers can decrease REE by 5%-10% (Welle et al. 1991); they also can influence EEA not only via their subjective negative effects on perceived "energy level," but by limiting heart-rate response to exercise.

Since exercise has been suggested as a way to raise both REE and TEE without undue side effects, several investigators have studied the effects of both aerobic and resistance training on REE. Unfortunately, the results are mixed. Poehlman et al. (1992) trained healthy elderly men and women (n = 18; mean age 66; mean body fat 25%; $\dot{V}O_2$max 1.9 L/min) for eight weeks using bicycle ergometers. At the end of the training period, the subjects had increased their REE by 7% (1,728 to 1,843 kcal/day, $p < .01$) and their $\dot{V}O_2$max by 11% (1.9 to 2.1 L/min, $p < .01$). Rates of fat oxidation (22%, $p < .01$) and norepinephrine production (35%, $p < .01$) also increased. These data suggest that—at least in healthy, elderly, nonobese subjects—aerobic training can increase REE. However, in a further study of 11 similar volunteers, Goran and Poehlman (1992) found that a reduction in physical activity during the rest of the day offset the increase in REE (11% in this second study), so that total energy expenditure did not change. Moreover, although body fat declined significantly, lean mass increased, so that total weight did not change. The intensity of the training is important if increasing REE is a goal. Light exercise (150 kcal/session, three times a week) did not increase REE, while moderate exercise (300 kcal/session, three times a week) increased REE by 9% (Poehlman et al. 1992).

Despite these encouraging results, other studies failed to demonstrate increases in REE in response to aerobic training (Broader et al. 1992; Wilmore et al. 1998). Meredith and coworkers (1989) found no change in REE after 12 weeks of endurance training in either young (mean age 24; mean body fat 21%) or older (mean age 65; mean body fat 37%) healthy adults. Broader et al. (1992) also found no change in REE in 15 healthy nonobese men (ages 18-35; mean body fat 18%) who trained aerobically for 12 weeks. More recently, a large and methodologically rigorous study of a 20-week aerobic cycling training program (60%-75% of $\dot{V}O_2$max for 30-50 minutes/day, three times per week) caused no change in REE in mildly overfat men (24% body fat) and women (35% body fat) despite a large improvement (18%) in aerobic fitness measured by $\dot{V}O_2$max (Wilmore et al. 1998).

Even if aerobic training can indeed increase REE in normal-weight individuals, there is reason to doubt that overweight adults can achieve similar increases. First, it is more difficult to achieve high absolute work loads in sedentary, obese adults, because they often have comorbid conditions (heart disease, lung disease, arthritis) that limit exercise capacity, and because they often must overcome a personal history of not exercising—perhaps even of disliking exercise. Second, there is evidence that obese adults have an impaired catecholamine response to exercise, with lower epinephrine (but not norepinephrine) production and greater postexercise insulin resistance compared to lean subjects (Yale 1989).

Effects of Weight Loss on Energy Expenditure

Loss of body weight leads to decreases in TEE, REE, and EEA. TEE decreases because its individual components decline. Although loss of metabolically active lean mass leads to a reduction in REE, the decrease is greater than predicted by simple loss of lean mass. As would be expected, the thermic effect of feeding decreases in proportion to the hypocaloric energy intake usually recommended for weight loss. Energy expended on physical activity also declines, in part due to the decreased energy cost of moving a smaller body mass, and in part due to other factors.

Negative energy balance achieved through a hypocaloric diet decreases REE substantially (often by 10%-15%). This drop is greater than would be expected from the loss of lean mass (Saltzman and Roberts 1995); and it is proportional to the actual caloric deficit (energy needed to maintain weight minus actual intake). Some researchers have observed that measured REE remains below that predicted by lean mass during weight stabilization following loss (Saltzman and Roberts 1995). Teleologically, we can view the below-predicted REE associated with weight loss as the body's attempt to defend its existing weight. While only a few studies have addressed the issue of whether exercise can overcome these decreases in REE, limited data suggest it is unlikely that aerobic exercise can completely overcome the metabolic down-regulation that underfeeding engenders.

An alternative approach, which has been studied to a lesser extent, is whether resistance training can increase REE. Unlike aerobic training, which is thought to increase REE (at least transiently) by increasing sympathetic nervous system outflow, resistance training may increase REE by increasing body cell mass—especially muscle mass. Ballor and colleagues (1996) compared 12 weeks of thrice-weekly aerobic or weight training in 18 men and women (aged 56-70 years) who had recently lost an average 9 kg by dieting. At the end of the 12 weeks, REE of the aerobic training group had declined 12 ± 41 kcal/day, vs. an increase of 79 ± 37 kcal for the resistance training group ($p < .07$). The aerobic training group lost more weight than the resistance training group (2.4 kg loss vs. 0.3 kg gain, $p < .05$)—but this is because the resistance training group gained 1.5 kg of lean mass and lost 1.2 kg of fat mass, while the aerobic group lost 0.6 kg of lean mass and 1.8 kg of fat mass (all $p < .05$). In addition, Van Etten et al. (1997) observed that resistance training increased not only REE but also energy expenditure of physical activity outside the training sessions—a phenomenon we have seen several times in our laboratory (Campbell et al. 1994; Rall et al. 1996). These studies indicate the profound differences between aerobic and resistance training in their effects (outlined in more detail below) both on metabolism and on body composition. Nelson (1998) has written a valuable book for the lay public, outlining how to reduce fat mass through strength training.

Negative energy balance also reduces EEA, which decreases to a greater extent than REE during weight loss (Leibel et al.1995; Saltzman and Roberts 1996; Weigle et al. 1988). To determine the role of lost body mass on EEA, Weigle and colleagues (1988) estimated EEA for walking before and after weight loss of 22% in obese men. After the weight loss, the men wore lead-filled vests to replace lost weight, permitting the authors to calculate the energy cost of carrying that weight. Weigle estimated that approximately 56% of the decline in TEE resulted from reduced energy cost associated with lower body mass. Other suggested reasons for lower EEA after weight loss include decreases in spontaneous activity and increases in the efficiency of movement. Given the reductions in energy expenditure during and following weight loss, exercise may compensate by contributing its own costs directly to EEA, by increasing REE (in the case of resistance training), and by helping to preserve lean mass. We further discuss these concepts below.

Exercise for Treatment of Obesity

In the absence of a hypocaloric diet, light to moderate exercise is unlikely to result in loss of *substantial* body weight or fat mass. The energy cost of such activity (see table 19.3) is unlikely to induce an adequate and uncompensated energy deficit over the long term—individuals create deficits sufficient to induce weight loss much more readily by reducing energy intake. However, exercise itself may induce *small* losses of weight. In comparing worksite-based exercise and diet programs, for example, Pritchard et al. (1997) found that the exercise program resulted in a decrease of 2.6 ± 3.0 kg of body weight.

Effect of Exercise on Weight Loss and Preservation of Lean Body Mass During Hypocaloric Feeding

In a meta-analysis evaluating the effects of exercise during dieting, Ballor and Poehlman (1994) found that exercise during dieting does not significantly increase weight loss. Although some researchers have observed improved weight loss when exercise accompanies dieting, the above meta-analysis increases the difficulty of interpreting these data. In trials where exercise increased lost weight beyond dieting alone, it is not clear whether the loss was due to the effects of exercise on energy output, the effects of exercise on REE, the effects of exercise on energy intake, or some combination of these factors.

While exercise does not appear to increase the amount of weight lost, it does appear that exercise while dieting helps to preserve lean mass. Just as accretion of lean mass accompanies gains of fat mass, loss of weight is characterized by loss of both fat and lean. In underfeeding studies that measured body composition changes during weight loss, approximately 25% of lost weight was lean mass (Saltzman and Roberts 1995). The meta-analysis by Ballor and Poehlman (1994) showed significant preservation of lean mass when exercise accompanied weight loss, in terms of absolute amount of lean mass and of lean loss as a percentage of weight loss. Sweeney et al. (1993) found that aerobic and resistance exercise were equally beneficial during weight loss (compared to no exercise) in preserving lean mass. While we need further effort to clarify the optimal nature and intensity of exercise to accompany hypocaloric diets, strong evidence suggests that exercise will allow preservation of lean mass with weight loss. This phenomenon may be especially important to those with **sarcopenic obesity**—i.e., reduced lean mass in the setting of increased fat mass—which often characterizes the obese state in older persons.

Effect of Exercise and Physical Activity on Weight Regain after Weight Reduction

Following loss of weight, maintenance of reduced weight is consistently associated with participation in regular supervised (Pace and Rathburn 1945; Pavlou et al. 1989; Sahakian et al. 1983; Saris et al. 1992; Vallejo 1957) or self-initiated (Schoeller et al. 1997) exercise. Klem and colleagues (1997) described factors associated with successful maintenance of lost weight in the National Weight Control Registry, a study of individuals who had lost at least 30 pounds and had maintained that loss for at least one year. These subjects reported, on average, energy spent on physical activity equal to walking 45 miles per week. Using DLW along with measurement of REE, Schoeller et al. (1997) observed

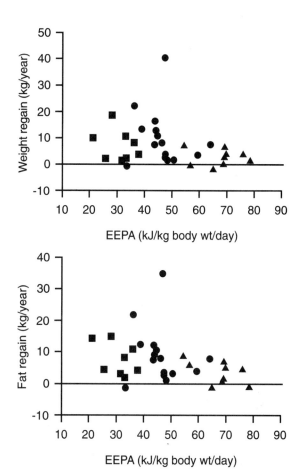

Figure 19.2 Weight gain (above) and fat gain (below) one year after weight reduction, plotted against energy expended on physical activity (EEPA). ■ = sedentary women; ● = moderately active women; ▲ = active women; 1 kcal = 4.2 kJ
Reprinted, with permission, from D.A. Schoeller et al., 1997, "How much physical activity is needed to minimize weight gain in previously obese women?" *American Journal of Clinical Nutrition* 66:551-556.

the relationship in women between energy expenditure and weight regain after an average loss of 23 kg (see figure 19.2). PAL was inversely related to weight gain. The relationship between energy spent on activity and weight regain was not linear, but showed a threshold effect. Note that in figure 19.2, there seems to be little correlation between energy expenditure of physical activity (EEPA) and either weight regain or fat regain until EEPA reaches about 46 kJ [11 kcal]/kg body weight/day—roughly equivalent to 80 minutes per day of brisk walking (Schoeller et al. 1997). All EEPA values above this level were associated with relatively small regains of weight or fat. Thus, exercise appears to have an important role in the maintenance of lost weight—but the amount of activity needed may exceed what has been previously recommended.

Effect of Exercise on Serum Lipoproteins and Glucose Metabolism

Weight loss per se is only one goal of weight reduction: amelioration of weight-related risk factors for diseases such as coronary artery disease and diabetes are also important effects of weight loss. Lowering serum LDL-cholesterol and triglycerides is an important benefit of weight loss, and even small changes in weight can markedly reduce the risk of heart disease. Several authors have examined whether exercise offers additional benefits beyond those conferred by weight loss through dieting. Schwartz (1987) showed that exercise could improve HDL-cholesterol and apolipoprotein A-1 levels in obese men, despite relatively little weight loss. Wood et al. (1988) studied the effects of weight-reduction diet (mean of 336 kcal/day lower intake after one year than at baseline, $p < .01$; n = 42) vs. a supervised aerobic exercise program (walking and jogging a mean of 18.9 km/week; n = 47) vs. a usual diet and activity control group (n = 42) over one year. All participants were men with 120%-160% of ideal body weight. There was no significant change in total or LDL-cholesterol in any study group, but triglyceride levels fell significantly in both groups (exercise: –0.16 mmol/L; diet: –0.27 mmol/L; control +0.08 mmol/L; $p < .05$ for both interventions vs. control). In addition, HDL-cholesterol increased significantly in both exercise and diet groups (see figure 19.3), and there was no difference between the two interventions in their ability to raise HDL-cholesterol.

In a follow-up study, Wood and colleagues (1991) examined the effect of adding aerobic exercise to a hypocaloric National Cholesterol Education Program (NCEP) Step 1 diet. This is a more realistic question to study, since most overweight persons are counseled to both reduce their food intake and exercise more. In the follow-up study, the authors randomly assigned 132 overweight men (BMI 28-34 kg/m²) and 132 overweight premenopausal women (BMI 24-30 kg/m²) to an NCEP weight-reduction diet alone, to the diet with aerobic exercise, or to a control group for one year. All subjects were between ages 24 and 49. The exercise intervention was brisk walking or jogging three times a week at 60%-80% of maximal heart rate for 25 minutes per session initially, increasing to 45 minutes per session by the fourth month of the study. After one year, both intervention groups had a similar mean decline in their total energy intake of about 470 kcal/day in the women and about 590 kcal/day in the men. There was a significant

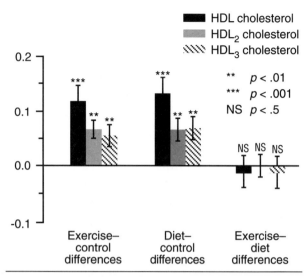

Figure 19.3 One-year changes in plasma concentrations of HDL-cholesterol, HDL₂-cholesterol, and HDL₃-cholesterol: differences in response between aerobic exercise, dietary restriction, or neither. Error bars indicate standard errors.

Reprinted, with permission, from P.D. Wood et al., 1988, "Changes in plasma lipids and pioproteins in overweight men during weight loss through dieting as compared with exercise," *New England Journal of Medicine* 319:1173-79.

reduction in body fat in both intervention groups (–4.3 ± 5.2 kg [mean ± SD] in the diet group; –7.8 ± 4.6 kg in the diet + exercise group; +1.2 ± 3.8 kg in the control group). As in the authors' previous study, HDL-cholesterol increased, but in the current study the increase was significantly higher in the diet plus exercise group compared to the diet alone group only among the men (see figure 19.4). Serum triglycerides fell in both intervention groups among the men, but not among the women. LDL-cholesterol fell with both diet and exercise in both men and women. This study confirms that both diet and exercise reduce lipoprotein risk factors for heart disease in men, but that the effects in premenopausal women are much smaller. In fact, the men in this study had significantly higher total cholesterol (5.41 ± 0.87 mmol/L in the men vs. 4.98 ± 0.73 mmol/L in the women) and LDL-cholesterol at baseline than did the women, whose premenopausal status further put them at lower risk of heart disease. Thus, the women with normal blood cholesterol at baseline showed less responsiveness to the intervention—but they were at lower risk of coronary artery disease in any case. The effect of diet or diet plus exercise in the men was to lower their cholesterol to the women's baseline mean level, while the women's response to the intervention lowered their cholesterol by an additional 10% or so.

As in the report by Wood et al. (1991) on premenopausal women, Fox and coworkers (1996) also observed limited effects of exercise and diet on serum lipids of postmenopausal women with relatively

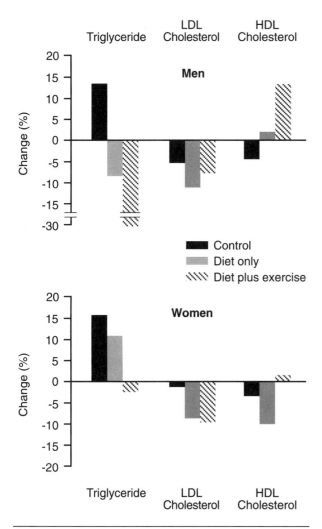

Figure 19.4 Percent change in plasma triglyceride and lipoprotein cholesterol concentrations in response to dietary restriction, diet plus aerobic exercise, or neither in men (top) and women (bottom). Reprinted, with permission, from P.D. Wood et al., 1991, "The effects on plasma lipoproteins of a prudent weight-reducing diet, with or without exercise, in overweight men and women," *New England Journal of Medicine* 325:461-66.

low risk for coronary disease. In this study, 41 healthy postmenopausal women (mean age 66 years; mean weight 120%-140% of ideal) were assigned to diet (500 kcal/day deficit) plus supervised exercise (aerobic exercise at 60%-70% of $\dot{V}O_2$max one day per week, plus resistance training using 12 major muscle groups at 80% of 1 RM two days per week); 500 kcal/day deficit diet alone; or 700 kcal/day deficit diet alone. The last group had an energy deficit equal to that of the diet plus exercise group. Assignment was evidently not random, as the availability of time to exercise was a factor in choice of study groups. The study lasted 24 weeks. All groups lost weight to a comparable extent (6.5 kg). None of the study groups exhibited changes from baseline in total cholesterol, LDL-

cholesterol, HDL-cholesterol, or triglycerides. However, all three treatment groups significantly improved their insulin responses to oral glucose tolerance tests, suggesting that the weight loss decreased insulin resistance both with and without exercise. Again, these data suggest that in overweight adults who do not have significant hyperlipidemia, there is little effect of diet or exercise on serum lipids. In contrast, persons who have elevated cholesterol levels appear to benefit from weight reduction, and have an additional benefit from exercise (Wood et al. 1991). The effect seen by Fox's group on glucose metabolism is larger in persons who have more severe insulin resistance at baseline, and can occur with exercise alone in the absence of weight change. Katzel et al. (1995) randomly assigned 170 men to weight-reducing diet, aerobic exercise (treadmill or stationary bicycle training three times per week for 45 minutes per session), or a weight-maintaining control group (figure 19.5). Only 111 men (65%) completed the study. For those in the exercise group, $\dot{V}O_2$max increased by 17%, and weight did not change; weight declined by 10% among the dietary restriction group, but $\dot{V}O_2$max did not change; neither measurement changed in the control group. Weight loss led to a significant 13% increase in HDL-cholesterol, decreased blood pressure, and improved glucose and insulin levels both in the

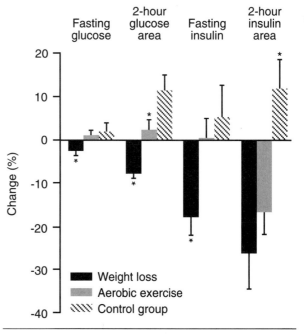

Figure 19.5 Percent change in fasting plasma glucose and insulin concentrations and 2-hour plasma and insulin concentrations during an oral glucose tolerance test, in men undergoing a weight reduction diet, aerobic exercise, or neither. Error bars indicate standard errors of the mean.
Source: Katzel et al. 1995.

fasting state and in response to an oral glucose tolerance test (OGTT). In contrast, the aerobic exercise group had a smaller improvement in OGTT insulin response, but without changes in fasting glucose or insulin resistance, HDL-cholesterol, or blood pressure. The authors concluded that weight loss was more effective than exercise in reducing coronary artery disease risk factors in obese men. However, the increase in aerobic fitness shown with the exercise intervention indicates that exercise causes unique changes in physiologic status that are independent of the effects of weight loss. In this sense, it is clear that weight loss and exercise prescriptions are synergistic and should be considered part of a complete package of lifestyle alterations to improve quality of life and prevent degenerative diseases in obese adults.

Summary

Over half of American men and women are either overweight or obese. Obesity is a risk factor for many serious disabilities and diseases—some of them fatal. It is natural and probably unavoidable that the ratio of fat to muscle will increase as adults age. Exercise, however, can significantly slow the rate of increase.

There appears to be an inverse correlation between total energy expenditure and subsequent weight gain, whether for infants or for adults. Preventing weight gain by increasing exercise levels appears easier than losing gained weight once it exists. High levels of physical activity—higher than most researchers have heretofore thought—apparently can largely prevent obesity.

Obese people have higher absolute values of total and resting energy expenditure than leaner people. It is difficult to create a negative energy balance (taking in less energy than that expended) through exercise alone. There is evidence, however, that increasing lean mass through resistance exercise can increase resting energy expenditure. And although neither aerobic nor resistance exercise appears to strongly abet weight loss—which primarily occurs through dietary restrictions—resistance exercise appears to help maintain weight loss by increasing lean mass and thereby increasing both resting energy expenditure and the general energy expenditure of physical activity.

Apart from weight loss, aerobic exercise has important effects on a number of cardiac risk factors, especially those related to blood lipids. Even in the absence of significant weight loss, in obese individuals with hyperlipidemia (but not so much in the nonobese or in obese individuals with normal blood lipids) aerobic exercise may increase levels of HDL and lower triglyceride levels.

Obese individuals are best served by well-designed hypocaloric diets and by exercise programs that include vigorous aerobic and resistance components.

Acknowledgments

This material is based upon work supported by the U.S. Department of Agriculture, under Agreement No. 58-1950-9-001. Any opinions, findings, conclusion, or recommendations expressed in this publication are those of the authors and do not necessarily reflect the view of the U.S. Dept of Agriculture. Also supported in part by NIH Grants DK45734 and AG15797, and General Clinical Research Center Grant M01-RR-00054.

References

Astrup, A., L. Breum, and S. Toubro. 1995. Pharmacological and clinical studies of ephedrine and other thermogenic agents. *Obes Res* 3:537-40S.

Ballor, D., J. Harvey-Berion, P. Ades, J. Cryan, and J. Callews-Escandon. 1996. Contrasting effects of resistance and aerobic training on body composition and metabolism after diet-induced weight loss. *Metabolism* 45:179-83.

Ballor, D.L., and E.T. Poehlman. 1994. Exercise-training enhances fat-free mass preservation during diet-induced weight loss: a meta-analytical finding. *Int J Obes* 18:35-40.

Broader, C., K. Burrhus, L. Svanevik, and J. Wilmore. 1992. The effects of either high-intensity resistance or endurance training on resting metabolic rate. *AJCN* 55:801-10.

Campbell, W., M. Crim, V. Young, and W. Evans. 1994. Increased energy requirements and changes in body composition with resistance training in older adults. *AJCN* 60:167-75.

Coakley, E.H., E.B. Rimm, G. Colditz, I. Kawachi, and W. Willett. 1998. Predictors of weight change in men: results from The Health Professionals Follow-Up Study. *Int J Obes* 22:89-96.

Cohn, S.H., D. Vartsky, and S. Yasumura. 1980. Compartmental body composition based on the body nitrogen, potassium and calcium. *Am J Physiol* 239:E192-200.

Colditz, G.A., W.C. Willett, A. Rotnizky, and J.E. Manson. 1995. Weight gain as a risk factor for clinical diabetes mellitus in women. *Ann Intern Med* 122:481-86.

Dash, A., A. Agrawal, N. Venkat, J. Moxham, and J. Ponte. 1994. Effect of oral theophylline on resting energy expenditure in normal volunteers. *Thorax* 49:1116-20.

Davies, P.S.W., J.M. Day, and A. Lucas. 1991. Energy expenditure in early infancy and later fatness. *Int J Obesity* 15:727-31.

Forbes, G. 1987. *Human body composition: Growth, aging, nutrition, and activity*. New York: Springer-Verlag.

Fox, A., J. Thompson, G. Butterfield, U. Gylfadottir, S. Moynihan, and G. Spiller. 1996. Effects of diet and exercise on common cardiovascular disease risk factors in moderately obese older women. *Am J Clin Nutr* 63:225-33.

Gardner, A.W., and E.T. Poehlman. 1993. Physical activity is a significant predictor of body density in women. *Am J Clin Nutr* 57:8-14.

Gardner, A.W., and E.T. Poehlman. 1994. Leisure time physical activity is a significant predictor of body density in men. *J Clin Epidemiol* 47:283-91.

Goran, M.I., and E.T. Poehlman. 1992. Endurance training does not enhance total energy expenditure in healthy elderly persons. *Am J Physiol* 263:E950-57.

Griffiths, M., and P.R. Payne. 1976. Energy expenditure in small children of obese and non-obese parents. *Nature* 260:698-700.

Griffiths, M., P.R. Payne, A.J. Stunkard, J.P.W. Rivers, and M. Cox. 1990. Metabolic rate and physical development in children at risk of obesity. *Lancet* 336:76-78.

Hubert, H.B., M. Feinleib, P.M. McNamara, and W.P. Castelli. 1983. Obesity an independent risk factor for cardiovascular disease: a 26-year follow-up of participants in the Framingham Heart Study. *Circulation* 67:968-77.

Jeffrey, R.W., and S.A. French. 1997. Preventing weight gain in adults: design, methods and one year results from the Pound of Prevention study. *Int J Obes* 21:457-64.

Katzel, L.I., E.R. Bleecker, E.G. Colman, E.M. Rogus, J.D. Sorkin, and A.P. Goldberg. 1995. Effects of weight loss vs. aerobic exercise training on risk factors for coronary disease in healthy, obese, middle-aged and older men. *JAMA* 274:1915-21.

King, N.A., A. Tremblay, and J.E. Blundell. 1997. Effects of exercise on appetite control: implications for energy balance. *Med Sci Sports Exerc* 29:1076-89.

Klem, M.L., R.R. Wing, M.T. McGuire, H.M. Seagle, and J.O. Hill. 1997. A descriptive study of individuals successful at long-term maintenance of substantial weight loss. *AJCN* 66:239-46.

Leibel, R.L., M. Rosenbaum, and J. Hirsch. 1995. Changes in energy expenditure resulting from altered body weight. *New Eng J Med* 332:621-628.

Leon, A., J. Courad, D. Hunninghake, and R. Serfass. 1979. Effects of a vigorous walking program on body composition and carbohydrate and lipid metabolism of obese young men. *AJCN* 32:1776-83.

Meredith, C.N., W.R. Frontera, E.C. Fisher, V.A. Hughes, J.C. Herland, and W.J. Evans. 1989. Peripheral effects of endurance training in young and old subjects. *J Appl Physiol* 66:2844-49.

Metropolitan Life Insurance Company. 1980. *The 1979 Build Study*. Chicago: Society of Actuaries and Association of Life Insurance Medical Directors of America.

Micossi, M.S., and T.M. Harris. 1990. Age variations in the relation of body mass index to estimates of body fat and muscle mass. *Am J Phys Anthrop* 81:375-79.

Nelson, M.E. 1998. *Strong women stay slim*. New York: Bantam Books.

NHLBI Obesity Education Initiative Expert Panel on the Identification, Evaluation, and Treatment of Overweight and Obesity in Adults. 1998. Clinical guidelines on the identification, evaluation, and treatment of overweight and obesity in adults. The evidence report. Bethesda, MD: National Institutes of Health.

Nieman, D.C., and L.M. Onasch. 1990. The effect of moderate exercise training on nutrient intake in mildly obese women. *J Am Diet Assoc* 90:1557-62.

Owens, J.F., K.A. Matthews, and R.R. Wing. 1992. Can physical activity mitigate the effects of aging in middle-aged women? *Circulation* 85:1265-70.

Pace, N., and E.N. Rathbun. 1945. Studies of body composition. III. The body water and chemically combined nitrogen content in relation to fat content. *J Biol Chem* 158:685-91.

Pavlou, K.N., S. Krey, and W.P. Steffee. 1989. Exercise as an adjunct to weight loss and maintenance in moderately obese subjects. *AJCN* 49:1115-23.

Pi-Sunyer, F.X., and R. Wood. 1985. Effect of exercise on food intake in human subjects. *Am J Clin Nutr* 42:983-90.

Poehlman, E.T., A.W. Gardner, P.J. Arciero, M.I. Goran, and J. Calles-Escandon. 1994. Effects of endurance training on total fat oxidation in elderly persons. *J Appl Physiol* 76:2281-87.

Poehlman, E., A. Gardner, and M. Goran. 1992. Influence of endurance training on energy intake, norepinephrine kinetics, and metabolic rate in older individuals. *Metabolism* 41:941-48.

Pritchard, J.E., C.A. Nowson, and J.D. Wark. 1997. A worksite program for overweight middle-aged men achieves lesser weight loss with exercise than with dietary change. *J Am Diet Assoc* 97:37-42.

Racette, S.B., D.A. Schoeller, R.F. Kushner, and K.M. Neil. 1995. Exercise enhances dietary compliance during moderate energy restriction in obese women. *Am J Clin Nutr* 62:345-49.

Rall, L., S. Meydani, J. Kehayias, B. Dawson-Hughes, and R. Roubenoff. 1996. The effect of progressive resistance training in rheumatoid arthritis: increased strength without changes in energy balance or body composition. *Arthr Rheum* 39:415-26.

Ravussin, E., S. Lillioja, and W.C. Knowler. 1988. Reduced rate of energy expenditure as a risk factor for body-weight gain. *New Engl J Med* 318:467-72.

Rising, L.R., I.T. Harper, A.M. Fontvielle, R.T. Ferraro, M. Spraul, and E. Ravussin. 1994. Determinants of total daily energy expenditure: variability in physical activity. *Am J Clin Nutr* 59:800-04.

Roberts, S.B. 1989. Use of the doubly labeled water method for measurement of energy expenditure, total body water, water intake, and metabolizable energy intake in humans and small animals. *Can J Physiol Pharmacol* 67:1190-98.

Roberts, S.B., W. Dietz, T. Sharp, G.E. Dallal, and J.O. Hall. 1995. Multiple laboratory comparison of the doubly labeled water technique. *Obes Res* 3(Suppl. 2):155S-63S.

Roberts, S.B., P. Fuss, M.B. Heyman, G.E. Dallal, and V.R. Young. 1996. Effects of age on energy expenditure and substrate oxidation during experimental underfeeding in healthy men. *J Gerontol* 51A:B158-66.

Roberts, S.B., J. Savage, W.A. Coward, B. Chew, and A. Lucas. 1988. Energy expenditure and energy intake in infants born to lean and overweight mothers. *N Engl J Med* 318:461-66.

Roubenoff, R., G.E. Dallal, and P.W.F. Wilson. 1995. Predicting body fatness: the body mass index vs. estimation by bioelectrical impedance. *Am J Pub Health* 85:726-28.

Roubenoff, R., and J.J. Kehayias. 1991. The meaning and measurement of lean body mass. *Nutr Rev* 46:163-75.

Sahakian, B.J., P. Trayhurm, M. Wallace, R. Deeley, P. Winn, T.W. Robbins, and B.J. Everitt. 1983. Increased weight gain and reduced activity in brown adipose tissue produced by depletion of hypothalamic noradrenaline. *Neurosci Lett* 39:321-26.

Saltzman, E., and S.B. Roberts. 1995. The role of energy expenditure in energy regulation: findings from a decade of research. *Nutr Rev* 53:209-20.

Saltzman, E., and S.B. Roberts. 1996. Effects of energy imbalance on energy expenditure and respiratory quotient in young and older men: a summary of data from two metabolic studies. *Aging Clin Exp Res* 8:370-78.

Saris, W.H.M., M.C. Koenders, D.L.E. Pannemans, and M.A. van Baak. 1992. Outcome of a multicenter outpatient weight-management program including very-low calorie diet and exercise. *Am J Clin Nutr* 56:294-96S.

Schoeller, D.A., K. Shay, and R.F. Kushner. 1997. How much physical activity is needed to minimize weight gain in previously obese women? *Am J Clin Nutr* 66:551-56.

Schulz, L.O., and D.A. Schoeller. 1994. A compilation of total daily energy expenditures and body weights in healthy adults. *Am J Clin Nutr* 60:676-81.

Schwartz, R. 1987. The independent effects of dietary weight loss and aerobic training on high density lipoproteins and apolipoprotein A-1 concentrations in obese men. *Metabolism* 36:165-71.

Sweeney, M.E., J.O. Hill, P.A. Heller, R. Baney, and M. DiGirolamo. 1993. Severe vs. moderate energy restriction with and without exercise in the treatment of obesity: efficiency of weight loss. *Am J Clin Nutr* 57:127-34.

Vallejo, E.A. 1957. La dieta de hambre a disas alternos in la alimentacion de los viejos. *Rev Clin Exp* 63:25.

Van Etten, L., K. Westerterp, F. Verstappen, B. Boon, and W. Saris. 1997. Effect of an 18-wk weight-training program on energy expenditure and physical activity. *J Appl Physiol* 82:298-304.

Van Pelt, R., K. Davy, E. Stevenson, T. Wilson, P. Jones, and D. Seals. 1998. Smaller differences in total and regional adiposity with age in women who regularly perform endurance exercise. *Am J Clin Nutr* 42:983-90.

Weigle, D.S., K.J. Sande, P.-H. Iverisu, E.R. Monsen, and J.D. Brunzell. 1988. Weight loss leads to a marked decrease in non-resting energy expenditure in ambulatory human subjects. *Metab* 37:930-36.

Welle, S., R.G. Schwartz, and M. Statt. 1991. Reduced metabolic rate during beta-adrenergic blockade in humans. *Metabolism* 40:619-22.

Williamson, D.F. 1993. Descriptive epidemiology of body weight and weight change in U.S. adults. *Ann Intern Med* 119:646-49.

Williamson, D.F. 1996. Dietary intake and physical activity as "predictors" of weight gain in observational, prospective studies of adults. *Nutr Rev* 54:S101-09.

Williamson, D.F., J. Madans, R.F. Anda, J.C. Kleinman, H.S. Kahn, and T. Byers. 1993. Recreational physical activity and ten-year weight change in a U.S. national cohort. *Int J Obes* 17:279-86.

Wilmore, J., P. Stanforth, L. Hudspeth, J. Gagnon, E. Daw, A. Leon, D. Rao, J. Skinner, and C. Bouchard. 1998. Alterations in resting metabolic rate as a consequence of 20 wk of endurance training: the HERITAGE Family Study. *Am J Clin Nutr* 68:66-71.

Wood, P.D., M.L. Stefanick, D.M. Dreon, B. Frey-Hewitt, S.C. Garay, P.T. Williams, H.R. Superko, S.P. Fortmann, J.J. Albers, K.M. Vranizan, N.M. Ellsworth, R.M. Terry, and W.L. Haskell. 1988. Changes in plasma lipids and lipoproteins in overweight men during weight loss through dieting as compared with exercise. *N Engl J Med* 319:1173-79.

Wood, P.D., M.L. Stefanick, P.T. Williams, and W.L. Haskell. 1991. The effects on plasma lipoproteins of a prudent weight-reducing diet, with or without exercise, in overweight men and women. *N Engl J Med* 325:461-66.

Yale, J.-F., L.A. Leiter, and E.B. Marliss. 1989. Metabolic responses to intense exercise in lean and obese subjects. *J Clin Endocrinol Metab* 68:438.

Part IV

Specific Patient Populations

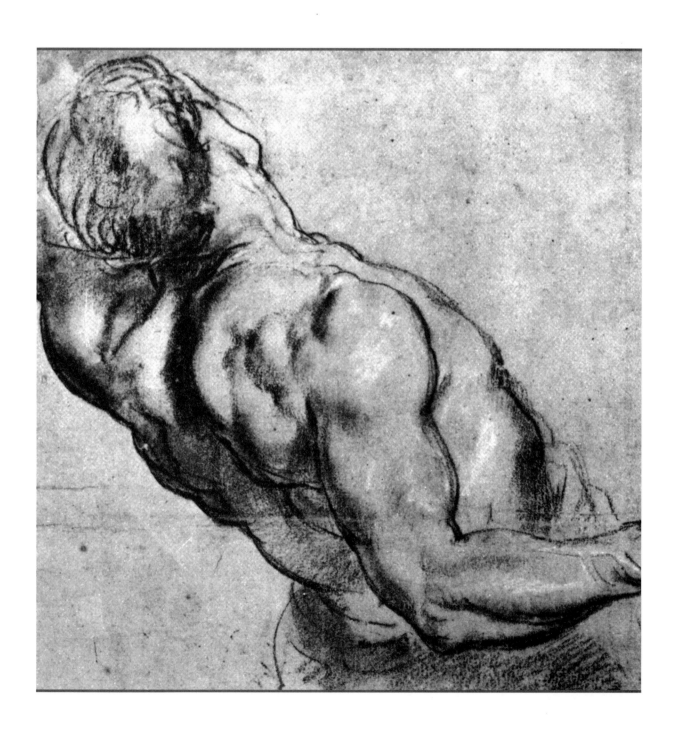

Chapter 20

Aging, Function, and Exercise

Charles T. Pu, MD, and Miriam E. Nelson, PhD

The goal of life is to die young, as late as possible.
—*Ashley Montague*

Unlike the preceding chapters, this section deals not with a specific pathologic condition, but rather with a process—the process of aging. As defined by Miller, "aging is a process that converts healthy adults into frail ones, with diminished reserves in most physiologic systems and an exponentially increasing vulnerability to most diseases and to death" (Miller 1993). No other condition or single category of illness comes close to approaching the impact that aging has on health and well-being. Perhaps most significantly, the process of aging brings dramatic declines in function that leads to physical impairment, disability, and loss of independence. One of the supreme goals of care for the elderly, therefore, is to prevent or reduce disability and maximize independence. This goal defines the primary objectives of both rehabilitation and geriatric medicine. In fact, a rehabilitative philosophy lies at the very heart of geriatrics.

Therapists increasingly look to physical activity—and exercise in particular—as an intervention that may maximize physical capacities, minimize declines, or even restore function in this population. This chapter explores the rationale for this interest. We first describe the significance of this topic from a demographic perspective. Secondly, we define the aging process from a functional point of view—specifically, that of physical frailty—and describe major forces associated with aging that contribute to frailty. We review the primary modes of exercise, as well as their specific effects on physiological and functional performance on older adults. Finally, we offer practical recommendations for exercising older adults.

391

Demographics of Aging

The U.S. population has been aging both relatively and absolutely. In the decade between 1980 and 1990, the population over age 65 quietly grew from 11.2% to 12.5% of the total population (Campion 1994). This rate of growth proved greater than that of any other group—more than double the growth rate of the total population. Barring major societal changes, the U.S. elderly population will continue its dramatic expansion. When the "baby-boom" generation begins to turn 65 around the year 2011, the demographic face of the U.S. will change even more dramatically. By 2030 the percentage of the population over age 65 will double, and one out of every five Americans will be "elderly." Within this population is a disproportionate growth in the group over age 85, the "oldest-old," who in 1990 numbered 3.3 million. Conservative estimates of the oldest-old from the Census Bureau, beginning in the year 2000, project growth from 4.9 million to a range of 8-13 million by the year 2030—as much as a 160% increase in that 30-year period alone (Campion 1994). More optimistic projections, in light of expected improvements in disease prevention and treatment, estimate the number of Americans 85 years and older in 2030 will be as high as 24 million (390% increase over the number in 2000) or even higher (Suzman et al. 1992).

Few if any changes in the coming century will affect our nation's health care system so profoundly as these demographic changes. Because health care services have not kept pace with this increase, many experts fear that these trends will stress the current health care system beyond its capacities. In 1989, the U.S. spent nearly $600 billion for health care, about 11.5% of the gross national product (Schneider and Guralnik 1990). The elderly, who constituted 12% of the population, accounted for nearly one-third of this cost.

Increasing life expectancy has been one of the forces driving these changes. Thirty years ago, average life expectancy at age 65 was about 15 years. Today, average life expectancy at age 65 years approaches 17.5 years (about 15 years for men and 19 for women) (Wylie 1984). On one hand, this extension in longevity is expected to bring heavy burdens of illness and/or disability as health care needs shift from acute disease processes to chronic disorders. On the other hand, the relatively long periods of remaining life after age 65 offer ample opportunity for efforts at risk reduction and health promotion to produce meaningful benefits. At present one

of the few viable solutions to the dilemma lies with strategies to prevent or delay age-related morbidity. Interventions that focus on reducing morbidity have great potential to influence future health care resource utilization.

The changing demographic landscape facing Americans and the challenge to develop preventive interventions apply globally as well. Of the planet's current 5.8 billion people, 7% are over the age of 65, somewhat less than the 12%-13% found in the U.S. As in the U.S., however, the global elderly population represents the fasting growing segment of the world's total population. In 1996 the number of people over age 65 grew by about 2.4%—one-third faster than the 1.8% growth reported for adults aged 20-64, and three times the 0.7% growth in the 0-19 year old age group (WHO 1997).

Global inequalities in the aging process exist between developed vs. developing countries. Individuals living in developed countries show longer average life spans than those in developing countries. Although many people in developing countries reach advanced ages, typically it is only the fittest who do so. Despite having shorter average life spans, developing countries were home to over half the world's elderly population in 1990. This proportion is projected to increase to over 66% by the turn of the millenium and to nearly 75% by the year 2020 (U.S. Bureau of the Census 1991). Perhaps the greatest concern is the fact that over half of the oldest-old—the fastest growing segment of the aging population in both the U.S. as well as the rest of the world—will be living in developing countries where resources for health care support are the most limited.

The Aging Process

The most common measure of aging, chronologic age, measures a person's quantity of life. **Chronologic age** offers a convenient basis for categorizations, but does not accurately portray the true picture of an older person's health or physical capacities. **Biologic aging** usually refers to the finite number of cell divisions that are genetically "preprogrammed," whereas **physiologic aging** often describes the gradual and progressive constriction of the homeostatic reserve of every organ system (Resnick 1997). This constriction, often referred to as **homeostenosis**, results in diminished "physiologic reserve" and limits the older individual's ability to adapt to stress. Although subtle age-related physiologic changes already begin by the third decade, the rate and extent of decline vary greatly—and the decline of each organ system appears to occur independently of changes in other organ systems. These declines eventually are influenced by disease, extrinsic factors such as diet, physical activity, environment, and lifestyle, as well as intrinsic factors such as genetics. Individuals, therefore, become more heterogeneous as they age, making it nearly impossible to stereotype someone who is "old." This heterogeneity underscores the complexity in deciding what information to obtain about the older adult and how to apply it in a way that relates meaningfully to clinical decisions.

A Functional Perspective

We believe viewing the aging process from a functional perspective most effectively addresses our needs as care providers. This approach not only addresses an aging individual's physiologic capacity as it relates to ability to perform tasks needed for independence, but also addresses the true problem of aging from the older adult's perspective—that of functional decline. Further, this approach provides caregivers a framework for tracking an individual's progression from independence to disability to dependence. The World Health Organization defines **disability** as a "restriction or lack of ability to perform an activity in the manner or within the range considered normal for a human being" (Chamie 1990). Surveys reveal that the elderly fear dying less than they fear becoming physically dependent, as evidenced by their strong desire to remain independent (Buchner et al. 1992). Forty-one percent of the "young-old" (64-74 years) fear depending on others, a number that increases to over 60% in the "old-old" (85 and older). Of the elderly who live alone, more than 75% fear becoming dependent on others. Eighty-six percent of this population cling toward remaining in their own homes even when faced with significant functional limitations (Commonwealth Fund Commission 1988).

Although many older persons maintain highly engaged and functionally intact lives into very late years, the rate of disability in the population increases markedly with age (Tinetti and Speechley 1989). Nearly all problems that result in disability are more prevalent in the elderly. Prospectively following noninstitutionalized men and women aged 55 to 84, the Framingham Disability Study showed that the risk of physical disability increased with advancing age as a greater percentage of elderly adults were unable to perform some of the most basic physical tasks (Jette and Branch 1981). One-fourth of the people in this study over age 65 stated that they were able

neither to lift 10 pounds nor to walk a half mile. Fifteen percent reported inability to climb stairs, and 7% were unable to walk across a small room. By age 85, the percentage of women unable to lift 10 pounds increased to 66%. Today, one in five persons of the old-old is institutionalized, compared to only 1.4% of those 65-74 years of age. Of the noninstitutionalized old-old, many are either close to being institutionalized or need increased social and medical support to remain independent. Although fewer than 5% of older adults over the age of 65 live in nursing homes at any given time, the lifetime risk of admission to a nursing home for this population is about 45% for women and 28% for men (Kemper and Murtaugh 1991). Finally, death in old age is usually preceded by eight to ten years with some disability and about a year of near-total to total dependency (Guralnik et al. 1991)

Frailty: The True Problem of Aging

As defined by Buchner, "frailty is a state of reduced physiological reserve associated with increased susceptibility to physical disability" (Buchner and Wagner 1992). Although most older adults with functional impairments are frail by this definition, some who are still functioning independently, though just barely, may also meet this definition. Frail older adults are those at highest risk of becoming disabled, although they may not be currently disabled. Older individuals who are physically disabled or dependent are by definition frail. Thus frailty, when defined in this way (a physiologic state of risk), is linked to, yet defined and measured independently of, disability (functional outcome). Figure 20.1 illustrates this conceptual model. According to this frailty classification, the non-frail or robust elderly (65-74 years) may be recognized as a group typically with no restriction of physical ability, the prefrail elderly (75-84 years) as having slight or few limitations, and the frail elderly (over 85 years) as facing severe limitations (Shephard 1990).

The growth in the elderly population will greatly increase health care needs as the prevalence of frailty and accompanying disabilities rises (Pendergast et al. 1993). Although it is difficult to measure frailty, it is the question of *function*—as reflected through the state of frailty—that is the main focus of this chapter, and that allows the fields of gerontology and rehabilitation to merge. Herein we discuss the age-related changes that contribute to frailty, and explore the extent to which these changes can be mitigated.

Frailty and Disability

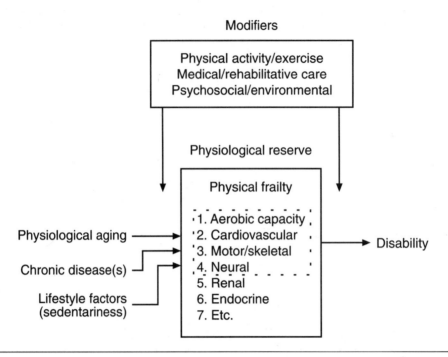

Figure 20.1   A conceptual model of frailty and disability. The losses of physiological reserve that are thought most to contribute to the state of physical frailty are represented within the dotted box.
Reprinted, by permission, from D.M. Buchner and E.H. Wagner, 1992, "Preventing frail health," *Clinics in Geriatric Medicine* 8:1-17.

Components of Frailty in Older Adults

Experts generally agree that physical frailty results from the interactions among three major forces: 1) the physiologic aging process itself, 2) the accumulation of chronic diseases, and 3) lifestyle factors; in particular, chronic sedentariness. Although all three will be discussed, we will devote the major focus of this chapter to the multisystem physiologic changes associated with typical aging.

Physiologic Aging Processes

The typical aging process is characterized by physiologic restriction in nearly all organ systems. Most declines in the absence of disease impose few restrictions on function for most of one's life span. Over time, however, even individuals spared from disease increase their risk of becoming frail as physiologic reserves drift downward and increasingly affect functional ability. The losses of physiologic reserve that most directly contribute to physical frailty are those

of aerobic capacity, cardiovascular endurance, motor/skeletal strength and endurance, and neural integrity.

Aerobic Exercise Capacity

The ability to exercise depends on the integration of cardiovascular, motor, and neural systems during physical stress. The standard physiologic measure used to determine one's overall ability to exercise is oxygen consumption or VO_2. Most cross-sectional studies demonstrate that peak VO_2 declines at a rate of approximately 10% per decade, or 1% per year, after the third decade of life in healthy, sedentary individuals (Anderson and Hermansen 1965; Åstrand et al. 1973; Grimby and Saltin 1966). The rate of decline varies greatly, however, and lifestyle factors such as physical activity may strongly influence it. Cross-sectional and longitudinal data show that VO_2 declines more slowly in habitually active compared to sedentary adults (Hagberg 1987). Using a cross-sectional study, Heath and colleagues (1981) first suggested that the rate of decline in VO_2 may be less for older individuals who continue to exercise regularly. By matching training regimens in younger and older adults and combining their data with other reports in the literature, they found a nearly twofold difference in the rate of decline in $\dot{V}O_2$max between habitual exercisers and sedentary individuals (5.5% vs. 9% per decade).

Rogers et al. (1990) confirmed these findings longitudinally when he showed both a higher initial $\dot{V}O_2$max and a slower rate of decline over an eight-year period. The $\dot{V}O_2$max of older master athletes who continued to train declined at about half the rate for age-matched sedentary controls (5.5% vs. 12% decline per decade). For men in the 50-59 year range, this difference is equivalent to a ten-year difference between physiologic versus chronologic aging. Although a few longitudinal studies in older adults have shown no declines in $\dot{V}O_2$max over a 10-year period when training was maintained, studies generally show some decline in VO_2 with advancing age regardless of training status (Kasch and Wallace 1976; Pollock et al. 1997). On the other hand, with continuous training most people should be able to achieve a higher initial peak VO_2 as well as a slower rate of decline.

Although physical fitness as measured by $\dot{V}O_2$max may predict mortality (Blair et al. 1996; Sandvik et al. 1993), it is less clear how declines in aerobic capacity (a physiologic measure of overall fitness) translate to functional outcomes such as activities of daily living. Some investigators have estimated the energy requirements of a broad range of physical tasks and compared them to the average $\dot{V}O_2$max of sedentary 75- to 80-year-old men and women as portrayed in figure 20.2 (Evans 1995). Theoretically, an individual cannot perform a task requiring more than or almost as much energy as can be produced. For example, a typical, sedentary older woman with a $\dot{V}O_2$max of 17 ml/kg/min (low) may have difficulty walking faster than 2.5 miles/hour for a sustained period of time and usually cannot climb more than 20 steps/minute. As these tasks of daily living represent an increasing percentage of the individual's maximal aerobic capacity, it becomes obvious why many older adults increasingly choose to avoid them, and thereby further exacerbate their decline in aerobic capacity.

Unfortunately, we have insufficient data to relate such laboratory-based measurements to outcomes such as functional capacity, functional status, or quality of life, perhaps in part due to the methodological challenges of obtaining these measures in the frail elderly. Cunningham et al. (1992), however, have shown that aerobic capacity is an independent predictor of functional performance such as gait speed, which in older adults has been independently associated with risk of falling and with functional status. More recently, Posner et al. (1995) demonstrated a curvilinear relationship between aerobic capacity and function measured by activities of daily living.

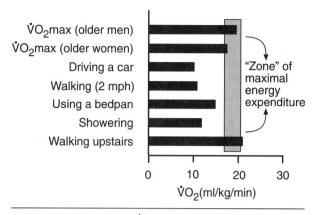

Figure 20.2   The average $\dot{V}O_2$max values of a typical sedentary 75- to 80-year-old man or woman, compared to the oxygen cost of activities of daily living. In the elderly many of these activities require near-maximal efforts with some requiring even supermaximal efforts.

Adapted, with permission, from W.J. Evans, 1995, "Effects of exercise on body composition and functional capacity of the elderly," *Journal of Gerontology* 50A (Special Issue):147-150. Copyright © The Gerontological Society of America.

Cardiovascular System

Because any type of physical work places stress on the heart to meet the metabolic demands of contracting skeletal muscle, the cardiovascular system plays a key role in exercise capacity. With increasing age, changes in cardiac structure and function result in an overall "stiffening" of the cardiovascular system (Lakatta 1990; Limacher 1994). Microscopic cardiac changes include increased fat, collagen, amyloid content, and lipofuscin. Myocyte numbers decrease, whereas myocyte size increases. Anatomically, although cardiac size does not change, there appears to be a mild increase in left ventricular mass and wall thickness. There are also vascular changes: the aorta loses elasticity as a result of increased collagen, calcification, and other degenerative processes. Furthermore, arterial pulse wave velocity increases with age, contributing to the overall decreased compliance of the cardiovascular system.

These cardiac alterations typically have minimal effects on resting individuals, but become significantly more apparent during physical exertion. The most consistent change that impairs exercise performance is the decrease in maximal achievable heart rate (Ogawa et al. 1992; Seals et al. 1984). Attributed to an age-related decline in sensitivity to myocardial sympathetic stimulation, this phenomenon occurs in all human populations, including elite athletes (Pollock et al. 1987)—$\dot{V}O_2$max appears certain to decline with advancing age even in maximally conditioned individuals.

The effects of age on other cardiac parameters such as stroke volume and cardiac output are more varied, and depend on the population studied. In an older population free of underlying coronary artery disease or hypertension, Rodeheffer and others have demonstrated that nearly all resting cardiac measures are maintained throughout one's life (Rodeheffer et al. 1984; Stratton et al. 1992). Even during peak physical exertion, peak cardiac output, although reduced, can still achieve high levels. Peak exercise stroke volume, in fact, increases more in older than in younger subjects, thus achieving some preservation of peak cardiac output with advancing age. To compensate for the inability to increase peak heart rate, aged hearts seem to maintain cardiac output during exercise by a greater dependence on the Frank-Starling mechanism via increased end-diastolic volume. Although exercise ejection fraction in this population increased, it was less than that achieved in younger adults mainly because older hearts could not achieve the same degree of end-systolic emptying (Stratton et al. 1994). This age-related dependence upon the Frank-Starling mechanism may contribute to reduced exercise capacity, however, since the myocardium must function at a larger volume—implying greater wall tension stress and therefore greater energy demand. The exertional ejection fraction often decreases in less rigorously screened older individuals, most likely due to underlying ischemia. As many as 30% of subjects over the age of 70 may have occult heart disease (Gerstenblith et al. 1980).

Motor Performance

Declining motor ability is one of the most obvious results of the aging process, and contributes to frailty. This decline is mediated by alterations in body composition that lead to losses in both muscle mass and bone density.

Changes in Lean Body Mass

Performance of physical work depends on the quantity, structure, and performance of skeletal muscle. Changes in skeletal muscle (the largest compartment of fat-free mass [FFM], or lean body mass) account for some of the most visible age-related changes. Cross-sectional studies consistently demonstrate that FFM progressively declines during adulthood, with a corresponding increase in fat mass—fat mass appears to steadily increase well into the eighth decade (Cohn et al. 1980; Parizkova 1974). Anthropometric measurements from male participants in the Baltimore Longitudinal Study, aged 20-92 years, revealed a slow progressive loss of lean tissue until age 65 years, followed by a more rapid

decline (Borkan and Norris 1977). Furthermore, the data of Cohn and colleagues showed that FFM—measured by the total body K:N ratio—declines primarily at the expense of skeletal muscle mass.

This loss of muscle mass with age has been demonstrated both directly and indirectly. Tzankoff and Norris (1977) confirmed that loss of skeletal muscle mass—declining approximately 6% per decade as measured by 24-hour urinary creatinine excretion—is largely responsible for the age-related decrease in resting metabolic rate. The human body may lose 30%-40% of its peak total body muscle mass by age 80. Recently more precise techniques to measure muscle mass, such as computerized tomography (CT), have confirmed a decrease in regional muscle density along with increased intramuscular fat (Evans 1995).

Skeletal Muscle Alterations With Age

Muscle mass as well as muscle structure and function—both of which are intrinsic to the performance of physical work—also change with advancing age. Most morphologic studies of aging muscle demonstrate both loss and predominant atrophy of type II, fast-twitch fibers. Type II fibers are recruited for actions requiring rapid or high-intensity muscle contractions, depending primarily on anaerobic metabolism. Controversy remains about whether the ratio of type I to type II fibers changes with age, implying a selective loss of one fiber type (Grimby and Saltin 1983; Larsson 1983). To gain insights into the mechanisms behind this age-related atrophy, Lexell and colleagues (1983a) examined the structure and fiber type composition of cadaver limb muscles. They found that limb muscles of older men and women were 25%-35% smaller, and have significantly more fat and connective tissue, than tissues from younger adults (Lexell et al. 1983a). Furthermore, comparative muscle biopsies revealed that fast-twitch fibers were smaller in the older adult. Electromyograms showing loss of entire motor units, as well as the occurrence of neuropathic changes in muscle biopsy specimens of old individuals with no history of neuromuscular disease, suggest that loss of the innervating motor neurons is a factor in this age-related atrophy (Lexell et al. 1983b).

The major physiologic consequence of aging atrophy, whatever the cause, is loss of musculoskeletal strength. Because muscle performance is directly related to muscle size, a decline in dynamic, isokinetic, and static muscle strength with advancing age is well documented (Aniansson et al. 1980). However, maximal dynamic and static strength and power—typically evident by the fifth decade of life—lag behind declines in muscle mass, which usually begin in the third decade (Pendergast et al. 1993). Thereafter, the extent and rate of decline in muscle strength with age become more pronounced, although highly variable. Several studies suggest that age-related weakness preferentially affects lower extremities (Aniansson et al. 1983; Culliname et al. 1986).

The greatest contributor to age-related decreases in muscle performance appears to be loss of muscle mass. Examining muscle strength and mass in 200 healthy 45- to 78-year-old men and women, Frontera and colleagues concluded that muscle mass is the major determinant of age- and gender-related differences in strength (Frontera et al. 1991). This relationship was independent of muscle location (upper vs. lower extremities) and movement (flexion vs. extension). Age does not seem to affect the quality of muscle contractions: when corrected for muscle mass, strength was remarkably similar in individuals no matter what their age. These and other data strongly suggest that a major component of age-associated loss of strength is sarcopenia (age-related decline in muscle mass) (Kallman et al. 1990). This relationship between strength and lean body mass pertains to even the frailest and oldest of individuals (Fiatarone et al. 1990).

Most importantly to the older adult, decreases in muscle mass and strength directly affect functional ability (Ory et al. 1993; Posner et al. 1995; Wolfson et al. 1995). Lower-extremity muscle performance, for example, is a critical component of walking ability, balance, stair-climbing ability, and getting up from a seated position (Brown et al. 1995; Judge et al. 1992). Several studies support the notion that muscle function affects selected functional activities of daily living (Buchner et al. 1992). Bassey et al. (1992) reported a significant inverse relationship between age and isometric strength of the plantar flexors; they also observed lower isometric strength in older women than in older men (Bassey and Short 1990). Declines in self-selected walking speed have been related to declines in lower extremity strength (Bassey et al. 1992). Older women with lower extremity weakness also have difficulty with very simple activities such as rising from a chair (Alexander et al. 1991). Finally, reduced lower extremity strength independently contributes to nursing home placement (Guralnik et al. 1994; Hubert et al. 1993) as well as to an increased risk of falling (Whipple et al. 1987).

Unlike in younger adults, alterations in body composition (in particular, the declines in skeletal muscle mass) directly affect basal metabolism and even overall exercise capacity of older people (Tzankoff and Norris 1977). Fleg and Lakatta (1988) showed that loss of muscle mass may account for nearly 30% of the declines in $\dot{V}O_2$max with advancing age when maximal VO_2 is normalized for muscle mass. Furthermore, loss of lean tissue body mass appears to affect disease outcome in patients with chronic illness (DeWyss et al. 1980). Given the clinical and functional significance of this age-related decline in skeletal muscle mass, the term "sarcopenia"—from Greek *sarkos* (flesh) and *penia* (poverty)—has been recently adopted to characterize this age-associated syndrome (Evans and Campbell 1993).

As with most age-related physiologic changes, there is great heterogeneity in musculoskeletal alterations with advancing age. Rather than being an inevitable part of the aging process, loss of muscle mass and strength may be more related to changes in habitual activity patterns. Klitgaard et al. (1990) reported that musculoskeletal strength and mass in older men (mean age 69 years) who had been strength training for 12-17 years was far greater than in age-matched swimmers or runners, and no different from those of young sedentary controls in their thirties. Furthermore, the muscle mass and strength of the older strength-trained men (but not the runners or swimmers) were indistinguishable from those of the young controls.

Changes in Bone Density

As reviewed elsewhere, sedentary adults over the age of 40 typically lose approximately 1% of bone density per year. Osteoporosis results in more fragile bones that are susceptible to fractures. Although the connection between bone density and physical function needs further study, osteoporosis and its consequences contribute significantly to physical frailty. Increasing the risk for disabling and fatal injury, osteoporosis carries tremendous personal, economic, and societal costs.

Exercise attenuates the risks for osteoporotic fractures in the elderly. Wolff's law states that remodeling of bone is directly related to the mechanical loads placed on it. One can therefore hypothesize that strength training could stimulate increases in bone density. Cross-sectional studies, indeed, have shown a relationship between muscle strength and bone density (Bevier et al. 1989; Pocock et al. 1989). Furthermore, recent controlled trials suggest that strength training can modify the physiologic declines in bone density associated with aging (Nelson et al. 1994).

Neurologic Control

Successful completion of physical tasks depends on the individual's ability to perform complex tasks in an integrated manner. Central and peripheral neural processing are needed for such optimal functional performance. When that system fails, often from disease, the consequences typically are devastating. Demographic data reveal that cerebrovascular disease has the greatest social and personal impact of all the most common chronic conditions, including cancer, cardiovascular disease, and hip fracture (Verbrugge et al. 1989).

In the absence of disease, reaction time generally lengthens with advancing age (Baylor and Spirduso 1988). Nerve conduction velocity slows approximately 10%-15% by the eighth decade in most people (Shock et al. 1984). Although an active lifestyle seems to delay the age-associated decline in reaction time, evidence that exercise improves reaction time in sedentary elders is less conclusive (Porter and Vandervoort 1995). It has also been suggested that decreased central nervous system recruitment of motor units, in addition to the age-related loss of motor units, may hinder neuromotor performance. Neuropsychological tests of timed manual performance strongly predict institutionalization (Williams and Hornberger 1984). Moreover, not only do more active older adults appear to have faster reaction and movement times compared to their sedentary peers—the order of reaction and movement times correlate more with subjects' levels of activity than with their ages, pointing to disuse as the major cause of this decline (Clarkson and Kroll 1978).

Accumulation of Chronic Diseases

In addition to diminishing physiologic reserves associated with typical aging, the elderly are at the greatest risk of developing chronic diseases that accelerate these declines, contribute to frailty, and lead to comprised function. Important examples are cardiovascular diseases such as coronary artery disease, congestive heart failure, hypertension, orthostatic hypotension, diabetes mellitus, chronic obstructive pulmonary disease, arthritis, obesity, and neurologic disorders such as Parkinson's disease, stroke, sensory deficits, or dementia. A review of each of these areas is beyond the scope of this chapter; but they are described elsewhere in this book. Moreover, disease processes do not exist by themselves as they often do in their younger counterparts, but accumulate and subsist as multiple, coexistent entities.

Because the elderly bear the greatest burden of disease, they also consume a disproportionate amount of medication and are prone to more adverse side effects than other groups. Although less appreciated than drug-drug interactions, drug-exercise interactions may assume increasing importance as exercise is prescribed for a wider range of the geriatric population. Many diuretics commonly prescribed for hypertension and fluid-overload conditions cause intracellular depletion of potassium and magnesium—which may lead to fatigue, muscle weakness, or arrhythmias (Dorup et al. 1988). Psychoactive medications such as antidepressants, antipsychotics, and sedatives can depress CNS function, which, in addition to increasing potential for falls, can lead to even more immobility and sedentariness. Beta-blockers, including ophthalmic drops for glaucoma, can diminish cardiac output by blunting the heart rate response to exercise. Finally, glucocorticoids used in chronic inflammatory conditions can induce their own form of myopathy and osteopenia.

Lifestyle Factors—Physical Inactivity

Because many physiologic changes associated with typical aging such as sarcopenia remarkably resemble changes seen with bed rest (the most extreme example of physical inactivity) (Harper and Lyles 1988; Muller 1970), chronic sedentariness is increasingly recognized as a major problem in the elderly. Bed rest can lead to dramatic losses of strength and aerobic capacity—as high as 1%-5% per day. Unfortunately, both cross-sectional and longitudinal studies of diverse populations show that individuals become less physically active with advancing age (Dishman 1994). This problem achieved recognition on a national level with the 1996 Surgeon General's Report on Physical Activity and Health (USDHHS 1996).

These observations give rise to two critical implications:

- First, because disuse syndromes closely resemble age-related changes in many organ systems, it becomes difficult to separate "usual or typical" aging from declines that result from chronic disuse or deconditioning. As we have seen, this point is supported by the fact that the long-term maintenance of high physical activity levels, as in the case of master athletes, often leads to an apparent separation of chronologic and physiologic aging (Rogers et al. 1990).

- Second, the resumption of activity at any point in one's life, even after a lifetime of sedentariness, may reverse certain deficits in physiologic structure and function previously ascribed to the inevitable consequence of the aging process. Table 20.1 summarizes some of the important physiologic similarities observed between typical aging and disuse that pertain to physical frailty as well as the potential ability for exercise to reverse these deficits. Despite the theoretical arguments for maintaining physical activity with age, most older adults are sedentary. Only about 22% of older adults engage in regular, sustained exercise (Dishman 1989; USDHHS 1996).

Chronic inactivity also contributes to subclinical disorders such as intra-abdominal obesity, glucose intolerance, osteopenia, hypertension, dyslipidemia, and coronary artery disease (Shephard 1990). The vicious downward spiral of further inactivity is further enhanced by the accumulation of overt disease and the medications used to treat them. Bortz introduced the concept that aging may be little more than a chronic disuse/inactivity syndrome. He em-

phasizes the possible role that physical activity, as reflected by active energy flow, may play in mitigating the age-related drift toward entropic decay (Bortz 1989).

In summary, the triad of (1) typical physiologic aging, (2) the accumulative effects of chronic diseases, and medications used to treat these conditions, along with (3) a typically sedentary lifestyle often places the older person on a path hurtling towards physical frailty. The myriad of possible dependent interrelationships among these forces, however, makes it difficult if not impossible to ascribe specific causality for the typical loss of physical vigor or function in many cases. On the other hand, the striking similarities between disuse syndromes and the typical aging process as well as the variability that these effects are seen in the elderly suggest that exercise, or more generally, the preservation or restoration of physical activity, can modify some of these aging effects. The next sections will discuss the varied exercise modalities that have been studied in the geriatric population.

Table 20.1   Physiologic Changes Associated With Typical Aging, Physical Inactivity, and Exercise

Physiological variable	Typical aging	Physical inactivity	Exercise
Aerobic capacity			
$\dot{V}O_2$max	↓	↓	↑
Arterial-venous O_2 difference	↓	↓	↑
Cardiovascular function			
Maximal heart rate	↓	↔	↔
Maximal cardiac output	↓	↓	↑
Maximal stroke volume	↓	↓	↑
Resting blood pressure	↑	↑	↓
Motor/skeletal function			
Fat mass	↑	↑	↓
Lean mass	↓	↓	↑
Bone mass	↓	↓	↑
Muscle strength	↓	↓	↑
Muscle fiber number	↓	↔	↔
Muscle fiber area	↓	↓	↑
Muscle oxidative capacity	↓	↓	↑
Neurologic function			
Nerve conduction velocity	↓	↔	↔
Motor unit function	↓	↓	↑

The similarities are striking between aging and inactivity as well as the potential ability of exercise to modify the deficits related to both factors.

Exercise and the Aging Process

The aging process as we typically know it is associated with reductions in physiologic capacity that contribute to declines in functional performance. These declines lead, in turn, to frailty and ultimately to dependence. Two of the most dramatic age-associated changes are aerobic capacity and muscle function. Because exercise is known to improve both variables in younger individuals, researchers increasingly look to exercise to attenuate age-related declines.

Aerobic (Endurance) Training

Aerobic exercise, also known as cardiovascular conditioning or endurance training, is characterized by many repetitive contractions of large muscle groups. Examples of endurance training include walking, jogging, cycling, climbing stairs, and rowing. Because chronic endurance exercise clearly improves cardiorespiratory fitness in younger individuals, researchers have studied aerobic training in older adults as a means to attenuate aging-related declines in maximal oxygen consumption and to improve cardiovascular efficiency at submaximal workloads. It is important when reviewing training studies to remember the components of an aerobic training program: intensity, frequency, duration, and length. **Training intensity** is usually measured as a percentage of maximal heart rate (HR) or heart rate reserve (HRR), both of which are attempts to reflect a percentage of $\dot{V}O_2$max. **Frequency** of exercise sessions is typically measured in number of sessions per week, with **duration** ranging from 30 minutes to 1 hour. The **length** of training ranges from weeks to years. Chapters 3 and 4 discuss endurance training in depth.

Effect on Aerobic Capacity

An increase in aerobic fitness is the fundamental physiologic response to endurance training. Table 20.2 summarizes several controlled studies of aerobic training in the elderly. Male and female subjects ranged in age from 54-84 years. The mode of training included walking, cycling, and in one study jogging. Training intensity ranged from low (30%-40% of HRR or HRmax) to high (>70% HRR or HRmax). Training frequency ranged from 3-5 times per week, with 30-90 minutes per session. The studies lasted from eight weeks to two years. Controls for these

studies usually consisted of sedentary, age-matched subjects or young participants. Although table 20.2 lists controlled studies, it should be noted that training studies have seldom been done as rigorously double-blinded randomized trials.

Several points from these studies deserve highlighting. The varied training protocols make comparisons among studies difficult; as expected, the response to aerobic training is heterogeneous. Despite earlier studies that found no change in VO_2 in elderly subjects after endurance training (Benestad 1965; DeVries 1970), most subsequent studies in older adults show a clear training effect, with improvements in VO_2 ranging from 7%-35%. Kohrt et al. (1991) found that 9-12 months of walking/running by 60- to 70-year-olds produced relative improvement in $\dot{V}O_2$max of the same magnitude (24%) as those observed in younger people. Similar increases of VO_2 were demonstrated by Hagberg (22%) and Seals (30%) in cohorts of men and women over a period of 6 months and 12 months, respectively (Hagberg et al. 1989; Seals et al. 1984).

Higher training intensities generally lead to larger increases in aerobic capacity. Sydney and Shephard (1978) assigned elderly subjects to low- vs. high-intensity as well as to low- vs. high-frequency protocols. The low-intensity groups showed no training effect. High-intensity training, on the other hand, resulted in average increases of $\dot{V}O_2$max up to 30%. Even the oldest and frailest populations who have typically led sedentary lives can demonstrate improved aerobic capacity after endurance training (Naso et al. 1990). Although more investigation is needed to determine the rate of improvement in $\dot{V}O_2$max with training in older age, it appears that elderly exercisers need longer periods of time to adapt (McDonagh et al. 1994).

In light of the heterogeneous responses to aerobic training, Green and Crouse (1995) used meta-analysis to more systematically delineate exercise-induced changes in the $\dot{V}O_2$max of older persons. Reviewing 146 studies, they incorporated 29 controlled studies representing 1,496 subjects into their analysis. On average, the subjects trained three sessions per week, 32 minutes per session, for 24 weeks. The authors concluded that endurance exercise training significantly improved peak VO_2 in the elderly. A more specific delineation of the analysis implied that, on average, a 68-year-old exercising for about 30 minutes, three times a week, might expect to improve $\dot{V}O_2$max by about 3.5 ml/kg/min—a 14% improvement from pretraining values. This absolute increase is slightly less than those found in younger subjects (Hagberg et al. 1989). Yet some studies on older individuals have yielded results similar in magnitude to those found in studies on the young. Using stepwise regression, Pollock and colleagues (1976) showed that the length of the training regimen contributed most to training effect (39%), followed by baseline VO_2 and then exercise session duration (8%). Unfortunately, they were unable to assess the effect of training intensity, which is thought by many to be the most important factor in training response. In summary, meta-analysis shows a clear training effect from endurance exercise; but the magnitude of the effect may decline with age.

Even if the elderly are not able to attain absolute increases in VO_2 similar to those of younger subjects, even modest increases in VO_2 are beneficial. An increase in $\dot{V}O_2$max as small as 3.5 ml/min/kg can benefit many older adults, and could mean the difference between independence and dependence.

Effect on Cardiac Function

Most research shows that aerobic exercise induces favorable cardiac adaptations, including improved cardiac output. Cross-sectional studies demonstrate higher cardiac outputs in older endurance-trained athletes compared to older sedentary controls (Ogawa et al. 1992). Although the specific mechanisms by which cardiac output increases have not been fully elucidated, both cross-sectional and longitudinal studies demonstrate that the improved cardiac performance following endurance training is not mediated through improved maximal heart rate (Heath et al. 1981; Seals et al. 1984)

The effect of endurance training on cardiac output is difficult to identify in longitudinal studies. Seals and colleagues (1984) found no improvement in cardiac performance when they estimated cardiac output indirectly during treadmill testing. Although there was a small but significant increase in estimated stroke volume, the associated small increase in maximal cardiac output was not enough to reach statistical significance. In contrast and in support of cross-sectional studies, research using direct methods provides evidence of enhanced cardiac output due to increases in stroke volume and perhaps ejection fraction. Schocken et al. (1983), in a 12-week training program, observed an increase in cardiac index mediated through increased end-diastolic volume, but not through systolic parameters such as ejection fraction or left ventricular end-systolic volume. Levy et al. (1993) supported the importance of diastolic adaptations in the heart: six months of aerobic training induced a 14% augmentation of peak LV filling, mostly explained by LV dilatation. Aerobic training

in older individuals, therefore, seems to improve stroke volume by augmenting diastolic function via the Frank-Starling mechanism. Two longitudinal studies have even demonstrated positive left ventricular systolic adaptations (Ehsani et al. 1991; Stratton et al. 1994). To attain such results, however, elderly subjects trained rigorously for one year. The maximal extent to which aerobic training can induce positive cardiovascular adaptations in the elderly has not yet been fully determined.

Effect on Skeletal Muscle

Aerobic training in older adults is also associated with adaptations in skeletal muscle (e.g., improved muscle oxidative capacity) that independently contribute to improved exercise capacity. It appears that vigorous exercise training in old age can lead to levels of muscle oxidative capacity as high as those in young individuals undergoing similar training (Cartee 1994).

Several longitudinal studies have shown that endurance training increases the capacity of skeletal muscle to oxidize substrates in older individuals. Training increases mitochondrial cytochrome oxidase (Orlander and Aniansson 1980) and Krebs cycle enzyme activity (Souminen et al. 1977) in the elderly to the same degree as in young subjects. Seals and colleagues (1984) attributed the improvement in peak VO_2 after aerobic training mainly to a better ability of the skeletal muscles to extract oxygen. Reduced systemic vascular resistance after training suggests increased capillary density as the mechanism by which this occurs. In support of these studies, Meredith et al. (1989) convincingly demonstrated dramatic peripheral musculoskeletal adaptations to endurance training in the elderly when compared to young controls subjected to a similar exercise protocol. After 12 weeks of aerobic training at 70% peak VO_2, muscle glycogen stores and muscle oxidative capacity increased 28% and 128%, respectively, while remaining unchanged in young controls. Although cardiac output was not measured, the dramatic increase in muscle oxidative capacity in older subjects (compared to no peripheral changes in young subjects) suggests that peripheral alterations may play an important role in improving peak VO_2 with training in the elderly. In contrast, younger subjects may be more dependent on cardiovascular adaptations such as cardiac output for training-induced increases in $\dot{V}O_2$max.

It is important to emphasize again the specific physiologic effects of exercise modalities: although aerobic training can induce oxidative changes in skeletal muscle (along with many other benefits), it generally does not improve muscle mass or strength in

Table 20.2　Controlled Aerobic Training Studies in the Elderly

Author	Study		Exercise protocol					Outcomes	
	Mean age (range) gender	Number (test/control)	Exercise type	Duration (wk)	Frequency (#/wk)	Intensity	Session length (min)	Physiologic outcomes	Functional/quality-of-life outcomes
Adams et al. (1973)	65.6 (52–79) F	23	Calisthenics, walk-jog program	12	3	60% MHRR	35–45	↑VO₂ 21%	
Suominen et al. (1977)	61.9 (52–70) M	31	Ball activities, jogging	8	3–5	HR up to 130–140 bpm	10–20	↑VO₂ 11% ↑Oxidative enzymes	
Badenhop et al. (1983)*	68 M/F	32 (8/24)	Cycling	9	3	Lo (30–45% MHRR), Hi (60–75% MHRR)	25	↑VO₂ 17% (lo) ↑VO₂ 14% (hi)	
Seals et al. (1984)*	63 (60–69) M/F	21 (13/8)	Walking, jogging, cycling	52 (26 wk lo, 26 wk hi)	3–4	Lo (40% MHRR), Hi (75% MHRR)	Lo (20–30) Hi (30–40)	↑VO₂ 12% lo ↑VO₂ 30% hi ↓Fat 13% ↑AVO₂ diff. No change cardiac output ↓Submax BP	
Thomas et al. (1985)*	63 M	188	Walking, jogging	52	3	65–70% MHRR	30	↑VO₂ 12% ↓Skinfolds	
Thompson et al. (1988)*	73 (64–83) M/F	35 (9 dropouts)	Dance	16	3	60–75% MHRR	20	No change in exercise capacity (METs)	

Study	Age/Sex	N	Mode	Weeks	Intensity	Min	Results
Hagberg et al. (1989)*	72.3 (70-79) M/F	47 (16 aerobic, 19 strength, 12 controls)	Walking, jogging, treadmill vs. upper/low ext. dynamic resistance training	26	50-70% MHRR Lo-mod strength	40	↑VO_2 22% in aerobic group only ↑Strength 9-18% in strength group only ↓Fat 6-8% in both groups
Sagiv et al. (1989)*	67 M	40 (20 aerobic/20 strength)	Running vs. strength	12	70% $\dot{V}O_2$max, 30% MVC	30	↑VO_2 12.5% in aerobic group ↓% fat
Meredith et al. (1989)	65.1 vs. 23.6 M/F	20 (10 old vs. 10 young)	Cycling	12	70% MHRR	45	↑VO_2 23% in old vs. 14% in young group ↑Oxidative enzymes
Blumenthal et al. (1989)*	67 (60-83) M/F	101 (50/51)	Cycling, jogging, arm ergometry	16	70% MHRR	45	↑VO_2 11.6% ↑AT 13%
Foster et al. (1989)*	78 (67-89) F	16	Walking	10	Lo (40% MHRR), Mod (60% HRR)	25-35	↑VO_2 12% lo ↑VO_2 15% mod
Naso et al. (1990)*	64-97 Nursing home	15 (4 dropouts)	Upper/lower extremity	52	80% MHRR (rarely achieved)	20	No change in VO_2
Ehsani et al. (1991)	64 (60-70) M	10	Walking, cycling, running	52	60-80% MHRR	60	↑VO_2 26% ↑Exercise cardiac function ↑Resting cardiac function

(continued)

*Randomized control trial

Lo = low; mod = moderate; hi = high

AT = anaerobic threshold; LVEF = left ventricular ejection fraction; MHRR = maximal heart rate reserve; MVC = maximal voluntary contraction; SV = stroke volume; VT = ventilatory threshold; HR = heart rate; AVO_2 = arterial-venous

Table 20.2   (continued)

	Study		Exercise protocol					Outcomes	
Author	Mean age (range) gender	Number (test/control)	Exercise type	Duration (wk)	Frequency (#/wk)	Intensity	Session length (min)	Physiologic outcomes	Functional/quality-of-lfe outcomes
Belman et al. (1991)*	68 (65-75) M/F	25 (13/12)	Walking	8	4	Lo (35% MHRR), Hi (75% MHRR)	30	↑VO$_2$ 7% in both groups	
Kohrt et al. (1991)	64 (60-71) vs. 25 (20-30) M/F	156 (53/57 old) (28/18 young)	Walking, jogging, cycling, rowing	36-52	4	60-85% HR max	30-50	↑VO$_2$ 24% with no gender or age effect	
McMurdo et al. (1992)*	65 (60-81) M/F	87	Combined	32	3	Lo	45	↑Knee/spine flexion ↑Back/leg strength	↑Life satisfaction, perceived health status, max physical exertion scores
Hamdorf et al. (1992)*	64.8 (60-70) F	80	Walking	52	2	Not specified	15-45	↓Resting HR 7.4% ↓Submax exercise HR 6.9%	↑Maximal activity level
Posner et al. (1992)*	68 (60-86) M/F	247 (94/153)	Cycling	16	3	45% MHRR	40	↑VO$_2$ 8.5%	

Study	Age	N (M/F)	Mode	Weeks	Days/wk	Intensity	Duration (min)	Outcomes	
Sheldahl et. al. (1993)	60-71 vs. (35-50) M	27	Treadmill, cycling	26	3	85% HR max	40	↑VO$_2$ 12% in both groups ↓Submax HR in both groups	No change in psych outcomes
Levy et al. (1993)	68 (60-82) vs. 28 (24-32) M	31 (14 old vs. 17 young)	Jogging, cycling	26	4-5	50-85% MHRR	45	↑VO$_2$ 19% in both groups ↑Resting and exercise cardiac function ↑Cardiac mass	
Warren et al. (1993)*	74 (67-85) F	30	Walking	12	5	60% MHRR	30-40	↑VO$_2$ 12.6%	
Stratton et al. (1994)	68 (60-82) vs. 28 (24-32) M	24 (13 old vs. 11 young)	Walking, jogging, cycling	26	4-5	5-85% MHRR	45	↑VO$_2$ 21% (↑17% in young group) ↑Resting SV 18% ↑Exercise cardiac function due to ↑ end diastolic volume in old group	
Barry et al. (1996)	70 (55-78) M/F	14 (8/6)	Cycling	12	3	Mod-hi	16-25	↑VO$_2$ 38%	
Fabre et al. (1997)*	64 (53-74) M/F	16 (6/10)	Walking, jogging	12	2	VT vs. 50% MHRR	60	↑VO$_2$ 20% in VT trained group ↓Submax HR	

the elderly (Harridge et al. 1997; Meredith et al. 1989). Those improvements come only from resistance training.

Resistance (Strength) Training

Resistance or strength training represents the other major exercise modality. In **strength training,** the resistance against which a muscle generates force is progressively increased over time. The tremendous clinical and functional consequences of declining muscle mass and strength have focused attention on the effects of strength training as a way to reverse sarcopenia. Progressive resistance training (PRT) has been consistently shown to increase muscle strength and mass in young individuals (Delorme 1945; MacDougall 1986). Despite studies showing that resistance training below 40% of the 1 repetition maximum (RM) results in no change in muscle strength, earlier investigators seemed reluctant to train older subjects at high intensities (>70% of the 1 RM) (Aniansson and Gustafsson 1981; Larsson 1982). Only in relatively recent years have investigators studied progressive resistance overload in older populations (Fiatarone et al. 1990; Fiatarone et al. 1994).

Effect on Musculoskeletal Strength

The most basic physiologic response to strength training is an increase in muscle strength, usually measured by maximal voluntary contraction. Table 20.3 summarizes a number of randomized strength-training studies in older individuals. Male and female subjects ranged in age from 42-98 years, using training modalities that included free or stacked weights, elastic tubing, or pneumatic resistance equipment. Training intensity, often measured as a percentage of 1 RM, ranged from low (30%-40% of 1 RM) to high. Training frequency typically was 2-3 times per week, each session lasting 30-60 minutes, in studies that lasted from eight weeks to two years. The muscles trained were the large muscles of the upper and lower extremities (since they are important for key functional tasks). Although varied protocols make comparisons among studies difficult, most investigators report increases in strength after resistance training in older subjects.

As with aerobic training, strength training effects depend on intensity, duration, frequency, and length. Higher intensities apparently lead to greater increases in strength (Buchner 1993). While studies involving low intensities in older adults have reported strength

increases of <20% (Fisher et al. 1991; Larsson 1982), high-intensity training has resulted in increases of up to 227% (Fiatarone et al. 1990; Frontera et al. 1988). These controlled trials strongly suggest that, if they engage in training of sufficiently high intensity, older men and women can attain strength gains at least similar to those of their younger counterparts. Overall, muscle strength gains have been the greatest when trained between 60%-100% of the 1 RM (Evans 1995; MacDougall 1986).

In addition to increasing muscle strength, strength training also improves submaximal muscle performance (muscle endurance) in older adults. Brown et al. (1990) showed that muscle endurance—defined in their study as the ability to lift the initial maximal 1 RM weight—increased from 1 repetition to 7-19 repetitions, changing a previously maximal activity to a submaximal one. This change theoretically could improve an individual's ability to perform activities requiring sustained submaximal effort (e.g., climbing a flight of stairs) rather than a single maximal effort (lifting objects whose weight is at the limit of the person's ability). Finally, the physiologic benefits of strength training can extend even to overall exercise capacity in the elderly (Grimby 1992). One randomized trial showed that submaximal walking increased 38% after strength training, while remaining unchanged in the controls (Ades et al. 1996).

Effect on Muscle Mass

An earlier study by Moritani and deVries (1980) in younger vs. older men showed no changes in muscle mass resulting from resistance training in older individuals. Although both groups increased maximal isometric strength following their eight-week training protocol, only the younger men demonstrated significant enlargements in muscle cross-sectional area as measured by girth. The authors concluded that neural factors alone might be responsible for the improvements in strength seen in older subjects. In contrast, Frontera et al. (1988) reported not only dramatic gains in lower-extremity 1 RM strength in older men following 12 weeks of strength training, but also an 11% increase in total thigh area as measured by computerized tomography (CT) and an increase in protein turnover. Subsequent studies confirmed hypertrophic responses, even in the oldest-old—in some cases even with a magnitude similar to that reported in younger subjects (Brown et al. 1990; Charette et al. 1991; Fiatarone et al. 1990).

In several studies reviewed by Porter and Vandervoort (1995) and by Hopp (1993), microscopic examination of skeletal muscle revealed enlargement of both type I (slow) and type II (fast) muscle fiber areas after strength training, with increases in fiber size ranging from 14% to 62%. When changes were small or nonsignificant, they were associated with small strength gains. The rate of protein synthesis in response to short-term resistance training appears to be similar regardless of age (Frontera et al. 1988; Yarasheski et al. 1993). These studies provide evidence that, even into old age, muscle retains the capacity for hypertrophy; but the limits of this response with long-term training remain to be determined.

Effect on Bone Density

Several randomized controlled studies support the notion that resistance exercises may directly counteract osteopenic processes and indirectly attenuate the morbid consequences of osteoporosis. Strength training directly increases bone density (Nelson et al. 1994; Menkes et al. 1993). Indirectly, strength training reduces the adverse effects of osteoporosis by improving balance, and thereby theoretically lowering the risk of falls and fractures (Nelson et al. 1994). Whether strength training or exercise in general reduces the risk of fracture has yet to be proven.

Neurologic Adaptations

Because the magnitude of muscle hypertrophy is relatively small compared to much greater strength increases, a large part of strength gains may result from neural adaptations (Sale 1988). Furthermore, strength gains are not fully transferable to different testing modalities (1 RM vs. isometric or isokinetic contraction)—suggesting that, for any given movement, formation of specific neural adaptations leads to a certain amount of skill or motor coordination. Brown et al. (1990) found that nearly complete (98%) motor unit activation was achieved before and after training in the elbow flexors during a maximal voluntary contraction (MVC), inferring that nervous system activation is not the problem. It is possible, therefore, that dynamic maneuvers depend more on central nervous system coordination or activation than isometric movements.

Miscellaneous Training Modalities

The importance of specificity of exercise modalities has been increasingly recognized in recent years, leading

to heightened regard for other modalities of exercise such as balance training (e.g., tai chi and yoga). Balance and its neuromuscular foundations deteriorate with age, but less predictably than strength does (Hindmarsh and Estes 1989; Woollacott 1993), and it is responsive to training (Wolfson et al. 1993; Wolfson et al. 1996). Table 20.4 lists results from controlled clinical trials that have included balance training.

There is no consensus regarding which of the critical elements of motor behavior must be trained to improve balance, or even how best to measure balance. Requiring central, peripheral, sensory, and motor input and coordination, balance turns out to be one of the most complex, multidimensional domains of function to study. A major problem is that few investigators have used randomized controlled studies in looking at balance (Wolfson et al. 1993). Of those studies that were randomized, most did not separate the effects of balance training, but included it as a part of the overall training program, making it impossible to isolate balance from other factors. To further confound matters, muscle strength independently contributes to balance (Wolfson et al. 1995). Studies that have attempted to improve balance in older adults have been characterized by highly variable subject compositions, study designs, and intervention descriptions.

Flexibility training represents the last but perhaps the most basic major exercise modality. A common complaint in the elderly, lack of flexibility may result both from connective tissue changes and from lack of frequent movements through each joint's full range of motion. Ideally, people should incorporate these actions into the warm-up and cooldown periods of both aerobic and strength-training regimens. For the frailest individuals, flexibility exercises may even form the mainstay of physical therapy.

Can Exercise Reverse Functional Decline Associated With Aging?

The problem of aging as it pertains ultimately to functional decline has been central to this chapter. Nagi (1965, 1991) defines this decline, the "disablement process," as a progression from *physiologic impairments* to *functional limitations* to *disability*. Because of the well-established ability of exercise to influence numerous age-related physiologic changes, exercise has held much promise as an intervention to modify the

Table 20.3   Recent Controlled Resistance Training Studies in the Elderly

	Study		Exercise protocol				Outcomes	
Author	**Mean age (range) gender**	**Number (test/control)**	**Exercise type**	**Duration (wk)**	**Frequency (sets/reps)**	**Intensity**	**Physiologic outcomes**	**Functional outcomes**
Charette et al. (1991)*	69 (64–86) F	19	Lower extremity	12	3 ×/wk 6/6	65–75% 1 RM**	↑Strength 28–115% ↑Muscle fiber size	
Meredith et al. (1992)*	(61–72) M	11	Knee	12	3 ×/wk 3/8	80% 1 RM	↑Strength 104% ↑MM 12%	
Nichols et al. (1993)*	67.8 F	30	Upper/lower extremity	24	3 ×/wk 3/(8–10)	80% 1 RM**	↑Strength 18–71% ↑Lean tissue ↓Body fat No change BMD	
Menkes et al. (1993)*	59 (50–70) M	18	Upper/lower extremity	16	3 ×/wk (1–2)/15	Hi**	↑Strength 45% ↑BMD	
Campbell et al. (1994)*	65 (56–80) M/F	12 (6/6)	Upper/lower extremity	12	3 ×/wk 3/8	80% 1 RM**	↑Strength 24–92% ↑Fat-free mass ↓Fat mass	
Fiatarone et al. (1994)*	(72–98) M/F (Nursing home)	100 (37/63)	Hip/knee extension	10	3 ×/wk 3/8	80% 1 RM**	↑Strength 26–216%	↑Physical activity, stair climb, gait speed
Pyka et al. (1994)*	67.2 (61–78) M/F	25 (8/17)	Upper/lower extremity	30 52 (n = 14)	3 ×/wk 3/8	65–75% 1 RM**	↑Strength 23–62% ↑Strength 30–95% (52 wks) ↑Muscle fiber size 20–62%	

Reference	Age (range) Sex	N (M/F)	Exercise type	Duration (wk)	Frequency	Intensity	Outcomes	Additional
Nelson et al. (1994)*	71 (50-70) F	39	Upper/lower extremity	52	2 ×/wk 3/8	80% 1 RM**	↑Strength 20-65% ↑MM 5.5% ↑BMD	↑Static and dynamic balance ↓Fall risk
Skelton et al. (1995)*	79.5 (75-93) F	40	Upper/lower extremity	12, home-based	3 ×/wk 3/4-8	Low**	↑Strength 22-27%	No change in functional performance
Morganti et al. (1995)*	59.9 F	39	Upper/lower extremity	52	2 ×/wk	80% 1 RM**	↑Strength 35-77%	
McCartney et al. (1995)*	(60-80) M/F	142 (63/79)	Upper/lower extremity	42	2 ×/wk (2-3)/ (10-12)	50-80% 1 RM**	↑Strength 20-65% ↑MM 5.5% ↑Treadmill time 18%	No change in functional performance
Lexell et al. (1996)	(70-77) M/F	35 (19/16)	Unilateral Upper/lower extremity	52 (3 phases)	1-11 (I): 3 ×/wk 12-38 (II): 1 ×/wk 39-52 (III): 3 ×/wk	85% 1 RM**	I: ↑Strength 49-163% II: ↑6% III: ↑32% ↑Muscle fiber size ↑% Type II fibers	
Jette et al. (1996)*	73 (66-87) M/F	93 (34/59)	Upper/lower extremity (therabands)	32, home-based	3 ×/wk 1/8	Low**	↑Strength 0-10%	↑Mood
Ades et al. (1996)*	70.4 (65-79) M/F	24 (11/13)	Upper/lower extremity	12	3 ×/wk 3/8	50-80% 1 RM**	↑Strength 29-65% ↑Fat-free mass	↑Walking time 38%
Welle et al. (1996)	(62-78) vs. (22-31) M/F	17 (9/8)	Upper/lower extremity	12	3 ×/wk 3/8	80% 3 RM**	↑Strength 21-64% ↑MM 1-9%	

*Randomized control trial

**Progressive resistance training protocol

BMD = bone mineral density; MM = muscle mass; RM = repetition max

409

Table 20.4   Controlled Balance/Combined Exercise Training Studies in the Elderly

	Study		Exercise protocol				Outcomes		
Author	Mean age (range) gender	Number (test/ control)	Exercise type	Duration (wk)	Frequency #/wk	Intensity	Physiologic outcomes	Functional outcomes
Crilly et al. (1989)*	82 (72-92) F (Nursing home)	50	Stretching Balance Strength	12	3	Low		No change in balance
Judge et al. (1993)*	82 (71-97) M/F	31	Strength Balance Tai chi	12	3	75-80% 1 RM	↑Strength 25-32%	↑Habitual gait speed 8%
Judge et al. (1993)*	68 (62-75) F	21	Walking Strength Tai chi	26	3	70% HRmax 70% 1 RM** (mod-hi)	No change in strength	Improved balance
Cress et al. (1991)	72 (65-86) F	27	Aerobic Strength (mostly aerobic)	50	3	60-70% HRR; Low-intensity resistance	↑VO$_2$ 16% ↑Strength 6-8% ↑Muscle fiber size	No change in functional performance
Lord et al. (1995, 1996)	72 (60-85) F	197	Aerobic Strength Balance Stretching	52	2	Low	↑Strength ↑Reaction time	Improved balance ↓Balance-related falls ↑Gait speed
Buchner et al. (1996)*	75 (68-85) M/F	105	Cycling Strength	24-26	3	75% HRR, 60-75% 1 RM (mod-hi)	↑VO$_2$ ↑Strength	Improved fall risk, health care use; no change in balance, gait, health status

Wolfson et al. (1996)*	79 M/F	110	Balance Strength Tai chi (phase 2)	36 (12 phase 1; 24 phase 2)	3(phase 1) 1(phase 2)	Mod-high	↑Strength 20%	↑Improved balance; no change in gait
Wolf et al. (1996)*	76 M/F	200	Tai chi Balance	15	TC: ≥2 Bal: 1	Low-mod	↑Grip strength; improved post-exertional BP	↓Fall risk ↓Fear of falling
Rooks et al. (1997)*	72 (65–95) M/F	131	Walking Strength	40	3	Low	↑Strength 65%	↑Improved balance, stair climb, physical performance, reaction time
Lan et al. (1998)	65 (58–70) M/F	38	Tai chi	52	5	Moderate	↑VO_2 16% ↑Strength 15–18% ↑Flexibility	Did not measure

*Randomized control trial

**Progressive resistance training protocol

BMD = bone mineral density; BP = blood pressure; HRR = heart rate reserve; MM = muscle mass; RM = repetition max; TC = tai chi

disablement process. The promise, however, has yet to be conclusively demonstrated. The challenges and evidence for exercise interventions to modify disability will now be presented.

How Is Function Measured?

The problem of aging as it pertains to physical function is central to this chapter. Because function comprises so many elements—including physiological, biomechanical, medical, and (perhaps most importantly) psychological components—measuring function proves to be one of the greatest challenges in gerontologic research. At present there is no standard way to measure function. Absent an agreed-upon standard, most researchers have measured function by using one or a combination of three variables, or "domains":

1. Physiologic capacity
2. Functional capacity
3. Functional status

Figure 20.3 represents these domains as a "functional measurement spectrum," the components of which correspond roughly to the components of Nagi's disablement process: physiologic capacity as a measure of physiologic impairment, functional capacity as a measure of functional limitation, and functional status as a measure of disability.

Physiologic capacity refers to the ability of the body's organs and organ systems to perform under physical stress. Examples are muscle strength, cardiac function, and $\dot{V}O_2max$. As reviewed earlier, the aging or disablement process is characterized by physiologic impairments or homeostenosis of many organ systems, although the rate and magnitude of decline is highly variable. Most clinical studies begin by characterizing physiologic changes in response to an intervention such as exercise.

In recent years, researchers have increasingly described functional declines according to changes in **functional capacity** or physical performance (Applegate et al. 1990; Guralnik et al. 1989). Corresponding to the functional limitations domain in Nagi's disablement process, this domain is assessed by observed tests of function and is generally viewed as a "transitional" domain along the functional measurement spectrum. Examples of functional capacity tests are stair-climbing power, chair stand ability, forward reach, gait speed, balance tests, or a battery of scored tests such as those proposed by Guralnik et al. (1994) or Reuben and Siu (1990). Tests of function—often timed, and usually administered by a trained tester—theoretically reflect tasks that are performed in daily life (Cress et al. 1995). Furthermore, functional capacity tests can independently predict disability and nursing home placement (Guralnik et al. 1995).

Functional status, corresponding to the disability domain in Nagi's disablement process, represents the

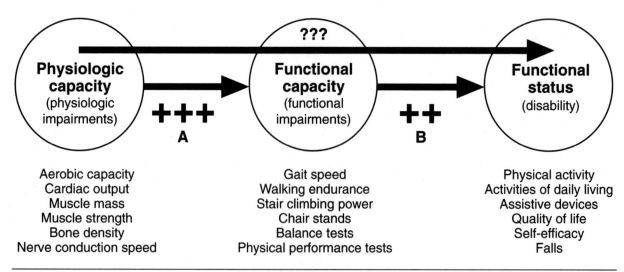

Figure 20.3 The "Functional Measurement Spectrum," showing the three major function measurement domains. These domains roughly correspond to the components (in parentheses) of Nagi's disablement process (Nagi 1965). Evidence supports an association between the domains of *physiologic capacity* and *functional capacity* as well as *functional capacity* and *functional status*. These relationships may be more curvilinear than linear. Whether exercise-generated improvements in physiologic capacity can translate to improvements in functional capacity **and** functional status (and, therefore, decreased disability) is the focus of ongoing clinical trials. *Source:* (A: Alexander et al. 1991; Buchner and deLateur 1991; Buchner et al. 1996; Bassey et al. 1992; Cunningham et al. 1992, Jette et al. 1998; B: Guralnik et al. 1994; Guralnik et al. 1995).

third major way to measure function. Behavioral factors—such as mood, self-motivation, self-efficacy, and even familial/societal roles expectations—become increasingly important as one moves into this domain along the "functional measurement spectrum." Self-reports and questionnaires provide most of the input for assessments of functional status, including such items as difficulties with and dependency on others for activities of daily living, use of assistive devices, falls, and nursing home residence. It is important to note that having or regaining the physiological or functional capacity to perform a certain task does not automatically translate into the performance of that task in daily life. For instance, most individuals use the escalator/elevator even when they have the physical capacity to walk up the stairs. This multidimensional characteristic of this domain highlights the difficulty in not only accurately measuring, but also effecting a change in, functional status. Until a universally accepted tool to measure function emerges, function will usually be assessed using a combination of all three domains.

The Relationship Between Physiologic Capacity and Functional Status

The theoretical relationship between physiologic capacity and functional status implies that exercise can improve functional status. Although many investigators conceptualize these relationships as being linear, they are probably better characterized as being curvilinear, i.e., physical function improves with improvements in physiologic capacity *up to a point*—a functional threshold, past which physical function does not improve further no matter how great one's physiologic capacity (otherwise weightlifters, whose physiologic capacity can be phenomenal, would walk at super speeds and veritably fly up stairs!). This curvilinear relationship between physiology and function has been supported by growing cross-sectional evidence in recent years (Posner et al. 1995; Buchner et al. 1996; Jette et al. 1998). The implication for older individuals then becomes to strive for their highest physiologic capacities so they can reach and exceed that minimum functional threshold—below which they are functionally impaired but above which they are acceptably functional (figure 20.4) (Buchner et al. 1992). And they reach that threshold through exercise. The curvilinear nature of the relationship between physical function and physiologic capacity may explain why correlations between function and physiologic capacity (e.g., strength) are sometimes absent

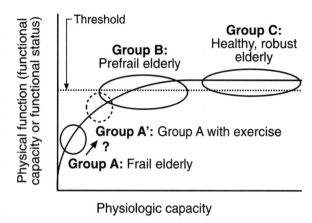

Figure 20.4 The theoretical curvilinear relationship between *Physiologic Capacity* and Physical Function (*Functional Capacity* or *Functional Status*). Here a threshold effect is shown where **above** the threshold, function is **not** influenced by changes in physiologic capacity; and **below** it, function **is** influenced by physiologic changes. This curvilinear relationship implies that the benefit from exercise depends on the group targeted, with the most impaired being **Group A**, the frail elderly, who hypothetically have the most to gain from improvements in physiologic capacities. The ability of exercise to improve function in **Group A** to **Group A'**, although promising, needs further study.
With permission, from the *Annual Review of Public Health,* Volume 13, © 1992, by Annual Reviews.

in cross-sectional studies of older, but healthy, nonfrail adults—if they are already above the threshold, improvements in strength should not bring corresponding improvements in function. For example, no correlation has been shown between leg strength and gait speed in healthy, independent older adults (Danneskiold-Samsoe et al. 1984).

Functional Benefits of Aerobic Training

Older adults respond to aerobic training with gains in aerobic capacity comparable to those of younger adults. Several classic prospective studies strongly support the benefits of aerobic activity on overall mortality (Paffenbarger et al. 1986; Sandvik et al. 1993). Lee and colleagues (1995) observed that men engaged in vigorous exercise training extended their lives on average by two years. The benefits extended even to individuals who began exercise programs after leading previously sedentary lives (Lee et al. 1997; Paffenbarger et al. 1993). Recently, Hakim et al. (1998) demonstrated in a 12-year prospective study that regular walking correlates with a lower overall mortality. Unfortunately, we have little information on the extent to which aerobic fitness as measured in a laboratory transfers to "real-life" functional outcomes. Cross-sectional studies, however, support the notion that individuals who have engaged in regular physical activity throughout their lives tend to maintain higher levels of function and experience fewer declines in functional status (Fries et al. 1994; LaCroix et al. 1996).

The simplest reason for older sedentary individuals to begin (or to continue) exercising is that sustained activities of daily living at submaximal levels of exertion will require less effort. Since the loss of aerobic capacity in sedentary adults can be as much as 1% per year, 80- to 90-year-olds may be functioning at or above their maximal aerobic potential during simple activities of daily living. Evans (1995) has estimated the oxygen costs of a number of daily activities, comparing them with the average $\dot{V}O_2$max of sedentary 75- to 80-year-old men and women. Because these tasks represent an increasingly large percentage of individuals' maximum potentials, it is not difficult to see why many elderly choose not to perform them. By improving $\dot{V}O_2$max, aerobic exercise training may substantially enhance quality of life by increasing endurance and thereby functional independence.

The long-term benefits of aerobic exercise on morbidity have also been shown. Fries et al. (1994) demonstrated that aerobic training attenuated morbidity, disability scores, and health care costs in an eight-year longitudinal study of 50- to 72-year-old runners who averaged 26 running miles/week. The difference in these outcomes between lifelong exercisers and nonexercisers was most dramatic in the oldest age group (>75 years). Hopkins et al. (1990) examined 53 sedentary elderly women participating in a dance-oriented fitness program. After 12 weeks of this low-impact aerobic-type exercise, the intervention group, compared with the control group, improved in cardiovascular endurance, body agility, flexibility, and balance. Although promising in its ability to mitigate the effects of aging on physiologic and functional capacity, the therapeutic efficacy of aerobic training on functional status and disability remains to be definitively proven.

Functional Benefits of Strength Training

Limited information is available on how gains in strength and muscle mass, as measured in the laboratory, apply to "real life." Most published data, however, support the notion that strength training can improve physical performance (Ades et al. 1996;

Fiatarone et al. 1994; Nelson et al. 1994). Some researchers have found little or no effect on functional measures (Buchner et al. 1997; McCartney et al. 1995). Different subject characteristics and levels of frailty may account for the differences in response. No study has conclusively demonstrated the effect of strength training on functional status, although there is anecdotal evidence for such an effect (Fiatarone et al. 1990). The theoretical benefits of strength training for function stem from the argument that the strength requirements for even basic tasks, such as rising from a chair or maintaining balance, exceed the capabilities of many frail individuals (Schultz 1992). Fiatarone et al. (1990) were the first to report functional outcomes in a randomized clinical trial, testing strength training in the frailest and oldest-old. The subjects dramatically increased in muscle strength, and noted positive functional changes for mobility—specifically, habitual gait velocity and stair-climbing ability—and spontaneous physical activity. Nelson et al. (1994) demonstrated that strength training not only improved bone density, but also improved static and dynamic balance and gait, thereby reducing risks associated with significant injurious falls. The increases in physical performance, however, were significantly less than the increases in measured strength (see figure 20.5). The impressive gains in strength may, therefore, only partially transfer to clinical or functional outcomes. Thus far no one has formally investigated why this is true. The research needs to be done. At present, we can say only that physi-

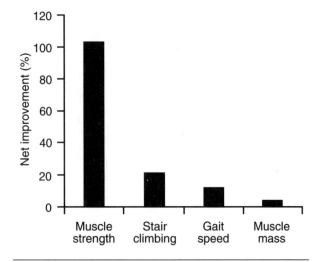

Figure 20.5 Differences in net percent improvement of leg strength, stair-climbing power, gait speed, and thigh muscle area following a high-intensity progressive resistance training program in very frail, elderly nursing home subjects.

From, J. Posner, and K. McCully. 1996. Exercise. In *Principles of geriatrics*, ed. D. Jahnigan. Cambridge, England: Blackwell Science. Reprinted by permission of Blackwell Science, Inc.

ologic capacity (e.g., strength) *contributes* to functional measures, but clearly does not determine the whole story.

Functional Benefits of Balance Training

Table 20.4 lists the functional outcomes of published exercise experiments that involved a balance component. Although earlier studies by Crilly et al. (1989) and Lichtenstein et al. (1989) showed no improvement in balance measures, the majority of published studies support the notion that exercise programs that include a balance component improve balance measures and decrease the risk of falls (Nelson et al. 1994;Wolfson et al. 1993). As with earlier aerobic and strength-training trials that showed negative results, the earlier balance training studies may have been limited by low training intensities. In a meta-analysis of exercise training in elderly patients, interventions that included general exercise reduced fall incidence by 10%; exercise interventions that included balance training had an even greater effect, with a 17% reduction in falls (Province et al. 1995). As noted earlier, there is still no consensus regarding which of the critical elements of motor behavior should be trained to result in improved balance, or what measures of balance validly reflect its complexity.

Summary of Effects of Exercise on Aging

In summary, the idea that exercise can improve functional status continues to show tremendous promise, but the evidence is still inconclusive. While many studies demonstrate positive effects of exercise on *physiologic* and *functional capacity*, most have lacked statistical power to detect changes in *functional status*. Adding to the methodological challenges is the heterogeneous nature of the elderly population and the difficulty in precisely targeting subgroups within this population, such as those who are frail or prefrail. Lack of adequate and sensitive instruments to test function has also been limiting. Epidemiological evidence, however, supports a strong correlation between physical activity, exercise habits, and functional decline (Harris et al. 1989; Kuta et al. 1970; Simonsick et al. 1993). We also know that functional capacity, as measured by tests that observe physical performance, correlates with and predicts functional status (Guralnik et al. 1994; Guralnik et al. 1995). Further, we know that exercise training has the potential to affect many of the "nonfixed" contributors to functional decline in the elderly, such as chronic disuse and morbidity from chronic disease. Evidence from controlled clinical trials shows that exercise of an appropriate type and intensity improves many measures of physiologic and functional capacity. Whether functional capacity reflected through performance-based test improvement translates to improved functional status, however, remains unproven but the focus of current ongoing clinical trials. Figure 20.3 summarizes the currently understood status of these relationships.

Practical Recommendations

We present here only general guidelines, since detailed guidelines are beyond the scope of this chapter and are found elsewhere (Barry and Eathorne 1994; Dishman 1994; Pollock et al. 1994). The key point is that age by itself should not be a deterrent to exercise—but, in fact, should be one of the most important indications to begin or to continue exercising.

Setting Goals

Older adults have widely differing goals, reflecting the heterogeneity of their population. On one end of the spectrum are the robust, nonfrail, healthy elderly who may have been exercising for many years. Goals for these individuals include preserving vitality, function, and independence for as long as possible. They should be challenged to extend themselves by increasing intensity or including other modalities such as resistance training. On the other end of the functional spectrum are the frail elderly who, by living at the limits of their physiologic and functional capacity, struggle with normal activities of daily living. Within this frail elderly group are some who are physically dependent and others who may still be independent, albeit marginally. The goals here should be to improve or restore functional capacity so that activities of daily living may be easier. Between these two extremes are the majority of older adults—the typically aging, sedentary elderly—the prefrail who are at imminent risk for becoming frail. While most of the elderly in this group have had minimal if any experience with exercise, it is they who have the most to gain by altering their sedentary ways. Reversing and preventing the downward functional spiral associated with the typical, sedentary aging process should be the primary goal for this group.

The Training Program

The ideal exercise program should be tailored to the older adult, using a combination of aerobic, resistance, stretching, and balance training. However, unlike training programs in younger adults that usually emphasize aerobic training, we believe that resistive exercises may be the most beneficial form of exercise, at least initially, for the frail elderly. An effective program will use all exercise modalities, and target large muscle groups of the upper and lower body such as the legs, arms, shoulders, calves, and back. As with younger adults, the elderly should train aerobically 3-5 days/week, 5-60 minutes/session. Strength training, on 2-3 nonconsecutive days/week, should include 2-3 sets of 8-12 repetitions for each muscle group, with short rests between sets.

Although studies show that the elderly can train safely at and respond to high-intensity exercise sessions, it is probably wise to begin at lower intensities (either by self-perception, 30%-50% 1 RM, or 40%-50% HRmax) and gradually work up to higher intensity levels. Frequent use of an exercise intensity scale such as Borg's Ratings of Perceived Exertion scale is strongly recommended.

Finally, an exercise program for the elderly should be progressive, although the rate of progression may need to be more gradual than with younger individuals. An improvement in physiologic capacity (strength or aerobic capacity) may occur just by increasing muscle repetitions or aerobic duration; however, most older people reach a limit where further physiologic gains are not possible without increased resistance or aerobic training intensity. On the other hand, intensity is not necessarily as important as participation for most elderly participants. No exercise program is effective unless the individual continues with the program. *The highest priority in regulating training intensity is to enhance exercise compliance.* A reasonable intensity goal for older adults is one that feels "somewhat hard" to "hard" on the Borg scale. Another guideline is the "talk test," whereby people know they are exercising excessively when they cannot carry on a conversation while exercising. A few missed exercise sessions are insignificant when the goals are long-term, and should not discourage the older participant from continuing.

Special Considerations

Although the same general principles of exercise employed for younger adults (e.g., intensity, training regimen, and frequency) apply also to the elderly, unique characteristics of the older adult require some special considerations.

"Start Low, Go Slow"

Reduced physiologic reserve, and therefore longer recoveries from injury, make the geriatric axiom "start low, go slow" perhaps the most important guideline for older individuals who begin exercising. Close supervision and attention to proper form are very important, given the risk for musculoskeletal injury. Pollock et al. (1991) have reported rates of soft tissue injury up to 57% among elderly participants in training programs that included a jogging component. Warm-up and cooldown calisthenics involving large muscle groups should initiate and end each exercise session. Older adults must avoid breath holding, which can cause great increases in blood pressure, especially during strengthening exercises where Valsalvas tend to naturally occur. Proper technique typically involves *inhaling* before the lift or during the eccentric contraction and *exhaling* during the lift (concentric contraction), and avoiding ballistic movements when stretching or lifting weights. Depending on a person's baseline physical state and past experience with exercise, training programs for the elderly may begin first with flexibility training, then progress to resistance exercises, and then to aerobic and balance exercises.

Pre-Exercise Evaluation

Most experts recommend a pre-exercise assessment, including a complete history and physical examination. There are few absolute contraindications for exercising, including the majority of chronic medical conditions that are most prevalent in this population. The most common reason against exercising is any acute or unstable medical condition; and even this contraindication is often temporary. In fact, aerobic and resistance exercise are now even being used as adjunctive treatment in severe but stable cardiopulmonary disease (Beniamini et al. 1997; Ghilarducci et al. 1989). The elderly are also the greatest consumers of medications. Anyone prescribing or overseeing exercise therapy for older people must have a clear understanding of their medications, and of the cardiovascular and neurologic effects of those medications; and should instruct patients to report all changes in their medications. Close monitoring of pulse, blood pressure, and symptoms is crucial at the beginning of an exercise program, and whenever the program is changed.

It is not clear whether a monitored, graded exercise stress test is warranted for every older adult about to embark on an exercise program. The substantial costs of such across-the-board evaluations would decrease the chances that local governments will adopt exercise as a public health measure; they would also limit the participation of many older individuals with limited financial means. Many older individuals on their own have probably participated safely in community-based exercise programs without formal screening. It is our belief that the certain risks of continued, chronic inactivity outweigh the possible risks of exercise.

Cardiac stress testing, however, may be appropriate for individuals with a known or suggestive cardiac history, even for the very old. On the other hand, stress-testing protocols may not be feasible—or even necessary—in the frail elderly for whom the test would present an overwhelming physical or even emotional challenge. For such individuals, close supervision during the exercise activity, with monitoring of blood pressure and pulse, may be sufficient to predict the risks of the proposed program.

Behavioral Issues Motivating the Elderly to Exercise

Young and old individuals generally share similar attitudes about exercise and physical activity, with some exceptions (Dishman 1994). Although both groups have a positive attitude toward exercise, the elderly feel less confident and fear hurting themselves more. A second major difference between adults under and over age 65 is that physically inactive older persons usually have no intention of becoming active. A third difference is that, despite the positive attitudes toward physical activity, most elderly consider it a low priority for leisure time. The unfortunate fact is that most older adults have been sedentary for most of their adult lives. Although it need not do so, beginning an exercise program often represents a major change. The first step usually involves transforming an older person's belief system. Behavioral modification programs developed for and successfully applied to smoking cessation may be increasingly applied to exercise programs as well.

For those who do begin to exercise, adherence is usually poor on the first try. More than 50% of individuals drop out of exercise programs within six months (Borg 1998). Adding counseling, education, or behavior modification, or changing the amount of exercise prescribed, may only modestly increase participation (Dishman 1994). Middle-aged adults are less likely to

begin and continue a vigorous exercise program designed for cardiovascular fitness than one involving less intense activities such as walking or gardening (Dishman 1989). The most successful programs include some combination of ongoing supervision and efforts to monitor and promote compliance.

Unfortunately, there are few guidelines available to help health care professionals increase participation in or adherence to exercise programs by older individuals. It is important to remember that training goals for the elderly often differ from those of younger persons. Rather than focusing on traditional exercise measures such as intensity, workload, or percent of maximal heart rate, programs for the elderly should target ease of mobility, maintenance of flexibility, and strength. It is these outcomes that maximize individuals' function and social integration. Creative, varied programs leading to sustained continuous involvement in exercise may be far more important than the specifics of the exercise regimen. Clearly, more research is needed in this area if we as a nation are to achieve the physical activity objectives set for older adults for the coming millennium.

Summary

The aging process presents challenges to health care systems throughout the world, centered mainly around problems of physical frailty and declining function. This property of function allows the geriatric and physiatric disciplines to intersect. The current aging paradigm attributes age-related declines to a combination of genetics, physiologic aging, chronic illness, medications, and lifestyle—although the degree to which each component contributes to frailty needs much further clarification. Exercise as an intervention, however, produces numerous physiologic changes that appear to counteract effects of the typical aging process. The extent to which these physiologic benefits do and potentially might mitigate functional disability needs further study.

While these and other issues are being clarified, there is little question that exercise is the single most effective way to preserve or even improve function in old age. As stated by Dr. Robert Butler, former director of the National Institutes on Aging, "If exercise could be put in a bottle, it would be the strongest medicine money could buy." With a few exceptions, the general guidelines for exercising apply equally to younger and to older individuals. Exercise programs should focus on long-term goals; and they should be individualized, to address the functional heterogeneity of the aging population Also rehabilitation specialists should not be afraid to "push" their patients to higher levels so long as it is done gradually and carefully. Studies have clearly demonstrated that older adults respond positively to progressive exercise training. Finally, while closely monitoring patients, therapists must exercise clear knowledge of both medication-exercise interactions and comorbid conditions. Ultimately, regardless of age or level of frailty, nearly all elderly persons can derive some physiologic, functional, or quality-of-life benefit from initiating an exercise program.

References

Adams, G.M., and H.A. DeVries. 1973. Physiologic effects of an exercise training regimen upon women aged 52 to 79. *J Gerontol* 28:50-55.

Ades, P.A., D.L. Ballor, T. Ashikaga, J.L. Utton, and K. Sreekumaran. 1996. Weight training improves walking endurance in healthy elderly persons. *Ann Int Med* 124:568-572.

Alexander, N., A.B. Schultz, and D.N. Warwick. 1991. Rising from a chair: effects of age and functional ability on performance biomechanics. *J Gerontol* 46:M91-M98.

Anderson, K., and L. Hermansen. 1965. Aerobic work capacity in middle-aged Norwegian men. *J Appl Physiol* 20:432-436.

Aniansson, A., G. Grimby, and A. Rundgren. 1980. Isometric and isokinetic quadriceps muscle strength in 70-year old men and women. *Scand J Rehab Med* 12:161-168.

Aniansson, A., and E. Gustafsson. 1981. Physical training in elderly men with special reference to quadriceps muscle strength and morphology. *Clin Physiol* 1:87-98.

Aniansson, A., L. Sperling, A. Rundgren, and E. Lehnberg. 1983. Muscle function in 75 year old men and women: a longitudinal study. *Scand J Rehabil* 9:92-102.

Applegate, W.B., J.P. Blass, and T.F. Williams. 1990. Instruments for the functional assessment of older patients. *N Engl J Med* 322:1207-1214.

Åstrand, I., P.O. Åstrand, I. Hallback, and A. Kilbom. 1973. Reduction in maximal oxygen uptake with age. *J Appl Physiol* 35:649.

Badenhop, D., P. Cleary, S.F. Schaal, E.L. Fox, and R.L. Bartels. 1983. Physiological adjustments to higher- or lower-intensity exercise in elders. *Med Sci Sports Exerc* 15:496-502.

Barry, A.J., J.W. Daly, E. D. Pruett, J.R. Steinmetz, H.F. Page, N.C. Birkhead, and K. Rodahl. 1966. The effects of physical conditioning on older individuals. I. Work capacity, circulatory-respiratory function, and work electrocardiogram. *J Gerontol* 21:182-191.

Barry, H.C., and S.W. Eathorne. 1994. Exercise and aging. *Med Clin N Am* 78:357-377.

Bassey, E.J., M.A. Fiatarone, E.F. O'Neil, M. Kelly, W.J. Evans, and L.A. Lipsitz. 1992. Leg extensor power and functional performance in very old men and women. *Clin Sci* 82:321-327.

Bassey, E.J., and A. Short. 1990. A new method for measuring power output in a single leg extension: feasibility, reliability and validity. *Eur J Appl Physiol* 60:385-390.

Baylor, A., and W. Spirduso. 1988. Systemic aerobic exercise and components of reaction time in older women. *J Gerontol* 43:121-126.

Belman, M.J., and G. A. Gaesser. 1991. Exercise training below and above the lactate threshold in the elderly. *Med Sci Sports Exerc* 23:562-568.

Benestad, A. 1965. Trainability of old men. *Acta Med Scand* 178:321-327.

Beniamini, Y., J.J. Rubenstein, and L.D. Zaichowsky. 1997. Effects of high-intensity strength training on quality-of-life parameters in cardiac rehabilitation patients. *Am J Cardiol* 80:841-846.

Bevier, W., R. Wiswell, G. Pyka, K. Kozak, K. Newhall, and R. Marcus. 1989. Relationship of body composition, muscle strength, and aerobic capacity to bone mineral density in older men and women. *J Bone Miner Res* 4:421-432.

Blair, S.N., J.B. Kampert, H.W. Kohn, C.E. Barlow, M.A. Macera, R.S. Paffenbarger, and L.W. Gibbons. 1996. Influences of cardiovascular fitness and other precursors on cardiovascular disease and all-cause mortality in men and women. *JAMA* 276:205-210.

Blumenthal, J.A., C.F. Emery, D. Madden, L.K. George, E. Coleman, M.W. Riddle, D.C. McKee, J. Reasoner, and R.S. Williams. 1989. Cardiovascular and behavioral effects of aerobic exercise training in healthy older men and women. *J Gerontol* 44:M147-M157.

Borg, G. 1998. *Borg's perceived exertion and pain scales*. Champaign, IL: Human Kinetics.

Borkan, G., and A. Norris. 1977. Fat redistribution and the changing body dimensions of the adult male. *Human Biol* 49:495-514.

Bortz, W.M. 1989. Redefining human aging. *J Am Geriatr Soc* 37:1092-1096.

Brown, A.B., N. McCartney, and D.G. Sale. 1990. Positive adaptations to weight-lifting training in the elderly. *J Appl Physiol* 69:1725-1733.

Brown, M., D.R. Sinacore, and H. Host. 1995. The relationship of strength to function in the older adult. *J Gerontol* 50A:55-59.

Buchner, D.M. 1993. Understanding variability in studies of strength training in older adults: a meta-analytic perspective. *Top Geriatr Rehabil* 8:1.

Buchner, D.M., S.A. Beresford, E.B. Larson, A.Z. LaCroix, and E.H. Wagner. 1992. Effects of physical activity on health status in older adults II: intervention studies. *Annu Rev Publ Health* 13:469-488.

Buchner, D.M., M.E. Cress, B.J. deLateur, P.C. Esselman, A.J. Margherita, R. Price, and E.H. Wagner. 1997. The effect of strength and endurance training on gait, balance, fall risk, and health services use in community-living older adults. *J Am Geriatr Soc* 52A:M218-M224.

Buchner, D.M., and B.J. deLateur. 1991. The importance of skeletal muscle strength to physical function in older adults. *Ann Behav Med* 13:95-98.

Buchner, D.M., E.B. Larson, E.H. Wagner, T.D. Koepsell, and B.J. deLateur. 1996. Evidence for a non-linear relationship between leg strength and gait speed. *Age Ageing* 25:386-391.

Buchner, D.M., and E.H. Wagner. 1992. Preventing frail health. *Clin Geriatr Med* 8:1-17.

Campbell, W.W., M.C. Crim, V.R. Young, and W.J. Evans. 1994. Increased energy requirements and body composition changes with resistance training in older adults. *Am J Clin Nutr* 60:167-75.

Campion, E.W. 1994. The oldest old. *N Engl J Med* 330:1819-1820.

Cartee, G.D. 1994. Aging skeletal muscle: response to exercise. In *Exercise and sports sciences review*, ed. T. H. Grayson. Baltimore, MD: Williams & Wilkins.

Chamie, M. 1990. The status and use of the International Classification of Impairments, Disabilities and Handicaps (ICIDH). *World Health Stat Q* 43:273-80.

Charette, S.L., L. McEvoy, G. Pyka, C. Snow-Harter, D. Guido, R.A. Wiswell, and R. Marcus. 1991. Muscle hypertrophy response to resistance training in older women. *J Appl Physiol* 70:1912-1916.

Clarkson, P., and W. Kroll. 1978. Practice effects on fractionated response time related to age and activity level. *J Motor Behav* 10:275.

Cohn, S., V. Yasumura, A. Sawitsky, I. Zanzi, A. Vaswani, and K.J. Ellis. 1980. Compartmental body composition based on total-body nitrogen, potassium, and calcium. *Am J Physiol* 239:E524-E530.

Commonwealth Fund Commission. 1988. Aging alone: profiles and projections. In *The Commonwealth Fund Commission on Elderly People Living Alone*. New York: Commonwealth Fund Commission.

Cress, M., D. Thomas, F.W. Kasch, R.G. Cassens, E.L. Smith, and J.C. Agre. 1991. Effect of training on VO$_2$ max, thigh strength, and muscle morphology in septuagenarian women. *Med Sci Sports Exerc* 23:752-758.

Cress, M.E., K. Shectman, C.D. Mulrow, M.A. Fiatarone, M.B. Gerety, and D.M. Buchner. 1995. Relationship between physical performance and self-perceived physical function. *J Am Ger Soc* 43:93-101.

Crilly, R.G., D.A. Willems, K.J. Trenholm, K.C. Hayes, and L.F. Delaquerriere-Richardson. 1989. Effect of exercise on postural sway in the elderly. *Gerontology* 35:137-143.

Culliname, E., F. Miller, S.P. Sady, B. Ribiero, and P.D. Thompson. 1986. Arm and leg exercise performance in healthy men 30-70 years of age. *Med Sci Sports Exerc* 18:596.

Cunningham, D., P. Rechnitzer, M.E. Pearce, and A.P. Donner. 1982. Determinants of self-selected walking pace across ages 19-66. *J Gerontol* 37:560-564.

Danneskiold-Samsoe, B., V. Kofod, J. Munter, G. Grimby, P. Schnor, G. Jensen. 1984. Muscle strength and functional capacity in 78-81 year old men and women. *Eur J Appl Physiol* 52:310.

Delorme, T. 1945. Restoration of muscle power by heavy resistance exercises. *J Bone Joint Surg* 27:645-667.

DeVries, H.A. 1970. Physiological effects of exercise training regimen upon men aged 52 to 88. *J Gerontol* 25:325-336.

DeWyss, W.D., C. Begg, and P.T. Lavin. 1980. Prognostic effect of weight loss prior to chemotherapy in cancer patients. *Am J Med* 69:491-497.

Dishman, R. 1989. Determinants of physical activity and exercise for persons 65 years of age and older. In *Physical activity and aging*, ed. W. Spirduso and H. Eckert. Champaign, IL: Human Kinetics.

Dishman, R.K. 1994. Motivating older adults to exercise. *S Med J* 87:S79-S82.

Dorup, I., K. Skjaaa, T. Clausen, and K. Kjeldsen. 1988. Reduced concentrations of potassium, magnesium, and sodium-potassium pumps in human skeletal muscle during treatment with diuretics. *Br Med J* 296:455-458.

Ehsani, A.A., T. Ogawa, T.R. Miller, R.J. Spina, and S.M. Jilka. 1991. Exercise training improved left ventricular systolic function in older men. *Circulation* 83:96-103.

Evans, W.J. 1995. Effects of exercise on body composition and functional capacity of the elderly. *J Gerontol* 50A(Special Issue):147-150.

Evans, W.J., and W.W. Campbell. 1993. Sarcopenia and age-related changes in body composition and functional capacity. *J Nutr* 123:465-468.

Fabre, C., J. Masse-Biron, S. Ahmaidi, B. Adam, and C. Prefaut. 1997. Effectiveness of individualized aerobic training at the ventilatory threshold in the elderly. *J Gerontol* 52A:B260-B266.

Fiatarone, M.A., and W.J. Evans. 1990. Exercise in the oldest old. *Top Geriatr Rehabil* 5:63-77.

Fiatarone, M.A., E.C. Marks, N.D. Ryan, C.N. Meredith, L.A. Lipsitz, and W.J. Evans. 1990. High-intensity strength training in nonagenarians. *JAMA* 263:3029-3034.

Fiatarone, M.A., E.F. O'Neill, N.D. Ryan, K.M. Clements, G.R. Solares, M.E. Nelson, S.B. Roberts, J.J. Kehayias, L.A. Lipsitz, and W.J. Evans. 1994. Exercise training and nutritional supplementation for physical frailty in very elderly people. *N Engl J Med* 330:1769-1775.

Fisher, N.M., D.R. Pendergast, and E. Calkins. 1991. Muscle rehabilitation in impaired elderly nursing home residents. *Arch Phys Med Rehabil* 72:181-185.

Fleg, J.L., and E.G. Lakatta. 1988. Role of muscle loss in the age-associated reduction in VO$_2$ max. *J Appl Physiol* 65:1147-1151.

Foster, V.L., G.J. Hume, W.C. Byrnes, A.L. Dickinson, and S.J. Chatfield. 1989. Endurance training for elderly women: Moderate vs. low intensity. *J Gerontol* 44:M184-M188.

Fries, J., S. Gurkirpal, G. Singh, D. Morfeld, H.B. Hubert, N.E. Lane, and B.W. Braun Jr. 1994. Running and the development of disability with age. *Ann Int Med* 121:502-509.

Frontera, W.R., V.A. Hughes, K.J. Lutz, and W.J. Evans. 1991. A cross-sectional study of muscle strength and mass in 45- to 78-yr-old men and women. *J Appl Physiol* 71:644-650.

Frontera, W., C.N. Meredith, K.P. O'Reilly, H.G. Knuttgen, and W.J. Evans. 1988. Strength conditioning in older men: skeletal muscle hypertrophy and improved function. *J Appl Physiol* 64:1038-1044.

Gerstenblith, G., J. Fleg, A. Vantosh et. al. 1980. Stress testing redefines the prevalence of coronary artery disease in epidemiological studies (Abstract). *Circulation* 62(Part II):III-308.

Gettman, L., M. Pollock, J.L. Durstein, A. Ward, J. Ayers, and A.C. Linnerud. 1976. Physiological responses of men to 1, 3, and 5 day per week training programs. *Res Q* 47:638-646.

Ghilarducci, L., R. Holly, and E.A. Amsterdam. 1989. Effects of high resistance training in coronary artery disease. *Am J Cardiol* 64:866-870.

Green, J.S., and S.F. Crouse. 1995. The effects of endurance training on functional capacity in the elderly: a meta-analysis. *Med Sci Sports Exerc* 27:920-926.

Grimby, G., A. Aniansson, H. Hedberg, G.B. Henning, U. Grangard, and H. Kvist. 1992. Training can improve muscle strength and endurance in 78- to 84-yr-old men. *J Appl Physiol* 73:517-523.

Grimby, G., B. Danneskiold-Samsoe, K. Hvid, and B. Saltin. 1982. Morphology and enzymatic capacity in arm and leg muscles in 78-81 year old men and women. *Acta Physiol Scand* 115:125-134.

Grimby, G., and B. Saltin. 1966. Physiological analysis of physically well trained middleaged and old athletes. *J Appl Physiol* 179:513-526.

Grimby, G., and B. Saltin. 1983. The ageing muscle. *Clin Physiol* 3: 209-218.

Guralnik, J., A. LaCroix, L.G. Branch, S.V. Kasl, and R.B. Wallace. 1991. Morbidity and disability in older persons in the years prior to death. *Am J Public Health* 81:443-447.

Guralnik, J.M., L.G. Branch, S.R. Cummings, and J.D. Curb. 1989. Physical performance measures in aging research. *J Gerontol* 44:M141-146.

Guralnik, J.M., L. Ferrucci, E.M. Simonsick, M.E. Salive, and R.B. Wallace. 1995. Lower-extremity function in persons over the age of 70 years as a predictor of subsequent disability. *N Engl J Med* 332:556-61.

Guralnik, J.M., E.M. Simonsick, L. Ferrucci, R.J. Glynn, L.F. Berkman, D.G. Blazer, P.A. Scherr, and R.B. Wallace. 1994. A short physical performance battery assessing lower extremity function: association with self-reported disability and prediction of mortality and nursing home admission. *J Gerontol* 29:M85-M94.

Hagberg, J. 1987. Effect of training on the decline of VO$_2$ max with aging. *Fed Proc* 46:1830.

Hagberg, J.M., J.E. Graves, M. Limacher, D.R. Woods, S.H. Leggett, C. Cononie, J.J. Bruber, and M.L. Pollock. 1989.

Cardiovascular responses of 70- to 79-yr-old men and women to exercise training. *J Appl Physiol* 66:2589-2594.

Hakim, A.A., H. Petrovitch, C. Burchfiel, G.W. Ross, B.L. Rodriguez, L.R. White, K. Yano, D. Curb, and R.D. Abbot. 1998. Effects of walking on mortality among nonsmoking retired men. *N Engl J Med* 338:94-9.

Hamdorf, P.A., R.T. Withers, R.K. Penhall, and M.V. Haslam. 1992. Physical training effects in the fitness and habitual activity patterns of elderly women. *Arch Phys Med Rehabil* 73:603-8.

Harper, C.M., and Y.M. Lyles. 1988. Physiology and complications of bed rest. *J Am Geriatr Soc* 36:1047-1054.

Harridge, S., G. Magnussen, and B. Saltin. 1997. Life-long endurance-trained elderly men have high aerobic power but have similar muscle strength to non-active elderly men. *Aging Clin Exp Res* 9:80-87.

Harris, T., M.G. Kovar, R. Suzman, J.C. Kleinman, and J.J. Feldman. 1989. Longitudinal study of physical activity in the oldest-old. *Am J Publ Health* 79:698-702.

Heath, G., J. Hagberg, A. Ali, and J.O. Holloszy. 1981. A physiological comparison of young and older endurance athletes. *J Appl Physiol* 51:634-640.

Hindmarsh, J.J., and H. Estes. 1989. Falls in older persons. *Arch Intern Med* 149:2217-2222.

Hopkins, D., B. Murray, W.W. Hoeger, R.C. Rhodes. 1990. Effect of low-impact aerobic dance on the functional fitness of elderly women. *Gerontologist* 30:189.

Hopp, J.F. 1993. Effects of age and resistance training on skeletal muscle: a review. *Phys Ther* 73:361-373.

Hubert, H., D. Bloch, and J.A. Fries. 1993. Risk factors for physical disability in an aging cohort: The NHANES I epidemiologic follow-up study. *J Rheumatol* 20: 480-488.

Jette, A.M., S.F. Assman, D. Rooks, B.A. Harris, and S. Crawford. 1998. Interrelationships among disablement concepts. *J Gerontol* 53A:M395-M404.

Jette, A.M., and L.G. Branch. 1981. The Framingham disability study: II physical disability among the aging. *Am J Public Health* 71:1211-1216.

Jette, A.M., B.A. Harris, L. Sleeper, M.E. Lachman, D. Heislan, M. Giorgetti, and C. Levenson. 1996. A home-based exercise program for nondisabled older adults. *J Am Geriatr Soc* 44:644-649.

Judge, J.O., C. Lindsey, M. Underwood, and D. Winsemius. 1993. Balance improvements in older women: Effects of exercise training. *Phys Ther* 73:254-264.

Judge, J.O., M. Underwood, and T. Gennosa. 1992. Exercise to improve gait velocity in older persons. *Arch Phys Med Rehabil* 74:400-406.

Kallman, D.A., C.C. Plato, and J.D. Tobin. 1990. The role of muscle loss in the age-related decline of grip strength: cross-sectional and longitudinal perspectives. *J Gerontol* 45:M82-M88.

Kasch, F., and J. Wallace. 1976. Physiological variables during 10 years of endurance exercise. *Med Sci Sports Exerc* 8:5-8.

Kemper, P., and C. Murtaugh. 1991. Lifetime use of nursing home care. *N Engl J Med* 324:595-600.

Klitgaard, H., M. Mantoni, S. Schiaffino, S. Ausoni, L. Gorza, C. Laurent-Winter, and P. Schnohr. 1990. Function, morphology and protein expression of ageing, skeletal muscle: a cross sectional study of elderly men with different training backgrounds. *Acta Physiol Scand* 140:41-54.

Kohrt, W., M. Malley, A.R. Coggan, R.J. Spina, T. Ogawa, A.A. Ehsani, R.E. Bourney, W.H. Martin, and J.O. Holloszy. 1991. Effects of gender, age, and fitness level on response of VO₂ max to training in 60 to 71-yr-olds. *J Appl Physiol* 71:2004-2011.

Kuta, I., J. Parizkova, and J. Dycka. 1970. Muscle strength and lean body mass in old men of different physical activity. *J Appl Physiol* 29:168-171.

LaCroix, A.Z., S.G. Leveille, J.A. Hecht, L.C. Grothaus, and E.H. Wagner. 1996. Does walking decrease the risk of cardiovascular disease hospitalizations and death in older adults? *J Am Geriatr Soc* 44:113-120.

Lakatta, E. 1990. Changes in cardiovascular function with aging. *Eur Heart J* 11 (Suppl. C):22.

Lan, C., J.-S. Lai, S.Y. Chen, and M.K. Wong. 1998. 12-month Tai Chi training in the elderly: its effect on health fitness. *Med Sci Sports Exerc* 30:345-351.

Larsson, L. 1982. Physical training effects on muscle morphology in sedentary males at different ages. *Med Sci Sports Exerc* 14:203-206.

Larsson, L. 1983. Histochemical characteristics of human skeletal muscle during aging. *Acta Physiol Scand* 117:469-471.

Lee, I.-M., C.-C. Hsieh, and R.S. Paffenbarger. 1995. Exercise intensity and longevity in men: The Harvard alumni health study. *JAMA* 273:1179-1184.

Lee, I.-M., R. S. Paffenbarger, and C.H. Hennekens. 1997. Physical activity, physical fitness and longevity. *Aging Clin Exp Res* 9: 2-11.

Levy, W.C., M.D. Cerqueira, I.B. Abrass, R.S. Schwartz, and J.R. Stratton. 1993. Endurance exercise training augments diastolic filling at rest and during exercise in healthy young and older men. *Circulation* 88:116-126.

Lexell, J., D. Downham, T. Larssen, E. Bruhn, and B. Morsing. 1996. Heavy-resistance training in older Scandinavian men and women: short- and long-term effects on arm and leg muscles. *Scand J Med Sci Sports* 5:329-341.

Lexell, J., K. Henriksson-Larsen, and M. Sjostrom.1983a. Distribution of different fibre types in human skeletal muscles. 2. A study of cross sections of whole m. vastus lateralis. *Acta Physiol Scand* 117:115-122.

Lexell, J., K. Henriksson-Larsen, B. Winblad, and M. Sjostrom. 1983b. Distribution of different fiber types in human skeletal muscles: effects of aging studied in whole muscle cross sections. *Muscle Nerve* 6:588-595.

Lichenstein, M.J., S.L. Shields, R.G. Shields, and C. Burger. 1989. Exercise and balance in aged women: a pilot controlled clinical trial. *Arch Phys Med Rehabil* 70:138-143.

Limacher, M.C. 1994. Aging and cardiac function: influence of exercise. *South Med J* 87:S13-S16.

Lord, S., J. Ward, P. Williams, and M. Strudwick. 1995. The effect of a 12-month exercise trial on balance, strength, and falls in older women: a randomized controlled trial. *J Am Geriatr Soc* 43:1198-1206.

Lord, S.R., D.G. Lloyd, M. Nirui, J. Raymond, P. Williams, and R.A. Stewart. 1996. The effect of exercise on gait patterns in older women: a randomized controlled trial. *J Gerontol* 51A:M64-M70.

Lord, S.R., J.A. Ward, and P. Williams. 1996. Exercise effect on dynamic stability in older women: a randomized controlled trial. *Arch Phys Med Rehabil* 77:232-6.

MacDougall, J. 1986. Adaptability of muscle to strength training: a cellular approach. In *Biochemistry of exercise VI*, ed. B. Saltin. Champaign, IL: Human Kinetics.

McCartney, N., A.L. Hicks, J. Martin, and C.E. Webber. 1995. Long-term resistance training in the elderly: effects on dynamic strength, exercise capacity, muscle, and bone. *J Gerontol* 50A:B97-B104.

McDonagh, T.A., S.B. Davison, J. Norrie, C.E. Morrison, J.J. McMurray, H. Tunstall-Pedoe, and H.J. Dargie. 1994. The effect of psychological depression on functional capacity. *Circulation* 90 (4, Part 2):I-162.

McMurdo, M.E., and L. Burnett 1992. Randomized controlled trial of exercise in the elderly. *Gerontology* 38:292-298.

Menkes, A., S. Mazel, R.A. Redmond, K. Koffler, C. Libanati, C. Gundberg, T.M. Zizic, J.M. Hagberg, P. Pratley, and B.F. Hurley. 1993. Strength training increased regional bone mineral density and bone remodeling in middle-aged and older men. *J Appl Physiol* 74:2478-2484.

Meredith, C., W. Frontera, E.C. Fisher, V.A. Hughes, J.C. Herland, J. Edwards, and W.J. Evans. 1989. Peripheral effects of endurance training in young and old subjects. *J Appl Physiol* 66:2844-2849.

Meredith, C.N., W.R. Frontera, K.P. O'Reilly, and W.J. Evans. 1992. Body composition in elderly men: effect of dietary modification during strength training. *J Am Geriatr Soc* 40:155-162.

Miller, R.A. 1993. The biology of aging and longevity. In *Principles of geriatric medicine and gerontology*, ed. W. Hazzard et al. New York: McGraw-Hill, Inc.

Morganti, C.M., M.E. Nelson, M.A. Fiatarone, G.E. Dallal, C.D. Economos, B.M. Crasford, and W.J. Evans. 1995. Strength improvements with 1 yr of progressive resistance training in older women. *Med Sci Sports Exerc* 27:906-912.

Moritani, T., and H.A. deVries. 1980. Potential for gross muscle hypertrophy in older men. *J Gerontol* 35:672-682.

Muller, E.A. 1970. Influence of training and of inactivity on muscle strength. *Arch Phys Med Rehabil* 51:449-461.

Nagi, S.Z. 1965. Some conceptual issues in disability and rehabilitation. In *Sociology and rehabilitation*, ed. M.B. Sussman. Washington, DC: American Sociological Society.

Nagi, S.Z. 1991. Disability concepts revised: Implications for prevention. In *Disability in America: Toward a national agenda for prevention*, ed. A.M. Pope and A.R. Tarlov. Washington, DC: National Academy Press.

Naso, F., E. Carner, W. Blankfort-Doyle, and K. Coughey. 1990. Endurance training in the elderly nursing home patient. *Arch Phys Med Rehabil* 71:241-243.

Nelson, M.E., M.A. Fiatarone, C.M. Morganti, I. Trice, R.A. Greenberg, and W.J. Evans. 1994. Effects of high-intensity strength training on multiple risk factors for osteoporotic fractures. *JAMA* 272:1909-1914.

Nichols, J.F., D.K. Omizo, K.K. Peterson, and K.P. Nelson. 1993. Efficacy of heavy-resistance training for active women over sixty: muscular strength, body composition, and program adherence. *J Am Geriatr Soc* 41:205-210.

Ogawa, T., R.J. Spina, W.H. Martin III, W.M. Kohrt, K.B. Schectman, J.O. Holloszy, and A.A. Ehsani. 1992. Effects of aging, sex, and physical training on cardiovascular responses to exercise. *Circulation* 86:494-503.

Orlander, J., and A. Aniansson. 1980. Effects of physical training on skeletal muscle metabolism and ultrastructure in 70 to 75 year old men. *Acta Physiol Scand* 109:149-154.

Ory, M.G., K.B. Schechtman, P. Miller, E. Hadley, M.A. Fiatarone, M.A. Province, C.L. Arfken, D. Morgan, S. Weiss, and M. Kaplan, for the FICSIT Group. 1993. Frailty and injuries in later life: the FICSIT trials. *J Am Geriatr Soc* 41:283-296.

Paffenbarger, R., R. Hyde, A.L. Wing, and C.C. Hsieh. 1986. Physical activity and longevity of college alumni. *N Engl J Med* 315: 399-401.

Paffenbarger, R., R. Hyde, A.L. Wing, I.M. Lee, D.J. Jung, and J.B. Kampert. 1993. The association of changes in physical activity level and other lifestyle characteristics with mortality among men. *N Engl J Med* 328: 538-545.

Parizkova, J. 1974. Body composition and exercise during growth and development. In *Physical activity: Human growth and development*, ed. G. Rarick. New York: Academic Press.

Pendergast, D.R., N.M. Fisher, and E. Calkins. 1993. Cardiovascular, neuromuscular, and metabolic alterations with age leading to frailty. *J Gerontol* 48(Special Issue):61-67.

Pocock, N., J. Eisman, T. Gwinn, P. Sambrook, P. Kelley, J. Friend, and M. Yeates. 1989. Muscle strength, physical fitness and weight but not age predict femoral neck bone mass. *J Bone Miner Res* 4:441-448.

Pollock, M.L., J.F. Carroll, J.E. Graves, S.H. Leggett, R.W. Braith, M. Limacher, and J.M. Hagberg. 1991. Injuries and adherence to walk/jog and resistance training programs in the elderly. *Med Sci Sports Exerc* 23:1194-1200.

Pollock, M.L., G. Dawson, and H.S. Miller. 1976. Physiologic responses of men 49 to 65 years of age to endurance training. *J Am Geriatr Soc* 24:97-104.

Pollock, M.L., C. Foster, D. Knapp, J.L. Rod, and D.H. Schmidt. 1987. Effect of age, training, competition on aerobic capac-

ity and body composition of masters athletes. *J Appl Physiol* 62:725.

Pollock, M.L., J.E. Graves, D.L. Stewart, and D.T. Lowenthal. 1994. Exercise training and prescription for the elderly. *S Med J* 87:S88-S95.

Pollock, M.L., L.J. Mengelkoch, J.E. Graves, D.T. Lowenthal, M.C. Limacher, C. Foster, and J.H. Wilmore. 1997. Twenty-year follow-up of aerobic power and body composition of older track athletes. *J Appl Physiol* 82:1508-1516.

Porter, M.M., and A.A. Vandervoort. 1995. High-intensity strength training for the older adult—a review. *Top Geriatr Rehabil* 10:61-74.

Posner, J., and K. McCully. 1996. Exercise. In *Principles of geriatrics*, ed. D. Jahnigan. Cambridge, England: Blackwell Science.

Posner, J.D., K.M. Gorman, L. Gitlin, L.P. Sands, K. Kleban, L. Windsor, and C. Shaw. 1990. Effects of exercise training in the elderly on the occurence and time to onset of cardiovascular diagnoses. *J Am Geriatr Soc* 38:205-210.

Posner, J.D., K.M. Gorman, L. Windsor-Landsberg, J. Larsen, M. Bleiman, C. Shaw, B. Rosenberg, and J. Knebl. 1992. Low to moderate intensity endurance training in healthy older adults: physiological responses after four months. *J Am Geriatr Soc* 40:1-7.

Posner, J.D., K.K. McCully, L.A. Landsberg, L.P. Sands, P. Tycenski, M.T. Hofmann, K.L. Wetterholt, and C.E. Shaw. 1995. Physical determinants of independence in mature women. *Arch Phys Med Rehabil* 76:373-380.

Province, M.A., E.C. Hadley, M.C. Hornbrook, L.A. Lipsitz, P. Miller, C.D. Mulrow, M.G. Ory, R.W. Sattin, M.E. Tinetti, and S.L. Wolf. 1995. The effects of exercise on falls in elderly patients: a preplanned meta-analysis of the FICSIT Trials. *JAMA* 273:1341-1347.

Pyka, G., E. Lindenberger, S. Chrette, and R. Marcus. 1994. Muscle strength and fiber adapatations to a year-long resistance training program in elderly men and women. *J Gerontol* 49: M22-M27.

Resnick, N.M. 1997. Geriatric medicine. In *Principles of internal medicine*, ed. J. Wilson, A. Fauci et al. New York: McGraw-Hill.

Reuben, D., and A.L. Siu. 1990. An objective measure of physical function of elderly outpatients: the physical performance test. *J Am Geriatr Soc* 38:1105-1112.

Rodeheffer, R., G. Gerstenblith, L.C. Becker, J.L. Fleg, M.L. Weisfeldt, and E.G. Lakatta. 1984. Exercise cardiac output is maintained with advancing age in healthy human subjects: cardiac dilation and increased stroke volume compensate for a diminished heart rate. *Circulation* 69:203.

Rogers, M.A., J.M. Hagberg, W.H. Martin III, A.A. Ehsani, and J.O. Holloszy. 1990. Decline in VO$_2$ max with aging master athletes and sedentary men. *J Appl Physiol* 68:2195-2199.

Rooks, D.S., D.P. Kiel, C. Parsons, and W.C. Hayes. 1997. Self-paced resistance training and walking exercise in community-dwelling older adults: effects on neuromotor performance. *J Gerontol* 52A:M161-M168.

Sagiv, M., N. Fisher, A. Yaniv, and J. Rudoy. 1989. Effect of running versus isometric training programs on healthy elderly at rest. *Gerontology* 35:72-77.

Sale, D. 1988. Neural adaptation to resistance training. *Med Sci Sports Exerc* 1988:S135-S145.

Sandvik, L., J. Erikssen, E. Thaulow, G. Erikssen, R. Mendal, and K. Rodahl. 1993. Physical fitness as a predictor of mortality among healthy, middle-aged Norwegian men. *N Engl J Med* 328:533-7.

Schneider, E.L., and J.M. Guralnik. 1990. The aging of America: impact on health care costs. *JAMA* 263:2335-2340.

Schocken, D.D., J.A. Blumenthal, S. Port, P. Hindle, and R.E. Coleman. 1983. Physical conditioning and left ventricular performance in the elderly: assessment by radionuclide angiocardiography. *Am J Cardiol* 52:359-364.

Schultz, A. 1992. Mobility impairment in the elderly: challenges for biomechanics research. *J Biomech* 25:519-528.

Seals, D.R., J.M. Hagberg, B.F. Hurley, A.A. Ehsani, and J.O. Holloszy. 1984. Endurance training in older men and women I: cardiovascular responses to exercise. *J Appl Physiol* 7:1024-1029.

Sheldahl, L., F. Tristani, J.E. Hastings, R.B. Wenzler, and S.G. Levandoski. 1993. Comparison of adaptations and compliance to exercise training between middle-aged and older men. *J Am Geriat Soc* 41:795-801.

Shephard, R.J. 1990. The scientific basis of exercise prescribing for the very old. *J Am Geriat Soc* 38:62-70.

Shock, N., R. Greulich, and R. Andres. 1984. Cross-sectional studies of aging in men. In *Normal human aging: The Baltimore longitudinal study of aging*, ed. N.W. Shock, R. Greulich, and R. Andres. Washington, DC: U.S. Government Printing Office.

Sidney, K., and R. Shephard. 1978. Frequency and intensity of exercise training for elderly subjects. *Med Sci Sports Exerc* 10:125-131.

Simonsick, E., M. Lafferty, C.L. Phillips, C.F. Mendes DeLeon, S.V. Kasl, T.E. Seeman, G. Fillenbaum, P. Herbert, and J.H. Lemke. 1993. Risk due to inactivity in physically capable older adults. *Am J Public Health* 83:1443-1450.

Skelton, D.A., A. Young, C.A. Greig, and K.E. Malbut. 1995. Effects of resistance training on strength, power, and selected functional abilities of women aged 75 and older. *J Am Geriatr Soc* 43:1081-87.

Souminen, H., E. Heikkinen, H. Liesen, D. Michel, and W. Hollman. 1977. Effects of 8 weeks endurance training on skeletal muscle metabolism in 56-70 year old sedentary men. *Eur J Appl Physiol* 37:173-180.

Stratton, J.R., M.D. Cerqueira, R.S. Schwartz, W.C. Levy, R.C. Veith, S.E. Kahn, and I. Abrass. 1992. Differences in cardiovascular responses to isopreterenol in relation to

age and exercise training in healthy men. *Circulation* 86:504-512.

Stratton, J.R., W.C. Levy, M.D. Cerqueira, R.S. Schwartz, and I. Abrass. 1994. Cardiovascular responses to exercise: effects of aging and exercise training in healthy men. *Circulation* 89:1648-1655.

Suzman, R., D. Willis, and K. Manton. 1992. *The oldest old.* New York: Oxford University Press.

Thomas, S., D.A. Cunningham, P.A. Rechnitzer, A.P. Donner, and J.H. Howard. 1985. Determinants of training response in elderly men. *Med Sci Sports Exerc* 17:667-672.

Thompson, R.F., D.M. Crist, M. Marsh, and M. Rosenthal. 1988. Effects of physical exercise for elderly patients with physical impairments. *J Am Geriatr Soc* 36:130-135.

Tinetti, M.E., and M. Speechley. 1989. Prevention of falls among the elderly. *N Engl J Med* 320:1055-1059.

Tzankoff, S., and A. Norris. 1977. Effect of muscle mass decrease on age-related BMR changes. *J Appl Physiol* 43:1001-1006.

U.S. Bureau of the Census. 1991. *Global aging: Comparative indicators and future trends.* U.S. Department of Commerce, Economics and Statistics Administration. Washington, DC: Government Printing Office.

U.S. Department of Health and Human Services. 1996. *Physical activity and health: A report of the Surgeon General.* Atlanta, GA: Centers for Disease Control and Prevention, National Center for Chronic Disease Prevention and Health Promotion.

Verbrugge, L., J. Lepowski, and Y. Imanaka. 1989. Comorbidity and its impact on disability. *Millbank Mem Fund Q* 67:450.

Warren, B.J., D.C. Nieman, R.G. Dotson, C.H. Adkins, K.A. O'Donnell, and B.L. Haddock. 1993. Cardiorespiratory responses to exercise training in septuagenarian women. *Int J Sports Med* 14:60-65.

Welle, S., S. Totterman, and C. Thornton. 1996. Effect of age on muscle hypertrophy induced by resistance training. *J Gerontol* 51A:M270-M275.

Whipple, R., L. Wolfson, and P.M. Amerman. 1987. The relationship of knee and ankle weakness to falls in nursing home residents: an isokinetic study. *J Am Geriatr Soc* 35:13-20.

Williams, M., and J. Hornberger. 1984. A quantitative method of identifying older persons at risk for increasing long term care services. *J Chron Dis* 37:705.

Wolf, S.L., H.X. Barnhart, N. Kutner, E. McNeely, C. Coogler, and T. Xu. 1996. Reducing frailty and falls in older persons: an investigation of Tai Chi and computerized balance training. *J Am Geriatr Soc* 44:489-496.

Wolfson, L., J. Judge, R. Whipple, and M. King. 1995. Strength is a major factor in balance, gait, and the occurrence of falls. *J Gerontol* 50A:64-67.

Wolfson, L., R. Whipple, C. Derby, J. Judge, M. King, P. Amerman, J. Schmidt, and D. Smyers. 1996. Balance and strength training in older adults: intervention gains and Tai Chi maintenance. *J Am Geriatr Soc* 44:498-506.

Wolfson, L., R. Whipple, J. Judge, P. Amberman, C. Derby, and M. King. 1993. Training balance and strength in the elderly to improve function. *J Am Geriatr Soc* 41:341-343.

Woollacott, M. H. 1993. Age-related changes in posture and movement. *J Gerontol* 48 (Special Issue):56-60.

World Health Organization. 1997. *The world health report 1997: Conquering suffering, enriching humanity*. Geneva: World Health Organization.

Wylie, C. 1984. Contrasts in the health of elderly men and women: An analysis of recent data for whites in the United States. *J Am Geriatr Soc* 32:670.

Yarasheski, K.E., J.J. Zachweija, and D. Bier. 1993. Acute effects of resistance exercise on muscle protein synthesis rate in young and elderly men and women. *Am J Physiol* 265:E210-E214.

Chapter 21

Elite Athletes With Impairments

Rory A. Cooper, PhD, Michael L. Boninger, MD,
Sean D. Shimada, PhD, and Thomas J. O'Connor, MS

Sports and recreation have changed the way in which people with disabilities perceive themselves and the way in which society as a whole perceives them (Cook and Webster 1982; Cooper et al. 1992a; Wade 1993). The concept that someone with a disability can be athletic and compete at high levels of sport has helped remove the stigma of being sick that was long associated with a physical impairment (Galvin and Scherer 1996; Loverock 1980; Rick Hansen Centre 1988; Snell 1992). Sports continues to be an important tool for social change as well as for individual rehabilitation. There is a growing trend towards integrated activities, in which people with and without physical impairments can participate in

sports and recreational activities side by side. People with disabilities participate in nearly every recreational activity that exists, in some cases using specialized equipment, in others using standard equipment (Asato et al. 1992; Cooper and Bedi 1990; Skinner and Effeney 1985). Figure 21.1 shows specialized equipment used by individuals for snow skiing. Recreation is an important aspect of peoples' lives, and good recreation habits can lead to a fuller and healthier life. People participate in a variety of recreational activities from gardening to skydiving. Recreational activities change over the life span as well. It is important for people with disabilities to learn healthy recreational activities during rehabilitation.

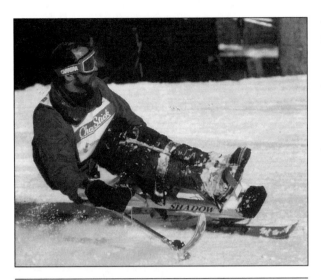

Figure 21.1   Using specialized equipment to snow ski.
Photo by Mary E. Messenger.

From Patient to Athlete

Shortly after World War II, Sir Ludwig Guttmann and his colleagues at Stoke Mandeville Hospital in England needed exercise and recreational outlets for the large number of young people recently injured in the war. Out of this need came wheelchair sports as a rehabilitation tool (Cooper 1990). News of Dr. Guttmann's success in rehabilitating his patients through sports spread through Europe and to the United States. In 1948, he organized "Games" for British veterans with disabilities. In 1952, the Games developed into the first international wheelchair sporting competition for people with physical disabilities, with participants from the Netherlands, the Federal Republic of Germany, Sweden, Norway, and Israel. During this event, the International Stoke Mandeville Games Federation (ISMGF) was formed to govern and develop wheelchair sporting competitions. The ISMGF established ties to the International Olympic Committee (IOC), thus expanding the scope of wheelchair sports. As the international sports movement for people with disabilities grew, and international multidisability events multiplied, the ISMGF expanded to include all wheelchair sporting events, renaming itself as the International Stoke Mandeville Wheelchair Sports Federation (ISMWSF). The first international games for the disabled held in conjunction with the Olympic Games took place in 1960 in Rome. The name "Paralympics"

was coined during the 1964 Tokyo games, and this competition still occurs every four years under that name (Cooper 1990).

In the early years of wheelchair racing, participants used bulky depot-type wheelchairs and did not compete in events with distances over 200 meters (Cooper 1989a, 1989b, 1989c, 1990, 1992a; Cooper et al. 1992). In the 1970s, athletes began to modify their wheelchairs for specific sports, and to take an interest in road racing. In 1975, a young man with paraplegia became the first person to compete in the Boston Athletic Association Marathon in a wheelchair. This opened the door for many future road racers, prompting Dr. Caibre McCann, a leading physician for the ISMGF, to say, "Running is natural, but propelling yourself in a wheelchair is an unnatural phenomenon. People never realize what a wheelchair athlete is capable of. This is a breakthrough in man's limits" (Cooper 1990). Within a few years, several recognized U.S. road races initiated wheelchair divisions, and more people with disabilities than had ever been anticipated began to train for these races (Cooper 1990). In 1976, the ISMGF started to coordinate with other international sports organizations to launch a unified international sports movement for people with disabilities (Cooper 1990). Racing wheelchairs began to evolve as special-purpose pieces of equipment easily distinguishable from everyday wheelchairs (Cooper 1992b; MacLeish et al. 1993). Distances on the track were extended to include races up to 1500 meters, and during this time the mile record dropped below five minutes.

The early 1980s saw the development of more sophisticated racing wheelchairs and training techniques (Cooper 1989c, 1992a; MacLeish et al. 1993). By 1985, most racing wheelchairs had no components in common with everyday wheelchairs (which had also improved dramatically), and George Murray became the first wheelchair racer to break the four-minute mile. In the years that followed, wheelchair racing continued to progress with improved equipment, training, and nutrition; consequently, world records were continually falling. Wheelchair racing began the path toward recognition as a legitimate Olympic sport in 1984, when the Olympic Games in Los Angeles included as demonstration events the men's 1500-meter and the women's 800-meter wheelchair races. Wheelchair racing continued to be an exhibition event at the 1988, 1992, and 1996 Olympiads. Athletes and organizers continue to work for further integration of wheelchair sports into the Olympic movement.

Organizational Structure of Sports for People With Disabilities

In the United States there are numerous sporting organizations for people with disabilities, five of which participate in the Paralympics. Figure 21.2 lists these organizations, with the exception of the Special Olympics. Special Olympic athletes participate in a separate international competition organized by Special Olympics International. The five U.S. Paralympic sports organizations are loosely linked through the United States Organization of Disabled Athletes (USODA). Formed after U.S. athletes and organizers experienced severe difficulties in raising funds for the 1984 Paralympic Games, USODA aims primarily to raise funds—it exercises no administrative power over the member organizations. The strength of USODA lies in its abilities to represent a large number of athletes and to speak with a unified voice.

The six organizations of athletes with disabilities presented in figure 21.2 also receive support from the United States Olympic Committee (USOC), via the Committee on Athletes With Disabilities (CAD) and through grant programs. The CAD distributes funds based on number of members, participation in international events, and number of elite athletes. These funds can be used for core support of organizations. Grants are also available from the USOC to support training camps, employ athletes, and support teams at Paralympic Games. Each of the sports organizations whose athletes participate in the Paralympics chooses its own teams and works directly with the international governing bodies.

Figure 21.3 illustrates the international structure of sports for athletes with disabilities. The IOC selects the sites of Olympic Games. Since Paralympic Games coordinate with the Olympic Games, the IOC and International Paralympic Committee (IPC) work together for the benefit of both. The IPC selects the sites for the Paralympics, determines the number of athletes, and approves the local organizing committee. The international governing bodies (IGBs) implement the decisions of the IPC, determining how many athletes from each organization and from each sport will compete. The IGBs also set the performance standards that athletes must meet in order to be eligible to compete. The IGBs also organize and sanction international events. The IGBs must work closely with the national governing bodies (NGBs) of each member country. The NGBs choose their team members, organize teams, and participate in the governance of the IGBs.

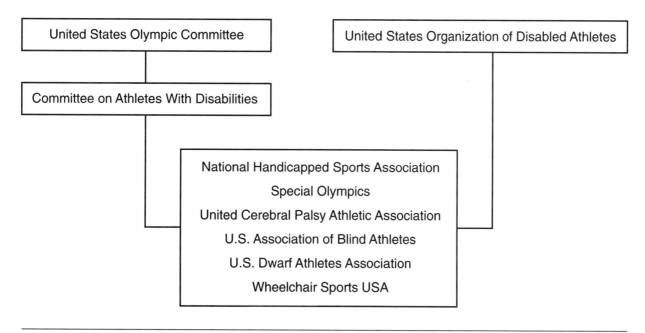

Figure 21.2 Structure of Paralympic Sports within the United States.

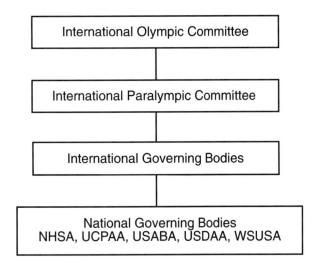

Figure 21.3 Structure of International Paralympic Sports.

Sports Equipment Technology and Use

A growing number of people participate in some form of wheelchair exercise or sports, including swimming, track and field events, basketball, rugby, and more. Along with expansion of the types of sports and exercise engaged in by individuals with a disability, there is a growth in assistive technology that helps these individuals participate safely in sports and exercise.

Racing Wheelchair Technology

The rules of wheelchair racing allow a wide variety of designs, the major concerns being safety, equity, and speed; however, most racing wheelchairs have some common characteristics.

Basic Construction

Racing wheelchairs are propelled by arm power only, and steered by the hands and/or arms. The frames are stiff and lightweight, typical frames weighing less than five pounds excluding the wheels. Athletes sit near rear axle height. Four-wheeled chairs commonly employ a rectangular main frame with a cross-member immediately fore and aft of the seat. Three-wheeled chairs are similar, but with a triangular main frame (as viewed from above). The rear wheels attach rigidly to the frame by a threaded insert welded either through the side frame tubes or into a cross-

member. The rear wheel inserts are aligned with 2-15 degrees of wheel camber, and no toe in/out (misalignment of the rear wheels), making the chair more stable and allowing the athlete to reach the bottom of the pushrims without hitting the top of the wheels or pushrim. Toe in/out causes problems for wheelchair racers: it can cause a significant increase in rolling resistance if not aligned properly, and may change with use (some manufacturers incorporate an alignment mechanism into the frame). Pushrims on racing chairs are smaller than those used on standard chairs, and they may be coated—usually with a tire or high-density foam—to achieve higher friction with the athlete's gloves.

Some elite racers use racing wheelchairs that incorporate seat and leg supports as an integral unit. Since they are more accustomed to racing wheelchairs, elite athletes usually prefer tighter fitting seat cages than do novice athletes. Seat and leg supports should hold the athletes solidly, so they can focus their energy on propelling the wheelchair rather than maintaining balance. Seat cages also offer greater chair control than conventional seats, and provide some protection in the event of an upset. Seat cages have side panels to provide support and to prevent the athlete's arms from rubbing against the wheels. Well-designed side panels follow the curvature of the wheel, and allow the athlete a large range of motion fore and aft. Most seat upholstery is made of nylon or cotton canvas slung from the seat cage. Some racing chairs use plastic or fiberglass seats. Athletes typically use low-profile foam or air-floatation cushions.

The frame and seat cage are made to fit each individual, and for different disability etiologies and levels. Both experience and disability etiology determine the location of rear axles with respect to the seat cage. While experienced athletes with paraplegia prefer 15-25 centimeters from the seat back to the rear axles' inserts, those with quadriplegia prefer 5-20 centimeters. Novice athletes generally choose more stable configurations. The seat cage upholstery adjustment and rear axle positions must be such that athletes can position their shoulders over the front edge of the pushrims and be able to reach the bottom of the pushrims with both arms.

Performance and Safety Features

Many racing wheelchairs have features that contribute to performance or safety—e.g., computers that aid in pacing and training; water bottles for fluid replacement; and caliper brakes (to help control the tremendous speeds attainable on some downhill sections). Brakes make training safer, and many races require their use. It is important that athletes be able to reach brakes from a comfortable position; and the brake levers must be long enough and at the proper angle so that the athlete can apply sufficient leverage to stop the racing chair. This is a critical issue for people with quadriplegia. Helmets have improved the safety of wheelchair racing, and most road and track races require them—athletes should purchase helmets when they purchase their racing wheelchairs. Helmets should meet national safety standards, provide good airflow over the head (which is a primary area for cooling the body), and fit snugly. Many helmets are adjustable. Aerodynamic helmets can enhance speed compared with that of someone wearing no helmet.

Customizing the Racing Wheelchair

It is important that a racing chair fit the user properly. Racing chairs are similar to shoes, in that a poorly fitted chair can be uncomfortable and awkward (Cooper 1989a, 1989b, 1989c, 1992a, 1992b; Cooper et al. 1992). They should fit as closely as possible without causing discomfort or pressure sores. Most manufacturers ask for a number of anatomical measurements when a chair is ordered (Cooper 1990)—most commonly hip width, chest width, thigh length, arm length, trunk length, height, and weight. It is important for the manufacturer to know of the athlete's special needs, such as asymmetry or limited range of motion. Knowing a rider's disability etiology and racing ability will help a manufacturer properly fit a racing chair to its rider for maximum performance with least risk of injury.

Because racing wheelchairs are very user-specific, and athletes vary greatly in their abilities, it is impossible to design a chair that is effective for every athlete. Racing wheelchairs often are handcrafted for individuals based on their specific needs. Getting into a racing wheelchair should be like slipping on a glove. Many new athletes make the mistake of getting a loose-fitting wheelchair. Top athletes can fit into their racers only when wearing racing/training tights. To push properly, athletes must sit properly. If they are flexible enough and feel comfortable leaning on their knees, they generally find kneeling to be the fastest position. If kneeling remains uncomfortable after a trial period, or if the athlete has very good trunk control, then a more upright posture is best. When seated in the chair and kneeling, or lying upon their knees, athletes should be able to touch the ground with both hands, and be able to reach all the way around both

pushrims. The center of each shoulder should line up with the front of each pushrim in the fully down position. The athletes should move their arms, simulating stroking, and test how difficult it is to breathe. They will need to synchronize breathing with stroking; but if it seems difficult to breathe, they should raise their knees.

Some personal considerations must be made when specifying a racing wheelchair, because athletes with paraplegia, quadriplegia, or amputated limbs have different preferences, and each person has unique abilities and anatomical structure. There are three basic seats to consider: kneeling bucket, kneeling cage, and upright cage. The kneeling position is very aerodynamic and has allowed paraplegic and quadriplegic athletes to make tremendous improvements in their performance. The kneeling bucket helps decrease the racing wheelchair weight. Athletes inexperienced with the kneeling position should use a kneeling cage, which affords them the option of sitting upright or kneeling and permits some adjustment of body position. Upright cage seats work well for athletes with lower limb amputations, and for athletes with low levels of paraplegia—i.e., those who have the trunk control to adjust their body position while racing. Athletes with contractures should order a cage seat, unless they have substantial experience. Athletes are held in their racing chairs with straps and webbing. Additional padding or extra width can be requested to reduce the risk of developing pressure sores for people who are prone to skin breakdown. Although many competitors do not use a seat cushion in their racing chairs, the danger of skin breakdown makes use of a cushion advisable.

Racing in a Wheelchair

The wheelchair racing stroke has two primary phases: propulsion and recovery. **Propulsion** is when the arms are applying force, and **recovery** is when they are off the pushrims getting ready for the next stroke. In order to effectively push a racing wheelchair, the upper body must rapidly apply a large force to the pushrims. Although athletes theoretically can achieve the greatest velocity by applying a large force over a long time period, it is difficult for them to effectively apply a large force during the entire propulsion phase. Ordinarily, athletes would tend to use the triceps and biceps muscles; by consciously learning and training to use the deltoids and pectoralis muscles, they can develop greater force over the propulsion cycle by using more of the upper body. The resulting larger force value and longer time of application create greater momentum. The price for this higher mechanical energy, however, is a higher consumption of metabolic energy.

Figure 21.4 illustrates the five phases of a racing wheelchair stroke:

1. Pushrim contact (a)
2. Pushing through to the bottom of the pushrims (b)-(d)
3. Push-off or follow-through (e)
4. Elbow drive to the top (f)-(h)
5. Drive forward and downward (i)-(j)

During the entire stroke the head should remain in-line with the trunk, with head movement kept to a minimum. Elbow height before the drive forward and downward is critical to generating propulsion force. Maximal elbow height requires strength and flexibility. Optimal force transfer from the body to the pushrim requires properly fitted and designed gloves, and a nonslip pushrim coating. The hand should be in line with the forearm at contact (i.e., wrist in the neutral position) to transfer maximum energy. The athlete must push continuously from contact through to the bottom of the pushrims. If the propulsion phase

is done properly, the hand will push off the pushrim with a flick. The momentum of the arms is used to carry the elbows upward. When the elbows are at their peaks, the athlete should contract chest, shoulder, and arm muscles to punch the pushrims.

Bicycles and Tricycles

People with mobility impairments want alternatives for recreational activities. Some people are interested in physically demanding sports such as marathons or triathlons. Others enjoy touring, and prefer the increased efficiency of levers and gears. Alternatives to wheelchair locomotion have been in development for a number of years (Engel and Seeliger 1986), but the commercial availability of arm-crank recreational equipment was delayed because

- people with mobility impairments lacked awareness of the equipment,
- insurance carriers have not been willing to purchase such devices,
- low-volume production of adaptive recreation equipment carried high liability risks for manu-

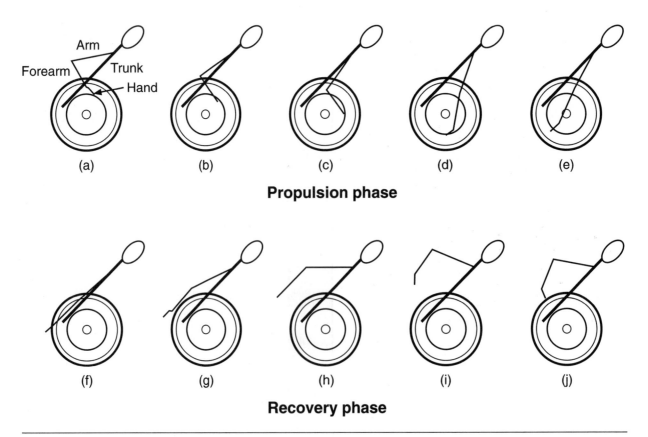

Figure 21.4 Schematic illustrating the phases of an efficient racing wheelchair stroke.

facturers (since appropriate liability insurance was very expensive), and

- building arm-powered vehicles at home was very complex.

Currently there are only a few restrictions on arm-powered vehicles for use in competitions: they can use no motors or external energy sources, and may have no structures that serve the sole purpose of reducing air/wind resistance.

Hand cycles are the bicycle of people with mobility impairments (figure 21.5). The present generation of hand cycles use from 15 to 21 gears. Whether going downhill or uphill, the rider searches for the gear ratio that best permits low effort and high pedal turnover—cadences between 80 and 100 revolutions per minute minimize both energy consumption and the risk of musculoskeletal injury. Before riding independently, people must consider several questions:

- Where will I do most of my riding (beach, neighborhood, country, city)?
- What kind of riding will I do (recreational, racing, touring)?
- Is the hand cycle appropriate to my abilities (disability etiology, physical function)?
- When the pedal(s) are fully extended (hands on the pedals, back against the backrest), are my elbows slightly bent?

Basic Construction

Arm-powered vehicles should efficiently convert the user's energy into motion, while permitting good control over the vehicle on normal surface streets. Ideally, arm-powered vehicles use as many standard bicycle components as possible, and fit into passenger cars without requiring disassembly. The vehicle frames are typically steel alloy (SAE 4130) tubing, with milled ends for best fit and stronger joints. Frames may be either brass-welded (simple and inexpensive) or inert gas-welded.

Balance Factors

A limitation of most arm-powered vehicles is the balance of the pilot. Accustomed to using a wheelchair for mobility, many people have unlearned their ability to balance. The loss of some kinesthesia and neuromuscular control of the trunk and lower limbs increases the difficulty of balancing a bicycle. A bucket seat as used on a racing wheelchair is effective in ameliorating these challenges for some people. In order to assure that the cranks clear the lower legs, some positions require placing the crank center farther away from the rider than is otherwise desirable. The result is a suboptimal center position and more difficulty steering at the front end of the crank cycle. Some bicycles position the rider low enough to the ground that riders may place their hands on the

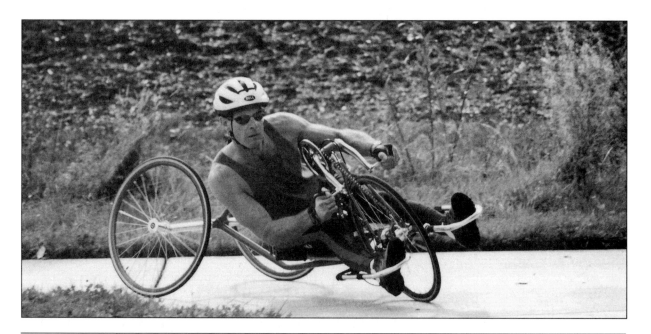

Figure 21.5 Handcycling can be a fun and exciting sport.
Photo courtesy of Freedom Ryder.

ground when starting or stopping. Some people prefer fully retractable side wheels. Riders power the bicycles through a combination of leaning and turning the crank about the steering axis. Side wheels may limit the rider's ability to lean the bicycle; when used, however, they must not interfere with normal lean steering. Since the height of the center of gravity, the user's balance, and the vehicle's steering geometry all interact, anyone designing an arm-powered vehicle must consider all these factors in order to make the device safe and efficient.

Steering

Since the steering and drive train are interconnected in many arm-powered vehicles, a primary design consideration is how the rider will both power the vehicle and maintain directional control. Arm-powered bicycles generally use direct arm steering because they require fine steering control to maintain balance. Some designers, however, have had moderate success in decoupling steering from the drive train by using the tilt (from side to side) of the seat for steering. These vehicles have a large turning radius for their size.

Crank-Arm Positioning, Gears, and Brakes

Crank arms may be adjacent or opposed. Opposite cranks provide greater mechanical efficiency. But because they create a moment about the head-set (the bearing housing that permits crank rotation), causing the front wheel(s) to turn from side to side as the rider cranks, the rider must waste energy in order to dampen the moment. A friction (nylon bushings in the head-set) or a viscous dampener can minimize the undesired turning moment. Bicycles and tricycles require different steering techniques: one initiates a turn on a bicycle by leaning with the front wheel turned opposite to the desired direction; the front wheels of tricycles go in the direction of the turn, and the rider does not lean.

Arm-powered vehicles must have a wide range of gear ratios, since the power output of the arms can be quite limited and fine increments are required to achieve optimal pedaling rates. Shift levers should be of the indexing type, and easily reachable. Chain guards are necessary to help keep fingers out of the sprockets, and to protect the rider in the event of an accident.

Standard bicycle brakes are acceptable, but with levers positioned so they can be grasped with one hand. Typically, the rider steers with one hand and brakes with the other. Some arm-powered vehicles use a cam-activated brake, which is engaged by reversing the crank direction. This simplifies braking, but prohibits back pedaling for balance at low speeds and when attempting to maximize leverage on inclines.

Alternative Arm-Powered Vehicles

Arm-powered vehicles do not exclude wheelchairs: **add-on units** can convert a wheelchair into an arm-crank vehicle. Some of these devices incorporate quick-release mechanisms that attach a self-contained front wheel-gear-crank system. Other devices— which may also be quick-release—attach cranks to each of the rear drive wheels. The clear advantage of quick-release units is that users can easily remove them in order to use their wheelchairs in the usual fashion. Add-on units are often easier to transport in an automobile. Although add-on units usually trade performance for convenience, they are relatively inexpensive and quite functional for recreational riders.

Tandems permit an ambulatory rider to use a leg crank while the other rider uses an arm crank. Tandems may be two- or three-wheeled, with the ambulatory rider sitting either in front or in back. When in the rear, ambulatory riders can sit higher and see over the other rider, providing both a clear view. With the ambulatory rider sitting forward, the wheelchair rider can use a carriage that permits cranking from the wheelchair. The ambulatory rider often does the steering and the shifting, in order to decouple cranking and gear changing from steering. Drive trains of tandems are most efficient when each rider can pedal at his/her own pace and coast independently.

Equipment for Field Events

The field events in which people in wheelchairs most often participate are the club, shot put, discus, and javelin. Only the most severely involved people (e.g., those with C4-C5 quadriplegia) compete in the club, in which individuals place the grip of the club (shaped like a bowling pin) between their fingers and then throw it.

Field event wheelchairs are not required to have wheels. Prior to the 1989 international athletics season, however, wheels were required. At that time most field athletes used old depot-type chairs that were as heavy as possible, since the weight made it stiffer and less likely to move while the athlete threw an implement (e.g., shot, discus, javelin). The rules describing the throwing chair were changed in order to modernize and revitalize the sport, leading to some interesting new features.

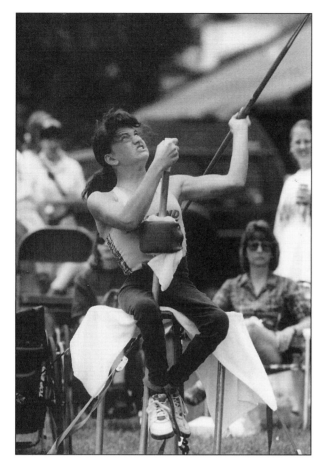

Figure 21.6 Athlete preparing to throw the javelin from a field event chair.
Courtesy of Sports 'N Spokes/Paralyzed Veterans of America.

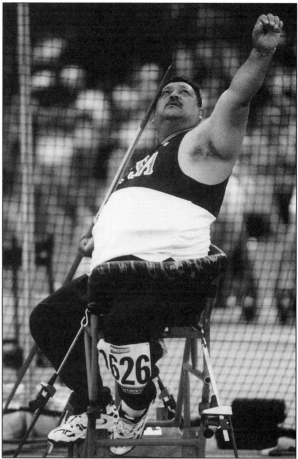

Figure 21.7 Note the supporting rails used by this athlete.
Courtesy of Sports 'N Spokes/Paralyzed Veterans of America.

Field event chairs provide a rigid base of support. The chair is strapped to the ground within a 1.5-meter throwing circle. Straps attach the chair to steel stakes that have been pounded into the ground. Although the thrower generally has the option of having the stakes moved, in many competitions the stakes are in a fixed location to expedite set-up. Throwing chairs include a means of leveling the seat, to help the thrower obtain the proper angle at release (40-50 degrees from horizontal). The seat of a throwing wheelchair usually has less than one centimeter of padding, because throwers desire maximum sitting height and the cushion is counted in the seat height. As throwers are not in the chair for very long, risk of pressure sores is minimal (but throwers should be cautious during extended training sessions). Figures 21.6 and 21.7 represent two different types of throwing chairs that individuals use for the javelin competition.

A large footplate supports the feet, permitting them to move as the thrower changes body positions.

Some throwers use the frame and straps of the throwing chair to restrict foot movement. In order for a throw to be legal, no part of the body may extend outside the throwing area until the judge signals. Rails guide the motion of the upper body through the throwing sequence, their shape customized to the size and abilities of the user. Those with lower impairments and high skills use the least restrictive rails to guide the trunk, whereas the rails are more restrictive (providing greater support) for people who are more severely impaired or less skilled. The rails are padded to protect the thrower's body from the impact received while moving through the throwing motion.

Since during major competitions the thrower and coach must move the chair into the throwing circle and secure it within a three- to five-minute period, most athletes add quick release wheels to the throwing frame for transport. This requirement has also led to simple attachment points and leveling mechanisms.

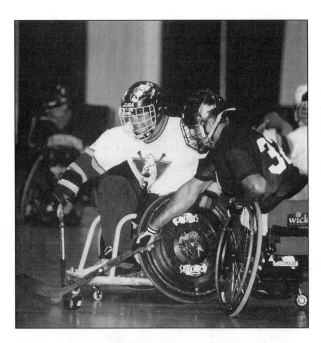

Figure 21.8 Athletes using court chairs to play floor hockey. Courtesy of Sport 'N Spokes/Paralyzed Veterans of America.

Equipment for Court Sports

Court sports wheelchairs are similar to ultralight wheelchairs designed for daily use, but with distinguishing features that make them more effective for use in specific sports (Coutts 1991; Golbranson and Wirta 1982). Court sports wheelchairs often display extreme camber in their rear wheels and small "roller blade"-type front casters. They use rigid frames. Many current features of lightweight wheelchairs were originally developed for wheelchair basketball and wheelchair racing. Figure 21.8 shows a version of the court chair that is used for floor hockey.

Basketball

Basketball wheelchairs must be lightweight so that players can accelerate and brake rapidly. Although basketball is not a contact sport, some incidental contact is inevitable. For this reason, spoke guards cover the rear wheel spokes. Exposed spokes can be broken during a game; sometimes, in fact, opponents may (illegally) try to disrupt play by ramming exposed spokes with parts of their chairs. Made of high-impact plastic, spoke guards provide several added benefits: they make it easier for players to pick up the ball from the floor by pushing it against the spoke guard and rolling it onto their lap; they protect hands and fingers when players are struggling for the ball; and they provide a convenient space to identify team affiliations.

Basketball wheelchairs are required to have forward anti-tip rollers or forward skids (commonly mounted to the footrests), both of which reduce the risk of forward falls and minimize damage to the basketball court. Some players use rear anti-tip casters, which help keep the wheelchair from falling over backwards (especially important for people with higher levels of impairment), but which can make it more difficult to accelerate the wheelchair by having the anti-tip wheels contacting the ground as a player pushes. Basketball wheelchairs have four wheels: two large wheels in the rear, used to push the chair, and two casters in the front for steering. The front casters are nearly always polyurethane with precision roller bearings, 5 centimeters (2 inches) in diameter. The rear wheels—commonly 61 centimeters (24 inches) or 66 centimeters (26 inches) in diameter—typically use high-pressure tires with no or very low-profile tread. High-pressure (120 to 200 psi) tires make it easier to push the wheelchair, and help to make it faster on the court.

Camber is an important feature of basketball wheelchairs, as it makes them more responsive during turns. Camber also protects players' hands when two wheelchairs collide from the sides, by limiting the collision to the bottom of the wheels and leaving a gap at the top to protect the hands. Refer back to chapter 15, figure 15.2, to see a front view of a wheelchair used for basketball, with camber on the rear wheels.

Basketball wheelchairs seats typically slope backwards about 5 degrees. Since the rules of basketball limit the maximum height of any portion of the seat, athletes usually try to make their seats as high as possible. Guards are an exception, as lower seat heights and greater seat angles can make chairs faster and more maneuverable for ball handling. Basketball wheelchairs often include loops for strapping the player into the chair. Strapping (the use of nylon or elastic straps) can be used to position a player in his wheelchair to improve performance. Positioning has been used so effectively by some players that it has changed their functional classification.

Tennis

Tennis is a very fast sport despite the two-bounce rule applied for wheelchair players. The wheelchair player must be able to cover the entire court. Many players focus on the baseline and move forward as

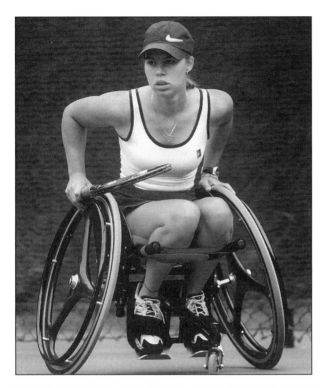

Figure 21.9 The tennis wheelchair includes several specialized features.
Photo © Curt Beamer.

necessary to make a shot. Winning play requires quickness, speed, maneuverability, and agility. For these reasons, tennis wheelchairs have evolved to include several specialized features: they use three wheels, the rear wheels typically being 61 centimeters (24 inches) or 66 centimeters (26 inches) in diameter; they use high-pressure tires (120-200 psi) to lower rolling resistance on the court and to increase speed; a single front caster, 5 centimeters (2 inches) in diameter, makes the chair light and more maneuverable; the rear wheels are cambered to increase lateral stability during side shots and to make the chair turn faster (figure 21.9). Neither front nor rear anti-tip casters are common on tennis wheelchairs.

Tennis players introduced the concept of radical seat angle: a steep seat angle, or "pinch," helps keep players against the seat backs, giving them greater control over the wheelchair and providing greater balance. The knees are abducted, with the feet on the footrest behind the player's knees. With the body in a relatively compact position, the combined inertia of rider and wheelchair is reduced (similar to figure skaters bringing their arms in to spin faster), making the chair more maneuverable. Tennis wheelchairs commonly use a rigid footrest so that the feet remain in place and do not touch the ground. Most players

strap their feet to the footrests. Handles incorporated into the front of the seat help the player balance while leaning forward or to the side to hit the ball; the handles also help keep the knees in place.

Quad Rugby

Quad rugby was developed by people with quadriplegia who can propel a manual wheelchair but who are not competitive at basketball. Because the rules of wheelchair basketball favor people who are not as severely involved (many of the top players do not even use a wheelchair as their primary source of mobility), people with low-level quadriplegia effectively had no team sporting opportunities prior to quad rugby. Quad rugby is a combination of team handball and rugby. Contact is permitted, and teams must carry the ball across their goal line to score. The ball may be passed or carried.

There is tremendous interest in quad rugby, whose rapid growth has led to the development of specialized four-wheeled chairs. The rear wheels are typically 61 centimeters (24 inches) in diameter, and the front casters 5 centimeters (2 inches) in diameter with precision roller bearings. The rear wheels are radically cambered to around 15 degrees, and protective framing is used around the wheels and the base of the chair (figure 21.10). This helps to protect the players from side impacts and glancing blows, and makes the chair turn faster. Guards wrap around the bottom front of the chair, from one rear wheel to another, and protect

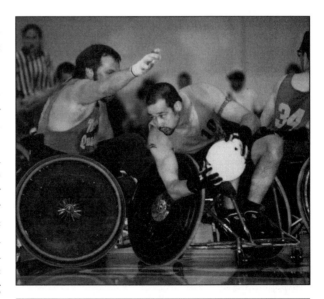

Figure 21.10 Note the protective framing around the base of the quad rugby wheelchair on the right.
Courtesy of Sports 'N Spokes/Paralyzed Veterans of America.

feet and legs against injury from other players' front casters. The guards also make it more difficult to hook the wheelchair—if a chair can be hooked, the player can be stopped and the opposing team gains an advantage.

In common with tennis wheelchairs, quad rugby wheelchairs use a radical seat angle—up to 20 degrees—that helps players maintain balance and maneuver more effectively. A highly stable seating position, with knees abducted and the feet behind the knees, provides the user good control over the chair. Because the rules for quad rugby restrict team members to wheelchair users who are more physically impaired, they require front and rear anti-tip casters that not only provide some protection from forward and rearward falls, but also help protect the court during impacts. Quad rugby chairs are a hybrid of basketball and tennis wheelchairs.

Prostheses

The major concern of people who undergo a lower limb amputation is whether they will be able to regain their previous level of physical activity (Czerniecki et al. 1991; Flowers et al. 1990; Gage and Ounpuu 1989; Gottschalk et al. 1985; James 1991). Prosthetic technology allows many individuals to achieve functional recovery nearly equal to preamputation potential (Krouskop et al. 1985; Krouskop et al. 1987; McDonnell et al. 1989; Michael 1989). People with amputations not only can participate in life's activities, but in many cases can participate with nondisabled people.

Foot Amputation Prostheses

Custom padding or inserts within conventional shoes often can treat partial foot amputation. Flexible shanks may prevent shoes from bending sharply at the end of the foot (Schneider et al. 1993; Suzuki 1972). Plastic laminate prostheses can provide functional ambulation for people with Syme amputations. With the aid of energy-storing feet—possibly the greatest advance in prosthetic design—people with lower limb amputation are able to move quickly and to run with a foot-over-foot gait (Wirta et al. 1991). These devices store energy via a flexible keel, which provides nonlinear spring action similar to the push-off phase of walking or running (Walker et al. 1985; Wirta et al. 1990).

The stationary attachment flexible endoskeletal (SAFE) foot is considered the first modern energy-storing prosthetic foot design (Wirta et al. 1991).

Since the introduction of SAFE, a number of other energy-storing feet have become commercially available. Energy-storing feet may be customized for an individual, or may be semi-customized. There are lightweight prosthetic feet with totally flexible keels to provide the appropriate dynamic elastic response for walking on uneven terrain. Lightweight graphite feet provide a strong push at toe-off for activities like running. Feet that provide a strong push-off are referred to as "super"-dynamic elastic response prosthetic feet (Torburn et al. 1990). These devices must have proper alignment for the leg to roll smoothly from heel-strike to toe-off (Nissan 1991; Wirta et al. 1991). This type of foot requires time to adjust to the spring action. A multiaxis foot provides motion in dorsiflexion, inversion, and eversion as well as plantar flexion. These features help to accommodate uneven terrain by having the foot conform to the terrain (Pinzur et al. 1991). Multiaxis feet can also store energy.

Swimming With Amputations

For a person with an amputation, swimming can be an important form of exercise because it is not traumatic to the residual limb. Although most people can enjoy swimming without a prosthesis, some choose to swim with one because it provides balance in the water. Both exoskeletal and endoskeletal prostheses can be used for swimming. Some prostheses are buoyant and may require the addition of weights. There are several types of swim legs: waterproofed walking prostheses, peg legs, stubbies, and hollow-chambered legs. Standard feet that are molded without an external heel cushion are less susceptible to becoming water-soaked. Any foot or standard prosthesis used in the water should be treated with a waterproof coating (e.g., New Skin, foot paint). Swimmers can add fins to stubbies or feet for added speed and control.

Factors to Consider in Choosing Leg Prostheses

The conventional patellar tendon-bearing (PTB) socket is adequate for activities of daily living, but not for active sports—it does not evenly distribute the impact impulse generated by active people. It is also uncomfortable to run with a prominent patellar bar. In contrast, a total surface-bearing socket provides for full contact, and dampens impact loading. Side joints and a thigh lacer can also reduce the forces on the residual limb by transferring some weight to the thigh.

Latex rubber suspension sleeves provide suction cup-type suspension, and help reduce pistoning for people with below-knee (BK) amputation. They may be used without additional support. A waist belt attached to a cuff suspension socket can provide additional suspension within the socket to prevent pistoning. Neoprene suspension sleeves can also provide atmospheric suspension. A silicone-suction socket (3S) can provide good suspension properties, and a socket interface that reduces shear forces. A simple "Muley" strap just above the femoral condyles—connected to smaller flexible straps pointing downward and backward along the medial and lateral aspects, and connected via a pivot to the shank—is effective for some people.

Computer-aided design and manufacturing (CAD-CAM) systems in prosthetics provide alternatives to traditional methods of producing positive molds used to make sockets. Several commercial CAD-CAM systems produce prosthetic sockets. Measurements intervals of 1.0 to 2.5 centimeters are satisfactory (Torres-Moreno et al. 1992).

Hydraulic knees allow stance and swing control, providing stability during single limb support (Popovic et al. 1991). Hyperextension of the hydraulic knee allows it to lock; otherwise, the knee provides hydraulic resistance to flexion. Force above a threshold at the prosthesis forefoot can be used to unlock the knee. Many hydraulic knees incorporate a manual lock for activities requiring maximum stability (e.g., driving an automobile, standing on a bus, standing at a work cell), and a release that allows maximum flexibility. Hydraulic knees typically incorporate a piston in a cylinder perforated with roughened holes that allow fluid to flow from one side of the cylinder to the other as the piston moves. Distribution of the holes within the cylinder determines the amount of dampening. Fewer holes are placed near the ends of the cylinder to provide terminal deceleration. The distribution of holes is asymmetrical. A consequence of using hydraulic knees is that some of the body's energy is dissipated through the hydraulic piston and cylinder.

Many knees incorporate several degrees of freedom. Flexible, or "bouncy," knees can reduce impact and provide knee stability. Friction and elastic components can be adjusted for an individual. However, fixed friction and elastic components of the knee are optimal only for the walking speed for which they are adjusted. Increases in gait speed may cause excessive heel rise and premature locking of the knee, while decreases in speed may result in toe stubbing due to inadequate knee flexion. Allowing friction adjustment by the user helps to alleviate these problems for some

people. The proper selection of the socket, knee, and foot can make possible such activities as heel-toe running for people with bilateral below-knee amputations.

Walking with a prosthetic limb varies substantially with surface inclination, camber, and roughness. Prosthetics designers must be familiar with all aspects of gait in people with lower limb amputations, as well as with the biomechanics of periodic events like stumbling, slipping, and falling. They must design prosthetics to minimize the occurrence and risk of injury associated with these events, while providing functional and efficient gait.

Biomechanical assessment techniques are not standard tools in most clinical settings. Most research has focused on level, steady-state walking; yet we very much need simple and easily measurable parameters related to various pathologies or misalignments. People can achieve normal prosthetic gait kinetics and kinematics using a variety of active muscles and neuromuscular control schemes—therefore level, steady-state gait analysis can miss many pathologies, prosthetic misalignments, or discomforts for which individuals compensate or which they hide. Electromyographic analysis provides little additional information usable by clinicians.

Classification

Classification of disabled athletes helps level the playing field for competitors with different disabilities or different degrees of the same disability. Competitions for athletes without disabilities use classification schemes for the same purpose (e.g., male and female competitions in marathons, and the senior PGA tour). The idea is that individuals with similar physical attributes compete against each other, allowing in the end for greater overall competition. The task of classifying athletes with disabilities is very complex because of the diversity of the populations.

An ideal classification system would

- be inclusive, including as many types of disabilities as possible;
- be fair, with no individual having an edge based solely on classification;
- enhance competition;
- enable individuals with different disabilities to compete on the same field;
- be easy to understand and apply.

Clearly no system can meet all the above criteria. Because there is no perfect system, there is also no uniformly accepted system. Each group representing a certain disability tends to have its own classification scheme. One example is the classification used by the United States Cerebral Palsy Association (USCPA), listed in table 21.1. This classification system is used in all individual sports, including track and field, swimming, cycling, and cross-country—where athletes compete only against athletes with their same classification. In the remaining sports, athletes are grouped in divisions according to classification as described in the web site **www.uscpaa.org**. Unfortunately, it is difficult to use this type of classification scheme to allow individuals with cerebral palsy to compete with other athletes with disabilities.

In the Paralympics, the largest sports competition for individuals with a variety of disabilities, several different classification schemes have governed competition. In earlier years, classification was based solely on type of disability such as blindness, spinal cord injury, amputation, and other orthopedic conditions. As the competition evolved, increasingly complex classification schemes resulted in a greater number of events—which, unfortunately, decreased competition by reducing the number of competitors

(Paralympic Spirit 1996). To assure that competition remains intense, the Paralympics have strict performance standards that must be met in order to qualify.

Recently the Paralympics have moved toward a functional classification system based on the athlete's ability to perform in a certain event. Wheelchair basketball, in which the wheelchair acts as an equalizer, is a leader in this movement: skills in the wheelchair determine competition level. Classifiers observe players' functions during competitions, and assign classifications based on their observations. Observed trunk movement and stability during actual basketball participation, rather than one's medical diagnosis or muscle function on an examining table, form the basis for a player's classification. Players are assigned a point value based on their classification. These points are summed during basketball play, with teams allowed only a predetermined maximum number of points on the floor.

Unfortunately, functional classification in basketball has made it harder for individuals with tetraplegia to compete. This situation led, in part, to the development of quad rugby. Moreover, functional classification cannot work for all sports: in many sports, com-

Table 21.1	Classifications Used by the USCPA

Class	Challenge
1	Severe involvement in all four limbs. Limited trunk control. Unable to grasp a softball. Poor functional strength in upper extremities, often necessitating the use of an electric wheelchair for independence.
2	Severe to moderate quadriplegic normally able to propel a wheelchair very slowly with arms or by pushing with feet. Poor functional strength and severe control problems in the upper extremities.
3	Moderate quadriplegic, fair functional strength and moderate control problems in upper extremities and torso. Uses wheelchair.
4	Lower limbs have moderate to severe involvement. Good functional strength and minimal control problem in upper extremities and torso. Uses wheelchair.
5	Good functional strength and minimal control problems in upper extremities. May walk with or without assistive devices for ambulatory support.
6	Moderate to severe hemiplegic. Ambulates without walking aids. Less coordination. Balance problems when running or throwing. Has greater upper extremity involvement.
7	Moderate to minimal hemiplegic. Good functional ability in nonaffected side. Walks/runs with noted limp.
8	Minimally affected. May have minimal coordination problems. Able to run and jump freely. Has good balance.

plex medical examinations are still needed to determine class. As in wheelchair basketball, many believe that use of prosthetics or adaptive equipment may make it easier to combine individuals with different disabilities. The current classification scheme used by the International Paralympic Committee is too complex to detail in this text. The full scheme is on the world wide web at the official site of the International Paralympic Committee: **http://www.paralympic.org** and the address of the IPC Headquarters is as follows:

International Paralyzed Committee
Adenauerallee 212 53113
BONN Germany
Telephone: +49 228 209 7200
Fax: +49 228 209 7209

Despite controversy over classification systems, each Paralympic game has been more inclusive and more successful then its predecessor. In addition, the Paralympics includes exhibit events that are open and have no classification system. It is anticipated that classification systems will continue to evolve with time, leading to systems that most closely meet the ideal.

Exercise Science and the Athlete With Impairments

Because the number of individuals participating in wheelchair sports and exercise is increasing, the need for research in this area is also increasing. Individuals with disabilities may have unique physiological adaptations to exercising or participating in sports activities. We need to investigate these physiological differences in order to help these individuals participate and succeed in their exercise and sport endeavors. Good research should lead to decreased injuries and health problems that stem from exercise or sports participation. If individuals with a disability can improve their health and fitness levels through exercise, they may be able to decrease their health care costs.

Physiological Studies

The history of exercise physiology in the United States dates back to the 1927 Harvard Fatigue Laboratory (Horvath and Horvath 1973). This laboratory,

directed by Dr. David Bruce Dill, laid the foundation for exercise and environmental physiology research within the university system. The early years of exercise physiology were dedicated not only to recruiting subjects for testing, but also to developing relevant instruments such as the classic Haldane analyzer for respiratory gas analysis. Advances in instrumentation have proceeded rapidly. Today we use sophisticated devices such as the computerized metabolic measurement systems that provide real-time oxygen and carbon dioxide measures.

The bulk of exercise physiology research since the late 1920s has focused on the nonimpaired population. Research on special populations has developed at a much slower pace. Several recent investigators, however, are doing significant work in exercise physiology research on physically impaired populations (Cooper et al. 1992; Cooper et al. 1993; Glaser 1989; Glaser et al. 1980; Janssen et al. 1994; Langbein and Maki 1995; Rodgers et al. 1994). The early stages of research focused on developing specialized exercise testing and training techniques for people with disabilities.

Several groups have studied the kinematics of racing wheelchair propulsion and its relationship to efficiency. Cooper and Bedi (1990) report that racing wheelchair propulsion has a gross mechanical efficiency over 30%, while Cooper et al. (1992) reported that 10K wheelchair racers have a maximum gross efficiency of 35%. Other investigators have studied physiological variables such as oxygen consumption, ventilation, and heart rate in elite wheelchair racers (Langbein and Maki 1995; Langbein et al. 1994; van der Woude et al. 1988). A common goal of exercise research today is to better understand the physiological responses of wheelchair athletes who seek to prevent or reduce secondary medical complications.

How Disability Affects Physiologic Control

Both the somatic and the autonomic nervous systems regulate the body during exercise. The **somatic nervous system** innervates and controls voluntary movements such as throwing a ball or propelling a wheelchair. The **autonomic nervous system** has two divisions. The **sympathetic nervous system** mediates the body's response to stress. It increases heart rate and blood pressure, mobilizes energy stores, and prepares to "fight or flee." In contrast, the **parasympathetic nervous system** works to restore homeostasis—it slows heart rate, reduces blood pressure, and prepares the body for rest. The somatic, sympathetic, and parasympathetic nervous systems together are a finely tuned network that prepares the body for every physiological need.

Physical impairments, however, significantly alter this finely tuned system. A traumatic spinal cord injury, for example, interrupts the **efferent** (motor) and **afferent** (sensory) pathways, so that communication between brain and the pathways below the level of injury generally does not occur. Damage to efferent pathways paralyzes the muscle fibers innervated by the damaged nerve: injury to the thoracic and/or lumbar region of the spine, for example, generally results in lower limb paralysis. Partial paralysis of the trunk muscles often occurs, depending on the level of the lesion. An injury to the cervical region typically results in both upper and lower limb paralysis, along with impairment to the trunk musculature. Injury to afferent pathways hinders communication to the brain regarding skin stimuli, muscle tension, muscle length, limb position, and rate of movement.

Skeletal muscle paralysis ultimately results in muscle atrophy. Atrophy of the skeletal muscles reduces functional capacity for voluntary exercise, especially since the primary movers below the level of injury, such as the leg and/or arm muscles, cannot be used for exercise. Many people, moreover, fail to consider how paralysis of the intercostal and abdominal muscles also diminishes physiological capacity. Because these muscles assist with ventilation, paralysis reduces one's ability to forcefully ventilate during exercise. The paralysis of primary movers and ventilatory musculature can greatly hinder athletic performance.

Injury to the sympathetic nervous system also hampers athletic performance. The sympathetic system strongly influences performance, because it is the "fight or flight" reflex. An impaired sympathetic system decreases the cardiovascular response to exercise, the effect during exercise varying with the level of injury. Impaired sympathetic systems influence athletic performance primarily by affecting smooth muscle regulation (for example, by impairing the ability to increase blood pressure) and by diminishing the capacity of the heart rate to increase during vigorous activity—in particular, individuals with high thoracic or cervical spinal cord injuries no longer have the capability of increasing the heart rate. This greatly hinders performance, since stroke volume and cardiac output cannot increase during exercise to meet the higher oxygen demands.

Spinal cord injury can also end sympathetic control of blood vessels. Injuries to the thoracic region have various effects on the sympathetic system, depending on the level of the injury. Individuals with cervical injuries lose the ability to constrict and dilate blood vessels—and the inability of arteries, arterioles, veins, and venules to dilate deprives active skeletal muscles of oxygen during exercise. Furthermore, the vessels can no longer shunt blood away from inactive organs and tissues (e.g., kidneys, stomach, intestines) to active skeletal muscles, further depriving them of oxygenated blood. These processes together greatly decrease one's ability to perform intense exercise.

Biomechanical Studies

Athletes with physical impairments—who participate in a variety of sports ranging from road racing to table tennis—constantly look for new ways to improve performance. But biomechanical studies of wheelchair sports are limited, as are studies of the biomechanics of tennis, rugby, basketball, field events, table tennis, weightlifting, rifle and pistol, archery, bowling, and swimming.

An exception is racing wheelchair propulsion. In order to increase athletic performance, investigators (Alexander 1989; Davis and Ferrara 1988; van der Woude et al. 1988) have extensively examined the biomechanics of this activity—especially such measures as segment angular and linear displacements, velocities, and accelerations. More specifically, they have studied the kinematics of the upper extremity during wheelchair propulsion in order to identify the most effective arm stroke pattern.

Training Techniques for Elite Athletes With Disabilities

The key to becoming an elite athlete is to attain peak performance at the appropriate time. Athletes cannot expect to be in peak condition during the entire season. It is best to focus on one event during the season, but this does not mean athletes should compete in only one event—in many instances, athletes must participate in preliminary events in order to qualify for larger events (e.g., Boston Marathon). In these cases, athletes should use the preceding events to train for the most important event, rather than attempting to win them. Because every game is important in team sports, however, such athletes should plan to peak immediately prior to the season and strive to maintain high levels of performance for the remainder of the season. They can do this by implementing a training technique called periodization.

Periodization is the technique of dividing the year into training intervals. Using team sports as an example, the year is divided into a preseason, in-season, main-season, and end-season. Even when training for one event, teams can use similar divisions: pre-competition, initial competition, main competition, and postcompetition. Athletes should implement the following five training regimens into their periodization program: endurance, speed, skill, strength, and flexibility.

Because each athlete and sport has different needs, time should not be allocated equally to each training program; implementing all five training regimens to some extent, however, will facilitate peak performance.

Endurance Training

Endurance training typically involves training for a particular event; a road racer would prepare for a 5K or 10K event, for example, by performing the event at least three days a week. Some athletes may train more frequently, others less, depending on their capabilities and levels of ambition. Training for a 6K event is a good way to prepare for an actual 5K event—the extra 1000 meters prepares the athlete for every weather condition and terrain, and also creates a psychological condition wherein the athlete, knowing he/she can easily complete a 6K, will push even harder during the competition.

Athletes should do interval training on days when they do not endurance train. During interval training, the athlete

- sprints a given distance,
- reduces his/her speed dramatically for a shorter distance, then
- performs the interval over again.

For example, a 400-meter sprinter would sprint for 200 meters, coast or lightly propel for 100 meters, then start the entire process over again, performing the intervals 5 to 10 times (depending on the distance of the intervals). As the athlete approaches competition, the sprinting portion of the intervals should increase while the "rest" interval decreases. This type of training stresses the cardiovascular and neuromuscular systems, preparing the body for competition.

Athletes who compete in endurance events should not focus solely on these two training regimens. They also should include training in speed, skill, strength, and flexibility in order to approach the highest possible physical condition. The following sections will discuss these training techniques.

Speed Training

Every periodization program should include speed training. Athletes who participate in sports such as basketball, rugby, track and field events, swimming, and weight training will benefit from speed training. Speed training increases reaction time—a fundamental element that separates first from second place.

Performing short sprinting intervals is the best method to train for speed. For an athlete who competes in 100-meter events, a single training session would be separated into four different distances. The following is a typical training day for a 100-meter athlete:

Distance (m)	Repetitions
80	3
90	3
100	3
110	3

The last set of repetitions is 10% longer than the event itself, so that the athlete will sprint for the entire 110 meters—which means he/she will drive through the entire 100 meters during competition. As athletes often slow down during the last portion of their workouts, this method assures that they will push through the entire event.

Another aspect of speed training is a technique called plyometrics. Plyometric exercise integrates strength and power into a single training session, resulting in explosive power. **Plyometrics** utilizes an external force to store energy within the musculature. The stored energy is immediately followed by an equal and opposite reaction, utilizing the natural elastic tendencies of the muscles to produce energy. Wheelchair sprinters can utilize a medicine ball or "plyoball" to perform upper body plyometrics. The athlete performs plyometrics by quickly catching and explosively passing the ball to a partner for multiple repetitions. The goal of plyometric exercises is to minimize the time the body has to recover from the external force (e.g., the thrown ball), thereby optimizing the amount of energy stored within the muscle. Because plyometric exercise is a very intense training technique, athletes should consult a certified trainer before performing these exercises.

Skill Training

Skill training in the context of this book is essentially equivalent to specificity training, which many athletes overlook because they think it encompasses only the competitive event. This is not entirely true. Although performing from a macroscopic standpoint is important, athletes should regularly examine events microscopically. For example, wheelchair sprinters should break down their stroking techniques into distinct phases—preparatory, propulsion, and recovery phase—with each phase examined for proper form and execution. This is the primary purpose for specificity training: proper form and execution of particular events will increase an athlete's performance. This chapter cannot cover every sport individually. Athletes should review relevant literature and consult coaches for training in specific activities. It is important for athletes to find third-party sources to consult rather than relying on themselves, since athletes almost universally find it difficult to criticize themselves.

Strength Training

Strength training typically refers to resistance training, which most commonly employs weight training. While noting that plyometric exercise and overspeed training (training at shorter distances with higher speeds) are often classified as resistance training, this book primarily covers weight training. Previous sections discussed plyometric exercise, while overspeed training techniques have not been widely used by athletes with physical impairments because of the lack of available commercial equipment.

Free Weights Versus Machines

Weight training can employ free weights or machines (e.g., Universal, Cybex, Nautilus). There are numerous advantages to using free weights:

- They permit small increments of weight.
- They teach coordination and balance.
- They allow creation of specific exercises for specific sports.

The primary disadvantage of free weights is that they require a "spotter" at all times. The advantage of machines is that they control the direction of movement—they do not allow for extraneous movements

that can contribute to injury. A disadvantage is that coordination and balance are minimized: an athlete can push entirely with one arm on a typical chest press machine, and the weight stack will still move. This is not true with free weights. Another disadvantage to machines is that they cannot be modified to become sport-specific, since they are usually are created to perform one basic exercise. Resistance training should not focus solely on free weights or machines—it is best rather to use both methods in order to provide a comprehensive workout. Figure 21.11 shows an individual strapped to the bench in order to compete in the bench press competition.

Popular Training Regimens

Opinions differ regarding optimal weight-training regimens. There is no one program that will suit every athlete. Athletes must consider their age, sex, weight, position, and particular sport when conditioning for the upcoming season. It is best initially to change training routines every few weeks in order to get an idea of what training program works best for an individual's particular needs—this should be done in the early preseason so that the athlete's training program will be established before the preseason is well underway, allowing the athlete to train hard for the greater part of the preseason.

Athletes use four common training routines. The first consists of training the entire body in one day: athletes perform fundamental exercises that train every major muscle of the body. A comprehensive weight-training program can include exercises such as the bench press, overhead/military press, seated rows, lat-pulls, squats, and standing calf-raises. To prevent overtraining, at least one day should be spaced between each workout of this type, with athletes devoting "off" days to training regimens for skill, flexibility, endurance, or speed.

The second training program consists of dividing the body into upper and lower portions. The individual dedicates one day to an upper body workout, with the second day focused on the lower body. Although this training program focuses on the fundamental exercises previously mentioned, it employs a more intense workout since only one-half of the body is exercised per workout. The higher intensity occurs via use of heavier weights or by performing more sets or repetitions (a later section will elaborate on the topic of sets and repetitions). The training program should include at least one "off" day to allow the body to recover from the more intense workout.

The third (and least commonly used) weight training program consists of exercising only one body part

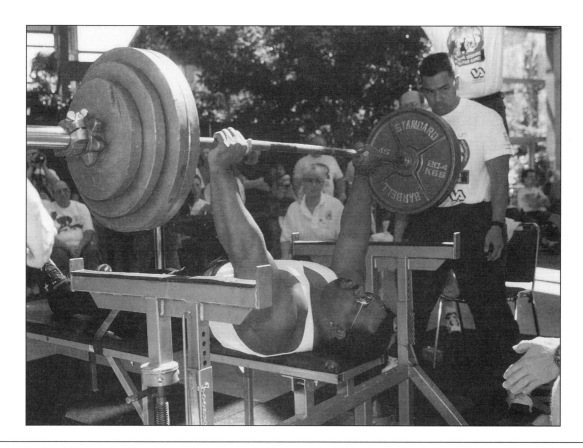

Figure 21.11 Athlete performing a competition bench press weight lift.
Photo © Curt Beamer.

per day. This type of program allows the athlete to focus his/her training routine on a single body part. A sample chest workout would include exercises such as bench press, incline press, decline press, and/or close-grip chest press, thus overloading the chest musculature in order to facilitate strengthening. The remaining days should be dedicated to the back, arm, shoulder, and leg musculature. Although this type of workout is every taxing to the body, it allows each body part to rest for at least three or four days, allowing for proper recuperation of the muscles. This program is useful not only for novice weightlifters because of its taxing nature—well-conditioned athletes also should use it when they are concentrating on building their strength.

The last (and very popular) program is commonly referred to as the "push-pull" workout. The push-pull workout divides the training program into three primary training days. The first day focuses on the chest and triceps area (the "push" day). The second day focuses on the back and biceps musculature (the "pull" day). The last day exercises the leg and shoulder musculature. This program permits very intense workouts, because each body part has at least three days to

recuperate—yet even with three days of muscle recuperation, individuals should dedicate at least one day to other training regimens after the last day of the entire push-pull routine.

Sets and Repetitions

The number of sets and repetitions per exercise depends on the purpose of the training program. Sets generally should remain between 2-5 per exercise, while repetitions should be between 6-15 per set. A general conditioning program should entail 3 sets per exercise, with 10-12 repetitions. The weight allocated to each set should be moderate. For strength training purposes, the repetitions should be reduced to 6 per set. The repetitions are reduced so higher weights can be used. Sets should typically be on the higher side (5), in order to properly overload the muscle. Endurance athletes should focus on lighter weights with higher repetitions (12-15), with the number of sets remaining around 3-4. It is important to remember that these are general recommendations. Each athlete should determine through experience the optimal number of sets and repetitions. It is best to begin a weight-training program by implementing a general conditioning program, moving to a more strenuous program only after general conditioning is completed. Most importantly, athletes should implement weight-training programs that complement their athletic events.

Flexibility Training

Flexibility training should be an integral part of any athlete's daily workout. Everyone should stretch before and after every workout, with static stretches held for at least 30 seconds. Everyone should avoid ballistic stretching, which can injure muscles.

Before each training session begins, the athlete should complete a warm-up session. This can consist of lightly pushing around the track a few times, or performing high-repetition/low-weight sets in a weight room. After the warm-up session, the athlete should perform a number of upper- and lower-extremity stretches, especially those specific to the competitive activity.

After every training session, athletes should cool down and stretch. Cooldowns can be similar to the exercises used to warm up, and can help alleviate muscle tightness and prepare the body for stretch-

ing. Stretching sessions after a workout should be comprehensive: both the upper and lower body require stretching after workouts. To insure that all muscles are properly stretched, a postexercise stretching session should last at least 20 minutes.

Injuries Experienced by Athletes With Disabilities

Since the inception of wheelchair athletics, health care providers have expressed great concern for the well-being of athletes with disabilities. Some early researchers argued against competition, stating that it could be harmful for the athletes. Yet Curtis et al. (1996), comparing two groups of individuals with spinal cord injuries, found that wheelchair athletes had fewer physician visits, and a trend toward fewer medical complications and fewer rehospitalizations, when compared with nonathletes. Sports participation did not lead to increased risk of medical complications and did not limit available time for vocational pursuits.

As in all sports, wheelchair athletes can be prone to acute injuries as well as repetitive strain type injuries (figure 21.12). According to Ferrara et al. (1992),

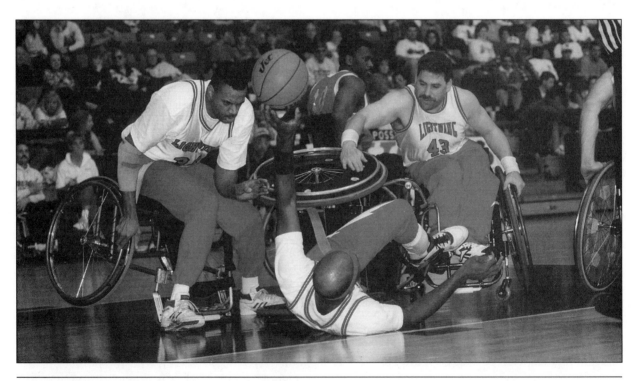

Figure 21.12 Wheelchair athletes do fall and sustain injuries.
Photo © Curt Beamer.

a wheelchair athlete is at no greater risk for acute injuries than any other athlete is. The most common acute injuries related to wheelchair sports are soft tissue injuries such as sprains, strains, muscle pulls, tendinitis, and bursitis (Curtis and Dillon 1985). The next two most common injuries are blisters and lacerations.

Treatment of these types of injuries is similar to that in the unimpaired population. The most common treatments are ice, nonsteroidal anti-inflammatory drugs, and relative rest. Relative rest is more difficult to achieve than in the general population, because wheelchair athletes use their arms for mobility and for all activities of daily living. For this reason, *prevention* of soft-tissue injuries is the best form of treatment. Selective strengthening and stretching, as well as appropriate warm-up exercises, are the mainstays of preventing injury.

Of special consideration for wheelchair athletes are the problems of hypothermia and hyperthermia, to which wheelchair athletes are more prone because temperature regulation is disordered below the level of a spinal cord injury. In addition, typical treatments for these conditions may not be as effective in individuals with spinal cord injury as in the general population. Standard techniques used to heat nondisabled athletes with hypothermia are ineffective: foil blankets commonly used after marathons do not work, because athletes do not shiver to generate the body heat necessary to rewarm inside a blanket. For this reason, it is important to remove wet clothing and use active methods to heat athletes, such as warm-water compresses. Unfortunately, clinicians who staff injury tents at the ends of marathons do not always know this information.

Athletes with spinal cord injuries bear increased risk of hyperthermia because of a decreased ability to perspire below the level of the injury. One way to check for hyperthermia in a distressed athlete is to feel beneath the arm (Bloomquist 1986): if it is hot, one should employ cooling techniques such as spraying water on extremities and removing layers of clothing. Adequate hydration is critical to preventing both hyperthermia and hypothermia.

As in acute injuries, research has shown that most wheelchair athletes are no more prone to repetitive-strain injuries than nonathletes. Boninger et al. (1996) and Burnham and Steadward (1994) found that neither elite wheelchair racers nor wheelchair basketball players had a higher incidence of carpal tunnel syndrome than that reported in the nonathletic disabled population. One exception may be weightlifters: all five competitive weightlifters whom Landsmeer

(1961) tested (using nerve conduction studies) had carpal tunnel syndrome, and most also had ulnar nerve injuries at the wrists. In light of this finding, it is prudent to monitor weightlifters for signs and symptoms of nerve entrapments.

Wheelchair athletes are by far the most studied group of athletes with disabilities. It is difficult to find studies assessing the risk to injury for athletes with dwarfism, visual impairment, or amputations. Although there is literature that shows increased risk to the contralateral limb in individuals with unilateral amputation, most researchers have studied individuals with dysvascular amputations. The pathology for the majority of athletes with amputations is traumatic or congenital; yet it is wise for athletes with amputation who participate in running sports to follow common-sense precautions in order to protect the contralateral limb from overuse injuries. Precautions include performing adequate stretching and strengthening exercises and choosing appropriate footwear. Many injuries occur when athletes are fatigued—appropriate conditioning training can prevent many of these injuries, reducing the likelihood of acquiring a secondary disability.

Summary

Advancements in the quality of emergency medical services, technology, and diagnostic tools have helped individuals with a disability to survive the initial accidents or illnesses and live longer lives. Individuals with a disability try to work themselves back into the general population, including all common aspects of life: work, everyday living activities, sports, and exercise.

Individuals with a disability are challenging many areas in regard to their participation in sports and exercise. Each individual can require different assistive technology in order for him/her to participate in a given sport or exercise and to obtain some success therein. Individuals need to achieve a certain level of success in order to maintain motivation to continue with sports and/or exercise.

Participation in sports and exercise leads to healthier and more fulfilling lifestyles. Advances in assistive technologies have enabled individuals with disabilities to participate increasingly in sports and exercise. There is need for much more research in this area, to help individuals with a disability to achieve their sport and exercise goals. Improvement in individuals' health and fitness levels may decrease their future health care costs.

References

Alexander, M.J.L. 1989. Aspects of performance in wheelchair marathon racing. *Journal de l'ACSEPL* 55:26-32.

Asato, K.T., R.A. Cooper, F.D. Baldini, and R.N. Robertson. 1992. Training practices of athletes who participated in the National Wheelchair Athletic Association Training Camps. *Adap Phys Act Q* 9:249-260.

Beck, K. 1992. Evergreen folding camper. *Paraplegia News* 46:31-32.

Bloomquist, L.E. 1986. Injuries to athletes with physical disabilities: prevention implications. *Phys Sportsmed* 14:97-105.

Boninger, M.L., R.N. Robertson, M. Wolff, and R.A. Cooper. 1996. Upper limb nerve entrapments in elite wheelchair racers. *Am J Phys Med Rehabil* 75:170-176.

Bosscher, R.J. 1993. Running and mixed physical exercises with depressed psychiatric patients. *Int J Sport Psych* 24:170-184.

Burnham, R.S., and R.D. Steadward. 1994. Upper extremity peripheral nerve entrapments among wheelchair athletes: prevalence, location, and risk factors. *Arch Phys Med Rehabil* 75:519-524.

Byrne, A., and D.G. Byrne. 1993. The effect of exercise on depression, anxiety, and other mood states: a review. *J Psychosom Res* 37:565-574.

Charles, D., K.B. James, and R.B. Stein. 1988. Rehabilitation of musicians with upper limb amputations. *J Rehabil Res Dev* 25:25-32.

Cook, A.M., and J.G. Webster. 1982. *Therapeutic medical devices: Application and design.* Englewood Cliffs, NJ: Prentice Hall.

Cooper, R.A. 1989a. Racing wheelchair crown compensation. *J Rehabil Res Dev* 26:25-32.

Cooper, R.A. 1989b. Racing wheelchair rear wheel alignment. *J Rehabil Res Dev* 26:47-50.

Cooper, R.A. 1989c. An international track wheelchair with a center of gravity directional controller. *J Rehabil Res Dev* 26:63-70.

Cooper, R.A. 1990. Wheelchair racing sports science: a review. *J Rehabil Res Dev* 27: 295-312.

Cooper, R.A. 1992a. Contributions of selected anthropometric and metabolic parameters to 10K performance—a preliminary study. *J Rehabil Res Dev* 29:29-34.

Cooper, R.A. 1992b. Racing wheelchair roll stability while turning: a simple model. *J Rehabil Res Dev* 29:23-30.

Cooper, R.A., F.D. Baldini, W.E. Langbein, R.N. Robertson, P. Bennett, and S. Monical. 1993. Prediction of pulmonary function in wheelchair users. *Paraplegia* 31:560-570.

Cooper, R.A., and J.F. Bedi. 1990. Gross mechanical efficiency of trained wheelchair racers. Paper presented at the 12th Annual International Conference of the IEEE/EMBS, Philadelphia, Pennsylvania.

Cooper, R.A., S.M. Horvath, J.F. Bedi, D.M. Drechsler-Parks, and R.E. Williams. 1992. Maximal exercise response of paraplegic wheelchair road racers. *Paraplegia* 30:573-581.

Coutts, K.D. 1991. Dynamic characteristics of a sport wheelchair. *J Rehabil Res Dev* 28:45-50.

Curtis, K.A., and D.A. Dillon. 1985. Survey of wheelchair athletic injuries: common patterns and prevention. *Paraplegia* 23:170-175.

Curtis, K.A., S. McClanahan, K.M. Hall, D. Dillon, and K.F. Brown. 1986. Health, vocational, and functional status in spinal cord injured athletes and nonathletes. *Arch Phys Med Rehab* 67:862-865.

Czerniecki, J.M., A. Gotter, and C. Munro. 1991. Joint moment and muscle power output characteristics of below knee amputees during running: the influence of energy storing prosthetic feet. *J Biomech* 24:63-75.

Davis, R. and M. Ferrara. 1988. The competitive wheelchair stroke. *National Strength Conditioning Association Journal* 10:4-10.

Engel, P., and K. Seeliger. 1986. Technological and physiological characteristics of a newly developed hand-lever drive system for wheelchairs. *J Rehabil Res Dev* 23:37-40.

Ferrara, M.S., W.E. Buckley, B.C. McCann, and T.J. Limbird. 1992. The injury experience of the competitive athlete with a disability: prevention implications. *Med Sci Sports Exerc* 24:184-188.

Flowers, W., C. Cullen, and K.P. Tyra. 1990. A preliminary report on the use of a practical biofeedback device for gait training of above-knee amputees. *J Rehabil Res Dev* 23:7-18.

Gage, J.R., and S. Ounpuu. 1989. Gait analysis in clinical practice. *Semin Orthopedics* 4:72-87.

Galvin, J.C., and M.J. Scherer. 1996. *Evaluating, selecting, and using appropriate assistive technology.* Gaithersburg, MD: Aspen.

Glaser, R.M. 1989. Arm exercise training for wheelchair users. *Med Sci Sports Exerc* 21:S149-S157.

Glaser, R.M., M.N. Sawka, M.F. Brune, and S.W. Wilde. 1980. Physiological responses to maximal effort wheelchair and arm crank ergometry. *J Appl Physiol* 48:1060-1064.

Golbranson, F.L., and R.W. Wirta. 1982. *Wheelchair III: report of a workshop on specially adapted wheelchairs and sports wheelchairs.* Washington, DC: RESNA Press.

Gottschalk, F., B. McClellan, A. Carlton, and V. Mooney. 1985. Early fitting of the amputee with a plastic temporary adjustable below-knee prosthesis. *Proceedings RESNA 8th Annual Conference.* Memphis, TN, 373-375.

Hinkle, J.S. 1992. Aerobic running behavior and psychotherapeutics: implications for sports counseling and psychology. *J Sport Behav* 15:263-277.

Horvath, S.M., and E.C. Horvath. 1973. *The Harvard fatigue laboratory: Its history and contributions.* Englewood Cliffs, NJ: Prentice-Hall.

Houtkooper, L. 1986. Nutritional support for muscle weight gain. *National Strength and Conditioning Association Journal* 8:62-63.

James, W.V. 1991. Principles of limb fitting and prostheses. *Ann R Coll Surg Engl* 73:158-162.

Janssen, T.W.J., C.A.J.M. van Oers, L.H.V. van der Woude, and P. Hollander. 1994. Physical strain in daily life of wheelchair users with spinal cord injuries. *Med Sci Sports Exerc* 26:661-670.

King, A.C., C.B. Taylor, and W.L. Haskell. 1993. Effects of differing intensities and formats of 12 months of exercise training on psychological outcomes in older adults. *Health Psychol* 12:292-300.

Krouskop, T.A., B.L. Goode, D.R. Doughtery, and E.H. Hemmen. 1985. Predicting the loaded shape of an amputee's residual limb. *Proceedings RESNA 8th Annual Conference.* Memphis, TN, 225-227.

Krouskop, T.A., A.L. Muilenberg, D.R. Doughtery, and D.J. Winningham. 1987. Computer-aided design of a prosthetic socket for an above-knee amputee. *J Rehabil Res Dev* 24:31-38.

Landsmeer, J.M.F. 1961. Studies in the anatomy of articulation: II. Patterns of movement of bi-muscular, bi-articular systems. *Acta Morphological Neerlando Scandinavica* 3:304-321.

Langbein, W.E., and K.C. Maki. 1995. Predicting oxygen uptake during counterclockwise arm crank ergometry in men with lower limb disabilities. *Arch Phys Med Rehabil* 76:642-646.

Langbein, W.E., K.C. Maki, L.C. Edwards, M.H. Hwang, P. Sibley, and L. Fehr. 1994. Initial clinical evaluation of a wheelchair ergometer for diagnostic exercise testing: a technical note. *J Rehabil Res Dev* 31:317-325.

Loverock, P. 1989. The athlete of the future. *Los Angeles Times Magazine,* March 12.

Maarlewski-Probert, B. 1992. The RV industry is meeting the challenge. *Paraplegia News* 46:21-23.

MacLeish, M.S., R.A. Cooper, J. Harralson, and J.S. Ster. 1993. Design of a composite monocoque frame racing wheelchair. *J Rehabil Res Dev* 30:233-249.

Maresh, C.M., B.G. Sheckley, G.J. Allen, D.N. Camaione, and S.T. Sinatra. 1991. Middle age male distance runners: physiological and psychological profiles. *J Sports Med Phys Fitness* 31:461-469.

McArdle, W.D., F.I. Katch, and V.L. Katch. 1991. *Exercise physiology: Energy, nutrition, and human performance.* 3d ed. Philadelphia/London: Lea & Febiger.

McDonnell, P.M., R.N. Scott, J. Dickison, R.A. Theriault, and B. Wood. 1989. Do artificial limbs become part of the user? New evidence. *J Rehabil Res Dev* 26:17-24.

Michael, J.W. 1989. Reflections on CAD-CAM in prosthetics and orthotics. *J Prosthet Orthot* 1:116-121.

National Academy of Sciences. 1989. *Recommended Dietary Allowances.* Washington, DC: National Academy Press.

Nissan, M. 1991. The initiation of gait in lower limb amputees: some related data. *J Rehabil Res Dev* 28:1-12.

Pappas, G.P., S. Golin, and D.L. Meyer. 1990. Reducing symptoms of depression with exercise. *Psychosomatics* 31:112-113.

Pelham, T.W., P.D. Campagna, P.G. Ritvo, and W.A. Birnie. 1993. The effects of exercise therapy on clients in a psychiatric rehabilitation program. *Psychosoc Rehabil J* 16:75-84.

Pinzur, M.S., P. Perona, A. Patwardhan, and R. Havey. 1991. Loading of the contralateral foot in peripheral vascular insufficiency below-knee amputees. *Foot Ankle* 11:368-371.

Popovic, D., M.N. Oguztoreli, and R.B. Stein. 1991. Optimal control for the active above knee prosthesis. *Ann Biomed Eng* 19:131-150.

Rick Hansen Centre. 1988. *Proceedings from a national symposium on wheelchair track and road racing department of physical education and sport studies.* Edmonton: University of Alberta Press.

Rodgers, M.M., W. Gayle, S.F. Figoni, M. Kobayashi, J. Lieh, and R.M. Glaser. 1994. Biomechanics of wheelchair propulsion during fatigue. *Arch Phys Med Rehabil* 75:85-93.

Rozenek, R., and M.H. Stone. 1984. Protein metabolism related to athletes. *National Strength and Conditioning Association Journal* 6:42-45.

Schneider, K., T. Hart, R.F. Zernicke, Y. Setoguchsi, and W. Oppenheim. 1993. Dynamics of below-knee child amputee gait: SACH foot versus flex foot. *J Biomech* 26:1191-1204.

Skinner, H.B., and D.J. Effeney. 1985. Gait analysis in amputees. *Am J Phys Med* 64:82-89.

Snell, F. 1992. Bringing prosthetics into the 21st century. *J Ark Med Soc* 89:337-338.

Stein, P.N., and R.W. Motta. 1992. Effects of aerobic and nonaerobic exercise on depression and self-concept. *Percept Mot Skills* 74:79-89.

Steptoe, A., J. Moses, S. Edwards, and A. Mathews. 1993. Exercise and responsivity to mental stress: discrepancies between the subjective and physiological effects of aerobic training. *Int J Sport Psych* 24:110-129.

Suzuki, K. 1972. Force plate study on the artificial limb gait. *Journal of Japanese Orthopaedic Association* 46:503-516.

Topper, A.K., and G.R. Fernie. 1990. An evaluation of computer aided design of below-knee prosthetic sockets. *Prosthet Orthot Int* 14:136-142.

Torburn, L., J. Perry, E. Ayyappa, and S. Shanfield. 1990. Below-knee amputee gait with dynamic elastic response prosthetic feet: a pilot study. *J Rehabil Res Dev* 27:369-384.

Torres-Moreno, R., J.B. Morrison, D. Cooper, C.G. Saunders, and J. Foort. 1992. A computer-aided socket design procedure for above-knee prostheses. *J Rehabil Res Dev* 29:35-44.

van der Woude, L.H.V., H.E.J. Veeger, R.H. Rozendal, G.J. van ingen Schenau, E. Rooth, and P. van Nierop. 1988. Wheelchair racing: effects of rim diameter and speed on physiology and technique. *Med Sci Sports Exerc* 20:492-500.

Wade, J. 1993. A league of its own. *REHAB Management* 6:44-51.

Walker, P.S., H. Kurosawa, J.S. Rovick, and R.A. Zimmerman. 1985. External knee joint design based on normal motion. *J Rehabil Res Dev* 22:9-22.

Wankel, L.M. 1993. The importance of enjoyment to adherent and psychological benefits from physical activity. *Int J Sport Psych* 24:151-169.

Wirta, R., F. Goldbranson, R. Mason, and K. Calvo. 1990. Analysis of below-knee suspension systems: effect on gait. *J Rehabil Res Dev* 27:385-396.

Wirta, R., R. Mason, K. Calvo, and F.L. Goldbranson. 1991. Effect on gait using various prosthetic ankle-foot devices. *J Rehabil Res Dev* 28:13-24.

Subject Index

Note: Page numbers in italics refer to the figure or table on that page.

Citation Index

Liebesman and Cafarelli 1994 84, 85
Limacher 1994 395
Lin et al. 1993 115
Lindeman et al. 1994 254
Lindeman et al. 1995 260
Linderman et al. 1995 259
Lindsay and Wyckoff 1981 355
Linsted et al. 1991 157
Lipetz et al. 1997 275
Lipman et al. 1972 218
Lipson et al. 1980 216
Lisboa et al. 1994 204
Lishman 1987 355
Logigian et al. 1983 298
Logsdon et al. 1989 131
Lohman et al. 1995 321
Lohmann et al. 1978 218
LoLorier et al. 1997 302
Lomo 1989 295
Londeree 1997 63
Long et al. 1996 138
Lord and Castell 1994 79
Lord and Hall 1986 298
Lord et al. 1991 165
Lord et al. 1995 410
Lord et al. 1996 326, 410
Loverock 1980 425
Lowey et al. 1993 6
Lucas and Koslow 1984 98
Luger et al. 1987 362
Lund-Johnson 1967 177
Lyngberg et al. 1988 230, 231
Lyngberg et al. 1994 229, 233, 235
Lysens et al. 1989 94

M

MacDonald 1987 219
MacDonald et al. 1987 355
MacDougall 1986 406
MacDougall et al. 1992 318, 335
Machover and Sapecky 1966 230, 231
Macko et al. 1997 306
MacLeish et al. 1993 426
Madsen 1993 361
Madsen et al. 1993 323
Maestro et al. 1990 200
Magel et al. 1975 64
Magel et al. 1978 64
Magnusson et al. 1994 298
Magnusson et al. 1996 93
Make and Buckolz 1991 196
Makrides et al. 1990 64
Malfatto et al. 1996 178
Maltais et al. 1995 198
Maltais et al. 1996 198
Mancini et al. 1991 179
Mancini et al. 1992 177
Mandel et al. 1990 302
Manson et al. 1991 159, 215
Manson et al. 1992 159, 176, 215
Marcus et al. 1985 317, 333
Marcus et al. 1992 320
Marcus et al. 1995 354
Margonato et al. 1986 217
Margulies et al. 1986 61
Markoff et al. 1982 62
Markovic et al. 1994 318
Marlatt and George 1990 136
Marrero et al. 1988 216
Marshall et al. 1980 85
Martin 1996 79
Martin and Notelovitz 1993 324, 339
Martin et al. 1979 58

Martin et al. 1991 200
Martin et al. 1992 271, 272
Martinez et al. 1990 200
Martinez et al. 1993 202
Martinson 1994 355, 356, 366
Martinson et al. 1985 357
Martinson et al. 1989 355
Massie and Holland 1990 355
Matsumoto et al. 1973 306
Maughan and Poole 1981 47
Mayou and Bryant 1993 187
Mazess and Barden 1991 320
McArdle et al. 1991 105
McArdle et al. 1994 274, 275, 278
McAuley and Jacobson 1991 355
McBride et al. 1992 153
McCain et al. 1988 61
McCann and Holmes 1984 62, 356, 357
McCartney et al. 1988 259, 260
McCartney et al. 1995 414
McCormick et al. 1990 5
McCrory et al. 1998 256, 259
McCulloch et al. 1990 319
McDonagh et al. 1994 400
McDonald and Hodgdon 1991 356
McDonald et al. 1995a 258
McDonald et al. 1995b 258, 259
McDonnell et al. 1989 436
McGavin et al. 1976 199
McLeroy et al. 1988 138
McMurdo and Burnett 1992 354
McMurdo et al. 1992 404
McPeak 1996 120
Melin et al. 1980 60
Mellah et al. 1990 283
Melton 1993 326
Melton et al. 1992 314
Melton et al. 1997 314
Menkes et al. 1993 407, 408
Menotti et al. 1990 294
Mense 1978 96
Meredith et al. 1989 48, 64, 381, 401, 403
Meredith et al. 1992 408
Merletti et al. 1978 304
Merlis and Watson 1949 280
Mertens and Kavanagh 1996 184
Merzenich et al. 1984 280
Messner-Pellenc et al. 1994 179
Metropolitan Life Insurance Company 1980 375
Metz et al. 1993 320
Metzger and Stein 1984 61
Meyer and Foley 1996 5, 9, 18
Meyer et al. 1984 4
Mezzetti et al. 1998 162
Michael 1989 436
Michel et al. 1989 322
Michel et al. 1991 322
Micheli 1983 85
Micossi and Harris 1990 375
Miglietta 1973 96
Mikines et al. 1987 60
Mikines et al. 1988 60, 222
Mikines et al. 1989 223
Milani et al. 1996 187
Miller 1993 391
Milner-Brown and Miller 1988 259, 260
Milner-Brown et al. 1973 282
Miniare et al. 1974 272
Minor et al. 1989 229, 232, 237, 242

Minotti et al. 1991 177
Mira 1982 270
Mitchell et al. 1988 220
Mitchell et al. 1992 64
Mizuno et al. 1994 7
Moens et al. 1993 255
Mogensen and Vittinghu 1975 217
Mogenson et al. 1993 359
Mogliner et al. 1993 280
Mohsenifar et al. 1983 196, 197
Moldofsky and Scarisbrick 1976 61
Moldover and Bartels 1996 109, 111, 115
Moldover et al. 1984 306
Mole et al. 1971 59
Mondin 1996 362
Mondin et al. 1996 362, 365
Monga et al. 1988 306
Moore and Blumenthal 1998 366
Moore and Hutton 1980 98
Moreland and Thomson 1993 299
Moretz et al. 1982 95
Morgan 1975 306
Morgan 1979 62
Morgan 1985 366
Morgan 1994 355, 356, 362, 364, 365, 367
Morgan and Goldston 1987 365
Morganti et al. 1995 409
Morgenson et al. 1993 360
Moritani and deVries 1980 406
Morris 1994 155
Morris et al. 1966 152
Morris et al. 1992 302
Morris et al. 1993 111
Morrison et al. 1986 56
Morse 1994 360
Moser et el. 1980 197
Moses et al. 1989 355
Mougin et al. 1987 61
Mroczek et al. 1978 300
Mulder et al. 1986 301
Muller 1970 398
Mundale 1970 112, 121
Murakami et al. 1996 254
Murray 1992 358
Mutrie 1988 357
Myburgh et al. 1990 317
Myburgh et al. 1993 317, 333
Myers et al. 1992 115

N

Nadel et al. 1974 59
Naeser et al. 1992 298
Naftchi et al. 1980 273
Nagi 1965 407
Nagi 1991 407
Nakamura et al. 1985 305, 306
Naso et al. 1990 400, 403
National High Blood Pressure Education Program, JNC VI 1997 156
Nelson 1998 382
Nelson et al. 1982 219
Nelson et al. 1988 321
Nelson et al. 1991 323
Nelson et al. 1994 79, 324, 339, 397, 407, 409, 414, 415
Nelson et al. 1996 299
Netz and Jacob 1994 354
Newsholme and Leech 1983 50
Newsholme and Start 1973 46, 48
Neylan 1995 358

NHANES III 374
NHLBI 1998 374
Nicholas 1970 95
Nichols and Glenn 1994 61
Nichols et al. 1993 79, 408
Nichols et al. 1994 164
Niebauer and Cooke 1996 158
Niederman et al. 1991 196, 198
Nieman 1996 165
Nieman and Nehlsen-Cannarella 1992 160
Nieman and Onasch 1990 379
Nieman et al. 1995 160
NIH 1995 268, 269
NIH 1996 56, 62, 63, 153, 155
NIH Consensus 1996 187
Nilsson and Westlin 1971 329
Nilsson et al. 1975 272
Nissan 1991 436
Nix and Hopf 1983 272
Nordesjo et al. 1983 230
Noreau 1995 366
Noreau and Shephard 1992 268, 269, 270
Noreau et al. 1995 354
North et al. 1990 358, 364
Notelovitz et al. 1991 324, 340
Nudo and Milliken 1996 296
Nudo, Milliken et al. 1996 296
Nudo, Wise et al. 1996 296
Nugent et al. 1994 296, 299
Nyberg-Hansen and Rinvik 1963 296

O

O'Connor and Youngstedt 1995 61
O'Connor et al. 1982 314
O'Connor et al. 1989 51, 186, 187
O'Donnell et al. 1993 197
O'Driscoll et al. 1978 244, 245
Ogawa et al. 1992 395, 401
O'Hara et al. 1984 199
Ohkubo et al. 1995 213
Ohlsson and Johansson 1995 296, 298
Okumiya et al. 1996 354
Olausson et al. 1986 61
Oldridge et al. 1988 186, 187
Oldridge et al. 1993 187
Olefsky et al. 1988 50
Oliveira et al. 1996 163
Orlander and Aniansson 1980 401
Ory et al. 1993 397
Owen and Jones 1985 118
Owens et al. 1992 378

P

Pace and Rathburn 1945 383
Paez et al. 1967 197
Paffenbarger and Hyde 1984 105
Paffenbarger et al. 1978 129
Paffenbarger et al. 1983 156
Paffenbarger et al. 1986 41, 413
Paffenbarger et al. 1993 413
Paffenbarger et al. 1994 167, 168, 350
Paivio 1986 283
Palmer et al. 1995 357
Pandolf et al. 1988 59
Panush et al. 1995 165
Pardy et al. 1981 204
Pare et al. 1993 115
Parizkova 1974 396
Pascual-Leone et al. 1994 296
Pashkow et al. 1988 181
Pashkow et al. 1995 187
Passmore 1971 131

Smith et al. 1995 176, 186
Smutok et al. 1994 159
Snell 1992 425
Snow et al. 1996 320
Snow-Harter et al. 1990 323
Snow-Harter et al. 1992 321
Snyder 1978 362
Sockolov et al. 1977 255, 258
Sonstroem 1984 62
Sorrentino et al. 1988 48
Souminen et al. 1977 401, 402
Sovijarvi et al. 1992 177
Spector et al. 1996 258
Spencer et al. 1984 73, 75
Stanescu et al. 1981 207
Staron et al. 1994 77
Stedman et al. 1991 258
Stefanovska et al. 1991 272
Steinberg et al. 1967 200
Stenstrom 1994 229
Stenstrom et al. 1996 229, 234
Stenstrom et al. 1997 234, 248, 249
Stephens 1988 350, 355, 364
Stern et al. 1970 298
Stevens et al. 1984 294
Stokols 1992 138
Stone 1988 78
Stone 1998 72
Stone et al. 1985 42, 44
Storstein and Jervell 1979 217
St. Pierre and Gardner 1987 75
Strand et al. 1985 294
Stratton et al. 1987 216
Stratton et al. 1991 187
Stratton et al. 1992 396
Stratton et al. 1994 396, 401, 405
Strawbridge et al. 1996 62
Streletz et al. 1995 280
Stremmel 1988 48
Stroke Unit Trialists' 1997 294
Stroud et al. 1989 94
Sudarsky 1990 326
Suinn 1984 283
Sullivan and Markos 1995 76, 77
Sullivan et al. 1989 177
Sunderland et al. 1989 305
Sunderland et al. 1994 299
Surgeon General 1996 63
Sutherland et al. 1990 38
Sutton 1978 60
Sutton et al. 1969 60
Suzman et al. 1992 392
Suzuki 1972 436
Sweeney et al. 1993 383
Swezey 1974 230
Sydney and Shephard 1978 400

T

Taaffe et al. 1995 316
Taaffe et al. 1997 317, 334
Tabary et al. 1972 87
Tamura et al. 1989 5
Tandon 1980 207
Tangeman et al. 1990 296, 299
Tangri and Woolf 1973 200
Tarnopolsky et al. 1992 48
Tate and Petruzzello 1995 357
Taub and Wolf 1993 296

Taub and Wolf 1997 299
Taub et al. 1993 298
Taylor et al. 1949 106
Taylor et al. 1955 46
Taylor et al. 1983 158
Taylor et al. 1990 87, 97, 99
Taylor et al. 1996 9, 88
Terrados and Maughan 1995 59
Tesch and Karlsson 1983 271
Tesch and Larsson 1982 78
Testa and Simonson 1996 187
Teylor et al. 1955 42
Thomas et al. 1985 402
Thompson 1994 74
Thompson et al. 1982 106
Thompson et al. 1988 402
Thompson et al. 1996 176
Thorstensson et al. 1976 72
Tiller 1992 355
Tinetti and Speechley 1989 393
Tinetti et al. 1988 326
Tinetti et al. 1994 326
Tipton 1991 129
Tipton et al. 1975 61
Topka et al. 1991 280
Topol et al. 1988 111
Torburn et al. 1990 436
Torres-Moreno et al. 1992 437
Tran and Weltman 1985 187
Treanor 1969 38
Treuth et al. 1995 79
Trexler and Fordyce 1996 353
Trombly and Quintana 1983 305
Trombly et al. 1986 298, 305
Turcotte 1992 48
Turner et al. 1991 258
Tzankoff and Norris 1977 397

U

UKPDS 1998 213
Ulrich et al. 1996 61
Urbsheit and Oremland 1990 306
U.S. Bureau of the Census 1991 392
USDHHS 1991 129, 130
USDHHS 1996 129, 135, 152, 153,
    155, 156, 160, 161, 163, 164, 168,
    294, 350, 398, 399
U.S. Preventive Services Task Force
    1996 132

V

Van Camp and Peterson 1986 185
van den Ende et al. 1996 230, 234,
    236
Vander et al. 1985 60
Vandervoort 1995 406
Van der Vusse and Reneman 1996 11
van der Woude et al. 1988 439, 440
Van Etten et al. 1997 382
VanGelderen et al. 1995 282
Vanlandewijck et al. 1994 115
VanLoan et al. 1987 274, 275
Van Pelt et al. 1998 376, 379
Veale et al. 1992 357
Verrill 1998 182
Verrill et al. 1992 182
Veves et al. 1997 49
Viberti et al. 1978 217

Vico et al. 1995 322
Vignos 1983 257, 259, 264
Vignos and Watkins 1996 259, 260
Viitanen et al. 1995 244, 245, 247
Virvidakis et al. 1990 316, 330
Vitanen et al. 1992 244
Vitug et al. 1988 49
Vodovnik and Karba 1992 272
Vollestad and Blom 1985 10, 13
Vongvanich et al. 1996 185
Vranic and Wrenshall 1969 49, 50
Vranic et al. 1976 47, 50
Vranic et al. 1990 49

W

Wade 1993 425
Wade et al. 1992 299
Wagenaar et al. 1990 298
Wahren et al. 1984 50
Walker et al. 1985 436
Walker-Batson et al. 1995 297
Wallberg-Henrickson 1987 50
Wallberg-Henrickson et al. 1986 216
Wallin et al. 1985 98, 99
Wang and Morgan 1992 284
Wannamethee and Shaper 1992 157
Wannamethee et al. 1995 160
Warren et al. 1976 230
Warren et al. 1993 405
Wasserman 1995 47
Wasserman and Cherrington 1996 11
Wasserman and Zinman 1995 50
Waterman-Storer 1991 85
Waters et al. 1979 38
Weber et al. 1982 177, 179
Weber et al. 1986 177
Weber et al. 1987 111
Weder et al. 1994 281
Weibel 1979 9, 13
Weibel 1984 9
Weigle et al. 1988 382
Weiner et al. 1981 186
Weiner et al. 1992 204
Welle et al. 1991 381
Welle et al. 1996 409
Weller et al. 1990 255
Wells et al. 1989 131
Welten et al. 1994 319
Werner and Kessler 1996 296
Wessel and Quinney 1984 230, 231
Westerblad and Allen 1993 16, 18
Westerblad et al. 1991 16
Westerblad et al. 1993 16, 18
West Virginia University 1988 131
Weyerer 1992 168
Wheeler et al. 1984 60
Wheeler et al. 1994 278
Wheeler et al. 1996 278
Whelan et al. 1991 363
Whipple et al. 1987 397
White et al. 1983 219
WHO 1997 392
Wigers et al. 1996 354
Wijkstra et al. 1994 197, 199
Wiley et al. 1992 51
Williams 1997 167
Williams and Goldspink 1984 75
Williams and Hornberger 1984 398

Williams and Klug 1995 14, 17, 18
Williams and Neufer 1996 19
Williams et al. 1984 61, 336
Williamson 1993 376
Williamson 1996 378
Williamson et al. 1993 376, 378
Willig et al. 1995 97
Wilmore et al. 1998 381
Wilson 1994 5, 9
Wilson et al. 1991 93
Wilson et al. 1994 93, 96
Wilson et al. 1996 177
Winchester et al. 1983 303, 304
Winder et al. 1979 60
Winstein et al. 1989 303
Winter 1990 26
Winters et al. 1987 35
Wirta et al. 1990 436
Wirta et al. 1991 436
Wiseman et al. 1996 14
Woledge et al. 1985 8
Wolf and Binder-Macleod 1983a 301
Wolf and Binder-Macleod 1983b 301
Wolf et al. 1989 296, 298
Wolf et al. 1996 411
Wolfson et al. 1985 407
Wolfson et al. 1993 407, 415
Wolfson et al. 1995 397
Wolfson et al. 1996 407, 411
Wood and Haskell 1979 216
Wood et al. 1988 384
Wood et al. 1991 385
Woolf and Suero 1969 197
Woollacott 1993 407
World Health Organization Expert
    Committee 1964 176
Worrell et al. 1994 96
Wosornu et al. 1996 185
Wright et al. 1996 256, 263, 264
Wylie 1984 392
Wyndham 1973 59

Y

Yahagi et al. 1996 284
Yale 1989 381
Yalom 1985 356, 364
Yang 1994 280
Yang et al. 1994 282
Yarasheski et al. 1993 407
Yarkony et al. 1992 272
Yates et al. 1983 365
Yki-Jarvinen and Koivisto 1983 222
Young et al. 1987 73
Young et al. 1994 316, 330
Young et al. 1995 62
Young et al. 1996 132
Yue and Cole 1992 282, 283, 284

Z

Zack and Palange 1985 196
Zatsiorsky and Seluyanov 1983 33
Zeni et al. 1996 65
Zinman et al. 1977 48, 216, 219
Zinman et al. 1984 49
Zinovieff 1951 77
Zubek 1969 280
ZuWallack et al. 1991 196

About the Editors

Walter R. Frontera, MD, PhD, is the Earle P. and Ida S. Charlton Associate Professor and Chairman of the Department of Physical Medicine and Rehabilitation, Harvard Medical School. He is Chief of Physical Medicine and Rehabilitation at Spaulding Rehabilitation Hospital and at Massachusetts General Hospital.

Dr. Frontera is board-certified in physical medicine and rehabilitation and has a PhD in exercise physiology. A recognized expert in both exercise physiology and rehabilitation medicine, Dr. Frontera has been published widely.

Dr. Frontera established The Center for Sports Health and Exercise Sciences at the Olympic Training Center in Puerto Rico. He is Secretary General of the International Sports Medicine Federation and Pan-American Confederation of Sports Medicine, and a fellow of the American Academy of Physical Medicine and Rehabilitation. He received the Erdman Lecturer Award from the Association of Academic Physiatrists.

Dr. Frontera attained his medical degree from the University of Puerto Rico San Juan, Puerto Rico, and his PhD in applied anatomy and physiology from Boston University, Boston, Massachusetts.

Dr. Frontera and his wife, Aida, live in Concord, Massachusetts.

David M. Dawson, MD, is Professor of Neurology and associate director of the Division of Rehabilitation Medicine at Harvard Medical School. He is board-certified in neurology.

Author of the widely-used text *Entrapment Neuropathies* (Little-Brown), Dr. Dawson has been extensively published. He served as director of residency training in neurology at the Brigham and Women's Hospital and Massachusetts General Hospital and has extensive experience in clinical neurology with particular interest in myasthenia, neuropathy, and multiple sclerosis. He has conducted clinical studies of outcome and experimental treatment of multiple sclerosis.

A Fellow of the American Academy of Neurology, Dr. Dawson is a member of the American Neurological Association, the American Society for Neurochemistry, and the Association for Research in Nervous and Mental Disease.

Dr. Dawson attained his medical degree from the University of Michigan in Ann Arbor, Michigan. He and his wife, Elizabeth, live in Concord, Massachusetts.

David M. Slovik, MD, is Assistant Professor of Medicine and associate director of the Division of Rehabilitation Medicine at Harvard Medical School. He serves as Chief of Medicine at Spaulding Rehabilitation Hospital and as an endocrinologist at Massachusetts General Hospital.

Dr. Slovik is board-certified in internal medicine, and endocrinology and metabolism. Well-known for his work with osteoporosis, he has clinical, research, and educational expertise in osteoporosis, as well as other metabolic bone diseases. He has worked in the rehabilitation field since 1975 and has been published widely.

Dr. Slovik is a member of the American Society for Bone and Mineral Research and The Endocrine Society. He attained his medical degree at the State University of New York, Downstate Medical Center.

Dr. Slovik and his wife, Lois, live in Newton, Massachusetts.

About the Contributors

James C. Agre, MD, PhD, is the Staff Physiatrist at Howard Young Medical Center in Woodruff, Wisconsin. Dr. Agre received his MD from the University of Minnesota and his PhD in Physical Medicine and Rehabilitation, also from the University of Minnesota. He has received numerous professional honors and awards including the Elizabeth and Sidney Licht Award for Excellence in Scientific Writing for 1988. He is a member of the American Academy of Physical Medicine and Rehabilitation, the American Congress of Rehabilitation Medicine, the American College of Sports Medicine, and serves on the editorial board of the *Archives of Physical Medicine and Rehabilitation*. He has published extensively and authored or coauthored over 40 papers, which have been published in a variety of professional journals.

Susan Aitkens, MS, is a Staff Research Associate in the Department of Physical Medicine and Rehabilitation at the University of California, Davis School of Medicine. She received her master's degree in exercise science from the University of California, Davis. For the past 15 years she has been an active researcher in the areas of physical activity and nutrition related to neuromuscular disease. She is particularly interested in evaluating the therapeutic benefits of exercise and nutritional intervention on physical functioning and quality of life. She is a member of the American College of Sports Medicine and has published in *Medicine and Science in Sports and Medicine, Heart and Lung, American Journal of Clinical Nutrition,* and the *American Journal of Physical Medicine and Rehabilitation*.

Thiru M. Annaswamy, MD, MA, is Chief Resident in Physical Medicine and Rehabilitation at Harvard Medical School. He received his MA in motor control and neuroscience from the Department of Kinesiology and Health Education at the University of Texas at Austin, and his Bachelor of Medicine and Bachelor of Surgery at Mysore Medical College in Mysore, India. He was a teaching and research assistant in biomechanics at the University of Texas, Austin, and a research assistant at the Gait Laboratory at Spaulding Rehabilitation Hospital in Boston. He has published articles in *Gait & Posture, Journal of Biomechanical Engineering,* and the *Archives of Physical Medicine & Rehabilitation*. Dr. Annaswamy is a member of the American Academy of Physical Medicine and Rehabilitation, the North American Society of Gait and Clinical Movement Analysis, and the Association of Academic Physiatrists (AAP).

Sang-Cheol Bae, MD, PhD, MPH, is an Assistant Professor at Hanyang University College of Medicine in Seoul, South Korea, where he also serves as an attending doctor at the Hospital for Rheumatic Diseases with the College of Medicine. Dr. Bae has served on the Board of Internal Medicine and the Subspecialty Board of Rheumatology in Korea, and as a Research Fellow and later as an Instructor in Rheumatology at Brigham and Women's Hospital in Boston. He is a frequent lecturer in medicine at Harvard Medical School, and serves as the Director of both the Section for Clinical Epidemiology and Economics at the Institute of Rheumatology, and the Lupus Clinic at the Hospital for Rheumatic Diseases with Hanyang University. Dr. Bae received both his MD and his PhD from Hanyang University, and he received his MPH from the School of Public Health at Harvard University.

Jonathan Bean, MD, MS, is the Director for Geriatric Physical Medicine and Rehabilitation at both Spaulding Rehabilitation Hospital and the Hebrew Rehabilitation Center for Aged in Boston, Massachusetts. He is also an Instructor in the Department of Physical Medicine and Rehabilitation at the Harvard University School of Medicine and an Assistant Professor in Research at Sargent College of Rehabilitation and Health Sciences in Boston. In 1998, he received the Director's Commendation from the Department of Veterans Affairs and the New Investigator Award from the Educational Research Fund-AAPM&R. In 1999, he received a research fellowship award from the Harvard/Hartford Center of Excellence in Geriatric Medicine. He is an active member of the American Academy of Physical Medicine and Rehabilitation, the Massachusetts Medical Society, the American College of Sports Medicine, and the North American Spine Society. Dr. Bean received his MD from State University of New York at Buffalo and his MS in applied anatomy and physiology at Boston University. His major research interests include geriatric rehabilitation, musculoskeletal medicine, and exercise physiology.

Michael L. Blei, MD, is an Assistant Professor and Director of the Electrodiagnostic Laboratory in the Department of Rehabilitation Medicine at the University of Colorado Health Sciences Center. He received his medical degree from Vanderbilt University and completed his residency in Physical Medicine and Rehabilitation at the University of Utah. He proceeded to continue his post-doctoral training in cellular energetics through the Department of Rehabilitation Medicine at the University of Washington. He is a member of the Association of Academic Physiatrists and the American Association of Electrodiagnostic Medicine. His work is supported in part through a K11 Physician Scientist Award from the National Institute of Arthritis, Musculoskeletal, and Skin Diseases.

Michael L. Boninger, MD, is an Assistant Professor and Research Director in the Department of Orthopedic Surgery, Division of Physical Medicine and Rehabilitation at the University of Pittsburgh. He also holds adjunct appointments in the Department of Rehabilitation Science and Technology and the Department of Mechanical Engineering. He graduated from Ohio State University with both a medical degree and a mechanical engineering degree. He is the Executive Director of the UPMC Health System's Center for Assistive Technology, which incorporates many disciplines in order to provide patients with the most appropriate assistive technology. Dr. Boninger serves as the Medical Director of the Human Engineering Research Laboratories. Dr. Boninger was honored with the 1998 Young Academician Award of the Association of Academic Physiatrists. He has published over 50 book chapters, journal publications, and extended abstracts.

Bartolome R. Celli, MD, is the Chief of Pulmonary and Critical Care at St. Elizabeth's Medical Center in Boston. He has been a member of numerous professional organizations in Venezuela and the U.S. and is currently the president of the New England Chapter of the American College of Chest Physicians. He is also a professor of medicine at Tufts University School of Medicine. Dr. Celli has held visiting professorships at over 20 medical centers and hospitals around the world, and has published more than 75 articles in such prestigious publications as the *New England Journal of Medicine* and the *American Journal of Medical Sciences*. He received his medical degree from Universidad Central de Venezuela, Escuela Luis Razzetti in Caracas. He was named one of the best specialists in pulmonary diseases in North America in *Town and Country* magazine in 1995. He received the Distinguished Citizen award from the city of Caracas, and the Citizenship Award for service to the Latino community from the city of Boston, among numerous other awards and honors.

Michael J. Cohen, PhD, is the Associate Chief of Staff for Research and Development at Veterans Affairs Healthcare System in Long Beach, California, and an Adjunct Professor with the Departments of Psychiatry, Neurology, and Pharmacology at the University of California, Irvine. He received his PhD in experimental psychology from Bowling Green State University, Ohio and did his postdoctoral work in neuroscience with the Brain Research Institute at the University of California, Los Angeles. Dr. Cohen is a member of the Society for Neuroscience, the American Psychological Society, and the American Paraplegia Society. He has published over 150 abstracts and articles in various professional journals and abstracts, and his most recent publications are in brain function and brain imaging of the spinal cord in injured humans. His teaching interests include research design, statistics, brain and behavior, learning and memory, and psychophysiology, while his research interests focus on cognitive psychology, brain imaging, motor learning, and alcohol effects on perception and cognition.

Rory A. Cooper, PhD, is Professor and Chair of the Department of Rehabilitation Science and Technology at the University of Pittsburgh, and Director of the Human Engineering Research Laboratories at the VA Pittsburgh Healthcare System. He received his BS and MEng degrees in electrical engineering from California Polytechnic State University, San Luis Obispo and his PhD in electrical and computer engineering from the University of California at Santa Barbara. He serves on the editorial board of the *Journal of Rehabilitation Research & Development*, the *Saudi Arabian Journal of Disability and Rehabilitation*, the *Journal of Neurologic Rehabilitation*, and the *Team Rehab Report*. He is the author of two books: *Rehabilitation Engineering Applied to Mobility and Manipulation*, and *Wheelchairs: A Guide to Selection and Configuration*. He has developed an ANSI-ISO Wheelchair Test Center. He was a consultant to the Office of the Vice President of the United States under Danforth Quayle, and in 1988, he was a bronze medalist in the Paralympic Games in Seoul, Korea.

Carlos J. Crespo, DrPH, MS, is an Assistant Professor in the Department of Health and Fitness at American University in Washington, DC. He received his MS specializing in sports health from Texas Tech University and his Doctor of Public Health from Loma Linda University, School of Public Health, California. Dr. Crespo received the U.S. Department of Health and Human Services Award for Distinguished Service in 1997 and is a member of several professional organizations including the American College of Sports Medicine, the American Society of Exercise Physiologists, and the American Public Health Association. He also served on the task force for promoting physical activity with the Centers for Disease Control and Prevention and is currently Chair of the Strategic Health Initiative for the National Health Objectives with the American College of Sports Medicine. He received the Mellon Travel Award from the College of Arts and Sciences at American University, and the 1997 Secretary's Award for Distinguished Service from the U.S. Department of Health and Human Services. He has served as a public health advisor for the National Institutes of Health and as a health statistician for the Centers for Disease Control and Prevention.

Allison M. Fall, MD, is a private practitioner of Rehabilitation and Performance Medicine with her practice focusing on spine, sport and industrial injury. She received her undergraduate degrees in mathematics and biomedical engineering from Vanderbilt University where she graduated *summa cum laude* and was co-valedictorian of her class. She received her medical degree from the University of Florida College of Medicine, Gainseville, and completed her residency training in rehabilitation medicine from the University of Colorado Health Sciences Center. She is a member of the American College of Sports Medicine and the American Academy of Physical Medicine and Rehabilitation. She maintains an avid avocational interest in aerobic conditioning and physical fitness.

Roger A. Fielding, PhD, is an Assistant Professor of Health Sciences in the Department of Health Sciences at Boston University's Sargent College of Health and Rehabilitation Sciences. He received his MA in physical education with a concentration in human bioenergetics from Ball State University in Muncie, Indiana and his PhD from Tufts University, School of Nutrition. He has been a member of the American College of Sports Medicine since 1982 and is a full member of the American Physiological Society. He was awarded the Brookdale Foundation National Fellow in 1997 and received the New England Chapter of the American College of Sports Medicine Scholarship Award in 1990. He has published extensively in such professional journals as the *Journal of Applied Physiology*, the *International Journal of Sportsmedicine*, and *Medicine and Science in Sports and Exercise*.

Bette Ann Harris, PT, MS, is the Program Director and Clinical Associate Professor of Graduate Programs in Physical Therapy at MGH Institute of Health Professions in Boston, Massachusetts. She also serves as a Clinical Consultant for Orthopedics/Outpatient Physical Therapy at the Massachusetts General Hospital. Harris acts as a manuscript reviewer for several professional journals including, *Physiotherapy Research International Journal*, and *Physical Therapy*. She is a Lecturer with the Department of Orthopedics at Harvard Medical School. In 1988, she received the Massachusetts Chapter APTA Award in Recognition for outstanding achievement in research. She received her BS with certification in physical therapy from Simmons

College and her MS in physical therapy from the MGH Institute of Health Professions in Boston. Her frequent publications have appeared in such magazines as the *American Journal of Sports Medicine* and *Physical Therapy*.

Gregory W. Heath, DHSc, MPH, is an epidemiologist and exercise physiologist in the Cardiovascular Health Branch, Division of Adult and Community Health with the Centers for Disease Control and Prevention in Atlanta. He received his Master of Public Health in epidemiology and his Doctor of Health Science in applied physiology from Loma Linda University in California. Among Dr. Heath's numerous awards and honors is the Secretary's Award for Distinguished Service for his 1997 contributions to the Surgeon General's report on Physical Activity and Health. He is a Fellow of the American College of Sports Medicine and a Fellow of the Council on Epidemiology and Prevention with the American Heart Association. His work has appeared in the *Journal of Applied Physiology*, *Medicine and Science in Sports and Exercise*, and the *American Heart Journal* among other publications.

Martin D. Hoffman, MD, is a Professor of Physical Medicine and Rehabilitation with the Medical College of Wisconsin in Milwaukee. He received his medical degree from St. Louis University School of Medicine and did his residency in physical medicine and rehabilitation with the Medical College of Wisconsin. He served as a team physician with the U.S. Biathlon Team from 1988-1995 and is currently serving as an Associate Editor with the *Archives of Physical Medicine and Rehabilitation*. He is a Fellow with both the American College of Sports Medicine and the American Academy of Physical Medicine and Rehabilitation and is a charter member of the American Medical Society for Sports Medicine. He has authored or coauthored over 40 articles, which have appeared in professional journals, and his work has been published in numerous chapters and reviews.

Edward S. Horton, MD, is the Vice President and Director of Clinical Research at Joslin Diabetes Center in Boston, Massachusetts. He received his medical degree from Harvard Medical School in 1957 where he is now a Professor of Medicine. His numerous honors and awards include the Robert H. Herman Award from The American Society for Clinical Nutrition in 1990, the Banting Medal for Distinguished Service from the American Diabetes Association in 1991, and the Mizuno Award and Lectureship, which he received in Nara, Japan in 1994. He has been a member of more than 20 committees, offices, and task forces associated with the American Diabetes Association and served as the Association's Vice President from 1988-1989 and President from 1990-1991. He also served as President of The American Society for Clinical Nutrition in 1986. Over the last four decades, he has published over 180 reports and papers in various professional journals.

Maura Daly Iversen, SD, PT, MPH, is an Assistant Professor in Physical Therapy at Northeastern University in Boston, Massachusetts and a Post-Doctoral Clinical Research Fellow in the Department of Medicine at Harvard Medical School. She received her BS and PT from Simmons College, her MPH from Boston University, and her SD from the Harvard School of Public Health. From 1986-1992, she served as a Clinical Researcher in Rheumatology at Brigham and Women's Hospital, Boston. She received the Doctoral Dissertation Award from the National Arthritis Foundation in 1994-1996, the Charles H. Farnsworth Trust Medical Foundation Grant in 1997, and the Arthritis Foundation's New Investigator Award in 1998. Iversen is an active member of the Association of Rheumatology Health Professions, the American Physical Therapy Association, and the National Arthritis Foundation. Dr. Iversen is a manuscript reviewer for *Physical Therapy*. She has published material in such journals as the *New England Journal of Medicine*, and the *British Journal of Rheumatology*.

Richard C. Kaiser, MD, is the Acting Director of Outpatient Psychiatry and the Consultant to the Complex Medical Rehabilitation Unit at Spaulding Rehabilitation Hospital in Boston, Massachusetts. He also serves as a Clinical Instructor in Psychiatry at Harvard Medical School and a Clinical Associate in Psychiatry at Massachusetts General Hospital. Dr. Kaiser received his medical degree from New York Medical College and participated in the Boston University Medical Center Psychiatric Residency Training Program from 1992-1995. He is a member of the American College of Sports Medicine, the American Medical Association, the American Psychiatric Association, and the Academy of Psychosomatic Medicine. In 1990, Kaiser received the JM Foundation Scholarship for Addiction Studies, and in 1995 he received the Murray Award for Resident Research in Psychiatry from Boston University School of Medicine.

D. Casey Kerrigan, MD, MS, is an Associate Professor and Director of Research in the Department of Physical Medicine and Rehabilitation at Harvard Medical School, and the Director of Center for Rehabilitation Science at Spaulding Rehabilitation Hospital in Boston, Massachusetts. She received her medical degree from Harvard Medical School and her MS in kinesiology from UCLA. Dr. Kerrigan is the Founder and Director for the Center for Rehabilitation Science, a founding member of the American Gait Laboratory Accreditation Board, and an active member of various other professional organizations including the American Medical Association, the Association of Academic Physiatrists (AAP), and the American Academy of PM&R. She has accumulated a long list of honors and awards for her research including The Young Academician Award from the Association of Academic Physiatrists and the Licht Award from the American Congress of Rehabilitation Medicine. Her research interests focus on the mechanics of normal and disabled gait, the relationship between clinical and quantitative gait assessments, and rehabilitative treatments to improve gait disability.

David D. Kilmer, MD, is an Associate Professor in the Department of Physical Medicine and Rehabilitation at the University of California, Davis School of Medicine. He received his medical degree from the University of California, Davis in 1985 and completed residency training at the University's Davis Medical Center in 1989. Dr. Kilmer is a member of the American Academy of Physical Medicine and Rehabilitation and serves as an Associate Editor for the organization's journal, *Archives of Physical Medicine and Rehabilitation*. He is also an active member of the American Association of Electrodiagnostic Medicine. Dr. Kilmer's research focuses on exercise and functional performance in persons with neuromuscular diseases with funding received through a grant from the National Institute of Disability and Rehabilitation Research. He has published in such professional journals as the *Western Journal of Medicine*, the *American Journal of Physical Medicine and Rehabilitation*, and the *American Journal of Clinical Nutrition*.

Lisa S. Krivickas, MD, is an Instructor at Harvard Medical School and has clinical appointments in the departments of Physical Medicine and Rehabilitation and Neurology at Spaulding Rehabilitation Hospital, Massachusetts General Hospital, and Brigham and Women's Hospital. She is also the Director of Electrodiagnostic Services and the Medical Director of the Assistive Technology Center at Spaulding Rehabilitation Hospital. Dr. Krivickas received her medical degree from Harvard Medical School in 1991. She is a diplomate of both the American Board of PM&R and the American Board of Electrodiagnostic Medicine. Her current research is in the area of muscle physiology. She is studying the effects of aging and various neuromuscular diseases on skeletal muscle contractile properties and function. Other research interests are in the areas of electrodiagnostic medicine and muscle fatigue. In 1997, Dr. Krivickas received one of only three New Investigator Awards from the American Academy of PM&R.

Martin J. Kushmerick, MD, PhD, is a Professor in the Departments of Radiology and of Physiology and Biophysics at the University of Washington and Adjunct Professor in the Center for Bioengineering. He is currently the Director of the Nuclear Magnetic Resonance (NMR) Spectroscopy Program at the University of Washington Medical Center. Previous positions held have included the Director and Head of Metabolic Research in the Division of NMR Research at Brigham and Women's Hospital, Boston. He received his medical and post-doctoral degrees from the University of Pennsylvania School of Medicine. He has maintained a very successful long-term research focus centered on the *in vivo* regulation of cellular bioenergetics.

Michael G. Lacourse, PhD, is a Professor in the Department of Kinesiology and Physical Education in the College of Health and Human Services at California State University, Long Beach. He received his MS in biomechanics and his PhD in motor control and applied statistics from Indiana University. Dr. Lacourse is a member of the American Statistical Association, the Society for Neuroscience, and the North American Society for the Psychology of Sport and Physical Activity. He appeared in *Who's Who in California* from 1989-1991. He also is a member of the Phi Beta Delta Honor Society for International Scholars. He has published in such popular press publications as *Strength and Conditioning, American Fitness*, and *Fitness Management*, as well as professional journals such as *Sport & Exercise Psychology, Journal of Applied Sport Science Research*, and *Medicine and Science in Sports and Exercise*.

Kristen E. Lawrence, MS, is a Research Assistant at Veterans Affairs Healthcare System in Long Beach, California. She graduated *magna cum laude* from the University of California in Los Angeles with a BA in psychology in 1993 and from California State University, Long Beach with her MS in kinesiology in 1999. She is a member of Sigma Xi (The Scientific Research Society), the National Strength and Conditioning Association, and the American College of Sports Medicine. Her current research focuses on the effect of delayed onset muscle soreness on the physiological response to endurance exercise.

Matthew H. Liang, MD, MPH, is a Professor of Medicine at Harvard Medical School and Professor of Health Policy and Management at Harvard School of Public Health. He is the Medical Director of Rehabilitation Services at the Brigham and Women's Hospital and the Director of the Robert B. Brigham Multipurpose Arthritis and Musculoskeletal Diseases Center. Dr. Liang is a trustee of the Massachusetts Chapter of the Arthritis Foundation, Chairman of the Research Advisory Committee of the Canadian Arthritis Society, and Chairman of the Board of the Medical Foundation. He received his medical degree from Harvard Medical School and his MPH from the Harvard School of Public Health. Dr. Liang serves on the editorial boards of *The American Journal of Medicine, Spine, and Lupus*. He is a primary care physician and rheumatologist and is a recipient of the Lawrence Poole Prize in Rehabilitation and the Lee C. Howley Sr. Prize for Research in Arthritis.

Ruy S. Moraes, MD, MSc, is the Director of FISICOR Cardiac Rehabilitation Center and Physician at the Cardiology Division in the Hospital de Clínicas de Porto Alegre in Brazil. He received his medical and his master degrees from the Federal University of Rio Grande do Sul, and did his cardiology training at the Hospital de Clínicas de Porto Alegre. His research interest is focused on the study of the autonomic nervous system.

Miriam E. Nelson, PhD, is the Director of the Center for Physical Fitness at the School of Nutrition Science and Policy at Tufts University. She is also the Associate Chief of the Nutrition, Exercise Physiology & Sarcopenia Laboratory, Jean Mayer USDA Human Nutrition Research Center on Aging at Tufts University. Dr. Nelson received her MS and PhD in nutrition from the School of Nutrition at Tufts University in Boston, Massachusetts. She is a member of the American Society of Bone Mineral Research, the American Society of Clinical Nutrition, and a Fellow of the American College of Sports Medicine. In 1998, Dr. Nelson received the Lifetime Achievement Award from the Massachusetts Governor's Committee on Physical Fitness and Sports for her work on exercise and older adults. Besides her numerous publications in professional journals, she has published two best selling books: *Strong Women Stay Young* (Bantam Books, 1997), and *Strong Women Stay Slim* (Bantam Books, 1998).

Thomas J. O'Connnor, MS, is a Research Associate with the School of Health and Rehabilitation Sciences. He received his BS in Physical Education and his MS in Physical Education/Exercise Physiology from California State University, Sacramento in 1995. He is currently pursuing his PhD in rehabilitation science and technology from the University of Pittsburgh. His current research interests include using computer video game play controlled by wheelchairs to motivate individuals confined to wheelchairs to exercise. Mr. O'Connor has a NIH Fellowship and is a member of RESNA.

Charles T. Pu, MD, is the Director of the Community-Based Transitional Case Program at the Massachusetts General Hospital in Boston, Massachusetts and is an Instructor in Medicine at Harvard Medical School. He received his medical degree from the Robert Wood Johnson Medical School at the University of Medicine and Dentistry of New Jersey and completed his clinical and research fellowship in geriatric medicine with the Division on Aging at Harvard Medical School. Dr. Pu is an active member of the American Geriatrics Society, the Gerontologic Society of America, the American College of Sports Medicine, and the American Medical Directors Association. In 1995, he received The Charles H. Farnsworth Medical Foundation Grant. His major research interests include sarcopenia, exercise, frailty, and heart disease in the elderly.

Jorge P. Ribeiro, MD, ScD, is an Associate Professor and the Chief of Cardiology at the Hospital de Clinicas de Porto Alegre in Brazil. He received his medical degree from the Federal University of Rio Grande do Sul, did his cardiology training at the Brigham and Women's Hospital, and received his ScD in exercise physiol-

THE
House
of
LANYON

VALERIE ANAND

MIRA

MIRA is a registered trademark of Harlequin Enterprises Limited, used under licence.

MIRA Books, Eton House, 18-24 Paradise Road, Richmond, Surrey, TW9 1SR

© Valerie Anand 2007

ISBN 978 0 7783 0230 8

59-0508

Printed in Great Britain by Clays Ltd, St Ives plc

ACKNOWLEDGEMENTS

I am most grateful to the many people who have helped me as I did the research for this book. My thanks go in particular to Dolores Clew and Father Garrett for information on the medieval church, and to Michael Grantham (Rector of St George's in Dunster), Laurie Hambrook (Churchwarden of St George's), Mrs Joan Jordan (local historian) and Dr Robert Dunning (County Editor) for information on west country families and fifteenth-century Dunster.

This book is dedicated, most affectionately and gratefully, to all members of the Exmoor Society, and in particular to the members of its London Area Branch.

PART ONE

FOUNDATIONS
1458

CHAPTER ONE 🙠

QUIET AND DIGNIFIED

Allerbrook House is a manor house with charm. Three attractive gables look out from its slate roof, echoed by the smaller, matching gable over its porch, and two wings, with a secluded courtyard between them, stretch back toward the moorland hillside which shelters the house from northeast winds. In front the land drops away gently, but to the right the slope plunges steeply into the wooded, green-shadowed combe where the Allerbrook River purls over its pebbly bed, flowing down from its moorland source toward the village of Clicket in the valley.

Allerbrook is far from being a great house such as Chatsworth or Hatfield, but its charm apart, it has unusual features of its own, such as a mysterious stained glass window in its chapel—no one is sure of its significance—and the Tudor roses, which nowadays are painted red-and-white as when they were first made, which are carved into the hall panelling and the window seats.

The place is a rarity, standing as it does out on Exmoor, between the towns of Withypool and Dulverton. There is no other house of its type on the moor. It is also unique because of its origins. The truth—as its creator Richard Lanyon once admitted—is that it probably wouldn't be there at all, if one autumn day in 1458 Sir Humphrey Sweetwater and his twin sons, Reginald and Walter, had not ridden out to hunt a stag and had a most distressing encounter with a funeral.

There was no manor house there when, in the fourteenth century, the Lanyons came from Cornwall and took over Allerbrook farm. Then, the only dwelling was a farmhouse, so ancient even at that time that no one knew how long it had stood there.

Sturdily built of pinkish-grey local stone and roofed with shaggy thatch, it looked more like a natural outcrop than a construction. Around it spread a haphazard collection of fields and pastures, and its farmyard was encircled by a clutter of barns, byres, stables and assorted sheds. Inside, the main rooms were the kitchen and the big all-purpose living room. There was an impressive oak front door, but it was never used except for wedding and funeral processions and the hinges were regrettably rusty. It was a workaday place.

On a fine late September evening, though, with a golden haze softening the heathery heights of the moors and gilding the Bristol Channel to the north, there was a mellowness. That mellowness seemed even to have entered the soul of the man whose life was now drawing to a close in one of the upper bedchambers.

This was remarkable, because George Lanyon's sixty-one years of life had scarcely been serene. He had been an aggressive child, apt to bully his two older sisters and his younger brother, for as long as they were there to bully. The Lanyons had never, for some reason, been good at raising healthy families. All George's siblings had ailed and died before they were twenty. Only George flourished, as though he possessed all the vitality that should have been shared equally among the four of them.

As an adult, he had quarrelled with his parents, dominated his wife, Alice, and shouted at his fragile younger son, Stephen, until the boy died of lung-rot at the age of eleven. The grieving Alice, in her one solitary fit of rebellion, accused him of driving Stephen into his grave, and she herself faded out of life the following year.

Only Richard, his elder son, had been strong enough to survive and at times to stand up to him or, if necessary, stand by him. George also quarrelled with their landlord, Sir Humphrey Sweetwater, when he raised their rent. George had refused to see that this was dangerous.

"The Sweetwaters won't throw us off our land. They know we look after it. They were glad enough to have us take it on when Granddad Petroc came here, looking for a place, back in the days of the plague when everyone who'd lived here before was dead."

"That was then. This is now, and I don't trust them," said Richard. He was well aware that the Sweetwaters, although only minor gentry, were on social if not intimate terms with Thomas Courtenay, Earl of Devon, which was a double-edged blade. On the one hand, they considered themselves so far above their tenants that they could scarcely even see them. But on the other hand, if the said tenants tilled the land badly or wrangled over a rise in the rent, they were as capable of throwing the offenders out as they were capable of drowning unwanted kittens. You never knew. Richard loathed the Sweetwaters as much as George, but he was also wary.

The quarrel passed over. George gave in and paid the increase, and the Sweetwaters continued to regard the Lanyon family with disdain. Quietly the Lanyons began to prosper, though Richard considered that they could have done better still if only his father hadn't in so many ways been so pigheaded.

But now…

Extraordinary, Richard thought as he stood looking down at his father's sunken face and half-shut eyes. *Extraordinary.* All his life he had fought this man, argued with him and usually given in to him. And now, would you believe it, George was making a good Christian end.

Betsy and Kat, the two middle-aged sisters who cooked and cleaned and looked after the dairy and were so alike in their fair plumpness that people often mixed them up, were on their knees on the other side of the bed, praying quietly. At the foot stood Father Bernard, the elderly parish priest. "He's safe enough," Father Bernard said with some acidity. He knew George well. "He's had the last rites. Luckily you fetched me while he was still conscious. Lucky you had that horse of yours, too, whatever your father thought!"

Richard Lanyon grinned, fleetingly. Father Bernard lived down in Clicket village, in a cottage beside St. Anne's, the elegant little church built of pale Caen stone imported from France for the purpose by some pious bygone Sweetwater.

There was a long, sloping mile of Allerbrook combe between the farm and the priest, but George had asked for Father Bernard with pleading in his eyes and begged his son to hurry, and

Richard had been able to do so, because he had a good horse at his command. George always said he had lost only three battles in his lifetime. One was the squabble over the rent. Another, a very long-running one, was the way Richard, once widowed, kept on refusing to remarry and make another attempt to raise a family. The third was over Richard's purchase of Splash.

"Why can't you ride a local pony like everyone else?" George raged when Richard went off to a horse fair miles away and came back leading a two-year-old colt with a most remarkable dappled coat. The dapples were dark iron-grey and much bigger than dapples usually were, overlapping and running into each other so that he looked as though someone had splashed liquid iron all over him. "The ponies round here can carry a grown man all day and never tire *or* put their feet in bogs by mistake. What did you spend good money on *that* for?" Master Lanyon senior demanded.

"He's well made. I'm going to break him for riding and call him Splash," said Richard.

"I give you your cut from any profits we make," George bellowed at his unrepentant son, "but I don't expect you to throw it away on something as ought to be in a freak show!"

But Splash, with his long legs and his undoubted dash of Arab blood, had proved his worth. He was as clever as any moorland pony at avoiding bogs and he could outdistance every horse in the parish and beyond, including the bloodstock owned by the Sweetwaters. He had got Richard down to the village and to the priest's house so quickly that by the time Richard was hammering on Father Bernard's door, the dust he had kicked up as he tore out of the farmyard still hung in the air.

"Get up behind me," Richard said when the priest opened the

door. "Don't stop to saddle your mare. It's my father. We think he's going."

And Splash, head lowered and nostrils wide, brought them both back up the combe nearly as fast as he had carried Richard down it, and before he drifted into his last dream, George Lanyon received the sacrament and was shriven of his sins and given, thereby, his passport into paradise.

"I couldn't have done it without Splash," Richard said, and glanced at his father, wondering if George could hear and secretly hoping so.

But if he did, he made no sign and when Peter, Richard's nineteen-year-old son, came quietly into the room asking whether the patient was better, Richard could only shake his head.

"Keep your voice down now, Master Peter." Betsy, the older of the two sisters, looked up from her prayers. "Don't 'ee be disturbing 'un. Your granddad's made his peace and he's startin' on his journey."

Peter nervously came closer to the bed. As a child, he had seen two small brothers die, and at the age of eleven he had been taken to his parents' bedchamber to say farewell to his mother, Joan, and the girl-child who never breathed, and every time he had been stricken with a sense of dreadful mystery, and with pity.

The pity this time was made worse by the change in his grandfather. Petroc, the Cornishman who was George's own grandfather, had died before George was born, but his description had been handed down. He had been short and dark, a very typical Cornishman. He had, however, married a local girl, said to be big and brown haired and clear skinned. The combination had produced good-looking descendants, dark of hair and eye like Petroc, but with tall strong bodies and excellent facial bones. In life, George had been not only loud voiced and argumentative; he had also been unusually handsome.

Now his good looks had faded with his vitality. He had been getting thinner for months, and complaining of pains inside, though no one knew what ailed him, but the final collapse, into this shrunken husk, had come suddenly, taking them all by surprise. To Peter it seemed that the man on the bed was melting before their eyes.

George himself had been drifting in a misty world where nothing had substance. He could hear voices nearby, but could make no sense of what they said. His body no longer seemed to matter. For a change, nothing was hurting. He was comfortable. He was content to surrender to whatever or wherever lay before him. But in him, life had always been a powerful force. Like a candle flame just before it gutters out, it flared once more. For a few moments the mist withdrew and the voices made sense again and his eyes opened, to focus, frowningly, on the faces around him.

Father Bernard. Sharp-tongued old wretch. But he'd provided the last rites. No need to fear hell now. With difficulty he turned his head, and there was young Peter, his only surviving grandson, looking miserable. Why did the Lanyons never produce big healthy families? As for Richard…

Wayward boy. Been widowed for years; should have married again long ago. Should have listened to his father. *I kept telling him. Obstinate, that's what he is. Big ideas. Always thinks he knows better than me. Always wanting to try new things out.*

Oh, well. Richard would soon be able to please himself. His father wouldn't be able to stop him. Didn't even want to, not now. Too tired…

Weakly he turned his head the other way, and saw the white-capped heads of Betsy and Kat. Beyond them was the window. It was shut, its leaded panes with their squares of thick, greenish glass denying him a view of the world outside. He'd had the windows glazed long ago, at more expense than he liked, but he'd always detested the fact that Sweetwater House was the only dwelling for miles that could have daylight without draughts. Yet even with glazing, the daylight was partly obscured and the view scarcely visible. "Open…window," he said thickly. "Now. Quick."

Betsy got up at once. Kat murmured a protest, but Betsy said, "No cold wind's a'goin' to hurt 'un now, silly. We'd be doing this anyway, soon." She clicked the window latch and flung the casement back, letting cool air stream into the room.

She meant that, once he was gone, someone would open the window anyway, because people always did, to let the departing soul go free. George knew that quite well. He wanted to see where he was going.

The window gave him a glimpse of Slade, the barley field, all stubble now, because the summer had been good and they'd got all the corn in and threshed, as well. The names of his fields told themselves over in his head: Long Meadow, Slade, Quillet, Three Corner Mead…

He had been proud of them, all the more so because they were really his. He knew that in many places fields were communal, with each farmer cultivating just a strip, or perhaps more than one, but compelled to plant the same crop as everyone else and changing strips each year. Here in the southwest, it was different. Here, a man's fields were his own.

Beyond the farmland was a dark green line, the trees of Allerbrook combe, and in the distance strode the skyline of the moorland's highest ridge, swimming in lemon light. There were strange mounds on the hilltops of Exmoor, said to be the graves of pagan people who had lived here long, long ago. He'd like to be buried in a mound on high ground, but he'd have to be content with a grave in the churchyard of St. Anne's. He wouldn't even be able to hear the sound of the Allerbrook…well, no, he wouldn't be able to hear anything, near or far, but…

He was growing confused and things were fading again. But how lovely was the light on those moors. He'd never attended to it in life. Been too damn busy trying to control that awkward son of his. Now he wanted to float away into that glorious sky, to dissolve into it, to be part of it….

His eyes closed. The voices around him became irrelevant once more and then were gone. Father Bernard, gentle now, spoke a final prayer and Richard, also gently, kissed his father's brow and drew up the sheet.

"It was a good passing," he said.

The priest nodded. "Yes, it was. I will make arrangements for the burial. Will you decide when the best day would be, and let me know?"

"Of course," Richard said. "I shall have much to do."

And organising the funeral would be only part of that. To Richard—and though he didn't speak of it aloud, he didn't conceal it from himself, either—the golden light of the descending sun was a sign of golden opportunity. He would give his father a respectful farewell, as a good son should. But his mental list of the people he would invite included some with whom he particularly wanted to talk, and the sooner the better. He had plans, and now, at last, he was free to put them into action.

But *certainly* the funeral itself would, he trusted, be long remembered as an example of well-organised, quiet dignity.

In the event, George Lanyon's funeral was unquestionably memorable and parts of it even dignified. But from that day onward, the conflict between Richard Lanyon and the Sweetwater family was more than a simple matter of dislike. That was the day when what had been merely dislike and resentment escalated into a feud.

CHAPTER TWO 🙰

SHAPING THE FUTURE

In the village of Dunster, a dozen or so miles away on the coast of the Bristol Channel, Liza Weaver, suitably grave of face, stood among other members of the extensive Weaver family and bade farewell to her father, Nicholas, the head of the house, and her mother, Margaret, as they set off on the long ride to Allerbrook for the funeral of George Lanyon.

She was a strongly built girl with warm brown eyes and hair that matched, although at the moment it was hidden under a neat white cap. Her big, florid father said cheerfully, "I'm sorry about George, and his family will miss him, but we'll likely bring back some good fresh bacon from the farm. It's an ill wind, as they say," and he leaned down from his saddle to kiss his eldest daughter. "Be a good wench. Help your little sister and—" he dropped his voice "—don't mind Aunt Cecy's tongue. She means no harm." He straightened up in his saddle, took off his hat and waved it to them all. "See you all soon!" he cried. Margaret smiled and turned her sturdy pony to follow him as he set off.

So there they went, thought Liza. Off to the funeral of George Lanyon. The two families were mostly linked by business, but there had been some social contacts, too. She had been to Allerbrook now and then—to Christmas and Easter gatherings as a rule—and she had met George. She had also found him rather alarming. She felt dutifully sorry for anyone who was ill, or had died, but she was young and the passing of Master Lanyon did not mean so very much to her.

On the other hand, the departure of her parents did mean something, of which they had no inkling. She had since childhood had a habit sometimes of going for walks on her own. Here in Dunster where everyone knew everyone else, it was safe enough and no one had ever stopped her, unless there was so much to do that she couldn't be spared. Aunt Cecy would probably say that with Nicholas and Margaret absent, there'd be too much to do just now, but it shouldn't be too difficult to give Aunt Cecy the slip after dinner.

And in the dell beyond the mill, where bluebells had been out the first time they met there, back in the springtime, a young man called Christopher would be waiting.

Autumn had declared itself. On the moors the bracken was bronzing and the higher hillcrests were veiled in cloud. It had rained overnight and there were puddles in the farmyard at Allerbrook. In the kitchen Betsy and Kat were busy by daybreak, preparing the food which must be served to the guests. When Richard came downstairs, the stockpot was already bubbling and there were chickens on the spit. The poultry population of Allerbrook had gone down considerably in George's honour.

Out in the byre Betsy's husband, Higg, was milking the cows while Kat's husband, Roger, fetched water from the well for the benefit of the kitchen and the plough oxen in their stalls. It should have been the other way around, since Higg was as broad chested as any ox while Roger was skinny and stoop backed from a lifetime of carrying full buckets and laden sacks. He carried buckets so lopsidedly that they usually slopped, but the cows, perversely, responded better to Higg.

Upstairs, guests who had had a long way to come and had arrived the previous day were still abed, but Peter was up ahead of his father and snatching a quick breakfast of small ale and bread smeared with honey. Richard sat down next to him. "Sleep all right? It'll be a long day."

"I didn't sleep much, no. It's strange without Granddad. Nothing's ever going to be the same again, is it?" Peter said.

Richard was silent, because to him, the fact that nothing was ever going to be the same again was a matter for rejoicing, but it would be quite improper to say so.

Under George's rule, life at Allerbrook had been the same for far too long. There were so many things that Richard would have liked to try, new ideas which he had seen put into practice on other farms, but his father was set against innovations.

It was always *Take it from me—I know best. No, I don't want to try another breed of sheep. Ours do well on the moorland grazing, so what do you want to go making experiments for? No, what's the point of renting more valley grazing? Got enough, haven't we? Nonsense, I never heard of anyone growing wheat on Exmoor, even if Quillet field does face south and the soil's deep.*

There were going to be changes now, and that was nothing to grieve about. He glanced at Peter again, and saw that the boy was hurrying his meal. "Take your time," he said. "Our guests'll be a while yet. Ned Crowham's never been one for early rising, I've noticed."

For a short time, Peter had been to school in the east of the county and Ned had been one of his fellow pupils. They had become friends, although they had little in common. A complete contrast to the Lanyons to look at, Ned was short, plump, pink skinned and fair as a newly hatched chick. He was also the son of a man as wealthy as Sir Humphrey, owner of several Somerset farms and a manor house twenty miles away, toward the town of Bridgwater. At home, young Ned was indulged. He had spent nights at Allerbrook before and shown himself to be a terrible layabed.

"And the Weavers didn't get here till after dark last night," Richard added. "Mistress Margaret was tired. It's only twelve miles from Dunster as the crow flies, but it's a heck of a lot more as a pony plods and she's not young. It was good of her to come. I hoped Nicholas Weaver would, for I've business with him, but I'm touched that his wife came, too."

"We'll have a crowd here soon," Peter said, swallowing his final mouthful. "Just as well Master Nicholas didn't bring his whole family! Poor Granddad used to envy the Weavers, didn't he, because of their big families? Father, why did you never marry again after my mother died? I've often wondered." Richard frowned and Peter hastily added, "I'm sorry. I didn't mean to say anything I shouldn't."

"I'm not offended, boy. I was just wondering what the answer was, that's all. I tell you," said Richard, man-to-man, "about three-quarters of the reason was that your granddad wanted me to marry again so badly! He kept on and on and the more he kept on, the less I felt like obliging him. So time went on, and it never happened. You'll gain! You won't have to share with others when you inherit the tenancy."

Another reason, although he was fond enough of Peter not to say this to him, was that he hadn't been very happy in marriage. Joan had been a good woman; that he wouldn't deny. Too good, perhaps, too gentle. He sometimes glimpsed the same gentleness in Peter and didn't like it. Peter was a Lanyon in looks but he had his mother's temperament, and that wasn't fitting for a man. It had even been irritating in a woman! He'd have liked Joan better if she'd spoken up more, the way Margaret Weaver sometimes argued with Nicholas: good-naturedly—there was no spite in it—but clearly, and often with very sensible things to say.

Joan was timid, scared of him and scared of George. She always had a bad time in childbirth and she was terrified of that, too. The fact that her last pregnancy had killed her had left Richard feeling guilt stricken. For some years now he had had a comfortable arrangement with a widow down in Clicket, a woman who'd buried two husbands and never borne a child. She did him good and he had done her no harm. He never discussed her with his family, though they all knew about Deb Archer.

"I don't think you'll be inheriting yet awhile," he said jovially to Peter. "I've a good few years in me yet, I hope. Do you want to see your grandfather again, for a last goodbye?"

George was in his coffin on the table in the big living room. After the funeral, the room would come back into use, with a white cloth over the table and the best pewter dishes brought down off the sideboard, but until then, the room was only for George.

Peter shook his head. "No. I…I'd rather not. I saw him yesterday but he doesn't look like himself anymore, does he?" He shivered. "I can't believe that what's in that box ever walked or talked…or shouted!"

"You're getting morbid, boy. Well, maybe before long I'll turn your mind in a happier direction. You just wait and see."

In another hour Father Bernard had ridden in on his mare, and shortly after that, Tilly and Gilbert Lowe arrived from the farm on the other side of the combe, accompanied by Martha, the plain and downtrodden daughter who was virtually their servant. The Lowes were followed by the Rixons and Hanna-combes from the other two farms on the Sweetwater estate, and then a number of folk from Clicket village straggled in, all soberly dressed, some on foot, some on ponies, to pay their last respects and escort George down to the churchyard and his final place of rest.

Among them came Mistress Deborah Archer, forty-nine now but still buxom and brown haired. Richard kissed her without embarrassment and Father Bernard greeted her politely. Like nearly everyone in the parish, he knew of the arrangement but accepted it without comment, just as he accepted the fact that neither Richard nor Deborah ever mentioned it in his confessional. He had had a lapse or two of his own. It was even possible that Geoffrey Baker, steward to the Sweetwaters, was his son. No one knew for certain.

The Sweetwaters didn't come and no one expected them, though some of their employees arrived, including their shepherd Edward Searle, along with his son Toby. Edward Searle was a local personality. Tall, gaunt, dignified as a king and able to tell every one of his sheep apart, he was one of the few in the district whose baptismal names had never, unless they were already short enough, been chopped into nicknames. In a world where Elizabeth usually became Liza or Betsy and most Edwards became Ned or Ed, Master Searle remained Edward and no one would have dreamed of shortening it.

The other exceptions included the Sweetwaters themselves, Richard Lanyon (who refused to answer to Dick or Dickon and had long since squelched any attempts to make him) and Geoffrey Baker, who arrived on a roan mare and gave his master's apologies with great civility though Richard knew, and Baker knew he knew, that Sir Humphrey Sweetwater hadn't actually sent any apologies at all.

Sir Humphrey, said Baker solemnly, had guests, connections of Thomas Courtenay, the Earl of Devon. The Sweetwaters had promised to show them some sport today. They were all going hunting.

"Sir Humphrey's showing off, as usual," Richard growled to Peter.

Friendship with the Courtenays had brought one very marked benefit to the Sweetwaters, since Sir Thomas was the warden of Exmoor Forest. Clicket was outside the forest boundary, but only just. All deer belonged to the crown and no one hunted them except by royal permission, but a Sweetwater had distinguished himself so valiantly at the Battle of Crécy that he and his descendants had been granted the right to hunt deer on their own land.

Normally, they would not have been allowed to pursue them into the forest, which was inconvenient because the deer, oblivious of human boundaries, very often fled that way. Sir

Thomas, however, had used his own considerable powers and granted permission for the Sweetwater hounds to follow quarry across the boundary. Sir Humphrey never missed a chance of demonstrating his privilege to his guests.

By ten o'clock all was ready at the farmhouse. The Clicket carpenter, who had made the coffin and brought it up the combe strapped to the back of a packhorse, had solemnly nailed it shut while Father Bernard recited a prayer. The Lanyon dogs—Peter's long-legged, grey-blue lurcher Blue, Silky the black sheepdog bitch who had belonged to George, and Silky's black-and-white son Ruff, who was Richard's special companion—knew that they were not invited on this outing and lay down by the fire. How much animals sensed, no one could guess, but Silky had been pining since George died.

The six bearers, Richard, Peter, Higg, Roger, Nicholas Weaver and Geoffrey Baker, lifted the coffin onto their shoulders. They would be replaced halfway by a second team of volunteers, since the mile-long Allerbrook combe which must be traversed to reach Clicket was a long way to carry their burden, but to put a laden coffin on a pack pony would be risky. Ponies could stumble, or take fright. Nicholas, whose hair and beard were halfway between sandy and grey and who had grown hefty with the years, grunted as he took the weight, and cheeky Ned Crowham, who was one of the relief bearers—he had been got out of bed only just in time to join the procession—said that at least Nicholas's pony could now have a rest.

"True enough," Nicholas said amiably. "My pony's stout, but I reckon the poor brute still sags in the middle when I get astride him. That's why Margaret's got her own nag. Not fair to any animal to put me on him and then add someone else."

Father Bernard smiled, but Margaret said seriously, "Oh, Nicholas. We shouldn't make jokes, surely."

Richard, however, easing his shoulder under the weight of the coffin, said, "Oh, my father liked a laugh as much as any man and he wouldn't grudge it to us now. Are we all ready? Then let's start."

The bearers carried George ceremonially through the front door—the hinges, as usual, had had to be oiled to make sure it would open—and took the downhill path into the combe. They trod with care. The sun was out now, but the ground was soft from last night's rain.

The voice of the Allerbrook came up to them as they went. It was a swift, brown-tinged peat stream which rose in a bog at the top of the long, smooth moorland ridge above and the rain had swollen it. Some feet above the water, the track turned to parallel the river's course down to Clicket. The trees met overhead and the light on the path was a confusing mixture of greenish shade and dazzling interruptions where the sun shone through. There was no other track to the village. The combe was thickly grown with trees and tangled undergrowth and on the far side, the few paths did not lead to Clicket. The track was wide but in places it was also steep, and in any case the coffin lurched somewhat because Higg and Roger were among the first team of bearers at their own insistence, and Higg's broad shoulders were four inches higher than Roger's bent ones.

Father Bernard led the way on his mare. The bearers followed him and the crowd formed a rough and ready procession on foot behind the coffin. They talked among themselves as they went, for funerals were not such rare events, after all. Death was part of life. Father Bernard, in church on Sundays, often spoke of the next world and told them to be ready for it.

Halfway down, a steep path descended the slope to the right, met the track, crossed it and continued down to a ford. Water was draining down the path from the side of the combe and the crossing was extremely muddy. "Carefully now!" Father Bernard called over his shoulder, and steadied his mare as one of her hooves skidded. "The rain's made this a proper quagmire. Mind you don't slip."

"Keep in step!" said Nicholas. "And take it steadily."

Somewhere on the other side of the combe they heard a hunting horn and the voices of hounds, but, being concerned with their uncertain footing, no one paid much heed to it. The horn sounded again, nearer. And then, out of the trees on the other side of the river, came the stag.

There were two ways of hunting deer. If the purpose was simply venison, the hunt could drive the quarry into a ring of archers who would mow them down like corn. But if the huntsmen wanted sport and the pleasure of the chase and maybe a fresh pair of fine antlers to decorate a hall, then they would look for a grown stag and bring him to bay after a chase. Sir Humphrey preferred the chase. The hall in his manor house bristled with antlers and he employed not only a huntsman to care for his hounds but also a harbourer to keep track of likely stags and lead the hunt to them on request.

The harbourer had found them a fine beast this time. The animal which burst out of the woods, splashed headlong across the stream and came up to the crossways like a four-footed hurricane was in full breeding array. He had twelve points to his crown, six each side, tipped white as if with pearl. His nostrils flared red with the effort of running and his eyes were rolling. The horrified bearers were passing the top of the slippery path down to the river when he hurtled up toward them, fleeing in such panic from the hounds on his trail that he was not aware of them until the last moment.

Then he swerved, with a huge sideways leap, sprang past the nose of Father Bernard's startled mare, which reared in alarm, and was gone, into the trees and on up the hill, and at the same moment the hounds, brown and black and patch-coated, giving tongue like wolves, poured out of the woods opposite, and hard behind them came Sir Humphrey's huntsman and then Sir Humphrey himself and his twin sons, Reginald and Walter, on their big horses, closely followed by three riders who were presumably their guests, all hallooing nearly loud enough to drown the hounds and the horn.

Hounds and horses crashed through the ford, water spraying up around them. They scrambled for footholds on the path and tore upward. The cortege had stopped where it was as if paralysed, everyone having unanimously decided to keep still and let the uproar flow around them as it would around a line of trees. Most of the hounds veered as the stag had done, but three of them took the shortest route and went straight under the coffin and between the legs of the bearers. One collided with Richard's ankles and another bounced off Nicholas Weaver's shins. Both Richard and Nicholas lurched and their burden shifted.

The lurches were small and the shift in the weight was minor, but feet slipped on the perilous ground and the uneven weight of the tilting coffin made them slip still more. There were shouts of alarm. The riders, coming hard after the hounds, swerved their mounts around the head of the cortege, but one of them came too close. His horse saw the coffin, shied to avoid it and kicked out, catching Higg's hip.

Higg, knocked sideways, held on but stumbled, and the tilt of the coffin became dangerous. Then Richard, who was one of the foremost bearers, lost his footing altogether and sat down, still holding on but pulling the front of the coffin down farther still. The tilt became a slide toward the ground, tearing the other bearers' hands and breaking their hold. There were more cries of alarm. Margaret Weaver and Betsy called aloud on God, and people crossed themselves. Kat and Deborah screamed.

In a shaft of sunlight through the leaves, the funeral party had a fleeting glimpse of tall horses, reins with ornate dagged edges, spurred boots, richly coloured saddlecloths and tunics, bearded faces, one with a hunting horn held to its lips, velvet cloaks and exotic headgear, twisted liripipes bouncing on their owners' shoulders, and then they were gone, leaping over the path and crashing up the hillside.

As they went, the coffin slithered right out of the bearers' grasp, came down slowly but inexorably onto the path to the ford and then, gliding on the mud churned by the hunt, set off on its own, straight toward the river.

Father Bernard was off his horse on the instant. He threw himself after the coffin, clutching at it as he landed facedown in the mud, but its weight dragged it out of his grasp. Others scrambled frantically down through the trees to help. Deborah Archer, exclaiming with horror, got there first, tearing her dark skirts on the underbrush. She flung herself on top of the coffin as it went into the water and somehow succeeded in hooking one foot around the trunk of an alder at the brink. Held by her weight, the coffin sank where it was, and grounded in the shallow water of the ford, Deb lying on its lid and spluttering with her face in the stream and her skirts floating to each side of her.

Roger, rushing after her, waded into the water to get to the other end of the coffin and push it back toward land. Other helping hands were there. They picked Father Bernard up, lifted Deb and grabbed the coffin, dragging it ashore and hoisting it up again.

Richard, white-faced, had got to his feet and reached them in time to help with carrying his father's casket back up the slope to the shocked procession on the path. "It's all right. It hasn't broken open. Deb saved it. If the water had moved it off the shallows…"

It could have done. The Allerbrook had a strong current and downstream of the ford it became quite deep. No one wanted to imagine what could have happened next.

"Father Bernard, you're covered in mud!" Richard looked at the priest in distress. "You must brush it off. You must call at your house and put on something clean before the service. Can you find Roger here some dry things, too? He's drenched to the knees. And Deb, oh Deb, I can't be more grateful, but you're wet through and shivering. Here!" He pulled off his cloak and threw it around her. "That'll keep some warmth in. You can hardly strip your wet things off just here, so go home, Deb, *run,* to keep some heat in you, and put on dry things. We'll wait for you in the churchyard. But you must get dry or you'll take a chill. Go on—*now!*"

"I'm past the age for running and it's over half a mile!" said Deb through chattering teeth as she wrung out her skirts and clutched the cloak to her. "But I'll get home fast-like and see 'ee in the churchyard." Holding her wet gown clear of the ground, she scurried off and Richard turned his attention to Betsy's husband, Higg, who was flexing his right wrist and rubbing his hip, a pained expression on his seamed brown face. "What's the matter, Higg? You've hurt yourself?"

"One of their damned hosses well-nigh kicked me off my feet

and then my wrist went when I was tryin' to keep a'hold of the coffin," Higg said. "Hip don't matter—that's just a bruise—but it feels like my wrist's been twisted half off. Don't think I can go on as bearer. T'wouldn't be safe, and we've had trouble enough for one day."

"It's time for the relief bearers, anyhow," Richard said, and raised his voice to call the volunteers forward: Ned Crowham, the Searles, Gilbert Lowe, Sim Hannacombe and Harry Rixon. Far away in the distance the hunting horn spoke again and the baying of the hounds once more drifted through the trees.

"Bloody Sweetwaters," said Richard through his teeth. "I hope they all fall off their damned horses and break their necks and I hope the hounds bring that stag to bay and it gores every single one of them to death!"

"It went well enough in the end," Nicholas Weaver said to Richard later that day as they stood together, partaking of the generous food and the excellent cider that was Kat's speciality, and yet very conscious of the space in the household, the empty niche in the air which once had been filled by George. "That accident could have been much worse!"

"I daresay," said Richard. "But I'll never forgive the Sweet-waters. Never!"

"Likely enough they hardly realised what had happened," said Nicholas. "It was all so fast. By the time they'd seen us, it was too late."

"They had time enough! Had to get across the ford, didn't they? And all of us up there on the path. Couldn't miss us!"

"Ah, well. The light under the trees is always dim and we were all in dark clothes. Can't come to a funeral in festive red and tawny!"

"You're a good-natured soul, Nicholas," Richard said. "I'm not so even tempered as you. The Sweetwaters behave as if this were still the days of serfs and villeins and we were nothing but animals with no human feelings. Before I'm done, I swear I'll teach them different. I'd like to kill every last man of them. It would be a pleasure to see every Sweetwater head on a chopping block."

"You're so fierce!" said Nicholas, and adroitly turned the subject. "Well, there's talk of war these days. Plenty of people will get chopped up if that happens!"

A good many of the gathering were talking about the accident to the coffin, some of them with amusement, some with anxiety for the health of Mistress Archer, who had been soaked to the skin and had had to go a good half mile like that in order to get home and dry herself. For others, however, talking about the Sweetwaters and their connections had led to conversation about the wider world in general. Here in this quiet corner of the southwest, the power struggles of kings and lords didn't often impinge, but it had been known to happen, and for years the news had been disturbing. King Henry VI was said to be ailing in his mind, and his relative, Richard, Duke of York, who like the king was a descendant of Edward III, had been made regent for a while, but it was an uneasy state of affairs.

"Ambitious, that's what I hear. He didn't much care for it when the king got better. Could lead to trouble…"

"Some say all that's a tale put about by the queen. She don't like him. They say he's sworn his loyalty but she don't believe it. I've heard no good of her. When I were in Lynmouth and there were a ship in from London way, the men aboard said folk in the eastern parts are calling her Queen She-Wolf, ever since her

French friends burned Sandwich port last year. Bloodthirsty, they say she is."

"Yes, I've heard that." Ned Crowham was unwontedly grave. "We had a queen over a century ago, a French-born one, that used to be called the She-Wolf of France. They must have named this one after her and it's hardly a compliment. You could be right. I can see war coming."

"Pray God and the saints it don't come near us or call any of us away. If the Sweetwaters go to war…"

Nicholas had heard things, too. "If war does come," he said to Richard, "then the Luttrells in Dunster Castle will go, for sure, and they'll take some of the young fellows in my family. We're their tenants."

"And I'm a Sweetwater tenant! The last thing I want to do is die nobly fighting at their orders!" Richard said angrily. "Oh, well, it hasn't happened yet. My friend, there's something else I want to discuss." He took Nicholas's elbow and steered him into a quieter corner. "I've something in mind that could do both of us a bit of good. You might think a funeral's no place for fixing up a marriage, but nothing'll bring my father back and this talk of war's unsettling. I'd sooner think of things that can be settled by you and me, here and now, and might give all our thoughts a happier turn. Your eldest daughter's still not betrothed. I've been thinking…"

The Sweetwaters lived at the eastern end of the village on a knoll, in a house with a battlemented lookout tower. The Allerbrook, running close by on its way to join the River Barle, provided the house with a half moat in front, and there was a good ford for the packhorse trains carrying wool to market, and a set of stepping stones maintained by the Sweetwaters for the convenience of travellers in and out of the village.

Richard envied the house and approved of the stepping stones, but his father had been sour. "They put all the village rents up when they put in the stones," George had said. "Lucky they didn't put the farm rents up again and all!"

In the great hall Reginald Sweetwater, the elder by twenty minutes of Sir Humphrey's twin sons, helped his father off with his boots while Walter did the same office for their guests, and Geoffrey Baker, who had returned to his duties immediately after the funeral, came in with two young pages and served mulled wine. He did not let the women servants wait on all-male gatherings. Sir Humphrey and Reginald were both widowers, and Walter's wife, Mary, preferred to remain in her solar with her young daughter when male guests visited without their own wives.

"That was a good run," said Thomas Carew, one of the guests—and an illustrious one, since his mother had been a Courtenay. "You'll have a fine new set of antlers for your wall, Sir Humphrey." He looked appreciatively around at the remarkable collection already there. "Twelve pointer, wasn't he? Not bad. They hardly ever go over fourteen points in England."

"That one did." Sir Humphrey, a heavily built man, stretched a large pair of feet toward the warmth of the hearth and pointed to the impressive trophy just above it. "My grandfather killed him. Eighteen points. Almost unheard of for this part of the world."

"It was a sixteen pointer that chased a friend of mine up a tree one September," said Thomas.

"Damned lucky to find a tree on these moors," said Walter Sweetwater.

"It was on the edge of Cloutsham vale, over beyond Dunkery hill. Plenty of tree cover there. Up there two hours he was, with the old stag parading around and going for the tree with his antlers every now and again. It was in the rut. Stag must have thought he was a rival. Do you reckon a male deer can tell male and female humans from each other?"

The conversation went on an excursion around remarkable hunting stories and anecdotes about animal sagacity, and an argument between Walter and his father about the intelligence of sheep, Walter maintaining that according to the Sweetwater shepherd, Edward Searle, they weren't as stupid as most people believed, and Sir Humphrey complaining that Walter spent too much time in the company of the shepherd and should concentrate on practicing his swordplay instead. "Edward Searle may look like a prophet out of the Old Testament and stalk about among his sheep with his head in the air as though he were royalty, but he's only a shepherd and ought to remember it, and so ought you," said Sir Humphrey, who was himself slightly intimidated by Edward Searle, though he would have died before he admitted as much.

Thomas's young son, whose mind seemed to have been elsewhere all this time, suddenly asked, "Who were those people we almost crashed into after we crossed the river? I could hardly see them in that bad light under the trees. What were they doing there?"

"George Lanyon of Allerbrook's funeral party," said Reginald contemptuously. "Our steward, Baker, attended it." He looked around, but the steward had withdrawn and was out of hearing. Reginald laughed. "He said they dropped the coffin and it almost went into the river. But they got it up and it was all right. There was no harm done."

"George Lanyon's no loss. Maybe deer know men from women, but George Lanyon never knew gentle from simple," said Sir Humphrey. His eyes, which were grey and always inclined to be cold, became positively icy at the thought of the departed George. "Had the presumption to argue when his rent went up, as if rents don't have to go up now and then—it's the course of nature. Let's hope the son—what's his name…?"

"Richard Lanyon, Grandfather." Walter's eleven-year-old son, Baldwin, was also in the company.

"That's it. Richard. Bigheaded peasant who won't let anyone call him Dickon. We can hope he's less bloody-minded than George, but I doubt it. There's something about him. He doesn't like taking his cap off to me. He'll very likely be even worse than his father was. Ah, here's Baker back again. More mulled wine, Baker."

When he brought the wine, Geoffrey said, "I've ordered a fresh basket of firewood to be brought in. The weather's turning colder. It feels as if winter's on its way early."

"That ought to cool the talk of war," Thomas said. "No fun campaigning in snow and mud. Wonder if it'll come to fighting?"

"That's anyone's guess," Sir Humphrey said. "What makes me laugh is the way they use roses as their badges! A red rose for the House of Lancaster, a white rose for the House of York! As though they were carrying ladies' favours at a tournament! Pretty-pretty nonsense."

"Their ambitions aren't nonsense, though," said Reginald. "They're fighting over the crown."

CHAPTER THREE

THE BUSINESS OF MARRIAGE

Nicholas and Margaret Weaver's home in the coastal village of Dunster had a characteristic smell, a mixture of oiliness and mustiness with a hint of the farmyard. It was the smell of sheep fleece, and it pervaded the whole house, even the bedchambers. Which was natural, for wool was their world.

Rents from sheep farmers accounted for much of the wealth of the Luttrell family, who lived in the castle overlooking the village. The spinning of yarn and the weaving of cloth were the main trades of the village, and the monks of Cleeve Abbey, a few miles to the east, close to a village called Washford, were industrious shepherds who brought their fleeces regularly to Dunster and did so much business there that they had a fulling mill at the western end of the village and a house of their own in North Street. The abbots of Cleeve spent nearly as much time in Dunster as they did in their monastery.

The Weaver family, who had taken their surname from their trade generations ago, were as prolific as the Lanyons were not. Nicholas, who had had some schooling and knew many well-travelled merchants, said that he had heard of people in far-off places who lived in communities known as tribes, which had usually grown from an original large family. His own cheerful, noisy, crowded family, he was wont to say, was almost a tribe.

It was a fair summing-up. They all knew how they were related to each other and they all, more or less, lived together, although sheer necessity had obliged them, eventually, to spread first of all into the house next door when the tenancy chanced to fall vacant, and later to rent the house opposite, as well.

By that time Nicholas's cousin Laurence and his richly fertile wife, Elena, had a family of formidable dimensions and it was their branch of the tribe that moved across the road, where they took to carding and yarn spinning as distinct from the actual weaving. At one time, like many other families, the Weavers had bought yarn from other cottagers, who made their living by spinning. Until it occurred to Laurence that they had hands enough to do both jobs, whereupon he set his side of the family to creating yarn. Only the fulling and dyeing had to be contracted out. Otherwise, the family bought raw fleeces and did the rest themselves.

Under Nicholas's roof, only Margaret now spun yarn. She had a knack for creating a thin, strong woollen thread which she sold, undyed, on market days, a small but useful addition to the household coffers.

Renting the third house was a wise move from every point of view. The various cousins, uncles and aunts who had been squeezed in with Nicholas and Margaret could now occupy the

next-door premises. Meanwhile, as time went on, Laurence and
Elena brought their family to ten, plus a daughter-in-law and
three grandchildren. As yet, the youngsters were too small to be
useful, but they would soon be big enough to learn to spin. They
would also take up space. Laurence eased the congestion as best
he could by building a workroom on to the back of his house.
Nicholas likewise constructed a weaving shed to the rear of his.
These additions made little difference, though. The Weavers
remained much as they always had been: amiably argumentative—and crowded.

With so many mouths to feed and three rents to be paid, their
prosperity had to be carefully nurtured. They grew vegetables
and reared poultry in the long back gardens of the three houses
and Nicholas now rented a meadow on a hillside at the seaward
end of the village, where he kept not only his three ponies but
also two cows. He had built a byre-cum-stable there as shelter
for the animals and somewhere to store tack and winter fodder.
Margaret was good at dairy work as well as spinning thread, and
they had cheese and cream for everyone.

It was also a family custom to marry their daughters off early,
taking their youthful appetites for food into other people's households. Sometimes even surplus boys were exported. Nicholas and
Margaret had two young sons and one of them, eventually, might
have to leave home. "A good rose bush needs regular pruning"
was the way Nicholas put it.

And the next one to be pruned, thought their daughter Liza, *is
going to be me.*

From the moment her parents arrived home from George
Lanyon's funeral, she had sensed that something was in the air,
though at first it wasn't clear what the something was. The

return of Nicholas and Margaret chanced to coincide with a busy time. New orders for cloth had come in, and there had been a problem at the Cleeve Abbey fulling mill, which the Dunster weavers used as well as the monks, to get their cloth cleaned with water and fuller's earth before dyeing. A thunderstorm on the moors had sent quantities of peat down the Avill River and polluted the water supply. "It's always happening. Nature wants us to dye all our cloth dark brown," Nicholas grumbled. "We'll have to send it somewhere else till the river clears. Can't go delaying orders from new customers. That's bad business."

But concerned though the family had been with these matters, there had been something else on their minds. Twice Liza had walked into a room to find her parents talking to other family members, and the conversation had stopped short the moment she appeared. And she had noticed her parents glancing at her, pleasantly enough, but thoughtfully, too, as though they were wondering…

Wondering what? Liza could guess the answer to that. Indeed, she had been through all this before and was fairly sure that she recognised the symptoms. They had a marriage in mind for her and were asking themselves whether she would be pleased with it or not.

She had been expecting something like this. After all, she was the eldest daughter. She was twenty-three now and should have been wedded long ago. Three of her younger sisters were married and the little one, Jane, the infant of the family, was single only because she was as yet only seven years old. Liza had stayed unmarried so far because first one thing and then another had interfered with her parents' plans. They had arranged a very good match for her when she was sixteen, but the young man inconsiderately died of a fever before the wedding day. Another proposal came in quite soon, but the prospective bridegroom, though well-off and good-natured enough, was nearly fifty. Liza objected and neither Nicholas nor Margaret were easy about the matter, either. The argument—put forward by Aunt Cecy, one of the older family members—that she would probably become a wealthy widow before long and could then please herself, failed to convince either Liza or her parents and the negotiations died away.

There had been others, too—a suitor who changed his mind and another whose parents changed it for him because they had found a better prospect. Time had gone on.

"And now," said Margaret indignantly when at last the business problems had been overcome and the family had gathered together—without Liza—for a full-scale discussion of the proposal which she and Nicholas had brought back from Aller-brook, "and now there's gossip. Folk have such vile minds."

She broke off to cough, because during the summer they did not light the fire in the big main room and now, when autumn had set in and they needed warmth, the chimney was smoking. She had pulled her spinning wheel out of the way of possible smuts, but was still using it, important though this gathering was. The steady whirr formed a background to the business in hand.

"Liza's a good wench," she said when the coughing fit was over. "And we've said naught to her about these hints we've heard, that she's been meetin' a man in secret, because hints is all it is, and we reckon they come from jealous old women with clatterin' tongues and naught better to do than make up nasty stories about young girls who still have pretty faces and all their teeth! But it's time we got her settled—that's true enough. She's got a right to depend on us for that."

★ ★ ★

I knew it. Flat on the planks of the floor overhead, with one ear pressed to a chink between two boards, Liza felt her stomach clench in fright. Earlier that day she had heard her name mentioned in a conversation among her elders and had without hesitation done some deliberate eavesdropping. She had guessed right, it seemed. Her marriage was being planned and it seemed that her future was to be discussed this morning, in her absence. Slipping away from duties in the kitchen, she had gone to her chamber just above the main living room, and then, having taken the precaution of bolting herself in, flattened herself to the floor to eavesdrop for the second time that day.

It wasn't the sort of behaviour her parents would have approved of in any of their daughters; in fact, they would have been appalled. But then, they would be even more appalled if they knew about Christopher, Liza thought, and by the sound of it, they had heard something. She could guess the source of the rumour, as well. That wretched woman who had the cottage down by the packhorse bridge. She had seen Liza and Christopher together and must, after all, have recognised them.

Lying flat, her left cheekbone in danger of being grazed by the floor, Liza felt tears pricking behind her eyes. She tried to blink them away. She had *known* this was coming. She had *known* that, sooner or later, arrangements would be made for her and all her dreams would be destroyed. She had thought she was prepared. But now…

Oh, dear God. Oh, Christopher, my dear love. I can't bear it.

A few feet away, below Liza, Aunt Cecy was staring coldly at Margaret, who stared back in an equally chilly manner. They all addressed Cecy as *Aunt,* but she was actually the wife of Nicholas's oldest cousin, Dick Weaver, who was the son of Great-Uncle Will, the most ancient member of the tribe. Her virtue was as rigid as her backbone, and her backbone resembled a broom handle. Her mouth and body were overthin, and alone among the women of the family she had had trouble giving birth. Her two daughters had been born, with great difficulty, eight years apart, with several disasters intervening. They had both been married off at the age of fourteen and had seemed glad to leave home.

"If that girl b'ain't wed soon," Aunt Cecy said now, "her pretty face'll get lines and her teeth'll start going. Margaret, do you have to keep on with that everlasting spinning when we're talkin' over summat as solemn as this, and what in heaven's name is wrong with that there chimney?"

"I think birds must have nested in it since the spring-cleaning. We'll have to clear it. The men'd better lop a branch off that birch tree in the garden to push down it. As for spinnin', I like keepin' my hands busy," said Margaret. "I can spin and talk, *and* listen."

Aunt Cecy snorted. Laurence, who had come across the cobbled road with Elena and others of his family, threading their way past the permanent market stalls which occupied the middle of the street, said reasonably, "Never mind the tales. Nicholas here says he's had an offer. If it's a good one, where's the problem?" He was very like Nicholas, with the same hearty voice and the same robust outlook on life. "Even if she has had…let's be charitable and say a friend—in secret—what of it? Who didn't, when they were young? All that'll be over. Who is it you've got in mind?"

"Peter Lanyon," said Nicholas. "Grandson of George, whose burial Margaret and I have just been to."

"Liza's older than Peter, isn't she?" Elena said. "Does it matter, do you think?"

"Er…" said their daughter-in-law, and her husband, Laurie, a younger version of Laurence, grinned. Laurence burst out laughing and so did several of Nicholas's cousins.

"Our Katy here's two years older than young Laurie and who cares? Didn't stop them having twin sons inside of a year!" Laurence said.

"Liza ought to be married," Nicholas said. "And I've called you all in here to discuss this proposal from the Lanyons. Peter'll do as far as I'm concerned. He's good-looking and good-natured, and Richard's offered me a deal. He got me in a corner at his dad's funeral and put it to me. I've a good dowry put by for Liza, but he's suggested something more. He wants to be cut in to our business. We've always bought about half his wool clip—he sells the other half when the agents come round from the big merchants. Now he says we can have the wool for a discount if he can have a regular cut off the profits when we sell the finished cloth and yarn. He asked a lot of questions and we went into another room and he clicked a few beads round his abacus, arriving at a figure. I reckon he's judged his offer finely. He'll come out on the right side more often than not. In effect, we'll pay more for his wool, not less, only not all at once, but…"

"Looks as if he's takin' advantage." Great-Uncle Will didn't like to walk far, so he spent his days sitting about. At the moment he was in a bad temper because the smoking fire had driven him from the settle by the hearth, where he liked to sit on chilly days, driving him back to his summer seat by the window. His voice was sharp. "We want to get Liza off our hands. He'll oblige if he's paid!"

"Quite. We'll have to look on his cut from our profits as part of Liza's dowry," said Nicholas. "Getting the wool cheap won't offset it, most years anyway. But he also pointed out that once we're all one family and one business, there are things we can do to help each other. Put opportunities each other's way—things like introductions to new customers, or brokering marriages. Word to each other of anything useful like new breeds of sheep. He's thinking to buy a ram from some strain or other with better fleeces. If he does, we'll gain from that after a while. Meanwhile, we'll have got Liza settled and she'll be eating his provender, not ours."

"You must admit the man's got ideas," said Laurence, and Dick Weaver nodded in agreement. "What of the girl herself?" he asked. "Has this been mentioned to her?"

"Why should it be?" demanded Aunt Cecy. "She'd be well advised to do as she's told."

"Not yet," said Margaret. "But she won't be difficult. When was she ever? She's a good girl, is Liza, whatever silly gossip may say."

"She'd better not be difficult. If 'ee don't get that wench married," said Great-Uncle Will, "she could get into trouble and then what'll 'ee do? Get her shovelled into a nunnery while you rear her love child? I've heard that there gossip, too, and if there's truth in it, the fellow can't wed her anyhow. In orders, he is. That's what the clacking tongues are saying."

The entire family, as if they were puppets whose strings were held by a single master hand, swung around to look at him.

"I've not heard this!" Nicholas said. "You know *who* this fellow is that Liza's supposed to be meeting? Well, who is he and how did you find out so much?"

"Gossip!" said Margaret, interrupting forcefully and snagging her thread in her annoyance. "Liza's a sensible girl, I tell 'ee!"

"She knows all the ins and outs of the business," said Nicholas. "I grant you that. She's handy with a loom and an abacus, as well. She understands figures the way I do and the way that the rest of you, frankly, don't! But she gets dreamy sometimes. Don't know where she gets that from. And now folk are asking why's she still single and is there some dark reason? Sounds to me as if there maybe is and the whispers have something behind them after all! Well, Uncle Will? What have you heard?"

"I sit here by this window on warm days and folk stop to talk to me," said Will. "I didn't want to repeat the talk. Not sure I should, even now. These things often fade out if you leave them be. Don't matter if she's had a kiss in the moonlight or a cuddle in a cornfield, as long as she don't argue now." The fire belched again, swirling smoke right across the room, and he choked, waving a wrinkled hand before his face. "Devil take this smoke!"

There were exclamations of protest from all around. "That won't do, Great Uncle!" said Nicholas bluntly. "If you know a name, then tell us. Who does gossip say the man is?"

"Young fellow working up at the castle, studying with the Luttrells' chaplain, that's who," said Great-Uncle Will. "I don't know his *name,* but I know the one they mean—he's stopped by to talk to me himself. Redheaded young fellow. In minor orders yetawhile, but he'll be a full priest one of these days. So he b'ain't husband material for Liza or any other girl. You get her fixed up with Peter Lanyon, and quick."

"I can hardly believe it." Margaret had stopped her spinning wheel.

Aunt Cecy gave her a look which said, *I told you you couldn't keep on with that and attend to this business as well,* and said aloud, "Where *is* Liza, anyway?"

"In the kitchen," said Margaret. And then stopped short, looking through the window. Liza, far from being in the kitchen, must have slipped out the front door only a moment ago. She was crossing the road, going away from the house on some unknown errand.

Uncle Will turned to peer after her. "There she goes. Well, let's hope all she wanted was a breath of air and that she b'ain't runnin' off with her red-haired swain yetawhile. You take an old man's advice. Say nothing to her about him. Pretend we don't know. No need to upset the wench. But get her wed, and fast. Get word off to Richard Lanyon tomorrow and tell him yes. That's what I say." Another wave of smoke poured out of the fireplace and he choked again. "Can't anyone do something about this? Put a bucket of water on that there fire and get to sweeping the chimney!"

CHAPTER FOUR

ONE MAGICAL SUMMER

Peter'll do as far as I'm concerned. When Liza heard her father say those words, she had heard enough. She sat back on her heels, miserably thinking, while the murmur of voices continued below her. At length she rose quietly from the floor, picked up a cloak, unbolted her door and stole out. The stairs were solid and didn't creak. She went softly down them, glad that in this house they didn't lead into the big main room as they did in many other houses, but into a tiny lobby where cloaks and spare footwear were kept, and from which the front door opened.

She could hear a buzz of talk and a clatter of pans in the kitchen. If anyone saw her, she would probably be called in to help and chided for having left it in the first place. She opened the front door as stealthily as she could, darted through, closed it and set off, crossing the road, trying to lose herself quickly behind the stalls in the middle of it, in case anyone should be looking from the window.

Bearing to the right, past the last cottages and the Abbot's House opposite, she hurried out of the village. Then she turned off the main track, taking a path to the left, crossed a cornfield and emerged onto the track that led to the next village to the west, Alcombe, two miles off.

She felt uneasy as she crossed the field, for here, as at Allerbrook, the corn had been cut and a couple of village women were gleaning in the stubble. Although they were some way off and did not seem to notice her, she was nervously aware of them.

Beyond the cornfield stood a stone pillar on a plinth, a monument to the days of the great plague in the last century. Villages then had kept strangers out in case they brought disease with them, but commerce had to go on; wool and yarn, cloth and leather, butter and cheese, flour and ale must still be bought and sold and so, outside many villages, stone pillars or crosses had been set up to show where markets could be held.

"I'll be by the plague cross at ten of the clock on Tuesday," Christopher had said at their last meeting. "I'll have an errand past there that day. The Luttrells send things now and then to an old serving man of theirs in Alcombe. He's ailing nowadays. They often use me for charitable tasks like that, and lend me a pony. Meet me there if you can. I'll wait for you for a while, though I'd better not linger too long."

It was only just past ten o'clock, Liza thought as she slipped out of the field, out of sight of the gleaning women. Had he waited? Would he be there?

He was. There was his pony, hobbled and grazing by the

track, and there was Christopher, his hair as bright as fire, sitting on the plinth.

"Christopher!"

He was looking the other way, perhaps expecting her to come along the main track instead of through the field, but he sprang up at the sound of her voice, and turned toward her. She ran into his arms and they closed about her. "Oh, Christopher! I'm so glad to see you!"

"Are you? What is it, sweeting? Something's wrong, isn't it? I can always tell."

"Yes, I know you can!"

That was how it had been from the beginning, when they met in the spring, at the May Day fair in Dunster. It had been a fine day, and the fair was packed and raucous. There were extra stalls as well as the regular ones, offering every imaginable commodity: gloves, pottery, kitchen pans and fire irons, hats, belts, buckles, cheap trinkets, questionable remedies for assorted ills, lengths of silk and linen from far away as well as the local woollen cloth, sweet cakes and savoury snacks cooked on the spot over beds of glowing charcoal. There were entertainments, too: a juggler, tumblers, a minstrel playing a lute and singing, a troupe of dancers and a sword swallower.

And, creating an alleyway through the crowd and inspiring a different mood among the onlookers, an unhappy man stripped to the waist except for a length of undyed cloth slung around his neck. Splashed with dirt and marked with bruises, he was escorted by the two men who that year were Dunster's constables. Ahead of them walked a boy banging a drum for the crowd's attention and announcing that by order of the Weavers Guild of Dunster, here came Bart Webber, who had been mixing flax with his woollen yarn to make his cloth, and selling it as pure Dunster wool, and had been fined for it at the last manor court.

It could have been worse. The hapless Master Webber hadn't been whipped or put in the stocks, and the crowd was good-humoured and not in a mood for brutality. Many of them knew him socially, which inclined them to restraint or even, in some cases, sympathy. He was still drawing a few jeers, though, and an occasional missile—handfuls of mud and one or two mouldy onions, which had caused the bruises. His situation was quite wretched enough and his face was a mask of misery and embarrassment. Liza, distressed, turned quickly away.

Her parents had often told her she felt things too deeply and ought to be more sensible. They clicked regretful tongues when she persisted in going for walks on her own or when they found her in the garden after dark—"mooning after the moon," as her father put it—or being stunned by the splendour of the constellation of Orion, making its mighty pattern in the winter sky. Yes, Nicholas said, of course the moon looked like a silver dish—or a lopsided face or a little curved boat, depending on which phase it was in—and yes, of course the stars were beautiful. But most people had more sense than to stand outside catching cold, especially when there was work to be done indoors.

Sometimes Liza felt that she was dedicating her entire life to appearing sensible when inside herself, she often didn't feel sensible at all, but wild and vulnerable, like a red deer hind, fleeing before the hounds.

Now she wanted to get well away from poor Bart Webber. Elena and Laurence, who were with her, stayed to stare but Liza, abandoning them, edged back through the crowd. Then she realised that a young man who had been standing next to

Laurence had turned away, too, and was beside her and seemed to want to speak to her. She looked at him in surprise, and he said kindly, "You didn't like seeing that, did you?"

She stopped and studied him. He wore a clerk's black gown and a priest's tonsure. The ring of hair left by the tonsure was an astonishing shade of flame-red. "I know him," she said. "Bart Webber. He's dined with us. No, I didn't like seeing him—like that." It occurred to her that the young clerk had been watching her and that this was impertinent of him. With a rush of indignation she said, "You were looking at me?"

"Forgive me," he said mildly. "But when I saw you move away alone—well, in such a throng, you shouldn't be on your own."

"I was with cousins, but they're still back there. I've other relatives somewhere about, though, and my home is over there." She pointed.

"Let me walk with you to your door, or until you find some of your family." His voice was intentionally gentle, cooling her flash of annoyance. "You never know. There could be cutpurses about."

She let him escort her and as they walked, they talked. He was Christopher Clerk, halfway to priesthood, studying with the chaplain at the castle. She was Liza Weaver, daughter of Nicholas Weaver who, with his family, owned three Dunster houses and was head of a business which carried on both spinning and weaving. "Our cloth's quite well-known, and so is my mother's special fine thread."

"You sound as though you're proud of your family," he said.

"I am! And you must be proud of your vocation, and of living in a castle! Is it very grand, with paintings and carpets from the east and silken cushions for the ladies?"

"All those things, but my quarters are plain, as they should be.

55

I wouldn't have it otherwise. I felt called to be a priest, and once that happens, a man doesn't seek to live in luxury."

"Do you mean you give it up even though you miss it, or you somehow don't miss it because you don't want it anymore?" Liza asked, interested. She often caught sight of the Abbot of Cleeve and his entourage of monks coming and going from their house and had many times wondered what made them choose such lives. Were they happy, always wearing such plain white wool garments and never marrying?

"Some of us cease wanting the pleasures of the senses," Christopher told her, "and others give them up. They are the price. But if you really value something, you don't mind paying for it."

"But which group are you in?" Liza asked acutely, and privately marvelled at her own outspokenness. He might well accuse *her* of impertinence! Yet it seemed easy to talk to him, as easy as though she had known him all her life.

"I'm among those who have to make an effort. But as I said, the price is worth it." She turned her head to look at his face and he gave her a grin, a tough, cheerful, entirely masculine grin, and she found herself smiling back. His eyes, which were the warm golden-brown of amber or sweet chestnuts, glowed with laughter, and without warning, her breath seemed to halt for a moment and her heart turned a somersault.

"I won't say it's always easy," he said, searching her face with his eyes, and she knew, without further explanation, with a certainty that would not be denied, a certainty as solid as the simple fact that two plus two made four, that now, this moment, was a time when it wasn't easy. That he was talking, obliquely, about her.

About them.

About us. But we met only five minutes ago!

At that moment she caught sight of her parents, apparently arguing and just going in at their door, for dinner no doubt, since it was past noon. With a few words of farewell and thanks for his company, she took her leave of Christopher and followed them into the house, to find that an argument was indeed in progress, and that it was about Bart Webber.

"To my mind, Margaret, it's enough, what he went through today. There's no need to keep on about it and say we can't have him and Alison to dine or ask them to Liza's wedding when it comes…."

"I don't agree, Nicholas. I can't. I'm sorry for Alison and I'd sooner lie dead and in my coffin than be in her shoes, but have them at my table…no, it won't do. It's makin' out we don't take honesty seriously and we do."

"But…"

Margaret would win, of course. When it came to social niceties she usually did, and as other households often followed the Weaver lead, Liza now felt sorry for Mistress Webber as well as for Bart. Her parents broke off their wrangle when they saw her and greeted her, and to her surprise, they seemed to notice nothing strange about her.

Liza herself gave the Webbers little further thought, for she was engrossed with the astounding experience she had just had, and amazed that it had apparently left no mark upon her. She felt as though it should have done; as though the wave of hair which always crept from under her neat white coif should have changed from beechnut brown to bright green, or as though luminous footprints should appear wherever she trod.

But after all, what had really taken place? Nothing that anyone could have seen, and nothing that could be repeated. Very likely she would never set eyes on the red-haired clerk again. *Whatever* had happened, it would never be repeated. She had better forget it. That would be sensible.

No doubt it would have been, but a perverse providence seemed determined to reunite them. Two mornings later, going to the herb plot at the far end of the garden to fetch flavourings for dinner, she discovered a small brown-and-white dog industriously digging a hole under the mint.

"Here, stop that! Where did you come from?" said Liza, advancing on the intruder and picking it up. It yapped at her indignantly and struggled, while Liza stood with it in her arms, wondering how it had got in. Then she saw that there was a hole under the wooden fence which bounded the end of the garden. Beyond, meadowland sloped away, down toward Dunster's harbour. It was silting up these days. Just now, the tide was out and a number of small boats from the Dunster fishing community lay aground, waiting for the sea to come back and refloat them. The sea itself was a band of iridescent blue and silver, far away, with the coast of Wales beyond.

To the right, however, the meadow was bounded by the castle hill and its covering of trees. The Luttrells' black cattle were in the pasture, and a man was hurrying across it from the direction of the trees and the castle. He saw her and waved, and came on faster. "You've got him!" he said breathlessly as he came up to the fence. "Wagtail! You wicked dog!"

"Is he yours?" Liza asked. "He shouldn't be let loose to scrabble in people's gardens. Someone might throw stones at him or kick him!"

Wagtail barked again and struggled in her arms. And then she recognised the man. He was once more in clerical black, though this time in the more practical form of hose and jerkin, and he had pulled a dark cap over his fiery tonsure. Some of his red hair was visible, though, with an oak leaf absurdly clinging to it. Christopher Clerk, the young man who had read her mind and knew that she was sorry for the swindler Bart Webber.

"I hope he did no serious damage," he said. "He belongs to Mistress Luttrell—he's her lapdog—but he's forever running off into the woods. I think he thinks he's a deerhound! Can you hand him over the fence to me?"

Liza went to do so and his eyes widened. "Don't I know you? Aren't you Liza Weaver? We met two days ago at the fair."

"Yes, yes, I am. And you're Christopher." At the fair they had stood and walked side by side. This was the first time she had stood face-to-face with him and really studied him. He had a snub nose and a square jaw with a hint of pugnacity in it, the effect both tough and boyish and remarkably attractive. His red-gold eyebrows were shapely above his smiling eyes, and once more she noticed how beautiful and unusual their colour was. That amber shade was quite different from the soft velvet-brown of her own eyes, as she had sometimes seen them when looking in her mother's silver mirror. There were a few gold flecks in the amber, and his skin, too, was dusted with golden freckles. There was a slightly denser freckling on his chin, adding an endearing touch of comedy to his face.

The hands that reached to take the struggling dog from her, though, were beautiful, strong without being coarse, the backs lightly furred with red-gold hairs, the bones clearly defined beneath the skin, the fingers and palms in perfect proportion. She found it hard not to keep gazing at them.

On his side, he was having his first clear view of her. He took in fewer details, but the little he did absorb was enough—the deep colour of the beechnut hair showing in front of the coif, the candid brown eyes, the good skin. She was tall for a girl, and within the plain dark everyday gown her body had a sturdy strength. Not that either of them felt they were studying a stranger. It was more as though they were reminding themselves of something they had known since before they were born but had unaccountably forgotten.

"The bluebells are still out in your garden," he said. His hands were now full of dog, but he nodded to the little splash of blue next to the herb plot. "There are wonderful bluebells in a dell on the other side of the castle. You can get there by the path past the mill. A few yards on, there's another little path that leads aside, leftward, to the dell. Do you know the place? Anyone can go there."

"Yes. Yes, I know it. But how do you come to know it?" Liza asked curiously. "I thought…I mean, you have your work."

"I came across it a week ago—chasing Wagtail again! He's always getting out, and whoever sees him slipping off usually goes after him—page, squire, man-at-arms, maid or cook or groom! Not the chaplain or Mistress Luttrell herself, though. They keep their dignity. I found Wagtail among the bluebells and I've been back since to see them before they fade. Father Meadowes—the chaplain, that is—gives me a passage from the Scriptures to meditate on each day, and three times I've done my meditating while walking about in the dell after dinner. At about two of the clock."

He shouldn't be saying these things. Liza knew it and so did Christopher. He shouldn't, either, have lain sleepless last night, while the girl he had met at the fair danced through his mind, glowing with light and warmth so that all thoughts of priesthood and his vocation had melted like morning mist before a summer sunrise. Now the words he ought not to say had come out, apparently by themselves.

"I walk out to take the air sometimes, too," said Liza. She smiled. "There's a leaf in your hair. Did you know?"

"Wagtail's fault. He tore straight off through the woods below the castle and I went straight after him. But it's hard going if you don't take a stick or, better still, a wood-axe along with you," said Christopher, grinning, and because he was still holding the dog, he leaned forward across the fence and let her remove the leaf from his tonsure. It was the first time they'd ever touched. It made her inside turn somersaults again.

"I must go," he said, and she watched him walk away across the meadow. He was almost a priest and her parents wouldn't like this at all, but it made no difference. Something had begun that would not be halted. At the thought of seeing him again, her spirit became as light as thistledown, dancing in the wind. Around her, the scent of the herbs, the green of the meadow, the azure of the bluebells, the distant sparkle of the sea all seemed enhanced, brighter, stronger, as though her senses had been half-asleep all her life and now were fully awake at last. She felt about as sensible as a hare in March, or an autumn leaf in a high wind.

She *would* see him again. She must.

In the afternoon she slipped away, through the village, along the path that led to the dell, and found him there and they walked together.

Three days later, although the bluebells were no longer at their best, they met there again and this time they kissed. Then they sat down on a fallen log and stared at each other in consternation.

"I'm going to be a priest. Well, I already am, in a junior way. I've been a subdeacon and six months ago I was ordained deacon. Becoming a full priest is the next step, the final one. If I…if I abandon my vocation now, my father won't take me back. He has other sons to settle. He's a merchant in Bristol, successful but not rich."

"I see. Well, you told me to begin with that you were going to be a priest. But…" Liza's voice died away in bewilderment, mainly at herself.

Christopher thrust his fingers through his tonsure. "Liza, my father and mother are both steady, reliable people. They expect their children to be steady and reliable, too, and I thought I was! And then—we met at the fair, and you smiled at me and all my good sense has flown away like a flock of swallows at the end of summer! You make me feel as though my feet have left the ground and my head's among the stars. I don't understand myself!"

He stopped running his fingers through his hair and reached out to take her hands. "What I do understand is that my world has turned upside down. Liza, as I said, I'm already in the priesthood. To get myself released from this would be horribly difficult. I'd have to go to my bishop and he'd probably say I was committed for life. I've heard of men who've bought their way out, but I have little money. I suppose I could borrow some. I know I could make my way in the world, given time, but it would be very hard at first and perhaps I'd be in debt. Would you wait for me? Would they let you wait?"

"I don't think so. They want to get me married, and they'd say that a priest can't marry and that's the end of it."

Liza knew her family. They were good-natured as a rule, though liable to shout loudly in times of crisis—if, for instance, a pot should be spilled in the kitchen or a piece of weaving be damaged or if Aunt Cecy discovered a spider in her bedchamber—but with no real ill feeling behind the uproar. Nevertheless, for all their seemingly easygoing ways, they took their work seriously; nothing slipshod was ever let past. And they expected their private life to be properly conducted, expected that parents would arrange their children's future careers and marriages and that the children would concur. The arrangements would be made with affection and consideration, but made, just the same, and with a very keen regard for respectability. What Liza was doing now would not be tolerated. She would be seen as a wanton who had tried to seduce a priest from his vocation. Her mother in particular would be horrified. Margaret prided herself on holding up her head among the neighbours.

"No, I see. I'd say the same, in their place. Liza, *what* has happened to us?"

"It's as if...this were meant to be. I was reared to be steady, sensible, like you. My father talks to me about cloth-making because sometimes I ask questions about it and he says he likes to see his daughter being interested in practical things and her family's business."

If you're taking the trouble to learn about my business, you'll do the same about your husband's business when you marry, whether he's in the weaving trade or no. I'd sooner see you with an abacus than mooning at the moon. Nicholas had said such things to her several times.

"He's taught me to keep accounts, with Arabic figures, and an abacus," Liza said. "I've always tried to be what he and my mother wanted of me. I think my parents are like yours in many ways. But now...my head's among the stars as well."

They looked at each other helplessly, two earnest young crea-tures who had suddenly found that common sense wasn't enough.

"Except that it can't come to anything. Dear heart. Oh, Liza, what have I done to you, letting you love me, letting myself love you? It really is like that, isn't it? I mean—love?"

To Liza's distress, there were tears in his eyes. "Yes. I don't see how I can ever marry anyone else, but they'll make me!"

"Oh, my poor Liza! *Oh!*" He cried it out in anguish. "Why can't a priest be a man as well and live as other men do? Why are we condemned to this…to rejecting human love, to being so alone? It's cruel! And there's nothing, *nothing* I can do about it, for you or for me!"

"Hold me," said Liza.

On the way home, aglow from the feel of his arms around her and the feel of his body as her arms closed around him, she came face-to-face with a small, wan woman whom she recognised as Alison Webber, the wife of the unfortunate Bart. Bart was at least forty, but Alison was his second wife and she was still very young; indeed, not yet married a year. She had been a rosy girl with bright eyes like a squirrel, but now she went about like a shadow, and Liza, troubled at the sight of her, paused to say good-day. Whereupon Alison's haunted eyes blazed at her.

"*You* wish me good-day? Your mother's the cruellest woman in all Dunster. Won't speak to me in the street, as if it was all my fault, and it isn't! Your parents should have dined with us yester-day and they cried off. And what the Weavers do, others do! If she'd put out a hand to us, it 'ud be different. She's pushed us into hell and she's done it a'purpose and I've no word to say to you. Just this!" said Alison furiously, and spat at Liza's feet before pushing past and going on her way.

No, thought Liza miserably, all the glow gone, no, there was no future for her and Christopher. Margaret would never forgive her if she knew. Never.

But all through the summer she and Christopher went on with their stolen meetings, most of them in the dell. One, by chance, was on the stone bridge which had been built across the Avill River for the benefit of packhorses carrying wool to and from Dunster market. On the bridge, shadowed by the trees that bordered the river, they hugged each other and then stood to talk and look at the water, and Liza saw someone in the garden of a nearby cottage looking at them. Alarmed, she dragged Christopher off the bridge without explaining why, which annoyed him because he thought he'd seen a trout and was about to point it out.

"A trout!" Liza gasped. "The woman who lives in that cottage has the sharpest nose and the longest ears in Dunster! If she recognised us…!"

"Never mind her nose or her ears. Unless she's got the eyes of an owl as well, she couldn't possibly have recognised us in the shade of the trees! Acting guilty like that, you've probably drawn her attention. She'll *think* about us now and start wondering who we were!"

"Oh!" Liza burst out, stamping her foot. "How I hate this secrecy!"

"Good thing we're off the bridge. You might damage it, stamping like that," said Christopher, and as he pulled her into his arms, there, once again, was that tough grin which had turned her insides to water at the fair.

They had other small squabbles later. Liza never told him of the feeling of guilt toward her family, which often kept her awake at night; nor did he tell her of his own wakeful nights, when he wondered what he was about, how it happened that the studies, the prospect of full priesthood, which had once, to him, been the meat and bread, the sweet water and glowing wine of the spirit, were now nothing but yesterday's cold pottage.

But sometimes their secret misery, forced to dwell side by side with this extraordinary thing which had come upon them and bound them together and could not be altered, seemed to turn them into flint and tinder and sparks of anger were struck, though only to be extinguished moments later by Liza's tears and Christopher's kisses and that sudden, enchanting grin as his temper faded.

They never went further than kisses, though. Their stolen embraces woke a deep hunger in them, but the common sense to which they had been bred, and the knowledge, too, that they would be breaking Christopher's solemn, priestly promise of celibacy, protected them.

"I think sometimes that we quarrel because I want you so much but I know I mustn't," Christopher said once, after one of their brief arguments.

Cautious caresses were all they would ever have of one another and they knew it. They would have this one magical summer, but never would the enchantment reach its natural conclusion, and the summer would soon be gone. As it now was. From what Liza had heard that morning, the woman with the sharp nose and ears apparently did have owl's eyes, as well. Talk had started somehow and almost certainly with her. Very likely she knew them both quite well by sight. Their secret was almost out. Only her family's kindly trust in her had kept them skeptical, but it wouldn't last.

Now, standing by the plague cross on the Alcombe road, they recognised that their time was done.

"They are arranging my marriage," said Liza. "And they've heard talk. We dare not ever meet again. It's over, Christopher."

"Oh, dear God. Don't say that!" He closed his fingers around her upper arms so tightly that she protested and he eased his grip, but his face had gone hard. "It can't be…so suddenly, so soon!"

"But we knew it was coming," said Liza miserably. "We've always known. I can't defy them and if I did—even if we ran off together—I shouldn't take you from your vocation. I know that. Only, I don't know how to bear losing you. I just don't know how to bear it."

"Nor do I!"

He drew her into the shelter of some trees, out of sight of the track, and pushed her coif back so that he could kiss her thick brown hair, and then for a long time they stood there, clasping each other so tightly that they could almost have been one entity, as they longed to be.

Parting was so painful that they did not know how to do it. Liza, gazing into his face as though she were trying to memorise it, had a sudden inspiration and pulled a patterned silver ring from the middle finger of her right hand. "Christopher! Take this! It's loose on my thickest finger, but it might fit one of yours. Please take it and wear it. I want you to have it!"

"But…how did you come by it? If someone gave it to you as a gift, should you give it away?"

"It belonged to my grandmother. When she died, Mother gave it to me. But it's always been loose, as I said. I can say I've lost it. Mother will scold because she'll think I was careless, but nothing more. Take it, Christopher, please."

He did so, trying it on his left little finger and finding that it fit quite well. Then, at last, after one final and furious kiss, they let each other go. Christopher, looking over his shoulder all the time, went to reclaim his pony, and Liza, putting her hair back under its coif, found her hands trembling. She saw him mount and waved to him, but then couldn't bear it anymore. She turned away, brushing a hand across her eyes, and started back across the field.

The women were still there, gleaning, nearer to the path now, and they looked at her curiously. One of them—Liza recognised her as Bridget, the wife of another weaver—said, "Are you all right, m'dear? You look a bit mazed and sad-like."

That was when she realised she was crying. She wiped her knuckles across her eyes. "It's nothing." They went on staring at her and she told them one small part of the truth. "I think I'm going to be married but I don't know him very well and…"

"Ah, that'll come right soon enough," Bridget said kindly. "Don't 'ee worry, now. Nicholas'll not agree to anything but what's good for thee. Don't 'ee fret a moment longer. You'll be as happy as a lark, and think of all they pretty babes that'll come!"

"Of course," said Liza, now determinedly smiling. "Of course I know you're right."

Whatever happened she mustn't have red eyes when she reached home. With a frightened jolt she realised she had been away without explanation for quite a long time, and that her parents knew there was gossip about her.

She must find an excuse for her absence. She could say she had wanted to go for a walk and when passing through the lobby had overheard her father talking about marrying her to Peter Lanyon. That she hadn't meant to listen but had accidentally heard that much. So she had walked to St. George's church to pray for happiness in her future, and then walked back across the stubble field. Yes, that would do, and if Bridget should ever mention seeing her, it would fit in.

CHAPTER FIVE 🔯

UNTIMELY AUTUMN

With an effort that felt like pulling her heart out of her body, Liza arranged another smile on her face as she approached her home, only to realise, on reaching it, that she needn't have troubled. Her family was in the middle of one of its noisy crises. Dirk, the younger of the two menservants in the Weaver establishment, was up astride the roof ridge along with her cousin Laurie, doing something to a chimney, and she could hear shouting within the house while she was still several yards away.

As she stepped inside, the smell of soot assailed her nostrils and the shouting resolved itself into confused cries of annoyance from women in the main room, and a furious bellowing from the back regions, which she recognised as the voice of one of the older cousins, Ed, declaring that soot was blowing into the fleece store and would somebody shut that accursed door before the whole lot had to be washed a second time!

She walked into the living quarters and her mother and one of the maidservants, both liberally smeared with dirt, turned from the business of sweeping up a shocking mess of soot and disintegrated bird's nest, which had apparently come down the chimney and mingled with the revolting remains of a fire over which someone had tossed a pail of water. Above it, the filthy and battered remains of what had once been a thin tree branch waved and waggled, presumably because Laurie and Dirk on the roof were agitating it. "What in the world…?" said Liza.

"The chimney were blocked," said Margaret. "Where've you been?"

"I just went out to take the air. I went to St. George's and—"

"You and your walks." But Great-Uncle Will had advised them not to challenge Liza, and Margaret, distracted by domestic upheaval, didn't at that moment want to. "Find a broom and help us out. Fine old muddle this is, I must say. Spring-cleaning in October. I never did hear the like."

No need after all for excuses or lies. She'd got away with it. Thanking the saints for her good luck, Liza made haste to be useful. Later in the day, when order had been restored and dinner eaten, her parents called her to their room, and she felt alarmed, but their faces were kind. They simply wanted to talk about her marriage. Nothing less, but nothing more, either. If her absence in the morning had aroused any doubts, they evidently didn't mean to mention them—unless Liza herself was foolish enough to be difficult. She knew her kinfolk very well indeed.

"The whole family has discussed it now," her father said, coming to the end of his explanation. "We've agreed it's a good thing for you. Peter Lanyon is young and healthy. The business side is not ideal, but it may work out well. Anyway, we intend to say yes."

"I understand," said Liza nervously. Since she had not had to invent an excuse for her absence in the morning, she had taken care, throughout the interview, to look as though the notion of Peter Lanyon as her bridegroom were a complete surprise. She added, "It's a big thing for me."

"Naturally. Have you any objection?" Nicholas asked. Her parents were both watching her sharply. Well, she'd better allay their suspicions before they voiced them. She dared do nothing else.

"No, Father. I…I'm sure it's a good thing." She must, *must* be the sensible Liza her family wanted her to be. She shuddered to think of the storm of wrath the truth would arouse, and besides, Christopher might suffer. She made herself smile again. Would she have to spend the rest of her life forcing the corners of her mouth upward when all she wanted to do was cry and cry?

Well, if so, so be it. She had no alternative.

Christopher, on his way to Alcombe, felt like crying, too, but except for that one uncharacteristic fit of emotion during their first meeting in the dell, he was not in the habit of shedding tears. He must face it. He had lost Liza for good and what had been between them must remain a secret for all eternity. They had known it would be like this one day. It felt worse than he had expected, that was all. It was like an illness, but he supposed he would recover someday. And so, of course, would Liza. At the thought of Liza forgetting him, he did find tears attempting to get into his eyes, but with a highly unclerical oath he repressed them and rode on.

At that very moment, at Allerbrook farm, another unsanctioned love affair was disturbing the air. It had been secret until now, and its emergence into the light had thrown Richard Lanyon into a dramatic fit of temper.

"*Marion Locke?* Who in God's name is Marion Locke? I've never heard of her! You're going to marry Liza Weaver—it's all settled! Who's this Marion Locke? Where did you find her? There's no Locke family round here!"

Richard Lanyon stopped, mainly because he had run out of breath. He stood glowering in the middle of the room, the same room in which George's coffin had lain awaiting its funeral. He had shouted so loudly that the pewter on the sideboard rang faintly as if trying to echo him.

"She lives on the coast. In Lynmouth, Father. I met her at the Revel there, in June."

"*Lynmouth?* That's as far as Dunster, the other way. I remember you went to the Revel. Well, half of Somerset and Devon go to it—young folk have to enjoy themselves. I've no quarrel with that, and if you've had a loving summer with some lass there, I've no quarrel with that either. Young men have their adventures. I did, in my time. But that's one thing and marriage is another. How have you managed to visit her since? Oh!" Richard glared at his son. "*Now* I recall. Two weeks back, we drove the moor for our bullocks and somehow or other you got yourself lost in a mist, you that's known the moor all your life. Came home hours late, after the cattle were all in the shippon, and said you'd mistaken the Lyn for the head of the Barle and thought you were going southeast instead of north. I thought your brains had gone begging, and all the time…"

Peter stood his ground. "Yes, I saw her then. Other times were when I said I'd ride out to see how the foals or the calves were doing. It came in useful that we're allowed to run stock on the moor. I've seen her twice a month since we first met. Marion visits relations—a grandmother and an aunt—in Lynton, at the top of the cliff, on the first and third Tuesdays of each month. We arranged it so I'd meet her in Lynton whenever I could."

"Who *is* she?" Richard spoke more calmly and with some curiosity. After all, if this unknown Marion Locke were a more profitable purchase than Liza Weaver, it might be worth indulging the boy. Nicholas would be upset, but maybe he could suggest someone else for Liza who would suit her parents better than Peter. He raised an enquiring eyebrow. Peter immediately dashed his father's hopes by replying, "The Lockes are fisherfolk. They run a boat—the *Starfish*—out of Lynmouth harbour. They—"

"Her father's a fisherman?"

"Yes, that's right. He—"

"Are you out of your mind, boy?" roared Richard. "When did fisherfolk and farming folk ever marry one another? Fisher girls can't make ham and bacon and chitterlings out of a slaughtered pig, or brew cider, or milk a cow, and our girls can't mend nets and gut mackerel!"

"Are those the things that matter?" Peter shouted back. "Marion's lovely. She's sweet. We love each other and—"

"When you're living day to day then, yes, they do matter, boy, believe me, they do! When a girl can't do the things you take for granted, that'll soon see the end of your loving summer! The autumn leaves'll fall fast enough then, take my word for it!"

"Liza Weaver's not been farm reared, either!"

"She can bake and do dairy work. She'll soon pick up the rest. *And* she'll bring a pile of silver and a cut into the Weaver profits along with her. What sort of dowry has this Marion got, I'd like to know? Well? Tell me!"

"I never asked. Not much, perhaps, but—"

"I'll tell you how much! Nothing! Fisherfolk never have a penny to spare. They put all their money into their boats. Marion Locke, indeed! You can forget this Marion, right away. I'll—"

"Father, she's beautiful. And we're promised to each other." Peter raised his chin. "We're betrothed and—"

"Oh no, you're bloody well not!" shouted Richard. "Not unless I say so and you needn't go trying to get Father Bernard on your side, either! I won't have it and that's that. I'll see this girl's father and see what he has to say about it, and I'll be very surprised if he doesn't agree with every word I say. Who is he? What's his name?"

"He's well respected in Lynmouth. He's Master Jenkin Locke and he lives by the harbour in the cottage with the birds made out of twisted thatch along the ridge of his roof. He made them himself. The *Starfish* is one of the finest boats—"

"Be quiet! Just forget about Marion Locke, as from now! And…what is it?" Hearing a sound at the door, Richard swung around and found a timid-looking young girl there with bare feet, a shawl wrapped around her and a lot of straw-coloured hair trailing from under a coif that was badly askew. "Who the devil are you?"

"I'm…I'm sorry, sir. But the mistress sent me—Mistress Deborah. I'm Allie, sir, her maid…."

"Allie! Oh, of course! But what brings you…is something wrong? With Mistress Deborah!" Suddenly he was taut and alert, his eyes fixed on Allie, Peter's vagaries for the moment quite forgotten.

"Yes, sir, dreadful wrong!" Allie was near tears. "She's so ill, sir. I've called the priest. She took a chill the day after the…the funeral, sir, when she fell in the river, for all you give her your cloak, and she's worse and she's sent me to fetch you, sir. She wants to see you…."

Richard turned at once to his son. "Go and saddle Splash for me, while I get my cloak. Allie, is anyone with your mistress now—any other woman?"

"Yes, sir, our neighbour. But she'll not be able to stay long. She has children and—"

"She won't have to stay long. I'll take you down to the village with me on my horse."

"But sir, I've never been on a horse."

"You'll get up behind me and hold tight and we'll be there in a trice. She'll need you. Go with Peter and wait for me. Go on!"

CHAPTER SIX 🙵
THE LOCKES OF LYNMOUTH

"I swore I'd never forgive the Sweetwaters for crashing into my father's cortege," said Richard Lanyon grimly. "Now there's something else I'll never forgive them for, in this world or the next. They as good as killed Deb Archer, that's what! If Humphrey Sweetwater ever meets me in a lonely place, he'll wish he hadn't!"

"Master Lanyon, I don't like to hear you talking like that." Father Bernard had conducted Deb's burial service with dignity, tacitly accepting Richard's presence as natural without making any reference to the reason for it. In the priest's eyes, however, this outburst went too far. It had also been too loud. In the group of mourners now moving out of the churchyard, heads had turned and brows had been lifted. Father Bernard put a hand on Richard's arm to halt him. "It's not wise to raise your voice so much," he said. "What if the Sweetwaters hear of it?"

"Maybe it'll stir their consciences!" Richard was unrepentant. "Poor, poor Deb. Never harmed a living thing and everyone who knew her was the happier for it." He was going to miss her more than he had dreamed possible. She had been friend as well as mistress—someone to talk to and laugh with as well as to sleep with. "And now I've watched her being put in the ground, all because of the bloody Sweetwaters!" Richard thundered.

"I'm sorry, too, Father." Peter, who had been walking with them, had stopped beside Richard. "Everyone is."

"Her little maid, Allie, said she was chilled when she came home all wet that day," Richard said. "But she still went out again after she'd changed, so as to come to my father's burial. Sun was out, but there was a sharpish wind. Allie told me she fell ill next day. Looked like a bad cold at first, but two days after that she started coughing and in two more days, she was in delirium and Allie was sending for the priest and for me, and she died that night, with me holding her. All because the Sweetwaters…!"

Fury choked him. Shaking off Father Bernard's hand, he jerked his head at Peter to follow, and strode out of the church-yard, not turning toward Deb's cottage where the other neigh-bours were going for the funeral repast, but turning the other way instead, evidently making straight for home.

"He's grieving," said Peter awkwardly to the priest.

"Yes, I know. You'd better go with him. Look after him."

"If I can," said Peter, and set off in his father's wake.

Kat and Betsy had a meal ready in the farmhouse. Richard ate it in a stormy silence, which Peter decided not to break. After-ward, when the two women had left for their own cottages, father and son repaired to the big main room where a good fire had been lit. Some saddlery in need of cleaning lay on the floor, to provide occupation for the evening. They lit candles, since it was October and darkness was closing down already. With only the two of them in the house, it had an echoing, empty feel.

"It's time we had more folk about this place, more helping hands and a mistress for our home." Richard broke his silence at last. He picked up a bridle and put some oil on a cleaning cloth, but fixed his eyes on Peter, in no kindly fashion. "Now I've something to say to you. What with Deb dying, I've not spoken to you again about Liza Weaver, but nothing's changed. You'll marry Liza and I'll hear no more talk of this girl Marion. Under-stand?"

Peter, in the act of reaching for a saddle, put it down again and drew a sharp breath. "I'm sorry, Father, I truly am, but…"

"Look here, boy!" Richard glared at him and his voice became aggressive. "I want to *make* something of this family, to wipe the lofty looks off those damned Sweetwater faces, even if we can't chop their heads off their shoulders. Last century, before my time, let alone yours, there was a big rising in the southeast of England. It got put down, but it left its mark. Higg and Roger would have been villeins then, with no right to leave Allerbrook and go somewhere else, but they're free men now and they can go if they want to. The rising was because—"

"I thought it was the plague that set men free," said Peter. "So many folk died that villeins were left without masters and no one could stop them going where they liked—and asking wages when they found masters who had no one to work the land and weren't in any position to argue."

"The plague and the rising together made the difference, so I've heard," said Richard. He moderated his tone, trying to be patient. "The one made the other stronger. But the rising was about people like us getting bone weary of having people like the Sweetwaters lord it over us. *When Adam delved and Eve span, who was then the gentleman?* That's what the rebels used to chant. What makes the Sweetwaters think they're so wonderful? My father sent me to school, though he could have used my hands on the land by then, because he wanted me to have a chance in life and not speak so broad that no one could understand me that wasn't born in the west country. Later I sent you, too—and paid through the nose for it!"

"Yes, Father, I know, and I'm grateful, but—"

"No buts, if it's all the same to you. We can read and write, just about; we can talk proper English and understand the Paternoster in Latin; we can add up our accounts and we know a bit of history. What have the Sweetwaters got that we haven't? Land and money, that's all. Well, that's what I'm after, and seeing my only son hitch himself up with a fisher girl ain't going to help. Liza Weaver's another matter. We could gain a lot from that, could start saving. I'm relying on you making a good marriage to give us a leg up in the world. You can just forget Marion!"

"But, Father…" Peter, too, was now trying to be calm and patient. "We've said the words that make it a contract."

"Without witnesses, and her a maiden in her father's house? Those words were never said, my boy, and that's that."

"But they *were* said, and they're binding."

"I see. You'll challenge me, will you? The young stag's lowering his antlers at the herd leader, is he?" Richard abandoned patience, rose to his feet, laying aside his own work, and unbuckled his belt. Peter also stood up. He was taller than his father and though not as broad, he had in him the coiled-spring vitality of youth. The two of them faced each other.

"Father Bernard told me to look after you," said Peter seriously. "So I wouldn't want to hurt you, but if you try that, I might. I'll fight. I mean it."

"My God!" Richard stared at him. The candlelight was shining on Peter's face. "You've had her, haven't you? There's nothing turns a boy into a man the way that does. She's let you…and you still want to *marry* her?"

Peter was silent, remembering. September, it had been; not the day of the heavy mist, which had been a brief and chilly meeting, but the time before, which was in warm, sunny weather. They had met as usual close to Lynton, the village at the top of the cliff, and wandered into the nearby valley, with its curious rock outcrops. He had left his pony to graze while he and Marion took a goat path up the hillside, through the bracken, untroubled by the flies which in summer would have surrounded them in clouds.

On a patch of grass, hidden from the path below by a convenient rock, they sat down to talk and caress. They had done as much before, but this time it went further. Marion made no protest and soon he was past the point of no return, far adrift on the dreamy seas of desire and at the same time full of energy and the urgent need for pleasure.

The memory of it, of Marion, of her curves and warmth and moistness, her murmurs and little cries of excitement, her arms around him like friendly ropes, the rustle of a stray bracken frond under his left knee, the scent of warm grass and Marion's hair, which she had surely washed with herbs, and then the splendour of his coming, were beyond putting into words and, in any case, they were not for anyone else to share.

"Yes," he said now. "I want to marry her. I intend to."

"We'll see about that," said Richard. "I'm going to Lynmouth tomorrow, to find the Lockes. I'll see what they have to say! And now I'm going to bed and you can damned well finish cleaning the saddlery. And you can tell that priest that I don't need looking after!"

His father, thought Peter bitterly as Richard stalked out of the room, was turning out as big a bully as George Lanyon had ever been.

The sky the next day was dull but dry and Richard left Allerbrook at dawn, a nosebag for Splash on his shoulder. He rode down the combe, through Clicket and then out over the moor, following the ancient tracks made by the vanished people who had buried their chieftains in hilltop barrows and had raised the strange standing stones one saw here and there amid the heather.

The tracks led across the high moor and brought him at last to the East Lyn River—which his besotted son could not conceivably have mistaken for the Barle, since the high ridge known as the Chains lay between them. He rode downhill beside the tumbling stream, on a steep path through bracken and trees, came to a fork, took the branch that bypassed Lynton village at the top of the cliffs and went on down to its sister village, Lynmouth, at the foot.

Here there was a harbour, with a quay and a square stone building with a smoking vent, where herring were dried. The tide was in and so were a couple of big ships and a fleet of small boats, which were being unloaded. Both men and women were bringing netting and baskets of fish onto the quay, and buyers were already clustering around them. Close by stood the thick-walled thatched cottages of the fisherfolk.

He looked for a roof decorated with birds made of twisted

straw, and found it at once. It was one of the larger cottages, which suggested that the Locke family was comparatively prosperous. But still nowhere near as well-off as he was, he thought grimly. This was not the place to find a new mistress for Allerbrook farm, even if the girl Peter had in mind was respectable, which he doubted.

There was a hitching post beside the cottage. He secured Splash, loosened the girth and ran up the stirrups, gave the horse his nosebag and went purposefully to knock at the door of the cottage. It was ajar and opened when he rapped, but he paused politely, waiting for someone to come. The door opened straight into a living room and kitchen combined; he could see a trivet and pot, set over a fire, and a woman stirring the pot. Another woman was standing over a whitewood table close to a window, no doubt for the sake of the light, and gutting fish with a ferocious-looking knife. A third, broom in hand, was now advancing to ask him his business. He knew at once that this was Marion.

Peter had said she was beautiful, but it was the wrong word. Inside his head Richard struggled to find the right one and found himself thinking *luscious,* like the pears and plums which grew beside the southernmost wall of Sweetwater House. It was sheltered there, with good soil, and the fruit was always so full of juice that it seemed about to burst through the skin.

Village boys were employed as bird scarers and when the fruit was ready to harvest, they were paid with a basketful each. Richard himself, as a lad, had sometimes helped to frighten off the starlings, and been paid with pears and plums, the taste of which he had never forgotten.

This girl called them to mind. Her working gown was a dull

brown garment, but within it, her shape was so rich and full that he had hard work not to stare rudely. He saw, too, that her hair, which was not concealed by any cap or coif, was extraordinary. It wasn't so much curly as wiry and it was an astonishing pale gold in colour. She had pulled it back and knotted it behind her head, but much of it was too short for that and stood out around her head in a primrose cloud. It was clean hair, too. She looked after it.

Beneath it, her face was round, but there were strong bones within that seeming softness and she had long, sloe-blue eyes, full and heavy with knowledge and an unspoken promise to impart it.

And she was aware of him, of his dark good looks, and young as she was—sixteen, seventeen?—she knew something about men. He couldn't blame Peter for falling for this. But all the same…good God, Peter was welcome to his wild oats. No one in their senses grudged a young man that. But marriage—that was different.

"Are you Marion Locke?" It came out harshly, as though he were angry with her.

"Yes, that I be." Her accent was thick. Her looks might be remarkable but he doubted if she knew *A* from *B*.

"My name is Richard Lanyon. I believe you know my son, Peter. Is your father at home?"

"Aye. Down on the quay, he be. You want to talk to 'un?"

"I certainly do…ah!"

The woman who had been stirring the pot had put her spoon aside and come toward them. "What is it, Marion?"

"Gentleman axin' for dad. Name of Lanyon." Marion smiled beguilingly, as though she imagined he was here to settle the marriage arrangements. *You're wrong, my wench,* said Richard to himself.

84

"Then go and fetch 'un," said the woman. "He'm unloading the boat. You can take over from 'un. And ax the gentleman in!"

"I'll want to come back with 'un," said Marion querulously, standing aside to let Richard enter. "With Dad, I mean. I've met the gentleman's son and it'll be about me."

"All the more reason for you to keep out of it. Send your father back here and you stop down there and get that there boat emptied. Go on!"

Marion clearly didn't want to go, and pouted. Her mother stared at her fixedly, however, and after a moment she left.

"I don't want to offend anyone, least of all a man and wife in their own home." Richard, sitting by the fire with his hat on his knees, was conscious of being on someone else's territory. Not that it was much of a territory. It seemed to consist of this main room, half the size of the one at Allerbrook, an upper half-floor, reached by a ladder, where he could see some pallet beds, and a small back room, partly visible through a half-open door. In there, he could see a workbench with what looked like some half-made garment thrown over it.

A wise arrangement, no doubt, if one wanted to keep bits of thread out of the cooking and bits of fish out of the stitchery. Dried fish hung from the beams above his head, and there were scales and innards all over the table. His farmhouse was plain, but it had a decent oak front door and two spare bedchambers and even a parlour. They weren't used much, but they were there. *This* place was squalid. It also reeked of fish. The smell was far stronger and much more disagreeable than the woolly odours of Nicholas Weaver's home.

Manners, however, were manners. "I'm here on an awkward errand," he said, "but likely enough, you'll feel the same way as I do. You'll be Master Locke, I think?" He addressed the elder of the two men who had come up from the quay shortly after Marion had left. The younger one had the same pale, wiry hair as Marion. The hair probably came from the father, if the older man were he, though his mop was turning grey. "And you—" he looked at the woman who had been tending the pot "—are Mistress Locke?"

"That's right," the older man said. "That's my wife, Mary, and this here's my son Art and this is my daughter-in-law Sue." Sue was the one who had been gutting fish. She had left her work and joined the rest of them on seats by the fire. She had a smiling pink face, and by the look of her, was expecting a baby in a few months' time.

"And the wench who came to fetch us," said Master Locke senior, "is my daughter Marion. I've a notion it's her you want to talk about. She said it could be. She said she knows your son."

Art said glumly, "Here we go again."

"She does know him," said Richard, plunging straight to the point, "and it's difficult. But I'm Richard Lanyon from Allerbrook farm, far over the moor. I rear sheep and grow corn and sell wool. It's a different life from yours. My boy Peter met your Marion at last summer's Revel and he says they've agreed to marry but…there's no use going all round the moor about it. I've other plans for Peter. Besides, I don't think he's right for your girl, or she for him. What do you think?"

"I suppose the lad claims they've betrothed themselves?" said Master Locke. He didn't sound surprised.

"More or less, yes."

"That'll be the third time," said Marion's mother crossly. "All the lads go after her, she's got such a pretty face." Richard heard this understatement with amazement. Did these people, who lived together as a family, never actually look at each other? *Pretty?* A girl as striking as Marion? You might as well say the sea was wet.

"Aye, she'll promise anything to anyone and go further, very likely," Art said. "Reckon she did go further last year, with that young sailor off that ship from Norway that had some foreign name. *Fjord-Elk,* that's it. Dunno what it means. She's in port again now. I wouldn't be surprised if Marion isn't on the lookout for that young fellow now this minute."

"You don't need to worry," Master Locke assured Richard. "She needs to be married and soon will be, but to someone like ourselves. There's a likely boy in Porlock, along the coast. Too many folk round here are cousins of ours and the priest won't have that. You did right to come and warn us, but nothing's going to come of this. Two silly young people get together and say things, but we don't need to take no notice. I say nothing about your son, but Marion's always saying things to young men, mostly the wrong ones. Will you take a dish of stew and a drop of ale with us?"

"I'll take our share down to Marion," said Art, "and we'll eat and drink together and I'll tell her I'm tired of her foolishness."

"It's natural, at her age. She's barely seventeen," his father said tolerantly. "We're an easy-natured lot," he said. "We don't watch each other. Marion's daft and the boys round here turn her head with their sweet talk, but I'll see it don't come to anything."

"She b'ain't in the family way yet," Mistress Locke said. "That I do know. And she'd better not be, till she'm wed."

"He meets her in Lynton when she goes visiting there, so my son says," Richard said cautiously, concealing his relief at learning that Peter had at least not got his sweetheart into trouble. He had wondered, but it was a difficult question to ask.

"Aye." Marion's father nodded. "My mother-in-law and my wife's sister that's crippled with the joint evil live up there—they've got a cottage and a bit of land at the far end, just outside that valley with the funny-looking rocks in it. Maybe you know it…?"

"Yes, I went there once," said Richard. It had been long ago, when he was young and had gone to the Revel, just as Peter had done in the summer. He'd taken a girl into the Valley of the Rocks, as many people called it. "I know where you mean," he said.

"Marion takes fish to my mother and sister twice a month and brings back eggs and goat cheese for us. They keep hens and pasture a few goats in the valley—there's others do the same—and their maidservant does the milking and makes the cheese," said Mary Locke. "I wouldn't like to stop Marion's visits. They'd be hurt if she didn't go regular, as they're fond of her, and they like the fresh fish. And *we'd* miss the eggs and cheese. I've no time to go up there, mostly, and Sue here can't just now. But don't fret. It'll lead nowhere. It don't do for fisherfolk and farming folk to marry. We don't understand each other's lives. That pot of stew's about ready. It's not fish." She grinned, displaying gaps in her teeth but a wealth of good nature. "Last time Marion went, she bring down a nice plump chicken as well, all plucked and drawn ready. Chicken stew, this is. Sue, get the ale."

Richard reached home to find that Peter's friend Ned Crowham had ridden in and that as usual, Kat and Betsy, impressed by his velvet doublet and silk shirt and the polish on his boots, had put him in the parlour, lit a fire especially for him and plied him with mutton pie and the best cider.

"Good day, sir," said Ned civilly as Richard walked in. "I thought you might be out driving ponies off the moor or something of that kind at this time of year, but I took a chance and I found Peter here, though he's had to go out to the fields now. Kat and Bet said I must eat before I set out for home again." He chuckled. "As though I hadn't flesh enough already! They said you'd gone to Lynmouth."

"Yes. You'd nearly guessed right about the ponies, though. We'll be bringing them in tomorrow. We fetched the cattle two weeks back." Richard helped himself to cider.

"I heard from Betsy that congratulations were in order and that Peter's going to marry Liza Weaver. I told him it was a good match."

"Did you, now? And what did he say?"

"He thanked me. What else would he do?"

"Hah! Well, if he's out on the land, he won't overhear anything." Richard planted himself on a settle and unburdened his soul. "You're his friend and I fancy you're no fool. I wish you'd try and talk sense into him. Liza's the right girl for him, but he doesn't think so. I've been to Lynmouth today to see the family of a girl—a fisher girl, would you believe it?—that he's got himself mixed up with. They agree with me that it won't do, but how the boy could be such a wantwit…!"

"Mixed up with? You don't mean…?"

"No, she's not breeding, though I've a feeling that that's just luck!"

"No wonder he was so quiet when I congratulated him," Ned remarked. "But I doubt if I can talk to him, you know, sir. I don't think he'd listen to me. I'm fond of him, but…"

"He's got an obstinate streak. You needn't tell me! You youngsters!"

"You're not so old yourself, Master Lanyon," said Ned with a smile. "Will you think me impertinent if I ask if you've ever thought to marry again yourself?"

"Not impertinent, though not your business either. I've been content enough single." Ned knew nothing of Deb Archer and Richard saw no need to tell him. "What brought you here today?" he asked.

"Why, to ask both you and Peter to my own wedding. My family have found me a lovely girl, from east Somerset, near where Peter and I went to school. We're to marry in the new year. If Peter and Liza are married by then, he must bring her, too."

The Luttrells heard Mass each day in the castle, said by Father Meadowes, but on Sundays they and their household came down into the village and joined their tenants in worship at the fine church which Dunster shared with the Benedictine monks of St. George's Priory. It was an uneasy partnership, with frequent arguments about who could use the church when, and who was to pay for what, but the Luttrells—mainly by dint of donations to the priory and regular dinner invitations to the prior—did something to keep relations smooth between the villagers and the monks.

To the villagers, they were familiar figures: fair, bearded, broad-built James Luttrell, putting on weight in his thirties; his wife, Elizabeth, who had been born a Courtenay, no longer a young girl but still good-looking because of her well-tended complexion and the graceful way she managed her voluminous, trailing skirts and the veiling of her elaborate headdress; their well-dressed young son, Hugh; their household of servants and retainers, and the castle chaplain, always known as Father Meadowes because he did not like the custom of addressing priests by their first names, along with his assistant, Christopher Clerk.

All the week, Liza had said to herself, *On Sunday Christopher will be in church. On Sunday I shall see him.*

She was seeing him now. The Luttrell family had benches near the front while the rest of the congregation stood behind them, but Christopher had placed himself to one side, and was able to glance over his left shoulder and scan the body of the church without it being too noticeable. He caught her eye and let a smile flicker across his face. Liza smiled, too, when her parents weren't looking.

Afterward, when the service was over, everyone trooped out as usual through the round-arched west door built by the Normans who had founded the priory, and gathered in sociable clusters among the graves, exchanging news and dinner invitations with neighbours. The Luttrells were accosted by the prior, who wished to complain that some unknown person, presumably from the castle, had carved a pattern into one of the benches and he wanted the miscreant brought to justice.

Mistress Elizabeth shook her head gravely, although the fact that she had her little brown-and-white dog under her arm, and he was struggling to get loose, somewhat spoiled the effect. Father Meadowes had also stopped to listen to the prior's complaint but Christopher, who had been walking respectfully in the rear, moved unobtrusively aside and stood looking up, as if studying a gargoyle on the church roof.

Her own family had fallen into conversation with a group of neighbours. Liza, grown cunning through desperation, drifted gently away as if to approach a group of chattering girls, all acquaintances of hers, but passed them and used them as a shield as she came to Christopher's side and paused, also looking upward.

"That gargoyle," said Christopher, pointing, "is supposed to be the face of the prior who was here when the church was being partly rebuilt, not so long ago. So Father Meadowes says. It isn't very flattering, is it?"

"No, it isn't. I should think the stonemason hated the prior."

"I think that, too, but Father Meadowes doesn't know any more. Liza, I can't bear it. I can't go on to become a priest. I've made some enquiries, discreetly. It's unlikely that I can get legally free of the church but I can still run away from it. Will you run away, too, and come with me?"

At any moment the group of girls might move away and her family would see her talking to a young man. Christopher, pointing up at the roof, was apparently instructing her on history or architecture, but that would be a poor protection if the whispers her parents had heard had hinted at the identity of her illicit suitor. But she couldn't answer him quickly, not over a thing like this. She must say, "Christopher, I need time to think." She must be sensible....

Christopher...

The sensible thing to do was to say, *No, we mustn't. It's wrong. The church would hunt us down. My family would never forgive me. I'm sorry, but I can't.*

Unfortunately—or fortunately, and only time would tell which estimate was the right one—she had lost the fight to be sensible. Liza-in-Love and Liza-the-Sensible had striven one with another all through the summer, and Liza-in-Love had won. She and Christopher belonged together. They had met as though they had been moving toward each other since the beginning of time and there was nothing to be done about it. And yet—to leave her family, to abandon her good name for an unknown future with a man she could never lawfully marry… that was as terrifying as jumping off a cliff. Even though she would be hand in hand with Christopher.

She stared at him, poised equidistant between two opposites and unable to speak.

"We could make for London," he said. "I'll have to shave this tonsure off on the way—and keep a cap on wherever I go till my hair grows again. I do have *some* money, if not much. I've been saving my pay all summer…half planning. We'll get to London. London's very big. We'll be lost in all the crowd. We might even marry eventually, though not yet because they'll be looking out for us. The church has a very long arm. We'll have to find a small church to attend on Sundays and stand modestly at the back. We'll take new names and for the time being we'll just say we're married. Or we might go to France. I speak French well. Sweetheart, don't be afraid. I'll make my way. I understand merchanting. I was brought up in the midst of it. I'll find a merchant somewhere who needs a clerk. Believe me, I *will* make a life for us!"

There it was again, that vigorous grin. "It'll be just lodgings at first, but one day we'll rent a little house. Here or in France, we'll manage. There'll be children. Just an ordinary, everyday life, but we'll be together. If that's what you want."

"It's all I can imagine wanting," said Liza. And closed her eyes for a moment, so as not to see the rocks at the foot of the cliff, and jumped. "Yes," she said in a low voice. "I'll come. But Christopher…even if we can't marry, can't we at least take vows?"

He glanced around. The girls were still chattering together; beyond them, the prior was still monopolising the Luttrells and Father Meadowes, and Liza's family was still deep in conversation with their friends. Rapidly, in a low voice, he said, "I, Christopher Clerk, promise before God that I take thee, Liza Weaver, as my wedded wife."

Also rapidly and in an undertone, Liza said, "And I, Liza Weaver, promise before God that I take thee, Christopher Clerk, as my wedded husband. There!"

"It's not valid," said Christopher. "Not in the eyes of the church. But it's valid for me, my love. When and where can we meet? I'm often free for a while after dinner, just as I always was, though I do more study now, so the best time would be later than it used to be. About three of the clock would be right, I think."

"Won't we need horses?"

"Horses!" For a moment he looked appalled. "Horses—of course! My wits are going, I think. Well, one thing I daren't do is steal horses from the Luttrells. Can you get hold of any horses?"

"My father has three ponies. We all use them. They're family animals...as much mine as anyone's. I don't think they'll come after us for horse theft! But Christopher, they suspect something—they watch me these days. Yesterday they wouldn't let me go out for a walk alone. I can go into the garden, though!" She was thinking aloud. "I could get away over the meadow at the back. That's easy for you to reach, too. You mean we'd set off at once?"

"Yes."

"We could meet and go straight to the paddock. Tomorrow?"

"No, Tuesday. Mondays I do some study with the chaplain after dinner and if I don't appear, he'll look for me. We need a head start if we're to get away safely. But Tuesday, yes, unless it's pouring with rain. If it is, then the first day when it's not. If Tuesday is dry—then that's the day."

CHAPTER SEVEN

FLIGHT

Ned stayed overnight but didn't broach the matter of Peter's love affair. Richard did not discuss his visit to Lynmouth, either, and Peter, though he knew well enough where his father had been, asked no questions. The next day Ned left. Peter still asked no questions. Richard, grimly, knew what the boy was up to. He was just going to blank Liza Weaver out of his mind and pretend she didn't exist. Well, that ploy wasn't going to succeed. Even if Liza had never been born, Marion Locke was an impossibly unsuitable bride for Peter Lanyon. It was time to talk to the boy again.

This, however, was the day when they and their neighbours went to fetch the ponies in from the moor, to check their condition, separate the foals from their mothers and choose the ones to be sold. It meant rising early and snatching breakfast on one's feet, with no time for family wrangles. Afterward they would dine with the Rixons, whose farm adjoined theirs farther down the hillside. It would be a late dinner and they'd come home tired, with a dozen chores to do before a hurried supper. There would be no good opportunity in the evening.

However, the matter was so urgent that Richard finally blurted it out when he and Peter were riding close behind the herd as it trotted, all tossing manes and indignant white-ringed eyes, through the narrow lane that led to the Clicket pound. Just then, they were out of earshot of their fellow herdsmen, who were some way behind. Richard seized his chance.

His son's reaction was pure outrage.

"You're lying!" Peter said fiercely. "Telling me that Marion's betrothed herself to others beside me! She wouldn't! She couldn't! Betrothal's serious—it's nearly as binding as marriage, and—"

"I've seen the girl and I've talked to her father. I don't blame you for going head over heels for her, boy, but she's not for marrying. What you've got," said Richard brusquely, "is an attack of sex. We all get it. It's like having the measles or the chicken pox. If you wed her, the day would come when you'd be sorry. She's a lightskirt. I tell you—"

"No, I'll tell *you*. If when you were betrothed to my mother someone had called her a lightskirt, how would you have felt? What would you have said?"

"No one would have said such a thing, that's the point, you damned young fool—can't you see it? Why, your mother'd hardly as much as kiss me until we'd both said *I will*. Can you say that of Marion?"

"I'm not going to talk about this. I'm betrothed to her and that's the end of it," said Peter, and spurred his mount up onto the verge alongside the track, shouting at the herd to hurry them up, his face averted from his father and likely, thought Richard bitterly, to remain that way for a very long time indeed.

It was all the more annoying because the fury emanating from Peter had almost intimidated him, and Richard was not going to tolerate being bullied by his own son. He knew he would be wise not to try physical force to make Peter obey him, but there were other methods. One way or another, Peter, that ill-behaved pup, must be brought to heel.

And he was beginning to see how he might achieve it. Since her death, he had more than once dreamed at night of Deb Archer, but oddly enough, last night she'd turned into Marion halfway through the dream.

Maybe that cheeky, overweight, well-bred friend of Peter's, Ned Crowham, was right. Maybe he ought to get married again after all.

There'd be no advantage, socially or financially, in marrying Marion Locke, but now that he'd seen her…

Peter hadn't got her with child, but probably that was because he hadn't had chances enough. That didn't mean she wouldn't have babies once she was a wife. It would be a pleasant change for Allerbrook to have children about the place. His and Marion's; Peter and Liza's. Peter's marriage would be the one to bring the material benefits. And it would show Peter who was master. Oh, yes indeed.

It wouldn't do to have Peter under the same roof as Marion, of course. No, that would be daft. But there was a good-sized cottage empty just now, over on the other side of Slade meadow, where Betsy's son and his wife and children had lived before the young fellow took it into his head to go off to the other side of Somerset because he'd heard life was easier there, away from the moors that were so bleak in winter. And off he'd gone, depriving Allerbrook of two pairs of adult hands and several youthful ones. George had been alive then and he hadn't been pleased. He'd said that all of a sudden he could see the point of villeinage.

Still, the cottage was there, and once Peter was installed in it with Liza, he needn't come to the farmhouse often. He wouldn't come at all, except when his father was there; Richard would see to that. Once the boy had settled down and seen what Liza was worth and got some youngsters of his own, and Marion had a few as well, wanting her attention, getting underfoot and thickening her midriff, Peter's infatuation would die away.

Marion would probably breed well. She looked strong, quite unlike his poor ailing Joan. It was an idea.

It was a most beguiling idea.

"Where's Liza?" Margaret called to Aunt Cecy as she came down the stairs from her bedchamber. "In the weaving shed? It's time we were talking of her bride clothes, and I must say I'm surprised that Peter Lanyon hasn't been over to see her. A girl's entitled to a bit of courting."

"Farm folk are different from us," said Aunt Cecy. She was patching one of Dick's shirts, though because her eyesight was faulty nowadays, she had Margaret's small daughter beside her to thread needles. "She'll have to get used to a lot that's different, out there on Allerbrook. She's not in the shed. She went into the garden with a basket—said something about fetching in some mint."

"I'll call her," said Margaret, and hastened out through the rear of the house.

Five minutes later she returned, frowning, and once more went upstairs. Great-Uncle Will, back in his familiar winter seat beside the hearth, remarked, "Looks as if Liza's not in the garden. Funny."

"She'll have slipped off somewhere," Aunt Cecy said. "She's always had a fancy for going walking on her own, but Margaret told her she wasn't to go out by herself anymore."

"I did indeed," said Margaret, reappearing on the staircase. "But she's not in the garden and not upstairs, nor is she in the kitchen or at her loom. I've looked. And I've just been into her chamber and her toilet things are gone—the brush and comb and the pot of goose grease she uses for her hands. So I opened her chest and I could swear some of her linen's missing. I don't like it."

Aunt Cecy said, "I can't see so clear as I used to, but I thought I saw her talking to a fellow in the churchyard when we came out of the service on Sunday. He were pointing out something on the church roof. Looked harmless, but…"

"She might have gone across to see Elena for something," said Margaret uncertainly.

"And she'd take her linen and toilet things for that, would she? Better look for her," said Great-Uncle Will. "And fast."

"So she's not in any of our houses," said Nicholas, who had been hurriedly fetched from the inn at the other end of the village, where he had been talking to a potential buyer of his cloth. "You've made sure, you say, Margaret. And she's not in any of our gardens and some of her things are gone." He turned to Will. "Great-Uncle, you said that according to the gossip that's going about, she's been meeting a red-haired clerk from the castle. I think I've seen him at church with the Luttrells."

"That's him. And that's what's being said, yes," said Will.

"The fellow I saw her talking to on Sunday were outside the church and he had his cap on. But he were all in black, like a clerk," said Aunt Cecy.

"I wish we knew his name," said Nicholas, "but I think we know enough. I'm going up to the castle. Now."

"Why is it," grumbled James Luttrell, standing in his castle hall, wishing he could sit down to a peaceful supper and irritably aware that any such thing was out of the question for the time being, "why is it that trouble is so catching? The whole world's disturbed these days and it spreads like plague. There's no good government in the land, with all this squabbling between the king and these upstart cousins of his, Richard of York and his sons. What's it matter if the king is weak in his mind? He's been crowned and anointed and that ought to be good enough for any man."

"But the point is…" began Father Meadowes, normally a stern and self-confident priest but unable to stem James's irrelevancies.

"No one has any proper sense of their duty anymore. Even priests aren't staying on the right path, it seems!" Abruptly James abandoned his excursion into national affairs and returned to the real matter in hand. "Are you *sure* Christopher Clerk has vanished, Father? He hasn't gone on an errand and forgotten to let you know? Something urgent, perhaps?"

"I regret to say this, but I don't think so," said Meadowes. "He went out to meditate in the open air as he often does, but I expected him to return later and there was a matter to do with his studies that I wished to discuss with him. He hasn't come back, and personal things are missing from his room. There has been village gossip concerning a girl. I took him to task and he assured me there was nothing in it, that he had merely escorted her home when she was accidentally separated from her family at the May fair and exchanged the time of day with her after church once or twice out of courtesy. Villagers do have a talent for making something out of nothing and I believed him then. I warned him to be careful and left it at that. Now, frankly, I wonder. Earlier this year he asked me some odd questions."

"What sort of questions?" Elizabeth Luttrell asked. She was seated, working at an intricate piece of embroidery while Wagtail snoozed at her feet. "He always seemed so earnest," she remarked.

"Yes, he did," Father Meadowes agreed. "But the questions he asked were about leaving the church if a man changed his mind about his vocation. I asked if he were having doubts about his own and he said no. Now I'm wondering!"

"He's always seemed very quiet and conscientious," said James. "Too much so, perhaps, for a young man."

"Yes, I felt that, too, sometimes," Elizabeth said. "He was— is—so very...very self-contained, yet I sometimes felt that there was a side to him that was hidden."

The two men looked at her with interest. Elizabeth, usually a quiet woman, had a knack of occasionally making very acute remarks. *Sharp as an embroidery needle,* her husband sometimes said.

She smiled at them. "All the same," she added, "need we be anxious so soon? There could have been a misunderstanding...or even an accident."

She broke off as the gatekeeper's boy arrived in the hall at a breathless run and barely sketched a bow before exclaiming, "There's a Master Nicholas Weaver from the village, zurs and mistress! He's axin' to see Father Meadowes and he says it's that urgent—can Father Meadowes see him now, at once. He looks that worried, zurs!"

"Nicholas Weaver?" said James. "I know him. Hardworking man and a hardworking family, that's him and his. It's you he wants to see, is it, Father Meadowes? Maybe he's got something to say about this mystery."

"Christopher was talking with a girl after the service on Sunday," murmured Elizabeth. "It looked quite innocent, but…I wonder…"

"The gossip," said Meadowes ominously, "concerned a daughter of the Weaver family."

"Fetch Master Weaver along, boy," said James.

Nicholas came in with a firm tread, which concealed a secret hesitation. He had never been inside the castle before, never hitherto walked up the steep track from Dunster to the gatehouse with the castle walls and their towers and battlements looming ahead of him, and although he was not a man with a poor opinion of himself, he felt intimidated. At the gatehouse the porter had greeted him politely, but with an air of surprise. Villagers, even well-to-do ones like Nicholas Weaver, didn't often call at the castle and certainly not to insist that they must immediately see men who held such dignified positions as castle chaplain.

Despite his secret misgivings, Nicholas had been resolute and he had been admitted, but now that he was actually inside, he was awed by the scurrying of the numerous servants and by the great, beamed hall, with its huge hearth and the dais where the family dined. Thick rushes underfoot silenced his footfalls, the rosemary sprigs strewn among them gave off their scent wherever one stepped and the walls were hung with tapestries: a huge, dramatic one of Goliath being downed by a gallant little David, and a pretty one with a background of flowers and a lady in the foreground with a unicorn beside her.

The fact that he had been led into the presence not only of Father Meadowes but of the Luttrells as well added further embarrassment. However, he bowed politely, murmured a conventional greeting and looked at the chaplain.

James took control. "This is Father Meadowes," he said. "At the moment something is making him anxious and we're wondering if your visit is to do with the same matter. Is your business by any chance connected with one Christopher Clerk, Father Meadowes's assistant?"

"It may be," said Nicholas. "If Christopher Clerk has left the castle. Has he?"

"Yes. He's vanished," said Meadowes. "He went out after dinner as he often does. I had set him passages of Scripture on which to meditate, and in fine weather like today he likes to do that out of doors. He went off across the pasture that slopes down to the sea. I saw him go. But he hasn't come back and we can't find him anywhere."

"Does he have red hair?"

"Very much so," said James. "A tonsure like a sunset, as a matter of fact."

"My girl Liza's vanished, as well," said Nicholas. "And so have two of my ponies! I thought to look before I came here. And there's been talk, about her and a young fellow with a red tonsure, possibly Christopher Clerk. We didn't want to make a to-do over a bit of flirtation, even with a clerk, especially as we weren't sure there was anything in it but silly tattle. We always thought Liza had some sense. We told her we'd found her a marriage and she seemed agreeable. We reckoned if there'd been any nonsense, it was just sweet talk and that she'd put it behind her. Now we think otherwise. We're afraid she's run away from home and if so, she'd hardly go on her own. Now you say this red-haired clerk…"

"He's a deacon," said Meadowes.

"Is he, indeed? Well, you tell me he's missing. Have they run off together?"

"It's possible," said Meadowes slowly.

"So what can be done? I want my girl back. The marriage we've arranged is a good one and by that I mean a happy one. I'm a careful father, I hope. I've got her welfare at heart and a runaway priest isn't what's best for her."

"And you want to get her back before anything happens and before the young man she's betrothed to finds out what she's done," said Elizabeth helpfully. "Father Meadowes, where might Christopher have taken her? Where does he come *from?* That might be a guide."

"Bristol," said Meadowes. "But his father's a highly respectable merchant there. He won't have gone near his father! He studied in Oxford, but—no, I doubt if he's gone there either. It's hardly the place for a runaway couple to go to for sanctuary. I'd guess they'd make for a city, but they'd be more likely to choose Exeter or London."

"Three directions," said James, thinking aloud. "London by way, to start with, of Taunton or Bridgwater, or south over the moor to Exeter by way of Tiverton. One of those."

"Bridgwater's likely," said Meadowes. "Christopher knows that road well. I've several times called on friends there and taken him with me. I doubt he's ever been to Taunton."

"I could be quite wrong," said Nicholas unhappily. "But Liza's *gone,* and taken linen and toilet things. There's been talk of her and a red-haired clerk, and we'd just told Liza about the marriage we'd planned for her. That could have been the spark in the straw. I *hope* I'm wrong. I want to be, but…"

He looked at James with a question in his face, and James answered it. "I'm sorry for you, Master Weaver, and I doubt very much that you're wrong. We'll go after them. Meadowes, are you joining us?"

"Of course. I can still sit a horse for a few hours, despite my grey tonsure," said the chaplain. "And the boy is my student as well as my assistant. I feel responsible for him. I should have pressed him harder over the rumours about Master Weaver's girl. I fear I've been remiss."

"The more helpers we have, the better," James Luttrell said. "Weaver, you and Meadowes can take one of my men and try the Bridgwater road. I'll send two men by way of Taunton, and myself, I'll take another two and ride for Exeter. Light's going, but the sky's clear and the moon's nearly full. We'll fetch them back, never fear. Young folk in love can be the very devil and their own worst enemies, but we'll see if we can't save these two from themselves. You can borrow one of my horses."

He turned to the gatekeeper's boy, who was still in the hall, listening openmouthed with excitement. "Get to the stable, my lad, and tell them to saddle eight horses. My Bay Arrow, Grey Dunster—he's hardly been out today—and whatever else is fit and not tired. Then send the garrison sergeant to me and after that, get back to your post. Hurry!"

CHAPTER EIGHT 🐚

HUNTERS AND QUARRY

The daylight was going. Grooms held up lanterns while the horses were brought out and saddled. Picking up the smell of urgency from the humans, the horses fidgeted and tossed impatient heads while their girths were tightened. James Luttrell, who seemed to have the entire map of the west country in his head, was giving final instructions, complete with landmarks, to the men who were going by way of Taunton. Nicholas, Father Meadowes and Gareth, the Welsh man-at-arms who was to accompany them on the Bridgwater road were all familiar with their own route.

The mood was that of a hunting party, albeit an unusually unsmiling one. Father Meadowes actually said as much to James Luttrell as they clattered down the slope to the village below. "If we had hounds with us, this would feel like a chase. Except that

I've never gone hunting after dark before and never had a man as my quarry before, either. It's a strange feeling."

At the foot of the slope they turned left, to circle the castle hill on its inland side. The first group to peel off was Luttrell's. "Good luck!" he called, taking off his hat to wave farewell to the others as he led his party away, bound for Exeter through the town of Tiverton on the south side of the moor. "I just pray somebody catches them before it's too late!"

Christopher and Liza rode eastward through the fading day. The Channel was dulling into a misty grey and shadows were gathering in the hollows of the inland hills. "You're safe with me. I hope you know that," Christopher said suddenly. "Believe me, I haven't quite abandoned my upbringing! There's a lot to be said for being steady and reliable, and I mean to be that for you. I shall take the greatest care of you. It was clever of you to think of taking the ponies. We'll send them back eventually."

"Yes, of course. I hated taking them, but we needed them so much." She did feel safe with him. They were doing a crazy thing, a wrong thing in the eyes of the world, but it was a right thing, as well. It was right because Christopher was Christopher and they belonged with one another.

"Will anyone guess where we've gone?" she asked. "They'll be after us as soon as they know."

"They might guess at London. If they do, they'll probably think we began by making for Taunton. It's the more usual road. But I know the Bridgwater one and just because it's not so usual, I think it's the safest one for us."

"I wish it could be different," said Liza. "I wish we could be married with everyone congratulating us and pleased with us, approving of us and wishing us luck. I feel like a hunted deer. I keep straining my ears to hear the hounds! But all the same, I'm so very glad to be here with you."

"And I am glad to be with you, sweetheart. I hate the thought of being hunted down, as well. We just mustn't be caught, that's all!"

At Allerbrook Peter was not exactly refusing to speak to his father, nor was Richard making it too obvious that he was furious with his son. Neither had any wish to expose their disagreement to the world. Conversation of a sort had taken place around the Rixons' table, mostly concerned with farming matters. It had been generally agreed that the field known as Quillet might well support a crop of wheat, but ought to be fenced.

"You've only got ditches there and wheat'll invite the deer in as if the Dulverton town crier had gone round calling them," cheerful Harry Rixon said. "You'll get they old stags lying down, the idle brutes, squashing great patches of it and snatching every ear of wheat within reach afore they get theirselves up and stroll off to find some nice fresh wheat to squash and gobble."

"The Sweetwaters won't like it," Gil Lowe prophesied glumly. "You've mostly used Quillet for pasture, haven't you? I've noticed they put their milking cows there now and then. Are they supposed to?"

"No, but when did that ever stop them?" enquired Richard sourly. "I pay rent on that land. I'll plant it if I like. Reckon you're right about the fences, though."

All that was normal enough, and if few words were actually exchanged between the two Lanyons, it was hardly noticeable, for the crowd was considerable. It included everyone who had helped in the pony drive, farmers and farmhands alike. Roger and Higg were there along with their employers. Higg alone seemed to sense something strange in the air. Higg looked and sounded slow, but he was nowhere near as slow as he seemed and Richard caught a thoughtful glance or two from him. He looked away. He was thinking.

All of a sudden Richard Lanyon was unsure of himself. All very well to decide that after all he ought to marry again and why not Marion, but there were things to consider. For instance, it was quite true that farm life would be strange to her, far stranger than to Liza, for Liza's father dealt a lot with sheep farmers and she knew farmers' wives and had some idea of how they lived.

Still, Marion was young enough to learn, and not squeamish. Fisherfolk were never that. Gutting a herring, or gutting a chicken; there wasn't much difference really, and Betsy could show her the dairy work.

The lack of any respectable dowry was a worse drawback, but that might be offset if she produced sons to help on the farm, and daughters to be married off into useful families. Taking the long view, even a Marion Locke might provide a step or two on the upward ladder.

Yes. He *could* take Marion to wife and still remake the future in the shape he wanted. And put Peter in his place.

What would be harder would be convincing her parents that the proposal was a good one, especially as he and they had already agreed that such marriages wouldn't do.

But, by God, he *wanted* her. He'd desired her from the moment he first set eyes on her. It was sheer desire that had overridden the old way of thinking, the taking it for granted that fisherfolk and farmers didn't intermarry, the lack of dowry, the embarrassing fact that his own son had probably had her first. The wench was by all the evidence about as steady as a weathercock in a gale, but he didn't care. He knew now that he wanted her more than he'd ever wanted Deb and about ten thousand times more than he'd ever yearned after Joan. He wanted to get his hands on her, to make her his, to surround and bemuse her so that she could see no other man, think of no other man, but himself.

The proper thing to do was to see her father, but instinct said no. Instinct said *win the girl over first*. Go hunting and bring her to bay; tame her to his hand and maybe she could help him tame her parents.

Today was a Tuesday, the second in the month. Next Tuesday was the third one, and she'd be going to Lynton to see her grandmother and aunt. Her mother had obligingly mentioned where her relatives lived—close to the mouth of that strange valley where he'd had a youthful romance long ago. He'd find the cottage easily enough. He meant to be open and honest. He'd call and ask to see the girl. Maybe he could coax her to stroll with him, alone, so that he could talk to her, persuade her…

And he'd make damned sure that Peter couldn't get away that day. Yes. One week from now. That was the thing to do.

It was a hunter's moon, shining ahead of the pursuers, low as yet, disappearing at times beyond shoulders of land as they came through the Quantock Hills, but when visible, bright enough to light the track in front of the horses, even to glint in the eyes of a fox as it darted across the path. They could see their way.

"Where are we?" Nicholas asked Gareth as they cantered their horses up a gentle hill and drew rein, looking down on the moonlit world. Somewhere in the distance was the fugitive twinkle of candlelit windows in a village. He knew the countryside east of his home, of course, but he had never ridden through the Quantock Hills after dark before.

"Nether Stowey, that is," said Gareth's Welsh voice at his side. "They'll have gone straight through there, I fancy, if they ever came this way. If I had all of us on my heels, I wouldn't stop till my pony fell over, indeed to goodness I wouldn't."

"Liza'd never push a pony too hard," said Nicholas, and to his own annoyance, found his eyes pricking. He had been proud of his daughter, proud of her glossy brown hair and her smile and her kindness. She was good with the ponies. Yes, and better at catching them than anyone else because they would come to the field gate to meet her! How could she have so misused her gift with them, and done this to her parents?

"We'd better do some pushing on ourselves," said Father Meadowes. "As fast as the moonlight will let us."

They pressed on. Presently, as they came into a shallow dip, he checked his horse again, and the others slowed down with him. "What is it?" asked Nicholas.

Father Meadowes pointed ahead, to the top of the little rise in front of them. "See? Against the skyline? Two riders…there, they've gone over the crest." As he spoke, his horse raised its head and whinnied. "If they're on the Nether Stowey road ahead of us," Meadowes said, "those two could be them."

"They've been dithering along the way if it's them," said Gareth with a chuckle. "I wonder what for?"

"You mind your tongue," said Nicholas.

Father Meadowes shook his steed up again. "Let's catch up. Heaven's been good to us—we can see where we're going, just about. We can gallop here."

"What are we to do tonight?" Liza asked. She was strong, but the day had taken its toll, and they weren't covering the miles as fast as they should. They had taken a wrong track three times, once heading for the shoreline by mistake, and twice in the fading light as they made their way through the Quantocks. Time had been particularly wasted on a steep, pebbly path which turned and twisted and finally tried to take them back westward.

They were on the right road again now, Christopher said reassuringly as they came out of the hills, but she was growing tired and she was very conscious of having left her home and all familiar things behind. This black-and-silver moonlit land was unreal, alien. And she was cold. There was a chill in the air after nightfall in October.

"We'll have to find somewhere to sleep, but if we can, we should avoid looking for lodgings or rooms at an inn," said Christopher. "We don't want to leave a trail behind. Maybe we should have gone another way, across to Devon, to Exeter. We'd have been that much harder to trace. But London will be easier to find than Exeter. I've been there before, as a lad, with my father. Exeter would be quite strange to me."

"But tonight, Christopher?"

"I think we should try to find a barn with hay in it. I've got some bread and cheese with me. I managed to take it from the kitchen when no one was looking. We can eat."

"But can we find a barn in the dark?"

"Oh, yes, I think so. Look, that's surely a farmhouse over there.

See—where the lights are? There'll be barns there. Let's walk the ponies. There ought to be a track turning that way."

"But what if we *can't* find a barn?"

"If we can't find one here, we'll find one somewhere else— on the far side of Nether Stowey. There are farms beyond it."

"Is Nether Stowey far?"

"Only a mile or a little more. Take heart, love. I know where we are well enough."

The search for a barn was unsuccessful. They found a lane to the right and before long they could distinctly smell a farmyard. But the lane seemed to be leading straight into it and if there were barns at a safe distance from the house, they couldn't be seen because the lane was a sunken way between high banks with brambles on top, which hid anything on the far side. To make things worse, the darkness became intense because the direction they had taken had put the moon behind a hill. They heard sheep bleating, and then, alarmingly, a dog began to bark. Christopher pulled up, reaching a hand to the bridle of Liza's pony, too.

"No good. If we go any farther we'll have people coming out to meet us and we'll have to explain ourselves. Turn round. We'll have to go back. Sorry."

"Oh, *Christopher!*"

"Don't let's have a wrangle here," he said wryly. "Let's quarrel later when we can enjoy it!"

"All right!" said Liza, and tried to sound as though she were laughing. She was beginning to feel frightened. They were losing so much time, and the pursuit must surely have begun by now.

They went back. Presently they were on the Nether Stowey road again and once more had the help of the moonlight. "Not far now," said Christopher. "I *think* I know where we'll find a barn, once we're through the village. And the bread and cheese are fresh. Take heart."

"I'm certainly hungry," said Liza, determined to be cheerful. "I'll enjoy our supper."

Her new, if somewhat forced, cheerfulness had five minutes to live. At the end of that time, as they cantered to the crest of a rise and paused briefly to look ahead, she saw her pony's ears flick backward, and then behind them, some way off but not nearly far enough to be comfortable, they heard a horse whinny.

"Christopher...!"

"Maybe it isn't them," said Christopher.

"It is! I know it is. I don't know how I know, but I do!"

"All right. Well, let's be on the safe side and assume it is, anyway," Christopher said. "Come on! Let's ride for it! We'll look for another side lane and try to dodge into it and let them go past. If it *is* them. Come on!"

It was the best plan he could make. He had kept his voice steady, but he too was now afraid, for her as well as himself. He could endure whatever they did to him for this, but what would happen to Liza? He had done horribly wrong in bringing her away, but what else was there to do, other than let her go forever?

Side by side, alert for a secondary track, they urged the ponies into a gallop, taking advantage of the moonlight. But providence wasn't with them. There was no break in the banks to either side, no escape from the track, and sturdy though their ponies were, their short strong legs could not match the stride of the Luttrells' big horses behind them. They heard the hoofbeats catching up, and then a rider swept past them and swung his horse right across the track to block their way. They found themselves looking up into a dark, square face which Liza did not recognise, though Christopher did. "Gareth!" he said.

"Look round," said Gareth, grinning, and they turned in their saddles to find that Nicholas Weaver and Father Meadowes had pulled up behind them.

Nicholas rode forward. To Liza's astonishment he didn't even look at her, but instead made straight for Christopher. "Have you taken her? Is that what slowed you down on the road? Come on! I want to know!"

"We kept missing our way and then turned aside to look for shelter," said Liza in a high voice. "We've taken vows to each other, but we haven't…Christopher hasn't…"

"I'm glad to hear it, but no doubt it was just a pleasure post-poned," said Nicholas. He spurred his horse right up to Christopher's pony and his fist shot out. It landed with immense force on Christopher's jaw and the younger man reeled sideways, out of his saddle. His pony plunged. Christopher, who had clung on to the reins, scrambled up again, his spare hand pressed to his face.

"Father, don't!" Liza cried it out in anguish. "Oh, please let us go! Let me go with Christopher! I can't marry Peter Lanyon. I can't. I tried, so hard, to make myself willing to marry him, but I can't do it. It has to be Christopher…and we've bound our-selves…oh, why won't you understand?"

"I understand that you're talking nonsense and one day you'll know it, my girl. I've come to take you home," said Nicholas.

CHAPTER NINE

REARRANGING THE FUTURE

"Go to her, Margaret," Nicholas said. "Bring her downstairs and get her thinking about her bride clothes. She's got to at some point. Saints in heaven!"

His normal robust heartiness was dimmed. He was sitting by the kitchen hearth while Margaret and Aunt Cecy helped the maids with supper, and he could hear his young sons, Arthur and Tommy, laughing over some game or other in the adjacent living room, but just now these pleasant things could not comfort him. His shoulders were hunched and his face drawn with misery, and the two maids, aware of it, were unusually quiet.

"We never had this sort of trouble with either of our girls," said Aunt Cecy righteously. "Maybe that was because we walloped them when they needed it instead of bein' soft, the way you two are."

THE HOUSE OF LANYON

"We haven't been soft this time!" Margaret snapped, and continued obstinately stirring a pan of pottage.

"No, we haven't!" Nicholas agreed irritably. "But at least we had good reason. Cecy, you used to slap your girls for a bit of careless stitching or a speck of flour dropped on the floor, as if there weren't worse things! Reckon they were glad to be pushed off when they was barely ripe!"

"Well, really!" said Aunt Cecy. Nicholas ignored her.

"There's never been anything really truly *bad* in this house in my time, till now. I never thought our Liza would do this to us! I never thought I'd... I've never raised a hand to her, all her life, afore this and to have to take a stick to her...it broke my heart and I'm half afraid it's broken hers."

"Then the sooner she's married and away, the better," Aunt Cecy said sharply. "We'll all be happier, her included."

"I wouldn't have believed it of her either," said Margaret, still stirring. "It's a mercy we got her back in time and that there's been no more gossip." She eyed the maids, who had become very busy about the cooking. "And if I hear of you tattling, either of you, you're out! I mean it."

"If you ask me, half of this business is Peter Lanyon's fault," said Nicholas. "And you've said it, too, Margaret. He should have come to see her and done a little wooing! Margaret and I hardly knew each other before we were betrothed, but once it was agreed between the families, I came courting, didn't I, Margaret? You had your share of stolen kisses. I don't know what young Peter thinks he's about, and that's the truth!"

"Bah! She ought to do as she's bid, with wooing or without. A few more days in the attic 'ud do her no harm," said Aunt Cecy. "And Margaret here thinks the same, even if she won't say so."

"I don't care what either of you think!" shouted Nicholas. "I'm her father and I'm the one who's giving the orders this time! She's had enough days up there, enough time to study her conscience and get over things, so do as I tell you, leave that damned pan you're stirring, Margaret, and fetch her down here, and let's *pretend* things are normal even if she don't ever smile at me again. Go on!"

"Oh, very well," said Margaret, threw down her spoon and went.

When she entered the small room under the thatch, where Liza had been locked in now for six days, she found her daughter, as she had found her every time she went up there to take food in or remove the slop pail, lying on the bed and staring at the wall. "Time to get up," she said. "Your father says so. He's heartbroken, let me tell you, over what he had to do to you. To run off like that, and with a priest…well, I always thought I was the one who cared about bein' respectable, but the state your father's in—sayin' he's heartbroken is hardly sayin' enough!"

Liza looked at her miserably but said nothing.

"Forget all about this clerk," Margaret said. "He's to finish his studies in St. George's monastery. Your father and I have seen him—went to the castle and all, and he said to us that he was sorry for the grief he's caused us all. So that's the end of it."

"We swore oaths, taking each other as man and wife…" Liza began, but her words sounded empty, even to her.

"Moonshine and you know it!" Margaret snapped. "A man in orders is no more free to swear oaths about marriage than a married man is. Now then. Master Richard Lanyon's sent us a message by that big hulkin' fellow of his, Higg. He's sorry that Peter's not been over to see you, but there's been so much to do on the farm. We've fixed a weddin' day in November. So you get off that bed, and put on fresh things and come down to supper. No one'll say anythin' to you. No one knows outside the family, or ever will. We've not gossiped and the maids daren't, believe me. Master Luttrell's promised he'll order his men not to talk. Everythin'll be just as usual. You'll see."

There was a long pause. Then Liza said, "You don't understand how it was between Christopher and me. What it was like. What it *is* like!"

"Maybe not, but there's something you don't understand either, my girl." Margaret's tone was kinder. She could not, she found, turn against her own daughter as she had turned against the Webbers. "You think you'll never love Peter, but you wait till you've lived with 'un awhile. The day'll come when he'll be tired and frettin' over something and you'll look at his weary face and your heart'll ache inside you with sorrow for him, and wantin' to put it right, whatever it is. Marriage has its own power. Now, you comin' downstairs?"

"I don't want to go to Allerbrook," said Liza dismally. "It'll never be home."

"You'll be surprised. Now, there's things to talk about—or do you mean to take your vows in old clothes?"

There was a silence. Then Liza sighed and, at last, sat up. She did it because she had to. To get up from this bed meant giving in; it meant yielding herself to the stream of wedding preparations and, ultimately, to Peter Lanyon, but she had known her fate from the moment her father had caught up with her and Christopher outside Nether Stowey. Nicholas hadn't had to explain; there were things one knew. If she refused to marry, she would either be shut up in this room until she gave in, or else she would be deposited in a nunnery. Those were the customary methods of dealing with wayward daughters. Her face was stiff with unhappiness, but nevertheless, she slid off the bed and stood up.

"All right," she said.

She didn't say it gladly or willingly or even submissively. It came out in a flat tone that might have meant anything. But she said it.

The week that Liza had spent in her parents' attic, Richard Lanyon had spent making his mind up and then unmaking it again.

It was all very well to rearrrange the future inside his head, but what if seventeen-year-old Marion didn't take to the notion of marrying thirty-eight-year-old Richard Lanyon? Or even if she did, *would* her parents allow it? And *if* she did and they did, what if Peter kicked up, refused to marry Liza, and set about wrecking his father's new marriage?

Well, let him do his worst! Good God, no decent lad ever made eyes at his own stepmother; it was against all the laws of God and man. Peter might rage and scowl and slam doors, but he'd know that Marion was out of reach. He'd come around.

At this point in his inner dialogue, something inside Richard would snap ferocious jaws, like a pike catching a minnow. Peter would damned well have to come around. Peter was going to marry Liza Weaver, and why should he object to her? He'd known the girl most of his life and she was a fine-looking, good-tempered wench. He was lucky to get her and it was to be hoped that he would have the simple good manners not to sulk to her face. Liza was for Peter and Marion was for Richard and that was that.

Whenever he thought of Marion, he felt as though a hot, damp hand had clutched at his innards, both maddening and weakening him. At the idea of approaching her, he became anxious, wondering what to do, what to say to her, how to please her. He was like a youth again, bewildered by those strange creatures, girls.

On the Monday following Richard's visit to Lynmouth they fetched the sheep in from the moorland grazing, and having done so, counted them, because on these occasions there were nearly always a few missing. Sure enough, the count was half a dozen short. *Good,* thought Richard. *I can make use of that.*

That evening, in the farmyard, he took Higg into his confidence.

"Tomorrow I'm sending Peter out to look for the strayed sheep and I want you to go with him and make sure he *looks* for the sheep and don't go slipping off anywhere. I've had a bit of worry with him. There's a girl in Lynmouth that he's being a bit foolish about."

"Yes, Master Lanyon," said Higg, and from his tone, Richard gathered that Higg, Roger, Betsy and Kat all knew the situation and were probably discussing it avidly out of his hearing.

"Most young men have their adventures before they get wed," Richard said offhandedly. "But Peter's getting married soon and it's time this stopped. Tuesdays are likely days for him to go dodging off to Lynmouth, so I'm charging you to see he doesn't. Understand?"

"Ah," said Higg, grinning, and added a comment for once. "Could work out well. A bride's best off with a groom as knows what he's about."

"I daresay," said Richard coldly. "Go over Hawkridge way and search there. I'm going the other way, up to the high moor. Between us, we'll find them, I hope."

In the morning he gave his orders, watching Peter intently. Peter glowered, opened his mouth as if to protest, but then shut it again as he met his father's stern eye. He shrugged, and after breakfast went off with Higg as instructed, taking Silky, the sheepdog bitch, with them. "She's still mournful, missing my father," Richard said. "The more work she does, the better. Leave Blue to guard the house."

When Peter and Higg were out of sight, Richard asked Betsy for some bread and cold meat—"I could be out of the house at noon, if the sheep have wandered far." He then saddled Splash, swung himself astride, called his own dog Ruff and set off westward, to the coast and Lynton.

It was a mild day, the sky a mingling of blue patches and good-natured brown-and-white cloud, carried on a light west wind. The rolling moors, which from a distance looked so smooth that their colours could have been painted on them, were patched pale gold with moor grass and dark where the heather grew. Here and there were the green stains of bogs, and in places there were gleams of bright yellow, for always there was gorse in bloom somewhere.

Splash was fresh and they made good time. Richard found himself almost at the Valley of the Rocks while the morning was still quite young. He drew rein and looked round. That must be the cottage where the grandmother and aunt lived, standing a little back from the road; he could see its thatched roof, just visible above some apple trees. He hesitated. Would Marion be here yet? She would have quite a long walk from home, up the steep path which linked Lynmouth to Lynton, and then through Lynton itself. Should he wait, or go straight to the cottage and knock, or…?

Then he saw her, walking toward him, her basket on her arm. He knew her at once. It was as though during that one brief meeting a week ago he had memorised her, head to footsoles, every line and movement of her. He rode toward her.

"Marion Locke!"

She stopped, looking up at him in surprise, and he saw that she didn't recognise him and was startled, although, as she looked into his face, he also saw appreciation there. Marion responded to the sight of a handsome man as instinctively as a flower opening in the sun. Ruff ran up to her, wagging his tail, and she stooped to pat him.

"I'm Richard Lanyon," he said. "Peter Lanyon's father."

She'd recognised him now. She straightened up and smiled and he doffed his cap. "You saw me last week, when I called at your parents' home. I brought you a disappointment, I think. My son is betrothed already, my dear. But I wish to talk to you. Will you ride with me a little way before you go to see your grand-mother?"

She got up behind him without the slightest hesitation and neatly enough, despite the basket on her arm, putting her left foot on his and accepting a hand to help her on. For the first time he touched her, and the contact burned him like white fire. More prosaically, a smell of fish arose from the basket and Splash snorted disapprovingly. "Your horse don't like the scent of herring," said Marion, laughing. "But they taste all right."

"Not to him," said Richard, also amused. "Hold tight!" He put Splash into a trot on purpose, so that she would have to hold on and he would feel her hands grip his waist.

"Where we goin'?" Marion enquired.

"Into the valley. We can get down and stroll awhile and have some private talk, if you will. It's a pleasant morning."

Marion laughed again. Bumping and jogging, they made their way along the rough track and into the valley, with Ruff running at Splash's heels. Once there, Richard drew rein again, dismounted and helped Marion down. He removed Splash's bridle and hung it on a small tree, eased the girth, hobbled the animal's forefeet and told Ruff to stay on guard. He offered Marion his arm. "Shall we walk?"

In the priory of St. George's in Dunster, Christopher Clerk stood in a small monk's cell, looking about him. He had made it plain that he had no intention of taking vows as a monk, but Father Hugh Meadowes hadn't cared.

"Take vows as a monk or not—that's up to you as long as you take vows as a priest. That's your business in life and you know it. You've a vocation, my son. I know one when I see one, and what will your father have to say if you abandon yours? He's proud of you! You're not going to let him down and you're not going to let me down and above all, you're not going to let God down. You young lunatic! If you hadn't been willing to swear on a crucifix that you didn't sleep with the girl, I'd have had to go to the bishop. Do you realise how serious that would have been? Forget her! Forget any oaths you thought you swore. Forget you ever thought you loved her. I doubt it, myself. What sort of a life were you going to drag her into? She's going to marry someone else, who'll give her a better future than you ever could!"

"I'd have made my way. I'd have made a life for both of us!"

"And one day your call to the priesthood would have risen up and poisoned it. I know about these things. You'll finish your studies in the priory and then you'll stay there and serve the monks and the parishioners. Liza Weaver won't be among them. She's leaving the parish. No more argument, my son. I don't want to repeat what I had to do when you were brought back to the castle, but if I have to, I will."

His back was still marked from Father Meadowes's whip. He could only hope that Liza had not been similarly treated. He had not dared to ask, not even when her parents came to see him, to hear him apologise and promise to put Liza from his mind forever. He had had little chance to say anything beyond the apology and the promise. Nicholas had done most of the talking. Some of his remarks had burned more bitterly than Meadowes's lash. *Callow young wantwit. Trying to lead my girl into a life of concealment and poverty. She doesn't know enough of the world to realise what was ahead. And you say you loved her. Bah!*

But all the time, all through that diatribe from Nicholas, and all through Meadowes's beating, he had prayed inside his head for Liza, hoping that God would let him suffer for them both.

He sat down slowly on the hard, narrow bed. He was thinking about the past. At the beginning it had been his own idea to enter the church. He believed he had been called. Their own parish priest, back in Bristol, had given a homily one Sunday on what a privilege a vocation was; how it was like a summons to a holy army, and how priests and monks followed the banner of Christ just as knights followed the banner of their overlord. The soldiers of Christ fought battles of the spirit, not of the body, and their purpose was to save the souls of their fellow creatures from damnation. There was no nobler calling on earth, said the priest ardently.

Christopher had thought about that homily many times during the following weeks and he had gone to talk to the priest privately, and before very long he had become convinced that he was among those who had been summoned to take Christ for his suzerain. His father had been delighted.

His mother, a practical woman, was less so, and expressed regret that her second son would not marry and have a family.

They were willing to help him, she said; he could go as an apprentice to another merchant and could in time become a merchant in his own right, could succeed in the world. But he shook his head and said he must leave the world, in that sense, behind, and his father told her to stop making objections; this was a great honour and he was proud of Christopher.

And he, Christopher, had been proud of himself, sure of himself, had thought of himself as a good soldier of God. And then, as he'd roamed through the fair at Dunster on that spring day, he'd stopped to watch as a dishonest weaver was paraded past for swindling his customers, and realised that the girl standing beside him hated seeing someone put on display like that. She had left the people she was with and walked off alone into the crowd and he had followed, concerned for her in such a gathering, with so many strangers about. She had suspected his intentions and looked sharply around at him, and he had spoken to her, meaning to show kindness, as a priest ought to do, and their eyes had met, and the whole world had changed.

He had known then, in that moment, that his vocation was a horrible mistake, that he was made for the ordinary life of a man, that he was on the wrong path entirely. He'd fought the knowledge off and might have won the fight if Elizabeth Luttrell's wretched little dog hadn't run away, and he hadn't found himself chasing after it and coming face-to-face with Liza Weaver once again. After that, there was no more resisting. His vocation had been nothing but a dream, a youthful ardour trying to find somewhere to put itself and making the wrong choice.

And there was no way back.

He looked around him, at the stone walls of the little cell, at the prie-dieu in the corner, with its embroidered cloth—the only splash of colour in the room. Whatever revelations had struck him when he met Liza, he had ended up here. His vocation might seem unreal to him now, might have faded into nothingness as far as his emotions were concerned, but he was bound to it just the same, a soldier plodding across an arid desert, sworn to the service of his lord whether he liked it or not.

Liza was lost to him and he had been a fool ever to think they could escape together and create any kind of life worth living. She had been rescued from that and from him and probably it was the best thing for her. He understood that now.

What none of them knew, however—though God presumably did—was that what he felt for Liza, and what she felt for him, was real and would remain real all the rest of their lives, even if they never met again. They were sworn to each other, whatever Father Meadowes and the Weavers might say. He said aloud, "I will go on praying for her all my days."

Yes, he would! And there was nothing anyone could do to interfere with either his private prayers or his memories.

Meanwhile, this priory and this cell were to be his home. Very well. His future had been ruthlessly reorganised and his life sold away. Soldier of God? No, he was a slave, and for life. But his love was unchanged and would remain so until he died.

CHAPTER TEN

CLOUD BLOWING IN

The Valley of the Rocks was a curious place. On the moor and among its surrounding, greener foothills, the water had sculpted the land and was still doing so. Streams ran through nearly every one of the deep, narrow combes that dented the hills as though a giant had repeatedly pressed the side of his hand deep into a collection of vast and well-stuffed cushions. The valley, by contrast, was dry.

It didn't run down to the sea, but lay parallel to it. Its floor was flat and broad, but on either side, hillsides of bracken and goat-nibbled grass rose steeply to curious crests where grey rock outcrops, weathered into extraordinary shapes, adorned the skylines. Richard knew that the hills to his right were a thin wall between valley and sea, with a drop of hundreds of feet from the hillcrests to the water, most of it sheer cliff with broken rock at its feet.

Ahead, the seaward hillside broke in one place, though even

from there, the drop below was still hair-raising. The heights resumed with a tall conical hill topped by an extraordinary mass of rock which looked, from a distance, so like the ruins of an old fortress that most people called it Castle Rock.

There was no one about, except for a goatherd encouraging his flock from one piece of grass to another, up on the slope to the left. He was high up and moving away from them, and showed no sign of having seen them. He certainly wouldn't disturb them. "Mistress Locke," said Richard, "as I said, I wish to talk with you. I came here today to find you. I have something to tell you and something to ask you. I hope you will listen."

"Well, what might all that be about?" asked Marion.

She said it with a smile in her voice, and provocation, too, and when he turned to look at her face, that provocation was in her eyes, as well. The white fire leaped again, shockingly, filling him up. Her hand burned on his arm. He hardly knew how to go on just talking to her. He wanted to throw words and politeness and every last vestige of civilised behaviour away and her clothing with them and his own as well and turn this bleak, lonely valley into a Garden of Eden, with him and Marion as Adam and Eve.

To steady his mind, he quickened the pace, leading her toward the foot of the goat path that wound its way up and around Castle Rock. With a great effort he kept his voice normal as he said, "Mistress Locke, you must understand, even if it disappoints you, that I've plans for my son Peter and that there can be no question of a marriage between you. However, I can see very well why he's lost his heart and his head over you. You are as lovely a wench as I ever saw."

It was a poor description of her, he thought, nearly as inadequate as when her mother called her pretty. Marion Locke was no conventional beauty. His first impression had been the right one. She was *ripe,* like a juicy plum. She gave off the very scent of ripeness, of readiness.

"Tell me," he said, still keeping his voice even with the greatest difficulty, "what if I asked you to think about me instead? I'm a widower these many years and I'd like a wife. Specially, I'd like a wife like you."

"Oh," said Marion, and dropped her hand from his arm.

"Why *oh?*" He caught her hand back and drew her to him. "Come! I'm older than you, but I'm hale enough. You'd get used to farm life, though it's different from what you know. Marion…"

"But I…no, please," said Marion, shaking her head and pulling her hand free. She edged away, arousing in him a sudden huntsman's instinct to give chase.

"Now, don't shy away from me, sweeting. There's no need. I just want you to listen to me." He stepped after her, repossessed himself of her hand and then changed his grasp to her elbow, drawing her back to him, clamping her to his side and walking her steadily on. "There's nothing to be afraid of. I'm not an enemy. Just listen, my dear."

Marion didn't know what to do. The young men she'd flirted with and, well, given way to once or twice—and she knew that she'd taken a risk and been lucky that no harm had come of it— had been easy to manage, even a little shy. She had never felt out of control. She had never encountered anyone like Richard Lanyon before. He was handsome, but he had an aura of danger, something new to her. Besides, this wasn't decent. She had made love with this man's son, and here in this very valley, at that. It wasn't *right.* Marion's morals were broad, but not broad enough for that.

But she couldn't break Richard's hold and if she did, she knew she couldn't outdistance him. She could still see the goatherd but he was far away; there was no help there.

They had reached the foot of the path up the Rock. "Let's climb a little way and see if we can see the coast of Wales," Richard said, and steered her upward. The path wound, bringing them to the seaward side of the Rock, giving them a view across the Channel and westward down it. He looked down at her, smiling, but then, unable to stop himself, suddenly swung her in front of him, bending forward to kiss her.

His forebear Petroc, the one who had brought the Lanyons to Exmoor, had started life as a Cornish tin miner. That meant a free man, even in the days of villeinage, but it was a hard life of digging and panning, which produced men with muscles like steel ropes.

Petroc had hated it and given it up to breed sheep, though with poor success at first, for Cornish pastures were thin and sheep reared on them grew poor fleeces. However, when the Black Death tore holes in the population and opened, for those who still lived, chances hitherto unimaginable, he had snatched his opportunity and travelled to Somerset, where the grazing, even on the moors, was far better. Here he found success at last with his sheep. But if he had left the harsh days of failure behind him, he hadn't lost his tin miner's physique. To those of his descendants who survived, he had handed it down. Richard Lanyon had the thick shoulders and knotted muscles of his ancestors and he scarcely knew his own strength.

Marion, feeling his fingers grip her like pincers of steel, cried out, turning her head away from him. "Master Lanyon, don't! You're frightenin' me!"

Realising that he must have hurt her, he let go. This was no way to go courting. "It's all right. Don't be afraid." Better keep walking; it gave his overheated body something to do. He turned her and guided her onward and up. "Watch your footing—the ground's rough," he said, and used that as an excuse to put a heavy arm around her shoulders. "I'd treat you kindly," he assured her, "and you'd eat well, on the farm. Not so much fish, but much more cream and good meat. The farmworkers' wives would show you how to do this and that, and…"

"Weather's changin'," said Marion.

It was. It was growing colder and the west wind was strengthening. There was no more blue in the sky and the high brown-and-white clouds had given place to low grey ones, flowing in from the far Atlantic. The path had brought them quite high up by now and wisps of cloud were blowing around them, bringing a hint of drizzle. Wales, which had indeed been visible at first though neither of them had paid any attention to it, had vanished.

Marion was shivering, partly with cold, partly with what was now serious alarm. When Richard had come to Lynmouth to see her parents, he'd been just Peter's father, a farmer in a brown wool jerkin and a hooded cloak, darker than most Somerset men were, and good-looking—she was never unaware of good looks in a man—but all the same, one of her own father's generation and not, in her mind, a potential lover. But now!

His dark eyes were like Peter's as far as shape and colour went, but their expression wasn't the same. Peter's eyes held an essential kindness, but Richard's were hot and demanding. He wasn't offering her love. What he wanted was possession. He wanted to hold and control and enter her, not for her pleasure but only for his own, and he meant to have his way.

Beneath the outer layer of sheer sexiness which enveloped Marion like a rich velvety cloak was a girl who not only had at least some moral sense but a knack of understanding people, too. It had been part of her attraction for young men. She always looked at them as though she knew them quite well already and longed to know them better still.

She said carefully, "You're kind, Master Lanyon, payin' court to me like this. But I couldn't. I mean, I don't think it 'ud be fitting. My father wouldn't like it!" The last sentence was an inspiration. It was surely the one thing that might impress this man.

"I'll talk to your father." They were nearly up to the rock outcrop on top of the Rock, although they could hardly see it, for the cloud around them was thickening swiftly. "I'll make him an offer he'll look at twice, or maybe three times. Marion!" He stopped and swung her to face him once again, grasping her upper arms. "Can't you see I've fallen as deep in love as a man can fall? I've fallen further than if I jumped off one of these here cliffs. Don't let me land on the rocks! Say yes!"

"I can't! I'm sorry, but I can't!" Marion was really petrified now. She could not have put into words what she sensed, but if someone had said the words *snapping pike* to her, she would have said at once, *yes, that's it.*

"Why not? *Why not?*" He hadn't meant to get angry but the anger rose up in him by itself. He'd never wanted anything or anyone in his life as he wanted this girl. He hadn't even known one *could* hunger like this. "What's wrong with me, eh? What is it about me that's not good enough for the likes of you?"

"Please! Please don't. Let me go!"

"No. Say yes. Marion, say *yes!*"

"Oh, please let me go. I want to go back. My grandmother

and my aunt'll be waiting!" She tried to free herself, and the basket of fish, still dangling from one arm, swung wildly to and fro.

"We're not going back yet. Not until you say yes. Not even if we have to stay up here all today and all tonight. I've got to have you, Marion. You're a temptress and I can't say no to you, any more than you can say no to me. Let me prove it!"

"No! Let *go!*" Marion shouted it at the top of her voice and jerked backward, kicking him on the shin in the process. Richard swore and released her, but remained planted like a wall between her and the downward path. She wanted to get away from him so much that she found herself turning and scrambling on uphill instead. He came after her and caught her up at the foot of the outcrop. It towered above them. There was grass beneath their feet, and a wide place to stand, safe enough close to the outcrop, but perilous at the edge, for here they were immediately above the sea and the grassy space ended at the edge of a cliff.

"I said, *let me prove it.* Let me show you!" He had hold of her again and when Marion tried once more to shout *no!* he muffled the sound by crushing her mouth with his. Not that there was anyone who could have heard her, anyway, for the goatherd was now out of both sight and hearing, even if the cloud all around them hadn't become as dense as a damp grey fleece. "There!" said Richard, lifting his head at last. "Doesn't that tell you all you need to know? Don't you know now that you can't refuse me?"

"No, I don't!" Marion shrieked, kicking him again. He pulled her hard against him and this time she lowered her head and sank her teeth into his wrist. He swore, and she stamped on his foot. They wrestled, swaying back and forth. The cloud, as much drizzle as vapour, got in their hair and their mouths and confused their vision. For one moment, with the greyness all around them, they couldn't even see the looming wall of the outcrop. It was only feet away, but they couldn't have told in which direction. Marion, struggling, kicking, shouting, "No, no, *no!*" at last broke free and threw herself sideways to avoid his clutching hands.

And then was gone.

It was as sudden, as total, as incredible as that. One moment she had been there, a crazed harpy, fighting him; the next, he was alone on Castle Rock, in a world that seemed to be made of blowing cloud and wetness. But not a silent world, or not immediately, for as she felt herself go over the edge, the rock and grass vanishing from under her feet, Marion screamed.

Till the day he died, he would never forget that scream. Throughout all the years to come, it would echo in his ears. It went on for what seemed an eternity, fading downward but continuing, continuing—and then abruptly ceasing, as though a blade had cut it off.

Seconds ago she had been here, with him, alive and shouting and struggling against him. He couldn't believe that she was just—gone.

And gone forever, at that. The capricious wind tore a rent in the vapours and he walked, trembling, to the edge to look downward. Stupidly, pointlessly, he shouted her name. "Marion! *Marion, Marion!*" There was no answer. Between the wisps of cloud blowing past beneath him—how unnatural, to look down upon cloud!—he glimpsed, briefly and horribly, the sea and rocks at the bottom. His head swam. He staggered backward to safety, before that yawning drop could drag him to oblivion, as well. It occurred to him, thinking of that final struggle, that it could have been him just as easily as Marion.

In which case, he would have been dead, as she was. No one could survive that fall. The tide at the cliff foot was rising; he had seen the white foam boiling in over the fallen rocks, which were a peril to ships all along this coast. Marion had fallen into that. The rocks had broken her and the sea had swallowed her up. She had been wiped out of the world, and if he hadn't actually pushed her, well, he had frightened her into falling. It was a poor distinction.

He slumped down with his back against the outcrop. The cloud closed in again. He still struggled with disbelief, but the silence slowly brought it home. He was, as near as made no difference, a murderer.

No one knew he was here, though. He had not told anyone he was coming here; he was supposed to be out looking for sheep. He had ridden over the moor, taking the shortest way, and not seen a soul on the way. He hadn't ridden through Lynton, either. And in this weather he wasn't likely to meet many people on the way back. In fact, he'd be glad of Splash's homing instinct. People got lost in mists easily, but horses didn't.

He could go home. He could pretend he had never come near Lynton or this valley. At least there was one thing. He couldn't marry Marion now, but neither could Peter. He almost felt a sense of relief, as though she had put a spell on him, which was now lifted. Perhaps she had been a witch, and in that case the world was well rid of her.

He repeated this to himself, firmly, several times. Then, careful of his footing in the bad visibility, he started down the winding path around Castle Rock. Down on the floor of the valley it was drizzling, but it was below the cloud itself and he could once more see where he was going. He glanced back once at the

Rock. It stood tall, wreathed in the drifting vapours, but with an air of menace, as though it was aware of him and was ill-wishing him. Hurriedly he turned his back and made off to where he had left Splash. Ruff was lying down but got up at his master's approach, whining with pleasure. Splash, too, seemed glad to see him. He bridled the horse, removed the hobbles, tightened the saddle girth and mounted, to begin the journey home.

It would take time but that was all the better, for his hands had trembled as he bridled his mount. He needed time to recover. Thank God no one had seen him. Thank God no one knew he had ever been here.

The goatherd, a lad of fifteen, had in fact seen Richard and Marion arrive, leave the horse and walk on along the valley to start climbing the Rock. He had noticed that the woman had remarkable hair, and a very attractive, not to say come-hither way of walking, and that they had a dog with them and that their horse was an odd colour, with dark grey dapples all running into each other. He had never seen any of them before as far as he knew. Most of his life was spent in the valley, along with his master's goats; even Marion had not hitherto crossed his path. Few people ever came into the valley. He wondered what they were doing there, but his business, after all, was to look after the goats.

The horse and dog had gone when, after settling his charges on fresh grass and attending to a cut on the leg of a limping nanny, he came down the hillside to escape the weather and eat his midday bread and cheese in a little shelter he had built for himself. The strangers had presumably come back, collected their animals and left.

A month or so later, local gossip reached him about a Lynmouth girl who had run away from home, but he made no connection between the gossip and the couple he had seen.

Richard's route home took him high onto the moors and back into the mist. He let Splash take his time and ate his bread and meat in the saddle. As at last he approached Allerbrook, he was both surprised and pleased to come across his own missing sheep, their fleeces spangled with damp, nibbling dismally at the thin autumn grasses and not at all unwilling to be rounded up by Ruff and shepherded home to the better pastures lower down.

Another half hour and he was there, riding in with them, a respectable farmer and shepherd who had gone out on the moor to look for missing stock, found them and brought them back.

Peter came home shortly afterward, complaining that he had not found any sheep. Richard described how he had searched in vain in the mist for hours and then discovered them just after he had given up trying.

All the rest of that day the talk was of nothing but sheep. In the morning, however, Richard remarked to Peter that they ought to ask Nicholas Weaver to bring Liza over for a visit to her future home, and a formal betrothal.

Peter, without answering, swallowed his final mouthful of breakfast and stalked out of the kitchen to go about his day's work. Richard glared at his son's retreating back, but for the moment held his tongue. Clearly he would have to think about this.

"The master's got something on his mind," Betsy said to Higg three nights later as they settled to sleep on the straw-filled mattress in their cottage. "He's been goin' around all grim-faced and hardly hears what's said to him. He don't look like he sleeps at night. And it's plain as the nose on your face that him and Master Peter b'ain't hardly on speakin' terms."

"Not much we can do about it," said Higg tersely.

"I don't like the look of things. Peter don't want this marriage the master's planned for 'un, and you know what Master Richard is like for getting 'un's own way. Just like his father, he's turning out to be. He'll have his way, mark my words, but whether it'll be a happy house afterward or not, I wouldn't like to guess."

"Let's worry about that when it happens," said Higg stolidly.

The fact that Marion no longer existed meant that she couldn't now marry Peter, but Peter didn't yet know this. Somehow or other he must be informed, and then coaxed into standing before a priest with Liza Weaver. But how? Richard asked himself, lying awake on his bed.

It was all too true that he was sleeping badly. Hour after hour, every night, slumber eluded him, while he relived that ill-fated walk through the Valley of the Rocks, and when at last he did sleep, he dreamed of it. Night after night, Marion's last scream echoed for him again. What had it been like for her, through-out that long fall, knowing that she was still herself, healthy and alive, but would in the next few seconds be smashed and dead and that there was no miracle in the world that could save her? Sometimes he dreamed that he was the one who was falling.

She had died because he had tried to force his will on her. It seemed that compelling people to do one's bidding could be di-sastrous. How then was he to force his will on Peter? Well, once Peter knew that Marion had disappeared, he might decide to be sensible of his own accord. With luck, he would. But how on earth was he to be told?

No one must suspect that Richard knew more than he should. Only, time was pressing and mustn't be wasted. The betrothal to Liza ought to happen soon or Nicholas would be raising his eyebrows, and he'd expect the wedding to take place soon after. How much time would Peter need to get over the shock of learning that Marion was gone forever?

He'd killed her...no, she'd died in an unfortunate accident last Tuesday. Bit by bit, a scheme emerged.

On October 27, the following Saturday, as he and Peter went out after a breakfast at which neither had spoken to the other, he said, "Look here, boy, I'm tired of your dismal face round here. So be it. You go to Lynmouth and see Master Locke and ask him for Marion if you're so determined. I don't fancy he'll agree and it'll be for him to say. But maybe after you've talked to him, you'll see that she's not for you, and you can stop treating me as if I were a leper."

"And what if he says yes?"

"Then he says yes. But you'd better bring her here before you handfast yourself to her. She might not like the look of Allerbrook. No betrothal until she's seen what she's coming to. Saddle your pony and go."

Fifteen minutes later Peter was on his way, with a leather flask of spring water and a rabbit pasty for his midday meal, and hope in every line of his retreating back.

He returned in the afternoon, riding slowly. Richard, who had arranged to be close to the farmhouse all day, wandered into the farmyard to meet him as he was unsaddling. "So you're back. How did it go?"

The face that his son turned to him was the face of grief, bloodless and stricken. "I can't believe it. I just can't believe it."

"Can't believe what?"

"She's gone! Just gone. The last time she went to take some herrings to her grandmother and her aunt, she never got there! But last year she was seen at times with a sailor from some Norwegian ship or other, and that ship's been back in Lynmouth harbour lately and Marion was seen talking to the sailor again, on the quay. Seems his ship sailed on the very day that Marion set out and didn't come back. They reckon she's gone with him. Her father said she was flighty. He said he'd rather she *had* married me—at least it would be an honest marriage into an honest family! But it's too late now. She's…*gone!*"

And you don't know how thoroughly and completely she's gone, Richard said to himself.

"And even if she ever came back…" Peter said, but couldn't finish the sentence.

Richard, carefully, said, "I'm sorry. You mightn't believe me, but I am. You're taking this hard and I'm truly sorry." *You have no idea how sorry or why, and pray God you never will.*

"She never…" Peter began, and then stopped short again.

"Never loved you?" Richard said it quietly, though.

"Can't have done, can she?"

"You'd best come inside. Did you eat your rabbit pasty?"

Peter took off the bag he had slung onto his back. It still bulged as it had when he rode away. "No."

"Let's see what Betsy can find for you. You need a hot meal."

"You're talking to me like a mother!" said Peter, half-angrily.

"Well, your mother's not here, after all. Come on, boy. You fill your belly with good victuals. The world won't look so dark after that." He did not mention Liza. There was no need. The right moment would come.

It came three days later. "I suppose," said Peter, late in the evening, when he and his father, having made sure that the poultry were shut up safely where foxes couldn't get at them, were lighting candles so as to see their way to bed, "I suppose I may as well marry Liza Weaver. She's a nice enough wench."

"Yes. She is. You won't regret it, my lad," said his father.

Nor, thought Richard, will you have a chance to back out, boy. I'll ride to Dunster tomorrow and have the Weavers and Liza back here the day after. We'll get the betrothal official and start having the banns called next Sunday.

CHAPTER ELEVEN 🙿

NEW BEGINNING

There came a time, Liza had realised, when one could no longer fight. Christopher was gone. Not far in the physical sense, since he was only a few minutes away in St. George's Priory, but it had been made clear to her that she would never see him face-to-face again, not if her parents and the Luttrells and Father Meadowes had any say in the matter.

She thought of Christopher often. Inside her head she talked to him, even raged at him for letting himself be knocked out of his saddle instead of somehow seizing her mount's bridle and getting them both away. But at other times he seemed unreal because everyone around her kept behaving as though he had never existed. She might never have fled through the night, never have been fetched back and dragged up to that horrible little room under the thatch, never have been made to weep with pain and grief, never bolted in as a prisoner.

She was a bride-to-be. The ceremony, her mother told her as they stood in the bedchamber Liza shared with her little sister Jane and looked at a roll of light blue silk, would take place in the third week of November. Her mother sounded as cheerful and fond as though Liza were insanely in love with Peter Lanyon and could hardly wait for the wedding day.

"When you've taken your vows, everyone'll come back here for the feast, and your father and I'll move downstairs for the night so as you two can have our chamber. It'll be too far to get back to Allerbrook that night. You'll ride off in the morning. Now, this silk is for you to wear to church. Cost a fortune, bein' silk and blue bein' such a costly dye, but we don't grudge it. I'm having a new gown, crimson, but using our own cloth and having it dyed by this new man Herbert Dyer who's come to Dunster from Taunton and taken over our old dyer's business."

"I heard that Hal Redman wanted to give up," Liza said listlessly.

"Yes, poor old man. He can live on the money he got for the business and this man Herbert charges less than Hal did. Now, the wedding feast. I'll need your help with the cooking."

"And Cecy can't make light pastry if her life depended on it. I can hear you sayin' it even if you *aren't* sayin' it," remarked Aunt Cecy, putting her sharp nose in at the door.

"Well, you can't," said Margaret matter-of-factly. "Though I never can see why not. It's not that difficult."

"I can never see why it matters. My weaving's good enough," said Aunt Cecy, and walked away.

It was all, Liza thought bemusedly, so normal, so ordinary. For as long as she could remember, her mother and Aunt Cecy had had exchanges like that. It was part of the atmosphere of home, of everyday life, the same everyday life which was rolling over the episode with Christopher Clerk like a team of harvesters scything their way across a barley field. When the harvesters were done, the field was nothing but stubble.

She went like a sleepwalker through the rituals of preparation for marriage. There was a flurry of coming and going between Allerbrook and Dunster. On the last day of October Richard Lanyon came to visit the Weavers, and on the following day Liza and her parents rode back with him to Allerbrook for the betrothal. They dined at the farmhouse and in the presence of Richard Lanyon and Liza's parents, who were all beaming, Peter took her hand, promised to marry her and kissed her. He was the Peter Lanyon she had always known, looking older now and oddly tired, as indeed did his father. She supposed the work on the farm had for some reason been extra hard this year.

They both said how welcome she would be at Allerbrook. "You won't have to work in the fields much," Peter assured her as they sat down to dinner, "except that everyone lends a hand at harvest time if they can. But otherwise, it'll be taking care of the chickens, and helping with dairy work and bread making. Betsy'll be glad of an extra pair of hands."

"Won't you mind me coming in and...well, interfering?" Liza asked doubtfully, looking at Betsy.

"No, that I won't," said Betsy, handing her a platter of oatcakes and cream. "I've got too much to do and so has Kat. If 'ee can make butter and set the cream, I'll see to the cheese. Can 'ee milk a cow?"

"Yes. Father has two cows and I often milk them."

"All the better!" said Kat, and gave her a smile.

They were kind, those two flaxen, middle-aged farm women who looked so alike. Perhaps it wouldn't be too bad.

The first banns were called the very next Sunday. Her parents were wasting no time in getting her to the church door, Liza thought ironically, unaware that Richard Lanyon was hurrying Peter to the point with equal anxiety and for similar reasons. On November 20, she changed her name to Lanyon.

Peter and his father spent the eve of the wedding at the inn in Dunster, and on the day itself, wearing their best clothes, were waiting in the churchyard amid a crowd of the Weavers' interested neighbours when Liza and her family arrived. Gleaming in blue silk, with a train which small Jane had been allowed to carry on the way to the church, Liza stood at the church door beside Peter and in front of the priest who had led the Sunday prayers for so many years of her life. Christopher was somewhere near, within these very walls, but another bridegroom stood at her side and there was no escape.

She said, "I will." Peter put a ring on her left hand, the priest pronounced them man and wife and another stone was added to the wall that divided her from Christopher, this one a wall of law and religion and society, not tangible like stone but just as strong. The priest was jocularly encouraging Peter to kiss the bride. Someone in the throng of well-wishers remarked that he'd be doing a lot more than that before another day dawned and everyone laughed, including the priest. Liza managed to smile. She even managed to smile at Peter. There was no point in being sullen. He would be a power in her life henceforth. Whatever went on inside her head must remain known only to her. Besides, she and Peter were old acquaintances, if not close ones. At least, she thought, trying her hardest to overcome the scared, lonely feeling which had been growing on her all day, she wouldn't be left alone tonight with a stranger.

The crowd that returned to the Weavers' home for the feast

seemed enormous. "If I've forgotten to invite anyone I should, they've turned up anyway," Nicholas remarked as the rooms filled up, the older folk occupying every last settle, stool and window chest while the younger ones sat on the floor.

Bart and Alison Webber were not there, but they were gone from Dunster anyway. Bart, only two weeks ago, had had an accident with an axe while chopping down a dead tree in his garden, or perhaps it hadn't been an accident. At any rate, he had sliced the great artery in his left thigh and died of it, and Alison had gone back to her parents in Dulverton. They were still subjects of gossip, but not today. Today everyone's attention was on Liza and Peter.

The feast was generous, including roast pork and a saddle of mutton, a fruit pudding with figs and raisins and honey (Margaret had gone all the way to the county town of Taunton for the figs), and another pudding made of bread, eggs, wine and spices, and with real sugar in it.

Cider and ale were on the board, and for the Weavers and Lanyons and their chief guests even some French wine. Liza's two little brothers acted as pages and helped to serve the guests. Liza was glad of the wine, because despite all her efforts to encourage herself, the sense of dread and loneliness was still increasing.

Dancing followed the feast. Nicholas's friends included people who could play pipes and lutes and drums and between them they formed an impromptu band. The bride and groom opened the dancing and then Liza danced with a dozen different partners at least, before the moment came when her mother and Aunt Cecy and Elena quietly cut her out of the gathering and led her up to the room where her parents usually slept. It was the wrong time of year for flowers, but it had been decorated with evergreens and some sprigs of gorse which were still in bloom, and the air had been sweetened with dried lavender. Candles were alight, and there were clean sheets on the bed beneath the white fleece coverlet.

"There's nothing to be afraid of. Just make up your mind you're goin' to be happy, and you will be," her mother whispered as they settled her in the bed. Liza, giddy with the wine she had gone on drinking between dances—though in her opinion, not nearly giddy enough—dutifully whispered, "Yes, of course. Thank you for everything." Then they went away and left her alone, but not for long.

All too soon she heard masculine footsteps and laughter on the stairs and then Peter was brought in, draped in what, so far as Liza could see in the flickering candlelight, looked like one of her father's loose bedgowns, a casual affair of brown wool that Nicholas tossed on if he wanted to move about the house before he was properly dressed.

The priest followed the men, and the women came back, too, for this final stage of the ritual. Peter was inserted under the sheets beside her and the priest said a short prayer, largely inaudible because of all the ribald jokes which were being thrown about. Like Liza herself, most of the company was rather drunk.

It was Peter, apparently less drunk than anyone, who, as soon as the priest had finished, proceeded to shoo everyone out of the room. He did it quite commandingly, even pushing his own father through the door. Having emptied the room, he slammed the door with vigour and shot the bolt.

"That's got rid of *them*," he remarked, coming back to her. "You must be tired out, Liza, and no wonder. I feel as if I'd been squashed in a cider press." He sat down on the edge of the bed and looked at her. "It's not as if we're strangers—there's that to be thankful for. This is a new beginning. I hope it'll be all right. I mean, I hope I can…"

He stopped. Liza studied him. The woollen gown had fallen open—she could see the paler brown cloth lining and yes, he had borrowed it from her father; there was the place where she herself had mended a small tear. She could see his bare chest with a scattering of dark hairs like the hairs on the backs of his hands. His hands were quite different from Christopher's—longer and narrower, though very sinewy, and browned by the weather. She wondered why he had stopped speaking in midsentence and noticed that he had turned his head away.

"Peter?" she said uncertainly.

He turned back to her. "I'm sorry," he said. "I've said *I will* to you, and I mean it. I'll be as good a husband as I can. I promise."

"But?" Liza pulled herself more upright. Through the haze of wine she had sensed that something was amiss, and knew she ought to find out what the something was, and try to put it right. "What is it? Peter, tell me."

"I can't do that, Liza. It wouldn't be right. I think we should…"

"Were you—are you—in love with someone else?" Liza asked bluntly, and the wave of scarlet that ran up into his face was answer enough. He did not have to speak.

"I'm so sorry," said Liza gently.

"I wanted to marry her. I thought we were betrothed, but her parents told my father that she'd promised herself to others before me, so her promises were empty. Then she ran off with another man. That's all," he said at last, with difficulty.

"Oh, Peter."

She was genuinely sorry for him. She of all people knew what it meant to be compelled to turn your back on the one person you truly wanted.

But she must never tell him about Christopher. He could speak of his girl, but she must not speak of Christopher. If she were to build any future with Peter Lanyon, and build one she must, then Christopher must remain her secret. She must be Peter's refuge, the rock on which his house could be founded. That was what a sensible girl would set out to do.

She shook herself inwardly, to disperse the wine fumes, and said, "I *am* most truly sorry. But here we are, together. I'll be coming back to Allerbrook farm with you tomorrow. I'll do my best for you. What else can I say, or do?"

"You can be my friend. Will you try to be that?"

"Yes, of course. But…"

"No, I know. We have to be man and wife as well and everyone downstairs is expecting us to get on with it. They're probably looking at the ceiling and listening for, well, interesting noises."

"If they're still drinking," said Liza, "they'll be too fuddled before long to listen for anything. Some of them won't get home tonight, or if they do, it won't be in a straight line. Soon we'll hear them going zigzag and singing along the street."

It worked. Suddenly he chuckled and Liza, thankful to see his face crease in amusement, chuckled, too.

She, like Peter, had said *I will*. This was indeed a new beginning, and yes, it was better not to look back through the gates of Eden. "I would like to be friendly," she told him, and, a little shyly, held out her arms.

Peter leaned forward. "I forgot to pack a loose gown. Your

father lent me this and the damned thing itches. Take it off for me, will you?"

She took it off. There was nothing unpleasant about his body. It was young and clean and hard and it would have been a very strange wench who didn't admire it. He took hold of her, strongly but not roughly, and his warmth was pleasant.

Peter himself was realising that Marion, who had hurt him so badly, had at least done him one service. She had taught him his business. He knew what to do, how to caress and persuade, so that when the moment came, it would be easy for Liza, and not frightening.

There was one absurd moment, about ten minutes later, when his left knee missed the edge of the bed and the two of them nearly fell off. Peter shot his right hand out, clutched at the bedpost behind Liza to check their fall, and hauled them both back to safety, whereupon they found themselves laughing aloud.

Downstairs, a number of people, including Nicholas, Margaret and Richard, did indeed hear the laughter, and smiled at each other.

"It'll be all right," Nicholas said. "Sounds as if it already is."

"God be praised," said Richard, rather overfervently, to Margaret's ears. She wondered why. She and Nicholas had reason to feel like that, but why should Richard? Had Peter been difficult?

Oh well, what if he had? He clearly wasn't being difficult now, and nor, thank heaven, was Liza.

PART TWO

BUILDINGS AND BATTLES
1458–1472

CHAPTER TWELVE 🍂

DEMISE OF A PIG

I t was all very well, borne on the emotional wavecrest of a
wedding day and more than slightly drunk on strong red
wine from France, to take resolutions about putting the
past away and dedicating one's life to being a rock and a refuge
for someone for whom you had no feeling beyond mild friendship.

At the time, Liza had thought *well, I have to do it, somehow,* and
believed that because she must, she could. She had roused up
her courage and for a while she felt brave, like a knight, ready
to sacrifice herself for a noble cause. But what it actually
amounted to was day-to-day life in Allerbrook farmhouse, and
getting used to that, she sometimes thought, was going to take
her a lifetime.

It would have been better if she and Peter had had a home of
their own, but although there was an empty cottage on the farm

which Peter's father admitted he had thought of giving them, they were living in the farmhouse after all.

"There's plenty of space here," Richard told them. "You two can have the room my father had. You'll be more comfortable and it's best if we're all together. I'd feel lonely, rattling around in the farmhouse with no family round me and I'm planning to plant some extra crops, so it's always possible I'll take on more farmhands one day. They might need the cottage. I could afford to pay them. Your dowry was generous, Liza."

Her father had increased it, perhaps to reward the family that had taken his erring daughter off his hands, perhaps to do what he could to see that she was valued by the Lanyons and well treated! Nicholas must have dug deep into his coffers, even though he had already agreed to share his profits with Richard Lanyon. She thought with longing of Christopher, but also, now, with guilt. Her father and mother had brought her up, loved her and cared for her and even given her some schooling, which many girls never had, and now her father had been very generous indeed with her dowry. Running off with Christopher hadn't been much of a way to repay them.

Christopher. What are you doing, now, at this moment? Are you thinking of me?

She must put such thoughts out of her head and knew it, but it was a tiring struggle and after only a few weeks at Allerbrook, she was already tired enough. Going to bed every night with Peter Lanyon, waking up beside Peter every morning and then working…*working*. She was strong and healthy enough, but despite Peter's reassurances beforehand, she had never, physically, worked like this.

At home she had helped with spinning and weaving, had

shared the task of milking the cows, had made cheese and butter and shaped bread. Here, although there was a loom, once used by Peter's mother, and a spinning wheel, too, she had so far had no time even to touch them. Here, the dairy work and the bread making were only a small part of a much more arduous regime, which involved carrying fodder to the oxen and buckets of swill to the monstrous pig that was being fattened in a sty next to the farmyard, caring for the poultry, searching for eggs and gathering firewood in the combe, as well as helping Kat and Betsy to get the meals and clean the house while, even at this season, the vegetable plot needed some attention. The onions and cabbages could be invaded by weeds at any time of year.

And at other times she would, she was assured, be busier still, for she would have to help with both the harvest and the lambing, and lend a hand in gathering the apples from the little orchard below the house, in order to make cider. Betsy would show her how, Peter said.

Even now, in winter, she was out of doors much more often than she had ever been at Dunster, at times in rain or bitter winds, with heavy leather boots on her feet to protect them from the mud. At night she was usually so weary that she swayed as she went up the stairs, and then Peter's embraces still lay between her and the blessing of sleep. She was often out after dark or before dawn, but she never, now, looked up to wonder at the moon or the stars. She hadn't the time.

The greatest relief came on Sundays when they went down the combe to attend the church in Clicket, after which, in dry weather, most of the menfolk would spend the afternoon at the archery butts set up on the green, close to Sweetwater House.

All able-bodied men were supposed to practise archery regularly, and although down here in the southwest they were well away from the quarrels between the ailing King Henry's warlike wife and his cousins of York, that could change. Families like the Luttrells and the Courtenays and Carews and the Sweetwaters, too, had their allegiances. For the moment, however, in Clicket, as in Dunster, the men—even though one at least of the Sweetwaters usually joined them, to make sure that their tenants attended—regarded the archery as sport, one of their few relaxations, except for occasional social gatherings at the various farmsteads.

Gatherings there had been, as the neighbouring farming families were friendly enough, and wanted to make the new bride at Allerbrook feel welcome. There had been Sunday dinners and Christmas celebrations with the other tenant farmers of the Sweetwater estate, the Hannacombes, the Rixons and the Lowes.

The Hannacombes, Sim and Anna, were quite young and had two small sons, one aged two years and another just two months. They were a good-humoured, broad-built, pink-complexioned pair who kept their fields well weeded and drained. The Rixons and their four children, whose ages ranged from two to eleven, lived squashed into a very small farmhouse but were jolly by nature and very musical. Gatherings at their home always meant singing and even dancing, cramped though their main room was. Harry and the elder of the two boys could play the guitar, Harry's wife, Lou, could perform on the flute and Lou's widowed mother would tap a hand drum to give them a rhythm. Going to the Rixons was enjoyable.

The Lowes, Tilly and Gilbert, on the other hand, were much less likeable, though they didn't seem to realise it. Tilly was skinny and as sour as turned milk, while Gil was an ugly little man with dirt seamed into the lines on his face and most of his teeth gone, the rest being mere yellow stumps. They had their byre and stable under the same roof as themselves, with only a central passageway between the humans and the animals, and hens wandering in and out of the kitchen. They were older than the others and had reared only one child, their daughter Martha.

"A very suitable name!" Richard said. "Poor wench is only in her twenties yet, but with no looks and no portion, she'll be an unpaid servant to those two, till either she dies, or they do."

The Lanyons had held a party of their own at Christmas. Liza found a stock of almonds in the house, and as she knew how to make and mould marchpane into simple shapes, she made a marchpane ram for the occasion.

"In honour of the shepherds who were visited by the angels and the sheep that matter so much to us," she said, which met with approval from all quarters. She was asked to make another as a gift when in January they journeyed across the county to attend the wedding of Peter's friend Ned Crowham. Those, at least, were occasions when she felt like a success.

Usually, however, any pleasure in these social get-togethers was limited because the talk was nearly all to do with farming, which as yet was not familiar to her. It was all so different from the wool trade society of Dunster that she sometimes felt she was listening to a foreign language.

She told herself not to complain. Peter was gentle in his love-making, and Kat and Betsy seemed to like her and had shown her how to cook dishes that Peter and Richard especially enjoyed, including the illicit rabbit pies which were a regular feature of the Lanyon table.

Rabbits were game in the eyes of the law and not to be taken without permission, but Richard and Peter, whatever their other disagreements, were as one when it came to hungry rodents in the cabbage patch. They set snares, made pies of the victims and carefully hid all the traces if anyone called who was employed by or simply too well in with the Sweetwaters.

Liza had worked hard to master the art of a good rabbit pie, and then achieved another small success when she showed Kat and Betsy her own recipe for verjuice, the sharp sauce made from unripe apples, which gave flavour to so many dishes.

Kat's husband, Roger, was a little shy of her but always polite, while Higg, who had some skill at woodwork, made her a Christmas gift in the form of a decoratively carved wooden platter for use at Sunday dinner. She couldn't say that she hadn't been made welcome.

But nevertheless, she knew that Peter's mind was still detached from her (as hers was from him, although she hoped she was concealing it better), and though he was always courteous, Richard Lanyon intimidated her. Everyone jumped to obey his orders just a little too quickly. And then, one cold, overcast January morning, she understood why.

Ever since Christmas, Richard had been talking about putting up fences around a south-facing field called Quillet, because he intended to use it for wheat this year instead of leaving it as meadowland, and it would need better protection from deer than the existing ditches could provide. The field sloped and the ditches drained rainwater off into the combe, which was useful, but they were hardly an obstacle and anyway, the ditches here and there ran through culverts so that people and animals could have a way into the field. Liza had already seen the ox team take the plough in to tear up the rich grass of Quillet. Henceforth, the entrances would be guarded by gates.

On that chilly winter morning, Richard and Peter, who had spent the previous two days in the wooded combe cutting poles, decided that they had enough for the first stretch of fencing.

"They'll be at it all the time it's light," Kat told Liza. "They won't want to stop till dusk, so you'd better take some dinner out to 'un. I've got some bread and hot chicken pasties ready. I'll put the pasties in a crock with a lid and wrap it in a cloth to keep them warm—and there's a drop of cider in this here flask."

Liza duly set off with a bag containing dinner for her husband and father-in-law and found them hard at work. "A hedgerow 'ud be better, like we've got round the fields near the house," Richard said as she admired the first few yards of fence. "But hedgerows take a man's lifetime to grow. Might plant some brambles or hazel, though, to get one started. We'd get nuts and blackberries that way, too."

Peter said, "I think we've got company. It looks like Sir Humphrey."

It was. Astride his big bay gelding, he cantered toward them, embroidered saddlecloth flapping and a brooch in his velvet hat gleaming in the dull light. He slowed to a trot, pulled up beside them, put one hand on his hip and then scowled. Liza hastily curtsied and after a moment's pause, her menfolk removed their caps. "Good day, sir," said Peter politely.

"I'm not sure that it is a good day," said Sir Humphrey. He pointed with his whip at the fencing. "What's all this, then? And why has this field been ploughed?"

"It looks to the south and the soil's deeper than in most places hereabout," said Richard. "It's more fertile, too. It's my belief that this field could rear a crop of wheat and I'm going to try. Only I've got to keep the deer out."

"You'll also keep my cows out, I see!" Sir Humphrey snapped. "And stop me riding over the land when I'm hunting. This *is* my land, let me remind you."

"I rent it from you, sir," said Richard, quietly, but with an undertone which Liza found alarming. "And it's my business to make the best of it. Wheat's a valuable crop."

"Barley's good enough for the likes of you. Wheaten bread's not for common folk. If any wheat's planted on Sweetwater land, it'll be on our home farm. We'll eat the bread and take the profit if any goes to market. Well, you've ploughed—you may as well plant. But make sure it's rye or barley and put the land back to meadow afterward. And take that fencing down. I'll have no fences getting in my way on my land."

Liza stared at him in astonishment and his cold gaze fastened on her face. "You're looking at me as though I had two heads, young woman. May I know why?"

"I just…wondered…"

"Yes, well? What did you wonder?"

"If a field has crops in it, Sir Humphrey…I mean…surely you wouldn't hunt across any crop, whether it's fenced or no," said Liza, quite seriously.

Peter gasped, but Richard laughed, although it was a mirthless sound. "My wench, a hunt goes where the hounds go and the hounds go where the quarry does, and find me the stag that solemnly runs round a field instead of across it!"

"Quite right." The bay fidgeted restlessly, but Sir Humphrey checked him with a rough hand on the curb. "I'll forgive her for her impertinence this time," he said. "She's new here, I believe.

But teach her to guard her tongue. Put your mind to breeding children, my girl, fine healthy sons to make the best of my land, but not to fence it. I'll be out here again tomorrow and I'll expect that fencing to be gone. My horse needs exercise, and standing here in the cold will do him no good. Good day to you all."

He swung the bay around, cantered it in a semicircle, jumped the ditch beyond the end of the new fencing and rode off across the ploughed field, veering away at the other side and heading downhill toward Rixons.

"What the devil," said Richard furiously to Liza, "did you want to go and say that for? We'll have no peace for months now. He's taken umbrage!"

"I think he'd taken it already," said Peter mildly. "The fencing's upset him much more than Liza did. We'll have to remove it, you know."

"I'm damned if we do! We'll finish the job, boy, and that's that."

"We can't," said Peter. "Do that and he'll send men up here to take it down for us. You know he will."

"God damn him and all the Sweetwaters. The only good Sweetwater is a dead one. Him and his two sons—I hate the guts of every single one of them. Why should they have everything and us hardly anything and not even the right to better ourselves? And why should he have two sons when it was all Joan could do to give me one? And when are *you* going to have some news for us, Liza?" His angry eyes appalled her. "Near eight weeks you've been wed and it's time there were signs. What have you to say for yourself?"

He took a step toward her and for a moment she thought he would strike her. "Father…" said Peter protestingly.

She did not know if he said more than that. Terrified by her father-in-law's fury, she dropped the dinner bag and cider flask on the ground and turned away and fled.

By nightfall the fencing was down, but Richard at the supper table was like a thunderstorm in human form. He shouted at Betsy that the pottage was too salty, which it was not, and berated Higg, who had hurt his wrist during the accident with George Lanyon's coffin and had wrenched it again while helping to cut fencing poles, as wrathfully as though Higg had done it on purpose.

Liza did not dare speak to him and scarcely even ventured to look at him. Next morning his temper seemed no better. Breakfast was nearly as frightening as supper had been.

When it was over, she fed the fowls and the pig and then went off to walk up the combe to the ridge above, abandoning the work of the house, taking—or stealing—one of the solitary walks she loved and hadn't had since she came to Allerbrook, desperate for escape from the atmosphere of rage which seemed to fill the house like smoke.

It was cold, but solitude was a blessing. She reached the top of the combe and paused, thankfully breathing the free air on top of the ridge, beside the bog where the Allerbrook rose.

The bog itself was a long stretch of virulent green amidst dark heather, with clumps of reeds here and there. It spread along the hillcrest in wet weather, sometimes even spilling over the edge, something Liza had witnessed in a rainstorm during December.

The slope of hill between ridge and farm was not smooth but undulated like the folds of a curtain. It wasn't perpendicular—sheep could find a footing there, and a few stunted trees clung to it, but it was certainly steep. During the December rainstorm, the overflow had poured down one of the creases and formed a new stream, which raced past the farmhouse about a hundred yards from the front door, to find its tumbling way eventually into the combe and the Allerbrook. It was quite a dramatic sight.

The bog was not overflowing just now, however. Liza turned northward along the ridge, climbing a little, and rounded an oval-shaped mound she now knew was called a barrow and was thought to be the grave of some ancient chieftain who had lived here before the name of Christ was ever heard in these parts. Peter had told her that there were many such barrows on the moor, and most were said to be haunted, at least after dark. This one seemed wholesome enough in daylight, though. Liza paused beside it, looking back and down, to the thatched roofs of Aller-brook. The place where she lived, though she did not think she would ever call it home.

She shouldn't be here, of course. If Richard noticed her absence, it wouldn't do much to improve his temper. But it was comforting to see the buildings of Allerbrook, where she some-times felt like a captive, dwindled by distance to the size of toys.

Raising her eyes from the farm, she looked northwest. There, in the distance, was Winsford Hill, where there were more sup-posedly haunted barrows, and far, far away beyond that rose the highest hill on the moor, Dunkery, where a beacon would be lit if any enemy invaded.

Just below Dunkery, though she couldn't see it, was the valley of the Avill River, which flowed to the sea through Dunster. Even though she couldn't, at this distance, glimpse as much as a trickle of hearth smoke, she knew where her home village was. Beyond it, lost in haze and therefore, today, just an emptiness, was the Channel. She missed it. At home, the sea had always been close at hand. If she was unhappy at Allerbrook, it was probably because she was homesick. Would she have been homesick living—in France, perhaps—with Christopher?

She didn't think so. Christopher was where she belonged. She had only to think of him and it was like a homecoming.

And she must not stay here too long, thinking about him. She was sure to be needed for something. She hoped to heaven that Richard was now out on the land and unaware of her idle wanderings.

As she took the path down the combe she noticed that while she had been out, someone had moved the cattle and horses from their housing in the farmyard and put them in a field, where they were making the best of the poor winter grass. She wondered why. A few moments later, as she neared the yard, she heard the scream.

It was the most hideous noise she had ever heard in her life, earsplitting and full of frenzied terror. Horrified, she began to run. As she rushed into the farmyard, the sound seemed to wrap itself around her. Raised voices were mingled with it now. That was Peter, shouting, "Not like that, you bloody fool!" and her father-in-law, clearly not out in the fields after all, bellowing, "Hold on, *hold on,* can't you? Damned slippery brute...*Higg!* What in hell's name are you doing? You've done this job before...."

"Can't hold 'un with this bloody wrist...!"

"You and your poxy wrist! Hold *on,* you and Peter, give me a chance...!"

The screaming crescendoed just as Liza arrived in the yard. It seemed to be coming from an outhouse which hitherto she had never entered. The door was half open. She ran to look inside and then stopped, staring, breathless and revolted.

Richard, Peter and Higg were all there, and so, hanging by its hind feet from a pulley in the roof, was the huge pig she had fed only that morning. The pulley rope stretched down and was made fast to a bracket in the wall, and immediately below the pig was a wooden bucket, empty. The pig was shrieking and struggling as Peter and Higg tried to hold it still. Richard was standing ready with a glittering knife in his hand. As she watched, the others finally stopped the pig from twisting its head and lunging with its front trotters, and Richard struck.

There was a final scream, which died away into a gurgle. Blood spurted all over the three men and then settled into a scarlet stream, which poured into the bucket. The pig jerked convulsively, not yet quite dead.

Richard, glancing around, caught sight of her and said quite amiably, "Oh, there you are. Stupid animal—put up a fight. Only made it harder for himself. But we'll get a good pork joint and some fine salted meat and chitterlings out of this one. Kat'll teach you to make chitterlings. She chops up some of the innards and fries 'un with bread crumbs and onions. She's a great one for them."

The pig was still now, dead at last. But the blood reeked, sweet and metallic and completely disgusting. Retching, Liza fled to the back door of the farmhouse, dashed inside and found a basin.

The kitchen was hot, full of steam from a vast cauldron bubbling over the fire. There was a bucket of fresh water under the table, however, and Betsy, clicking her tongue in concern, dipped a beaker into it and brought it to Liza as she leaned against the wall, basin in hand, and threw up what, to her, felt like her entire insides.

"Here, when you're sure you're done, wash your mouth out with this. What was it, seein' the pig killed? Meant to warn 'ee they were plannin' that for today since they can't go on with the fencin', but 'ee'd slipped off somewhere. Never seen it afore, I expect. You'll get used to it."

"Get *used* to it? It…it shrieked!"

"Who wouldn't?" said Kat, unconcernedly beating eggs for a pudding. "It's mostly quicker and quieter than that. Get it right and piggy's dead afore he knows he's even been hoisted off the ground. You only get that racket when whoever's holding 'un b'ain't got a proper grip. Roger ought to have helped instead of Higg, until that wrist's properly better. Pig should have been killed back afore your wedding, anyhow, to my mind, but Master always keeps one goin' till the New Year, so as to have fresh bacon and hams still hanging when everyone else has run out."

"Why isn't Roger helping?" Liza asked, and then retched again. When the spasm was over, she added, "Where is he?"

"Out clearing a ditch. Higg said holding a pig would be easier if he strapped his wrist, but it looks like he was wrong," said Betsy. "Dear Lord, you do be upset. Here, sit on this stool."

Liza was still sitting on the stool and sipping water when Richard came in, carrying a stack of empty buckets. She looked around once at his bloodstained form and hurriedly turned away, swallowing.

"Kat, is that cauldron boiling yet? Liza, you'd better come and learn how to get the bristles off a pig…what's the matter?"

"She's been sick. Gave her a shock, walkin' in on that," said Betsy.

"Oh, I see. Well, having something to do ought to put that right. Come along, Liza. Come and help. Betsy, Kat, that water."

He and the two women between them scooped water from the cauldron and bore the buckets away. Liza emptied her beaker, wiped her mouth on her sleeve and followed them reluctantly back to the outhouse. No one seemed to have noticed how long she'd been gone—there was that to be thankful for, at least. The cattle and horses must have been moved in case the screaming and the stench upset them.

Inside the shed, the pig still swung from the hook in the roof, but the bleeding was over. The pail of blood had been put aside and a piece of wood placed over it, while a large barrel had been placed under the pig instead. Peter had climbed, by way of a ladder, onto a stout timber ledge in the nearby wall and Higg was standing sulkily at the ladder's foot, saying that this was his job rightly and his wrist would be all right. "Bucket won't clobber me with its trotters and twist about."

"We're not risking you losing hold and emptying boiling water over us by mistake," said Peter brusquely. "Ah. Here's the water. Hand me up that bucket, Kat."

"Stand back," said Betsy to Liza—unnecessarily, since Liza had halted nervously in the doorway. Kat passed her pail up to Peter, who emptied the contents over the pig. The water sloshed down into the barrel and Peter handed the empty pail down through clouds of steam to Higg. Betsy gave him her full one and he doused the pig again. Liza found the first empty pail being passed to her.

"Fetch another lot of hot water," Richard said. "Quick! It needs to be boiling. It strips the bristles off. Didn't you know?"

"No. What…what do we have to do after this?"

"Scrape him down, get any leftover bristles off, right down to the skin. Couple of days and we'll start cuttin' him up and getting his meat salted and whatnot. Betsy and Kat'll show you what to do."

Liza slept badly that night, dreading the tasks that lay ahead. Her parents had bought their meat from a butcher who did his slaughtering out of sight and sound of the village. This close contact with it was something for which she hadn't been prepared. "I wish someone had warned me," she said that night to Peter.

"It's just the first time that's upset you," said Peter calmly. "Next time, you won't mind so much and the time after that, you won't mind at all. You'll see." Liza, who had eaten little that day and still felt nausea clenching at her stomach, hoped he was right, but doubted it.

But two days later, when the next stage of the work began, her tasks weren't too unpleasant after all. The good-hearted Higg had said that morning that the gutting and cutting up should be done out of Liza's sight. "The mistress b'ain't used to such things yet. It'll take a while."

Liza therefore stayed in the kitchen while the pig was dealt with in a barn. Under instruction from Kat, Liza peeled onions and grated bread for the mysterious product called chitterlings. Presently, Betsy brought in chopped-up intestines for the purpose, but they didn't look much like insides and therefore weren't particularly horrid. When they were fried with the crumbs and onions, the smell was appetising.

Nor, when larger cuts of pig were carried in, did she mind the business of laying down hams and bacon in troughs of salt with juniper berries and dried bay leaves. However, all the chopped intestines hadn't gone into the chitterlings. When Kat, quite forgetting Higg's warnings, went to the icy-cold shed where she had left the bucket of blood, after stirring barley and oatmeal into it, fetched it in, added the rest of the chopped-up innards and tipped the whole lot into a pan, saying that this would make a fine black pudding, Liza was overtaken anew with uncontrollable sickness, and Richard, once more choosing the wrong moment to walk in, said, "Oh, for the love of heaven! Not again! What's wrong with the wench? You're on a farm now, my lady. These fine airs won't do!"

Liza, sitting miserably on a stool and clutching another basin, said, "I can't help it!" and burst into frightened tears, punctuated with further heavings. Betsy, coming over to her, leaned down and whispered a question.

Liza looked up. The nausea subsided a little. "Oh! I'm not sure. I think it should have come three days back, only it hasn't."

Betsy asked another question and Liza nodded. "Yes. Always regular, till now."

Kat had come over as well and was listening. She and Betsy then turned to Richard and surveyed him unitedly and with so much authority that Richard actually subsided and said quite quietly, "What are you women muttering about?"

"Babies," said Betsy shortly. "I'd bet the next clip on it. It's got nothin' to do with putting on airs. She's expectin' or I'm Queen She-Wolf, and that I'm not."

"You are? Oh, Liza! *Liza!*"

For the first time, Liza found her husband looking into her eyes with something like joy, as though she actually mattered to him. "I'm sorry I upset everyone over the pig," she said. "I'll be more sensible another time—I'll get used to things."

"Never mind about any of that. We've got to look after you now. This is the best of news."

Peter himself was surprised by the comfort it brought him. Marion had enchanted him and then failed him, but here was this sensible, honest Liza, trying to please him, trying to please everyone, and carrying his very own child. Liza wouldn't betray him and nor would their offspring.

Richard, his temper now magically restored, said that Liza must do no work at all that was in the least heavy. It wasn't the time of year for butter making, but when the cows were in milk again in the spring, Liza was not to do any churning, nor was she to help with the lambing, not this time.

"You were brought up to weave, weren't you?" he said. "Try and get my wife's old loom and spinning wheel working again. You'll come to no harm with that. Nor with making rabbit pies," he added with a grin.

For two weeks there was peace in the house, albeit with a little nervousness because Richard had decreed that wheat would be planted, whatever the Sweetwaters said; he had the seed and would brook no argument. Then came the morning when Liza woke to find an all too familiar ache in her lower stomach, and by the end of the day she knew the hope of a child was gone.

CHAPTER THIRTEEN

THE HOWL OF THE SHE-WOLF

"So that's that! Twice!" said Richard furiously, standing beside Liza's bed and looming over her, his face dark with fury. "Twice! You've gone and lost another and before you'd got well started, at that! The wheat's sprouting in Quillet, but what's the good of the wheat growing if the family doesn't? You've let us down, wench!"

Liza, her hair tangled and streaks of tears on her pale face, shrank away from him, wishing she could bury herself in the sheets. It was May, and warm, and she felt not only wretched but feverish. But there was no pity in her father-in-law's angry eyes.

"I'm sorry. How could I help it?" she said wretchedly.

"What's wrong with you," Richard demanded, "that you can't do a simple thing like this? You're as bad as my wife Joan was. You were a good strong girl, I *thought*. You do your work and you go off walking on the moor as well—funny sort of habit, that, but it looked as if you were healthy. All right, you lost one, but it was the first—these things happen. I reckoned that this time it 'ud be all right, but no, it's hardly begun and then this!"

"It wasn't my fault!" She made herself try to fight back against the bullying. "You tell me how I could have helped it! What did you expect me to do?"

"Father!" Peter strode into the room. "What's this? Leave Liza alone! Betsy and Kat say she's had a nasty time and she's still bleeding. I won't have you shouting at her and blaming her! Go away!"

"You don't order me out of a room in my own house, boy!"

"Out of this room I do!" Peter retorted. "She can't get better with you standing over her, shouting. Do you think she did it on purpose? It'll be all right in the end. Betsy had the same thing happen to her, but she had children later."

"All right. I hope you're better soon, girl, and I hope next time'll be different." Richard gave Liza a last glare and walked out of the room. Peter followed him and tramped angrily down the stairs behind him. At the foot, Richard turned to face him.

"Sometimes I almost wish I'd let you marry Marion Locke."

"It's not Liza's fault! She's heartbroken. She prays each night, on her knees by our bed, asking God and Our Lady for a healthy child. We thought her prayers had been heard when we knew she'd quickened again. It's no help when you say things to her like *hope you'll finish the job this time* and *what we need is half a dozen sons.* You ever thought it might be something in us? Happens sometimes with animals, so why not people? Remember that ram that kept siring weakly lambs?"

"You're strong enough." Richard's voice, however, was suddenly tired. He had realised that his feelings had just betrayed him into mentioning Marion, and that was something he should never do, ever. The trouble was that now and then, he didn't seem able to help it.

He still sometimes dreamed of her death and heard her scream inside his head. Again and again he told himself that in the eyes of Peter and her family she had run off with another man and that he should tell that story to himself until he believed it. Except that he would never believe it. Always and forever he would know it for the lie it was, and one day he was afraid he would talk in his sleep and somebody would overhear.

More quietly he said, "You can tell her I spoke in the heat of the moment, and that I mean it when I say I wish her better." He led the way into the living room and added, with a change of tone, "Seen the wheat in Quillet? Looks good, if we can keep the deer out. The ditches just aren't wide or deep enough."

"Let's go and look at it," said Peter, willing to make peace if his father would, and also thankful to get his father away from Liza.

Long ago, when the Norman conqueror, William, first made Exmoor a royal forest, the land now occupied by the Sweetwater farms had been already under cultivation, and at that time it had lain outside the boundaries of the forest, as it did now. But in between, another Norman king, King John, had greedily en-larged the forest, moving the boundary so that the farmers on what was now the Sweetwater land found themselves inside, and subject to forest law, under which fences were forbidden. Deer must be able to move about freely and if this inconvenienced anyone, Norman kings didn't care.

When the boundary was changed again and the Sweetwater estate once more fell outside it, the law against fencing lapsed, but the Sweetwaters had made it plain enough that they held the same views as the Norman kings had done. Richard and Peter stood beside the growing crop, looking at the ditches which were allowed for purposes of drainage but which weren't nearly enough to discourage hungry and determined deer. "When the corn starts to ripen, could we tether the dogs out here?" Peter suggested.

"Deer aren't stupid," Richard said. "They'll soon work out how far the tether stretches. Then they'll take whatever they can out of the dogs' reach. It's growing well, though. I was right about the soil." He hesitated and then said, "Think Liza'll be well enough to get to church in Clicket on Sunday? It's the May Day competition, if the weather'll let us shoot this time. A bit late, but we'd have drowned if we'd tried to have the contest *on* May Day. Wettest first of May for years, I'd say."

"I hope she'll be up and about in time. I worry about her."

"So do I! I like the wench. If only..."

"Let's drop the matter." Peter did not wish to start the quarrel again and his eye had been caught by something in the sky, high above the barley. "There's a falcon up there, hovering. Can you see?"

"Where? Oh, yes. It's not a kestrel. Looks like a peregrine. There it goes! It's after that wood pigeon! Look at that! What a strike!"

The falcon had swooped, vertically, headfirst, a living arrow, straight onto the back of an incautious pigeon and borne it down to the ground. At the same moment there came a thunder of hooves and two riders came tearing up from the combe.

"Oh, damnation!" said Richard.

Coming level with the Lanyons, they checked and curvetted around them, colourful scalloped reins gripped in gauntleted hands, spurred boots gleaming, fantastic headgear on well-barbered heads. Richard and Peter gritted their teeth but removed their caps, since arguing with these two arrogant young men was unwise.

Then Reginald and Walter Sweetwater laughed, swung their horses away and put them at the ditch. The big horses leaped it side by side, manes and tails flying, and galloped on, headlong, this time across the wheat, to slow down in the middle and stop, while one of them dismounted and went to pick up the falcon.

"They did it on purpose!" Richard snarled, glaring across the field at them. "They know wheat when they see it and I daresay they know their father told me not to plant it! So they trample it for their sport and to put me in my place. Showing off with a damned great peregrine falcon, too. I swear," he added, "I *swear* that one of these days I'll turn things round. One day *they'll* take off their caps when they see *me* coming!"

"You won't be well enough to go to Clicket on Sunday." Betsy said. "You lie flat and still and, except when nature calls, you stay in that bed until that there bleeding stops. Wretched time you've had."

"And nothing to show for it," said Liza, turning her head away. *"Nothing!"*

"Sleep you need," said Betsy firmly, "and no goin' to church this week, let alone hangin' round they butts watchin' longshafts fly!"

Liza tried to take an interest in the archery. "I think they're having a crossbow contest, as well. Father-in-law is good with the crossbow."

"We'll bring 'ee all the news. Kat's said she'll stay here on Sunday, so she'll be within call." Outside the room, encountering Kat, who had just come up with a posset, she said, "The mistress is brightenin' up. Showin' interest in the shootin' next Sunday. That's a good sign. Just keep Master Richard out of there, that's all."

Liza thanked Kat for the posset, and once left alone, tried to sip it quietly and be what she knew her mother would have called "sensible." Tears and self-pity would worry Peter and annoy his father more than ever. She was grateful that Peter had not been angry. After Betsy had told him that it was all over, he had come to ask how she fared and done so in a kindly tone of voice. Later he had ordered his father to leave her alone, and got Richard out of the room, for which she was infinitely grateful.

If she had never set eyes on Christopher she could easily have loved Peter, and in a way, she did. The glittering spark that had been between her and Christopher wasn't there and nothing could put it there, but Peter was her real world, the company she would have to keep until one of them died, and there was much in him to value. Except that nearly all the time, Peter was ruled by his father. It was Richard who counted most in this house.

She lay there, puzzling over her own feelings, wondering why what she felt for Christopher was so very different from the mild affection she had for Peter. It was the difference between a leaping waterfall and a placid meandering stream; the difference between a bright fire and a dull red ember.

With Christopher she could have had a healthy child. She knew it.

The spring had been wet, but the following Sunday began with sunshine. Liza, lying on her bed after everyone except Kat had gone off to church and the archery competition, taking midday food with them, imagined how the grass and the cow parsley would be springing along the sides of the sunken lanes. In the most sheltered places there might even be some early foxgloves, adding their soft red to the green and white of the verges. Birds were singing. They were nesting.

Oh, dear God, they were nesting, rearing their young. Only Liza Lanyon, apparently, was not allowed to do that. She heard Kat coming to look in on her and turned on her side, closing her eyes. Kat was apt to want to talk and Liza didn't feel like it. Better look as though she were asleep.

She let Kat give her a meal at noon, but said she was still drowsy and put on another pretence of sleep to keep Kat at bay. The sunshine had gone by then and rain was beating on the windows. She wondered if it had spoiled the archery competition. She fell asleep in earnest then, but woke later to find that the bleeding had almost stopped, and that there were hooves and voices in the farmyard below. Then came the tramp of feet on the stairs. Pulling her pillow up behind her, she propped herself into a sitting position just as Richard and Peter came in.

As cheerfully as possible, she said, "I am better. I'll be up soon. Did you have your archery in spite of the rain?"

"I won the crossbow competition," said her father-in-law. "Harry Rixon won the longbow final, with Sim Hannacombe second. Peter here only got third. The rain started just afterward. We've something to tell you, though."

They came to her bedside and looked down at her, their faces solemn. Richard said, "Father Bernard made an announcement at the end of the service. He said that news has come that the king's mind has gone cloudy again but the queen, Queen Marguerite, is raising a host in his name, to keep the York family out of power. The She-Wolf is howling for the pack to gather, that's what Father Bernard said, and the Sweetwaters will answer the call. Sir Humphrey and Reginald are going, Reginald being a widower with no children, while Walter's got a wife and young-sters. Walter's staying home. But Master Humphrey's calling up men from the Sweetwater tenants."

Liza stared at them.

"They all came to the archery butts—the Sweetwaters, I mean," Peter said. "They watched the competition and then called us together. Just then the downpour started, so they hurried us all off the green, just as if they were herding a flock of sheep, and right into Sweetwater House to talk to us in their great hall."

Richard nodded. "I've never been inside that house before. From outside, you can see the gatehouse and that lookout tower with battlements round the top, and there are all those windows like lance heads, all with glass in, but it's plain inside. The hall's quite small! There's panelling, but nothing fancy about it, and only a couple of tapestries. The rest of the wall's full up with a lot of antlers, and weapons hanging in patterns. I got the feeling the Sweetwaters aren't as rich as they'd like us to think. Just hanging on the skirts of the gentry, that's them."

Liza, wondering if her father-in-law had paid any attention whatsoever to what was said or done inside the Sweetwaters' hall, or had spent all his time there memorising his surroundings, said, "But when you were in there, what happened?"

"They sorted us out," said Peter. "They still want their land tilled and the village trades to go on, so they're not taking all the men. But they're taking Edward Searle's son Toby. Geoffrey Baker's going and so are Harry Rixon and Sim Hannacombe, and some of their farmhands and from here at Allerbrook, either I must go, or Father. They don't want Higg or Roger."

"Both too old," Richard said, "and Roger too bent-backed

anyhow. But even with Higg and Roger still here, we'd be short-handed if Peter and I both went. We haven't men enough on this farm as it is, since Betsy's boy took his family away. All Kat's young ones were girls. The Sweetwaters know all that. We'll just take one of you, Sir Humphrey said to me, meaning me or Peter here. We can choose which. Generous of him! Dear God, we've got to follow the Sweetwaters to war whether we like it or no, just because we rent their land! It's enough to make a man puke."

"But which of you…?" Liza's mouth had gone dry. Peter was the younger man, the stronger one. The thought of being left at Allerbrook with her father-in-law and no Peter for an unknown length of time was terrifying.

"I said I'd go," Richard told her. Relief flooded through her, only to be stemmed a moment later when he added, "I'm fit enough and Peter's got work to do here. I said to him, you stay home and make a few more efforts to get this place populated. I'll do the fighting. My father went to war a couple of times and there's an old helmet of his somewhere. I've got my crossbow and I've been given a dagger. They handed out weapons from the ones they had hanging on their walls. We leave in two days."

It was more than two years before he came back, and by then they had all but given him up for dead.

T hroughout those two years they rarely had reliable news. They never knew for sure what was happening or where. Scraps of information filtered in sometimes, of course. Since her marriage, Liza had managed to get away from the farm only on rare occasions, and before Richard went away she had visited her parents in Dunster only once. However, Nicholas came to Allerbrook each year to collect his wool, sometimes bringing Margaret, too. They both came during the first summer of Richard's absence, a couple of months after his departure, and they had a little news.

"We get ships in Dunster harbour," Nicholas said. "Smaller than they used to be, on account of the silting up, but some of them have come from London. The rumour is that Queen Marguerite means business and hates the Yorkists and wants to see every last man of them dead. King Henry's woollier than your sheep and has nothing to say in the matter, and the Yorkists claim they're loyal to him, but if they can't convince Queen Marguerite of that, it won't help them. Our cousin young Laurie has gone to join her forces, my dear," he added to Liza, "and two of his brothers and a couple of our other cousins. The Luttrells called them up. She-Wolf or no, Luttrell said, while the king's ill, the queen represents him and the Luttrells follow their legal lord. Or lady, as the case may be."

But none of that amounted to much, and after it came a long silence until Walter Sweetwater received word from his father and brother, and passed the information on to Father Bernard to announce from the pulpit. It was unhappy news. There had been fighting in the southeast of England and Harry Rixon would not return to his home. Nor would the two farmhands who had gone with him.

A full two years had passed before Father Bernard announced one Sunday that the war was over, that they were now ruled by Yorkist King Edward IV, that King Henry VI with the wandering wits was a prisoner in the Tower of London, that the She-Wolf had fled the country with her son and the conflict was at an end. But still no word came from or about Richard Lanyon of Allerbrook, and the Sweetwaters did not come home, either.

Meanwhile, a number of things had happened.

The depredations of the deer at the first wheat harvest were nearly disastrous. They sold every last ounce of what was salvaged but made a loss, and even Liza understood why Richard had been so angry at being denied fences. Shortly after that, however, Walter Sweetwater told Peter that he could plant wheat in Quillet and fence the field, provided he didn't put up any other new fences. The results were highly satisfactory.

"We're making money from the wheat now," Liza said. "Walter Sweetwater's not all bad."

"No," Peter agreed. "I suppose not. The new bridge is useful, I must say."

Another innovation for which Walter Sweetwater was responsible was a packhorse bridge he had had constructed over one of the streams to the northeast of Allerbrook. The stream in question was deep, and the ford which had been its previous crossing place was unreliable. The area was so apt to flooding that packhorse trains from the Sweetwater manor usually took the long plod down the combe when they wanted to take their wool to Dunster, always the best market, if not the nearest.

The new bridge was built of stone and looked very like the one at Dunster, being long and narrow but high sided, to protect the packs when the river was in spate, and solid enough underfoot to reassure the most jittery pony. It made the journey to Dunster much shorter. Every time Liza saw it she recalled the Dunster bridge and knew a secret heartache, for it reminded her of the time she and Christopher had met there by chance and had their first tiff.

"I grant you," Peter said, "that there are things on the credit side of Walter Sweetwater's account." Then they both laughed, because Liza had learned double-entry accounting from her father, and introduced it at Allerbrook, which had impressed Peter considerably.

"Just as well your father-in-law's away," Margaret had said during the visit to pick up the wool. "Now you and Peter can settle down without him pokin' his nose in."

Liza knew very well what her mother meant, but it was a long time before she had any fresh hopes of a child. Peter at least refrained from nagging, for which she was grateful, and he tried to be considerate about the amount of work she had to do. She knew that although to her the outdoor work of Allerbrook was hard, the Lanyons—Richard included—expected less of their womenfolk in that way than most of their neighbours did. Everyone helped with the harvest, but Lanyon women weren't expected to do the winnowing, which meant standing on an upland field in the wind, no matter how chilly it was, and tossing grain into the air. Nor did the Allerbrook women carry manure to the fields on their backs as Tilly and Martha Lowe, Anna Hannacombe and Lou Rixon did, but loaded the smelly stuff in panniers and took them out on the backs of the oxen.

Not that Lou Rixon would be carrying any more manure out to the fields, for she had left the district, taking her children and her aged mother with her. She had been in despair when she heard of Harry's death, having already found that she could not manage the farm with the two elderly hands who were left. She had, however, been offered a chance to marry a widowed farmer on the other side of the moor who had somehow avoided having his helpers taken away to the war, and she seized the opportunity.

"I've been thinking about the Rixons' farm," Peter said to Liza after Lou's departure. "I reckon we should take the place on and pay the rent to Walter Sweetwater."

"But we can't look after Allerbrook *and* Rixons, as well!"

"We won't," said Peter, grinning. "We sublet it and make it pay its own rent. The Rixons ran sheep and Lou's selling the flock. Your father knows every family on the moor that runs sheep. Somewhere there'll be a young couple wanting a place and willing to buy the flock and work like demons to see that it pays. And so it will."

"But why shouldn't this young couple of yours just pay rent to Walter Sweetwater? You'll have to, and if you're to make a profit, you'll need to charge them higher, won't you?"

"I might let them have Three-Corner Mead in the bargain. It's our smallest field and we never use it much, but it marches with Rixons. We can do without it and they can pay extra for it. It won't be a big profit, but it'll be one just the same."

At lambing time a year after Richard went away, the weather was unkind and some of the ewes had trouble. Peter had bought a new ram with a magnificent fleece but, unfortunately, a magnificent set of horns as well and a massive skull to support them. Some of his lambs were too big in the head to give their mothers an easy time.

Liza, taking part in this year's lambing, found that she had some instinctive skill. Her fingers were sensitive to the shapes and movements of lambs which had got themselves into awkward positions, or tangled up with their twins, inside the ewes. She could very often free a little leg that was caught up with one from another lamb, or feel a tiny hind hoof which had come forward too soon and guide it gently back so that the lamb could slide safely into the world.

But halfway through that lambing season she was overtaken with sickness, just as she had been at the pig killing, and messy as lambing could be, the reason was nothing to do with that. Once more, Betsy was asking questions and passing the answers to Peter, who said, "No more getting up in the night for you, my girl. We'll see to the ewes without you."

This time let it be a success. Liza was never sure what she thought about God, and had been less sure still since He'd taken Christopher away from her. It did not seem right to her that strong young men should give all the urges of nature away to this invisible deity, or what the said deity wanted with the said discarded urges when He'd got them.

"You didn't time this too well," Betsy said, poking up the brazier that heated Liza's bedchamber, making sure that the window was fast and trying to cheer Liza along with jovial talk. "Nearly Christmas, and who's to make the marchpane fancies, with you abed like this? And what weather! Just look at it out there!"

"Well, who can choose these things?" said Liza between gasps. The thick window glass didn't reveal much of the world outside, but she knew well enough what it looked like: smooth-backed hills covered in snow, with only the tops of banks and bushes showing here and there, and a sky the colour of lead. Beneath it, the white covering was as bleak as a shroud. Nearer at hand, rows of icicles hung from the eaves of the outhouses and the water trough was frozen like stone. More snow was on the way.

"If it's a boy," said Betsy, "you'd best call 'un Jack, for Jack Frost."

"If it's a girl, we'd better call her Jill, then," said Liza, and then cried out as another pain seized hold of her. "Maybe he or she's in a hurry!" she panted hopefully when the spasm had passed.

The child was not in a hurry. It was the evening of the next day when Liza's exhausted and anguished body surrendered its burden at last. "Just in time," Betsy muttered to Kat as she lifted the little thing away from the bed. "The mistress couldn't have stood much more."

"Is it breathing?" asked Kat. "Which is it?"

"A boy," said Betsy sombrely. "And he's not."

They did their best with warm towels and massage, but it was no use. Jack Lanyon had been dead before he left the womb.

"But he was formed, a proper boy child." Peter tried to hide his disappointment, and indeed, it wasn't so hard, because only a monster would have denied pity to such white-faced misery. "You went your full time with this one. The next one'll live. You'll see."

Liza, speechless, just nodded. There would be a next time; of course there would. A man like Peter couldn't live like a monk. There would be another time and then another and then another…

Or would there? Next time she might well die! She tried to stop them, but the tears squeezed themselves out of the corners of her eyes and ran down her temples onto her pillow. Peter looked at her in consternation. "Liza? Are you in pain?"

"No. Not much, not now."

"What is it, then? Liza, you mustn't grieve like this. There'll be another time." Liza shook her head from side to side and the tears came faster. Peter, frightened, strode to the door and shouted for Kat and Betsy.

They pounded up the stairs and arrived breathless. "What is it? Is the mistress worse?"

"She's upset. I can't comfort her. She'll make herself more ill than she is now!"

Betsy went to the bedside. "Now, what be all this, then? These things be the will of God, and there are more babes born than ever live to grow up—we all know that. Hush, now. Hush."

"I'm so tired," Liza sobbed. "I wish I could go home."

"She's wandering in her mind!" Peter burst out. "She *is* at home. You're here in Allerbrook, Liza. *This* is your home!"

Liza, speechless once again, closed her eyes but the tears went on oozing from under her eyelids.

"You'd best leave her now, Master Peter. Worn right out, she is. You're feelin' let down, but she's been let down more than you have, let me tell 'ee. If she don't feel this is her home, it's because she's got no living child here. Where she rears her family, that's the place a woman calls home. She needs her children. But like I said last time, she needs a rest first and it's for 'ee to see she gets it. Longer than last time. You know what I mean!"

"We're doing very well indeed," said Liza. She was sitting at the parlour table with a small abacus in front of her. On the table were several tally sticks and also a writing set consisting of ink, paper, quill and sander. Her father had not only taught her to keep accounts by double entry (which the Lanyons had never heard of until she joined them, but which Nicholas had said was invented by Venetian merchants, long ago), he had also taught her the modern Arabic figures, which had begun to seep out of the east in the days of the crusaders and were now making rapid headway. Peter still recorded weights of fleeces and pounds of cabbages and bushels of grain by cutting notches in tally sticks, but Liza would translate them into figures on paper and have them totted up on the abacus the very same day.

"The wheat's promising again," she said, "and the bit of extra rent that comes in from Three Corner Mead is very useful, and the wool we kept for ordinary sales to merchants' buyers has brought in more than it normally does. I wish our new ram didn't have such a heavy skull. That's lost us two lambs. But I fancy that when we get our share from the cloth making, it'll be a healthy one this year. If only the weather holds for the harvest."

July had brought hot weather. The window was open on a vista of ripening grain, peacefully grazing cows and blue-hazed hills, but the room was stuffy, all the more so because it was slightly cluttered. Liza had acquired a bigger loom and put it in the corner of the parlour, and beside it was a basket of carded wool and her spinning wheel. She spun and wove whenever she got the chance and the Lanyons had both yarn and cloth to sell at Dunster market.

Wool and hot weather didn't mix, however. The mere presence of wool in quantity seemed to create heat. Liza herself was wearing a thin undyed linen gown and had thrown her crimson overdress aside. She had woven the crimson material herself, from yarn so fine it was more like silk than wool, but it was still too hot in weather like this. Even the linen gown had a damp and crumpled air. She rubbed a hand over her wet forehead, failed to notice the ink on her fingers and left a dark smear across her brow.

Peter, who had just come in with some extra figures for her to include, from the sale of surplus hay, burst out laughing. "You look so funny! You have ink in your eyebrows!"

"Have I?" Liza rubbed again and made things worse. Peter laughed again and looked at the discarded overdress, which Liza had tossed over the back of a settle.

"Why were you wearing your best overdress in order to do the accounts?"

"Because it isn't my best any longer," said Liza. "I washed it, very gently, after the Easter party Anna Hannacombe gave, because there was a gravy stain on it, and now it's gone streaky. The dye didn't hold as it should. See?" She reached out to pick it up and Peter saw that in places its colour had faded to pale red with pinkish streaks.

"That's a pity. Who did the dyeing for you?"

"Herbert Dyer of Washford, Father's usual dyemaster. He used to be in Dunster, but he moved to Washford a year ago. He does a lot of work for the monks of Cleeve and says he likes to be near them, though in his last letter Father says he can't understand why because the Cleeve monks send their wool to Dunster for weaving and fulling anyway! Herbert Dyer does good work as a rule. I must have been unlucky. Father still uses him, though nowadays it means taking cloth and yarn to Washford. I'm making another overdress for best and I'll have it dyed green. This will do for everyday when it isn't too hot to wear it! How much did we get for the hay?"

She picked up her quill again, added in the amount that Peter gave her and studied her totals. "I think that when your father comes back, the amount of money in our coffer will please him."

"If he comes back at all," said Peter. "Where is he? There's been no news of him or anyone else from round here, for months. They should all be home by now. If any of them are still alive. I've heard," he added, "that Walter Sweetwater is ailing with worry over his father and his twin."

"News must come in the end," she said. "Surely it must. *Someone* will let us all know what's happened. Won't they?"

"Who's to say? We're a long way from the heart of things here. I've heard of men going off to war in times past, and no more was ever heard of them, and no word ever came back." He stopped, gazing past Liza as though into some imagined scene. She looked at him enquiringly.

There was a long silence, though it was friendly enough. Since the loss of poor little Jack, Peter had slept in his father's old room instead of with Liza and oddly enough, the absence of lovemaking seemed to have brought them closer as friends. She was relieved because she need not watch for signs of pregnancy, to dread the outcome if they appeared or dread, with equal force, Peter looking disappointed when they didn't. She and Peter talked to each other more easily than they had ever done before.

"What is it?" Liza asked at last.

"I'm making a fair success of being master of Allerbrook, I think," Peter said at length. "Aren't I?"

"Yes. You are. That's very true." Liza studied him gravely. "Oh, Peter, I don't want any harm to come to your father and I know you don't, either, but I rather dread the day he comes back and takes the reins away from you."

"So do I," said Peter glumly. "It's a dreadful thing to say, but so do I. Better not to think about it, Liza. Better not to talk about it, either."

"Then we won't," said Liza, and then became alert, cocking her head. "The dogs are barking. Someone must have ridden in…Peter!"

"What is it?"

Liza had risen and gone to the window that faced toward the yard. She turned to Peter, her eyes wide. "The day has come, anyway. It's your father," she said.

CHAPTER FIFTEEN 🌀

DEAD DRUNK ON A HALF-STARVED HORSE

S pringing up, Peter ran to join her. "He's still riding Splash! But why is he lurching in the saddle like that? He's sick or hurt!"

Together they made for the kitchen and the back door, shouting to Betsy and Kat, who were cleaning the dinner things, to come with them. As they all spilled out into the farmyard, Higg and Roger, who had been in the fields and had recognised Splash from a distance, rushed in to join them.

Richard was still sitting on Splash, who was standing still, head drooping. Except that his curious dark dapple coat was the same, the horse would have been unrecognisable, so gaunt had he become, with ribs and hips jutting. Richard too was as lean as a pole, burnt brown by wind and sun, and his clothes were patched and dusty. He had gone away with a crossbow slung on his back but must have lost it somewhere, although his father's helmet hung behind his saddle and he had acquired a sword.

"Father!" Peter gasped. "You're home…but what's wrong? Are you ill…wounded?"

"Neither. Jusht worn out," said Richard in slurred tones. He breathed out as he spoke. Liza and Peter exchanged quick glances and Richard emitted a short laugh. "Yesh, drunk as well. Shtopped at the White Hart in Clicket. Got some shider…cider. Had money. Picked up two sh…swords on the field at Towton. Sold the other. Walter Sweetwater gave me shome money, too. For bringing the news. No one else to do it."

They helped him down, and then Higg and Roger, one on each side of Splash's head as though he might fall down without their guidance, led the horse to the trough to drink while the others took Richard indoors.

Kat, eyeing his condition with disapproval, shook her head at him when he ordered her to bring cider, and said she'd brew a herb-and-honey posset. "More cider on top of what he's had already," she muttered under her breath to Liza, "or even a cup of my elderflower wine, and he'll drop unconscious. Wouldn't be surprised if he does that anyhow!"

"Shorry about this. No way for your father to come home, dead drunk on a half-starved horse," Richard said as Peter steered him to the parlour settle. "I've come from the north. I—we were with the queen. God'sh…God's elbow, is that what queensh are like? Winning, losing, going here, going there. Up to Shropshire, down to the Midlands, westward to Harlech, back east again to Yorkshire, shouth…south to attack London, back again north… zigzagging round the country like a bluebottle in a panic, and the thingsh she let happen!"

"Let me get your boots off," said Peter, kneeling to ease his father's feet free of their worn footwear, while Liza fetched some slippers and Betsy adjusted cushions behind Richard's back.

"I was ashamed, I tell you," Richard said as the slippers were put on his feet. "Queen She-Wolf and no mistake! Army wanted food—men just took it. Army wanted billets or horshes or wine, men took them. I did, too. Shtole…stole food, drink, fodder. Got to eat. Horse got to eat. I didn't rape any women, but some did. Anyone argued, he'd get his home and fields burned and a pike through his innards. Granaries emptied, fieldsh burned…no getting away, though. I was an archer with the Sweetwaters and deserters got hanged if they were caught. What'sh this muck?"

"Camomile and honey," said Kat firmly, presenting her posset. "That's what 'ee needs, after ridin' in that hot sun."

"We've seen to the horse," said Roger as he and Higg came in. "He'll be all right, given time and a few good feeds."

Richard was suddenly seized by aggression. "I hope sho. It'll take more than that to put me right!" His voice went up to a shout. "Bring me cider!" he bellowed and struck out, knocking the goblet from Kat's indignant hand.

"No cider, and none of my elderflower wine either. I'll brew 'ee another," she said, picking up the goblet. "Lucky this is pewter and not damaged," she added.

"You'll bring what you're told, woman!"

"Bring the elderflower wine," whispered Liza, "but water it."

This seemed to work. Richard growled but accepted the homemade wine in lieu of cider and didn't seem to notice that it was weak. More quietly, and more clearly, he said, "There were battles. I got through 'em all and so did the Sweetwaters, right till the end. It was in Yorkshire, Towton it was called. That's where the Yorkish…Yorkists did for us. The queen got away, went to Scotland, took her son—Prince Edouard, they call him, French-fashion—with her. We've got a King Edward now—so they shay…say."

"Yes," said Peter. "King Edward the Fourth. But there was no word of you, or Sir Humphrey Sweetwater or Reginald."

"No. They won't come back." Richard leaned back and closed his eyes for a moment. When he opened them again, he said, making a determined and obvious effort to speak clearly, "Sim Hannacombe's come home with me—Toby Searle, too. We were together—parted just outside Clicket. They couldn't face Walter Sweetwater. Us three, we're the only ones to come back. Sir Humphrey, Reginald, all the other men they took, they're dead and…Liza, I'm sh…sorry to carry bad news here as well, but five of your kinfolk went to war along with the Luttrells, and they won't come home, neither."

"Young Laurie?" Liza whispered. She had always liked Laurie, the son of her father's cousin Laurence and his prolific wife, Elena. Laurie and his own wife, Katy, had been a fond couple, both skilled at the yarn making which was the speciality of their side of the family and anxious to teach their trade to their own three children.

"Katy'll live on and find another, I daresay!" Richard snapped harshly. "What else *can* she do? Harry Rixon died early on and most of the others at this place Towton. Geoffrey Baker, too." His voice grew heavy and slurred again. "I shaw his body and Reginald Shweetwater's. They were on foot, not in heavy armour. Dear God, what a big axe can do to a man! I didn't know. Never 'magined. Horrible! Reginald…chopped near in half. Baker'sh head two yards from his body. I saw the Weavers, too, when I was getting away afterward. They was all together, in a heap. As for Sh…Sir Humphrey…"

He gulped at his drink and once more forced his speech to clear. "I used to want to murder all the Sweetwaters. Once said I'd like to see all their heads on chopping blocks. Don't feel like that now." He fell silent, apparently lost in some dreadful memory.

"What happened?" Peter asked at length.

"The Yorkist soldiers, they did Humphrey and Reginald in for me," Richard said, "and Walter Sweetwater can stay alive, far as I'm concerned. Death like that—it's shick…sickening. I didn't know! But someone had to tell Walter Sweetwater. See now why I want this wine? I went to Father Bernard first. They were in his flock, and it put off seeing Walter—only I didn't say much about Geoffrey Baker, just in case that old tale's true…."

"What tale?" asked Liza.

"Oh, you didn't know about that?" Betsy, with a sudden chuckle, interrupted. Richard didn't seem to mind, but closed his eyes again. "Geoffrey Baker's mother—Annet her name was—was widowed young, went to work as housekeeper to Father Bernard, and there was talk. Then all of a sudden she says yes to Jimmy the Baker, who'd been askin' her for months and bein' stood off, on account of he got hisself done for putting chalk in his bread flour the year before."

"Probably true, too." Richard's eyes opened again. "Too well dressed for a baker. Made more money than he should by the look of him."

"Jimmy got away with it for a long while," Betsy said, "but in the end he went too far, put too much chalk in and folk could taste something wrong. Harry Rixon's dad was parish constable then, and had Jimmy marched through the village with a loaf of chalky bread hung round his neck and put him in the stocks for half a day. Annet said he was no man for her. But all of a sudden she changes her mind, and less'n eight month later she tripped over a step goin' into her house and Geoffrey was born. Who's to say? He didn't look like either Father Bernard or Jimmy, but that's the tale."

"Father Bernard believes it, I reckon," Richard said. "Turned the colour of old cheese when I told him Baker was dead, and I didn't say about his head being cut off, even. I think I hoped he'd go to the Sweetwaters for me, but he looked so stricken...couldn't ask him to. I had to be the one. Not pleasant, bringing news like that to a man's son, a man's brother, even Sweetwaters! Walter's wife and youngsters were there, too. The boy Baldwin's an arrogant brat, but he's only about thirteen and his sister Agnes is younger. She was there, with her mother. She's pretty...."

He paused, plainly unwilling to come to the point of Sir Humphrey's death. Then he said, "Mary Sweetwater and Agnes both cried, hearing the news. They're decent enough women-folk, I suppose. Baldwin just went white. Cocky, like I said, but I pitied him then. Didn't tell them all of it. Couldn't. Must tell someone, though."

They were listening intently now, and in silence. Richard braced himself. "Sir Humphrey, he was up on a great big charger, in full armour. Horse was killed and he tried to run. Can't run fast wearing a lot of iron plates. Pack of Yorkist infantry caught him. Knocked him over, took his armour off. Hardly took 'em a minute—they knew how to do it—then one of them shtuck... stuck...a sh...sword in his guts and...and dragged it...he screamed and screamed. Like drawing a pig but not killing it first. I saw his insidesh spilling out...."

"Oh, no. Oh, don't!" Liza was appalled. Kat stood with a hand clamped over her mouth. But Richard had begun at last to empty the horror out of himself and now couldn't stop. His voice grew slurred again as he remembered. "Shaw…saw…his legs jerking about and the blood shoot up. I wash…was…hiding in a ditch, quite near. Didn't see the finish. Cowered down, let the long grass droop over me. Couldn't help him. Eight or nine of them, there were. Told his family he died quick. Thass what you have to shay. Everyone sh…says it, breaking news like that. Shometimes it's true. Sh…sometimes not."

Liza was trembling. Betsy had an arm around her. "Master Walter looked sht…stunned when I told him his father and his twin wouldn't be coming back," Richard said. He tried to steady his voice again. "Messengers bringing bad news aren't welcome mostly, but he was polite—I'll shay that for him. Paid me for my trouble. Gave me a drink and I gave him back the dagger his father lent me. Me and Sim and Toby, we've been monthsh…months— three or more—getting home from the north. Didn't have much money then—everything'd been in a muddle for so long; Sweetwaters couldn't pay us. Toby got sick on the way, too. We had to stop. Sold the spare sword to buy food—didn't like shtealing, but some places, where we'd passed through before, there weren't much left to buy *or* steal! Folk were trying to get back on their feet. Twice we stopped to help on farms where there was some provender going, got our keep and a bit more to take with us, moved on. That way I could keep shome of the money I got for the sword. Slow journey…dead shlow…"

He fell silent again and seemed about to fall asleep, but roused himself. "Give me your arm upstairs, Peter. I'm giddy and I want my bed."

Liza's stomach turned over and she saw Peter gnaw his lip, but Richard was already getting shakily to his feet. There was nothing Peter could do but help him up the stairs. Liza watched them go, hoping that Richard was too fuddled to notice that someone had been using his room, and that while he lay asleep, Peter could tiptoe around him and remove his own belongings.

It didn't work. Even when drunk and dazed with sleepiness, Richard was still remarkably observant. Liza, waiting nervously downstairs, flinched when she heard the roar of rage.

"What's this here, boy? Looks like one of your jerkins! You been using this room while I've been gone?" Then heavy footsteps—under the influence of fury, Richard had evidently recovered his sense of balance—and a door banging and another roar. "But Liza's still in here, seemingly! Ain't you two been shleeping together?"

She heard Peter's voice, quieter, trying to explain. A word or two reached her. "…last December…nightmare business…born dead…Betsy said…"

"To hell with Betsy, interfering old cow! You get your things and get back where you belong and do your duty and see Liza does hers! Fine sort of a stud you make, boy! Bad enough she's made a pig'sh ear of it again and again, but if you're not even trying…should have let you wed that Marion! Wager she'd have had a baby nine months after the wedding!"

Peter was annoyed enough to raise his voice in answer and the reply came clearly down the stairs. "I daresay Liza can hear you, Father. Just as well that she knows about Marion…."

Richard rumbled something, on a questioning note.

"Yes, I told her myself! And I'm damn glad I didn't marry Marion. Maybe she *would* have had a baby straightaway, and I'd never have been sure it wasn't fathered by a Norwegian sailor off a ship called *Fjord-Elk!*"

Betsy and Kat came to stand beside Liza at the foot of the stairs. "Now, don't 'ee worry," said Betsy, while Roger, embarrassment written all over his lined face, scurried out of sight. Higg stood where he was, shaking his head in concern. "Master'll calm down after a sleep," said Betsy, "and as for the other, well, a man needs his wife. Nice rest 'ee've had. Likely enough everything'll go right next time."

"I've one piece of good news for you." Peter's voice drifted down the stairs.

"Have you indeed?" Richard barked. "And what might that be?"

"Money. We're doing well and Liza's got more to offer than you think. You need new clothes and she's weaving cloth now, from our own wool and she'll see to it without paying a tailor—not that we couldn't pay a dozen tailors if we wanted. You wait till you see inside our coffer!"

"Really? Bloody good news, boy, given you and she provide us all with somebody to leave it to!"

"*Oh!*" said Liza in a desperate voice. Betsy put an arm around her. "Crying's no use," Liza said. "I know that. But just what does he think I can *do* about it?"

The Lanyons were not the only ones to receive news that day.

"My lady," said the gatekeeper's boy—a younger one this time, since the youth who had once announced the arrival of Nicholas Weaver had followed Sir James Luttrell to join Queen Marguerite's army—"my lady…there's a man to see you. He's got a string of knights with him."

Lady Elizabeth Luttrell knew that already. She had been in the grounds, not doing anything in particular, just roaming here and there and thinking about the past. Her son, Hugh, was at his studies. Her husband, James, Sir James, knighted at the end of the previous year after distinguishing himself in the service of the Lancastrians, had enjoyed his knighthood for seven weeks and then died in his next battle.

She was still struggling to grasp the two great changes in her life—the fact that she was now Lady Elizabeth Luttrell and the fact that she was also a widow. She had had no say in her husband's choice of allegiance, but she knew enough about the kind of passions which swayed both York and Lancaster to be afraid.

Then she heard the horsemen arrive, hooves clattering and striking sparks from the cobbles of the steep road up from the village to the gatehouse. She hastened to the walls, to a place from which she could see what the visitors looked like. One glance at the standard-bearer who led the way was enough to tell her that her fears were justified. The new king himself wasn't likely to be calling upon her in person, but his representative most definitely was. The standard displayed the badge of York, the spectacular Sun in Splendour.

She made for the hall to take her seat on her dais, the lady of the castle in her own kind of splendour, ready to receive defeat and dismissal with dignity.

Her visitors marched in, clanking as they came, since they were all in armour, with swords at their sides and spurs on their heels. Their leader gave her his name and rank, which was high, but somehow she was never afterward able to remember who he was. It didn't matter. It was what he said that was important.

"By order of King Edward, fourth of that name, the estates of the late Sir James Luttrell are forfeit to the crown. They will be granted to those who have shown loyalty to the house of York during the past few years."

"You are disinheriting my son?" said Lady Elizabeth.

"His father disinherited him, my lady. Blame him, if you wish to blame anyone."

"Frankly," said Lady Elizabeth, sitting very still and keeping her voice very calm, "I blame this new king, who takes vengeance on a young boy who has done him no harm and is not responsible for the actions of his father. Is that justice?"

"You have a right to your opinion, my lady. It makes no difference. You are required, forthwith, to pack your belongings, take your maid, your chaplain and one manservant and your son's tutor if he has one…"

"Father Meadowes tutors him."

"All the better. You and the boy and three companions, then. You must leave this castle. You may take horses for your son and the two men. You and your maid must travel pillion. You may take a pack pony."

"One pack pony only? There will be clothes, plate…."

"No plate or valuables beyond a little personal jewellery are to be taken. What you can't put in saddlebags or on the pony, you must abandon."

He looked with dislike at the woman sitting in the carved chair on the dais. She was more slender and softer of feature than Queen Marguerite, but reminded him of Marguerite all the same. She had the same knack of leaning regally back in her chair, with her forearms resting on the chair arms and her hanging sleeves sweeping the floor. Marguerite always had a thronelike chair, complete with arms and high pointed back, in her baggage so that she could hold court impressively wherever she chanced to be, even in the middle of a field. Lady Elizabeth looked as though she were holding court now.

He did not know that behind the dignified facade Lady Elizabeth Luttrell felt as though her inside were weighted with lead, and was holding back tears of longing for her husband, wondering tormentedly whether he had suffered much before he died, and making such an effort to hide her feelings that her body was rigid from crown to toes.

After a silent moment, however, something of the anguish in her still figure communicated itself to him, and more civilly he said, "You have somewhere to go? Kinfolk?"

"Yes. I have kinfolk."

"Good. You have today to prepare. You must leave tomorrow."

Edward Searle, his shepherd's crook in his hand and Drover, his black-and-white dog, at his heels, strode down the path from the moor where the Sweetwater flock was grazing, toward the home farm where three ewes he had recently bought for Walter Sweetwater were in a field along with their lambs. He would introduce them to the flock on the moor in a few days' time. A good year, except...

At the gate of the field he found Walter, standing with one foot on the lowest rung of the gate and resting his elbows on top. He was staring at the ewes and their frisking offspring, but not as though he was really seeing them. Searle moved quietly alongside him and also leaned on the gate.

After a while Walter said, "My father and my brother, both

gone. And from what I hear, it could be my home as well, when the Yorkist king gets round to it. I have my son, at least. Thank the saints that we all agreed Baldwin was too young to go to war. But what will happen to his inheritance, God only knows. You may have to work for a new master, Edward."

"Aye. It's a strange new world we're living in," said Searle.

As a boy, Walter had made friends with the shepherd, who was only eight years older than he was, but then they had talked only about sheep. Now, however, their conversation moved as smoothly into the sphere of power politics as though they had met there in the first place.

"Seems to me," said Searle, "that it's nothing to most of us whether it's York or Lancaster sits on that old throne in London. All we want's a bit of peace to get on with things as matter, like shearing and reaping and all of that. Pity they can't settle their squabbles without dragging us into 'em."

"It seems that they can't. My father and brother were dragged in and now see what's happened. They fought for Lancaster but York won, and this Edward of York is vengeful. He even wants revenge on the dead."

"If I were you," said the gaunt man at Walter's side, gazing straight ahead, blue farseeing eyes fixed on the distant outline of Dunkery Beacon, "I'd get in first. You'll know who to tell. I wouldn't, but you do, likely enough. Tell 'un you never went with your father and brother because you didn't agree with 'un. Say you're Yorkist and offer to…what's the way you folk put it? Swear your fealty. Offer 'un your sword for the future. See what happens."

"Hmm," said Walter. The ache of bereavement did not ease, because only time would ever relieve that, but the despair which had settled on him as word got out concerning the way the York-ists intended to treat those who had upheld the enemy thinned a little. "I've not much to lose, when all's said and done."

At breakfast on his first morning at home, Richard was silent and Liza found herself eyeing him nervously, but he seemed pre-occupied rather than angry. After the meal, he went out with Peter to ride around the farm. Peter came back ahead of him and walked into the parlour where Liza was weaving. His mouth was tight. Liza glanced at him and stopped her shuttle. "Peter? What is it?"

"My father," said Peter, "ought by rights to be lying in bed with a wondrous hangover. Instead, he's out on the land finding fault with every decision I've taken while he's been away—my God, I've made Allerbrook prosperous and not a word of real thanks has he uttered! I tell him our coffers are full and all he says is *bloody good news, boy, given you provide somebody to leave it to!* Sometimes I think that if he calls me *boy* again, I'll…I'll…*burst!* And now he's having revelations!"

"*Revelations?* Whatever do you mean?"

Peter rolled his eyes heavenward and cast himself into a settle. "I left him outside that old cottage—the empty one he thought of giving to us at one time. He has plans for it now. The sight of it has inspired him. After what he saw during the fighting, es-pecially at Towton, he no longer wants to see all the Sweetwa-ters dead, and anyway, two of them already are! But that doesn't mean he likes them. He's pleased that Walter's given us permis-sion to grow wheat on Quillet and fence it round so that he can't ride across it, but why, Father wants to know, should we need his permission or have to be grateful because he won't be tram-pling it down anymore? Walter, he says, has just as much conceit of himself as his father and brother—he just shows it differently. And as for what happened at my grandfather's funeral, and to Father's friend, poor Deb Archer—you know about her?"

"Yes, you told me long ago."

"Well, for her, he'll never forgive any of them. Trampling our wheat was nothing by comparison."

"They can't have meant any harm to Mistress Archer," said Liza. "That was just misfortune."

"He says it doesn't matter, that it was their fault and that's that and he's going to get the better of them for it. Not by killing them, no, not now. He's thought of another way. We're going to prove ourselves as good as they are. We're going to rise in the world. He said aloud, the day they rode across the wheat field, that one day they'd take off their caps when they saw *us* coming! He's been brooding over ways and means ever since, apparently, and now he's made up his mind. The first step, he tells me, is to build ourselves a fine house. Folk judge a man by the house he lives in."

"But we can't afford—"

"No, we can't afford to do it all at once, he says, but we can make a start, and to begin with, that old cottage is built of very good stone. It was looking at that cottage that gave him the idea. He wants to knock it down and use the stone, along with some more that he'll have to buy—saying thank you chokes him but I think he's a *little* bit grateful to us for tending our finances so well—and build a new wing for the farmhouse."

"But we don't need a new wing!" Liza protested.

"You try telling him that. It'll contain a hall, a proper dining hall like the one the Sweetwaters have. And one day he'll build on more rooms so that the hall will be part of the splendid new house he's inventing inside his head. He's as excited as a child going to a fair for the first time. Walter Sweetwater's going to hate this, he says, but we're not asking permission, and though the Sweetwaters ride across our land as if they owned it—"

"They do own it," said Liza reasonably.

"—they don't come right to the house or ride into the farmyard and with luck, the wing'll be finished and ready before they realise it's there. It'll cost the earth. We'll be begging alms from the parish by then, if you ask me," said Peter bitterly.

CHAPTER SIXTEEN

HOUSEWARMING

"Beginning to look like something, that is," Richard Lanyon, feet astride and hands on hips, said to Peter as they surveyed the new wing of the farmhouse. One day, as he had told his disapproving son, he hoped it would form part of a much bigger house, but this would do as a first step and as far as it went, it pleased him.

His satisfaction wasn't total, because Liza never these days bulged around the middle and was never sick at a pig killing. Nagging her was useless—he'd grasped that, and he couldn't help liking her, but his disappointment was still there. Betsy said it was the will of God. Richard would have liked a few words with God.

Peter found no satisfaction in the building work at all. "This new wing, it's got hold of him like a disease," he had complained to Liza, back in the early days of the work. "And according to him, this is just the start. And it's all because he wants to make a show in front of the Sweetwaters. Even if Walter Sweet-water does ride round with his nose in the air as though he were a lord of creation, what of it? He's less trouble than his father was!"

To Richard, that made no difference. Walter had been in that hunting party which had disturbed George's funeral and led to Deb Archer's death, and if Deb had lived, dear Deb, who had meant more to him than he knew until she was gone, perhaps he himself would not have become entangled with Marion and doomed to a lifetime of guilt. Only, that was not something that could be told to anyone. Ever.

"Well," Liza had said, "we'll have to help *your* father, whatever he does, to keep him happy. Life's easier that way."

She and Peter had been out in the yard during that conversation, watching while Richard prowled around the site, making sure that the masons were following their instructions properly. She had spoken distractedly, because something about that late October, the feel of the autumn weather, the look of the drifting clouds and the way their shadows moved across the hillsides had reminded her unexpectedly of the day she and Christopher had tried to run away together.

She had had no idea what kind of life lay ahead for the two of them, but she had believed that it would be a life with Christopher, and not with Peter and Allerbrook. But here she was, and it looked as though she always would be, but somehow or other, to her surprise, she wasn't miserable. Christopher's memory was always there, but the commonplace happiness of day-to-day living had come to lie over it, like a warm coverlet over tired limbs. She sometimes thought that it wasn't so much a matter of missing Christopher as missing her own longing for him. She didn't long for him much now. It felt like disloyalty, but it was true. She had too many other things to do, for one thing.

And one of the things she had to do was keep her father-in-law in a good temper as far as she could. Her husband, and for this she was grateful, had not blamed her for failing to produce the much-wanted family, but she knew very well that it was always in Richard's mind, a provocation ready to break out into temper at any moment.

She would be wise to be as helpful as possible over this unnecessary new wing. Anything, as long as it kept Richard Lanyon sweet.

As time went on, she discovered that she actually had a knack for good ideas. Richard admitted as much, and thanked her for them quite graciously. There was plenty of time to discuss her suggestions and put them into effect, because building the new wing took much longer than anyone expected. It was five years from the beginning to the day when Richard planted himself in front of it, put his fists on his hips and said that it looked like something now.

After studying the ground, Richard had settled that the new building should extend from the old farmhouse at right angles, along the side of the farmyard closest to the hill above. The farmyard sloped a little, and the new wing should stand at the higher, drier end. There was ample room, as the ground flattened out just there, extending back some way before the hill soared up again. The new wing, being a little higher than the rest of the house, was linked to it inside by a short flight of steps. It contained a single high-roofed hall, over thirty feet long, which as far as Richard could reckon from memory was longer than the one inside Sweetwater House.

The stone from the demolished cottage was pinkish-grey like

that of the farmhouse, which was as well, for Richard had decreed that the new wing and the old house must match. This, however, concerned more than just the colour of the stone. In George Lanyon's time the door to the dairy had been widened, revealing that the farmhouse walls were actually double, the space between being filled in with rubble. Richard could remember looking at it.

The new wing must be exactly the same, he said, which meant that after the hired workmen had dug out the foundations, rubble and extra stone had to be bought and fetched over the moor from a quarry six miles away.

Wheeled vehicles were of so little use on the moor that no one bothered with them as a rule. Stone could hardly be moved any other way, but it was half a century at least since any new building had been done locally and Richard's ox-drawn waggons therefore aroused great interest, not to say hilarity.

It was summer at the time, but the waggons still managed to get bogged down in muddy patches and wedged in narrow sunken tracks. On steep uphill stretches, loads had to be brought up piecemeal, which was slow, and one waggon lost a wheel while crossing the ford two hundred yards below Walter Sweet-water's packhorse bridge, the bridge itself being too narrow for any kind of cart. The vehicle had to be unloaded and hauled onto the bank and a wheelwright fetched from Taunton to repair it. After that the stone had to be loaded once again. It meant two days' delay and the farmer who accommodated the oxen in a field meanwhile cheerfully charged for the grass they ate as though (complained Richard) it had been best-quality oats. "As if I haven't had expense enough, buying stone and hiring the waggons and extra oxen, the loads being so heavy," he grumbled.

"Aye, the stone's heavy," Peter growled to Liza. "Which is more than you can say for our coffers nowadays!"

Once the shell of the building was in place, the next stage involved oak timbers for the roof beams, and slates for the roof itself. "Won't thatch do?" said Peter, but Richard would have none of it. "Good modern slate, that's what I want, boy!" he declared. "And planks for the floor. A thatched roof and floors of cobbles and earth are good enough for the old house, but not for this."

Work stopped once the walls, roof and floor were in place, because at that point the money ran out altogether. The next stage had to wait for a year, while the Lanyon coffers were replenished.

It was Liza (if only she functioned as well below the belt as she did above the neck, Richard thought but had the consideration not to say) who pointed out that if they were to eat meals in the new hall, then the kitchen ought to be next to it. Was food to be carried from the existing one at the other end of the old house, either through the rooms or across the farmyard when dinner was to be eaten?

"We shall just end up doing all our eating in the kitchen," she said.

"We do that now," Peter pointed out.

"But I don't want us to go on doing it," Richard snapped. "I want us to eat in the hall. Liza, what's in your mind?"

"Well, we won't just eat in the hall, surely, Father-in-law? Won't it be our place for living, whenever we're indoors? Like the big living room is now? We'll want to use it, enjoy it, won't we?"

"Yes, of course. Go on."

"Our cider press room is at the end of the house that joins the new wing. It's at the front. Why not turn it into a dairy, and make most of the present main living room into a kitchen and larder? The rest of the main room and the present dairy can all be knocked into one and if you agree, I can put my spinning wheel and loom in there and my accounts table and make a really good workroom of it. Then the parlour can be a proper parlour again. In case any ladies ever come to call! Any house of standing should have a good parlour, but I've fairly ruined ours, with my baskets of wool and my ledgers and all the rest."

"Where's the cider press to go, then?"

"Where the old kitchen is now. The new hall will still only need two doors—one into the farmhouse, and now it can lead straight into the new kitchen, and one into the farmyard."

"It's going to mean more trouble and more expense," said Peter.

"It's a good idea, though," said Richard, and went ahead with it.

It did indeed mean trouble and expense, and on top of all that, Richard insisted on glazing for the windows. This meant another delay while yet more funds were gathered. The glazing was made in Taunton and delivered with each window entire, wrapped in fleeces and roped on pack ponies, which could use packhorse bridges. But there were still places where streams had to be forded, and fords could mean trouble for ponies as well as waggons. Early in one journey a pony lost its footing while crossing a stream and fell. That was the end of one whole window. It had to be made again and transported again.

Peter, this time, said outright to his father that if only Richard didn't dislike the Sweetwaters so much, the new wing need never have been built and think of all the money they'd have saved. Richard retorted that he was just sorry that the new king hadn't thrown Walter Sweetwater off his land.

Walter was still on his land because he was a sprat compared to the Luttrells, who were much bigger fish. Sir Humphrey's title had not been hereditary and Walter had never been knighted. He was still only plain Master Sweetwater, a fact that in itself made him unimportant in royal eyes.

Before the king's clerks had worked their way far enough down their list of possible victims to reach Walter Sweetwater, Walter had reached the royal secretariat with a respectful message of submission, willingness to uphold the house of York henceforth, with his sword if need be, and the offer of a healthy fine in return for being left where he was.

King Edward was not particularly anxious to snatch a manor of Clicket's modest proportions. He accepted the fealty and the fine. Walter was left hard up and cursing, but still in possession of his property, and he even managed to negotiate a marriage for Baldwin, which would bring four farms, scattered around Devon, into Sweetwater hands.

After the fiasco with the glass, however, the Lanyons were hard up, too. There was another wait, another shearing and another payment from the Weaver profits before any furniture or panelling could be installed. Panelling was essential, Richard said, and so was a big new table with benches to go around it, plus a high-backed chair for him to use at the head of the table, and so, too, were three lidded chests-cum-settles, with lift-up seats and storage beneath, to go into the window nooks. The Lanyon coffers just barely succeeded in paying the Clicket carpenter.

"Well now," said Richard, turning to his son and daughter-in-law, when at last, after five stop-and-go years, the work was finished. "What about a housewarming?"

"Do we invite the Sweetwaters?" Liza asked, but Richard shook his head.

"Not yet! Not just for this. One day…but that's far ahead. This time," said Richard, "just our friends. There's a long way to go before we bid the Sweetwaters to dine."

"Richard Lanyon's invited us to a feast," Margaret said. "Because of this new hall he's added to the farmhouse. Will you feel up to going?"

"I'd like to," said Nicholas. "Only…"

His decline had started, Margaret thought, at the time of Liza's marriage, though the death of five family members during the recent fighting had assuredly made things worse. He had mourned especially for Laurie, of whom he had been very fond, literally mingling his tears with those of Laurie's wife, Katy, because when she heard of her husband's death, she had cried in his arms.

But Katy had left the household now, having married a saddler who had a workshop in West Street, at the other end of Dunster. He was a widower, much older than herself. His own children were grown and gone and as he hadn't wanted to take on her two boys, though he didn't mind her little daughter, the boys were still with the Weavers, learning to work looms. They were welcome, since so many pairs of hands had been lost, but Katy's departure had been another blow to Nicholas, who had had a tenderness for her.

But Liza's behaviour had begun the damage, of that Margaret had no doubt. "I feel betrayed," he said to her, not once but frequently. "If she'd fallen for a proper fellow, with a proper future, I'd have listened to what she wanted, but to lose her head over a half-fledged priest—and then to bolt with him! I never would have believed it of her, never, and what I had to do to her, it went to my heart, Margaret."

He had worried about it, wrinkled his brow over it, stayed awake at nights over it. Margaret tried to distract him by pointing out how well the business was doing, which it was. Despite the dividends that had to be paid out to the Lanyons, the union between the families was working. The Lanyon fleeces were so good these days that they were set aside for the manufacture of a particularly light, warm cloth, much of which was dyed red and yellow, because Master Herbert Dyer, whose competitive rates had so pleased Nicholas, specialised in those shades.

Herbert Dyer seemed to be a restless man, since he had come to Dunster from Taunton and then moved on to the village of Washford. Nicholas was not the only one to wonder why, and a member of the local Dyers' Guild, which watched over standards of work in Dunster, had been heard to say that he'd heard a thing or two from the Dyers' Guild in Taunton. "It's been hinted that he cut prices for favoured customers by charging others too much and that all his work wasn't good. Could be that a few folk in Dunster have started noticing things," he said. "We've had no formal complaints, but I've a feeling we might have started enquiring if he'd stayed. Well, he's someone else's problem now."

Nicholas, however, had no complaint of him and he was a large, genial soul who visited the Weavers quite often and made cheerful conversation. Margaret, who liked him, was grateful for it. After one of his visits, Nicholas always seemed more like his old self.

The effect never lasted, though. Gradually Nicholas's hair had changed completely from flaxen to grey and he had begun to lose weight and complain, at times, of odd pains. Margaret, worrying about him, tried to encourage him to take life quietly, but he preferred to go on attending to his business, and still tried to fill his normal place in the family.

"It's just that I get tired the way I never used to, and Aller-brook's such a long ride away," he said as they lay in bed the night after the arrival of the invitation. "It's good of Lanyon to ask us, considering."

"Considering what?" Margaret asked. "They don't know about Christopher Clerk."

"Considering that there's been no child. Richard Lanyon wanted grandchildren. I know that."

"It could still happen. Cecy went four years once with nothing—after she had such a time with that first little girl and then that string of miscarriages—and then, all of a sudden, there was another little girl."

"Girls won't please Richard Lanyon either," Nicholas said. "Though he ought to be grateful for anything by this time! How long have they been wed? Getting for eight years come November, surely? I often fret about her, wondering whether we did right, pushin' the marriage on like that, and not givin' her more time. Still, she and Peter seem to get on, what I've seen of them. I wish we could see her more often, but there's hardly ever time for ridin' out all that way and I reckon it's the same for her. Women on farms always have work to do. I've decided, Margaret. We'll go."

The work on the new wing had been finished in early August, before the corn harvest but comfortably after the haymaking and the shearing. It was a convenient time for a feast. The weather was sultry, however, and Kat and Betsy, working with the kitchen door wide open, grumbled as they swatted flies, trapped wasps in a bowl of honey and water, and sweated over the creation of rabbit pie and a mighty pan of custard. However, by the previous evening, most of the work was done; all that remained was to roast the chickens and the saddle of mutton next day. The household retired early.

That night, Richard slept badly. The heat plagued him, forcing him to leave the window wide so that gnats came whining into the room, looking for blood, and the light of a full moon streamed in with them. When at last he fell asleep, he was again on Castle Rock, in swirling mist, and Marion Locke was there. As in real life, he had hold of her, but this time she didn't struggle against him but laughed in his face and made him angry and he threw her from him.

She fell backward through the vapours and then she was gone and only her scream remained, echoing in his ears, jerking him awake, except that he wasn't awake but had only been jolted into another layer of dreams. He was in his bed, but he was lying in a shaft of moonlight that held him down, like a mouse under the paw of a cat, and he knew it was holding him there so that Marion could come back and find him. In the mysterious way of dreams, he was in two places at once, both on his bed and staring down from Castle Rock at what, this time, was a clearly visible moonlit sea, from which Marion, white as bone, was rising toward him, coming for him, fingers curved as if to strangle him, with droplets of moonlit water falling from her fingertips.

He tried to call Deb's name, but his voice wouldn't work and Deb didn't come. Then he was really awake, heart pounding and sweat pouring off his body, but safe in his bed, though he was indeed lying in the moonlight. He got up and went to the window. The world lay hushed and still, a vista of shadows and whiteness, blanched corn, dark moorland marching against a silvered sky. Castle Rock was far away. Yet what would that matter to a ghost? It would be easy to believe that Marion's pallid shade was travelling toward him, floating over moor and peat stream, farm and woodland, just as birds did, searching for the man who had killed her.

He went back to bed and lay facedown, shuddering, waiting for the sanity of dawn.

It was a good gathering, even if everyone who accepted the invitation hadn't done so out of admiration for the new wing, or affection for the Lanyons, as the Lanyons would have known, had they been in the White Hart tavern in Clicket the previous evening.

"Can't think who he thinks he is, buildin' a great hall, as if he were a Sweetwater," said Sim Hannacombe.

"Vyin' with them, that's what he's up to," said Gilbert Lowe, spluttering slightly through his yellowed stumps of teeth. "'Member when they knocked his dad's coffin into the Allerbrook?"

He then added (because Gilbert always considered that his own personal grievances were the most interesting topics imaginable, and was skilled at twisting any conversation around to them) that it was a pity some folk couldn't stop where God had put them.

"That girl of mine, Martha, thirty-four she is now and you'd think she'd be past any girlish nonsense, but do you know, she went and took a shine this year to a travelling minstrel that stayed over one night with us! He hung round the district awhile and she took to slippin' off to meet him! Tilly followed her one day and found them having a cuddle, of all places, in St. Anne's Church, here in Clicket. We soon had her home and made her understand she'd got to stop there. Would you believe it!"

"Yes. Sounds natural to me. You should have got her wed years ago," said Sim disapprovingly.

"We need her at home and there she'm stayin'," retorted Gilbert.

"I daresay. Does the work of three, don't she?" said Sim.

"What's this about a coffin being knocked into the Aller-brook?" Young Will Hudd, who was now the tenant of what was still called Rixons, hadn't heard the story and thought it sounded more intriguing than the details of Martha Lowe's shattered romance. Information was duly supplied from several willing sources, including Edward Searle, who, along with Toby, often called in for a tankard of ale.

"I was at George Lanyon's funeral," Edward said. "I'd have offered to be a bearer, only I'm taller than most and I'd have unbalanced it. It was bad enough with Roger and Higg being different heights!"

"Then the hunt came by and unbalanced it well and truly," said Toby, amid laughter.

"If you ask me," said Adam Turner, who was the landlord of the White Hart and responsible for its name, which was in honour of an albino deer that had appeared in the locality twenty years ago, "the Lanyons have always thought they were above the rest of us, or ought to be. George Lanyon, he sent Richard to school and Richard sent Peter, and because they can read and write, they think they're special. Why, even Liza Lanyon can read and write and how many women can do that? But I wouldn't go challengin' the Sweetwaters—no, I would not. Do that to the gentry and you get trodden on, soon or late."

Turner, unlike most of his customers, was an indoor man, as his pale complexion and his stringy build clearly showed. He was a morose individual and none too fond of his fellow men. He wasn't even particularly fond of his own wares. His long nose had no red tip or broken veins. He was a good businessman, however, and the White Hart provided him with a steady living.

"I've been invited," he remarked. "But an innkeeper can't go gaddin' here and there, though I doubt I'll get much trade tomorrow. You'll all be drinkin' for free at Allerbrook."

"Don't grudge us a free mouthful of cider for once, Adam." The Clicket carpenter had joined the crowd, his day's work over.

"You've made more'n enough out of they Lanyons, what with panelling and furniture," said Turner glumly, and everyone laughed again.

Nicholas and Margaret were the first to arrive next day, having stayed a night with friends in the village of Winsford, which was on their way. "It made the journey shorter for Nicholas," Margaret explained as they were getting out of their saddles in the farmyard.

"I can't ride any distance nowadays," Nicholas explained, "and it's that hot and sticky. Thunder soon, I'd say."

Others presented themselves within the next hour or two: the Hannacombes, the Lowes, the Hudds, a number of villagers and Father Bernard. Betsy and Kat strove in the kitchen, mopping wet brows as they turned the chickens and the mutton on the spit, prepared sauces and sharpened carving knives. There was no breeze and the sky was beginning to dim from blue to a curious shade of bronze.

Liza and Peter put finishing touches to the new hall, decorating it with garlands of wildflowers made by Liza, spreading the table with white cloths and setting it with bowls and platters, spoons, ladles and an elaborate silver salt, a marvel of little salt and pepper pots and tiny engraved spice trays, which Ned Crowham had sent.

The Crowhams couldn't come, but this, said the letter their

messenger had brought along with the salt, might make up for that. It was the most handsome piece of tableware that Liza had ever seen. They had plenty of tableware otherwise; harvest suppers were always big occasions with most of the parish there, and the Lanyons were proud of the fact that they had ample spoons and dishes and didn't have to ask people to bring extra.

Shortly after midday the feast was under way and Richard, seated with dignity in his high-backed chair at the head of the table, with Peter and Liza one on each side of him, regarded the scene with complacency. They had got it right. He had thought of having a dais for the family, but both Peter and Liza had objected, saying that it would cut them off from the others, on days when everyone ate together.

"I wouldn't be easy," Liza had said. "I'd feel uncomfortable." And Peter had added that even if the dais were there, he probably wouldn't be able to bring himself to sit on it.

For a moment Richard had been angry and inclined to tell the pair of them that they'd do as he told them and like it, but realised in time that at heart he didn't want to cut himself off from Higg and Roger and Betsy and Kat, either. For one thing, farm-house meals were opportunities for useful conversation. *Should we slaughter that cow that isn't giving good milk anymore? When do we decide to cut the hay? The bay pony's had colic again—how much root ginger have we got? The rain's getting in at the corner of the big barn— better see to it, Higg.*

Decidedly, it was better to keep the household together, maintain normal farmhouse life but with a bit of extra dignity. Liza was admirably dignified, in a long green linen gown with hanging sleeves. It could have come from the finest dressmaker in Taunton, but hadn't, because Liza had bought the undyed linen, had it dyed to her own choice of colour, made the dress and embroidered it herself. She'd chosen green, she said, because crimson always seemed to run in the wash and she'd had much the same trouble with a tawny-yellow gown, too.

The green didn't suit her as well as the warmer shades, but she still looked handsome in it. She could have had silk for best; he and Peter wouldn't have minded. She'd chosen a good linen instead because she was thrifty and sensible. She'd be an ideal daughter-in-law, except for...

No use thinking of that now. He looked around at his guests instead and saw with satisfaction that they were making short work of the roast meat, the big rabbit pie, the beans in sauce and the cold ham and salad, and were interestedly eyeing the bread pudding that would follow, adorned with clotted cream and a sharp-tasting preserve which Kat made from the barberries that grew up on the dry part of the ridge, north of the barrow. The guests were enjoying themselves. Even Father Bernard, who had grown frail since he'd heard of Geoffrey Baker's death, was talking animatedly to his neighbour.

Richard reached for the cider jug, replenished his tankard, recommended his guests to try the elderflower wine as well, and was wondering whether to propose a toast to the future prosperity of Allerbrook Farm or whether he ought to ask Father Bernard to propose it instead, when beyond the new leaded windows, all of them open to let in some air, a movement caught his eye.

"Who's that coming up from the combe?" he said. "Thought we were all here."

Peter stood up to look, gazing across the farmyard to its open gate and the path beyond, which led down to the combe. He sat down again with a thud. "It's the Sweetwaters," he said.

CHAPTER SEVENTEEN

ONE COMES, ONE GOES

"The Sweetwaters?" Richard was indignant. "They weren't asked. Have they gone and invited themselves?"

"They've a nerve. Which of us got invited when Walter's son got wed last year?" said Sim Hannacombe. "And Sir Humphrey never even put his nose in at mine and he *was* asked to that."

"That's right. They don't goo axin' us to their affairs or come to ours." Gilbert Lowe's sTluttery voice was heavy with disapproval.

His daughter Martha, who was wearing a plain dull gown as she always did, even at church, probably because she had no others, muttered, "What affairs do we have for them to come to? We don't build halls *or* have weddings," and was silenced by her mother Tilly's sharp elbow.

"Well, they've come to the feast this time," said Peter, standing up again to look. "There's Mistress Mary on Master Walter's pillion, and Baldwin with Mistress Catherine behind him, and a groom on a pony."

"I'll go out and welcome them," said Liza, and hurried off, murmuring, "Get that rabbit pie out of sight" into Betsy's ear on the way. Betsy hastened to obey. Peter, rising to his feet, said, "I'd better go with Liza, hadn't I? Father…?"

"Yes, you go, boy," said Richard. "And you, Higg. Give the groom a hand with the horses and bring him in for some food and drink."

The three Allerbrook dogs—descendants of Silky, Blue and Ruff—who had been panting in the shade of the stable all got up and barked as the newcomers rode into the farmyard, and Liza and Peter had to quieten them before turning to their guests. The groom was already helping the ladies down. In the farmyard surroundings the Sweetwaters looked incongruous.

They had dressed for the occasion or, possibly, just to put their hosts at a disadvantage. Mary and Catherine were in flowered brocade gowns that had to be held clear of the farmyard dust, and headdresses draped in white silk which would be ruined if the threatened storm broke while they were out of doors, while Walter and Baldwin, both fleshy and perspiring in velvet doublets, had jewelled brooches in their caps and gems in their dagger hilts, and looked as though they had come from a world unknown to the Lanyons.

Peter and Liza, both feeling demoted by these unwanted guests of honour, bowed, curtsied, were graciously polite and secretly angry.

There were other difficulties, too. Welcoming the Sweetwaters involved some hasty rearranging of people around the table. Roger beckoned to Sim Hannacombe and Will Hudd, and between them they brought an extra table and benches from the parlour to extend the hall table so that space could be made near the head for the landlord and his family. Betsy, returning from the kitchen where she had hidden the illicit rabbit pie, moved the salt so that Margaret and Nicholas should not find themselves unexpectedly below it, which would never do. "Thank you," said the flustered Liza as she passed Betsy while leading the unwanted guests to their places.

"So," said Walter Sweetwater once he had been seated, "this is the new Allerbrook hall that the whole village has been agog over these past five years. If you thought we didn't know about it, you were mistaken, Master Lanyon. A most ambitious project. To tell you the truth, I didn't think you'd ever manage to finish it, which was why I left you alone. There's a saying about give a man enough rope and he'll probably hang himself. But you've confounded me and done it after all, and all without ever dreaming of asking my permission."

Walter had the same bushy brown hair and thick brows as the other Sweetwater men, though he was not quite as heavily built as his father and his twin had been, or as Baldwin already showed signs of becoming. He was more subtle than his father and his twin, and now it was hard to tell whether he was sneering or admiring or both of them at once.

Baldwin, however, just turned nineteen and full of himself, looked about him and said, "It's a fine hall enough, but at home we have two pages to serve us, kneeling, with linen towels over their arms so we can dry our hands after using finger bowls, and we have rose-scented water in the bowls."

His father nodded in agreement, and Baldwin's quiet little wife, Catherine, who, with her small pointed chin, the dark hair

VALERIE ANAND

just showing under her headdress and her almond-shaped blue eyes, looked like nothing so much as a kitten, gazed at him in admiration. Baldwin caught her eye and preened. He was fond of her and had actually been heard to call her Kitten, in tones of real affection.

Of his family, only his mother eyed him reprovingly, but he paid no attention. There were no finger bowls on the Allerbrook table, with or without rose water, and certainly no pages on bended knee with towels.

Neither Richard nor Peter seemed sure what to answer. Liza found that she was now frightened, to the point of feeling trembly and actually rather unwell. These Sweetwaters were dangerous. They had too much power.

Drawing a deep breath, she remembered that long ago, as a child, she had heard her mother say that it was the duty of a hostess to keep guests content. The idea of even trying to intervene made her feel more trembly than ever, but Margaret had always been particular about the details of hospitality. She was looking at Liza now, obviously expecting something of her. Shakily Liza rose to her feet, picked up a dish of carved mutton slices and offered it to Walter, saying, "We meant no offence by building this hall. We're plain farming folk with plain farming ways. We just wanted a good-sized room for our harvest suppers."

Richard almost glared at her, since this was not at all how he saw his hall, but realised that she was trying to smooth a difficult moment over, and checked himself. Liza did not notice the momentary scowl, indeed could hardly have seen it, for the bright noonday was rapidly fading to a livid half-light. Beyond the window the sky had turned leaden and, in the distance, there was a flicker of lightning. Nicholas's storm was on its way.

Liza's effort won her a little smile from Catherine and an approving nod from Mistress Mary, but these too were lost in the gathering gloom and her valiant attempt hadn't, unfortunately, managed to impress Baldwin.

"This new wing has added to the value of the farm, whatever the reason for building it," Baldwin said to all the Lanyons impartially, and then addressed his father. "I don't say we should order them to pull it down, but shouldn't their rent go up to reflect the increase in the worth of the place? Wouldn't you say?"

There was a startled hush, except for an intake of breath, a communal gasp, which seemed to go right around the table. Richard, in the act of lifting his cider tankard to his lips, banged it down again. Then he broke the hush. "I paid for every last stone, every slate, every inch of timber in this hall. *I* paid for it. No Sweetwater did."

"My son has a point," said Walter, though his voice held a hint of mischief. He took some of the meat Liza was still patiently holding out to him and began to eat it. He had an air of private amusement.

"It's Sweetwater property, though," said Baldwin, persistently and quite seriously. "Rents should be charged to fit the nature of the property. It'll come to me one day and to my son John after me," he added, and there was a trace of self-satisfied emphasis on the word *son*.

"Baldwin. We are guests here!" His mother spoke quite sharply. Catherine glanced from her mother-in-law to her husband and back again, bit her lip and clearly didn't know which opinion to hold. She looked down at her platter and kept silent.

"If I've put up the value of your property, Master Sweetwater," said Richard, "Master *Walter* Sweetwater, that is, for your son has nothing to say in this matter—if I've raised the value of your property, that's no good reason to fine me for it! You do that, and I *will* pull it down! I'll burn this damned hall to the ground again and take my biggest hammer and knock down what won't burn! What do you say to that?"

"It might be as well for you to remember," said Walter Sweetwater, "that I am indeed your landlord and that your right to occupy Allerbrook rests with me, and therefore to remember your manners."

There was a pause. The light by now was very bad, except for the flicker of the distant lightning. Thunder growled, low but almost continuous. The air felt scanty in the lungs, so that breathing seemed difficult. It was full of a huge tension, half of it nature's contribution and the other half emanating from the people at the table.

Betsy, seated below the salt, said frankly, "Now, that's not fair!" and another voice, male and anonymous, muttered audibly, "Aye, remember poor George Lanyon's coffin goin' in that there river?"

Walter peered along the table, but could see only a row of expressionless bucolic faces. He had sense enough not to ask who had said that last sentence. No one would tell him. All the same, he couldn't let the insult pass.

"I'll need to think this over," he remarked. "I must consider how much the value of the house has been raised by this addition, offset, of course, by how much the stock could have been improved if you had spent your money differently, Lanyon."

"The animals are mine, same as the hall!" said Richard angrily.

"But the right to run stock on the moor goes with the farm. Pretty sight you'd make, Lanyon, if you had to leave here. There you'd be, driving them along the tracks, with no idea where you were going or how to feed them on the way."

"Master Sweetwater," said Liza, getting in quickly before Peter could join in, "please...you surely don't mean any of this?" She had put the meat dish down on the table and resumed her seat, rather quickly, because her legs now felt very weak indeed. "You wouldn't harm us, would you?" She looked at him pleadingly. "We've been good tenants, have we not?"

"Yes, we have!" Peter snapped, joining in anyway. "And if anyone tries to turn us off our land—yes, I did say *our* land because we till it and seed it and cut the corn and it's our hands that work it, no one else's—then we'll find some authority to appeal to!"

"And if we left, you'd be hard put to find folk as good and hardworking as us to replace us!" Richard shouted.

"Don't speak to my father like that!" Baldwin was on his feet. He had had his dagger out to cut his meat. Now his fist was holding it at a threatening angle, straight toward Richard Lanyon.

He was not within arm's reach of Richard, and it was a gesture rather than a threat, but Richard, infuriated, instantly shot to his feet as well, pushed back his chair and started around the table. Mary Sweetwater looked horrified and Catherine, her eyes enormous, clapped her hands to her mouth to stifle a shriek.

Then several things happened, in rapid and shocking succession. A huge flash of lightning filled the hall with blazing blue light, causing people to cry out in alarm. It was followed almost instantly by a gigantic crash of thunder, so loud that the building seemed to shake.

And Liza Lanyon, tilting slowly forward, slumped over the table, slithered sideways off her bench and fell to the floor in a faint.

"It's all right. It's all right!" The lightning and the noise had passed and the hall and its occupants were all apparently undamaged. Richard, forgetting Baldwin, had dashed to the outer door to look at the rest of the house and that, too, was still standing, even its chimneys unharmed. As he stood there, rain came down, sudden and heavy, as though the lightning had released something inside the dark sky. He shut the door and came back. "Can't see any damage. It was just a big flash. I'll have to look at the cattle when the rain stops, though…. What's amiss with Liza?"

Betsy had already gone to Liza's aid and so had Margaret Weaver. She was coming around. They helped her up and settled her once more on the bench and Kat, who had hurried out to the kitchen, came back with a jug. "Well water. That's what she needs."

"I'm sorry," said Liza. "Sorry." She looked at the three women and suddenly smiled. Then she said something, very quietly. Margaret, her eyes widening, also whispered something, and Liza replied.

Standing up again, Margaret turned to the worried gathering, most of whom, now that they had realised that the lightning hadn't killed any of them, were looking at Liza in consternation. She turned to Richard. "Master Lanyon, pour me some wine! Quickly, now! There's a reason!"

Richard, bemused by her sudden air of command, did as she asked and handed her the goblet. Taking it, she raised it high.

"Everyone, listen! You, too, Master Sweetwater and you, Master Baldwin. This is no time for threats and quarrelling. It's a time for congratulations to the Lanyons, especially to Liza and Peter. God willing, there will be a child in this house by next spring."

"What? What's this?" Nicholas had gone scarlet with excitement, looking more like his old self than he had in years. "Is Liza…are you saying…?"

"Yes, I am," said Margaret strongly, "and I hope there'll be no more talk of turning folk out of their homes because they've toiled like slaves, which they're not, to grow good corn and improve their houses! What's wrong with that?" She gave a fierce glance to Walter and Baldwin, but then swung her attention back to the rest of them. "Fill your cups, every one of you, and drink to their health and to the baby's safe arrival and to good luck to this house!"

Mary Sweetwater unobtrusively put a persuasive hand on her husband's arm. Walter Sweetwater looked at it and at her, and then said, "Oh, very well. This changes things—I grant you that. I'll drink the toast, and so will you, Baldwin." Catherine, who had clearly been wondering what to do, took the hint and filled her own goblet. Goblets and beakers were raised all around the room.

"To Liza and Peter!" Richard bellowed.

The thunder rumbled, like an echo. Kittenish Catherine giggled. Walter looked at her and then laughed. Around the table, the atmosphere lightened.

Richard, thankful enough to find friendly relations restored, played the genial host until all the guests had gone, except for Liza's parents, who were staying the night. But when Liza had been put to bed by her mother, and the Weavers had retired, and Richard was alone in the parlour with Peter, he gave voice to his real feelings.

"They could have killed her! With the trouble she's had in the past, those threats could have made her miscarry again and who's to say she'd have come through?" he said furiously, sounding for all the world as though he had been Liza's earnest defender and protector since the day she'd come to Allerbrook. "That would have been Liza as well as Deb! How dare that young devil Baldwin point a dagger at me, here in my own home, at my own table?"

"He's just young," said Peter, wishing his father would calm down.

"He's the same as Sir Humphrey and that bully Reginald were, and so is Walter—just not so crude, more sly. I reckon most of all that talk about throwing us out was just cat and mouse, reminding us of his power. Inviting themselves, pushing their way in, throwing their weight about…"

"The storm's lost us two cows," Peter said, trying to change the subject. "I was afraid that lightning would get something."

"Yes, and one of them was Clover, our best milker," Richard growled. "It would be! See here, Peter, it's good news about Liza and that was a clever move that Margaret made, proposing that toast, but considering what's happened in the past, it's too soon for rejoicing. I just hope we don't have any more storms or trouble from the Sweetwaters."

"We'll take good care of Liza," said Peter. "We'll all pray for a good healthy child this time and may it be a son. There's still a long way to go."

"And not only as far as Liza's concerned," Richard remarked.

"How do you mean?"

"I'm talking about the Sweetwaters. So we've got a hall as good as theirs. But that's just the beginning, boy. I've told you before. One day we'll have a house as good as theirs, as well. That's my next step, however long it takes."

"Father, we've no need of such a house. We—"

"Don't make any mistake," said Richard grimly. "I mean it."

"As easy as though she'd been oiled," said Betsy joyfully, coming down the stairs to give the good news to Richard and Peter. "Not a problem in the world. Wish mine had come as quick and smooth. The mistress'll be ready to see 'ee soon, Master Peter. Kat's givin' her a wash. And the baby's as pretty as a newborn lamb and I don't know what's sweeter than that. She's got a tuft of brown hair, just like her mother's."

"She?" queried Richard.

"Yes, it's a wench," said Betsy with an air of challenge. "But strong, healthy, bawling her lungs out."

"Now that there's been one child, there could be another. Maybe a boy next time," said Peter. "After what's happened in the past, I'm glad there's just a strong baby and that Liza's safe."

"Humph!" Richard shrugged. "What do you want to call her?"

"We'd have called a boy either after you or Master Weaver, but if it was a girl, Liza said her mother's mother was called Quentin and she liked the name and could we use that?"

"Margaret Weaver's mother? I met her when I was a boy, I think." Richard was mildly interested. "Carroty-haired woman. Good thing Liza didn't inherit that. I don't call it pretty. Call this one Quentin if you like. If you ever get that boy, call him Nicholas. We don't want two Richards under one roof—too confusing. But get on with it. Time's going by."

★ ★ ★

"At least he lived long enough to know about Liza's daughter," said Margaret, struggling to find comfort as she looked down at the emaciated image which had been her husband. He was only three hours dead and already a terrible remoteness had laid hold of him. "One comes and one goes—b'ain't that the sayin'? Well, I'm glad that it was over quick, when it came to the point. Only three days from when he was took ill, to this."

"I fancy he'd had pain he didn't talk about. He was gettin' thin and lookin' drawn and not eatin' right, for a long while," said Aunt Cecy.

"What a cheerin' soul you are," Margaret said. "Always ready with a few words to make folk feel better. Did your mother make a habit of walkin' through graveyards when she was carryin' you?"

"No need to be nasty, just because this is a sad day. Oh, what is it?"

The last sentence was addressed not to Margaret, but to Elena, who had poked her head around the door of the bedchamber where Nicholas lay, awaiting the arrival of the coffin maker.

"It's Master Herbert Dyer from Washford. He'd like to see Aunt Margaret, to give her his condolences."

"How did *he* get to hear of all this, away in Washford?" demanded Aunt Cecy before Margaret could speak.

"Laurence called at Cleeve Abbey two days ago," said Elena, who wasn't intimidated by Aunt Cecy. "He called on Master Dyer as well, out of courtesy, and must have let on that Cousin Nicholas's illness looked serious because Master Dyer set out today, to see how he was faring. I've just told him what's happened."

"I'll see him," said Margaret.

She was glad, on descending the stairs, to find Herbert waiting alone in the main room. He was so big and cheerful, darker than the flaxen Nicholas but similar in type and he had a wide, kindly smile.

It seemed quite natural to say, "Oh, *Herbert,* this is dreadful. Nicholas is gone and I can't believe it!" and walk into his arms for comfort.

CHAPTER EIGHTEEN

DREAMS ARE SECRET

"You have a fine place here," Herbert Dyer said, standing respectfully in the Allerbrook hall, velvet cap held politely in his hand. His lavishly pleated tawny doublet was probably meant to conceal his well-fed stomach, but didn't quite succeed. Shrewd blue eyes scanned his surroundings.

"Those fine horses that I saw in the pasture along with some ponies are yours, I take it? Very unusual colouring, I noticed— one's a striking dark dapple grey and the other's piebald. They were never bred out on the moor."

"No, they weren't," said Richard, rather shortly. "They're both mine. I like a horse with looks. The grey's old now. He's never rightly got over being half-starved on the way south when I came home from Towton. He lives out at grass except in bad weather and takes his ease. Magpie, the piebald, is a Barbary horse.

Four years old and full of fire is Magpie, though he needs a stable and corn after a day's riding. Peter prefers a moor pony. Plume, he calls his, because of its great thick tail. Surely you didn't come here to talk about horses?"

"No, I came to talk business, but it's a chance to see Mistress Liza, too. You weren't at the wedding, Mistress, and I did wonder…"

"I'm not upset," Liza assured him. "I'm sure Mother knows what she's about. But it's a long way in lambing time. We're always busy then."

"My daughter-in-law has a way with ewes in trouble," Richard said. After considering the matter, he had decided that the birth of Quentin, even though she was only a girl, was a sign that Liza might yet fulfil her real purpose as a wife. Where there was a healthy daughter there might in due course be a son, as well. He had warmed very much toward Liza. Quentin was now two, and so far there had been no hint that a brother for her might be on the way, but it wasn't all that long since Liza had stopped feeding her. For the time being, he was willing to be patient.

"We did send a gift," Peter said mildly. "There's been no bad feeling here, sir, don't fret about that."

"I always liked your mother, in the most proper manner," Dyer said to Liza. "And after my Bess died, I used to think, well, Nicholas is a lucky man. But he's gone and there are things you very likely don't know, things your mother told me. I'm family now, so I suppose I can talk of them to you—I wouldn't otherwise. But your aunt Cecy as you all call her fairly made your mother's life a burden to her after she lost your father."

"Aunt Cecy?" said Liza. "Yes. I can imagine."

"Your father," said Herbert, "was the eldest son in a line of eldest sons. He was the head of the house, since your great-uncle Will sat back and said he was tired of running it, and that made your mother the first woman in the house, as well. But after Nicholas went, Aunt Cecy started saying she was the senior woman and she took to giving orders and countering what Marge—"

"Marge?" said Liza.

"My name for your mother, my wench. My pet name." Herbert Dyer's luxuriant brown beard fairly bristled with merriment. "Aunt Cecy would change Marge's orders—over what to cook for dinner, and who was to work at which looms and who was to tend the garden. All sorts of things. It was hard for Marge to bear."

"Aunt Cecy always did have an edge on her tongue," Liza agreed.

"Edge! Like a saw. I was glad to take Marge out of it. I gave her time to mourn, but then I went courting and she was happy to say yes. I'm six years younger than she is but that doesn't worry either of us. She's got a good home with me and no heavy work, and her younger children are off her hands. Your two brothers, Arthur and Tommy, are both grown up and working in the weaving shed. Tommy's so handy there, everyone marvels at it. And your little sister Jane's been married to a weaver in Timberscombe, just up the valley from Dunster."

"Yes, I know," Liza said, somewhat acidly. "I hear news of my family often. After all, we work with them, supplying fleeces and so on."

"Well, then. Your mother's well-off with me, I promise." The glance his deep-set eyes gave to Liza, who had come from the dairy in an undyed gown and the old, streaky pinkish-red overdress she used when working, and with her hair pushed into a creased coif, suggested that in his opinion, Liza might well envy her mother.

"I've got servants," Herbert said, "and my sons are grown up and gone, except for the eldest, Simon, and he's my partner in the dyeing workshop. I'll take care of Marge, I promise. Well, I'm your stepfather now, and if you ever need anything…"

"She won't need anything while she's here with us." Peter had noticed that disparaging glance and his tone was stiff.

"I'm sure of it. That was just a few words of goodwill. And now perhaps we can talk business. That's what I came for, mainly. My workshop and the Weavers' workshop and your sheep are linked together, after all, like a chain. I've been thinking. Now, I've always tried not to overcharge my customers. I'm not a greedy man," said Master Dyer. Peter's eyes roamed over Herbert's stomach, but its owner, oblivious to this cynical scrutiny, swept on.

"As it happens, though I get a good weight of cloth and yarn through my workshop, I could handle more. To tell the truth, business has dropped a little in the last few months. If the amount of cloth from the Weavers' place could be increased, I might be able to offer them a discount and still come out on the right side myself. I've had a word with them on the matter and we reckoned that since it's my scheme, I ought to be the one to come and see you and talk to you about fleeces. They said they could manage extra work, but you can't weave extra cloth without extra wool. Now, you supply a regular quantity of wool to the Weavers at a competitive price. If that quantity could be increased…"

Richard frowned. "I think we need to take a good hard look at what it all means when it turns into money."

"I've got some estimates here." Dyer produced a roll of parchment from inside his doublet. "I worked out my costs and prices before I came. You were bound to want them. We're all men of business."

"Very well." Richard nodded. "Come this way. Come along, Peter. And you, too, Liza."

"But this is business," said Dyer, disconcerted. "It'll hardly interest a lady."

"Liza is better with figures than either of us," said Richard unconcernedly. "And handier with the abacus. This way."

Some time later, when business had been discussed at length and Peter and Liza had gone out to the lambing pen, Richard called Betsy to bring some cider, and then sat down to drink it in private with his guest.

"I think our deal should work well," Herbert said, "if you can withstand the delay in income at the very beginning. Normally, you'd have sold those extra fleeces for their full value. But there should be a better profit for you when the finished cloth is sold—profits for all of us. I'm glad to see that you're prosperous, I must say. You have a good family life, too, I notice. Your son and his wife seem well suited. I've had trouble with my son Simon, though it's over now."

"Indeed?" Richard said, refilling Herbert's tankard.

"God's teeth, yes. I've got him married now to a good wench, but before he was wed, he was always getting wild notions about impossible girls. There was a Gypsy lass, going about with her wandering folk, hawking silly gewgaws and playing a tambourine, and then there was a milkmaid over at Withypool, pretty enough but not a penny piece to go with her…no one knows the struggle I had to bring him to his senses."

"Young men are like that," said Richard. "Peter had wild ideas, too, at one time—fell in love with a fisher girl at Lynmouth. Marion Locke, her name was." It still happened. From time to time he found himself impelled to speak of Marion, as though she were an itching scab he felt he had to pick. "I went to see her family," he said in offhand fashion. "I had a look at her. She was pretty, in her way. Extraordinary hair, she had. Close up, it was like gold wire but from a distance like a pale mist."

He managed to laugh. "It isn't only young men who have wild fancies. I wasn't going to let Peter throw himself away on her, not with Liza there, ready to marry him, but do you know, I had a notion for a while of marrying her myself. She ran off with someone else before I could do anything about it, though. Peter and I were both well out of that, I think."

"He didn't want me there," Liza remarked later, when Master Dyer had taken his leave and the Lanyons were gathering in the hall before supper. "He didn't like talking to me about my accounts, or watching me use the abacus. I think he couldn't really believe that I understood figures!"

"Well, most women don't understand them," said Richard, willing to be amused, and wondering, within himself, *why,* now and then, he still had this frightening need to speak of Marion. Why in the world had he, this time, actually admitted that he had once thought of marrying her? Saying that, he had stepped dangerously close to the edge of a cliff. The trouble with cider was that it mellowed a man and loosened his tongue.

"I can't really like Master Dyer," said Liza, "though no doubt my mother does. I hope she'll be happy. I didn't say so at the time," she added, "but some of his figures puzzled me. I learned a lot about these things from my father. He said once that I was better at figures than anyone else in the family except himself, and he's gone now. I think Master Dyer could have shown those estimates to my folk in Dunster and they might not have seen how odd they were. But some of the prices he was assuming for dyes and mordants…"

"Mordants?" said Peter. "I saw those listed on his estimates, but what are they?"

"Things to stop the dye from running. Yarns and cloths are soaked in mordants before being dyed. The amount he expects to pay for them struck me as low, and his estimates for what our cloths and yarns will fetch seemed rather high. They vary each year and if you're trying to work out profits in advance, it's best to be careful." Liza frowned. "There have been a few stories about Dyer, you know. My father never complained, but…"

"What stories would those be?" said Richard sharply, forgetting all about Marion Locke.

He and Peter listened thoughtfully to what Liza had to tell them. "So that's why you prefer green gowns to red or yellow ones!" said Peter.

"I don't, really. But in the cloth trade, everyone knows everyone and if I sent cloth to be dyed red or yellow to anyone but Herbert Dyer, and then my family heard of it, they'd wonder why. I didn't want that, because, as I said, my father never had any complaint. But it looks as though he's lost a few customers lately. He said business had dropped, didn't he? And now, of course, my mother's caught up in it. She's married to him! But this deal he's offering to my family, those figures of his—I don't like them. I don't believe he ought to be able to afford that discount. I think," said Liza sternly, "that he's trying to pull wool over all our eyes!"

Richard laughed. Peter said, "Go on."

Awkwardly, Liza said, "Look, here at Allerbrook we've done well, so far, out of the arrangement you made with my father. We sell fleeces at low prices and then have a percentage paid to us when the cloth's made and sold. Sometimes we gain and sometimes my family in Dunster gain, but mostly we're the lucky ones…." She hesitated, and Richard grinned.

"Your father saw it as part of your dowry."

"Yes, he did," Liza said. "Anyway, the market's been good. My family in Dunster haven't lost much by it. But if Herbert Dyer is up to something, well…I've a feeling that we'll be selling more wool at a discount and relying on good cloth sales to make up for it. And my family may be selling cloth that…I shouldn't be saying this without proof, but…"

"This is a private conversation," said Richard. "Speak your mind."

"What if my family find themselves selling cloth that isn't all it should be? What will that do to their good name, to their sales in time to come?"

"Just what is it you suspect?" Peter asked.

"I'm not sure," said Liza slowly. "I could make guesses—but I just think something's not right. Those figures weren't right."

"We'd better be cautious," Richard agreed. "Especially since that crafty bugger Walter Sweetwater put our rent up!"

Liza smiled. "There's rabbit pie for supper again. I hope you won't mind."

Her father-in-law threw back his head and laughed. "Liza, I'd never go calling you a vixen, but you're damn near as foxy and cunning as Master Sweetwater is."

"We ought to recoup if we can," said Liza reasonably.

Walter Sweetwater had exacted his toll for the building of the hall. Since the housewarming, the Sweetwaters, when hunting, had three or four times cut a swath through the Lanyon barley and once, after a gale had blown some of the fencing down, even galloped across a corner of the wheat. Richard swore it was intentional. Nor was that all.

"You built the hall at your own expense, as you said," Walter had said, stepping to Richard's side one Sunday as they came out of church. "Well, I accept that. You're entitled to benefit from it. In fact, I think a man with a hall so handsome should have some special rights to match."

The right he had in mind, it emerged, was permission to kill and eat rabbits on Allerbrook land.

Only, of course, such permission didn't come free. The rent had gone up ostensibly to cover it, and since rabbits had been on the Allerbrook menu since the fall of man in any case, everyone there was furious. For a time, in order to get their money's worth, the outraged Lanyons had eaten so much rabbit—stewed, roasted, fried, minced up to be seethed in cream and spread on toasted bread, and of course served in the familiar pies, mixed as usual with onions and mushrooms—that Peter said if they didn't stop it, they would all grow long furry ears.

After that, their diet returned to something like normal, but not quite. Rabbits still featured oftener than in the past.

After a pause for laughter, and Richard's agreement that as they hadn't had rabbit pie now for nearly a week, no one would object to it today, they reverted to the subject of Herbert Dyer. "I'm truly worried about Mother," Liza said. "I keep thinking of that story that Betsy told, Father-in-law, when you came back from

Towton. About Geoffrey Baker's father or stepfather or whatever he was."

"No one knows for sure which," said Richard. "But what's he got to do with Herbert Dyer?"

"Betsy said he got into trouble for putting chalk in his bread flour. And I remember once in Dunster seeing one of our own neighbours shamed for putting flax threads in his woollen cloth—"

She stopped short, while they all looked at her enquiringly. To her own surprise, the memory of Bart Webber had sprung into her mind with such vividness that for a moment she had been transported back to that day. When she had turned away in distress from the spectacle of Bart, and found Christopher beside her. She had believed herself reconciled. She hadn't thought that a reminder like this would hurt so much, as though it had opened an old wound.

"What is it?" Peter asked. "What's the matter, Liza?"

"I *hated* seeing that happen, to a neighbour, to someone we knew!" Well, so she had; it was true enough. "And it caused misery to his wife. I couldn't bear to see Mother embarrassed because her husband had been been put in the stocks for cheating his customers. I'm afraid for them," she said unhappily. "I keep thinking of the trouble I had with his red and yellow dyes. He wouldn't play games with my father, but he may have cheated me—just one farm woman sending home-woven cloth. Oh, I may have been born Liza Weaver, daughter of one of his best customers, and later on his stepdaughter, but I'm a Lanyon now, and I'm living out on the moor, away from my family, and he thinks women are all fools. He'd take advantage of me the same as he would of any woman among his customers. I fancy there may have been many of us."

"This hall should have made him think again about farming folk," said Richard.

"It did," said Liza. "So did Splash and Magpie, when he saw them in the field. I think Allerbrook made him uneasy. I don't trust him. It seems to me that he wants to increase his business and is trying to use family connections to help him. I fancy he's waved figures in front of my family and got them to believe that he has benefits for all of us in mind, but all he's really after is benefits for him, at our expense if it comes to it. And I just don't see how he'll get really worthwhile benefits even for him, unless there's some sort of trickery going on."

"I think," said Peter slowly, "that when the lambing's over, we should pay him a visit and look round that workshop of his. No reason why Liza shouldn't visit her own mother and take an interest in the workshop while she's there, now, is there? And she knows something about the business. Liza's the one who must go. I'll take her."

"You'll do that?" Richard asked, looking at Liza.

"Yes, I will," said Liza. "We'd better find out, though what we can do about it, with my mother caught up in it now, I can't think."

"Leave that to me," Richard said. "Let's get at the truth first."

It's strange. I'm really not unhappy. I care about Allerbrook, and having Quentin makes a difference. A great difference! She's beautiful. I tried to do what Mother said, to make up my mind to be happy, and now I more or less am, and even Father-in-law has stopped saying things, though if I don't conceive again soon I suppose he'll begin again. But Peter is kind. I'm as well-off as most women. Mother was right. Only, talking about

Bart Webber reminded me. It all came back. I thought I'd left Christopher behind, but…it seems I haven't. Will I ever? Can I?

It was now suppertime on the day of Dyer's visit, and Liza was not at table eating rabbit pie but instead was lying flat in a muddy lambing pen, with a bucket of water and a pot of goose grease beside her and one arm inside a distressed and bleating ewe, trying to work out through her fingers which of the tangle of legs she could feel belonged to which lamb. There were certainly two of them, and sorting them out without being able to see what she was doing was always a challenge, and she was hungry and this was as messy a job as God ever invented.

It was useful work, though, and she seemed to have a talent for it, and if she succeeded this time, there would be beaming faces everywhere. Hence the thoughts now coursing through her head.

She had little to complain about. She was the wife of Peter Lanyon, a respected farmer of Clicket parish. Her home was better than most farmsteads were, now that the hall was part of it; she had plenty to eat and clothes to wear; she even, now, had a child—not the son everyone had hoped for, but the son might follow yet.

And Peter was a good man. Many women, bullied women, beaten, overworked women, envied her and she knew they did. It was shameful to discover that deep within her the little flame was still there after all, still burning, the flame that was not for Peter. When first she came to Allerbrook she had dreamed of Christopher at night, quite often. That hadn't happened for a long time, but she had a feeling now that the dreams might return, wakened by talk of Bart Webber and the reminder of that day at the fair.

Well, dreams were secret. If Christopher did come to her in her sleep once in a while, no one need know except herself…ah! She had traced that little foreleg back to its rightful owner, and got it out of the way of the lamb lying in front…now, if she let the ewe push…poor thing; she was bleating so. If she were human, she would be crying out for help. The lamb was coming forward, sliding toward the light. Here it came. And its twin was following. "All done, you poor thing," said Liza to the ewe. "Look, lovely twin girls."

The ewe, much relieved, was struggling to her feet, turning to inspect her progeny, and Peter came into the pen just as Liza was plunging her greased and bloodied arms into the bucket of water.

"You've done it!"

"It was a difficult one. I was afraid we'd lose them all."

"Far from it, by the look of that." The ewe was nosing at her offspring and beginning to wash them and the lambs were already attempting to stand up. Peter fetched the towel Liza had hung over the gate and handed it to her. "You really have a way with you, Liza. Liza…"

"Yes, dear?" said Liza, rubbing her arms as clean as possible.

"I'm not one for too much talking about such things, but I really love you. It's a wonderful thing, having a wife one can trust, really trust."

"I'm just ordinary," said Liza, very busy with drying herself. "Not special in any way."

"Oh, but you are," said Peter, laughing.

Dear God, said Liza inside her head, *make the flame spring up for Peter. Make it! Why won't it? I thought all this was over. Why is it that after all, I still burn for Christopher?*

★ ★ ★

"I have no objection," said the prior of St. George's Benedictine monastery. William Hampton was a calm individual, not given to making objections for the sake of it. "I don't own the man. He has never taken vows as a monk, although he has become a priest. In that capacity, he's useful to the brothers and to our vicar, Will Russell. He takes services on occasion when Russell is away, or falls sick. We sometimes send Father Christopher out to other churches as well, when their vicars need help. In fact, we've lent him to the castle once or twice. There are chantries attached to this church—not based here, but controlled from here—and when there's a vacancy, the vicar and I had intended to recommend him as a chantry priest. But you say you really need him at the castle for good?"

"Instructions from my lord of Pembroke, sir," said Master Miles Hilton, the steward of Dunster Castle, sipping wine in the prior's sanctum. He was elegant and relaxed, legs stretched out in front of him, ankles crossed. "We have no chaplain at the moment. We have had difficulties with chaplains ever since the Luttrells left and took their own man, Father Meadowes, with them, and the Earl of Pembroke became the landlord."

"Yes, your chaplains do come and go, don't they?" said Hampton. "Every time I dine at the castle there seems to be someone different in the chaplain's seat."

"We've had three!" said Hilton with feeling. "The first was a career man who soon found himself a deanery in Gloucestershire. The second one went on an errand to Winsford, lost his way in a moorland mist, found himself on Winsford Hill instead, thought he saw a ghost on one of the old mounds up there, came back hysterical—his horse brought him…sensible animals, horses—and left next morning."

"Did he really see a ghost?" asked Hampton, intrigued, offering his guest some more wine.

"Possibly," said Master Hilton. "People say that ancient kings are buried under the mounds—barrows, they call them hereabouts—and that they don't like to be disturbed. Or he may just have caught sight of some deer-poaching peasant slipping out of sight, or even merely a deer. Mist makes everything look strange. Anyway, he couldn't get back to what he called civilised parts quick enough."

"And the third one?"

"Went on an errand to Porlock, up the coast, took a path over Dunkery, got thrown by his pony, fell into a bog and came home on foot, hours later, soaked to the skin. Dead in a week of lung fever. And that's when I remembered hearing that you had a one-time chaplain here in this very monastery and I thought, my lord of Pembroke's the landlord of Dunster and has a right to him if anyone does. And at least your man knows the district. Presumably, *he* won't get panic-stricken if he's caught in a mist on Winsford Hill, or go falling into bogs on Dunkery."

A belated sense of responsibility overtook the prior. "You do know how Father Christopher comes to be here?"

"Oh, yes. The servants left at the castle when I first came spoke of it now and then. Some trouble with a girl, wasn't there?" Master Hilton didn't sound as though he attached much importance to this.

"It was quite a serious matter," Hampton said. "He was a deacon at the time, studying with Father Meadowes, and helping him. He and a local girl ran off together, though they were caught before they'd gone far and it seems that they did not actually commit fornication. Still, as I said, it was a serious piece of misbehaviour for a man in orders."

"Where's the girl now?"

"Oh, she was married off and left Dunster. I think she went to Clicket—you know where that is?"

"Right out on the moor, I believe. Has Father Christopher given any trouble since?"

"None whatsoever. He keeps the Rule more carefully than some of the brothers do and when he prays, he looks as if he means it. I'd call him a devout man. We'll miss him," said the prior, refilling their goblets for the third time. "But as I said, I don't object if you don't. It's for him to say."

"I can but ask him. My lord is right—there should be someone to hold daily prayers in the castle. It's only proper. We'll all still come to church on Sundays."

Prior William Hampton, who dined at the castle fairly often, thought privately that though it was admirable of the unknown Earl of Pembroke, to whom King Edward IV had presented the Luttrell lands, to concern himself about the souls of those who looked after his Somerset castle, it wouldn't be at all a bad thing if he concerned himself a little more about the castle itself. The earl had never as much as visited it. He took the rents from the village and the farms attached to it, but the castle, it seemed, could fall down from neglect for all he cared.

In the time of the Luttrells, black grapes had ripened on a vine on its southern wall and it had been customary to send a few bunches to the priory each year. Nowadays, no one bothered to harvest them and the walls around the vine were streaked with the droppings of glossy and gluttonous starlings. The prior itched to let a hawk loose among them. The harbour was silting up faster than ever, too, and no one was even trying to do anything about it.

"I'll send for Father Christopher," the prior said.

Christopher was in the small walled garden where the monks grew their herbs, culinary and medicinal. During his years within the priory he had discovered in himself an unexpected knack for gardening. It was peaceful to be here, weeding, on a soft spring evening like this, with the rooks circling and cawing above the trees on the tall hill, Grabbist, that overlooked the village, and hearing the sound of someone in the church, practising the organ.

While he worked, his mind could drift as it would. He had become quite learned by now in Latin and Greek and theology. The novices regarded him with awe, and the novice master said that when Father Christopher toiled alone in the garden, he shouldn't be disturbed, for he was surely meditating on a theological problem or seeking the truth behind an ambiguous translation of a Greek text.

Sometimes he was. The years had made his enforced vocation easier, even against his will. He had resisted at first, wanting to grieve, to yearn, to remember Liza every moment of every day, but gradually reality and day-to-day living had their effect. When he'd believed himself to have a vocation, he had perhaps not been entirely mistaken. He had, eventually, begun to find satisfaction in his studies, and had embraced priesthood with something like sincerity. If he could not have Liza, well, there was much to be said for this—the beauty of ritual, the fact that he could offer help and comfort to others, the intellectual pleasure that Greek and Latin and theological problems could give.

Always, though, before going to sleep, he said a private prayer for Liza. He had promised himself he would do that, on the day that he came to the abbey, and sometimes, especially in this garden, especially in the evening, especially on one such as this soft, green April evening, with the scents of mint and lavender so very disturbing to the senses, then Liza's memory would come to him, clear and vivid still and not blurred by time.

When her parents had come to see him, after he and she had been brought back from Nether Stowey, they had told him of their plans for her. What kind of life did she have now, Liza Weaver who had become Liza...Lanyon, wasn't it...and gone to a farm out on the moorland? Was she happy? Did she have children? Did she love her husband? Were the Lanyons kind to her?

Did she still remember Christopher Clerk or was he just a youthful escapade, even, perhaps, embarrassing to remember? He hoped not, and at this point in his thoughts he would slip a hand inside the habit he wore although he had not taken a monk's vows, and find the thin silver chain he kept hidden under his clothes, and trace it down to the patterned silver ring which hung from it. No one knew of these hidden thoughts, of course. Dreams like this were secret.

He was in the depths of one when a novice came hastily but nervously through the gate to call him to the prior's lodging. "I'm so sorry to disturb you, Father, and of course I wouldn't, except that Father Prior sent me. I don't know what it's about, but he wants you to come at once. The steward of the castle is taking wine with him."

"The steward?"

"Yes. Shall I clean your tools and put them away for you?"

"If you would. Thank you." He stood up, brushed some earth

and bits of weed off the habit and hurried to answer the summons. He found, on arriving, that the castle steward, whom he had met when, now and then, his services were borrowed by the castle, was sitting with Prior Hampton, and that there were three goblets on the table, along with a flagon of wine.

"Here he is," said the prior. "You know Master Hilton, of course, Father Christopher. What have you been doing, Father? Gardening?"

"Yes. Weeds sprout overnight, at this season. Good evening, Master Hilton."

Hampton filled a goblet and handed it to him. "Sit on that settle there, Father. Master Hilton wishes to make you an offer. How would you like to go back to the castle as the official chaplain?"

"Go…and live there, you mean?"

"Most certainly you would have to live there," said Hilton, and began to explain, all over again, about the instruction received from the Earl of Pembroke, and the misfortunes of the chaplains he had employed hitherto. There was more, about the stipend he would receive, and the fact that he would have a free hand in restoring the castle chapel. He listened as attentively as possible, but his mind was leaping ahead, on a path of its own.

He would be living outside the monastery. Not just making occasional excursions, usually with a lay brother as servant and companion—or guardian—but living, all day and all night, right outside.

He had probably been free to go ever since Father Meadowes went away with Lady Elizabeth, but he wasn't sure. Meadowes had said that if he set foot outside the priory unaccompanied, he would find his behaviour with Liza reported both to his father in Bristol and to higher church authorities as well, and he did not know whether, before leaving Dunster, Father Meadowes had, as it were, passed the threat into the hands of the prior.

He had made no attempt to find out. He couldn't, in any case, see the point of going out into the world again when he had an assured and very comfortable life where he was. The Dunster Benedictines never had interpreted their vows of poverty too literally, for which Christopher was grateful. In his opinion, deprivation wasn't as good for the soul as some believed. It often made people unhappy, and unhappy people, in his experience, were often unkind ones, too.

So he stayed where he was, made no protests, kept the Rule and never made enquiries about a young woman who had once lived in Dunster, just in case the prior found out, and had, as it were, been left on guard.

Now, however, Hampton was setting him free. The castle would be very different from the priory. Hilton was in charge there and he couldn't see Hilton bothering to act as watchdog.

At the castle, no one would supervise him. He wouldn't approach the Weavers directly, but there would be people, in the castle itself, no doubt, who knew them but knew nothing about Christopher and Liza's little scandal. It was more than ten years ago now. At last he might come by news of Liza. That was all he wanted. Just to know that all was well with her. Then he could forget that he had ever let his feet walk on air, forget he had ever had his head among the stars, and give his heart and mind to being a good priest for the rest of his life, as was now his duty and his wish.

The steward had stopped talking and was looking at him expectantly. So was the prior. They wanted his decision. "But of course," he said. "If I am wanted at the castle, naturally I'll come."

CHAPTER NINETEEN

A GOOD SENSE OF SMELL

A crow, flapping steadily across the moors and the tangle of lower hills and combes between the heathery heights inland and the Bristol Channel, would have found the distance between Allerbrook and Washford to be about fourteen miles. Earthbound riders, who had to go over hills or, on occasion, around them and take detours to find fords and bridges and avoid bogs, needed to travel half as far again.

"We ought to take Quentin," Liza said. "Mother's never seen her."

"With Quentin along, you'll want the quietest pony and you'll be tied down to a walk," Richard said. "Take Mouse. And I think you'll need to spend a night on the way."

"Ned Crowham owns a farmstead about halfway," Peter said. "They'll put us up."

The farmstead was somewhat farther than halfway. It seemed

a long ride the first day, going at the slow pace imposed not merely by Quentin but also by Mouse, who from a filly had been the gentlest and most responsible of ponies, and seemed well aware that the woman on her back had a two-year-old child in her arms and must be treated with care. But it was a pleasant ride through the May sunshine with lark song sparkling in the sky, and by putting in the extra miles, they shortened the second day's journey. It was only just after noon when the little party rode past the gatehouse of Cleeve Abbey and on along the track to Washford village, where Herbert Dyer's combined home and workshop stood, a little back from the road.

The house, recently thatched and looking as though it had a golden pelt, was in front, with the slate roof of the workshop rising behind. There was a patch of front garden, with a few flowers coming into bloom.

"And someone's weeding," Peter remarked as the ponies plodded toward the gate.

"It's Mother!" said Liza.

Margaret had heard the approaching hooves and straightened up to look over the fence. "Liza! Peter—my dears! What brings you here? Nothing's wrong, is it? Oh, is that my granddaughter? You've brought her all that way?"

"Yes. We…we just came on a visit because I wanted to see you and I thought you'd like to see Quentin," Liza said carefully. "The weather's good and she's been no trouble. The pony's pace just sends her to sleep."

"Oh, give her to me!" Margaret held out her arms and Quentin, waking up, laughed. "Come along, poppet, let your grandmother look at you. You named her for my mother—that was sweet of you. But she hasn't got my mother's hair," said

Margaret, laughing, too. "She has yours, Liza, the very same pretty brown. I am very well, I'm glad to say." She lowered Quentin to the ground. "Good girl. Nice and steady on your feet. Oh, you're all so welcome. Down you get. I'll call someone to see to the ponies and you can come in through the garden."

She hurried to the right-hand fence and shouted, and a groom appeared around the side of the house, presumably from a stable-yard somewhere. He took charge of the ponies and the Lanyon family followed Liza's mother indoors.

"She looks happy," Liza whispered to Peter when they had been shown into a low-beamed parlour with padded settles and an agreeable smell of beeswax, and Margaret had bustled off to tell Herbert they were there. "I'm grateful to Master Dyer for that, but if, after making her happy, he goes and spoils it all…!"

"He's never got into trouble yet."

"I smelled trouble in those figures. I couldn't see how he was turning a profit. I *know* that some of the materials he was buying in should cost more than his estimate. Why did he leave Taunton and then Dunster, I wonder?"

"The Guilds?" said Peter.

"Yes, maybe. They keep a close eye on the tradesmen in both places. My father was part of the Dunster Guild of Weavers and used to attend meetings and have other Guildsmen to dine. But…" Liza frowned. "I do remember them saying sometimes that the Guilds weren't active enough in some villages. Maybe Washford is one of them and maybe that's why he came here! And isn't it true that the longer folk get away with things, the bolder they get? Like the man who was supposed to be Geoffrey Baker's father and…and the clothier I mentioned, in Dunster.

I've sometimes thought maybe we snared a few rabbits too many and Walter Sweetwater somehow got to hear of it."

"Sssh. They're coming back."

Margaret came in, pink and excited, followed by Herbert Dyer, who was calling over his shoulder for someone to bring wine and pork pasties to the parlour. He strode in, beaming, and also burping slightly; clearly he had only just finished his dinner. "Welcome! Have you dined? No, don't tell me, you haven't. Why would you, when you were nearly here? I'll see you right. And what about the little lass, eh? What would she like?"

"She likes oatmeal porridge and minced meat and little squares of bread with fruit preserves on it."

"Say no more." He went to the door and shouted a second time, which produced a bobbing maidservant. Herbert gave instructions. "And now," he said, turning back to his guests, "all your family news, if you will. Marge here will want to hear everything. She often talks of you, Liza, and she's as proud of your girl as if no little wench was ever born before…."

"I should have ridden out to see her long ago, but first there was Nicholas and I just never could get up the heart, and then there was Herbert's proposal, and arrangin' the weddin'…" said Margaret.

"So we've come to you, instead," said Liza.

Overwhelmed with hospitality, it was an hour and a half before Peter finally managed to say, "Now that we're here, could we look at the workshop? I'd be very interested to see what goes on and I know Liza would. After all, she was born into the Weaver family."

The meal was finished and Quentin had gone outside, where she was playing in the garden with one of the maidservants. Herbert glanced through the window at them and smiled. "All your family spin and weave, don't they, Liza? When she's a little older, I suppose you'll have Quentin sitting at a loom, instead of toddling about being a household pet. But surely, even in your family, the womenfolk didn't concern themselves with what went on when the cloth left the premises for fulling and dyeing. Why should they?"

"My wife," said Peter, "takes an interest in everything round her. She's learned the work of the farm better than some girls who're born to it."

"Ah, well, farming folk are different. Everyone has to join in. But Marge here, why, she's hardly set foot in the workshop and I wouldn't want her to. I want her to have a life of ease and luxury, unless she likes to embroider, or maybe spin and weave a little for her own amusement."

"I'd be *very* interested to see the workshop," said Liza in steely tones. "And so would Peter. Please show us."

"Well, if you're sure. Excuse me, I'll just go and see what's being done in there now, and tell my men to expect visitors."

He went out. With Margaret there, Peter and Liza couldn't turn to each other and say *what's he hiding?* out loud, but they could and did exchange glances which said it silently.

Herbert came back a few minutes later. "Well, if you'll come with me… Marge, are you coming, too?"

"No, I thank you," said Margaret comfortably. "I've weeding to finish and I want to play with my granddaughter. She's a pretty one, Liza, no doubt about it. And I'll see the kitchen knows there'll be extra mouths for supper. You'll stay the night, of course."

They reached the workshop by a covered passage. "I had the works adjoining the house in Taunton and again in Dunster, but the smells used to get in," Herbert said. "I used to think I was drinking alum soup."

"Alum?" Peter queried.

"A sort of clay. Comes from the Mediterranean and it's scarcer and more costly than it was," Herbert said, pushing open the door at the end of the passage. "It's used to make a mixture—a mordant, we call it—to soak cloth or the yarn before it's dyed."

"To make the dye stay put?" said Peter, airing his recently acquired knowledge.

"Exactly. Then it won't run when it's washed. As I was saying, when I came here and had this workshop built, I thought, this time, things will be different. I put it away from the house, but I made this passage in between so as to get in and out without getting wet in the rain. Here we are."

The workshop was big, built of stone, with three louvred roof vents, beneath which were big open hearths where cauldrons full of strange substances were bubbling. Materials were apparently soaking in them, and perspiring youths—all the workforce seemed to consist of youths except one young man who appeared to be in his twenties—were pushing them about with poles. From one cauldron, a couple of lads were lifting red-dyed cloth on their poles and draping it over a rack. Crimson drops, looking rather gruesome, fell into a drip tray below. Over another rack, some hanks of scarlet yarn had been draped.

Built into the wall was yet another hearth, which seemed to be heating a giant oven, and also, set into the floor so that they were completely stable were a number of wooden vats, most of them full of liquid of some kind and some of them steaming. Materials were soaking in these, as well. The heat was colossal and an extraordinary mingling of smells, some nasty and some merely peculiar, filled the air.

"No," said Peter thoughtfully. "You'd hardly want your soup smelling like that!"

"Now this dye," said Herbert instructively, leading them to a bubbling cauldron, "is made from madder, *rubia tinctoria* a scholar would call it."

"Latin," said Peter. "Meaning red colouring."

"You know Latin?" Dyer looked surprised.

"I learned some at the school I went to for three years or so."

"And where was that?"

"It was run by a schoolmaster in east Somerset. He used to take a dozen boys or so at a time, house and feed them and give them a bit of learning. My father was sent to him and he was still in business when I was growing up, so I was sent there, too. Some schools wouldn't take boys from an ordinary farm, but he did," Peter added.

Out of courtesy to Liza, he didn't also add that according to Richard, though the schools run by churches were often less particular, they were apt to turn boys into monks and priests and keep them from breeding families.

"Seems you remember what you learned," said Dyer, not sounding over-pleased about it. "So. I buy the madder root ready dried and ground and it creates the shade of red you see here. The cloth inside is being moved around to make the colouring even."

"What's in there?" asked Liza, pointing to the sunken vats.

"Oh, those are the alum tubs. That's the first stage, before the dyeing proper begins." Herbert, however, did not offer a closer inspection but led them instead to another simmering cauldron. "Now, this dyebath is a different shade of red. Madder was the basis but it was mixed with brezil wood. That's costly—comes from India. Mix it with madder and you get a stronger red that wealthy folk'll pay for. We're not doing yellows today. Simon, come here and tell my guests all about our work!"

He beckoned to the one fully adult member of the workforce. "This is my son Simon, who'll take over from me one day when I get too old. He knows all the jobs in the workshop and sometimes fetches consignments of dyes for me that come from abroad by ship. Simon, meet my stepfamily. My stepdaughter, Liza, and her husband, Peter Lanyon."

Greetings were exchanged. Simon was a solidly made fellow, with a beard which, although fair, grew in exactly the same way as Herbert's. At the moment he was dressed in red-splashed and sweat-stained garments, and was crimson with heat. He seemed glad enough to desist from prodding linen around a tub with a long pole in order to talk instead.

"I heard Father telling you about madder and brezil wood. There's a very rich scarlet dye made from insects, too—see those hanks of scarlet yarn? That's what we used for them. We don't do much work with it, though. It's too expensive. Uses up fuel, too. You literally have to boil the material in it. That comes from an island to the south of India. Yellows we're not doing today, as Father says, but for them there's a berry that's said to come from Persia or else there's saffron from India. The best dyes nearly all come from faraway places—that's why they're so expensive."

"Where do you keep your ingredients for dyes?" Liza asked Herbert.

"Oh, over there in that press against the wall. Not that they'll mean much to you. Half of them don't look like much, raw. You'd hardly guess what colours are hidden in them."

Liza wandered off, peering into cupboards and then into the mordant vats, before coming back to join her husband and step-father as they left Simon to his poling and moved on to a door at the far end of the workshop, which opened onto a drying yard, where what seemed like miles of cloth swung on lines, in the breeze.

"Nothing like a natural breeze for drying," Herbert said. "In bad weather there's space enough at the end of the workshop to hang cloth for drying and it's warm there, but give me God's good winds any day."

"It's so interesting," said Liza. "I really must thank you. I knew a little about your work before, but I didn't know the dyes had to be brought from such distant lands."

"Yes, I've got contracts with a couple of merchant captains based in Lynmouth and meeting ships there is part of our lives. They send word when they're in port. Minehead or Porlock would be nearer, but the captains I use know my trade and can do the buying for me. Simon and I don't mind the journey. It saves paying for the ship to make an extra call and it's an outing for us now and then," said Herbert Dyer cheerily.

Christopher set foot inside the hall of Dunster Castle and for the moment forgot about Liza, or any notions he had had of making enquiries about the fate of his former love. It was some time since he had last come to the castle, and though he hadn't liked what he found even then, it hadn't been his business. Now, however, he had come here to live, and things had clearly dete-riorated further. His scandalised and cringing nasal tissues were protesting.

In the days of the Luttrells the castle had been kept sweet, with lavender and rosemary always strewn among the rushes on the floor of the hall and beeswax rubbed into the furniture. Applewood had burned in the hall fire, and Elizabeth Luttrell liked rosewater perfume.

The present landlord, the Earl of Pembroke, had been absentee from the start, though not entirely through his own fault. At the moment he was said to be in attendance on King Edward and not likely to leave the court, as Christopher knew. Prior Hampton received news regularly and Christopher was aware that the court had been in an uneasy state for the past few years, ever since Edward had wrecked his cousin Warwick's scheme to arrange a marriage between the king and a French princess by blandly announcing that he had married a widow called Elizabeth Woodville.

"He's poked Warwick in the eye and no mistake," the prior had told Christopher in a gossipy moment. "And now, it seems, the new queen's got enough relatives to populate a city and they're out for all they can get. Edward's giving them good positions with one hand and wealthy marriages with the other and I heard that Warwick's as mad as a forest fire. There'll be trouble one of these days. As if the land hasn't seen enough of that!"

No, the state of Dunster Castle was probably not Pembroke's fault, but that of his steward, who had done nothing to correct the bad habits of the slovenly caretaker servants. No one had polished the furniture for years and years, or put as much as a single sprig of scented herbage among the rushes. It seemed doubtful that anyone had even changed the rushes.

The place stank, of dogs, dead mice and something suspiciously like ordure, and whatever was smouldering in the hearth of the great hall certainly wasn't applewood. The fire was smoking, and it reeked as though someone had tried to dispose of canine droppings and old chicken bones on it. Christopher looked down and saw that there actually were bones among the rushes, tossed to the dogs, no doubt. He had nothing against dogs, but the Luttrells had made sure that someone cleared up after theirs.

He stood looking around him, appalled. The beautiful tapestries were still there, but they were dimmed, unbrushed, and the pretty flowered one with the unicorn and the lady had moth holes in it. He had been brought in and told to wait for the steward. He wandered up to the dais to look more closely at the table. Its dull surface was not only dusty but also marked. Careless people had been putting hot serving dishes down on it without a cloth in between.

Well, he wasn't here as a steward. But God's teeth, this was a disgrace. Very well! Steward or not, his name wasn't Christopher Clerk if he didn't, somehow, kick and prod the idle louts here into doing their jobs better than this. A few homilies on the virtue of doing the work you were paid for, a few clipped ears when the steward wasn't looking…. Well, someone ought to bring this crowd of lazybones to heel!

"So," said Peter when at last he, Liza and Quentin were alone in the spare bedchamber they were to occupy that night. Quentin was asleep, in a crib beside the curtained bed. "This is the first time I've been able to talk to you without anyone else listening. You've been very quiet, as if you were thinking. Were you?"

"*Thinking!* I've been seething since we came out of that workshop. I've been longing to talk to you, as well. Never in all my life…!"

"Never what?"

"Alum!" said Liza witheringly. "Alum indeed! There were

three mordant vats and maybe one of them had alum in it. One of them had vinegar—cheap cider vinegar by the smell of it—and what was in the other, well, I hardly like to say!"

"I think you must, love. What was it?"

"Fermented piss."

"What?"

"I really do know something about the cloth-making business. Much more than I let Master Dyer realise! I was always interested, more than some of the boys in the family were, and Father used to talk to me, and he'd talk frankly. Before people found out about alum, which is much better, they used fermented urine or vinegar to fix cloth so that dyes would hold, except that neither of them worked all that well. They're out of date now because alum's much better."

"But…are you sure that Master Dyer is…?"

"When I went poking in that press," said Liza, "there were three vinegar barrels stowed under the lowest shelf. I put my nose down and sniffed at them. And as for what was on the shelves! Persian berries and Indian saffron, indeed! He had barberries there."

"Barberries? What Kat makes that bitter jam from sometimes?"

"Yes. They're another out-of-date thing. They used to be used for making yellow dyes, but no good dyeing works uses barberries now! Oh, there were Persian berries and saffron there as well, but I suspect that somebody's paying for good dyes and getting cheap ones, and that a lot of people are getting cloth where the dye's not fixed as it ought to be. I think that's what happened to me, when I used to send cloth here to be coloured red and yellow. He's making a profit—and offering my family a big discount because he's saving on dyestuffs and mordants. He's getting away with it because whatever local Guild keeps an eye on Washford, it isn't very thorough. Father would never believe any ill of him, though there were whispers when he was in Dunster. Well, I think the whisperers were right! No wonder he keeps moving from place to place!"

"Dear saints. But what are we to do? If he's really cheating his customers like that, then it's only a matter of time before he's caught! It's a wonder he hasn't been caught before."

"He was more careful at first, probably."

"Well, it can't last!" said Peter, horrified. "It won't even need a Guild to find him out. All it needs is one resentful customer with enough knowledge to work out what he's doing! Then a complaint will be lodged with the parish constable. And that will be the end of him."

"I don't know *what* to do, Peter. He's married to Mother now! I wish we hadn't come here. Or that we'd found out long ago and reported him ourselves, before she was tangled up in it. We can't do that now! I thought we'd find something amiss, yes, but not this much! This is…it's *awful!*"

"My father wanted us to find out what we could. Well, we have. Now we have to tell him what we've found and leave it to him, like he told us. He'll do his best to protect your mother; I think we can trust him for that. Don't upset yourself. Maybe we can make Herbert stop this. Then he'll be safe and so will your mother. Think of it that way. You're a marvel. My nose would never have told me half what your nose has told you!"

"Your nose can smell different things. I think you can smell a rabbit in the cabbage patch from the other side of Winsford Hill."

Peter laughed. Quentin made a little squeaking noise as though she were dreaming and then settled quietly again.

"Liza…?"

"Dear love." Liza moved against him, feeling the hard pressure of his need, pushed back the covers, which were heavy, and drew him on top of her.

"If you're not tired…"

"I'm not tired."

"Dear, dear, clever Liza…"

Good kind Peter, whom I ought to appreciate much more, whom I ought to love, really and truly, from the very depths of me. He protected me from his father when Master Lanyon was angry with me. And he trusts me to love him. Oh, God, I've tried to love him. Make it so! Help me to be what he thinks I am. Let me have a son for him. Let us make a son tonight. Please.

CHAPTER TWENTY

ESTRANGEMENT

"So now," said Liza to her father-in-law, "we know what he's doing. I'm as sure as I can be that he never swindled my father. Father was an important client. But I suspect he's battening on smaller clients. Like me! He's been getting away with it because it takes time for this sort of thing to become obvious. Any dye will run sometimes—if the water's too hot or the soap's too strong. It takes a while for the word to get round that cloth dyed in such and such a workshop runs more easily than cloth dyed somewhere else! It does get round in the end, of course. I'm quite sure that's why he moved from Taunton to Dunster to Washford!"

"Yes." Richard was grim. "So far he's kept one step ahead of the hunt, so to speak."

"Yes, just that!" Liza was animated and indignant. "And now I think he wants to prop up his business by getting work from my family, who'll do it because now they're his family as well, in a way, and he can pretend to be doing them a favour with his discount while he makes up the difference—and probably more, by a nice little margin—by charging for mordants he didn't use! My family's reputation, or their profits, in the end, don't matter to him. Oh, it makes me so angry!"

"Did you say anything to him?"

Liza shook her head and Peter said, "Not with Liza's mother there, but we're worried for her sake. If he gets caught, and he will if he goes on like this, she won't be able to look her neighbours in the eye."

"It would matter so much to her. She'd never get over it. We had to tell you, but don't go to the parish constable. Please, Father-in-law, don't do that!" Liza pleaded.

"Don't worry," said Richard grimly. "There are other ways of dealing with Master Dyer, without the constable. Well done, Liza. Very well done indeed. I'll saddle Magpie in the morning."

Richard, riding alone on a long-legged horse, left home early the next morning, used shortcuts over the moorland and covered the miles to Washford easily by midday. There was an inn in the village, where he dined and Magpie could have a manger. "I doubt if Master Dyer will ask me to dine," he had remarked to his family before starting out.

He was back by nightfall, though he had lengthened his journey by travelling via Dunster and at first seemed more inclined to talk of Dunster and the Weaver family than to report on his meeting with Herbert.

"There's a steward in the castle these days. The Earl of Pembroke—he's the castellan now—has never been near the place and the farmland's going back to the wild. I saw two great fields with brambles spreading out from the hedges and clumps of bracken where there ought to be crops, and as for the harbour! Nowadays the sea's going back so fast that half the quay's out of use altogether. If the inside of the castle is as bad, then it's nothing by now but a great big hovel."

"But what about…?" Peter began.

"And I thought," said Richard, refusing to be interrupted, "that you'd like news of your family, Liza. Your cousin Laurence seems to know what he's about. He's looking after it for your brothers while they learn the business all through. Your great-uncle Will's still alive, though frail as thistledown nowadays, poor old fellow, and hardly stirs from his chair."

"How does Elena manage Aunt Cecy, I wonder?" Liza said, setting his place for him at the table in the hall, while Betsy fetched his supper. The rest of them had eaten theirs.

"Laurence told me all about that," said Richard, grinning. "Said Elena just got on with her spinning and told Aunt Cecy if she wanted to run the household, she was welcome. Left it all to Cecy, and the old girl soon got tired of having to work out what was to be cooked for dinner, listing what was to be bought and worrying over whether the flour bin was going down too fast, and chivvying the maids on washday. Cecy's handed the task back to Elena and the worst she does now is carp now and then just for the sake of it, and Elena takes no notice. If your mother had thought to pull the same trick, she'd maybe still be in Dunster and Herbert Dyer could take his own road to hell and do no harm to her."

"Well, it didn't turn out that way," said Peter. The weather had turned chilly, as it sometimes did in May, and he was sitting by the fire with his favourite dog, Rusty, who had been the most beautiful puppy in Silky's last litter, between his knees. "Father, *did you see Master Dyer?*"

There was a moment of silence. Betsy came in with food and put it in front of Richard, who took a spoonful of broth and broke some bread before saying, at length, "Yes, I saw him, and it weren't pleasant. I made him take me round the workshop and I did a bit of sniffing at this tub and that and then I said to him, let's talk outdoors. Why, says he. You'll see when we're out there, I told him. So we went into that drying yard he has at the back and I said my piece. Then he said his. I won't repeat it."

"About us?" said Liza. "Well, what else could we expect?"

"He didn't give in easy," Richard said. "Blustered and shouted and swore and called us the sort of names that would make the air stink if I spoke them. And—I'm sorry, Liza—but in the middle of it all your mother came out to us. She'd heard the noise. He told her I was insulting him and making up slanders about his work, and he said that you two had been prowling and sniffing round when you came to visit and then she started calling us—all of us—names as well…. I don't like telling you this…."

"Calling *Liza* names?" said Peter indignantly.

"Herbert's her husband," said Liza, her face stiff. "If only my mother hadn't heard the shouting. What happened next?"

"I'm sorry for her," Richard told her. "She's a decent woman and she'd had a shock, but when I heard her saying things about you…well, I lost my temper. I reckoned she ought to know who was telling the truth and who weren't. My nose told me what yours told you. I could tell which vats had piss and vinegar in them and you've explained the meaning of it. I grabbed her by the arm and walked her into the workshop and told her, you just sniff at that there vat. Pushed her head down to make her breathe the smell in, as a matter of fact. And this one as well, I said…"

"Father-in-law, you didn't!"

"Yes, I did. Herbert had told her what I was accusing him of and he'd denied it. I made her know it was true. I tell you, I wouldn't stand hearing you and Peter abused like that. She started crying and broke away and ran into the house and I finished dealing with Herbert. I told him what he could expect if the constable got to hear of it, and said that if it didn't stop, the constable *would* hear of it, from me. And I said, don't think you can fool me. I'll know if you cheat. I'll be visiting once in a while, unexpected like, and I'll look at this workshop and you'd better let me in because if you don't, that'll send me straight to the parish constable, too. He said he'd do no more business with me, but then I said, well, that means not doing business with the Weavers either, which might be quite a loss, and what'll folk say when word gets round that you've parted company with your wife's own family?"

"I wish I'd been there," said Peter.

"I'm glad *I* wasn't," said Liza.

"Anyway," Richard said, "I told him, if you refuse to work with us, maybe that's another thing might send me to the authorities. I left him cursing but not before I'd made him swear, on the crosshilt of my dagger, to give up using cheap dyes and mordants and stop charging customers for what they hadn't had. I swore, too, that I wouldn't tell on him, as long as he stayed honest. That was for your mother's sake."

"She'll be saved from trouble in the end," Peter said to Liza. "Whatever she feels now, think how it would be if he were taken up for cheating! Why, the men in his workshop must all know. What if one of them were to turn nasty?"

"They were all very young, didn't you notice?" said Richard. "Hardly a boy over fourteen and one or two of them almost simple, I'd say. I doubt if they know what's in the mordants, or what ought to be, either. Cunning bugger, that man Dyer is. He guards his back."

Liza looked miserable. "I know it's best for my mother that he stops cheating. But I hate to think how it is with them now. They may be quarrelling. I wish I knew she was all right."

"He was scared when I started talking about penalties," Richard said, reaching for a chicken leg. "He's quite a personage in Washford. He didn't fancy having a vat of bad dye poured over him and then being marched through the village covered with it."

"Please, don't!"

"It won't happen now," Richard reassured her. "There's nothing to worry about, Liza."

Margaret arrived the following day, tearful and furious.

They were at dinner, all the household, eating quickly because in May cows needed milking three times a day, weeds grew in the fields between dusk and dawn, and paths vanished under overhanging grass if left untended for a week. The day was dry and most of them would be out of doors again the moment the meal was finished. It was Richard, busily mopping up gravy with the last of his bread, who glanced through the hall windows and said, "We have visitors. Got a packhorse with them, too. Liza! It's your mother!"

"What?" Liza, who had been helping Quentin with her food, twisted around to stare through the window. Quentin, perched in a high chair Higg had made for her, wailed. "There, there, you've finished anyway," said Liza. Hurriedly she wiped her daughter's mouth and ran out just as Margaret and Simon Dyer, leading a pack pony, came to a halt.

Simon was better dressed than when they had seen him last, but with a face as hard and closed as a bolted oak door, while Margaret had tear streaks on her face. The pack pony was hardly visible under the bundles and hampers strapped on its back.

"What on earth…?" Liza began.

"Here you are." Simon ignored her and spoke over his shoulder to Margaret. "Get down." He made no move to assist her. Margaret, who had been riding astride but without breeches to protect her legs from the stirrup leathers, scrambled painfully off.

"What *is* all this?" Liza hurried forward and Simon, acknowledging her existence at last, thrust the pony's leading rein at her.

"Here. The pony's your mother's, same as the mare she's on. I shan't take them back. I've brought Mistress Dyer safely here. I'll go home and say I've done my errand. Good day to you."

"But won't you come in? There's water in the trough for your horse and—"

"No," said Simon shortly. "I won't. The Allerbrook's good enough for any horse. *Good day!*"

"Ohhhh!" wailed Margaret, and burst out crying, though in a way which sounded as much like rage as grief.

The others were outside now, some of them with their mouths full, all exclaiming. Higg led the pony and the mare away and Liza went quickly to Margaret's side. "Mother? What's the matter? What's wrong?"

"Wrong?" screamed Margaret, and struck her an openhanded blow in the face, with such force that Liza staggered away with a cry of pain and bumped into Roger, who grasped her support-

ingly and said, "Here, what's all this? There's no call to go on like that, Mistress!"

Peter got in between mother and daughter just in time, as Margaret lunged after Liza and tried to hit her again. "Stop it! What's the matter with you? Mistress *Dyer!*"

"Yes, none of that!" Richard grabbed Margaret's upper arm, shouted, "Get inside!" and hustled her roughly through the door into the hall. He bundled her to a settle and shoved her into it, not letting go of her until she was seated and more or less imprisoned because he had planted himself in front of her. "Now then!" Richard bellowed. "Let's hear the meaning of this!"

Margaret, scarlet in the face and rubbing her arm where Richard had gripped it, let out a screech of fury and misery mingled, and then stopped rubbing in order to point a shaking finger at the horrified Liza, who had stumbled through the door after them, with Peter's arm about her. "It's her fault! Interfering, nose-poking, smug, righteous, nasty little bitch!"

"Mother!" Liza was weeping now and holding her face, and to add to the chaos, Quentin, abandoned at the table, began to howl. Kat and Betsy, hurrying indoors on Liza's heels, hastened to her, clucking.

"What the devil are you talking about?" Richard thundered.

"I was happy! I was happy bein' Mistress Dyer and she's gone and spoilt it all. I can't stop there anymore. I can't bear it!"

"Can't bear what?" demanded Richard.

"It's because of *Herbert,* you fool!" shrieked Margaret. "First of all, *they* came to see him, Liza and your Peter, and they pried and peered and asked questions and then you came and…and… all because that little…"

"Don't call my wife names!" shouted Peter.

"Because *Liza,* dear, sweet, adorable little Liza, my favourite daughter, with her saintliness and her base-metal halo, sniffed round the workshop and found that my husband was…was…"

"Using cheap methods and materials while charging for expensive ones," said Peter coldly.

"And now I can't stay there anymore! I can't! Nicholas was always honest and I can't live with a man who isn't. I was always that proud that there wasn't a word anyone could say against me or mine! But I'd have been happy if I'd never known about this and it's broken my heart but I can't stop with him, I can't, I can't, and it's all her fault and…"

"No, don't, please!" begged Liza as Richard's right hand came up.

"She's hysterical. *Mistress Dyer!* Be quiet or I'll make you!" The threat was enough. Margaret subsided, hiccuping and glaring at Liza.

"You would have known before long," said Liza, sobbing. "He'd have got caught. We've saved him from that, and saved you, too. No one knows what he's been doing except us."

"You ought to thank Liza," said Richard. "Her keen nose and her knowledge of cloth making told us the truth and you ought to be grateful!"

"Grateful? *Grateful!* My life's ruined and I should be *grateful?*"

"Yes, you should. If he'd been caught, half Somerset would have known," said Richard. "You couldn't have held your head up, ever again."

"He'll be honest from now on," Peter added. "He swore to that and we'll keep him to it. It's all right, Mistress Dyer. You can go back and live with him…he wants you to go back?"

"Not now! I said such things to him, I was so angry with him. I never thought—there had been stories, but Nicholas always said he'd treated us fairly and I never dreamed…he said if I hated him so much, I'd better go. I wish I'd never found out! He's been kind to me. I didn't *know*. I never went into the workshop. But *she* used to ask her father questions and he told her more than he ever told me. I'd never have known but for her—it's all her fault!" wailed Margaret, from whose mental processes any kind of logic had clearly taken wing.

"Didn't you hear what Peter said? You would have known before long. I'd take my oath on it," Richard snapped.

"But where are you going now?" said Peter icily. "Because I tell you frankly, Mother-in-law, you're not welcome here, not after this. Are you going back to the Weavers in Dunster, or to your own kinfolk, or where?"

"Stop here? With her? I'd sooner die!" Margaret bawled.

"I did it *for you!*" shouted Liza, and was rewarded with a shriek of fury. Margaret, still virtually imprisoned in her seat by the looming Richard, actually drummed her feet on the floor in rage.

"How can I go back to Dunster?" she screamed. "They'd ask why, and I can't tell anyone—he's my husband! Folk would point fingers, and anyhow, a woman can't betray her husband, even if he sprouts horns and a tail and she can't stand to live another day with him! As for my kinfolk, there's none left that I mean anything to and if I had, I couldn't tell them either! I can't be like that Alison Webber was, sayin' it's nothing to do with me! She got wed again, we heard, in Dulverton. Well, I can't do that either. I'm still wed and there's no gettin' away from it. I just wanted to come here to tell *her* what I think of her and her nosy ways! I'd like to kill you, Liza, I'd like to…!"

"*Where do you want to go?*" demanded Richard. "Just tell us and we'll see to it!"

"There's a women's abbey in Devon. They've a guest house and Nicholas and I stayed there sometimes, when I travelled with him. They'll take me in. Herbert gave me money. He said I'd better go but he'd make it easy for me. At the last minute he said he'd take me back if I liked, but I won't like! I can't!"

"Very well," said Richard. "You'll take some food and a night's rest, I trust?"

"I'll neither eat nor sleep under your roof. I brought food with me. We left at dawn and I ate in the saddle. Simon's gone to the inn at Clicket and then he'll go back to Washford. He hates me for his father's sake and I don't want to ride another yard with him and I told him as much. You'll just have to lend me a man and I'll start for Devon at once. Now!"

"You won't," said Richard. "Your horse is tired. You'll rest here till we say you can leave. Betsy, come here. Let Kat look after the child for a minute. Take Mistress Dyer upstairs…."

"There's one more thing," said Margaret. Her voice now was quiet, but in an ominous fashion. "Something I think you should know."

"And what might that be?"

"Dear Liza, that you think I ought to be grateful to, sweet Liza, that's wrecked my life, my whole life…"

"It was Herbert Dyer if it was anyone!" shouted Liza. "Stop blaming me!"

"You all think she's such a good girl," said Margaret nastily to Peter and Richard. "But afore she was married, she tried to run off with a half-baked clerk from Dunster Castle. Oh, we got them back in time. There was no harm done, but she was seein' him in secret, all that summer. And him in the priesthood! She'd have shamed us all if we hadn't stopped her. She's not quite the perfect angel you think. What have you to say about *that?*"

Richard swung around. "Is this true, Liza?"

"Yes." Liza had gone very white. "I was a young girl. I fell in love. But we were never…never lovers. I just tried to do a silly thing but I was brought home and—"

"God knows, I was sorry for her when her father beat her," said Margaret. "Now I wish he'd knocked the smugness and the cleverness out of her, too. I wish…"

"Mistress Dyer," said Peter, "I too fell in love with someone else before I married Liza. I've told her about it. My girl wasn't suitable, any more than I suppose this clerk was. What was his name, by the way?"

"Christopher Clerk," said Liza in a low voice. "But it was just a young girl's fancy. I've tried to be a good wife to Peter and forget all about Christopher."

"I wish you'd told me," said Peter. "I told you about Marion!"

"I wanted to!" cried Liza. "But I was afraid to! Men get forgiven more easily than women, and later on, it didn't seem to matter. Nothing *happened* between him and me! It *doesn't* matter, not now!"

"No, it doesn't," said Peter firmly. He looked his father in the eye. "She is telling the truth when she says that nothing happened. I can vouch for that."

"I'm glad to hear it. Ah, well, it's all over, years ago," said Richard. He was aware that he ought to be angry, to complain that he and Peter had been deceived, but there was no bigger deceiver in this hall than Richard himself and he knew it. "Young folk will be young."

He turned back to Margaret, who was gaping, astounded to see the aggressive Richard Lanyon, who should have turned on Liza in a fury, behaving like a lamb instead of a dark-maned lion. "If you thought I'd throw Liza out of the house because when she was a dreamy lass, she let some young fellow make up to her for a while, you don't know me. Now let Betsy take you to a bedchamber. You can stop there till tomorrow. I won't have you sharing meals with us down here. Betsy'll fetch food and hot water for you, all that, and tomorrow I'll escort you to this abbey of yours. It's a bloody nuisance this time of year, but I'll see you get there safe. You ought to be grateful to Liza instead of abusing her, yes you ought. But I damn well don't feel grateful to *you!*"

"What sort of place is it?" Liza asked when Richard returned two days later. "Will Mother be safe there? Happy?"

"I doubt if she'll ever be happy again," said Richard sombrely, "but that's her fault, not ours. The place is well enough. It's small—no more than a dozen nuns, but they look well fed, and they seem kind. They've given your mother a room in the guest house and a lay sister to wait on her. Your stepfather did give her some money and he's willing to send a yearly payment for her support. He's fond of her, I think. He's not entirely wicked."

"I'll have to visit her later. When she's settled. Maybe…"

"I wouldn't," said Richard. His nerves were still rasped from some of the bitter things Margaret had said about her daughter on the way to Devon. "I should leave her be. Your home's here, my girl. You're a Lanyon now. Come, don't look so downhearted. There's work to be done."

"Yes, of course," said Liza, and went to do some hoeing, putting a good deal of energy into it because physical effort sometimes eased the discomfort of the monthly nuisance, which had come upon her that morning. Her downheartedness was only partly due to the estrangement with her mother. She and Peter had loved like mad things that night in Washford, but all in vain. There would be no child.

CHAPTER TWENTY-ONE

REBELLION

The year of 1469 wore uneasily on. Liza fretted a good deal. She had made up her mind that she must not think of Christopher, that he must indeed be consigned to the past, but instead she worried about her mother. Also, there was disturbing news from the outside world. From his pulpit one Sunday, Father Bernard announced that trouble had broken out in the north of England. In Yorkshire there was a rising against the king.

"It's a small affair," said Father Bernard. *"As yet,"* he added ominously. "But things could worsen. Just in case, every man who can shoot at all *must* be at the butts every Sunday, unless he's injured or ill. Those are the orders of Master Walter Sweetwater."

At first, matters rested there. June came, with sheep to be sheared and hay to be scythed, and Liza, her mind still on her mother's troubles, made an attempt to mend the breach. Following Richard's advice, she did not try to visit Margaret, but she sent Higg with gifts—a honeycake and a length of her own green homespun cloth, accompanied by a loving letter. Margaret could not read, but one of the nuns might read it to her. Higg came back with the gifts untouched.

"And the letter? Did someone read the letter for her?" Liza asked unhappily. Higg looked at her mournfully.

"Tell me," said Liza.

"Mistress, she…she tore it up."

"She needs more time," said Liza, trying to be calm, trying to be sensible. "Did she look well?"

"She said she wasn't ailing, Mistress. I didn't see her for long."

Liza worried afresh, but at this point, Father Bernard's gloomy forecast came true. The situation was indeed worsening. A new rebellion had started in Lancashire. "So far," said Father Bernard, "men have only been summoned to arms from the districts where the troubles actually are. We can but pray they come no closer."

The next report said that the rebellion was bigger than expected and was led by a relative of the powerful Earl of Warwick. The king had taken refuge in Nottingham Castle and the rebels had issued an alarming proclamation, condemning the queen and her family, the Woodvilles, and claiming that the Earl of Warwick was one of their own supporters.

July brought the news that Warwick had fled to France and that George of Clarence, King Edward's younger brother, had gone with him and had been married to Warwick's daughter Isabel. The air was full of danger. The southwest was still not caught up in it, but trouble was coming closer, like an incoming tide. The king had summoned the Earl of Devon to him, and the Earl of Pembroke, too, the same Pembroke who was lord of

Dunster Castle. The Duke of Somerset, however, was reportedly supporting Warwick, which now meant supporting the king's enemies. The Sweetwaters, who were now Yorkist and therefore on King Edward's side, came to the butts at every practice, and were seen watching the men of the parish with keen eyes, picking out the good marksmen.

The next reports were still more grave. Warwick and Clarence had landed in southeast England. They had marched through Kent, gathering men, entered London with a swagger and then set out northward to join their supporters. There had been fighting. And the Earl of Pembroke had been taken by the Lancastrians and beheaded. Dunster's absentee landlord would be an absentee forever now.

"I don't like it," Richard said over Sunday supper the day that Father Bernard made that announcement. "It's as if we're perched on a rock on a beach, watching the sea roll in!"

Further news was brought to Clicket by a seaman called Ralph Stubb, whose parents lived in the village. He had been granted leave from his ship, which had put in at Porlock, bringing goods from London. Having greeted his family, he had repaired to the White Hart to renew his acquaintance with old friends—Adam Turner's ale counted as one of these—and also to enjoy holding forth to a fascinated audience.

"Seems," Stubb said, "that whatever Warwick and Clarence are up to, King Edward's in London, and reigning. Only," he added, "there's another tale going round. It's old news now but some folk hadn't heard it before and it does make a man think. Some of them on the rebels' side…well, looks like they had a point."

"What do you mean?" demanded Father Bernard, who,

although now very pale and thin and assisted by an energetic curate who would take over from him eventually, was still, as yet, in charge of his parish, still liked his ale once in a while and was in the tavern that evening.

"Two years back," said Stubb, "that's when it happened. It's about the Earl of Desmond. You've not heard?"

"Nothing about anyone called Desmond. The Sweetwaters don't tell us everything they hear," said Father Bernard. "Not if it's against the Yorkists, anyhow."

"Well," said Stubb, "it's like this…"

It was an unpleasant story. The king's controversial marriage to the widow Elizabeth Grey, whose family of origin, the Woodvilles, now occupied so many splendid posts, was probably much of the driving force behind the rebellion, and with reason. The Earl of Desmond, who two years ago had been Deputy Lieutenant of Ireland, had paid a visit to England at that time. He had talked with the king and he had criticised the queen, who had learned of it and been angry.

Later Desmond returned to Ireland and lost the post of Deputy Lieutenant to the Earl of Worcester. "A friend of the queen, it seems," said Stubb. "He had Desmond arrested, for no good reason as far as anyone knows, and then had him beheaded. Worse! He had Desmond's two small sons beheaded, as well."

There was a stir, and a horrified murmur.

"One of them were no more than six years old and didn't understand," said Stubb. "Had a boil on his little neck and said to the headsman to mind it. That's what's being said."

"Wicked, that is," said Turner.

"We shouldn't be speaking evil of the king's own wife," said Father Bernard uneasily, but he was frowning. "But if that tale's true," he said slowly, "then it's a shameful thing. To murder two little boys!"

Father Bernard did not care for children in person, because he liked to read and pray or—these days—snooze undisturbed, and every child in Clicket knew better than to play near the vicarage. One incautious shriek and Father Bernard, who could still move surprisingly fast for someone of his age, would shoot out from his door, waving a stick. He would, however, have given his life without hesitation to protect any one of them from real harm. "This is ugly news," he said. "Pray God it's *not* true."

"But it is," said Stubb. "We gave passage to some of Warwick's men last year, had 'em on board for a week, going up north. They'd been at court the year before, when word got to the court from Ireland. They said the court was buzzing with it."

For the time being, however, quiet seemed to have fallen, even though Warwick and Clarence were presumably still at large. In the autumn Liza tried again to make peace with her mother, and sent Roger with two big mutton hams and two large cheeses. Another letter accompanied the offerings, this one not only loving, but pleading. When Roger returned, however, he brought the hams and cheeses back with him.

"I won't ask what happened to the letter," said Liza bitterly.

"Best not try again," said Richard. "You'll only upset yourself. Maybe it's because of all this that Quentin's still the only one."

He had begun, once more, to make digs. This was not the first. "Perhaps you're right," said Liza dejectedly. She felt heavy and tired and her head ached. The last thing she wanted just then was to be harried over her poor showing as a brood mare.

In fact, her out-of-sorts feeling was the harbinger of illness.

The autumn was damp and cold and it brought an epidemic—a cross, it seemed, between an ordinary cold and the sweating sickness. The sufferers were feverish and ached all over with violent coughs in the later stages. Liza was the first person at Allerbrook to succumb, but everyone there took it in due course, one after the other, and in the village there were deaths.

At Allerbrook they all recovered, although Higg never quite shook off the cough. In Clicket, however, just before Christmas, Father Bernard died. His erstwhile curate, Father Matthew, conducted his funeral and was confirmed by the Sweetwaters as Clicket's new vicar.

The winter closed in and a heavy snowfall cut off the higher farms and villages. Richard, these days, wasn't the good shot that he used to be with either crossbow or longbow though he was still accurate over short distances, but Peter's eye was straight enough, and he had the idea of putting out a few vegetables on the snow to tempt rabbits, or even deer, within range of his arrows. The rabbits, of course, were now legal, but the deer were not.

"Only, if we can't get down the combe to church through the snow, I doubt any Sweetwaters'll be clambering up it to see what we're up to," Peter said cheerfully, stepping into the kitchen one morning with a dead hind on his shoulder. "See what you can do with this, Liza."

The thaw made the Allerbrook spate and flooded some of the field, but at least it became possible once more to get down the combe from Allerbrook, attend church and hear Father Matthew give out the latest news, whenever there was any.

Father Matthew was a learned young man who believed in education and had started a small school for the Clicket children, though he was much given to homilies about the sinfulness of pleasure and the fires of hell, and his pupils found their lessons more depressing than inspiring. His face, though, had never been as sombre as it was when in March he announced that the time of quiet was over. Lincolnshire had risen on behalf of the imprisoned King Henry VI.

After that, for months, the news was a continual muddle as the warring factions went up and down on the wheel of fortune. "It's enough to make you dizzy," Richard said in disgust. "First one side's on top, and then the other. Where will it end?"

Everyone was relieved to hear that Warwick and Clarence had fled the country again, but in September the conflict at last rolled its first waves into the southwest, as the two of them brought fleets to Devon and landed.

"But they have set out straight for London," said Father Matthew. "Once more, the worst has passed us by."

It seemed to be so. King Edward and his youngest brother, Richard of Gloucester, were now the ones in exile. They had gone to Burgundy and King Henry was back on his throne. The queen was in sanctuary at Westminster.

"No business of ours," Richard Lanyon said as the winter once more clamped down. "I don't care who sits on the throne as long as they leave us alone. Let anyone have it!"

In March 1471, Father Matthew stood up in his pulpit once more and said the words they had all been dreading to hear. "The king is in England again. He is in the north, but he is mustering men and this time calling for aid from every able-bodied man in the country. All men of this parish are to assemble at the butts as soon as they leave this church. The women should go home.

The men who are to go will return home for one night before setting out with Master Walter Sweetwater and his son Baldwin Sweetwater tomorrow."

"I argued with them!" Richard said furiously to Liza as she stood, stricken and horrified, in the hall, while Peter, grim faced, put his arm about her. "I told them, take me, I've been soldiering before and I'm fit enough for all I'm fifty-one this year. But no! That sly Walter Sweetwater said he'd been watching me at the butts and I don't aim as true as I did over distances. Peter's to go and there's no appeal. God's teeth! If only we weren't Sweetwater tenants! I'm sick of being in their power, sick to my stomach of it!"

"I may not have to be gone long," said Peter. "It may be all over quite soon."

Liza, biting her lip, saw little Quentin looking at them wideeyed from the doorway to the kitchen, with Betsy hovering behind her. For Quentin's sake, she mustn't give way. If ever there was a moment to be sensible, it was now.

"I...I must help Peter put his things together. Peter, you must have clean things...shirts, hose...."

"Yes, he must. Could find himself sleeping out in the damp. You've always got to have dry things to get into." Richard, though still burning with fury, hauled useful memories into the light. "And you'd better take the old helmet, and that sword I got at Towton."

"I don't know how to use it!" said Peter. "I'll have my bow."

"I daresay the Sweetwaters'll put you through some drilling before you get to the king. You take the sword, anyhow."

Liza, slipping from Peter's arm, went to Quentin and picked

her up. "Your dad's got to go away for a while, sweeting. You and I have to send him off with plenty of good stout clothes. Come and help!"

As she went out, taking Betsy with her, she heard Richard say to Peter, "I suppose there's no chance that you've left her with child?"

She didn't hear the answer, but the proof that no such thing had happened had come only two days before. It looked as though Quentin would be the only one forever. After all, she was now nearly thirty-six. If only, if only her father-in-law would just forget about it.

CHAPTER TWENTY-TWO

SHE-WOLF AND CUB

When men came home from war and sat warming their feet at the hearth and drinking ale and talking about their exploits, their descriptions of how armies met on the field made pictures in the minds of their families and friends. In their imaginations, these admiring hearers saw squadrons of horsemen with lances and swords, or a mass of determined foot soldiers grasping pikes, all shouting war cries and racing toward a cringing enemy.

What their mental pictures didn't contain was a confused collection of men, some in full plate armour, some light-armoured, some in chain mail handed down from bygone generations, and a number of unfortunates not in mail at all, some riding a variety of horses from massive destriers to wild-eyed ponies, and many others on foot, trying to keep out of the way of the horses, all sweltering hot and cursing the month of May for producing such a heat wave, and all so lost in a tangle of sunken lanes between banks and ancient hedgerows that they couldn't even find the enemy, let alone charge him. By the look of things, the Battle of Tewkesbury was going to be a disaster, though it wasn't yet clear for whom.

Peter Lanyon, in the middle of it all, was a horseman without armour, except for his helmet. He had his sword. He also had a destrier, which he had acquired just over two weeks ago at the Battle of Barnet, by grabbing the leg of the knight who was riding it, yanking him off and then sticking a dagger through a gap where his victim's armour was falling apart. This enabled him to fight on horseback, since ponies like Plume weren't used in battle, and anyway, he was fond of Plume and didn't want the poor animal to come to harm. Plume had been left behind the lines with the baggage.

He was now wondering, however, whether the enormous liver chestnut destrier was quite the prize he had thought. After Barnet, when the Captain of Archers he had been following saw that Peter now had a charger, he had been transferred to a mounted troop, but he had ridden Plume and led the destrier during most of the march from Barnet to Gloucestershire, and hadn't had much practice in handling his new mount.

He was now discovering that although he was strong and accustomed to horses, a trained war stallion was very different from even the most wilful pony. It had several times tried to bite him, even when he was offering it food, and now, with ears flattened back, it seemed to want to bolt, a desire he could understand but couldn't, just now, allow.

Richard of Gloucester, the king's youngest brother, the loyal one, who was in charge of this wing, had ordered them all to have their weapons ready, which meant that Peter needed his right hand for his sword. He had only his left hand for controlling the horse, and his left shoulder felt as though it were about to come out of its socket.

A pretty state of affairs it would be if he fell off the moment they met the Lancastrians. He would probably be killed and the Sweetwaters wouldn't care. Walter Sweetwater and his son Baldwin were both in this same company, among the lightly armoured riders but mounted on hefty chargers, which they handled with contemptuous ease, and they had already laughed to see him trying to manage his new steed.

It was a wonder he hadn't been killed already. This whole expedition was a nightmare, and not only that. Something completely unexpected had happened to him.

He was, after all, a vigorous man of thirty-two, a long way from boyhood. He hadn't expected to be seized with homesickness when he had been gone from Allerbrook only a matter of weeks. He was suffering from it now, and all the more because these deep lanes and high banks, where the grass was thick and the cow parsley was already in bloom, reminded him so much of the lanes of Somerset.

He kept on remembering Somerset. He was haunted by images of wooded combes with steep sides plunging down to swift peat rivers, of high moors where the wind whispered through the grass and gorse and over the dark heather and there were larks and curlews and ravens and now and then hovering kestrels or buzzards, searching the moor for prey.

He longed with all his heart to be back there, tending the sheep, watching the crops sprout, watching the calves and lambs grow, repairing ditches and fences. He was a farmer, not a soldier, but here he was, with no means of escape, trying to manage this horrible horse with one hand and wondering if Gloucester was ever going to get them out of this maze of lanes. He hated war, hated being away from home, and he was afraid.

Somewhere a cannon boomed, and just ahead of him a shower of arrows swished over the hedgerow to the left. Men fell, toppling from saddles; those with bows and quivers tried to return the compliment, shooting wildly over the hedgerows. Gloucester, who had already ridden past the place, turned back, shouting, and the trumpeter at his side blew a signal telling them to close up against the left-hand bank and use it as shelter.

Peter's stallion reared, snorting, and Peter stayed on only because he had acquired the saddle along with the horse, and a knight's saddle, with its high pommel and cantle, fore and aft, was designed to keep the rider in place. But he still wouldn't bet a single penny piece on his chances of ever seeing his home, or Liza, again.

They had set out as quite a sturdy force, fifty men all told from the parish of Clicket, led by Walter and Baldwin Sweetwater, who did indeed make opportunities along the way to drill them all in the use of various weapons, and bullied them pitilessly in the process. Long before they reached the king, north of London, Peter, whose dislike for the Sweetwaters was strong but had never hitherto been quite as violent as that of his father, found it becoming positively virulent.

They were part of a bigger company by then, having fallen in with others on the way. Ned Crowham had joined them for a while, still very much the same old Ned despite his added years— still pink faced, fair-haired, overweight and a terrible slugabed, much given to complaining when obliged to rise at dawn. They had skirmished with a few bands of men who were trying to link up with Warwick, but there were not many of these. They were small groups and easily routed.

As they went, they gathered news of the king's whereabouts, and by April 10 they had found him at St. Albans in Hertford-shire. There they found themselves being reorganised and allo-cated. Ned Crowham was sent to a force under the king's direct command and the Clicket contingent was handed over to Richard of Gloucester.

This was interesting, even rousing Peter at times from his fog of homesickness. The king, of whom he caught several glimpses, was a tall, blond, good-looking man with considerable presence and a broad smile, but the Duke of Gloucester was spare and dark and hazel eyed and though he was now the youngest brother of a king, in his boyhood he had more than once been a fugitive and at the age of twelve he had been riding around the country in armour, raising men and arms for Edward.

The result was that he looked older than his years. Gloucester had a worried face which rarely smiled and an overdeveloped right shoulder, usually visible because he preferred lighter armour, for the sake of mobility. He said that the thickened shoulder came from being determined from boyhood to learn to handle a sword as big as Edward's. He was known to have a great devotion to Edward. His motto was *Loyalty Binds Me*.

The news was that Warwick was on his way south to enter London, and had sent orders to the London City Council to be ready to receive him. Edward had sent spies into the city, who reported that the City Council were in a frightened dither and the mayor had taken to his bed with a (presumably) diplomatic illness.

"We'll see what they all do when I'm at their gates," said King Edward, addressing his troops, and when he tried it, what the City Council did was fling the gates open and welcome the king inside.

After that, Warwick arrived, and Easter Sunday, which should have been a day of rejoicing and church bells ringing and happy congregations singing praise for the resurrection, instead was the scene of the Battle of Barnet, outside the city to the north.

When he'd left Allerbrook, Peter had said to himself that if he had to fight in a battle, he would do his best. But he had never imagined either the horror or the sheer confusion of the reality. The Battle of Barnet, which had taken place in a thick morning fog on the edge of a marsh, had been as chaotic as this present campaign at Tewkesbury was.

Peter had been brought along as an archer, but archers were of little use in such bad visibility and when their lines were attacked, all sense of order was lost. Everything dissolved into mist and muddle. Standards appeared and disappeared and were mistaken for other standards. Friend and foe could hardly be distinguished in the confusion and men on the same side attacked each other. The fully armoured knights, who should have been kept back ready to ride down enemy foot soldiers once they were running, somehow got into the fray. It was at that point that Peter seized his chance and an armoured enemy leg and acquired the horse he now wished he'd left alone.

At the time, he was glad to get into the saddle because it felt safer. On foot, one was too vulnerable and too near, much too near the horrors that kept appearing and echoing out of the murk: the wet puddles which were not water but scarlet blood, the severed limbs, the piles of entrails, the trampled bodies, the maimed things that crept and wailed; all the dreadful sounds of despair and agony and death.

Then, somehow or other, Richard of Gloucester, though wounded in the arm, materialised from the vapours with his trumpeter and standard-bearer still beside him. Familiar trumpet calls pulled his men together and there was something like an organised charge on the part of the royal forces, and as the sun at last struggled through the mist, King Edward was triumphant.

And Warwick was dead.

Thank God for that, had been Peter's main thought. Now we can all go home. In a day or two, the king will disband us.

Forty eight hours later a frantic messenger rode headlong into London with the news that no one wanted to hear. There was another army to fight. Queen Marguerite had landed in Devon, with her son Edouard of Lancaster and a force of French soldiers. There would be no disbanding. They must march for the west, and at once.

Here at Tewkesbury they were supposed to be confronting the Lancastrian right wing, led by the Duke of Somerset (which to Peter felt odd, since he was a Somerset man himself). Still, unless they could escape from this labyrinth of sunken lanes, he couldn't see how they were ever going to confront anybody. However, a surge of movement ahead and a glimpse of Gloucester, his waving right arm beckoning them onward, suggested that their leader at least had some idea of where he was going. He was taking them into a lane going westward, toward a small wooded hill.

With a tightening of the stomach muscles, Peter saw glints of metal among those trees. There were armed men up there.

Then they were out of the lane, with almost open meadow between them and the hill, except for a few elm spinneys and clumps of bush. Trumpets spoke. Men sorted themselves out— horsemen this way, foot soldiers that way, fully armoured knights to the rear, archers to one side, front row down on one knee, back row standing, all with bows drawn or wound. Peter found himself near Gloucester, with the two Sweetwaters only a few yards away. "See you give a good account of yourself!" Walter Sweetwater shouted at him across the gap. "Seeing you've got yourself a warhorse when you ought to be on your feet like the rest of my lot!"

The stallion, sensing battle, plunged against the bit and Peter nearly replied that Walter could have the damned animal and welcome, but thought better of it in case he was taken at his word and summarily ordered out of his saddle so that Walter or Baldwin could have a spare mount and Peter be left once more among the foot soldiers, who in the eyes of mounted warriors were corn to be cut down.

There was no time for more. There were other trumpets, distant ones, among the trees. The glints of metal were moving, were coalescing, were emerging from the green shadows… were charging straight down toward them. There were enemy archers hidden somewhere, too, the same, no doubt, whose volley into the lane had done such damage. From a spinney to the north came another flight of arrows, intended to wreak havoc in Gloucester's forces before the main charge reached them. A shaft bounced off Peter's helm. Another went straight into the flank of Gloucester's horse, which reared with a scream and was at once struck by a second arrow, which went into its throat.

The horse fell, kicking, and Gloucester extricated himself just in time, snatching his legs clear and throwing himself aside before the horse could roll on top of him. He rolled almost under the hooves of Peter's stallion, which curvetted sideways to avoid him. Walter Sweetwater was one thing. Richard of Gloucester was quite another. Without pausing to think, Peter was out of his saddle. "You need a horse, sir. Take this one."

"My thanks!" Gloucester gasped, getting to his feet and grabbing the reins that Peter was offering him. "Who are you?"

"Peter Lanyon, sir, of Allerbrook farm in Somerset."

"I won't forget," said Gloucester, already up and astride. Then he was gone, shouting to his trumpeter, and a moment later the enemy was on them. Peter, dashing aside to join the foot soldiers after all, wondered why he had done it, but found himself more relieved to be rid of that diabolical horse than afraid of his fate on foot.

"Did you see that? Typical Lanyon!" Walter Sweetwater shouted to his son as the charge crashed into them. "I was going to give Gloucester my horse!" With a savage swipe of his heavy sword, he swept an enemy horseman out of his saddle. "Likely enough I'd have got another! Now Peter Lanyon's going to get commended instead of me...!"

"None of the Lanyons know their place!" Baldwin shouted back.

The scrimmage was short. Somehow or other Gloucester's forces held their shape, giving ground a little but not enough to matter. At the end of it, the Lancastrians retreated, Richard of Gloucester's trumpets sounded yet again and this time it was Gloucester who was charging.

Ten minutes later Edward of York's standard, The Sun in

Splendour, appeared behind the Lancastrians, borne at full gallop, with Edward and his standard-bearer leading a shouting, weapon-waving force straight at the Lancastrian rear.

The Duke of Somerset's forces wheeled in disorder, beset before and behind, broke and fled.

It was over. Peter was not at all sure how he had managed to survive but here he was, still alive, with dents in his helmet, other men's blood on his sword, a lot of bruises but otherwise a whole skin. On this warm, velvety May night he was not lying dead on the field, but sitting by a campfire with half a dozen other men, including Ned Crowham, who had been with the king in that final charge from the rear, and Sim Hannacombe, who had stayed with Gloucester's archers. Both had come through unscathed. They had all found each other afterward and as dusk fell, they had made their own campfire and were frying veal steaks in a pan along with chunks of bread, knowing that no further battle awaited them tomorrow.

A figure loomed up from the twilight, cloaked and unremarkable except that its right shoulder was bulkier than its left. It squatted down beside Ned, who started, peered at the stranger's face and then hurriedly got up and bowed, exclaiming, "My lord of Gloucester!"

"Oh, sit down, all of you," said Gloucester as the rest of them started to follow Ned's example. "We're all tired soldiers, aren't we? We've all been frightened half out of our wits and wondered if we'd finish the day with our heads still on our shoulders." He touched his left hand to his right upper arm and Peter realised that the bulkiness under the cloak was partly due to a padded dressing, over the wound that Richard had received at Barnet.

He had marched to Tewkesbury and fought this long day through with a swordcut still not healed.

"The news will be proclaimed tomorrow," Richard said, "but I can tell you now that Edouard of Lancaster, the son of Queen Marguerite, is dead, and that the queen herself has been taken. She had fled to a house of nuns. The She-Wolf is caged and her cub is slain. The Duke of Somerset is a prisoner, too. Meanwhile, I am looking for a man called Peter Lanyon, of Allerbrook farm in Somerset."

"I am Peter Lanyon," Peter said.

"You gave me your horse."

"Yes, sir."

"It's a good horse and it's still alive and well. Do you want it back?"

"Frankly, no, sir. I am not a knight. I found the beast nearly unmanageable," Peter said, amid laughter from the others.

"I'll give you its price, then. Here." A hand came out from under the cloak, with a leather bag in it, and Peter heard the coins inside clink before he felt their edges through the bag. "But there'll be more, when we get to London. In giving me that horse, you rendered service far beyond the animal's value in the market. I've spoken to the king and there'll be a reward in accordance. We ride for London soon. You'll ride with us."

It was an accolade but also a command.

He was still homesick for his native combes, but he wouldn't be seeing them again yet. Ned Crowham, who knew him well enough to guess at his feelings, said softly, "It'll keep you from Allerbrook a while longer, but you won't be empty-handed when you get there. Well done."

"Thank you, my lord," said Peter to Gloucester.

"That's Lanyon that Gloucester's talking to." Baldwin Sweetwater, seated by a neighbouring fire with his father, nudged
Walter and pointed. "I saw Gloucester's face in the firelight just
now when he went to join them."

"And he's making a pet of Lanyon. God rot the Lanyons," said
Walter. "Richard Lanyon's already got a hall the size of ours and
a swollen head to go with it and the talk round Clicket is that
he has dreams of one day building himself a house to outdo ours,
never mind a mere hall!"

"I've heard that," Baldwin agreed. "But you're his landlord.
You can forbid it."

"I certainly will! You know," said Walter, "it's high time we
finally got your sister Agnes married. A good marriage for her
could carry us up in the world and put us beyond the reach of
any Lanyon impertinence. Negotiations have fallen through
twice, but somehow or other it's got to be done. If I'd been quick
enough to hand my horse to Gloucester before Peter Lanyon did,
I might have asked for a rich marriage for her as a reward!"

"The Courtenays or the Carews might have a connection in
the marriage market," Baldwin remarked. "Or there are the
Northcotes in Devon—they're a wealthy family. We haven't tried
in that direction, have we? We'll enquire when we get back."

"I wonder," said Walter thoughtfully, "what will happen now
to poor deposed King Henry? If I were King Edward, I'd get rid
of him. Just by existing, he's a breeding ground for trouble, like
a corpse collecting flies."

"Poor old Henry," said Baldwin cynically. He added, "I
wonder if the She-Wolf ever loved him?"

"I shouldn't think so. Love's for peasants—if it ever really
happens at all, which I doubt," said Walter Sweetwater.

★ ★ ★

At Allerbrook the last tasks of the day were finished. Liza wanted to go to bed and made for the stairs, which meant crossing her workroom, since the stairs came down into one corner of it. She found Richard sitting at her desk and drawing something by candlelight.

She knew what he was doing, for she had seen him at this before. She sighed a little. Like her quarrel with her mother and her lack of a second child, this was one more thing to worry about. Richard had been doing this a good deal in Peter's absence and it would upset Peter if he knew. No, she silently corrected herself, *when* he knew. When he returned. "Are you designing another house, Father-in-law?"

"Yes." He didn't look up but with his quill and the straight edge of a box, began to draw a careful, straight line across the paper in front of him.

"But we have our beautiful hall." She spoke very gently and with caution, afraid of annoying him, but impelled to speak through sheer anxiety. "Do we really need any more than that? We...we're not..."

"Not gentry like the Sweetwaters, you mean? But I intend us to be one day, my lass." He tapped his drawing with the end of the quill. "I had some new ideas last night. If I can't sleep, I often refresh my plans for the house I'm going to build one day. I mean it, you know. It's the best way I can think of to make the Sweetwaters pay for the things they've done. In gnashed teeth, if nothing else!"

"But even if you do build it, Father-in-law," said Liza cautiously, "won't it cost a lot? And won't the Sweetwaters put up the rent? Or forbid you to build, even!"

"It won't be cheap, but I'm saving. It might take years but I'll get there in the end. You're right to fret about the Sweetwaters, though. I've been cudgelling my brains over them, my girl. Walter Sweetwater let me build my hall because he didn't think I'd ever finish it! When I did, he made his gesture with that rabbit rent, damn him, and left it at that. But a whole house…yes, he might well forbid me."

In view of the likely cost, Liza rather hoped so but wisely held her tongue.

"What I need to do," said Richard, "is buy Allerbrook from the Sweetwaters—buildings and land. The freehold, in fact. Then I can put up what buildings I like. Only I've still got to find a way of making them sell!"

CHAPTER TWENTY-THREE

OUT OF THE PAST

"Is there any news of my mother?" Liza asked across the supper table.

Richard Lanyon, who had just returned from visiting Dunster, shook his head as he sat down. "Your brothers say they send gifts to her sometimes and get messages back—by word of mouth. She says she's well. But they have to send by a servant. She won't see family. Her messages say that she has a call to religion and is living in permanent retreat."

"She has a kind of loyalty to Herbert Dyer, I suppose," Liza said. "It's plain she hasn't told them what really happened."

"He still sends money to support her, to be fair to him," Richard said. "I fancy she's afraid to see her family in case they worm the truth out of her. Not that he's stepped out of line since then. How he hates the sight of me when I turn up in Washford.

I laugh to myself, watching him curdle like milk in thundery weather with the effort of being polite to me."

"Did all go well in Dunster, Master?" Roger wanted to know as Betsy and Kat served out the food.

"Aye, good enough. The Weavers are pleased with our clip and they've got two extra looms. I fancy our share of the profits could go up. I took a look at our hay meadow before I came in and it's about ready for scything. We'll have a surplus to sell if the weather holds. Pity Peter's not here to lend a hand."

There was a silence. Richard glanced across the table at Roger and Higg. Higg had lost weight in the past year or two. He was not the oxlike individual he had once been and his formerly tow-coloured tangle of hair was grey. As for Roger, his stoop was more pronounced than ever and his back was humped at the top of the spine.

"Peter ought to be here!" Richard said abruptly. "Fighting's over, so we heard, finished last month, and the Sweetwaters are home and so is Sim Hannacombe, but all we've had is Sim telling us that Peter hasn't been released from service yet. He's alive at least, which is a mercy. I'm thinking to ask Sim if his two younger sons could come and work here. They'll have to leave home anyway once they're grown. They're thirteen and eleven now and big enough to be useful and I'd pay 'em something. Not much because I'm saving, but something."

"That 'ud help," Higg agreed.

Richard started to say, "If only…" and then stopped, glancing at Liza and then to where four-year-old Quentin, who had had supper earlier, was seated in one of the hall window seats, solemnly experimenting with a spindle. A kitten was beside her and she was gently discouraging it from wanting to play with the thread. At four, Quentin already had a way with animals. Liza, recalling how the ponies at Dunster had come to her call, thought that Quentin was very much a Weaver, in more than one way.

Richard's mind seemed to be running on similar lines. "Looks like Quentin's going to be handy at spinning and weaving, Liza," he was remarking. "Just like you. She's getting to look like you, too. She's a good child. Maybe if that elder Hannacombe boy shapes well, we could make a match between them one day. Sim would like that. The boy's future would be made and if he and Quentin stop here, the Lanyon blood'll go on, if not the name."

"I think it's a good idea," Liza said. He had said no words of censure aloud, but she had heard them, just the same. Since Peter had ridden away she had tried hard to keep her father-in-law happy, and on the whole, by working hard, making sure that there was good food on the table at the right times and trying to agree with everything he said, she had succeeded. But the undercurrent was always there. *I like you well enough, Liza, but you should have had a son.*

Well, she would have liked one, as well, she sometimes thought rebelliously. What a pity Richard Lanyon never seemed to realise that.

However, he spoke amiably enough now as he said, "By the time Quentin's old enough to marry, I hope she'll have a fine house as her inheritance. Every time I see the Sweetwater place, I get new ideas."

Betsy said, "Well, well." Kat clicked her tongue, Roger grunted and Higg shook his head as if in sorrow at the insanity of an old friend. Liza decided to introduce a new topic.

"It's time I went myself to see my mother and tried to break through this…this wall she's put between us," she said. "I've been afraid to go in person before, but a lot of time's gone by. Maybe she's not so angry now. I can see why she won't see the rest of the family, but I know all about Master Dyer. She has nothing to hide from me, and after all, I'm her daughter. I ought to try, anyway. Father-in-law, may I go?"

"After the haymaking," said Richard. "Higg can go with you and you can come home by way of Dunster if you like. See your family and give them firsthand news. But don't go upsetting yourself over it, if your mother wants to keep up the feud. Just let her."

"Is that the place?" Liza said to Higg as the two of them rode their ponies over a low hill and came in sight of the little abbey in the Devon valley below. It was indeed small; a tiny church beside a cluster of thatched buildings. There was a vegetable plot where two or three black-clad figures were working and a patch of fruit trees, hardly big enough to be called an orchard. It was all encircled by a wall with a gatehouse at the nearer side, but a few fields, which probably belonged to the abbey, lay on the gentle slope of the hillside beyond.

"Yes, Mistress," Higg said. "That be St. Catherine's, where your mother is. Let's get on. Don't like this sticky heat. It takes it out of me."

The gate was closed but there was a bell rope, which Higg tugged. After a moment they heard footsteps, and then a shutter in the middle of the gate was opened and an elderly nun peered out. "Visitors, hey? Who might you be wantin'? Seen you afore," she added to Higg.

"I am Liza Lanyon, daughter of Margaret Dyer. She is living here. I've come to ask after her welfare," said Liza.

Bolts were pulled back. They dismounted and, leading their

ponies, they entered and followed the porteress along a path to one of the thatched buildings, where she knocked on the door. It was answered promptly by another nun and the porteress announced them. The second nun went away briefly and then reappeared. "Mother Abbess will see you. This is her study time, but she is willing to interrupt it for you. Mistress Lanyon, please come this way. Dame Porteress, show the lady's manservant the stables and then take him to the kitchen and see he's given food and drink."

The abbess's room was cool and dim, its stone walls and floor unadorned, but for that very reason it was a welcome haven in weather which, as Higg had said, was over-warm and sticky. Built into an alcove were shelves laden with parchment scrolls and several books and a supply of unused paper. Another book lay open on the plain walnut desk.

"You wish to see your mother?" It was hard to guess the abbess's age. Her pale face was unlined but her hazel eyes were knowledgeable and there were knotted veins on the backs of the thin hands folded at her waist. She had risen to greet her visitor and did not sit down again or invite Liza to do so.

"If I can," Liza said. "If she will not see me, at least, please, tell me how she fares."

"I will ask if she will see you." The abbess was a small woman and had to look up to talk to Liza. "But I can tell you that if she does, what you find may disquiet you. Oh!" Seeing Liza's alarm, she raised a hand in reassurance. "She is not sick. She sometimes occupies herself with spinning, which is useful, since we own sheep which are cared for and sheared for us by the brothers of a monastery not far from here, and we make woollen cloth to sell. But…well, let me take you to her. She lives in our guest house."

Much concerned, Liza followed the small, black-draped figure out of the room and then out of the building and across a cobbled space to another house. Again it was necessary to knock, but again a nun came at once and with a murmured "*Benedicite, Mother,*" she stood aside to let them in.

The abbess led the way up a twisting stone stair. The guest house was built around three sides of a small courtyard and a covered gallery, overlooking the courtyard, ran around all the first-floor rooms, which opened onto it. The abbess knocked at one of the doors and announced herself. A voice called to her to come in. Signalling for Liza to wait, the abbess did so, but moved a little to one side, so that from where she stood on the gallery Liza could still see into the room.

The room looked comfortable, with a bed and a table and stools, a window seat and, in one corner, a spinning wheel with a basket of wool beside it. Margaret Dyer was not using it, however. Dressed in a robe of unbleached wool, and with a plain coif on her head, she was seated, hands folded, on the window seat, half turned so as to look out at the rolling Devon country-side beyond.

"Mistress Dyer!" said the abbess, rather too heartily. "I am sorry to see you so dispirited again. On such a day it is pleasant to walk in the grounds. Sister Honoria would go with you gladly."

"I know, but I don't want to go walking," said Margaret, not rudely, but despondently. She turned from the window and caught sight of Liza, hovering just outside the door. "Oh, so you've come. Thought 'ee would one day. All right. You may as well come in. I no longer care enough to get up and throw you out."

"Mother—how are you?" Liza entered the room and wanted

to go to her mother and embrace her, but somehow dared not. Margaret's eyes, both dull and unfriendly, repelled such affectionate gestures. "I've thought of you so often," Liza said timidly. "And I've worried about you and so have the family in Dunster. I had to come, to know how you were, whether you needed anything…."

"I never wanted to set eyes on you again," said Margaret tonelessly, "but I knew it' ud happen in the end. Here you be, and here I be, and you can see I'm well. I'm doin' penance for my husband's sins. Someone must, since I know he won't. It eases my mind. I'm still a wife, even if I can't bear to live with 'un, nor he with me."

"Doing…?"

Margaret looked at her coldly and then undid the lacing which held the neck of her unbleached robe together. She pulled out a fold of the garment under it. "Come here and feel this."

"Oh, no!" said Liza as her finger and thumb told her the miserable truth. "Not a hair shirt. Oh, *Mother!*" She tugged the fold out farther and looking below, saw the pricks and scratches on Margaret's skin. "Oh, why, why? He's not worth it. Don't do this to yourself, *please!*"

"I'll do it while I live and you've no say in the matter. Don't go tellin' them in Dunster what Herbert did. That's between him and me." She pushed Liza's hand away, tidied her clothing and did up the lacing with fingers that fumbled. Then she turned her head away, to resume her contemplation of the outside world. "Go away. I can't talk long to anyone. It's too much effort."

"But…Mother…" Liza was at a loss.

"Go away!" said Margaret.

The abbess took Liza's arm and drew her gently out to the

gallery, closing the door after them. "Sister Honoria, the lay sister who looks after her, will bring her midday meal soon. She often sits with your mother, although she says they talk very little because Mistress Dyer seems to have no energy, no spirit. We do what we can. We pray for her and with her. I have told her that it may well be sin to give way so to melancholy, and that she cannot take her husband's sins, whatever they are—she won't tell us that—on herself. But she only says she's doing what she must. Come."

They walked back to the steps and went down them. "You are welcome to dine with us," the abbess said. "But it might be better not to try to see your mother again. I promise you she is safe with us."

"But—something's wrong with her!" Liza expostulated. "You said she wasn't sick, but…"

"She isn't, in the usual sense, but I know what you mean. I have seen it happen before. No one can explain it. Mostly to people growing older, but not always. They fall into a lethargy and there is no getting them out of it. Some physicians say it is a thing of the body, some say it is of the mind and some call it an affliction sent by God, and perhaps they're right. But no one knows the cure. Sometimes people recover, sometimes not. We will look after her as long as she needs it, that I can promise."

"I brought things. They're in our saddlebags. A mutton ham and some money and a big round cheese. Please keep them and use them and let her have a share without telling her where they came from."

As they walked back across the cobbles to the nuns' house, side by side now, the abbess turned her head and for the first time, she smiled. "We will do that. Don't fear for her. We *will* take care of her."

"Thank you," said Liza miserably. She added, "I'm travelling back by way of Dunster, where my brothers and my sister live, to give them what news I can. At least I can say that she's safe—if no more."

The sticky heat dissolved into a downpour as they started for Dunster, and lasted for the two days of their journey. On open hillsides they rode with heads bent against the west wind and the rain blowing in from the sea; in the lanes, the mire was hock deep and the ponies were splashed with mud above the girth.

"We're goin' to arrive wet through and with news about as cheerful as this here weather is," Higg said as at last they emerged from the woods above Dunster and crossed the packhorse bridge where once Liza had quarrelled with Christopher. "I'm that sorry about your mother, Mistress Lanyon. Only maybe she's better off there than in Washford. A busy workshop and a man like Dyer, all jolly and hearty, mightn't be best for someone that just wants to be quiet. Though I'm not sure," said Higg doubtfully, "that we shouldn't have called at Washford to give Master Dyer news of her. He's her husband, after all."

"No, Higg! I don't want to go near Master Dyer. Master Richard deals with him when it's necessary, but I can't bear the thought of even seeing him in the distance," said Liza angrily. "If he wants to know how his wife is, let him go to the abbey himself! If it hadn't been for him and his dishonesty, she'd be happy with him now."

"Well, the illness might have come on her anyhow," said Higg mildly. "Who's to know? It could be the abbey's the best haven."

"I hope you're right," Liza said, pulling her cloak more firmly around her. She glanced anxiously at Higg, who had sneezed twice since that morning. He was a healthy man normally, but he still had the cough he had acquired during the epidemic, and he had had several feverish colds since then, when he'd had to keep to his bed in his cottage. She hoped he wasn't going to fall ill now.

Liza had been at Allerbrook now for over twelve years and had visited Dunster very rarely since her marriage, but the woolly, unmistakable smell of the overfull Weaver household, the clack of looms from the weaving shed at the back and the usual air of domestic confusion still meant home. The moment she set foot in the house, she could hear one of the menfolk upstairs complaining that he wanted to change into a clean shirt and hadn't got one, and a protesting female voice, pointing out that things weren't yet dry from the wash. "It b'ain't ideal drying weather, now, be it, zur?"

The sound of the argument made her laugh. It welcomed her as much as the smiling faces of her family. Yes, this was her home, even though her parents were no longer here, even though Aunt Cecy was among the first to greet her, and her first words were "Well, Liza, you look fine and healthy and I'm glad to see it, but still only the one daughter, I hear?"

However, someone had called her brother Tommy from the weaving shed and he came to her rescue, although for a moment she hardly recognised him. She had missed her father's funeral, being still abed after Quentin's birth, and had last seen Tommy when he was only fourteen. He was twenty-one now and disconcertingly like his father. He, however, knew her and seized her in a delighted hug. "Liza! We thought you'd forgotten us! Oh, we're glad to see you."

"I've been visiting Mother. The news isn't happy, I'm afraid.

But first, we need to get dry and warm. Higg here has been sneezing and we're both wet through."

"Elena's here in the house. She and Laurence are supping here tonight. She'll look after you. I'll take care of Higg. Come in, man. I'll get someone to take those ponies down to the stable and rub the mud off them. They look as if they've been rollin' in it! You get that cloak off—God's teeth, it's drenched, right enough. There'll be mulled ale before you've time to turn round. We've news of our own that's not so cheerful, either, but that can wait. *Joss!*" He turned to shout up the stairs, where the altercation about shirts seemed to be getting noisier. "Help yourself to one of my shirts—we're the same size! And stop makin' such a to-do. Liza's come to see us! That's Joss, one of Laurence and Elena's boys," he added to Liza. "Not a boy now—he's grown up since you last saw him. Well, let's get you and Higg here dry and settled."

Before long the whole family, including cousin Joss in his borrowed shirt, had gathered in the big main room to drink mulled ale and exchange news. Liza told them of Margaret's strange malady, though she did not mention the hair shirt. Her mother had said she was not to tell the Weavers why she had really left Herbert, and Liza would not disobey her. Besides, even to think of her mother in that self-imposed discomfort was anguish and she knew she couldn't speak of it without crying.

"The nuns seem to be looking after her as best they can," she said. "Now, tell me where my brother Arthur is."

"That's the thing we've got to break to you," said Tommy. "When all the trouble broke out, the lord of Dunster Castle, Lord Pembroke, I mean, sent someone round to do some recruiting. Or conscripting, rather. He took Arthur, and another of

Laurence's sons—the youngest one, Dickon. Twenty-seven, he was. Good job neither of them was married. They didn't leave widows and children crying for them and that's something. I'm sorry, Liza. They were killed in the fighting before Pembroke was captured. There's a lot of families in Dunster that have lost men. We didn't send word to Allerbrook because the news was all muddled at first. We kept hoping maybe it was wrong. We didn't get firsthand word until a Dunster lad came home a month ago."

"Arthur—dead?" She had not let them see that she wanted to cry for her mother, but the tears pricked now, for her brother. "Oh, *no!*"

"Aye." That was Great-Uncle Will, still in his familiar chair although by now he was over eighty-five. "Tommy's your dad's heir now, Liza."

"Better not send word to St. Catherine's," said Liza. "It would do Mother no good to hear of it. Oh, this cruel war! My husband's away, too, though we've heard he's alive, but when he'll come home I've no idea!"

"More mulled ale for you, my girl," said Tommy. "Try not to be too sad. The lad who came home said he saw Arthur die and it was quick. One sword slash and it was over. Let's hope it was the same for Dickon."

"I'm glad of that," said Liza in a strained voice, and did not repeat what Richard had once told them, that people reporting such deaths always said they had been quick, whether it was true or not.

Laurence and Elena were both at supper and Liza thought that although they were of course not young, they looked older than they really were. They had lost two sons now to the fighting between Lancaster and York and grief had left its mark.

The supper was generous and as good in quality as ever it had been under Margaret's skilled guidance. Higg, who had been given dry clothes from the skin outward, while his own steamed in the kitchen, partook like everyone else, although Liza noticed that he didn't seem to be eating much.

"Aren't you hungry, Higg?" she asked, leaning forward to speak to him down the table.

"Seemingly not so very, Mistress," Higg said. Or rather, croaked.

"Higg! What's wrong with your voice?"

"I'm sort of husky, Mistress. It'll be the damp that's done it, I daresay."

Liza got to her feet and walked down the table to put a hand on his wrist. It almost burned her fingers.

"You have a fever! You should be in bed."

"How is he?" Liza asked next morning, encountering Tommy as she climbed up to the attic room where Higg had been put to bed.

"Not too well, Liza. Go in and see for yourself. Elena's brewing him a draught—she's handy with herbs. Horehound and honey, she says, for his throat and feverfew to cool him."

Liza went on and into the room, not without a shiver because although it was so many years ago, this was the very room where she had been not only imprisoned but beaten. But the memories fled when she saw Higg lying on a pallet, his face flushed and his breath coming harshly.

"Sorry, Mistress. Can't talk much."

"Elena will bring you something. Then you must try to sleep." He was warm enough; coverlets had been placed over him and the weather was sunny again. If only it had been sunny on that two-day ride! "I'm sorry I dragged you on this journey. But we shall get you well again and I'll stay here until you are. I'll send a message to Allerbrook to explain."

Higg looked at her unhappily and coughed. When he had finished coughing, he said, "Wish Betsy were here. Can't 'ee send for Betsy?"

Liza found Tommy at the foot of the attic stairs, waiting for her to come down. "He shouldn't be left alone," she said.

"He won't be. We'll see someone watches by him. How do you think he is?"

"Very ill. He wants his wife. Tommy…"

"We've a customer staying at the inn and setting off today for home—and that's in Hawkridge. Allerbrook's hardly out of his way. I'll ask him to take a message."

"Thank heaven," said Liza, "that the shearing's over and we've got the hay in."

"There's my sensible sister! And now," said Tommy, scanning her thoughtfully, "I think you've had misery enough, what with our mother, and hearing the news about Arthur and Dickon, and now all this worry about Higg. We'll look after him. You go out and walk the way you did before you were married. I remember even though I was so young! Take the air and leave Higg to us. I'll see that word goes to Allerbrook, never fear."

"I still like to walk," Liza said. "At Allerbrook, when I have a little time to myself, I go walking on the moor and I enjoy gathering bilberries there when it's the season. Yes, I'll go out. Just for a while."

The air was fresh after the rain, as though the two wet days had washed the air clean. If she were not so anxious about Higg, walking through the village would be a delight and it was pleasant even as things were. She knew her family could be trusted to give Higg the best of care for an hour or so. Stepping out briskly, Liza made her way through the narrow street around the foot of the castle, and wandered on over the crossroads where the track came down the castle hill and continued on to Alcombe.

She had set out with no particular aim but her feet, as if they knew where they were going, took her down West Street, and turned off across the flat little bridge over the mill leat, which had been made before William the Norman ever set foot in England. She walked on beside the gurgling water in its narrow channel, passing the mill, its wheel turning slowly in the leat which farther on rejoined the Avill River. Crossing another small bridge, she found herself turning into a tiny path on her left. It led into a dell that earlier in the year would have been full of bluebells. It was just a grassy place now, with a few daisies and yellow dandelions in it.

On the far side was a fallen tree, not the one on which she and Christopher had once sat, but very like it. It wasn't recent, though, for its bark was gone, exposing the smooth grey wood below. Being sheltered by overhanging trees, it was also dry, despite yesterday's rain. It was just as good a seat as the other had been and a man was sitting on it now, studying a book. The sun had laid a shaft on his head, as if deliberately. He had a tonsure, but it was ringed with thick, springy hair the colour of fire.

It was as though she had known he would be there and had come to meet him.

"Christopher?" she said.

CHAPTER TWENTY-FOUR 🌀

LOVE AND DEATH

Christopher stood up, closing his book. "Liza!"

They stood for a long moment, speechless, until he said hesitantly, "It is Liza, isn't it? It's been so long…."

"Of course I'm Liza. Have I changed so much?"

"No. Hardly at all. It's just that…I come here quite often. I think I do it so as to sit and read in a place where the memories would keep me company. But now the memory has become real and taken me by surprise. What brought *you* here?"

"I think I was looking for memories, too. Or did I know you'd be here? I can't tell. My feet just brought me."

"How are you? You're married, of course? Yes, I can see your wedding ring. Are you happy? With—Peter Lanyon, is that the name?"

"Yes. He's kind and I'm fond of him. He's away at the war now."

"And you pray for his safety every night?"

"He is safe. We know that now. He just hasn't been released from service. But yes, I prayed every night and every morning until the fighting was over," said Liza.

She walked across the dell and they sat down, side by side, on the log. Christopher put his book down at his feet and turned to her. "I'm glad things have gone well for you. Have you children?"

"A daughter, four years old. Quentin, we called her, after my grandmother. I had...some bad luck with children."

"Some families do, and no one knows why. I sometimes think God doesn't want the human race to multiply too fast."

"Are you still at St. George's?" Liza asked.

"No. I'm back in the castle now, chaplain to the steward and servants there. When I first left the priory I thought, perhaps now I can make some enquiries—find out how you were. But I kept hesitating, wondering if I should. I'm a full priest now. I have been for years."

"Yes. I supposed that would happen. Is the castle very different, without the Luttrells?"

"The castle is a disgrace!" said Christopher with energy. "That's how it always is when landlords stay away. I've urged the servants to attend to their duties better, but I'm not the steward and the man who is is bone idle. The land is nearly as bad and so is the village. So many roofs in need of repair! You're visiting your family, I suppose? Are they well?"

"Not all of them." Liza began to explain. With kindness in his eyes, Christopher listened to her account of her mother's illness and the deaths of her brother and cousin, and now of Higg's illness, too. She did not mention Herbert Dyer's dishonesty but kept to the story her mother had chosen to tell, of a desire to retire from the world and take refuge in an abbey. Christopher asked no awkward questions.

"Everything hasn't gone well for you, after all. You have many troubles," he said. "I am sorry. I will pray for Higg's recovery."

"Christopher, are you happy as a priest? Was it the right thing for you after all?"

"I suppose so. I've given myself to it. Sometimes I think that what I took to be a call, back when I was a boy, was just a case of a passionate youth looking for somewhere for passion to go. Like a river seeking the sea. I'm not sure I found the right sea in the end, no. But I have done my best. There's no going back, Liza. Not for me, or for you."

"No, I know. I'm glad we've met again, though. Oh!"

"What is it?"

Liza was looking at his left hand. "You still have my ring. You're wearing it on your little finger."

"Yes. I had it on a chain round my neck while I was in the priory, but now I wear it openly. No one has ever questioned it."

There was silence while she absorbed the significance of that. "I've often thought of you, you know, wondered what you were doing, whether you were in good health and if…whether…"

"Whether I ever thought of you?" Christopher asked, and suddenly there it was again, that tough grin which had always made her insides turn somersaults. "Well, now you know that I have. As your ring testifies."

There was another silence until Liza said, "I've been over twelve years married and I've no complaint of Peter. And you're a priest. I'm glad we've met again, glad you didn't forget me, but…"

"I know," said Christopher, and stood up, holding out his hand to her. "Come. Let us part as friends and remember each other in our prayers. I am happy to know you're safe, and loved by your husband."

"I wish you well in your efforts to make the castle servants work properly!"

"Hah! Absentee landlords!" Christopher said, and they parted, with a handclasp, an exchange of smiles and one backward glance from Liza as she walked away.

Her step was light and her heart sang all the way back to the Weavers' house, although her mood changed quickly when she got there, for Tommy met her at the door, his normally cheerful young face unnaturally solemn.

"Higg is very unwell indeed," he said. "I didn't use our customer as a messenger to Allerbrook after all. I've sent one of Laurie's boys to Allerbrook to fetch his wife, at once."

Betsy was in Dunster by suppertime that same evening. She was well over fifty now and she was drawn with exhaustion by the time she arrived, on a broad-backed Allerbrook pony from which she toppled rather than dismounted. She refused, however, to sit down or take any food or drink or even remove her cloak before she had seen Higg. Liza took her to the attic.

Higg was lying on his back, his mouth half-open and his face sunken. He was barely conscious and his breathing now was very bad, in spite of all Elena's herbal remedies and the steam inhalations recommended by the physician who had been called.

"He's all dry-skinned. He b'ain't sweating," said Betsy, feeling his forehead. "He did ought to sweat. Higg, can you hear me, love?" His eyes half opened and a weak hand stretched out to her. Betsy seized it. "You got to sweat. It'll mean being very hot but it's best for 'ee. We'll put more covers on 'ee and see if that does it, that and this June weather."

"If only we hadn't been caught in that rain," said Liza desperately. "I feel it's my fault."

"He could of got wet through out in the fields, just the same," said Betsy. "He often has, only it never used to matter. Thirty-five years we've been wed. Oh, *Higg!*"

Her face creased suddenly, and Liza put an arm around her. "We'll get him through. Come. Let's fetch some more covers."

Elena helped to carry extra rugs up to the attic and spread them over the patient. "I'll brew some more medicines and fetch another bowl of hot water. The physician gave us something to put in it, some sort of balsam, he says it is, to clear the chest. And I've an ointment to rub in."

"And water," said Betsy. "He should have water. Feverish like that, he'll have a thirst. Have you got well water?"

"Yes. I'll fetch a jugful. Now, you take off that cloak and come down for some supper, even if you eat it quick. You've had a long journey. You can sleep up here if you want. We'll put another pallet down. But one of us'll be here and awake all night. Don't worry."

The warm June night descended, with stars in a sky so clear that the recent downpour seemed unbelievable. The window was closed against draughts and a candle was set on the sill to light the vigil.

Betsy, wearied beyond bearing, slept on the second pallet alongside Higg's, while Liza sat up, relieved by Elena at half past three in the morning. From time to time they gave Higg water to drink, or doses of Elena's medicine, and Elena, coming on duty, brought a towel and a basin full of hot water mixed with the physician's aromatic balsam. Deftly she sat Higg up so that with his head under the towel to keep the steam in, he could breathe the scented vapour.

Liza returned in the morning after a snatched breakfast. She found Betsy and Elena sitting one on either side of him, their faces anxious. "Has the fever broken yet?" she asked.

Miserably, Betsy shook her head.

It went on all that day and all the next night. Betsy kept vigil that night, refusing to rest although Elena was there with her. At daybreak both of them took some hurried food and then collapsed into exhausted sleep while Liza, who had slept, took over. This, the third day of Higg's illness, wore wretchedly on. Hot and dry, drawing breaths that sounded as though they were rattling over shingle, he lay and tossed but no sweat came. Toward evening, Tommy went to fetch the parish priest.

The last rites were spoken over Higg, who managed to croak some weak responses. The priest was still there when Higg, who had been propped up on pillows to ease his breathing, was seized with a paroxysm of coughing and could not stop. It grew worse and worse and his eyes became huge and dark as he fought for breath. When he began to cough up blood, spraying the covers and the wall beside him, the priest said, "Take his wife away," and Liza, though Betsy resisted her, somehow persuaded her out of the room and kept her out until it was all over.

When he had been tidied by some of the other women and moved to another room where there were no bloodstains, Elena and Liza took Betsy, weeping, to say goodbye to him. She clung to his hand and called his name as though still hoping that he would answer, and it took some time before they could coax her to leave him. They took her to the bedchamber Liza was using, where they induced her, though still with difficulty, to eat something, and gave her a drink of honeyed wine which Elena said would help her to rest. Then they put her to bed and stayed with her until she slept.

Liza shared the bed with Betsy that night, and when they both woke in the dead hours of the night, shared her tears.

In the usual course of events, Higg would have been buried in Clicket, with people who knew him well to gather at the graveside. As it was, he was laid in the churchyard of St. George's, and few of those present knew him at all. There were plenty of them, however. The Weavers turned out in force and so, in neighbourly solidarity, did many other Dunster folk.

"Well, he went off with an escort I'm proud of," Betsy said to Liza when the funeral refreshments, arranged in the Weavers' house, had been consumed and the crowd had gone. She had got over her tears and borne herself with dignity all through the ceremony, though Liza saw, with sadness, that overnight she seemed to have grown bent and lined. "Now we'll have to go home, I suppose. Can't leave Kat and Roger and your father-in-law to manage all alone."

"Father-in-law was talking of bringing in the two younger Hannacombe boys," Liza said. "They're old enough to be useful."

Betsy sat heavily down in the window seat of the Weavers' big room. "I can't do the ride tomorrow, not so soon. I've got to do it sometime but I'd be that thankful for another day, to get my breath back, like."

"Of course you shall have another day," said Liza. "Spend tomorrow how you like. Sleep, or walk in the garden, whatever you want. My family won't mind. We'll go home the day after."

The weather, as though that one rainstorm had cleared the air of trouble, had since then remained pleasant—warm without being hot. In the morning Betsy went back to the churchyard to stand for a while beside the filled grave. "I want to be near 'un. Can't help thinkin' he'll be lonely when I go home."

Liza went with her, but sensing that Betsy wanted to be alone, said that she would go for a walk by herself and call at the churchyard on the way back, to see if Betsy were still there. "We can go back to dinner together," she said.

"All right. Just let me be. I want to cry a bit on my own."

"I'll come back soon," Liza said, and moved away toward the churchyard gate into West Street. Presently she reached the lane by the mill leat and once again, she took the track toward the dell. Once again, it was as though her feet were choosing where she should go.

And once again, Christopher was sitting, reading, on the fallen log. As before, he stood up as she came toward him, and another shaft of sunlight shining from behind Liza's head turned the ring of springy hair around his shaven poll to the colour of flame.

"I hoped you'd be here," Liza said and her voice shook, so that he came to take her arm and steer her to the log, to seat her on it.

"Liza, what's happened? Something is wrong. I can tell."

"Higg died. We buried him yesterday."

"Ah. Yes, I wondered. I visited the monks yesterday—some of them are my friends and I wanted to see how their herb garden did now that I'm not there to look after it—and when I left them, I passed the churchyard and saw that a burial was taking place. I suppose it was his. I'm sorry."

"He was kind. He was always kind. When I first went to Allerbrook—that's the name of our farm—I felt so strange, so far

331

from home. He made me a carved wooden platter as a gift, my first Christmas. His wife, Betsy, is kind, too, and she's heart-broken. She's sitting by his grave now. She didn't want me to stay with her. They'd been married for thirty-five years. We tried so hard to save him. We tried and tried but…"

"Liza. Dear Liza. Don't you go breaking your heart. You're still too young for that."

"Everyone's dying!" Liza cried out. "My brother Arthur's been killed, and my cousin Dickon and though I know now that Peter is alive, it seems to me that I spent forever wondering if I'd see him again. And my mother…I'm afraid for her! I didn't tell you everything. She's not *herself* anymore. She's turned her back on life while she's still living it. I know she's in good hands. I know I should be more sensible. I'm fortunate in so many ways. I'm alive and well and have a good home and a daughter and Peter will come back. But it's all so dreadful. If I'm breaking my heart, I can't help it. Sometimes one just *can't* be sensible."

"No, I know," said Christopher, and his arms went around her instinctively. She never afterward recalled deciding to put hers around him in turn; they went there by themselves. She and Christopher clung together as they had done in the old days, but more strongly, more intensely. Their mouths locked. He pushed her coif off just as he used to do and his fingers were in her hair and hers deep in the circle of his thick red locks, rejoicing in their texture, their vitality.

The grass in front of the log was short and soft. They slid down to it easily. Liza found herself staring into his eyes, thinking once again how beautiful, how rare was that warm amber brown, those golden flecks. She freed her mouth and said, "We shouldn't, we mustn't, but I need you to hold me. I need someone…"

"And I need you. Liza, my only love, there has never been a day when I didn't think of you. My dear and my sweetheart, we should have been married. We were meant to be married. They shouldn't have dragged us apart."

"There's been too much death," said Liza brokenly. "Just too much."

"I know."

All the time their bodies, driven on by the need to outwit death, to perform the one act which could create life, to fling a challenging gauntlet at the old man with the skull face and the scythe, were finding ways to reach each other. Clothing was pushed aside, untied. As they glided together, a tangle of unspoken emotions blazed into life; all the old desire, all the old frustration at its denial; all the bitter grief and secret rage they had felt at being wrenched away from each other. Their union began with a vigour which was near to violence, with anger in it as well as passion; almost a vengefulness.

The storm passed, dissolving into simplicity and love; Christopher nuzzling, comforting, murmuring endearments, giving himself as a gift; Liza laughing and crying, clinging and giving herself in reply, seeking to engulf him as he sought to be engulfed.

Never had it been like this with Peter. Peter had given her satisfaction and sometimes enjoyment, but not like this, this fury melting into tenderness, this growing, spreading tree of joy within her and this unbelievable bursting into bloom at the finish; a flowering the colour of fire, which flamed and died softly away, to leave her marvelling.

They lay entangled, holding each other, until at last it seemed

time to get up, to resume their garments and to sit down, won-
deringly, side by side on the dry grey log and look into each
other's faces.

"I didn't mean that to happen," said Christopher. "But…"

"I'm glad it did. Glad. I've wanted it to happen ever since…I
think ever since we met at the fair. Do you remember? Oh,
Christopher, how can I go back to Allerbrook now? Though
I must," said Liza, bewildered. "I can't, but I must. There's
Quentin, my daughter. I've a life there. And…you must go back
to the castle. There's no way forward for us. There was just
this…this one morning."

"It's real, you know," said Christopher. "What I feel for you.
It always was. It's as though it comes from outside, drawn up into
me as a tree draws up sap from the earth. Today it burst into leaf
and blossom."

"You see it as that? I had such a picture in my mind just now,
when we were together!"

"Did you? It seems we think together. Our minds must be
linked. I believe they would be linked even if one of us were
removed to Cathay."

"I shall have to remove to Allerbrook soon. Darling, I must
go. How long have we been here?"

"I don't know. Half an hour? Most of eternity?"

"Do I look dishevelled? Am I fit to be seen?"

"Your coif isn't straight and there's mud on your face!"

"There's mud in your *hair!*"

They parted, clasping hands once more in farewell, looking
at each other with longing but managing, bravely, to smile. Liza
made her way slowly back up West Street, wondering how it was
possible to be filled with loss and sorrow but also to be insanely

happy, all at once. She found Betsy still sitting alone beside Higg's resting place.

"Betsy, please come. I'm sure that grass is damp, out in the open like this." *The grass in the dell wasn't damp. It was cool and soft and a perfect bed for lovers. Don't think about that!* She helped Betsy up, took her arm and led her out of the churchyard by the main gate.

"Where did you walk to?" Betsy asked as they went.

"Oh, just down to the river. I stood there awhile and looked at the water. One can watch flowing rivers for hours, though I don't have much spare time to watch the Allerbrook, of course."

"We won't have much spare time now Higg's gone, Mistress."

"No," Liza agreed, "I don't suppose we will."

They walked on, arm in arm, two unremarkable women with their plain headdresses and workaday dresses. One of them was still in a nightmare of bereavement and the other had just been to heaven and back, but no one would have guessed it.

Christopher, returning to the castle, knew that he should be racked with guilt. He had betrayed his vocation, his priesthood, his celibacy. Shame should be drowning him. Instead, he felt as though strength and energy were pouring through him. Liza was gone. They might never meet again. But they *had* met; just once in their lives they had met as fully as two human beings ever could and he was glad, glad, *glad*. Whoever thought he should feel guilty did not know what living was.

The castle's state of neglect struck him anew as he went into the hall. He had made repeated attempts to stir the servants up, but Master Hilton never gave him any support and they always slid back into their old ways before long. Eventually he had given up. This, he suddenly decided, was going to change.

Catching sight of the steward, Christopher advanced on him. "Master Hilton!"

"Ah. Father Christopher. I have been looking for you. I have heard of a most interesting devotional book for sale, which—"

"Never mind that now," said Christopher. "There's something I want to say to *you*. The Earl of Pembroke is dead, but he has heirs. One of these days, a new landlord may well descend on this castle. What do you imagine he will think of it?"

"I don't understand," said Hilton disdainfully. He had sought the services of Father Christopher, but since Christopher's arrival, he had sometimes wished he'd chosen differently. There was something positively crude in Christopher's energy. Priests were supposed to be gentlemen and they should be quiet, refined, devoted to prayer and worthy conversation. Priests shouldn't stride about pulsating with red-headed vitality. It was not the way either a man of the cloth or a gentleman should behave.

Christopher, on his side, eyed the elegantly dressed Hilton with annoyance, wondering how a man so plainly fastidious in his person could tolerate such squalid living conditions.

"What he or they will think," said Christopher, kicking the mouldy rushes at his feet, "is that these rushes stink, that the hangings are rotting and no one has as much as brushed them, let alone repaired them, for the last hundred years. That every floor in this place needs a broom and every cooking pan needs some sand and a whole lot of elbow grease, and every table and settle and chest needs a taste of beeswax! The only decently kept room in the castle is the chapel! The rest is something a half-witted peasant wouldn't want to live in!"

"My good man, I've said to you before, you're here to lead us in prayer, not to set us a housewifely example! You have no authority to speak to me in this fashion."

"Authority? Well, if necessary, I can and will write to Pembroke's family and report the lax way you perform your duties. I expect they'd be interested, whoever read the letter. I've got another form of authority, too."

"Which is?"

Christopher grinned. Liza would have recognised that grin. "I'm not taller than you are," he said sweetly. "But I'm stronger and sturdier than you. It's probably due to all the gardening I did at the priory." He flexed a biceps and regarded it complacently. "I advise you to cooperate with me."

CHAPTER TWENTY-FIVE

A MATTER OF A DOWRY

"So once again," said Agnes Sweetwater bitterly, "I am not good enough. It's always the same. They come and look me over, as though I were a mare they might want to buy. At times I expect them to look at my teeth and feel my legs! And then comes the little matter of money—and land."

Walter Sweetwater regarded his daughter unhappily. She was a good girl, with no foolish, romantic notions. She was a Sweetwater through and through—cool grey eyes, bushy brown hair which her maid had to thin out and shave at the front, a build that would one day turn to flesh but not, please God, until after she had produced a flourishing family of brown-haired, well-built, cool-eyed youngsters. Unluckily, before she could start producing the family she needed a husband, and the kind of man he wanted for her always expected more dowry than the Sweetwaters could provide.

The ladies' solar at Sweetwater House was upstairs, at the southwest end of the building, with windows on three sides, providing views of farmland, river and village. It possessed a wide hearth, comfortable, cushioned seats, a table and some shelves to hold such things as lutes, packs of cards, workboxes and a backgammon set. The beamed ceiling was high and the light was good. The room was big enough for a dozen ladies, but at the present time it was used by only four, for Agnes Sweetwater's mother had been dead for a year or more, and two girl cousins who had lived with the Sweetwaters for a time had been retrieved by their parents and married off. Married well, moreover. Their parents had been more skilled at such negotiations than the Sweetwaters were, it seemed. The remaining four were Baldwin's kittenish wife, Catherine, Agnes herself, and their maids. Catherine, head bent over her embroidery, was keeping out of the conversation and her maid was not there, but Agnes's woman, Maude, was seated by her mistress.

"I am sorry for your disappointment," Walter said awkwardly. He was never quite at ease in the feminine surroundings of the solar. They always made him want to be out practising martial skills on his warhorse, or else in the fields discussing sheep with Edward Searle. "Young Northcote is half a Carew and both families are rising in the world and have an eye to gain, it seems. They want land. I would settle land on you gladly if I had it to spare, but I haven't. You liked Giles Northcote, then?"

"Yes, Father. I did, as it happens."

Maybe his daughter wasn't as free of romantic nonsense as he had supposed. Her voice was sad and the maid gave her mistress a worried glance. Maude was attached to Agnes and had done much to comfort her during the sad days after the death of his wife. She was also pockmarked and gossipy and he didn't, personally, like her much, but when Agnes did marry, Maude could go with her and then he wouldn't have to see that pitted face about the place anymore. If only there were a way to bring this marriage off!

"Do you think Giles took to you, as well?" he asked.

"I think so, yes," Agnes said.

Well, and why not? Agnes had good health, clear skin and a pleasant smile. Any young man might find her attractive. But Giles Northcote, like Agnes, was only twenty-one and his parents expected him to do as he was told. If Agnes's dowry were not up to standard, he would be told that he couldn't marry her and he would have no say in the matter.

If only that damned Peter Lanyon hadn't got to Gloucester's side with his confounded horse so quickly at Tewkesbury. If only Walter Sweetwater had got in first!

Three days overdue, Liza thought. She had checked over and over again, counting on her fingers, but there it was. Seventeen days ago she and Christopher had made love in the dell at Dunster, and seen, in their minds, an image of a flowering tree. The flowers, it seemed, had seeded.

Had Kat or Betsy noticed anything? Neither of them now needed the cloths which younger women required at regular intervals unless they were carrying, and Liza looked after hers discreetly, soaking used ones in a lidded pail of salt water which she kept in a corner of the kitchen, changing the salt water night and morning, wringing out cloths when the salt had done its work and putting them in a pail of clean water, and finally, when it was all finished this time around, boiling the whole lot with some soap and drying them on some bushes at the back of the farm-house if the weather was good, or around the little hearth in her room if not.

Liza didn't think that the other women had realised the long gap since last time. Betsy was too sunk in her grief to notice anything at all and Kat was distracted by anxiety about Betsy. Neither was much good at keeping track of time, anyway. If either of them did mention it, she would say that all the distress over her mother, and Higg, and the news of her brother's death had upset her. That would stave off disaster for a while.

But what then? Discovery was bound to come in the end unless nature released her. That was possible, even likely, given her history. But if nature failed her...

So many times she had prayed to God, to the saints, to let her carry a child to term. Now she must pray that she would not and that she would lose it soon enough to pass the matter off as a normal course, keeping secret the pain and the violence of the bleeding. If nothing happened...

If nothing happened, then there would be no shelter any-where, no hope, no future. She would be cast out by the Lanyons and the Weavers alike, perhaps paraded through Clicket as a whore. She would do better to make some excuse to go out on a pony one day, and ride to the distant coast, where there were cliffs, and cast herself into the sea.

Meanwhile, she must appear as normal as she could. It was natural that she should seem downcast, of course. Seeing her mother in such an unhappy state *had* distressed her; so had the news about Arthur and Dickon, and so had Higg's tragedy.

"But life goes on," Richard had said at breakfast, only that morning. "No use looking so dismal, my girl. Death's always with us. If it isn't war, it's illness and if it isn't illness, it's accident. Will Hudd managed to be down with a fever when the Sweetwaters were mustering, so he didn't have to go off to fight, but then what happened at the very next haymaking? He gets careless with a scythe and takes the top off his left forefinger. Life's full of trouble. I've got those two Hannacombe lads—Eddie and Jarvis—coming before the harvest, by the way. You'd better think about where they're to sleep."

Liza spent much of the day planning for them. They could lodge with Betsy, which would give her something to do. She need not feed them; they could have meals at the farmhouse. Betsy, approached on the matter, was *agreeable,* if agreeable were the word for mere acquiescence.

"Just as you say, mistress. Just as you say." Every word that Betsy spoke sounded like a clod falling on a coffin. It would be an even chance whether the young Hannacombes brought cheerfulness back to Betsy, or Betsy's sorrow crushed their youthful high spirits forever. Even Peter's lively dog Rusty looked depressed when Betsy was about.

Liza tried to laugh about it with Richard. It was a huge effort, but he said with approval, "That's better. You sound more like yourself. You're a sensible wench."

Sensible. That word again! Her parents had reared her to be sensible; then one day at a fair in Dunster a redheaded young man had noticed that she didn't like seeing Bart Webber being exhibited as a cheat, and there went common sense, wiped out of existence like food stains from a dish. She'd tried to be sensible over the matter of Herbert Dyer, and look what had come of that! But if only she'd been sensible seventeen days ago in Dunster! Maybe tomorrow…

On waking next morning, she checked herself. There was nothing, except a tightness in her stomach and a slight sense of nausea.

Eighteen days since she and Christopher had been together. Four days overdue.

"I've heard some pretty gossip down in Clicket," Richard announced, arriving back from a foray into the village to meet Sim Hannacombe and Will Hudd in the White Hart and discuss details of whose barley was going to be reaped first when the time came. He sauntered into the kitchen, where supper was giving off fragrant smells. "What's this? Pottage with fresh meat in it?"

"Chicken," Liza said. "That hen that seems to have stopped laying. I decided we'd better eat her. I've put her in a stew and cooked cabbage to go with her and there's fresh cheese and dumplings, too." *Sound cheerful, Liza. Why, oh why won't nature set me free when she's done it so often before?*

"Get it on the table, and I'll tell you my tale," Richard said. "Betsy, leave scraping those pots and come and help me off with my boots, and don't burst into tears this time because you'll never take Higg's boots off for him again. Mourning's one thing, but it can't go on forever."

"He's not been gone a month," said Betsy resentfully, though she wiped her hands and went to help him as he sat down by the hearth.

"It feels like a year. Never seen such a lot of long faces in all my life. You ought to be happier, Liza. We know that Peter'll be home one of these days. Thanks, Betsy. Just let me get some supper inside me, and then I'll tell you my tale."

A few minutes later, breaking bread into his stew, he said, "It's more than one tale, as it happens, but they're both about marriage. Gilbert Lowe was in the White Hart today, in a vile temper. That put-upon daughter of his, Martha, well, for all she's not far short of forty, she's run off with a sheepshearer, a widower fellow, about her own age. Gone off with him to Barnstaple, where he comes from, and wed him, too, all right and proper, and left Tilly Lowe to do all the work of the house unless Gilbert loosens his purse strings and takes on a maid or two. Whole tavern was laughing, except for Gilbert!"

"Well!" said Liza, determinedly showing the interest that would be expected. "I never would have thought Martha would have so much spirit! But you said there was more than one tale?"

"Indeed there is. Before Gilbert came in with his long face as though his girl were dead instead of wed, the talk in the Hart was that the Sweetwaters have had another try at marrying off their girl, Agnes, and been turned down again. Same reason as before—her dowry's too small. Adam Turner said they aim too high, and I reckon he's right."

"How did all that come to be known?" Liza asked. "Who spreads the Sweetwater business round the tavern?"

"Agnes has a maid with a tongue that wags like Rusty's tail—or at least like Rusty's tail when he hasn't got it between his legs because Betsy's making him sad. We all valued Higg, Betsy, but he did die cared for and with a priest at hand and that's not so for everyone."

It hadn't been so for a girl on Castle Rock, years ago, but better not think of that.

Betsy, on the verge of weeping, rose and went to the kitchen, banging the door after her. Richard looked after her and sighed.

"I suppose she'll get over it one day. Getting back to my story—Agnes Sweetwater's chatty tirewoman is partial to a tankard of ale now and again and that's the way word gets round the White Hart. It seems that the man they had in mind is a Northcote—they're a wealthy Devon family—and he's related to another one, the Carews. His people want land as part of the dowry, but though Walter has more than just Clicket and the farms round here, he still hasn't enough going spare and he can't afford to buy more. That'll be the third time the girl's been said no to." He sounded pleased about it.

"Well, I be sorry for her, if you're not." Kat didn't care for Richard's ruthless attitude to Betsy's grieving and seized the chance to argue. "'Tweren't her fault that her men went huntin' and crashed into your dad's funeral. It's no good thing for a wench to be left unwed, like a dusty old bowl on a potter's shelf that no one wants to buy. Martha Lowe was lucky to escape. Another couple of years and she'd have been past praying for. Agnes Sweetwater's got as much right to a good man as any other, and once 'ee've got one, it's the best thing in the world, even if it don't last forever." She gave a kindly glance toward Roger, who was so stooped now that his nose was almost in his pottage. "Better to have and lose than never have at all."

"As long as you don't lose too soon." Betsy, returning from the kitchen with a dish of dumplings, sighed heavily. She put the dish on the table and set about providing little Quentin with some stew and a chopped-up dumpling.

"I'll have some more stew," said Richard, ignoring her. "It's good. Who'd have thought that hen would be this tender? What's the matter, Kat? You've gone rigid like a standing stone out on the moor. Pass the stew to me, can't you? What are you staring out at the farmyard for?"

"Look!" said Kat, and at the same moment Liza, who had also risen to see what had caught Kat's eye, let out a cry, abandoned her own food and ran for the door into the yard.

A moment later, exclaiming joyously, she was in Peter's arms, even though one of them had Plume's reins looped around it. Peter, in turn, was clutching his wife as though afraid she might vanish if he let her go.

"Liza! My sweet Liza, I've missed you so very very much."

"And I you," said Liza, holding him just as tightly. "And I you!"

"Let me put Plume in the stable and see to him, then I'll be with you. I'm not tired. I've got used to riding for hours on end, but Plume's feeling it, poor fellow."

Richard came out to greet his son and help with the pony. By the time they came in again to the stew, which Betsy, looking more animated than she had in weeks, had hurriedly heated again, they had exchanged a good deal of news. Peter condoled with Betsy, shaking his head at the place where Higg used to sit. "And I'm sorry to learn of the troubles in Liza's family. Maybe a bit of good news will help—well, Father, tell them what I told you just now, out in the stable."

"No, you tell it, boy. It's your story."

"I've been in battles," said Peter. "Two big ones especially. I'm lucky to be still alive but here I am, none the worse except for a nick or two that healed easy. That's by the way. I was made to go with the Duke of Gloucester's men—"

"Who'd he be?" Kat asked.

"King Edward's youngest brother, the loyal one. The one in

the middle joined Warwick at one time, though I think he's back supporting his own kinfolk now. That's not the point. I didn't take Plume into the field. I fought on foot, to start with. But in one battle, in a lot of muddle and a thick fog, I got hold of a big horse, got myself put amongst the mounted soldiers. But in the next battle I saw Gloucester's horse fall under him and I gave him mine. He was grateful. That's why I'm late back. After the king had won, he and Gloucester went to London and I had to go as well, and be there at a ceremony—in front of the Tower of London, it was—where rewards were presented to men who'd pleased the king or Gloucester during the war. I had an award! The deeds are in my saddlebag. I've shown them to Father."

"Two farms and a village, just to the south of the moor." Richard couldn't contain himself after all. "We'll get the rents for all of them."

"It was a parcel of land someone left to Gloucester," Peter said. "It's good land, too. I visited it on my way back. It's all let to tenants, but I am the landlord. I have the freehold."

"Freehold…" said Richard thoughtfully. "You know, that's making me think…. Betsy, bring out your best elderflower wine and we'll drink to Peter's reward, and we'll drink to what we might do with it, too." His mouth curved in a satyrlike smile which startled Liza because it looked so alarming. "If you do as I say, boy, like a good son should, maybe poor Agnes Sweetwater'll get her man after all, but if she does, her father'll be beholden to me for it and oh, how he won't like that!"

"But are you really going to agree? After all, the award's yours, not your father's," Liza said when she and Peter were at last alone. She was glad to see him come into the bedchamber, for he hadn't hurried, and when she looked out the window, wondering where he was, he was chopping firewood in the farmyard with excessive violence, though there was plenty of firewood and no need for a man, who had come home only that day from fighting battles, to create more. She was perplexed.

"I won't have much say in the matter," said Peter dryly. "But it will keep him happy, if it works." He was stripping off his hose and shirt as he spoke. The light of the long summer evening streamed into the room. His body, kept muscular from continual riding and frequent fighting, was in fine trim. Even to Liza, with the splendour of Christopher's body still fresh in her memory, this man was beautiful. It seemed that she loved them both, though differently.

There was a sheen of sweat on his skin, from his efforts with the chopper. He found himself a linen towel and rubbed it dry. "*If* it works," Peter said, "we'd be free of the Sweetwaters. No more landlords! I wouldn't mind that, I admit. We'd own Allerbrook outright. Allerbrook can be sold—that's been so for a good century, since the boundary of the Royal Forest was last moved. You can't buy property inside the forest, of course, but that doesn't matter to us now. We can purchase Allerbrook if the Sweetwaters will sell."

"And your father wouldn't need their permission to build the new house he wants so much," said Liza. She hesitated and then said, "He's very serious about it. While you were away—well, I know he gave it a lot of thought."

"And drew plans. I know. He showed them to me," said Peter.

"Yes," Liza said. "And I know he's afraid that if he had to ask them, the Sweetwaters might say he wasn't to build anything that could challenge their own house."

"Exactly!"

"But Peter, you don't *want* a fine new house and I don't think we need one, either."

"Quite right, but Father thinks otherwise. He talked to me and brought out those plans of his while you were doing your evening chores, and I saw just how determined he is. In fact, I'd say that slightly crazed would be nearer the mark! All the same, there *is* sense in breaking free of the Sweetwaters. What Father wants to do is to keep the village and one of the farms I've been granted, and sell the other farm, the bigger one, and then make an offer for Allerbrook. There's a chance that Walter Sweetwater will sell, because he needs money so badly. With it, he may be able to provide Agnes with enough dowry. Father said he and I could share ownership. We won't have to pay rent—or for the right to eat rabbit—and the Sweetwaters couldn't order any of us to follow them to war, ever again, either!"

"I see that. But—oh, I wish your father didn't keep calling you *boy*. You're not a boy. You're—what—over thirty, and you've just come back from a war and been rewarded for your service!" Liza found that her indignation on his behalf was entirely genuine.

"He likes to feel he's the master," said Peter. He spoke quite calmly but then, as though a surge of rage had overtaken him, hurled the towel away, to land in a heap on the floor. "He *has* to feel he's the master. Damn him, damn him! Do you remember the time he went away to war and I was the master of Allerbrook while he was gone? I did well, I know I did. Did he ever say thank you? Did he ever say as much as well done, thou good and faithful son? Did he? *Did he?* No, he bloody well didn't. It was *Out of the way, boy. I'm back now, I'll take charge.* I'd looked after the place for two years but all of a sudden I was supposed to accept that I knew nothing and he knew it all. Liza, there are times when I think I hate him!"

"Oh, Peter!" said Liza inadequately.

With a groan, he sat down on the edge of the bed. "I didn't mean that. Well, maybe I hate him some of the time. He takes after his own father. I remember *him* well enough! It's best if I let him have his way. One day I'll come into my own and meanwhile, letting him pretend I'm still a boy is a small price to pay for peace. When I feel angry with him, I can always go and chop firewood, and put some effort into it!"

"So that's what you were at just now! I saw you from the window."

"Er…yes." Peter laughed, rather awkwardly. "Yes. He's made me angry today, that's true enough. What the Duke of Gloucester has given me is rightly mine and my father's laying claim to it, as near as makes no difference. But I decided not to quarrel with him. I'd rather my wife and child lived in a peaceful household, my love."

"Yes. You think your own thoughts in secret," said Liza. "I understand."

If anyone had gone in for secret thoughts, she had.

Peter had become calm once more. "If Walter Sweetwater's really desperate for money," he remarked, "there's a real chance he'll agree to sell—after a bit of cursing. And there's something else. I've told Father, and now I'll tell you. It's how we decided which farm to keep and which to turn into money."

"What do you mean?"

"I mean," said Peter, "that one of them, the one we mean to keep, isn't just a farm. The Duke of Gloucester did well by me." He smiled, remembering the moment when the deeds were handed to him by the sparely built young man who had known danger and responsibility from an early age, whose right shoulder was a little too big for the rest of him, whose face was lined before its time, but was now lit by a smile of gratitude. The smile widened his thin mouth and gleamed in his hazel eyes, making him almost handsome.

"There's a stone quarry on that piece of land as well," Peter said. "And a profitable one. As I said, I've visited the place." He frowned. "Of course, Father said that when he builds his house, a stone quarry of our own would be useful! Slightly crazed, as I said. But the quarry ought to be a good source of income and perhaps Father won't go on with this notion of building a house, not when he really sees how much it would cost. He'll still have to do a deal of saving and it'll take years, and perhaps by then he'll have changed his mind. Meanwhile," he said, standing up in order to turn back the coverlet, "I'll chop firewood when I feel the need, and keep him happy."

"Well, it's for you to decide," Liza said, pulling off her own clothing. She slipped into the bed. "Peter, I'm so very very glad to see you back."

"I've ached to *be* back, sweetheart."

He came to her, eager and hungry, pulling the covers right off to look at her and then pouncing joyfully, to meet with a response which made him laugh aloud and shout her name and roll across the bed with her, kissing her frantically. Later, the tiredness of the long road from London finally overtaking him, he fell asleep with his nose pushed into her shoulder and Liza, holding him, silently sent up prayers of gratitude to heaven.

She was safe now. If the child within her prospered, no one, least of all Peter himself, would question its parentage. It would be the child of this night; what else? Even if anyone took to counting on their fingers, and they wouldn't, they would take it for granted when the baby came that it had arrived a little early and there was nothing odd about that, not with Liza.

She was a hypocrite, faithless, a liar, a deceiver, an adulteress, probably damned, probably destined for hell. She might well die in bearing this child. That would be heaven's revenge.

But the baby, if it were born and lived, would be safe and so would her good name. Peter had come home in time.

"Buy Allerbrook?" howled Walter Sweetwater, stamping up and down his hall. "Freehold and all? Those damned Lanyons! First of all Peter Lanyon wrecks my chance of getting a reward out of Gloucester and now…"

"We can't do it." Baldwin was as angry as his father. He stood staring out the window, at the hill and the combe above Clicket. He blocked the light from the window like a thundercloud. "It's unthinkable. They just want to thumb their noses at us! We know that Richard Lanyon wants to build himself a big house! Most of Clicket knows—he talks about it in the White Hart. If he gets his hands on Allerbrook, he'll do it! We won't be able to stop him. No one has a bigger head than a prosperous peasant!"

"If we sell to him, would there be enough?" Agnes asked.

Her father and brother turned around. She had been sitting in a window seat, listening, with Catherine beside her.

"What?" said Walter.

"If we sell them Allerbrook for the best price we can get, could we buy enough dowry land to please Giles Northcote's family?"

"There's no question of it!" Baldwin shouted.

"My dear loving brother, it isn't for you to say. Father?"

"You really do want to marry Giles Northcote?" said Walter. "I mean, *want* him?"

"That isn't the point!" Baldwin bellowed.

"Shouldn't it be considered?" said Catherine. "My dear, did you not *want* to marry me?"

"What? Yes, of course I did, my Kitten, but there was no bar, no difficulty. No one asked me to insult my family for your sake."

"But is it such a dreadful insult? They want to buy something from us for a fair price, that's all. And look what it would mean to Agnes!"

"What it could mean to all of us!" Agnes's head was high and her voice proud. "It is not *only* that Giles Northcote and I liked each other when we met. The Northcotes are a good family and so are the Carews, from whom his mother comes. They mix with people in high office. If Giles and I have children, they would have the chance of good marriages. They might go to court. Our sons might be appointed to good positions. So might you, Baldwin! All that, just for Allerbrook!"

"I wish I'd had the sense to find Peter Lanyon and kill him in the fog on Barnet field!" said Baldwin furiously.

"I want to marry Giles Northcote," said Agnes obstinately. "And I think he wants to marry me, and I don't think any of you would regret it. Father, I wouldn't urge you to this if I didn't believe that! If Giles Northcote were a stable boy, I wouldn't ask to marry him, even if he were as pure as a saint and as beautiful as an archangel! I know my duty. But this is a *chance* for us—if there's enough money. Would there be?"

"There could be…yes. I have some in my coffers that I could add and if Catherine will agree—for I wouldn't do this without her agreement—we could part with one of her dower farms…."

"There are four altogether. Two could go," Catherine said at once.

"That's generous. They could be sold and with that money, and some of my savings and whatever I get for Allerbrook, I could buy an estate worth having," Walter said. "There's one in Devon that would do. I heard of it while I was with the king. It may well be for sale. The owner and his heir were both killed at Tewkesbury."

"No!" shouted Baldwin. "Think of the income we'll lose! Rents from two farms as well as Allerbrook! *No,* Father!" Catherine opened her mouth to speak again, but he glared at her and she stopped. "This isn't your business!" Baldwin snapped at her. "Keep out of it!"

"I'll go to the solar," said Catherine. Looking exactly like a dignified kitten, she slipped off the window seat, but before she left the hall she put a kind hand momentarily on Agnes's arm.

Baldwin saw it. "Women!"

"You were crazy for Catherine," said Walter coldly.

"Yes, you were! And now you want to stand between me and Giles just for spite against the Lanyons!" Agnes shouted. "Because that's what it is. We can live without the rents. We could gain much more than we lose! Which is more important, anyway? Your quarrel with the Lanyons or the future of this family and *my whole life?*"

"Stop that! Shouting like a woman selling yarn in a market! I don't expect my sister to raise her voice. Ladies should be soft-spoken, gentle."

"Father!"

"Your sister cannot remain unwed much longer," Walter said seriously to his son. "As for the Lanyons…I detest them as much as you do and the loss of the rents will be a nuisance, but I can see the advantages of this marriage. No, Baldwin. If this makes you lose your temper, then go out and ride your horse till it founders, or get a couple of the stable boys to fight a round or two with you, bare fisted. That'll take the fury out of you. I've made my mind up. I don't like it either, but I am responsible for settling Agnes in life and we could indeed gain from a link with the Northcotes and the Carews. Those two families are very much on their way up. I'll sell."

"And that upstart Richard Lanyon will be digging the foundations of his house before we know it," said Baldwin indignantly.

"Not he," said Walter. "Allerbrook will cost him enough to keep him short for a long, long time. I'll see to that!"

Allerbrook was indeed expensive. Even with the profitable quarry (of which Walter was comfortably unaware), the new Lanyon house might never have come into being at all if nature hadn't taken a hand.

PART THREE

STORM DAMAGE
1480–1486

CHAPTER TWENTY-SIX

BOULDER

"I want to go out!" said Nicky crossly. He was sitting on a chest-cum-settle under one of the hall windows, expressing his view of the weather by kicking the front of the chest. A squall of wind rattled the window and Liza, going to it, saw that it wasn't properly latched. She raised the latch, intending to secure it with a firm push, and the gale tore the window from her grasp. Rain blew into her face. The moors were invisible, lost in the cloud and the downpour, and the sound of the swollen Allerbrook deep in the combe came with it, audible even from here, so high on the hillside.

Nicky kicked the chest again as she snatched the window back. She slammed and latched it and turned a stern face to him. "Stop that. Why are you not at your books? Did Father Matthew give you nothing to study until your next lesson with him?"

"I've done it," said Nicky. There had been no need to send

Nicky away to school as Peter and Richard had been sent, not with Father Matthew in the village and willing, at Richard's request, to give Nicky private lessons three times a week. "He gave me some Latin to put into English and some sums and they're all finished. And now I want to go out and I can't!"

"Well, I don't order the weather, and if you went out in this, you'd probably drown," said Liza with vigour.

"Father and Grandfather went out in it this morning! So did the Hannacombes!"

"They're grown up and they had to fetch the animals in and even at that, Roger didn't go. He says he's too old. Kat came over to say he was staying in the cottage, and we sent her back to him. I've never seen such weather. It's just as well this is November and the stock's not out on the moor, except for the pony herd, and they seem able to find shelter from anything. I'd like a walk on the moor but I can't have one. Why don't you make another try at learning to weave?"

"I hate sitting at a loom. It goes clatter, clatter, clatter and every moment's just like the one before and it's dull."

"And you're clumsy. You break threads and I'm always afraid you'll break the loom, as well."

Nicky laughed, and Liza, unable to help it, laughed with him.

It was always happening. She would try, for his own good, to be severe, to tell him he must study his books or be patient about bad weather, be a good child, like his sister, Quentin—who was at this moment in the workroom, busy at the loom, weaving the first piece of cloth she had ever made completely by herself.

Quentin was hardly ever disobedient. She was a responsible little girl with a gift for soothing people. Once or twice, when Peter had been angry about something and marched out to vent his fury by chopping wood or digging a ditch with ferocious energy, Quentin had gone out to him and restored his good temper simply by being there and chattering to him about some everyday matter.

Nicky was the wayward one, and Liza knew she ought to be firmer with him. But then Nicky's astonishing resemblance to Christopher would overwhelm her with love as though a great wave had broken over her, and if he came to her for comfort because his father had rebuked him, she would give him an apple or a honeycake because she couldn't bear that little snub-nosed, freckled face to look unhappy. Wayward he might be, but he was affectionate, too, which made giving in to him all the easier.

She was thankful that none of the Lanyons had ever met Christopher and that in the present Weaver family, there was no one now who knew him except as a distant figure occasionally glimpsed in church. She shocked herself sometimes by admitting privately that it was just as well that her parents, who actually had met him, were both gone.

It was six years now since Margaret had finally taken to her bed in the guest house at St. Catherine's and slipped out of life. Liza had mourned her deeply, but was also relieved that Margaret had never set eyes on Nicky and now never would. There was only one source of danger left, and that was the risk that one day, somehow or other, Nicky and Christopher would be seen together by a member of the family. There, she must hope for the best and pray, although it seemed unlikely that God and his angels, or even the merciful Virgin, would collude in hiding her guilt.

Yet her path of deception had certainly been marvellously smooth. Nicky had been born, as far as Liza could calculate, a few days later than he should have been; certainly no one had ever questioned that he was the result of her reunion with Peter. He had emerged straight into a patch of spring sunlight, and that had been the worst moment because there on his newborn head was a tuft of hair as red as fire.

Whereupon Betsy had said, "Look at that! Mistress, didn't you say when Quentin was born, and the master said to name her for your grandmother, that your grandmother was carrot-haired? This one's going to be more like her than Quentin is!"

"Yes," said Liza faintly. "Yes, he will. There was a little red in my mother's hair when she was young and there's just a glint of it in Quentin's, in some lights."

"Maybe he did ought to be named for your side of the family, Mistress."

"Yes," Peter said, when his opinion was sought. "Call him after your father, Liza. Didn't my father suggest that once?"

Never, for a moment, had there been suspicion. Yet every time she looked at Nicky, Christopher was there again for her, fiery hair, shapely eyebrows, eyes the colour of amber or sweet chestnut—quite unlike her own soft brown ones or Peter's Lanyon eyes, which were so dark that from only a short distance away they looked black. He had Christopher's dear snub nose and even a cluster of freckles on his square little chin.

Christopher was still, as far as she knew, at Dunster Castle. She hadn't seen him since that day in the dell and probably would never see him again, for she didn't go to Dunster now. Nicky occasionally did, because his father had decided when the boy turned eight that he was old enough to be taken along when wool was delivered to the Weavers. Sometimes he had stayed there for a week or two, helping to wash fleeces at the river, and being instructed in the craft of weaving, though his Dunster relatives, like Liza, all agreed that he had little aptitude for it.

Liza was uneasy at the idea of Nicky and Christopher being in the same village, but she knew that he should get to know his mother's family. This was a gamble she must accept. For her, Nicky's resemblance to his father was a blessing. He kept Christopher's memory green for her. Christopher lived in her mind, unknown to all others, a quietly flowing underground river. It was enough.

She wished the Allerbrook were flowing more quietly. The noise of it worried her. The wind was increasing, too, and when she peered through the window glass she saw that still darker weather was approaching from the west. Something worse was on the way.

The door to the kitchen swung open and Peter came in, wrapped in a blanketlike robe and rubbing his hair on a towel. The robe was one of a set created by Liza after Higg's death. In farm life, people were always getting drenched in bad weather but she didn't want anyone else to die as Higg had done, and she had woven and sewn a set of thick robes for the purpose of getting wet bodies warm and dry in a hurry.

"What a day! Betsy's put our clothes to dry and the Hannacombe boys are wandering about in a couple of your woolly gowns, looking like a pair of monks."

"I don't see them as monks!" Liza said. "I've been meaning to mention this to you. Quentin's thirteen now. She's growing up. What do you think about Eddie Hannacombe? Your father mentioned the idea once. When Quentin's seventeen, say. Eddie'll be about twenty-six by then. Jarvis is younger, but I'd prefer Eddie. He's is quiet and responsible and Jarvis already has a bit of a name for flirting among the village wenches."

"Father mentioned it to me as well, not long ago. As a matter of fact, Eddie's in the workroom now, talking to Quentin. They're good friends, those two. I fancy the idea will appeal to them. Well, I'm agreeable if they are—and Sim, of course. And yes, it should be Eddie—you're right about Jarvis, I'd say. We could arrange a betrothal party soon, I think—when the rain stops. I've seen plenty of wild weather, but I've never seen rain like this in my life. We've lost a sheep. The bog on the ridge has overflowed and there's a torrent down the hillside out in front of the house, and a sheep lying on an outcrop in the middle of it. Must have been caught and swept away when the water came over the edge."

"I hope it's the only one," Liza said anxiously.

Nicky, who had now climbed up to stand on the window seat so that he could look out, said, "Oooh! Look at that cloud! I've never seen one like that before!"

Liza went to look and was alarmed. The dark weather from the west was now an advancing inky mass that seemed to be wiping out the world below it. "Nicky, go and fetch Quentin, and take her to Betsy in the kitchen and ask for honeycakes. She made some yesterday. Say I said you could both have one. Go along now."

As soon as Nicky had gone, she turned to Peter. "That sky's frightening. There's no thunder. But—*look* at it."

"There's nothing we can do about it," Peter said. "But there's nothing to be afraid of. There's been a house here for centuries. The stock's safely in now, all but that sheep. It'll pass and meanwhile, we're safe, too, in here. We'd better have some candles. It'll be as dark as night in a moment."

They were lighting candles when the monstrous cloud reached

them, taking the last of the daylight, and the wind and rain suddenly doubled. The windows streamed as though water were being poured down them by the bucketful. A mass of water tumbled down the chimney, putting out the fire with a noisy sizzle and causing Liza to spring around in alarm, taper in hand. Then, her eyes widening, she cocked her head and said, "What's that?"

"Nothing," said Peter calmly. "It's just the wind. It…"

A fearful roar and crash from outside interrupted him. The very walls of the hall, stout as they were, shuddered. A chorus of frightened cries rose from the kitchen and the door to it crashed open. Eddie came in at a run with Quentin and Nicky. Eddie and Quentin were both pale with alarm though Nicky, by contrast, had gone red with excitement.

"What's happening?" Liza rushed to meet them. "What…?"

"Mistress, it's terrible! There's water in the back of the house—"

"Right inside!" Nicky squealed.

"And a great big tree's come down with it!" Quentin was clearly terrified.

Jarvis Hannacombe arrived in haste, and his normally stolid pink face was also unwontedly pale. "It's the bog on the ridge— I think! It's overflowed in a new place, close above here. It's pouring down the hillside like a new river. It's—"

"It's in the dairy!" screamed Betsy, lumbering in at the nearest approach her aged legs could make to a run. "There's filthy water in the dairy! The window's burst in and so's the outer door! A tree came down and smashed them in! It's sticking its branches through into the dairy and the apple store up above. And there's water in your parlour, Mistress!"

Incredibly, as they stood there exclaiming, the wind and rain strengthened yet again. A shower of slates hurtled off the hall roof. From the stable, faintly audible through the din, came frightened whinnying.

"I'm going to look at the damage to the rooms in front," Peter said. "Betsy, Liza, stay here with the children. You lads come with me!" He beckoned to the Hannacombes and they all hurried off through the kitchen. Quentin ran to her mother and stood trembling in the curve of Liza's arm but Nicky shook himself free and ignoring his mother's protesting shout, ran after the men.

"Quentin," said Liza, "be good and stay here. It's all right. It's just a loud noise and a lot of rain and some damage to the front of the house, and it's let water in. But I must fetch Nicky. Betsy, take care of her!"

Lifting her skirts, she sped off through the kitchen and almost collided with Richard, who had been upstairs and had now rushed down, to stand aghast at the door into the dairy. "Where's Nicky?" Liza panted.

"I don't know. Wasn't he with you?"

"Nicky!" Liza shouted. "Where are you? *Nicky!*"

"The whole front of the house is flooded!" Peter came striding back through the workroom with Eddie and Jarvis behind him. "I've never seen anything like this before, never!"

"God's teeth, nor have I!" Richard gasped.

The dairy was several inches deep in brown peaty water, but it was on a lower level than the kitchen, with two steps down to it, and so far, the kitchen and its adjoining larder had escaped. But wind and rain were now driving in through the broken window and the shattered door and the thing that had done the damage, one of the shallow-rooted trees from the hillside above the farm, was thrusting vicious twigs and branches in through the holes. The inrush of water had knocked over a table where a row of pans had stood, full of cream which was setting. The pans were afloat in the water, and a milky swirl was all that remained of the cream. Several cheeses, swept from their shelf by an intrusive tree branch, wallowed dismally beside them.

"Where is Nicky?" Liza wailed. *"Nicky!"*

Her redheaded son appeared in answer, in the doorway from the storeroom next to the dairy. "Isn't it exciting? The tree's trying to get in!"

"Nicky! Come here! No, don't wade across through that water. It's disgusting! Go round by the workroom but then come to me at once! What do you mean by running off…?"

There was a renewed roar and rumbling from outside and Nicky, not obeying orders but plunging excitedly knee-deep into the flooded dairy, kicking pans and cheeses aside, made toward the broken outer door. *"Look!"*

They did look, and Liza cried out. The worst of the cloud was passing and grey daylight was returning to the stricken world. Even from the inner side of the dairy, they now had a view of the landscape beyond the smashed outer door and what they could see was terrifying. High on the slope above the farmhouse, a great boulder, one of the outcrops which dotted the hillside, had been torn loose by the flood from the overflowing bog. It was rolling, bouncing, straight toward the house, and another surge of water was coming with it, as though the uprooting of the boulder had released it.

"Nicky!" Liza screamed.

But Nicky, wildly excited, did not even hear her. Eager to see better, he splashed right into the broken doorway, clinging to the doorpost.

Peter and Liza shouted his name again, in unison, and started forward, stumbling down the submerged dairy steps, but Eddie Hannacombe, younger and quicker than either of them, brushed past and threw himself across the room. In the brief seconds before the boulder arrived, he grabbed Nicky, picked him up bodily and hurled him back across the room toward Peter and Liza. Liza flung her arms around him, and Peter, grabbing her arm, dragged them both back up the steps into the kitchen. Eddie waded after them, the skirts of his thick robe spreading out around his knees.

The boulder struck.

The kitchen survived because the inner walls of the old farmhouse were as strong as the outer ones and the outer ones took the brunt, slowing the monstrous missile down. As it was, the dairy's outside wall shifted under the impact and then gave way in a tumble of rubble and stone slabs. The huge rock, crashing through it, crushed the tree as though its sturdy trunk were nothing but a twig and then fetched up against the far wall while the flood that came with it poured across the dairy in a murky brown wave and on into the kitchen, knocking everyone there off their feet.

Like the boulder itself, however, it had lost impetus on the way through the dairy and they scrambled back to their feet, choking and spluttering. And then clung to each other in terror as they saw a second boulder coming. It thundered into the front of the house farther along, striking the parlour by the sound of it, and the entire building shuddered. Then there was stillness except for the sloshing of water.

In the kitchen, though soaked and terrified and standing in two feet of water, everyone was still alive. But Eddie Hannacombe had not been in the kitchen when the boulder hit. He had still been wading across the dairy and had been caught between boulder and wall. They found him there, his body crushed and his head lolling, the blood flowing out and staining the water all around him. The only consolation was that he had probably died at once.

CHAPTER TWENTY-SEVEN 🌀
THE RISING HOUSE OF LANYON

News found its way around the moor in the days that followed, news of farmhouses and cottages swept completely away; of villages flooded by rivers which had always hitherto been friendly brooks; news of sheep and cattle, ponies and wayfarers, caught and drowned; of meadows under water which had never been flooded before; of uprooted trees, of landslides, of peat streams which had changed their courses.

The Lanyons swept the water out of their farmhouse and considered the damage. The outhouses around the yard were unscathed and so, because it was on higher ground, was the hall. The cottages were safe, too. Kat and Roger had crouched, petrified, by their hearth, but their sturdy stone walls had stood firm in the wind and rain, and only their thatch would need repair. Betsy's cottage, sheltered by a spur of hillside, was altogether untouched.

The farmhouse itself, however, had been badly hit. The rooms facing the yard had survived, though their floors had been flooded, but the second boulder had smashed right into the parlour and also destroyed the rusty hinges of the disused front door. The front of the house was a wreck, the upper storey sagging dangerously on unsteady beams, and the thatched roof half gone.

Worst of all was the death of Eddie Hannacombe, and among the most urgent tasks, as well as the most distressing, was his retrieval and burial. Once the water had been swept out, Peter took Plume down the mired path through the combe to see the carpenter and the sexton and bring a coffin back, strapped to Plume's back. The carpenter usually had one or two in readiness and Peter returned two hours later, bringing not only the coffin but Father Matthew, who did his best, offering physical aid as well as prayer, to help them through the horrible business that faced them.

To do it, they had to clear away the rubble of the smashed dairy wall, and then hitch their own and some borrowed oxen to the boulder to drag it away, and even at that, the men, including Father Matthew, had to add their strength to the ropes. Then they lifted the crushed thing that had been Eddie, laid him in the coffin and placed the lid over him, in haste.

The burial was the next day. When the pitiful remains were safe in the churchyard, the Lanyons turned their attention to Nicky.

Since the disaster, no one had said much to him. He had been given jobs to do and had done them, but it had been made unsmilingly clear to him that the adult world was merely dealing with more immediate matters before it dealt with him. Once he found Quentin crying in the workroom, and gathering from her tearful explanation that she was grieving for Eddie, he cried, too, and said he was sorry, and Quentin, surprisingly, actually attempted to comfort him rather than the other way around, saying that she knew he hadn't meant any harm, that it wasn't his fault. The only friendly words he heard during those frightening days were hers. Everyone else, his mother included, was chilly and remote.

The morning after the funeral, Nicky found himself in the hall, facing what amounted to a tribunal.

Liza had dreaded this moment, though she knew it was coming. She knew that Nicky had been in the wrong, but her heart ached for him.

"He's still only eight," she had said that morning when Peter and his father told her in detail what to expect. "I've made it clear to him that he's behaved very badly, but it was just ordinary naughtiness, after all. It was bad luck that it led to something so awful."

"Nonsense!" Richard barked. "He ran off when you told him to stay with you in the hall, and he ran to look out of the dairy door instead of coming back to you when you called him. He ignored you when the very tone of your voice should have told him that it mattered. He knows that Eddie saved him and was killed in doing it. He knows what death means. He saw Eddie's body. I made sure he did! He's been spoiled, Liza. We've all spoiled him, myself included. We've all been so overjoyed to have a Lanyon son."

"I agree," Peter said. "I'm sorry, Liza, but it's true. No one's ever raised a hand to him. He's never been more than mildly scolded. But what sort of man will our son be if he doesn't learn to behave while he's still young enough to learn?"

"I suppose you're right," said Liza unhappily.

If only he didn't look so like Christopher. Oh, my poor little Nicky. All this for just only a moment's disobedience. Every boy has those. Father-in-law and Peter both did in their time—I'd take an oath on it!

But Eddie is dead. I can't deny that.

The table had been pushed out of the way. Liza sat in a window seat, with Quentin and Betsy. Betsy sat grimly, with folded arms. Quentin, on the other hand, looked nearly as frightened as Nicky. Nicky himself stood in midfloor, confronted by a stern row of men: his father, his grandfather, Roger, Jarvis Hannacombe and Sim, father of both Eddie and Jarvis, who had come over for the occasion. There was an ominous air of formality.

His father recited his misdeeds to him, much as Richard had recited them to Liza, and reminded him of the tragedy to which they had led. "What have you to say?" he asked at the end.

Nicky looked from one face to another, finding no comfort anywhere. He looked toward his mother, but her gaze was on the floor. Betsy's face was like flint. Quentin was watching him with huge, worried eyes but her obvious fear only made him feel worse. "I'm sorry. I only wanted to see what was happening. I just wanted to look. I didn't mean…"

"Because of you," said Richard, "as we have just pointed out, Eddie had to snatch you from the path of that boulder and it caught him. You saw what it did to him. It could have been you. Eddie saved your life. And died for it."

"But I didn't mean to hurt Eddie. I didn't think…"

"Nevertheless," said Richard, "you were responsible for his death."

Just as the Sweetwaters were responsible for Deb Archer's death; just as I was responsible for the death of Marion Locke. Never mind that they didn't mean it, that I didn't mean it. They killed Deb and I killed Marion and that's the truth. And Nicky killed Eddie and he's got to know it.

None of that could be said aloud, not to Nicky and not to

anyone else, but it put an implacable look on Richard's face and made his voice as hard as rock.

Nicky's mouth was trembling. His knees had begun to shake. Something dreadful was going to happen to him, though he didn't know what.

"I didn't mean…" he said again. His voice faltered. Then he saw his father glance toward the table and he saw the riding whip that lay there.

Quentin had followed that glance as well and cried out, "Oh, Father, no, please. Nicky's only little. He couldn't have known—"

"Liza," said Richard, "take yourself and your good kind daughter away. There is no need for either of you to witness this."

"Oh, no, don't, please!" Quentin jumped down from the window seat and ran to Nicky's side, but Peter picked her up bodily and carried her back to Liza. She kicked and struggled and then, as he thrust her into Liza's arms, burst into tears.

"Take her away, Liza. Go on."

"Come, sweetheart." Liza, herself trembling, set Quentin on her feet and with an arm about her, steered her toward the door. "Don't cry so. We can't change anything and we mustn't stay here. We'll wait upstairs."

"Eddie was as good as a son to me," said Betsy grimly. "Cheered me up in the days when I was that miserable over Higg. I'd sooner stay here."

The two main bedchambers were now suspended perilously over space, but the ones at the back of the house were usable. When Quentin and Liza were in the one farthest from the hall, with door and windows closed, Quentin said, "Mother, did you and Father have some idea about…about me and Eddie one day?"

"Yes, dear. We did." Liza sat down on a stool. "How did you know?"

"I liked Eddie. He often came to talk to me when I was spinning or weaving—and once or twice I saw you and Father notice it and smile. It made me wonder."

"You're a sharp little thing! There was talk of it, but Eddie's gone now, Quentin." Had the child cared very much for him? Well, she was still little more than a child, after all. "He died very bravely," said Liza, doing her best to say the right things. "There'll be someone else, one day. You're still very young and you'll stop thinking about him in time. Try not to blame Nicky. He didn't realise what might happen, and at this moment he is learning to do as he's told, and learning the hard way." Liza herself knew how hard a way it was.

"I know." Quentin nodded a serious brown head. "He's so unhappy about Eddie. I've talked to him. I told him it wasn't his fault. Only, Mother…I don't like Jarvis so much."

"Oh!" This at least was easy to deal with. Liza drew Quentin to her and put an arm around her. "If that's what's worrying you, put it out of your mind. We don't think Jarvis would be suitable either. You would never be asked to marry someone you didn't like, anyway."

No, indeed you won't. And if there's someone you really want, one day, I'll do all I can to help you. I know what it's like.

Despite the shut doors and windows, sounds were escaping from the hall. "Oh, no!" said Quentin miserably. Liza held her closer still and sat with bowed head until at last there was the sound of a slammed door, and then feet were running up the stairs, accompanied by a pitiful wailing. Nicky, tears streaming down his freckled face, burst in and rushed to clutch at Liza.

"Father beat me! Why did you let him? Grandfather *held* me, held me down…Betsy and Jarvis and Master Hannacombe watched and they were…they were *pleased*. I'll never forgive them, not any of them! It wasn't fair!"

"It was fair," said Liza. She spoke gently, but as she did so, she detached his hands and held them while she looked into his reproachful golden-brown eyes. Christopher's eyes. "Eddie died because of you. I am sorry for you but it was for your own good."

"No!" screamed Nicky, and sobbed more wildly than ever.

"Yes, Nicky. I mean it."

Nicky, in answer, wrenched himself away from her. He would have run from the room, except that Quentin, slipping from her mother's arm, caught hold of him and pulled him to her.

"Oh, Mother, you said it yourself—he never meant anything dreadful to happen. He never meant Eddie to be hurt. I know he didn't." Her voice shook as she said Eddie's name, but her arm around Nicky was gentle. "Hush, Nicky. Mother, can I use some of your salves to help him?"

"Yes, of course you can. You're a good girl." Liza stood up. "I'll leave him with you for a while. The salves are in my chest— the elderflower ointment's in a little glass pot and the yarrow and woundwort one is in the earthenware box. Quentin will look after you, Nicky. I must go to your father."

She found her husband alone in the hall, sitting by the table with his head in his hands. "Peter?"

"That was the hardest thing I've ever had to do," he said. "My own son. It was as though I were hurting myself. Where is he now?"

"I've left him with Quentin. She's taking care of him. She's very fond of him. She was fond of Eddie, but she has sense enough not to blame Nicky. We're lucky in our daughter. Nicky will be all right soon. Don't think about it anymore."

With a shaky smile Peter said, "Did you give him an apple or a honeycake?"

"No. Not this time."

"Wise of you. Oh, dear God," said Peter miserably, "I want to be proud of my boy. But why did I have to do that to him to make him into the son I want?"

Liza, for a whole tumult of reasons, had no answers and simply, silently, held him fast.

The day after that, while Nicky, lying on his stomach, stayed in bed and Quentin continued to minister to him, Liza joined her husband and father-in-law as they went around the property, discussing how best to repair it.

"It looks," said Richard, "as if I'll have to go in for some new building whether I like it or not, so I've been looking in my coffers and talking to Peter here about the yield from that quarry. We've been saving the rents all these years, too."

"We'll certainly have to build something," Peter said, "but I think we can repair the old house. After all, this is a farm and we're not lordlings."

"I don't agree, boy," said his father. "What do you think I've been saving *for*? Seems to me that fate's telling me to get on and build the fine house I've dreamed of. I was putting it off, thinking of the expense, but I reckon we can do it if we want to."

"I don't want to," said Peter frankly.

"Well, I do. We can demolish what's left of the old house bit by bit, as we go along, and use the stone—the way we did with the stone from that old cottage when we had the hall built. We won't put the new place where the old house is—a flood that can happen once can happen again—but behind the hall, where it's higher. The ground there is flattish for quite a way before the hill rises again. I've plenty of ideas. I've been working them out for years. Come with me."

Peter caught Liza's eye and rolled his eyes in annoyance but Richard, oblivious, marched them both into the hall and began to expound on his ideas.

"You know my plan always was to have the hall as a part of the new house. We can lift the roof higher and put bedchambers over the top with windows looking out of gables, like the ones at Sweetwater House. It'll look fine. And perhaps instead of leaving the outer door of the hall in a recess as it is now, we could have a little porch jutting out, with another small gable over the top, to match the ones over the hall. And see, come here and look through this window…there's room enough between here and the hillside for a couple of wings, going off at right angles…."

"Father, what *is* all this going to cost?" said Peter, aghast.

Richard ignored him. "One wing can have the kitchen, dairy and cider press in it and we'll make a spiral staircase going up to an apple store and servants' rooms above. Liza will need more help in the house—I realise that. The other wing can lead from the other end of the hall—over here…."

He led the way, gesticulating. "We can have a workroom in this one, on the ground floor—or two rooms, a study for doing accounts and a room for weaving, if you like, Liza—and some spare bedchambers above. We'll have a straight, wide staircase here, in this corner of the hall, going up to the spare rooms and a door leading into the workrooms below. And I think—yes,

come this way, back to the other end—I'll have a chapel built
onto the hall with a little tower above it...."

"Father!"

"We'll put stained glass windows in the chapel," said Richard,
unheeding, "and Father Matthew will come and say Mass there
once in a while and Liza, you can have a parlour or a solar, as
the Sweetwaters would call it, above the chapel, looking out
across the combe to the moor. The tower can have battlements
at the top, just like the Sweetwaters have...."

"Father, this is absurd!" Peter was really angry now. He moved
in front of Richard and stood there, hands on hips, glowering.
"We shan't have a coin left to call our own at the end of it and
what's it all for? Just to show off, to score off the Sweetwaters!
All we really need is a house to replace the one that's been
damaged."

"Don't argue with me, boy. I'm master of Allerbrook and I
know what I want and I mean to have it!"

"No!" Peter, by now, was shouting. "No, we don't need this
and we shouldn't waste money on it. I've hoped, all these years,
that you'd just forget this idea! Well, I've decided to stand my
ground, just for once. The money you're proposing to use will
come mostly from that quarry, and that's *my* quarry, presented
to me by Richard of Gloucester for *my* services on a battlefield.
You've no right to be so free with it and for such a useless
purpose. I am telling you—"

"You'll tell me nothing, boy. You'll do as I say or leave Allerbrook."

"Oh...*no!*" whispered Liza, pulling at Peter's sleeve.

"If I leave Allerbrook," said Peter dangerously, "I'll take with
me the deeds to that land with the quarry on it."

"I think not," said Richard. "Sons should do as their fathers tell them and any property that comes into this family is for me to control. The deeds are locked up in my personal chest. I put them there long ago. It was after we sold that other farm to get the Allerbrook freehold. You left them out on the workroom table and I put them away. I told you I'd put them away safe. You never questioned it."

"They still belong to me!"

"To us," said Richard. "Now let be. You're upsetting Liza here. She don't want to be made to leave Allerbrook, do you, Liza?"

"No, I don't!" Liza stared at him, wide-eyed with alarm. For the first time, it struck her that in spite of everything, Allerbrook, once so alien, once nothing but a place of exile from Christopher, had somehow become home. "No, of course not! *No!*"

"And nor does Peter here, not really, do you, boy?"

Peter ground his teeth.

"I need my fine house," said Richard. "I've saved every penny I can, these nine years past. I've drawn plans and then torn them up and drawn new plans. I tell you, the whole thing's been growing in my head. Peter will like it well enough once it's built. Oh, yes, you will, boy. Before I'm done, I'll put those damned Sweetwaters in the shade for good and all."

"I despair of you," said Peter. "No, I don't want to leave Allerbrook, and since you're my father, I can't fight you. But before God…!" He left the sentence unfinished and strode away. Presently Liza heard him chopping firewood, with all the vehemence and fury he could not direct against Richard.

CHAPTER TWENTY-EIGHT

WHIRLIGIG

"So there it is," said Walter Sweetwater to his son and grandson, finding them in the stable yard when he came in from exercising his horse. He dismounted and handed his reins to a groom. "I've just been up Allerbrook combe to see for myself, and yes, Richard Lanyon's finished his house and there it stands. Bah!"

"Well, we knew what he was up to. I've taken the odd glance at it myself," Baldwin said. "Though not lately. I hoped it would all come to a stop, that Lanyon would be standing below when a lump of badly placed masonry fell off the wall, or at least that he'd run out of money halfway."

"He managed it quicker than when he built the hall, by a good bit!" said Walter irritably. "Though no doubt he had his troubles. Last time I caught sight of him, I saw his hair had gone white. I've also heard he's had a noisy quarrel or two with his son about the cost. Peter Lanyon seems to have more sense than his father. It must have taken every farthing they've got. But he's done it. There's smoke rising from the chimneys and I saw a couple of windows open."

"I wonder what the inside is like?" said his sixteen-year-old grandson.

"My dear John, I doubt if we'll be invited in!" Walter said. "They don't challenge us when we ride across Allerbrook land, but I've seen a few dirty looks from men in the fields. It still feels weird, knowing it isn't my land anymore. I made sure today that I got a good view of the outside of the house, anyhow. It's an imitation of ours—gables, crenellated tower and all."

"I'd heard that," Baldwin said. "From Denis."

Denis Sawyer, the stocky, quiet-spoken former archer who had replaced Geoffrey Baker as steward after Towton, drank regularly in the White Hart. Unlike the talkative Maude, who had now gone away with her mistress to Agnes's married home, he didn't gossip about Sweetwater business. What he did do was listen to other people gossiping, and then report what he heard.

"I sometimes think I'd like to sit in a corner of the White Hart and watch Denis collecting news," Walter said. "I think he sits there, quiet as a cat at a mouse hole, paws folded and ears twitching. But—" he grinned suddenly "—I wonder if he picked up this titbit? Gables and battlements or not, the front rooms upstairs, under the gables, look straight onto the farmyard, complete with hens and a cattle byre and a very good view of the pigsty. Likely enough they're the best bedchambers. I suppose you could say it has a comic side to it!" He glanced around him. "Where is Denis now, by the way? Not back from Dunster market yet? Your Catherine will be wanting her new cloth and her spices, Baldwin."

"They're not urgent. No, he's not back." Baldwin, scowling, was not interested in Denis, cloth or the household supplies of pepper and ginger. "Whatever the Lanyons can see from the windows, that house is like a glove thrown in our faces. One day, one of us will pick up the gage."

John said mildly, "Does it really matter? They're not our tenants now so why should we care what kind of house they build for themselves?"

His seniors regarded him with irritation. He was a Sweetwater as far as his solid build was concerned, but he had Catherine's dark hair, and his well-shaped blue eyes were hers, too. He also had something of her sweet-natured temperament, which was becoming in a woman but completely unsuitable in a Sweetwater male.

"He's an upstart," said Walter. "It doesn't do to have peasants saying they are gentlemen and gentlemen forced into penury." The amount he had spent to get Agnes married and the means by which he had acquired it would rankle for the rest of his life. Also, the Sweetwaters had gained nothing from the marriage. Agnes had become wholly a Northcote and had brought no valuable contacts or lucrative posts within reach of her blood relatives. She wrote to them now and then; that was all.

"A man should stay where God has put him," said Walter virtuously. "Social whirligigs are unhealthy. They make plain men restive, and who will till the fields if the labourers think themselves too grand?"

"That whole family has pretensions," said Baldwin furiously. "I hate the Lanyons. One day, our chance will come."

"But…" John was clearly about to express a point of view not in accordance with Sweetwater tradition. His father and grandfather, recognising the symptoms, turned to him frowning, but the threatening argument was disarmed by the clatter of hooves as Denis Sawyer rode in, followed by a groom leading a well-laden pack pony.

"Ah, here's Denis," said Walter, not altogether displeased by the interruption. He was now fifty-six, and sometimes, to his own annoyance, felt wearied by things which in the past had stimulated him, and his dislike of the Lanyons was on that list. Heartily as he loathed them, he no longer had the energy to do more than abuse them verbally, and he didn't like family disputes, either. Baldwin was the one with the violent passions now.

"Sir!" Sawyer began to talk while he was still in the saddle. "Sir, there's news! It's running through Dunster like fire in peat. There's not much doubt that it's true! King Edward is dead!"

The news was brought to Allerbrook by Ned Crowham, who rode from his home on purpose to tell them. "Because you live so far from anywhere—I wondered if you'd heard," he said as they welcomed him in. "I don't visit you often enough myself. It's twenty miles of wilderness and I feel I'm travelling to the moon. In winter I don't even try. It's only when spring arrives that I can face the thought of it. Isabel the Second sends her kind greetings," he added with a smile.

Except for putting on yet more weight he was still, at nearly forty-four, recognisably the Ned Crowham he had been at nineteen when he came to George Lanyon's funeral, even though he had long since lost his own father and was now Sir Ned Crowham of Crowham in east Somerset, and had added substantially to his family estates through a couple of wealthy marriages. His first wife had died young of a wasting sickness, leaving him with no children but in possession of the valuable Dorset manor which had been her dowry. His second wife had presented him with three sons and another valuable manor in Nottinghamshire. He travelled a good deal between the three counties where he owned land.

As it happened, both his wives had been named Isabel, for which reason Ned usually referred to his present spouse as Isabel the Second. He was still fond of a joke, though he took life more seriously now that he was a man of property and had served at court. On his occasional visits to Allerbrook, both Peter and Liza had noticed how, now and then, if some political subject arose in conversation, his eyes would become expressionless and his face very still, as though he were thinking over things that he knew but did not wish to share.

He had come to share knowledge this time, however, and when Peter said, "But how did the king die? What happened? He wasn't an old man," Ned knew the answer.

"He went fishing, got wet, caught cold, was gone in a week," said Ned. "Spring weather can be treacherous. Ninth of April, that was the date…" On the verge of taking a seat, he turned away and went back to the door, pushing it open. "Listen!"

"What is it?" Peter came to his side.

"Church bells, down in Clicket. Father Matthew is tolling a death. The news was hard behind me, clearly."

"I'll send Nicky to tell my father. He and Jarvis are out seeing to the lambing. Where's Nicky?" Peter asked as Liza, who had gone to fetch food and drink, came back into the hall with a tray.

"In the stable cleaning harness with Hodge. I'll give him the message."

"Oh, send Hodge and let Nicky finish his work." Peter took

his friend's arm and led him back to the comfort of a seat by the fire. "Hard work's good for him. How do you like our new house, now that it's finished, Ned? We've got extra people to help us run it, too."

It wouldn't, Liza knew, be wise to say as much to Richard and she never had, but the two years and four months it had taken to bring the new Allerbrook House into being had, in her opinion, been two years of purgatory.

It had been bad enough at the beginning, when they just lived in the few habitable rooms of the old house. They were squeezed for space even though they cleared a barn to use as a dairy, and the ominous creaking every time they trod on certain upstairs floorboards which extended into the damaged rooms at the front had worried her badly. It was impossible to hold any gatherings or even invite the Hannacombes to dine. But as time went on, things became still worse. Richard had held to his plan of knocking the old house down bit by bit in order to use the stone. He had decided to buy from the quarry he had used when building the hall, rather than bring supplies in from Peter's, partly because it was a better match in colour, and partly to save on transport costs.

"Though five miles is quite far enough," he said. "And stone's costly to start with. We'd better not waste our ruined farmhouse."

They could not knock the farmhouse down and simultaneously live in it, and before long the Lanyons had been obliged to camp—there was no other word for it, Liza said bitterly to herself—mostly in the hall. She arranged beds at one end, pushing tables and seating to the other. The place still looked congested, especially as her loom had to be put in the hall, as well. No guests could be asked there, either.

The process of demolishing the farmhouse was difficult, too, for the massive walls could be broken only by levering the stones loose one at a time, with crowbars. Or, as Peter said grimly, by a boulder crashing down a steep hillside with a flood to help it on its way, but they couldn't conjure that up to order.

The masons were not a problem. When the hall was built, they had been accommodated in the farmhouse; this time they took lodgings in Clicket. Once again, however, there were hitches with the waggons which brought the stone. No wheels came off this time, but the brakes on one waggon broke on a steep downhill stretch of track and the driver prevented a bad accident only by turning his ox team and urging them up a bank. The waggon stopped but toppled sideways, spilling half its load. Neither the oxen nor the men in charge were harmed, but once more there was a long delay while repairs were carried out. Richard's curses when he heard of it bordered on the blasphemous.

When the work was finally finished, Liza ventured one complaint, half a joke. "The air's still full of stone dust and sawdust. I doubt I'll ever get it out of the linen, or even out of my lungs!"

There was a grim truth behind the jest, for Roger never did get the dust out of his lungs. He and Kat, of course, had their own cottage, but they were often at the farmstead and the haze that continually hung over the site made Roger cough. Before the new house was finished, he took to his bed and died of a choking phlegm. Kat, after a few angry words flung at Richard's head, went to live with a married daughter in Lynmouth.

"I'll stop on," Betsy said. "I've been here so long I don't want to move. But it seems to me that 'ee've paid for this here house with lives, Eddie's and Roger's, and it'll bring bad luck in the end, mark what I say."

"Don't talk nonsense!" Richard barked, but added that he knew the house and farm couldn't be run with so few people, and ordered Peter to find two more men and two more maidservants. "We've room for them now that we've moved in, as it were."

It was September, the time of year for hiring fairs, so Peter went to one and came back with two farmhands called Hodge and Alfred, and a pair of jolly young sisters named Phoebe and Ellen.

Alfred was stolid, amiable, a sound worker and not given to wenching, but Hodge and Phoebe were now married, of necessity, since Hodge, far from being stolid, was good-looking and silver-tongued, and almost the first thing he did at Allerbrook was to get Phoebe with child.

"Bad luck, like I said" was Betsy's comment.

"Bloody careless," said Richard, and Jarvis Hannacombe, who—because the girl preferred another swain and passed her condition off as his responsibility—had narrowly escaped enforced matrimony with a lass in Clicket, put on a prim face and said, "Not the right thing at all, fouling his own doorstep, like."

"He's good with the sheep," said Richard, "and Phoebe's a wantwit to let it happen. But she's handy with a broom, I'll say that for her. They can have Kat's cottage, and no more talk of bad luck, Betsy, if you please!"

The new Lanyon household had shaken down together and they had been in their completed new home now for a week. To Liza, it was an immense relief.

It was even possible, she thought, now that life was returning to normal, that everything else would return to normal, too.

Maybe Nicky would even become his trustful, affectionate, if sometimes disobedient self again.

The beating after the death of Eddie had been reinforced at times by further beatings from his grandfather. Peter took no part in these but did nothing to prevent them, either. "My father may be right. I just don't want to do it myself," he had said to Liza when she protested.

The outcome was that Nicky had now become more or less what Richard and Peter wanted him to be—respectful, hardworking and courteously spoken. Only Liza was aware that the loving side of his nature seemed to have died. He rarely laughed these days, and sometimes she had seen him do something she thought he had learned from Peter (who had demonstrated it frequently after arguments with his father about the expense of the new house), which was to chop wood or do some other physical task with furious violence, as though to relieve a secret rage.

Well, the news of the king's death ought to distract all of them. "What will happen?" she asked when she returned from sending Hodge with the message.

"The king's elder son is in Ludlow, up in Shropshire," said Ned. "He will be brought to London and crowned, I suppose. Richard of Gloucester is the Protector of the Realm until the prince comes of age. He's in Yorkshire, but I imagine he'll be sent for. There may be trouble."

"Why trouble?" Peter asked. "The succession's clear enough."

"Gloucester will control the country and Gloucester loathes the queen's family, the Woodvilles," said Ned simply. "And they've got half the good posts in the kingdom. They've also had charge of the elder prince until now. His maternal uncle, Anthony Lord Rivers, is his guardian. It's an interesting state of affairs. Let us hope it doesn't lead to fighting."

★ ★ ★

"If it does lead to fighting," said Herbert Dyer to his son Simon, "you might have to go. You're only thirty-five. We'd better pray for peace. I don't like these rumours that the Woodvilles tried to keep control of the king's person."

"Gloucester seems to have dealt with them. The queen's in sanctuary, one of her sons has fled the country and her brother Lord Rivers is under arrest. Though I don't suppose Prince Edward is any too grateful for that," said Simon. "Rivers looked after him in Ludlow. However, if it comes to the point and the Protector calls for extra men, I'll do my duty, as all honest men should."

It was a sour joke, understood only by the two of them. Since Richard's ultimatum, years ago, their workshop had been so extremely honest in its dealings that Herbert Dyer and his son had acquired a shining reputation for miles around. They had been complimented on it often and publicly. On the whole, it had been worthwhile, since it had brought in business enough to compensate for the money that virtue had lost them.

But Herbert, lying at night in his solitary bed, missed Margaret so intensely that he rarely spoke of her, because to do so made the wound of her loss throb so very badly. He would never forget the bitter words with which they had parted. To his life's end, he would regret the things he had said to her, and shrink from remembering the things she had said to him. It had been the interfering Lanyons' fault. He would never forgive them for dividing him from Margaret.

Nor would either he or Simon ever forget or forgive the threat that Richard held over them. Simon's wife, who knew nothing of the threat or what had led to it, sometimes heard them make sardonic jests about honesty and was often puzzled. She remained puzzled to the end of her days, for they never told her the truth.

★ ★ ★

News usually reached Dunster Castle promptly. The son of the Earl of Pembroke who had died before Barnet and Tewkesbury were fought, another William Herbert who was now Earl of Huntingdon, took marginally more interest in the castle than his father had. He had never set foot in the place, either, but he styled himself Lord Dunster and he recognised a political crisis when he saw one and wished to be prepared for trouble if it came. That meant preparing any castles which happened to be in his charge.

When he learned, firstly, that Richard of Gloucester had executed Lord Rivers, the young king's maternal uncle and erstwhile guardian, and then, astoundingly, that someone (rumour pointed fingers at Gloucester himself and also at Robert Stillington, the Bishop of Bath and Wells, a diocese which included Dunster itself) was casting doubt on the lawfulness of the late king's marriage and therefore on the legitimacy of his two sons, Lord Dunster sent his orders. These were accompanied by money with which to carry them out and a squad of men to reinforce the skeleton garrison at Dunster.

The castle was to be put into a state of defence, with crossbows and cannon; the storerooms were to be filled with nonperishable food, the walls were to be checked and trees which might help an enemy gain entrance were to be cut down. Father Christopher and Miles Hilton, who had been in charge of the castle hitherto, and to some extent still were because they knew it thoroughly while the captain of the new garrison did not, found themselves extremely busy.

On the day Christopher had so graphically pointed out the shortcomings of the castle maintenance, adding the fact that he was strong enough to put pressure on Master Hilton in a most direct and physical manner, Hilton had been furious. However, time and some diplomacy on Christopher's part had eroded this somewhat.

"I don't mean that *you* ought to get behind a broom or take to mending tapestries," Christopher had said reasonably. "Only that you ought to make other people do it."

As it chanced, a few months after that Hilton found himself a wife, the bright young widow of a Dunster woodworker. The woodworker had been much older than she was, well established in his trade, and of a saving disposition. Dying, he left her with a coffer full of silver. On her side, Mistress Anne Fry was accustomed to keep her house neat and when she joined her new husband at the castle, saw no reason that shouldn't be kept neat, as well. Mistress Anne had done a great deal to smooth the friction between priest and steward.

Now, while the political news turned into a whirligig, with power spinning from boy king to Woodvilles to Richard of Gloucester, Christopher and Hilton worked in double harness in something like accord. Both were equally horrified when, at length, a messenger on a tired horse clattered up the long slope to the gatehouse to announce that the Duke of Gloucester was now King Richard III and that the young ex-king Edward and his brother were lodged in the Tower of London out of the public eye, and King Richard's coronation would be on July 6.

"There'll be risings, sooner or later," said Hilton as he and Christopher stood on the walls looking out over Dunster High Street and watching the everyday traffic below, of people on ponies and people on foot, coming and going. For all his idle airs, Miles Hilton was politically sharp enough. "Boys turn into men. The princes have been dispossessed and they won't forget it and nor will a good many others. A party will gather round them as they grow up. There are still Woodvilles in influential places and they'll lead the way. Trouble's coming, for sure. That is, *if* the boys grow up."

"You mean…but they're King Edward's sons!" Christopher was scandalised. "Gloucester was always faithful to Edward. *Loyalty Binds Me* is his motto."

"King Edward's dead," said Hilton. "But Gloucester may prefer to stay alive, and if there were to be a successful rising on behalf of those boys, I doubt if he'd live long. Besides, he's inured to such things. King Henry VI died very conveniently, after Tewkesbury. Very conveniently. Nothing could have drawn the She-Wolf's teeth as effectively as that. All her wars were to put him back on the throne so that she could be the power behind it, and in the fullness of time, behind their son. But the son was killed on the field, and as for King Henry—do you remember the proclamations? That he had died of displeasure and melancholy? No one believed a word of it. King Edward only let the French king ransom *her* because she could do no more harm."

"Yes. I heard that she died a year or so back," Christopher said. "As King Louis' pensioner, and apparently it wasn't much of a pension. But the boys would be a different matter. Dispossessed kings are likely to turn into dead kings—that's what you mean, isn't it?"

"Yes, I do. Those boys are lodged in the Tower. What if something happened to them there? Who, outside it, would know exactly what? No one knows for sure what happened to the other royal brother—George of Clarence—the one who kept betraying King Edward. He was shut in the Tower and supposed to have drunk himself to death on Greek malmsey, but how does anyone know?"

"It's horrible," Christopher said. "Those two boys have done no wrong, apart from being born to a king who died before they were old enough to fight for themselves. Their poor mother!"

"Ah, well. Some people still remember the Earl of Desmond's two little sons," Hilton said sardonically.

"But these boys weren't responsible for that!" Christopher drummed his fingers on top of the wall, and then sighed. "There'd be public fury if word got round that the boys had come to harm, but without a rival to put up against King Richard, what could anyone do? There are no Lancastrian claimants left."

"But there are," said Hilton.

Christopher was startled enough to step back from the wall and turn to the steward in astonishment. "Are there? Who?"

"Well, there's one, anyway. Descended from John of Gaunt, Edward III's third son. It's a senior line to the house of York. His mother's Margaret Beaufort, Gaunt's great-granddaughter." Hilton seemed to have royal genealogy at his command. "That line's been attainted and cut out of the succession but attainders can be reversed—by law or by force. The last Lancastrian's got royal blood on his father's side, too, though not English blood."

"But who are you talking about?" asked Christopher.

"Did you ever hear about Catherine of France, queen to King Henry V? When he died, she married a Welsh minstrel called Owen Tudor. She was a French princess by birth. The Lancastrian claimant is her grandson. He's in France now, in exile. Henry Tudor, that's his name."

CHAPTER TWENTY-NINE 🌀
HEATHER, GORSE AND HENRY TUDOR

The news that England was now ruled by King Richard III rather than King Edward V, caused both surprise and disapproval at Allerbrook.

"Can it really be true?" Liza wondered. "If it is, then he's stolen the throne from his brother's children!"

"That's what's being said in Dunster, and they get their news from the castle and the priory." Richard, primed with information, had just returned from a visit to Dunster.

"If the children aren't lawful..." said Liza doubtfully.

"Bah! All this gossip that the old king had a precontract before he married his queen!" said Richard. "That's been used as an excuse often enough when someone wants to break a marriage, but as an excuse it's never been all that good." Peter had tried to lay claim to it once, he remembered. "Both the parties are dead," he said, "and the only witness, seemingly, is this Bishop Stilling-ton. Bishops have been bribed before this."

"I can't see Gloucester wanting to snatch power and bribing his way to it," protested Peter. "I've met him. I think…"

"Power goes to men's heads, boy," said Richard. "Gloucester was generous to you once, but you weren't standing in his way! Well, he's got the crown. I wonder if he can keep it on his head. There've been rumblings already, from what I hear."

They heard more before long. Ned Crowham might say they lived out in the wilderness and might as well be on the moon, but the years of peace under King Edward had made it easier for news to travel. Time had brought a sense of security, giving people the confidence to move about because they no longer feared they would ride straight into a battle, or be cut off from home by one.

The roads had grown busy with travelling merchants and wool buyers, itinerant pedlars, tooth-drawers and strolling players, and the ships sailing into Bristol Channel ports came from every-where from Plymouth to Palestine. These travellers carried news with them. Sometimes it seemed to be borne on the air like dan-delion seeds, spreading through the population even before well-connected families had heard it from contacts at court and given it to priests like Father Matthew to announce.

"I can see what happened, I think," Peter said, returning one July evening from a fair in Dulverton, where rumours were cir-culating briskly. "The dowager queen's family, the Woodvilles, apparently tried to hold on to the person of the young prince so as to rule through him. Richard stopped that, and there were exe-cutions. Well, one of them was Prince Edward's favourite uncle! People are saying that if the boy had been crowned, the first thing he'd have wanted when he was old enough to take power—and it wouldn't have been long—would have been his uncle Richard's head on a nice silver platter, and *that's* why Gloucester stepped in and took the crown himself. It was self-defence, not ambition."

"Well, it's no business of ours," his father said. "A bit of peace and stability, that's what we all need. And plenty of demand for stone," he added. Despite the cost of the new house (and Peter's dire predictions that they would all end up as beggars), the quarry was doing so well that the Lanyons had been able to afford some extra land, in Hampshire this time. Two farms and a village stood on it, and the rents would repay the price of it in due course. Meanwhile, the quarry went on making money. "I told you so," said Richard to Peter, rather too often.

The name of Henry Tudor was spoken in rumour quite frequently and at one point was more than a rumour. Baldwin Sweetwater in fact rode off once to join the defence of the south Devon coast after Tudor had tried to land in Dorset, been driven off and was then said to be approaching Devon. But the attempt failed and Baldwin came home without having drawn his sword. Tudor had been repulsed; the Duke of Buckingham, hitherto King Richard's friend, had tried to raise a rebellion to support Henry Tudor and had been beheaded for his mistake. The trouble faded away.

For the time being.

Two years after the crown had been placed on Richard of Gloucester's head, Henry Tudor landed in earnest.

The day the news reached them, the Lanyons were immersed in a private combat of their own. Unintentionally started by Liza.

It was August 13, and sunny. Crops were ripening and the

cattle grazed contentedly, enjoying the warmth on their backs; every lane was edged with musty pink foxgloves and the moorland glowed with the purple and deep gold of heather and gorse in full bloom, patched here and there by the paler gold of the long moor grass, rippling in the breeze.

Peter and Richard, coming into the hall one morning, found Liza there already, staring at a patch of sunlit panelling and frowning.

"What's amiss, Liza?" her father-in-law asked.

"I was thinking that I wished we had just one tapestry to hang on that wall. There are merchants in Dunster who sell them."

"Not tapestries, not yet," said Richard. "The Sweetwaters don't have much in that way, I believe, so we needn't either. First of all, I want that panelling replaced by something better, with carving on it, and I still haven't managed the stained glass I want for the chapel."

"Well, if we ever do have tapestries," Peter said, "let us have some lively colours. The hues of the moor are worth seeing at this season. The heather's as purple as an emperor's mantle, and the gorse is bright gold. Let's have those."

"God's teeth, what poetic marvellings!" Richard snorted. "Heather? Emperor's mantle? Bright gold gorse! Since when did any of us have time to stand about like gape-mouthed images, gawping at things like that! Tapestries will have to wait!"

Over the years Liza had grown very used to acting as a buffer between her husband and his father, though it was sometimes a tiring business and she was glad that she had kept her health, although she was nearing fifty, and thick around the middle despite her active life. "Perhaps one day," she said pacifically. "What kind of carving had you in mind, Father-in-law?"

Peter cut in before Richard could answer. "Since we *do* have this fine house, though I've always said we didn't need it, we may as well do justice to it. And I'd like to decide something once in a while and not be shouted down. This is my home, too, and Liza's!"

"I've told you before—don't lower your antlers at *me!*" retorted his father. "In this house, I'm the one who says."

"Or shouts," said Peter coldly. "Or strikes."

"Oh, so that's what this is about, is it? So I gave my grandson a reminder or two when I caught him slipping off after he'd been told to help Hodge cut back those brambles. He came running to you, did he?"

"No. I saw, from a distance. You went too far. It wasn't a reminder or two, it was more like a reminder or twelve."

"Don't get clever with me."

"Oh, *please!*" said Liza.

They continued, however, to stand glowering at each other and in the end she decided to seek peace in her workroom. This sort of thing had happened more often of late; it was as though Peter was losing patience after holding himself in for years, and as though her father-in-law's wish to rule his son as if Peter were still a boy was growing on him, like a bad habit.

She never reached the workroom, however, for Quentin, who had been outside collecting eggs, rushed suddenly into the hall without her egg basket, breathless and alarmed. "The beacon on Dunkery's been lit! There's smoke going up!"

"What?" Richard was out in the yard in a moment, the rest of them at his heels. Quentin was right. To the northwest, from Dunkery's purple crest, a column of smoke was pouring into the blue sky.

"But why…what's happened?" said Liza.

Peter said, "I can hear hoofbeats!"

Half a minute later Ned Crowham came in at a gallop, threw himself off his horse and said peremptorily, "It's a call to arms. You've seen the smoke? There go the church bells in Clicket. I was at home in Crowham and a messenger reached me late last night, from my place in the Midlands. Henry Tudor's landed in Wales, with an army. He's marching on to England. I'm gathering my able-bodied tenants and I thought of you, as well. Peter, will you come and bring a man or two with you? We'll have to be quick. Come back to Crowham with me now!"

"You're going? Just like that?" Liza said. "But…"

"I must. Listen—we wouldn't have this house, wouldn't be able to afford half the things we have afforded, but for Gloucester, that's King Richard now, and what he did for me after Tewkesbury. I have to go," Peter said. "Jarvis says he'll come, as well. He's a good shot at the butts. Hodge and Alfred can stay here—someone must get the harvest in. Besides, Hodge is married with two children now and Alfred's courting a girl in Clicket. But I'll come and so will Jarvis. What do you say, Father?"

"Yes, you'd better go, and take one fellow with you at least. Liza, stop standing there looking as if someone's banged you on the head, and go and put his things together. I'll look for the old sword and helmet for you, Peter."

"What's happening? Is it a war?" Nicky, who had been in the fields, ran into the yard. "I saw the smoke from the beacon!" He looked in wonder at Ned and his sweating horse.

"Not for long," said Ned. "King Richard will see the Tudor off if he has men enough. Your father and Jarvis are coming with me. The king's at Nottingham and that's where we're going."

THE HOUSE OF LANYON

"Can I come? I'm big enough to fight. I've got a bow of my own now and a dagger, too!"

"Certainly not!" Liza, turning to go indoors as Richard had bidden her, swung around again in a swirl of skirts and clamped a hand on her son's shoulder. "You're far too young! Ned! Peter! Say something!"

"King Richard was riding about raising help for the king when he was younger than this lad is," Ned remarked. "And we always have boys looking after the baggage. He could be useful."

"No!" said Liza passionately.

"I agree. He's too young," said Peter. "Go inside, Nicky, and help to find my war gear."

"But I don't want to be left here with Grandfather!" Nicky shouted.

"Oh, so that's it! Well, you'd find a battle a lot more frightening than your grandfather is," Peter said frankly. "You stay home and practise doing as you're told. Go and help your granddad. *Now!*"

"Why didn't you leave us alone?"said Liza furiously to Ned. "Why must Peter go? He's not a tenant of yours, or anyone's! The Sweetwaters will go, I expect, but we don't have to follow them now!"

"I'm not following them," said Peter. "I'm following Ned, if you like, but it's out of gratitude to King Richard. I never wanted this house, but our prosperity made it possible and yes, I do like the prosperity. Well, it's due to him. Now, Liza, don't let your face crumple like that. Let us get my packing done."

It had happened so fast that Liza felt giddy. One moment they had been arguing about tapestries. The next, Peter was wearing a helmet and a sword, saddling Plume and saying farewell. Plume, though old, was still very much alive, unlike Magpie, who had died a year ago. Richard had a new horse now, another piebald, called Patches. Peter, however, was content with his pony and didn't intend to go into battle on horseback anyway. Jarvis, he said, could take one of the other ponies.

That suited him, Jarvis said. It looked to Liza as though Jarvis regarded the whole expedition as an adventure, an interesting break from his normal routine. Peter said goodbye with a grave face, but when, saddlebags bulging, the two of them rode away with Ned Crowham, Jarvis went off smiling.

They were gone, and who was to say when they would ever eat at the Allerbrook table again? Peter was forty-six now, not a young man anymore, not as fit for fighting as he was. Richard was irritable, probably because he was worried about Peter though he wouldn't actually say so.

Quentin was tearful and Nicky, angry because he had been left behind, sulked all evening and she made him go to bed early to keep him out of Richard's way.

She and Quentin went to bed not long afterward. Whether Quentin slept or not, Liza didn't know, but she herself did not. The long, slow hours of darkness went by and she hoped that Peter was at least in a comfortable bed in Crowham this night. She missed his presence, the comfort of his body next to hers. They no longer made love frequently; as the years went on, their daily work drained them more and at night they were usually content to embrace briefly and then fall asleep, but they gave each other company. The empty place beside her ached.

She began at last to drift toward sleep but then woke, abruptly, to find the world dark and silent, and yet with the certainty that she had been roused by a noise. The dogs weren't barking, but they had been out all day and were now asleep in the kitchen. She sat up, listening. Yes, the hens were cackling. Something was wrong. Flinging off her covers, she went to look out the window.

She and Peter had one of the best bedchambers and, as Walter Sweetwater had so disparagingly remarked, it overlooked the farmyard. As she pushed the window open, the noise from the henhouse grew louder. At the same moment, the window in the neighbouring gable opened and Richard's white head peered out of it. He noticed her and turned toward her, pressing a finger to his lips and then pointing.

Liza, peering accordingly, saw a slinking shadow close to the henhouse and then, momentarily, the brush of a fox showed in the moonlight. Glancing sideways, she saw that Richard had disappeared, but even as she looked, she saw a crossbow protrude from his window instead. He took aim and loosed the bolt. The Sweetwaters had said that he didn't aim as true as he used to do, but he was as good a shot over short distances as he had ever been, and the fox had come unwisely close. There was a screech from below and something flopped out of the shadows into the moonlight, twisted, cried and then lay still.

"I'll go down and finish it off if need be," said Richard, sticking his head out again. "Go back to bed."

Liza went back to her couch and this time slept, until she was awakened early in the morning by Quentin anxiously shaking her. "Mother—wake up! Please wake up!"

"What is it?" Liza sat up again. It was just dawn and time to milk the cows, but that was work, these days, for Quentin and Ellen. Liza allowed herself a little longer to rest in the morning now.

Quentin's face was worried. "Mother, I went out with Ellen to see to the cows, but as we passed the pony field I couldn't see

Nicky's pony, Sunset! Sunset's the only bay pony we have just now, and it wasn't there! I sent Ellen on to fetch the cows and I went to the harness room. Nicky's saddle and bridle are gone, as well."

"What?" Liza was already out of bed. "Have you looked in Nicky's room?"

"Yes, I did that at once, as I came in, before I came to you. His door wasn't quite shut. I called but he didn't answer, so I looked in. I don't think he slept in his bed last night and his clothes weren't there! You know how he just tosses them across a stool."

Memory flooded back. The sound that had woken her had been mixed up with a dream and only now was she recalling the dream, a muddled fantasy of searching for Peter through a strange, dark house. He was always ahead of her, sometimes in sight, but she couldn't catch up and he kept going through doorways and shutting doors in her face.

Nicky, creeping out, had left his own door ajar for the sake of quietness, but he must have shut the harness-room door after fetching his pony's tack. In the hushed moonlit night, the sound had carried. And then the fox had come and upset the hens, providing another explanation. Meanwhile, Nicky had got away.

"But where can he have gone, Mother?" Quentin was asking.

"I would guess," said Liza, "that he's gone to Crowham. He could be there by now. Is your grandfather awake? I think he'll have to go after Nicky."

In the big stable yard at Ned Crowham's manor house, horses were being groomed and saddled, armed men were talking in clusters and the air was full of a sense of departure. Isabel the Second and her women servants were walking among them, offering stirrup cups. Isabel was pale, but she came of a family whose menfolk went to war as a matter of course, and she knew how to seem cheerful. Ned would have his way, she knew. He wanted to fight and had gathered men to go with him, and all she could do now was wait for news and his return, if return he did.

They were all astonished when a solitary redheaded figure on a very tired pony rode in through the gate, paused to look around and then spurred his pony over to where Peter and Ned stood in conversation, and said, "Hullo, Father, Master Crowham. I've come to join you after all."

"What?" Peter stared at him in horror. "Nicky, what are you doing here? How did you get here? Your mother never gave you permission. I know she didn't!"

"No, I slipped out at night and just rode here. Are you setting off today? Can I have something to eat before we go? I'm awfully hungry."

"You must be tired, too," Ned said. "Can you face a day's riding after a night with no sleep? We're going north to join William Berkeley, Earl of Nottingham. I've land in his earldom and he's my natural leader if there's war in the Midlands. We'll find you something else to ride, because even if you can keep awake all day, you can't ask the same of your pony."

"Ned! What are you talking about? He must eat and rest and then go straight home!" Peter said indignantly. "Haven't you got some older man here, who isn't going with us, who could take him back? Nicky, how dare you behave like this? What your mother and your grandfather will say I dread to think. Come. We must speak to Mistress Crowham and—"

"He'd certainly better snatch some food," Ned said. "We shan't be riding for half an hour or so. There's time."

"What are you talking about? We're not taking Nicky!"

"And I don't want to go home. Grandfather will be angry."

"You'll see angrier men on a battlefield! I told you as much before! Why didn't you listen?" Peter thundered. "Ned, he's not to come. I can't understand why you seem willing to take him!"

"You may understand presently," said Ned, and to Peter's astonishment, that curious, closed expression which he had sometimes noticed before on Ned's face, when some matter of state was being discussed, was there again. His friend's blue eyes were blank and even chilly. "Oh, yes." He put a hand on Peter's shoulder. "I have a reason. Nicky could be very useful. I'll do my best to see he comes to no harm. But there are other boys of his age coming with us. A lad should start learning men's business as soon as he's old enough to understand it. We'll take him along."

Richard came back in the evening on Patches, leading Nicky's pony, but with an empty saddle.

"They'd already left Crowham," he said as soon as he came into the hall. "They'd ridden away long before I got there. The pony was tired and they wanted to go fast, so they'd given Nicky something else to ride. Isabel told me. I hadn't a hope of catching up. But he'll be all right! The boys stay behind to guard the baggage when an army goes into the field. Nicky will come back all right and he'll find me waiting for him."

The unspoken message was *but Peter may not come back.* Richard's face, under his snowy hair, was drawn with worry but not for Nicky. Liza on the other hand was terrified for them both and fear made her flare into anger. "Why didn't Peter send him home? *Why?*"

"God knows. I don't," said Richard, sitting down on the nearest seat and presenting his dusty boots to be removed. Liza brushed tears from her eyes and helped him off with them. If Peter were to walk in at that moment, she didn't know whether she would run to him or throw something at him. What if she lost both husband and child?

Suddenly and quite unexpectedly, she was seized with a need to get away from Allerbrook. It was home now, had been for many years, but without Peter it lacked human sympathy. She needed her kinfolk. She wanted to go to Dunster and be with her own family again, with people who would sympathise. She knew Richard was afraid for his son and grandson, but she knew, too, that he would never seek comfort, or give it, either, and she was frightened as well and could have done with comforting.

As she returned to the hall, Richard expressed a wish for some cider. Liza fetched it, carrying the tankard to him with a smile of deceptive sweetness. After all, if she were to visit Dunster, she would need her father-in-law's permission.

CHAPTER THIRTY

THE RED DRAGON

"No!" said Peter. "I can't believe what you're saying, Ned. I've met Gloucester—King Richard. It's just rumour, wicked tattle, and it's no reason to…what you want us to do is treachery, don't you understand? I can't and I won't. Nor will Jarvis."

"Jarvis Hannacombe, I have no doubt, will do what you bid him."

"Then I shall bid him stay with me and fight on the side of the king of England and the house of York. I'll take him and Nicky and leave this inn at once. We'll find the Earl of Nottingham and—"

"Inform him that there's a little detachment of forty men under Sir Edward Crowham, occupying the Sign of the Azure Dove outside Leicester, and they intend to slip off to join Henry Tudor tomorrow morning? I'm sorry, Peter, but I think not."

"You…!" Peter looked about him. They were outside in the innyard, where Ned had brought him, saying that he wanted a private word. The rest of the company, two score or so strong, were inside the inn, which they had virtually commandeered, eating a late supper and drinking ale. The only guests at the inn who were not part of Crowham's following were a small party of tumblers, who were seizing the chance to earn a few pence for entertaining the rest. The light was fading and candles gleamed within the hostelry. Beyond the stone arch of the gateway the dusty road was empty, and opposite were quiet meadows.

They were still some miles short of Leicester, where the king and his lords were, but Ned had halted them here because he said the men must be fresh for the morning. He had sent just two galloping ahead to Leicester and they had returned to say that the royal army would march westward from the city in the morning to meet Henry Tudor, who had advanced through Wales.

As Peter had at first understood it, William Berkeley, Earl of Nottingham, was with the king and his was the banner Ned proposed to follow. They could cut across country tomorrow and join him during the march. Baldwin Sweetwater and his son, John, who had overtaken them on the way, had been pushing on faster, and were probably with him in Leicester already.

But now…

"I don't think you've been listening to me," said Crowham. "Do you think I do this lightly? Don't you know me better than that?"

"I've known you, or so I thought, since I was ten and now I feel I've never really known you at all!"

"King Richard," said Ned, in the very patient voice of one who has tried to make the same point fifty times, without success, "or the Duke of Gloucester as I prefer still to call him, has murdered his brother's sons to keep himself safe on his throne.

He was supposed to be the Protector of the Realm, but he has had the boy who should have been King Edward the Fifth assassinated and the younger brother, too. He put them in the Tower over two years ago and they haven't been seen since. On Exmoor you may hear news but you're still off the main track and you never hear all of it. Every London tavern has seen grown men shed tears, thinking of the fate of those two lads."

"I don't believe it. I will *not* believe it!" Peter struggled for words, remembering the tired, prematurely aged face of the man to whom he had given his horse at Tewkesbury, and the smile in Gloucester's hazel eyes as he'd handed over the deeds which had created Allerbrook's prosperity. "I understood why he had to take the throne—but this! I *can't* believe it. He was devoted to his brother King Edward, and the princes were—are—Edward's sons! His motto was loyalty!"

"Not any longer, I think," said Ned.

"Well, I shall stay loyal! I tell you this, we Lanyons owe him too much to abandon him for a…a…rumour."

"It's more than a rumour. Where *are* those boys? No one has heard or seen them for two years. And Richard, they say, sleeps ill at night."

"I daresay, with filthy slanders being spoken about him and his own troubles. We heard that his wife and his son had both died. That's enough to keep anyone awake at night."

"The elder boy, Prince Edward," said Ned, "had good reason to hate his uncle Gloucester. After the old king died, the Woodvilles tried to snatch power and oversee the boy's crowning. Once the crown was on young Edward's head, the Protectorship would legally have lapsed, though a new one would have had to be set up until the lad was of age. The Woodvilles by all accounts meant to make sure that the new Protector was one of them-selves, and not Gloucester. To stop that, Gloucester beheaded the boy's Woodville uncle, Anthony Lord Rivers, because he was the head of the Woodville family. No doubt he thought he was doing the right thing, but Rivers had been the prince's guardian and there was affection between them. I've been to court, close to the heart of things."

"Believe it or not, I've heard all this, as well!" Peter protested. "I understood why Gloucester took the throne. If the prince became king, he probably wouldn't have left his uncle Gloucester alive for long. I realise *that!* But he didn't become king, did he?"

"You haven't thought it out properly. The boys would grow up—no doubt the younger one would have backed up his brother—and supporters would inevitably gather round them. That could start another civil war. I daresay," said Ned coolly, "that Gloucester felt he had no choice but to rid himself of them. In his place, I might even have done the same. But I'm not in his place and I don't greatly care for the murder of young lads who can't protect themselves."

"And I can't believe it, not of the Gloucester I knew."

"Really? He and King Edward certainly got rid of old King Henry," said Ned. "And of their own brother Clarence, I suspect. None of those were young boys, of course, but they were all helpless prisoners and if you ask me, King Henry was weak in the head. King Richard is much more used to such things than you are. You're only used to killing pigs."

"I was at Tewkesbury," said Peter firmly. "And I intend to be at this battle and *not* on the side of Henry Tudor."

"You will fight for Henry Tudor," said Ned, and now there was nothing at all left of the Ned Crowham who had been

Peter's schoolfellow. A plump, joke-loving, layabed chrysalis had cracked open and out of it had stepped a lethal, subtle dragon-fly. "You will," he said, "because if you do not, you may never see your son Nicholas again."

"*What?* Are you out of your mind, man? What do you mean, I may never see Nicholas again? He's here in the inn. What the devil are you talking about?"

"A number of my men have a regard for you—I've noticed it. If you go to Leicester to join William Berkeley and Gloucester—"

"The king!" said Peter savagely.

"Berkeley and *Gloucester,* some of them might slip off, as well. Also, you'd deliver a warning and the rest of us might be intercepted. I won't have it, Peter. I won't see swords denied to Tudor and extra soldiers going to Gloucester's side. They would strengthen the hand of a murderer, and Tudor has need of swords—and archers and axemen. His forces are too small, even though the Earl of Oxford has joined him now. His stepfather Thomas Stanley may decide to back him up, but Richard is holding one of Stanley's sons as hostage. It's plain enough that he doesn't at all mind making war on mere boys!"

"Neither do you, by the sound of it! What did you mean about Nicky? Tell me!"

"If he prevails," said Ned, ignoring this, "Henry Tudor has sworn to marry the Princess Elizabeth of York—the princes' sister. I suppose you didn't know that. That will unite his line to that of King Edward. York and Lancaster will lie down together in peace at last—literally."

Ned smiled his old familiar smile, now horribly out of place. "Nicky is no longer in the inn," he said. "I had him removed an hour ago. You will not know where he is until the battle is over.

When it is, whatever the outcome, provided you accompany me to Tudor's camp, he'll be sent home. He'll be safe, even if we are not. But you must buy his freedom by lending your sword arm to the Red Dragon."

"To the what?"

"The Tudor's standard is a red dragon. If you refuse to fight beneath it…"

"You…you…" Peter could not think of any epithet which did justice to this. "You talk of young boys being murdered or held hostage by Richard, but in almost the same breath you threaten to kill Nicky! Nicky's a young boy—he's only thirteen! He—"

"I'm not going to kill him! Don't be a fool. I own ships. Three of them, to be precise. They ply in and out of Dorset, where I also have land. If you fail me, Nicky will be taken to Dorset and sent to sea as a ship's boy. He may flourish or he may not, but it's no easy life for a lad fresh from loving parents, on a peaceful farm. My people in Nottingham have had their orders and will see that Nicky is taken to Dorset or sent home in accordance with my wishes—and your behaviour. Whether I live or die, and whether you live or die. Our fates will make no difference."

Peter's sword was at his side. He drew it instinctively, and then saw that after all, he and Ned were not quite alone in the innyard. Four figures came out of the shadows by the stable and seized hold of him.

"No, Peter," Ned said. "You will not harm me. You will sleep tonight on a wide pallet that these trusty fellows will share with you. If you stir, so will they. They are Crowham men. I've known them all my life and they're the best of human watchdogs. They will see that you don't come near me. They won't stop you from slipping out of the inn. They won't even stop you from collect-ing Jarvis and taking him with you. But if you do, you know what will happen."

The curse that Peter now pronounced on Ned was compre-hensive, and most men would have flinched from it. Many would have stepped backward, crossing themselves or making the sign against the Evil Eye. Ned Crowham did not move. "I mean it," he said. To his men, he said, "Watch him. You know what to do." With that, he turned away and walked back into the inn.

"Now, better just come along and take some supper and get some sleep," said one of the watchdogs amiably. He had a Somerset voice, burring and good-natured, tending to turn *s*'s into *z*'s. His advice actually sounded like *take zome zupper and get zome zleep.* It was an accent Peter had heard all his life; indeed, it was his own, though his was not so marked. To hear it under these circumstances was like seeing Dunkery Beacon turned up-side down and balanced on its summit.

But there was Nicky. His son and Liza's and the only son that Allerbrook had. He went into the inn.

It was very difficult to believe that this was happening. What on earth, Peter asked himself despairingly, was he doing here, marching among the foot soldiers behind the stars and streams of the Earl of Oxford's banner, about to fight against Richard of Gloucester, for Henry Tudor? How had he ever been dragged into such a position?

Because Nicky, confound him, had never learned to do as he was bid, not even under the heavy hand of his grandfather. Because Nicky had run away to join the army and was now Ned's captive and the lever by which Peter was to be forced to fight where Ned wished.

It was the second morning after the confrontation at the inn. Ned had marched them all out at daybreak, leading them westward across rolling country. Dusk was falling when they reached an encampment, where cooking fires burned and there were tents with banners flying above them. The stars and streams of Oxford flew over one tent. Over another, and the sight of it sent a thrill of sheer horror through Peter, was a scarlet dragon. To Peter, it was the enemy, the banner of Treason. And willy-nilly, Ned was leading him and Jarvis to it.

Jarvis understood the situation, but was bemused by it. "This b'ain't no way for a friend to treat a friend," he had said as they rode. "Nicky bein' made a prisoner, and by Crowham. That b'ain't right."

"No, Jarvis, it b'ain't right at all," Peter said. "But it's happening."

"I'm with you, sir, wherever you go, whoever you fight for, but if we all come out of this, maybe Master Crowham and me'll have a reckoning one of these days."

"I might get in first," said Peter grimly.

But the fighting was still to come, and he had been forced, so far, to do Ned's will. At the camp, Ned had gone to present himself at the Tudor's tent and presently Henry Tudor himself came out to inspect the reinforcements Ned had brought.

Peter, seeing him close to, was startled. Tudor, although he was wearing a breastplate and a sword, didn't look even remotely like a warrior. He was certainly nothing like Richard of Gloucester, who, though not big, was tough and muscular.

Gloucester had had a determined air, too; there had been resolution in that careworn face. Henry had the face of a conscientious clerk and the beginnings of a scholar's stoop and looked somewhat bewildered, as though he, as well as Peter, were wondering how in the world he had got here. He thanked Ned Crowham for bringing him forty more men, and his thanks were so heartfelt that they verged on the undignified.

"We've got to fight for *him?*" Jarvis whispered in Peter's ear.

"Looks like it. Be quiet," Peter growled in reply.

They had been assigned to the Earl of Oxford, whose name was John de Vere. Peter was a competent archer but Oxford had enough archers, apparently. Peter had retained his sword, but his bow had been given to someone else and in its place he had been presented with a fearsome weapon called a poleaxe. It was long, like a pike, and sharply pointed, and a few inches from the point a blade, savagely sharp and with an edge six inches long, jutted out from one side. A smaller but equally disagreeable blade with teeth like a saw jutted out from the opposite side.

Henry had a mounted escort on good chargers but ponies weren't wanted, and he had been able to leave Plume in safety. Now he and Jarvis and Ned's other men were marching with Oxford.

Ahead of them was a hill, which the man beside him had said was called Ambien Hill. It was occupied now by the king's army and Oxford was leading them toward it. He had sent archers on ahead and already their shafts were flying toward the foe, who were retaliating. Suddenly a cannon boomed. Cannonballs crashed into their midst and a crossbow bolt struck the man who had told Peter the name of Ambien Hill. His blood, hot and stinking, splashed up into Peter's face and screaming broke out all around him. Cursing, sidestepping, he clutched his poleaxe more tightly and felt the sweat of fear on his brow and temples and running down his spine.

Henry Tudor was keeping back. With his mounted escort he was behind them, on another hill. Farther back still and slightly to the right, with a distinct air of not belonging to either faction, was a mounted force in scarlet, the followers, Ned had said when they all set out that morning, of Thomas Stanley, Henry's stepfather.

A front line from the king's army had started downward toward them, flourishing a standard with a silver lion on it. "Norfolk," shouted Ned over his shoulder. "He's leading the charge! We have to deal with him first!"

He slowed down and Peter found himself striding up alongside. "We'll engage in a moment," said Ned rapidly. "It's too late for you to change your mind so I can tell you now—I've put Nicky in the village of Stoke Golding, in an inn called The Seven Stars. He will be returned to Allerbrook after this, even if you fall."

There was no time for more. They were almost face-to-face with Norfolk's men now. Both forces halted. Curses and taunts were exchanged; weapon hafts were pounded on the ground. Peter shouted with the rest, thinking of the man who had fallen to the crossbow bolt and those who had been struck by cannon-balls. He couldn't see them as enemies now. Like it or not, he was their comrade. He had become a Lancastrian, regardless.

A trumpet rang out and the advance began again. The arrows and the cannon fire had ceased, because in a moment, friend and foe would be indistinguishable.

The two lines met.

Up on Ambien Hill, in the mounted reserve, Baldwin Sweet-water said to his son, "It looks as if we won't see any action today. The peasantry's going to see to it on foot."

"It just looks like a mess to me," said John.

Peter, caught up in the collision between Norfolk and Oxford, would have used stronger words than *mess* to describe what was happening. It was a vile chaos of kill or be killed. Trumpet calls from both sides kept drowning each other out and since many of the men in Oxford's following seemed to be Welsh, their captains were bellowing orders in the Welsh language, causing confusion because the English couldn't understand them and didn't therefore know what their Welsh allies were supposed to be doing. The Welsh were probably having the same problem in reverse.

Peter lost sight of Ned Crowham, lost sight of Oxford's standard. People collided with him. Blades rang on his helmet. A furious man, his face distorted with rage, attacked him with a sword and Peter swiped with his poleaxe, taking his assailant in the throat and thankful that the poleaxe had a longer reach than the sword had.

The cry went up that the Duke of Norfolk was slain. Peter found himself in the midst of a melee around Norfolk's body. There was one moment when he had a clear view of Ambien Hill and there, high above, saw King Richard, the sunlight flashing on a gold crown worn over his helmet, seated on a white charger, watching. Suddenly he was alongside Ned again. They could see the Stanley forces, in their vivid livery, also watching the conflict, but keeping aloof.

"Buggers want to see who's winning before they join in!" Ned gasped, wiping sweat out of his eyes and wiping blood into them instead from a gash on his arm.

On Ambien Hill a trumpet spoke and Baldwin Sweetwater said, "Action after all!" as their section of the mounted reserve started downhill to help Norfolk's men. They were halfway down when a squad of crossbowmen rose up, apparently from nowhere, and a hail of bolts drove them back. John Sweetwater, uninjured but struggling with a frightened horse, lost sight of Baldwin for a moment. Then his father reappeared beside him, still in the saddle, but with the armour over his left arm smashed and blood seeping through. "You're hit!" John shouted.

"Flesh wound!" Baldwin shouted back. "I'll live!" Another shower of crossbow bolts swished into the air, but the horsemen had veered out of range by now and the bolts fell short. Glancing back, the Sweetwaters caught sight of the king on his white courser. The king, however, was no longer merely watching. "God's teeth!" gasped John. "Look at that!"

Down in the melee, Norfolk's son had taken over command from his fallen father. He was fighting with the fury of an ancient Viking berserker. But a handful of Norfolk's followers had panicked and were fleeing, and with Ned and others, Peter found himself in pursuit. Before they had time to realise it, they were on the outskirts of the fighting, in the open, with a solid phalanx of armoured Yorkist horsemen bearing down on them from Ambien Hill. Just in time, Ned grabbed Peter's arm and threw them both down under a bush, with a hillock between them and the charge.

It missed them and tore past to slay with fine impartiality the men who had been fleeing and those who like Peter and Ned had been chasing them. Then, as though going on an outing after finishing a few dull chores, they made for the scrimmage around Norfolk's fallen body and plunged in, weapons swinging.

Peter, crawling out from the bush and peering around the hillock, glimpsed a flash on the hill above, looked upward and, like John Sweetwater, gasped at what he saw. The king was on the move. With a small squad of men behind him, he was riding down the slope of Ambien Hill, gathering speed, turning it into a charge, aiming straight for the opposite hill where Henry Tudor still sat, an onlooker, among his mounted guard. There was less than half a mile between them.

"Is that King Richard?" gasped Ned, crawling out beside Peter. "Has he gone mad?"

The king and his followers were clear of Ambien Hill already, and Henry's guard were starting down to meet them. The Stanley banner—it was a white hart, like the name of the Clicket tavern—was moving, too, and the red-jacketed Stanleys were following and not, it seemed, to attack the Tudor forces. Swords out, lances lowered, bellowing war cries which reached Ned and Peter faintly despite the roar of the fighting behind them, the Stanley contingent was thundering headlong straight toward King Richard.

The din of the struggle between Oxford's men and the Yorkists crescendoed. Peter and Ned, suddenly and guiltily aware that they ought to be in it, began to run toward it. A charger whose rider had fallen broke away in panic from the struggle and came galloping toward them. It saw them at the last minute, veered away, all but lost its footing, regained it and then skidded to a stop, sweating, trembling, white-ringed eyes rolling and ears flat back. It tossed its head and a rein swung, lashing Peter's arm. He caught hold of it. "Steady! Easy! Easy now!"

He saw Ned looking at him, and realised why. He could get away if he wanted to. He could scramble astride this gift from heaven, cock a snook at Ned and be gone from this arena of horror. He knew where Nicky was now, after all.

But he had lost sight of Jarvis and he couldn't leave him behind, couldn't, somehow, even leave Ned Crowham. A man didn't run from a battlefield, at least not until the Retreat was sounded or all his fellow soldiers decided to run, as well. Ancient instincts, forged in battles through countless aeons of time, forbade it. You stood by your comrades, even if you didn't like them, even if you'd been forcibly co-opted into their midst.

Peter had hated his previous experience of battle chargers. He was about to fling the animal's reins to Ned, who was more used to such things, when, veering around as the horse sidled and dragged him with it, he again caught sight of King Richard's sally and suddenly understood. Richard of Gloucester had chosen to settle the outcome in the most ancient and formal of ways, by single combat with his challenger. He was trying to reach Henry Tudor, to cut him down personally.

At that moment King Richard and his men crashed into Henry's guard. The Stanleys had farther to go and deceptive dips in the ground had slowed them down. They were still on their way. Peter could see the crown flashing on the king's helmet, see Richard's arm rising and falling as he plied his battle-axe like a man hacking his way through a forest. Or a man possessed by a demon of rage. If he could get through, then the invading Tudor would be cut down for sure. But he wouldn't get through; he couldn't, not through so many; no man could...

At Tewkesbury, Peter had given Richard of Gloucester a horse and Gloucester had given him riches in return, and in Peter, a loyalty had been forged which could not now be wiped out, not even for Nicky.

He could not leave the battlefield, but he couldn't go on fighting for Lancaster either. Once more he would dedicate a loose horse to Gloucester's service. He was in the saddle. The horse, steadied by the familiar feeling of weight on its back and strong hands on its reins, let him turn it and put it into a gallop. Peter drove in his heels, crouched over the tossing mane and grasped his poleaxe as though it were a lance. He was only one man and he would probably do nothing more than get himself killed but he would die with Gloucester, and Nicky must take his chance.

As he put the horse to the slope, he could still see Richard ahead, still fighting, still alive. He spurred on, in among Richard's followers whose charge had been checked by the head-on collision with the enemy. At the same moment the Stanleys arrived, bursting into the confusion, trying to get at the king. King Richard, with bitterness, had recognised his betrayal. Peter could hear him shouting *"Treason!"* over and over again.

A man beside Peter shouted a warning and he ducked just in time as a Stanley sword swept through the space where his head had been. The warning had been given in a voice with a distinct west country burr and he wondered briefly whether the Sweetwaters were in King Richard's escort, but he had no time to think about it, for at that moment King Richard fell. He saw the gold-crowned helmet vanish beneath a tide of scarlet Stanley jackets. And saw the blades that rose and fell with hideous intent.

Then Peter's horse trod on a still-living body, plunged away with a squeal, tangled its feet among the legs of a dead horse and went down, throwing Peter to the ground headfirst. His helmet, already badly battered, failed him and fell off. There was an explosion of light and pain mysteriously combined into one sensation and then oblivion.

He came around to find someone shaking him. He tried to

raise himself, but a bad-tempered blacksmith was wielding a fourteen-pound hammer inside his head and his stomach felt queasy. He sagged back. A Welsh voice above him said, "He's coming to. Who is he now, for the love of God? He has no red Stanley jacket, but he's not one of Richard's—proper armour they have, all of them. Horse is his, though. See, he still has a foot stuck in a stirrup." He felt a hand on his ankle, releasing it from something. "Here, fellow, up you come. What's your name?"

For one dreadful moment he couldn't remember. Then his sense of identity came muzzily back. "Peter." He got it out with difficulty. "Lanyon."

"What's that mean, bach? Who are you?"

Another voice, English this time, said, "I think he's that lunatical fellow we saw tearing across on horseback just before Richard fell. Speak up, man! Who's your commander?"

They had hauled him into a sitting position. The demonic blacksmith redoubled his efforts and his stomach heaved. The two men stooping over him seemed enormous and threatening. He struggled to focus his blurred eyes. He seemed to be still where he had fallen. He could see Ambien Hill and fighting still going on below it, and close to him, all around him, were dead men and horses. He could smell blood. It was everywhere, congealing in pools and rivulets, a hell of butchery.

Men were moving about amid the carnage. He saw a group tearing battered armour off a body only a few yards away, tumbling the corpse as they did so. For a moment he saw its face. Its helmet was half off and the golden crown was gone, but he knew those features; even stained with blood and grey with death, he knew them. It was King Richard.

"Who are you?" Hands on his shoulders were shaking him, to get an answer out of him. The hammer in his head almost made him scream.

He ought to say he was Richard's man, and face whatever vengeance that brought on him, but if Peter Lanyon had an aching head, he also had a hard one. He might annoy his father by marvelling poetically at golden gorse and purple heather, but at times he was very much his father's son. Gloucester was dead and no longer needed his allegiance. Where was the sense in dying for a corpse, in sacrificing his son for an empty gesture? He'd sooner stay alive and go home with Nicky.

"I was with…Earl of Oxford," he said mumblingly. "We were in a battle. That way." He made a vague gesture toward Ambien Hill. "I saw…Gloucester trying to get at Henry Tudor. There was a loose horse. I got onto it and tried to get here to help." At the last moment he left it ambiguous and didn't say who, precisely, he had wanted to help, but he had used a fuddled voice and he had already spoken of following Oxford, and nobody queried it. "Got here but…my horse fell. Can't remember anything else."

"He's one of ours, bach," said the Welsh voice. "Give me a hand with him. Best get him to a tent."

"Thank you," said Peter faintly, and was then very very sick.

CHAPTER THIRTY-ONE 🙚

FRIENDS UPON A BRIDGE

I'*m getting too old for riding,* Liza told herself as her pony carried her down the final stretch of track around the hill which formed the southwest end of Dunster Castle's private chase. She rarely rode these days and now every bone ached.

Richard refused to admit that he was anxious about Peter and Nicky but he quite clearly was and at first he was unwilling to let Liza visit her family. He'd finally agreed after two weeks of persuasion.

"I can see you're fretting. But harvest's not far off—don't you be gone long, now."

"I won't do that," Liza promised. She was glad to set off, for she found it wearisome to be constantly in Richard's company without Peter there, even though when Peter *was* there, she often had to mediate between them. She was happy to be returning to these familiar surroundings. Nearly there now. Here was the path around the edge of the Luttrell chase, overhung by trees as ever, and here was the turn to the packhorse bridge and there was the bridge, with the Avill flowing serenely beneath.

She and Alfred, who was with her, used the ford below the bridge and let their mounts drink from the stream, while a couple of horsemen riding toward them and already on the bridge finished crossing it. It was too narrow for horses to pass each other. Then they rode gently on, through the village, into the broad cobbled North Street where the stalls in the middle of the road were still doing business. Alfred, who came frequently to Dunster, since he often escorted the wool clip there, leaned from his saddle as they came level with the Weavers' house, and took her rein.

"I'll take the ponies to the Weavers' pasture, Mistress, and walk back. You go on in. You'll be tired, I reckon."

"Thank you, Alfred." She got down, stiffly. Their arrival had been seen; doors were opening on both sides of the street and there was Laurence coming across from his house, with Elena hurrying after him, and there was Aunt Cecy—*dear heaven, is Aunt Cecy still alive? She must be over eighty*—at the opposite door. She was swathed in black, except that her headdress, a curious affair shaped like the door of a church, had white beads around its edge. Within it, her face had a grim expression and her greeting was characteristic.

"Well, well, Liza! What brings you here?"

"It's good to see you!" Laurence himself must be about seventy and Elena not much younger and they both looked tired and old. Laurence had lost most of his hair, except for a few grey wisps. But unlike Aunt Cecy, he and Elena were smiling in welcome. They embraced Liza joyfully.

"Nothing's wrong," she said, "except that Peter's gone to the war and Nicky's gone with him. But…"

"Oh, my dear! I wondered why Nicky wasn't with you," Elena said. "Come. Let's go inside."

Aunt Cecy moved aside to let them pass. "If you've come for the funeral, my girl," she said sourly, "you're too late."

Liza stopped short. "The funeral? What funeral? Whose?"

"Dick, my husband. Died nine days back and buried a week since," said Aunt Cecy. "It comes to us all. Well, come in, no need to stand there."

Liza and Elena followed her indoors. The house, to Liza, now seemed both familiar and strange. Familiar because there were the same rooms, with the same furniture and the same woolly smell, and from the kitchen, the sound of an argument. A mislaid crock of butter was causing recriminations. Faintly, just as always, she could hear the clack of looms.

But Dick, Cecy's husband and Uncle Will's son, was gone, and Uncle Will too had departed. He had died at eighty-seven. Richard had brought her the news, after a visit to Dunster. The corner where he used to sit looked empty. This was the house that she remembered, yes. But…how odd. She really *had* put roots down at Allerbrook. What was it she had once heard Betsy say? She had been lying with her eyes closed after the birth and death of poor little Jack. *Where she rears her family, that's the place a woman calls home.* Quentin and Nicky had both been born at Allerbrook. Her other relatives were here in Dunster, but her home was not.

Her relatives, however, were gathering eagerly around her. Many of them had changed: grown up or grown older. Her brother Tommy was very much a family man now, with a sensible-looking wife called Susannah, and two small children. They were all full of sympathy when they heard that both Peter and Nicky had ridden away with Crowham, and that Nicky had gone after his father.

"No one's gone from Dunster this time," Laurence said. "And a good thing, too. If only this battle can be the last one. It's high time it was settled once and for all who's going to sit on the throne." His lined face became suddenly red with anger. "The whole of England is sick to the stomach of their squabbling and the way they take our sons and use them and never bring them back. It's a disgrace!" He stopped, breathless.

"Gently, my dear," said Elena, looking at him worriedly. She turned to Liza. "We lost Laurie and Dickon to the wars and now Jem's dead, too, though not through war. He got something wrong with his innards two years back." Liza nodded sadly. Richard had brought that news to her, too. "We've still got Luke and Joss, for which we're grateful, but we don't forget," Elena said.

"Yes, there's death enough without battles creating more. I say it's a bitter shame that folk can't live their ordinary lives in peace," said Laurence. "All we want to do is weave our cloth, bring up our families, look after our homes. But are we ever left alone to get on with it? No, we're not, and more shame to those who call themselves our betters and take our sons away."

"When little Joanna there was baptised," said Susannah, pointing to her five-year-old daughter, "our priest was sick and the castle chaplain came to the church to do it—Father Christopher." Susannah, clearly, had not been told about Liza's past indiscretions and to judge from her casual tone, no one had stared at the priest and exclaimed that he was exactly like Nicky Lanyon. Liza herself gave no sign that Christopher's name meant anything to her, though it had gone through her like a crossbow bolt.

Susannah was continuing. "He gave a little homily afterward, congratulating us, and he quoted a psalm. *Like as the arrows in the hand of a giant, even so are the young children*—that's what he said. Well, that's just how the great men have been treating ordinary folk like us. They just want our lads as arrows to be used and spent. It's true!"

"No one took Peter and Nicky," said Aunt Cecy. "Peter's a free man and from what Liza here says, Nicky just ran off as silly boys do. Nicky *is* a silly boy. We've tried to teach him weaving when he's been here, but he's that mutton fisted he'd break threads even if he was making chain mail. But Peter's no better, going off like that. Men have no sense. If they get spent like arrows, half the time it's because they've spent themselves."

Aunt Cecy had decidedly not mellowed with age. Before supper was over, Liza was beginning to think that she had better not stay too long. Not only was Dunster somehow unfamiliar, but also, she had come to be soothed by the company of her family, only to find that all the news seemed to be unhappy and Aunt Cecy's contributions to the talk were anything but soothing, and no better for being oblique.

Aunt Cecy did not actually say outright that if Liza had had more authority over her son, he would not have defied orders and run off after his father; she merely said that nowadays young people lacked respect for their parents and that parents should insist on it more. Nor did she remark outright that Peter and possibly Nicky as well could be killed. Instead, she asked who would inherit Allerbrook after them, and then added that it was a great pity that Liza hadn't had a good healthy family of boys.

The Weaver family as a whole was used to her and most of them seemed hardly aware of her comments, while those who were, such as Laurence and Elena, tried to change the subject or rephrase Aunt Cecy's remarks for her, in a kinder form. This usually failed, as Aunt Cecy, more than once, said, "No, that's not what I meant," and then repeated her remark in the original wording. Long before the end of the meal Liza was wondering why Aunt Cecy had not been banished to retirement in the guest house of some convenient women's abbey. She understood now why her mother couldn't tolerate life with Cecy after her father's death.

As they left the table, Susannah put a hand on her arm, and said, "Please don't mind Aunt Cecy. She's unhappy without her husband and he hasn't been gone two weeks. She's bitter but she doesn't mean it. She's old and doesn't realise that she upsets people."

Her brother had married a likeable woman, Liza thought, glad for him. She gave Susannah a smile. And wondered if her aching bones could endure riding back to Allerbrook the very next day.

Next morning, as the Weavers gathered just after daybreak to take their breakfast of bread and honey, cold meat and small ale, the talk turned to the state of Dunster harbour.

"If it goes on silting up at this rate, Dunster will end up two miles inland and someone will be planting wheat where the fishing boats are moored now," Tommy grumbled.

"That's right enough." Joss, the younger of Laurence and Elena's two surviving sons (though he was no longer young but was now a widower aged forty) was a weaver and had moved across the road, as he put it, to live with his loom. "No one's even trying to do anything about it. The big ships can only get halfway in these days. Minehead's not much better. Porlock, Lynmouth and Watchet'll all end up more important."

"Dunster'll do well enough," said Aunt Cecy. "Everyone

comes here to buy cloth and yarn and fleeces, too, and there are good roads for the packhorses, in and out."

"That's not the same as having a good harbour," Joss objected.

"From all I've heard, if this Lord Dunster as he calls himself—"

"Pembroke's son," said Tommy aside to Liza.

"If this Lord Dunster," said Aunt Cecy, more loudly, "wants the harbour dug out, he'll put up all our rents to pay for it and even then, from what I've heard, the sea'll bring trouble in faster than any gang of men could dig it out."

"Nonsense," said Tommy robustly. "There's a whole garrison up at the castle, doing nothing most of the time but swagger round the village eyeing up the wenches. That there harbour could be dug out for the cost of a few spades and an ox team."

"You think so? They're soldiers and they'd say digging and ploughing, whether it's fields or a harbour, is beneath them. It's only for common folk like farmers," said Aunt Cecy, achieving further depths of tactlessness. "I've lived a long time," she added. "There's always changes, and never for the better as far as I can see."

"Oh, be quiet, you croaking old raven!" snapped Tommy.

Tears appeared in Aunt Cecy's weak blue eyes and Susannah said mildly, "My dear, Aunt Cecy is in mourning."

"Well, I'm sorry," said Tommy. "But…"

He left the sentence unfinished. However, when breakfast was over, Liza grew restless. The kitchen wrangle about the mislaid butter still seemed to be continuing and this time she found it not amusing, but tiresome. Neither Richard nor Peter would have tolerated such a haphazard atmosphere at Allerbrook and Liza now discovered that she, too, found it irritating. She didn't think she could bear the journey back so soon, but she couldn't stay within earshot of Aunt Cecy a moment longer.

"It's a sunny day," she said. "I want to walk round the village."

"You were always one for walking," said Aunt Cecy. "And no one ever knew who you met or talked to."

"I just liked walking," said Liza coldly.

She left the house and set off along North Street. As she went she took note of changes. She knew none of the people she saw. They were all younger than she was, a new generation, and their clothes were different. Hers had changed very little; on a farm in the midst of the moor, no one followed fashion. But now it seemed that women wishing to appear well dressed had adopted fuller gowns and shorter headdresses, and that the young village men were going in for the kind of elaborate caps which once had been the prerogative of folk like the Sweetwaters. They seemed to like a lot of pleating in their tunics, too. Liza began to feel dowdy.

But the sunshine was pleasant; even the castle towering up at the end of the street looked more hospitable than grim. She followed the lane around the foot of the castle hill, turned into West Street and presently took the lane to the packhorse bridge. The trees were in full and heavy leaf, meeting above the river and rustling softly in a light wind.

She stopped on the bridge to look down at the water, and gazed at her reflection in it, wondering if she had really become dowdy. Since the Lanyons now had a fine house, they ought to dress accordingly. Weaving for long hours was tiring these days. Perhaps she should buy some good cloth in Dunster and get some modern patterns for gowns.

The water rippled into rings as a trout came up. When the ripples settled, there were two reflections in the river. She swung around. "Christopher!"

Like her, he was older. The fire had died in his tonsure, although it was not grey but had faded from flame to sandy, though a few traces of the original flame colour remained. There were lines in his face. But the rest was the same—snub nose, freckled chin, amber eyes smiling and, resting on the parapet beside her own, shapely hands with sandy hairs on them. It was a little surprising that at Joanna's baptism no one had noticed his resemblance to Nicky, but the church was often shadowy, and a man always looked different in full priestly vestments.

Astonished at seeing him, she gazed at him in wonder and he laughed. "There's no magic. I never go to the dell now. It has…memories of something I value very much but know must never be repeated. I come here instead. I come nearly every morning and linger for a while. We argued here once, but it was only because we were so much in love and knew we had no hope of marrying. Do you remember?"

"Of course I remember."

"If you came out walking, on any day when it's not raining, at this time and came to this bridge, you'd be almost sure to find me here. Just as once you'd have been almost sure to find me in the dell. As I said, there's no magic."

"How are you? I heard you were still at the castle. You…you baptised a child in my family not long ago."

"Ah. Yes, I did. I wondered if any of the Weavers would remember our—escapade. But if so, they didn't mention it. You were mentioned, though. I heard you had a son."

"Yes. Named Nicholas after my father. We call him Nicky."

Does he know? Shall I tell him? Liza did not know what to say until Christopher said, "Is he with you? You are visiting your kinfolk, I suppose."

"Yes. But Nicky isn't here. He and my husband…they've both gone to the war, to fight for the king."

"Your son as well? How old is he?"

"Thirteen."

He might work it out from that, but he showed no sign of doing so, and Liza's racing heart had quietened. She would not tell him. It would disturb his peace, and he did seem peaceful; reconciled, at least. She said again, "How are you? Are you well—happy?"

"You know, I think I am. I live at the castle and hold services for the servants and the men in the garrison. I have conducted weddings for some of them, given the last rites to others. Sometimes I run errands here and there."

"If you're really happy, then I'm glad."

He leaned on the parapet, looking down at the water. "It's a quiet life but not dull." He paused and then said, "I ride out quite often on the errands I mentioned. As far as Withypool, sometimes. There's a woman in the castle who sweeps and dusts and she has parents there. They're old and not well and she sends them comforts by me, and money when she can spare some of her wage. I add a little to it. I like the old pair. He used to be the Sweetwaters' harbourer, before he got too old. Faulkner, that's their name. I do jobs about the cottage and garden for them because they're both lame. Liza, you must be very anxious, with your husband and son away at the war, but apart from that, I hope your life is good."

"Yes. I think it is."

There was a silence. Then he said, "It's over, isn't it? The storm and the passion. No more lightning in the air between us. No more agony. I just feel I am standing on this bridge beside a very old friend."

"So do I. As though we hadn't really been parted all this time. As though we'd been together often, only I've forgotten it, as one forgets dreams. Oh!" A wave of guilt had poured over her. "I shouldn't say such things! Not with Peter and Nicky both in danger. I don't know if I shall ever see them again. Aunt Cecy—did you see Aunt Cecy at the baptism?"

"Was she the very elderly lady with the sharp tongue?"

"Yes! She was hinting last night that they might both be killed, and I hate her for that but it's true and I should be thinking of nothing but them. Yet I'm standing here with you and saying… thinking…feeling…"

"You are talking to a friend. I am sorry for your fears and I wish I could reassure you. All I can do is pray for you and for them."

"I'm going home again tomorrow, if I can bear the thought of the saddle. I can't face staying near Aunt Cecy!"

There was another silence, until at last he said, "I pray for you anyway, every single night. I am happy. *My* life is certainly good. Yet there's something missing and always will be. I shall always miss *you,* Liza. I always have. I can't help it."

"I know. I feel the same. Exactly the same."

"There's another dell," said Christopher, "half a mile, perhaps, from the packhorse bridge the Sweetwaters built on their land, on the Allerbrook side. It's lonely, well off the track. It doesn't grow bluebells but there are foxgloves there. I found it one day when I was coming back from the Faulkners and tried to take a shortcut to Washford. I needed to call on the monks there with a message from the steward. He arranges to buy fleeces from the monks, to be turned into cloth by a Dunster weaver—not one of your family. It's to provide livery for the garrison."

"Yes?" Liza was puzzled.

"My shortcut wasn't a shortcut at all. It was a sheep track and it wandered in all directions, but I found the dell on the way. The sheep path turns off the main track just by a standing stone, a small one, the only one in that part of the moor. Liza, I visit the Faulkners every second Tuesday and I'll be there on Tuesday of next week. In the afternoon, if the weather is kind, I may go out of my way and take a rest in that dell. I'll be there every Tuesday fortnight, given fair weather."

"Should you be saying this to me?" said Liza.

"Perhaps not, but aren't we old enough now to be—just friends? It would warm some part of me that has always been left chilled, if we could once in a while meet and talk, just talk. Would it be so wrong? Friendship is a happy thing."

Liza did not know what to answer. The words *some part of me that has always been left chilled* had come home to her. Within her, too, was something that had longed for warmth, for comfort, and never had its wish granted, a secret poor relation longing to hold out its hands to a hearth fire but forbidden to draw near.

She said nothing and he did not ask for an answer. He kissed her before they parted, but just in kindly fashion on the forehead, and then walked away, but he glanced back, just once. He wanted to see her again and she wanted to see him. The old longing for each other's company had not faded, although now it was no longer physical. They didn't want to make love, only to be together and talk, but yes, they did want that. It hadn't changed. And he hadn't been able to stop himself from offering them a way.

She knew even before she had turned to go home that as long as the skies were dry, she would be in that other dell next Tuesday.

CHAPTER THIRTY-TWO 🙢

COMING HOME

Peter was too giddy to walk, but the owner of the Welsh voice took charge of him. He found himself being carried to a tent in the Tudor encampment. Someone gave him something to drink and he fell asleep. When he woke in the evening he felt easier, although his head still throbbed and when he gingerly fingered it, he found a tender lump.

It was another full day before he could stand up without the world swimming around him, but he told the Welshman who had helped him that he ought to get word to his leader, Sir Ned Crowham, who was one of Oxford's captains, and this called forth some startling news.

"The Earl of Oxford's gone to Leicester with King Henry. Leicester's the nearest city and the king's making a triumphal entry." The Welshman gave Henry Tudor's new title without a flicker of hesitation. He grinned. "Richard of Gloucester had a crown on over his helmet. King Henry has it now. He'll ride into Leicester in style, indeed he will. But the earl set some sorting out in hand before he went. Well organised is John de Vere, and King Henry, too. He made lists of names—all his lords and captains and most of their followers. If you're Peter Lanyon… that's what you said?"

"Yes, I am."

"Did you have a man along with you, by the name of Jarvis Hannacombe?"

Peter sat up more sharply than was good for him, but he ignored the thud of pain in his skull. "Yes, I did! Is there news of him?"

"It is not good news," said the Welshman sympathetically. "Nor is there good news of Crowham. They're both dead."

"Oh, dear God."

"Crowham was found lying on his back with his breastplate smashed in, and a wound in his chest. Hannacombe was facedown on top of him, with his head half off and a bloodied dagger in his hand. Looks as if he threw himself on top of Crowham when he fell and tried to defend him, only Crowham's wound was mortal already. Meant something to you, did they, Crowham and this Jarvis Hannacombe?"

"Yes," said Peter, feeling his mouth shrivel as he said it, as though he had taken a gulp of verjuice. Ned Crowham was a friend who had turned into an enemy. What he had meant, in the end, was as bitter as any crab apple. But Jarvis was a country lad who hadn't cared a straw for York or Lancaster. He'd come because Peter had told him to and, perhaps, for the sake of an adventure. And died for it.

"It was an honourable end," said the Welshman, kindly enough, seeing Peter's face. "For them both."

THE HOUSE OF LANYON

"I'm sure it was."

"And you had a pony in the horse lines. One of your comrades knew which one it is and he's taking care of it. He was pleased you'd been found alive."

Peter said, "I must get myself on my feet. Are we free to go home, or not?"

"If you want. We're all small fry and you're walking wounded. But a whole lot of men have gone to Leicester, following the king. You come from the southwest, don't you?"

"Yes."

"Not many of you in the fighting," said the Welshman. "But there were two in Gloucester's pack, that came across to try and kill King Henry. Father and son, they were. They're prisoners. They'll hang."

"What? What are they called?" said Peter.

"Brecher, that's the name, so I heard."

Not Sweetwater, then. He detested the Sweetwaters, but he didn't want to think of either Baldwin or John pinioned, terrified, swinging and choking on the end of a rope. He was surprisingly glad it was neither of them. "Poor devils," said Peter, and lay back once more, closing his eyes.

He heard the Welshman leave the tent, and let himself release a sigh of thankfulness that he had had the sense to lie at the right moment. Otherwise, he would probably have found himself hanging beside that luckless father and son.

As it was, he was alive and free. Where had Ned said he would find Nicky? In a village called Stoke Golding, at the sign of The Seven Stars. He must get there as soon as he could. He wouldn't need to search for Jarvis as well, not now.

Had young Hannacombe really died trying to defend Ned

Crowham? Jarvis had been angry on Nicky's behalf. He had said that one day he and Crowham might have a reckoning. In the confusion of the battle, thought Peter as he lay there, physically weak but privately seething with impatience, had Jarvis seized his chance and made Crowham pay? Very likely, but he'd never know for sure.

The Seven Stars inn at Stoke Golding was the most unpleasant hostelry he had ever seen. It was a rickety timber building that looked as if it might fall down at any moment and the groom who offered to take Plume did so with a slouch and a scowl which caused Peter to insist on stabling and unsaddling the pony himself. The stable was dismally dark and badly needed mucking out, but while he was seeing to Plume, he realised that the animal in the next stall, a chestnut pony, about fourteen hands, with white socks and a blaze, looked familiar. Surely it was the pony Ned Crowham had given Nicky to ride when they set out from Crowham's manorhouse.

With, Peter observed in alarm, an empty manger and a coat that hadn't been groomed for days. He began to feel afraid. He had taught Nicky to take care of his pony. Why hadn't he?

You cared for your horses before yourself, or even other people's horses if necessary. He put fodder in the chestnut's manger as well as in Plume's before he went hurrying into the inn. It was as bad inside as outside—gloomy and smelling of mice and mildew. He stood, nostrils twitching, in a cobblestoned room with a sagging wooden ceiling, and shouted until the landlord came, a thin man with an air of despair about his bent shoulders and watery eyes, as though life had long since defeated him. Oh yes, he had a boy called Nicky here. Brought in by three elderly fellows two days back. *Marched* in was what it looked like, with one of them holding the lad's arm good and hard.

They'd paid in advance, he said, a week's money for each of the four, and the old men had watched the boy like cats watching a mouse hole. Looked as if they thought he'd run away. In fact, he had an idea they had him tied to the bed in the room they'd taken. "Not my business," said the landlord when Peter wanted to know why he hadn't offered Nicky any help. "Thought maybe he'd done something wrong."

"Well, are they still here?" Peter demanded.

"Not the old ones. They came from up Nottingham way. Someone brought a message to them, about the battle and how the Tudor had won the day, and then they were off. Just left the boy behind, as he'd fallen sick…."

"Fallen sick?" shouted Peter. "Where is he?" He wanted to grab the landlord's bony shoulders and shake him.

"Up there," said the landlord, pointing to an unreliable looking staircase. "Something wrong with his stomach." Peter went up it two at a time. It made his head thump again but he didn't care.

Nicky was in a tiny room under the thatch, lying on a straw pallet beneath a grubby coverlet. If he had been tied up at first, he wasn't tied now but the place was filthy and the contents of a bucket by the bed stank horribly. Nicky's hair was soaked with sweat and his eyes had the look, both filmed and bright, of fever. But he struggled to sit up when Peter came in.

"Father! I thought I heard your voice but I'd been dreaming…I thought I'd dreamed that, too…. It really is you? Father, I'm so sorry. I shouldn't have come after you. Please don't be angry! I couldn't help being brought here. I couldn't…"

Relieved and panic-stricken both at once, Peter strode across to the bedside. "I've found you and that's all I care about. But I had no notion you might be sick! I know you couldn't help being captured. Ned Crowham died in the battle, by the way," he said.

"I know. There was a message for the old men that brought me here—"

"On Ned Crowham's damned orders!"

"Yes. The message was about the battle, but the messenger said Crowham had been killed. Then the old men said they wanted to go home, and I could go home, too, when I felt ready, but they didn't want to stay here till I was well. So they just left me. They came from Crowham's Nottinghamshire place, I think."

"What's wrong with you?"

"I've got a fever and I keep being sick. I think it was the salted pork the second night here. It tasted funny. The old men didn't have it—they had pottage. I tried to get away, Father, I really did, but they gave me no chance. I was roped to the bed at first, until I got ill…." He gagged suddenly, and reached in haste for the bucket.

"I'm not surprised. This place is a disgrace. Now, listen. I'm going into the village to fetch some clean, fresh milk and whole-some food for you. And I'll find someone to make you up a cooling draught. Don't worry."

It took Nicky over two weeks to recover. Not wanting to move him while he was still so feverish and liable to fits of nausea, Peter ordered the inn's only maidservant to clean the attic room and change the bedding, while he himself scoured the district for trustworthy victuals. He compelled the landlord to prepare them under his eyes. He also found a village woman with a name for making medicinal herb infusions, who supplied a purge and a febrifuge. The purge made Nicky wretched for several hours, but it seemed to clear his system. After that, the cooling medicine took effect. His fever dropped and he began to eat again, while Peter groomed Plume and the chestnut and bullied the groom into cleaning the stable and feeding its occupants properly.

Ned Crowham had at least done one thing right. He had not expected his followers to bring their own subsistence money as some men did, but had paid them. Peter could buy what he needed—oats for the ponies as well as food for himself and Nicky.

There came a day, at last, when he could pay their bill, put saddles on the two ponies and, with Nicky, leave thankfully for home.

Henry Tudor, in a sense, was home already.

He had been firstly an exile at the French court and then an adventurer trying to seize the estate of England by force, with backing from French troops and a handful of English Lancastrian nobles and some Welshmen who owed allegiance to his Welsh ancestry, but with very little real support in the land he wanted to conquer. All this had turned him into an impressive-looking but privately petrified armoured figure sitting motionless on a large horse and glad of the ironclad fence of French and Welsh knights in front of him.

They had destroyed his enemy for him and he had metamorphosed again, this time into a triumphant new king, riding into Leicester, meeting dignitaries, getting to know those English lords who had fought for him but had hitherto not met him personally, presiding over meetings and banquets, sending out proclamations to announce the outcome of Bosworth Field all over the land, and also attending a few hangings, which he didn't enjoy though he kept his countenance and didn't look away.

This was followed by another triumphal march to London, and a formal reception with entertainments and more banquets. Here he ordered new silk shirts and embroidered doublets, had his hair washed and trimmed and purchased a new cap of soft velvet to put on top of it. His plate armour and helmet were, he trusted, laid away for good and he hoped he would never have to hang a sword from his belt again as long as he lived.

In London he was reunited with his mother, Margaret Beaufort, whose descent from Edward III was his strongest claim to the throne. He also had his first meeting with King Edward's daughter, Elizabeth of York, having summoned her from the north, where she had been living. He had sworn to marry her, to unite at last the warring clans of York and Lancaster, and was relieved to find her a pleasing girl, quiet and biddable. He did not wonder whether they would ever come to love each other. Henry wasn't accustomed to love.

Now, at last, in the quarters he had been given at the house of Thomas Kemp, the Bishop of London, he had embarked on the business and administration side of kingship and that was his true moment of homecoming. Living in tents, marching and riding, warfare and physical danger were not at all to his taste; nor was he truly at ease with ceremonies or making speeches or thinking of pretty things to say to young women. Desks full of papers and parchments, the scratching of quill pens, deferential clerks in decent black gowns, offering him things to sign and seal; this was the world where he belonged.

"Men who stood by me should be rewarded," he said to one of the chief clerks. "And a few examples should be made of the major figures who stood against me. Gloucester was a usurper and never a legitimate sovereign and to fight on his side was an act of treason."

Several stacks of parchments were on the desk in front of him. He picked up a set, leafed through it, hesitated and then removed one or two sheets before shaking the remainder into tidy order and handing them to the clerk. "These estates are to be confiscated and we require the necessary documents to be drawn up, ready for our signature after Parliament reopens at the end of October."

"There should be no difficulty, sir. There is sufficient time."

"Such confiscations will of course require an Act of Parliament before they can go into effect." Henry's voice was formal. "We trust that the act will go through smoothly. We have made notes on each of these pages, suggesting the dates by which the present occupants must leave. Time must be allowed, of course. We are not a barbarian. These, on the other hand…"

He reached for another set of parchments. "These concern families which are to be rewarded or, in some cases, reinstated. For instance, this one refers to a Lady Elizabeth Luttrell, whose husband was killed fighting for the Lancastrians. She was ordered out of her home at Dunster Castle in Somerset. The castle and its estates are to be restored to her and to her son—Hugh Luttrell. He must be grown up by now. Again, the documentation must be prepared for my signature. And these…"

He paused, frowning, considering yet another pile. The chief clerk waited. "These are small ale, as it were," Henry said. "Minor gentry who fought for Gloucester, but did so of their own choice and not because they were tenantry who had to follow their lord. We don't wish to persecute them too savagely but on the other hand…although these properties aren't large, the sale of a fair number would add up to a useful sum, and the exchequer needs money. War is expensive. We will consider each case with care. But we do need to make a profit," he added thriftily.

★ ★ ★

For Nicky and Peter, the journey home was slow, for Nicky was still not strong. It was a week before, at last, they saw the track underfoot turn from brown to the familiar pinkish-red, and Exmoor's hills rose before them and the people to whom they spoke used the familiar accent of home.

"The very air smells different," Peter said, and was grieved anew for the two unknown westcountrymen, the Brechers, who would never draw a breath of it again. The Sweetwaters might well have fallen in that last conflict; but that was better by far than hanging.

"Are you sure you ought to ride yet, with your arm not healed?" Walter Sweetwater said to his son.

Baldwin, whose left sleeve still bulged with the dressing beneath it, merely snorted. "I'm well enough. It's taking time to mend, but Catherine's comfrey ointment is doing its work. I rode all the way back here! And now Blue Lyn needs exercise again."

"But you were feverish when you came home." Catherine had brought some mending into the hall because in the morning the light was better there than in her solar. "You should take care," she said with concern.

"I'm well enough now, Kitten!"

"I wish John could go with you," said Catherine doubtfully.

"So do I, but as John is out heaven knows where, training a hawk, he can't," said Baldwin testily.

"At least he came back safe. I was so thankful to see the two of you home again, even though you were wounded. I prayed for you every morning and every night, believe me. You don't know what women suffer when men are away at war."

"You don't know what we suffer on the march or on the field," retorted Baldwin. "You at least can sleep warm and safe while we try to get to sleep in draughty tents or out on the ground, under the sky at times! It was our duty to go and yours to keep Sweetwater House in order till we came home. That's the way life is. And now I'm going to take the air."

As she watched him ride out of the courtyard, Catherine said, "I think his arm still pains him. It makes him irritable."

"It's more than that," said Walter. "I think I should warn you. There's been a rumour. I heard it when Giles Northcote called on us yesterday. He didn't go to the war but he has well-placed friends who did, who fought for King Henry and went with him to London. He is planning heavy fines for families that supported King Richard, and in some cases, confiscations of land. It's possible that we are on his list."

"Oh, no!" said Catherine, horrified.

"I hope the rumour's not true, but only time will tell. Oh, and the Lanyons won't be on the list. We heard, just before the battle at Bosworth, that Ned Crowham was going over to the Tudor and taking all his followers with him, Lanyons included. There were some travelling tumblers in the same inn as Crowham and his companions, two nights before the battle. They overheard them talking, it seems. Anyhow, they turned up in Leicester next day with information to sell to the Earl of Nottingham. They didn't reach him soon enough for anything to be done, but word got round. So we can assume that even if the Lanyons were important enough to be robbed by Henry, they won't be, whereas we might. *That's* why Baldwin is so angry."

"But…we only fought for the reigning king!"

"This man Henry Tudor," said Walter, "seems to be fond of

money. According to Giles, he has an abacus where other men have hearts. He'd rather shuffle papers and count coins and wield a pen than ride in battle with a sword in his hand. King Richard at least died fighting! Henry never struck a blow. I can't blame Baldwin for his short temper. I'm badly worried myself. But at least his wound is much improved, for which we must both be thankful to you."

"But if we lose our home, John will lose his inheritance!" Catherine cried. "The rumour can't be right. Men can't be called traitors if they fight for an anointed king!"

"I wouldn't place any wagers on it," said Walter Sweetwater grimly.

CHAPTER THIRTY-THREE 🐚

FOES UPON A BRIDGE

"Nearly home now," Peter said to Nicky as they left the town of Dulverton, where they had crossed the River Barle, and set off northwestward through the moorlands.

"Your Plume knows he's going home," Nicky said as the ponies lowered their heads to tackle a steep rise. "Look at the way his ears are pricked."

"Of course he knows it," said Peter. "He can smell it!"

They rode steadily onward, over a hillcrest thickly grown with bracken and then by way of a winding pebbly track down into a valley wooded with oak and beech, to emerge beside Walter Sweetwater's packhorse bridge over the small river at the boundary of the Sweetwater land. Nicky fell back, because it was too narrow for them to ride across abreast.

Stepping onto the bridge, Plume tossed his head and whinnied and Peter turned to call over his shoulder that he reckoned his mount was saying, "Nearly home!" in the language of horses.

But before he had framed the words, there was an answering whinny, and out of the trees on the other side of the bridge rode Baldwin Sweetwater, astride a big blue roan stallion.

By rights, since Peter was already on the bridge and the nearest ford was some distance away, Baldwin should have drawn rein and waited for him to finish crossing. Instead, to Peter's surprise and indignation, Baldwin came straight on.

Baldwin himself could not have said clearly why he didn't follow established custom and allow right of way to the rider already on the bridge. All he knew was that within him there was a seething anger, like a lidded pan boiling over a fire, and that he longed, somehow, to relieve the pressure, to let the lid blow off. His wounded arm had been badly infected and though Catherine's treatment was gaining ground, it still had pus in it and it throbbed when he tried to use his left hand. On top of that, the warning his brother-in-law, Giles Northcote, had brought yesterday, that the Sweetwaters stood in danger of a heavy fine or even confiscation of their land, had outraged him.

It hadn't helped that Giles, though outwardly sympathetic, had been unable to hide his smugness when he admitted that no such threat hung over his own family. He had kept out of the war, and his property, including the estate that formed most of Agnes's dowry, was safe. Giles was proving a good husband to Agnes, who seemed, judging from her letters, to be well content, but he clearly considered himself to be a wiser man than either her father or her brother, as well as several social rungs above them. Baldwin would very much have liked to encounter Northcote on that bridge, and force him to leave it backward.

He had, however, recognised Peter Lanyon, and failing Giles, a Lanyon—any Lanyon—would do nicely as a substitute. The Lanyons had gone Lancastrian along with Ned Crowham, so no one was going to take their home away from them. What if the Sweetwaters were compelled to leave their fine house while the Lanyons stayed in untroubled possession of theirs? They were nothing but peasants who thought themselves equal to him, and that was an impertinence.

He did not mentally put any of these things into words. They merely boiled inside his head, in bubbles that came and went, but one thing did emerge plainly and that was that he was damned if he would draw rein and let Peter cross that bridge in peace.

Peter was already two thirds of the way over. Baldwin, however, rode onto the bridge at his end, blocking the way, and halted. So did Peter. Across the intervening space they glowered at each other.

"Lanyon," called Baldwin, as one who identifies the face of a foe. "Go back, if you please!"

"Why? I was on the bridge first!" Peter retorted. Not long ago he had actually been glad to think that Baldwin and Walter had escaped from Bosworth, that they were not the two west-countrymen who had hanged for supporting their crowned king. Now all his normal dislike of the Sweetwaters and his resentment of the things they had done to his family surged up in him. He sat still, Plume's reins in his left hand and his right hand placed aggressively on his hip.

"Just go back!" Baldwin barked.

"No, it's my right of way. I'll be across and out of your road in a matter of seconds. Back off yourself, Sweetwater!"

To turn on the bridge would be difficult if not impossible, but though two thirds of the bridge was a long way for a horse to back, any pony bred wild on the moor, as Plume had been, could get out of trouble tailfirst if necessary. Baldwin's mount had only just set hoof on the bridge. Either could have moved out of the other's way quite easily. Neither did so.

There was a pause, during which the fury inside Baldwin mounted, wiping out, for a moment, not only the throb of his wound but even the memory of it. Here, at last, was the thing he wanted: an enemy with whom he could engage, hand to hand, as murderously as he chose. Suddenly, violently, he swung himself to the ground, removing his sword belt, which he tossed over his saddle. He walked toward Plume.

"Get down and fight it out. Put your weapons aside. I'm not crossing swords with you. That's the way gentlemen settle their accounts and you're merely a peasant with feet too big for his boots. Besides, it wouldn't be a fair fight," he added disagreeably. "I've had real training in arms and you have not."

"So courteous," Peter said coldly. "Such knightly manners, just like your grandfather had." He glanced over his shoulder. "Nicky! Get down, tether your pony and come here. Take charge of Plume and my weapons."

Nicky obeyed but looked worried. "Father! Should you?" he asked as he came forward to take Plume's bridle.

"I'm going to, anyway," said Peter, handing his sword and dagger to Nicky. The Earl of Oxford had given his bow to somebody else and the poleaxe was probably still lying on Bosworth Field. He hadn't seen it since the moment he was knocked out. "Take those, and move Plume back."

"You Lanyons always did think far too much of yourselves. This is where I show you your place," said Baldwin, and launched himself.

It should have been a fairly even contest. It was true that Baldwin had been trained in arms and he was the younger of the two by some years. Peter, however, had spent his life plodding behind ploughs, herding stock on horseback, cutting down trees, shearing sheep, scything corn and slaughtering pigs. Had Baldwin not been injured, they would have been virtually equals.

Peter, unaware of the injury, assumed that they were, and Baldwin had briefly forgotten his wound. Both threw their strength into the fight. It was all in a confined space, the narrow width of the bridge. Blue Lyn, accustomed to human beings fighting one another, stood solidly. Plume, already being coaxed backward by Nicky, flattened his ears and backed faster, dragging Nicky with him. Baldwin's preference was to use his fists, Peter's to wrestle. Nicky tried to soothe Plume, but was himself nervous, afraid for his father.

The combatants made little noise, beyond grunts, until the moment when Baldwin's right fist on Peter's chin sent Peter reeling backward and Baldwin tried to follow it up with his left. Then the wound in his left arm blazed into agony. He cried out and his arm dropped. At the same moment Peter recovered himself and leaped forward again, grabbing for Baldwin's arms and closing powerful fingers right on top of the injury.

In the brief struggle that followed, Baldwin's curses sent birds flying in alarm from the trees. Somehow he broke that agonising grip, wrapped his arms around Peter and tried to heave him backward over the parapet of the bridge. Peter, savagely resisting, once more unknowingly closed his fingers over the wound and Baldwin, one arm suddenly paralysed, could not stop him from turning them both over so that now Peter was on top.

They hung, struggling, half over the parapet and the ten-foot drop below. The parapet was grinding into Baldwin's back and his left arm was useless. Peter, realising this though he didn't understand it, used the edge of his left hand to chop at Baldwin's right arm, momentarily paralysing that, as well. Twisting aside, he tried to shove Baldwin over and Baldwin, shaking life furiously back into his right arm, clutched at Peter and swung his legs up to encircle Peter's calves. For one terrible moment it seemed that they must both go into the river.

Then Nicky let go of Plume and ran to Peter's aid, yanking Baldwin's crossed ankles apart, seizing Peter's feet and dragging him back. Baldwin finally slithered from under his enemy and fell, his heavy body hitting the water with a loud splash while Nicky hauled his father to safety.

"You shouldn't have done that, Nicky!" Peter said, gasping, as he sat down with a thud on the floor of the bridge.

"You could have been killed. I wasn't going to let you be! And he started it! Oh, *Father!*"

Peter got up and looked over the bridge. The river was fairly deep, certainly sufficient to break a fall. It wasn't lethally deep, however, and it was mercifully free of boulders. Baldwin, dripping, had got to his feet. His right hand was clutching at his left arm above the elbow. He stumbled to the bank, but seemed unable to climb it. He stood there, head drooping, thigh-deep in cold peat water. At a run, Peter left the bridge.

"Here." He slithered down the bank, grabbed at Baldwin's right elbow and hauled. Baldwin swore and shouted at him, but Peter merely retorted, "Don't be a bloody fool. What do you take me for?" And as Baldwin was now too shaken and hurt to resist, Peter succeeded in dragging him up to dry land again. Once there, however, his opponent angrily wrenched himself free.

"I'm all *right*. I've got wet, that's all."

"Then go home and get dry!" said Peter, and went himself to fetch Baldwin's horse. By the time he had brought it, Master Sweetwater had pulled himself together. He glared at Peter, face suffused with angry crimson under an interesting array of red bruises from Peter's fists. He snatched Blue Lyn's reins, although Peter noticed that he seemed able to use only his right hand, and tried to mount. He was so awkward, his left arm evidently useless, that Peter gave him a helpful leg up, which produced more curses. Once up, he gathered his reins in his right hand and rode off without ceremony, going back the way he had come, leaving a trail of drops from his wet clothes like a spoor behind him.

Plume had backed himself right off the bridge and into the comforting company of the chestnut. Their owners went together to get them. "I think Master Sweetwater hurt himself, falling," Nicky said.

"It looked like it," Peter agreed as he mounted, somewhat stiffly.

"What about you?" Nicky asked with concern.

"Only bruises and scrapes. He'll have made for home by the straightest track, I suppose. We'd better use a different one! If he's hurt, he might slow down and I don't want to overtake him."

"All right," said Nicky, getting into his saddle.

They took a path they knew would bring them home, although it wasn't straight, since it was a sheep track and meandered a good deal. Plume was still upset, tossing his head and pulling. He cantered ahead until a sharp drop in the ground ahead slowed him down. The path led down into a cup-shaped hollow thickly grown with golden moor grass, with the soft red of fox-gloves here and there.

It was dry and sheltered, a pleasant place, and others clearly thought so too, for it was occupied. A bay horse and a mealy-nosed moor pony, both saddled, were grazing quietly on the farther bank, tethered to the same small bush. Close to them, a man and a woman sat on the grass, side by side. They were not young and they were not making love. His arm was around her and she was leaning back into it as though against a pillow, but it was in a most companionable fashion. They had the air of friends, content to sit together.

Peter halted his pony and looked at them. They saw him and looked back, their eyes widening in shock. They stood up, just as, with a thudding of hooves, Nicky rode up beside his father and halted there.

Peter stared across the dell at the man with whom his wife Liza had been sitting, in that attitude of such hateful intimacy and peace. He turned his head and looked at his son.

His world ended.

CHAPTER THIRTY-FOUR

FALLING APART

So it has happened, Liza thought. She watched Peter as he looked, again and again, from Christopher to Nicky and back, and stared at her husband's face, and knew that the long deception was over. There was no escape now. Without warning, not giving her even a moment in which to prepare, the truth had sprung from the grass to confront them all. She felt the blood drain from her face, knew that her very features had shrivelled.

Nicky and Christopher themselves, as yet, only looked puzzled. Well, how often did Nicky gaze into a mirror? Presumably Christopher, as well, saw his own reflection only rarely. But they, too, were seeing Peter's horror as he glanced between them and understanding had begun to dawn.

Peter felt as though the breath had been punched out of him. The stranger at Liza's side was in middle life, and what was left of his tonsured hair (*tonsured*—dear God, Margaret had said that

Liza had once been in love with a priest of some kind!) was mostly a faded sandy, but there were a few traces of the original colour and they were a blazing red, just like the red of Nicky's hair.

Nor was that everything; far from it. The well-defined eyebrows, the unusual golden-brown eyes were identical. There was something dreadfully familiar about the shape of the man's left hand, which had been curved around Liza's shoulder. Peter's eyes, drawn to the little finger by the silver ring which encircled it, recognised that shape at once. Familiar, too, were the planes of the face, the snub nose, the freckles—faint, as freckles usually were in older people, but there—the strong chin, *and even the cluster of freckles on the chin*. Nicky had them, too. This was Nicky's face, as it would be, half a century hence.

The awful silence had to be broken. Liza, with a dry mouth, took it upon herself to break it. "This…this is…is Master Christopher Clerk," she said. "We met by chance." She heard the defiance, the lie, in her own voice. "We are friends, that's all," she said desperately.

"This is the man you once tried to run away with?" Peter asked coldly. Liza, shivering, put a hand to her mouth to stop herself from uttering a wail. Tears sprang into her eyes.

"You, I take it, are Master Peter Lanyon?" said Christopher.

"Yes. You had your arm round my wife. Not for the first time, I think." There was a silence. Then Peter said, "Nicky was born as soon as was even remotely possible after I came back from Tewkesbury. I suppose you were carrying him already, Liza, my love. You must have been so relieved to see me ride in. In fact, now that I look back, you were."

Christopher had grasped the full situation by now. His wide

eyes were fastened on Nicky's face with an aching intensity. "But…" he said. And then stopped.

"You are a priest," Peter remarked.

"Yes." Christopher recovered himself. "Priests are men, you know."

Before he could stop himself, Peter had remembered Father Bernard and the tales about the parentage of Geoffrey Baker. He passed a hand across his face, and touched the places where Baldwin's fists had landed.

"Peter," said Liza, "what's wrong with your face?"

"It doesn't matter."

Nicky had not been as quick-witted as Christopher. "I don't understand," he said. Peter turned to him. It hurt, far more than the bruises did. He had loved Nicky, for himself as well as because he was an heir for Allerbrook. He had sold his integrity at Bosworth to protect this boy—and on that bridge, not half an hour ago, this son of his had seized his feet and saved him from crashing headfirst into the river. Only, it seemed now that Nicky was no son of his at all. It felt as though something inside him were being slowly dragged apart by oxen pulling in opposite directions.

Sooner than fling himself out of his saddle to hammer his fists on the ground and scream, sooner than abandon all pretence of dignity, he took refuge in extreme formality.

"Nicky," he said politely, "let me introduce you. This is Christopher Clerk, your mother's lover and your natural father. Ride over to him and shake his hand. He is entitled to courtesy from his son."

Once more Christopher opened his mouth and then shut it again, this time without even uttering one syllable.

"Peter," Liza pleaded. "You can't…it isn't Nicky's fault…!"

"I haven't said it is. I have only suggested that Nicky should show respect to his father, as is proper."

"I still don't understand," said Nicky hopelessly.

"Let the boy alone," said Christopher sharply. "If...even if I really did sire him, and I admit that he looks as if I did, you are still his father, sir. You have reared and educated him all these years. He looks like a fine boy and I thank you for your care of him." He looked at Liza. "I'll go now, unless your husband wants to knock me down. He can do so if he wishes. I won't object."

It was an invitation that Peter almost accepted, but the fight with Baldwin, coming so soon after Bosworth, had drained that kind of violence out of him. Besides, the misery of this moment, of the loss, at the same moment, of both wife and son, was too great to be assuaged in such a commonplace and useless manner.

"Just go," he said. "Mount your horse and leave. But tell me first, where is your home?"

"Dunster Castle. I'm the chaplain there."

"And a splendid example of priesthood to all your flock, I feel sure. You will see me there before long. For the time being...just go."

Christopher turned to Liza and held out his hand. "Farewell," he said. "With all my heart, I mean it. Both halves of the word. Fare well."

"And you, you fare well, too," said Liza.

They clasped hands briefly. Peter watched but did not interfere. They let each other go. Christopher picked up a cap which he had put down on the grass beside him, clapped it on his head, went to the bay horse, attended to stirrups and girth, mounted and touched his heels to his horse's sides. With a scramble of hooves the bay climbed out of the dell. A dark tail flicked as he vanished over the top and then horse and rider were gone.

"You had better get on to your pony," said Peter to Liza. "And we'll go home."

"Father, what's happening?" pleaded Nicky. His eyes were wide and frightened but Peter, looking into them, no longer saw the eyes of his son, only those of his rival, the man Liza had loved before she married him, and, it seemed, had never ceased to love, through all the years between.

"I'm not your father," he said sharply. "Haven't I just said so?" The horror mixed with the dawning comprehension in Nicky's face did touch him then, and he spoke more quietly as he added, "Your real father has just ridden out of the dell. You are his living image."

"You are out of your mind, boy!" Richard shouted at Peter. "Beat her and throw her out, the whore!"

"If you call Liza a whore again," said Peter, "I shall punch you on the nose."

He had called her that himself at first. After riding home in stony silence, the three of them had ridden into the yard, where Alfred, who was forking old straw out of the stable, had started to exclaim in welcome. Cutting him short, Peter had dismounted, gestured for Liza and Nicky to do the same, ordered Nicky to help Alfred see to the ponies, seized Liza's arm and hustled her into the hall. Then, throwing her into a window seat so that he could stand over her, he let his rage explode into cursing and accusation.

Liza, staring at him with huge, frightened eyes, said nothing until at last, when the need to breathe had made him pause, she said tremblingly, "I'm making no excuses. I love you, whether you believe it or not—"

"Oh, yes! It's easy to believe, of course!"

"But I loved Christopher before I was married to you and… some things just don't die."

"I wish *I* had died! I wish I had died at Tewkesbury or at Bosworth! Anything so as not to find out what I found out today!"

"We met by chance not long ago and…then we met twice in that hollow, to talk. Only to talk, as friends."

"Friends! You were more than that in the past! Once, at least!"

"Poor Nicky," said Liza, and that was the moment when he came nearest to striking her.

But at that moment he realised that his father had come in, presumably from the fields, since he was in dusty working clothes. He was listening from the doorway. Now Richard, turning crimson, burst into fury as well, hurling terrible invective at Liza, and would certainly have attacked her, except that at that moment, something in her terrified, tearstained face, had a startling effect on Peter.

Ever since being hit on the head at Bosworth, he had had occasional headaches. They were growing fewer, but the force of his emotions now had brought one on and it felt like a jagged crack in his skull, through which an unbearably bright light was pouring. That light seemed to illuminate pictures inside his brain. They were pictures of Liza, his Liza: Liza in his arms, Liza weaving, cooking, tossing hay, laughing, crying, nursing babies; Liza young, Liza growing older and broader around the middle…*Liza*. Part of his life, which was unimaginable without her. And she wasn't a whore. She was *not*. It made no sense. The word didn't fit Liza, not *Liza*.

As Richard strode forward, his right hand upraised, Peter seized his father's arm. "Liza! Go to a spare bedchamber and bolt yourself in! Go! *Quickly!*" Liza slid from her seat and fled to the stairs, and as she did so, he saw Quentin staring, horrified, in the kitchen doorway. "Quentin, go and look after your mother. Take food to her and whatever else she needs!"

Then he dropped Richard's arm and went out, passing a scared-looking Nicky, who was just coming in, without even glancing at him. He went up to his own bedchamber and lay on the bed and although he was a grown man in middle age, he cried.

It went on, the misery and wretchedness, for three interminable days. The loss of Jarvis, over which everyone grieved, made the misery worse. Peter spent one whole day with the Hannacombes, talking about him and condoling with them. Otherwise, he worked on the farm but took meals alone in his room, making Betsy and Ellen, who by now knew all about it, bring food to him there. He avoided the children, though he sometimes saw Quentin looking at him anxiously. Glimpses of Nicky's white, closed face appalled him, because he didn't know what to do about it. He turned away.

He tried to avoid his father as well, but couldn't do so entirely and whenever they met, Richard would break into another stream of fury against Liza, demanding that Peter throw the whore out of the house.

Now, as the third day neared evening, Richard, coming face-to-face with him in the hall, had attacked once more, striding about, storming and threatening, his face scarlet and an engorged vein pulsing in his temple.

And now, to his own surprise, Peter found that the fury inside him was directed more at Richard than at Liza. All his life he had lived in his father's shadow, obeyed him, allowed himself to be addressed as *boy*. Now Richard was trying to tell him how to deal with his own wife, and that was enough. That was private territory.

"If you call Liza a whore again, I shall punch you on the nose."

"You dare to threaten me for telling the truth?" Richard bellowed at him.

"Yes. You call her a whore, but what was Deborah Archer? You remember Deb?"

"Of course I remember Deb! My poor Deb that the Sweetwaters as good as murdered! She was a widow! Her husbands, both of them, were in their graves. That's different! I won't have that woman here for one more night! I won't…!"

"Liza isn't a whore," said Peter. "I called her that at first but I know it isn't true. All these years! So many years. I can't throw them away."

"Send her home! I keep telling you! Send her back to Dunster!"

Peter said, "Do you remember Marion Locke?"

He hoped the name might induce his father to pause for a moment. He didn't expect it to bring Richard's outraged pacings to a complete, frozen halt. "Yes, I do! A fisher girl you had a fling with, in Lynmouth! She ran off with someone else!"

It was hard for Richard to get the words out. He had never broken free of Marion's haunting memory and now, forced to speak of her—worse, to lie about her—he saw her again in his mind and heard her, as she fell backward into the mist….

Only with an effort could Richard keep from raising his hands to grip his temples, to crush her memory out of his head by force.

"I was mad for her," Peter said, "and even after she'd gone…I still didn't want to marry Liza. Only, I had to marry someone and so I agreed to it, and did my best. But maybe…I can… *just*…imagine what it was like for her, since she, too… If I were to meet Marion again, even now…"

He had never spoken of it, but three years after his marriage to Liza he had made an excuse to be out on the moor all day, had gone to Lynmouth and asked if the *Fjord-Elk* was expected to dock there any time soon. Someone directed him to a harbourside tavern where men from another Norwegian ship were drinking, though the ship was not the *Fjord-Elk*. "They might know something about her. She's not been here of late."

And one of the Norwegian sailors had known something. The *Fjord-Elk* had been lost at sea, with all hands, just two years before. If Marion had gone away on her, she was probably in Norway, maybe as a widow, maybe married to a second husband, maybe not married at all but making a living as a whore. He had tried not to think of her again, but had never been able to keep the resolution for long at a time.

"It's different for women!" Richard shouted. "And there's Nicky to tell you why! Most people know who their mother is, but if women aren't honest, how can men be sure their children are their own? Get rid of her!"

"If Mother goes to Dunster, or anywhere else, I go with her." Quentin had joined them. Peter looked at her, thinking that she at least was an unmistakable Lanyon. The beechnut hair and the apple-blossom skin were Liza's but the dark eyes, the shape of the face were entirely his own. He saw, too, that she had left childhood behind. She was a young woman now, eighteen years old, and she was courageous.

"She lies on the bed in that room all day, sobbing," Quentin said. "Grandfather, I don't believe she's any of the horrible things you've called her, but that doesn't matter, not to me. She's still my mother and if no one else will help her, I will."

"You can't leave unless your father and I say so!" shouted Richard.

"You can't chain me up forever," said Quentin reasonably. "And if Mother and I are both gone, who'll see to the accounts?" She looked at Peter. "Oh, *Father!* Are things never to come right again?"

Her voice had always had a calming quality. The crimson faded somewhat from Richard's face. Awkwardly Peter said, "Quentin, I'm sorry. I hate seeing you distressed." He turned to Richard. "For years and years Liza and I have dwelt in peace together, even though we were not each other's first loves. I wish her to stay. I want to mend the breach…."

Quentin's soothing tones could achieve only so much. Richard lost his temper again. "I repeat, you're out of your mind! Look how she's deceived us all! Going for walks on the moor! We thought they were harmless. I wonder how many times she's *really* met this red-haired lover of hers? I wonder how many others there've been besides him!"

"There have been *no* others! Of that I'm sure."

"Oh, are you indeed?"

"Yes, I am! I *know* Liza. As for the red–haired lover, I intend to visit Dunster Castle and see that Christopher Clerk leaves the west country and never returns. I also intend to keep my wife, and I would remind you, Father, that Liza is *my* wife and not yours. It's for me to say."

"Very well," said Richard grimly, quietening down once more but this time becoming, in the process, somehow more menacing, more alarming than ever. "But I'll tell you one thing, boy. If I have to tolerate that woman here, there's one thing I *won't* stand for. Try making me and you'll regret it. Listen to me!"

"It's not right. None of this is Nicky's fault. Please, Father, please, please think again," Quentin implored him, but Peter, accosted as he sat at the study table, only shook his head and sanded the new will he was preparing.

"No, my dear. Nicky is not my son or my father's grandson and he can't inherit the Lanyon property. There, sadly, my father is right and he had no need to threaten to disinherit me as well if I argued. Allerbrook and all the rest of our property will be for you instead. You'll be an heiress!"

"I don't want to be an heiress! I'll…I'll…give it away to Nicky when the time comes. I will!" said Quentin passionately.

"You'll be married by then, I trust," Peter said, "and your husband won't let you, not if he has any common sense."

"But Nicky! What will he do? How will he live, where will he go? It's *Nicky,* Father! *Nicky!*"

"I know. Quentin, my dear girl, I'm not going to abandon him just like that. I shall ask him what he wants to do with his life and help him as far as I can. I know I must do that."

His head was aching again. He found it intolerable to be in Nicky's presence. Every time he looked at the lad, he seemed to see him double—the Nicky he had always known as his son, with an interloping stranger weirdly superimposed on top. But Nicky had followed him to war, and on that packhorse bridge Nicky had saved him from, at the least, a disagreeable accident. And if he had thought of Nicky as a son all these years, Nicky had regarded him as a father. None of these things could be thrown onto the midden. They were reality.

"He can't be the Lanyon heir, but he won't be flung out to starve, Quentin, my dear. I will explain to him. Don't tell him yourself. Leave it to me and to my father. But now I have to go to Dunster. I have one last item of business to deal with."

★ ★ ★

"I have been expecting you," said Christopher, showing Peter into his room at the castle. It was no more than a small stone cell with the plainest of furnishings and coarsely woven blankets on the narrow bed. The only touches of luxury were a prie-dieu with a very beautiful silver crucifix above it, and two or three books on a shelf. By the look of them, they were printed, Peter thought. Father Matthew had a printed Latin Bible in the church at Clicket and Peter had handled it sometimes. A man called Caxton had brought the art of printing to England, Father Matthew said. Printed books were precious.

Christopher offered him a stool, but Peter remained standing. He was studying his rival, wondering what it was in this unremarkable tonsured individual that had so enchanted Liza. Even as a young man, he hadn't been that handsome, surely. Well, Nicky wasn't going to be particularly handsome and Nicky was a good enough comparison. Too good. Practically identical! "Do you know why I've come?" Peter said.

"To make sure I'm thrown out of Dunster Castle, I daresay. Well, rumour says that Lady Luttrell is to return soon and she may not want me here in any case. I daresay she hasn't forgotten the trouble I caused once long ago. I was already making plans to leave. Believe me, I have no wish to disturb Liza's life, or yours, any more than I already have."

"You can hardly outdo the disturbance of finding that I've been saddled with another man's son!"

"I had no idea," Christopher said. "None at all. Liza never told me, never sent me word. She just…did her best, I expect, for you and for the child. What else was she to do?"

"She's no concern of yours now. When do you intend to go? And where?"

"I leave tomorrow. I have already informed the bishop's office that I wish to give up this chaplaincy and seek a new position somewhere in northern England. I told part of the truth. It is on record that as a deacon I behaved in a most unfortunate way and I said that by chance, the woman concerned had crossed my path again and I thought it best to put a distance between us."

"And that was accepted?"

"Yes. I spoke to the bishop's deputy, as a matter of fact. This is the diocese of Bath and Wells, and the bishop's Robert Stillington, the man who stood up in council just after King Edward died and said he was sorry to upset everyone just as they were planning to crown the young Prince Edward, but young Prince Edward wasn't legitimate. He almost put Gloucester on the throne himself! He's now in London, attending King Henry's council and no doubt earnestly promising his utter devotion to the Lancastrian dynasty."

"And has bigger fish on his line than your bygone sins anyhow? I take it," said Peter, "that you have never confessed what must have happened fourteen years ago!"

"No. I prefer to trust in the understanding of God rather than men for what I did, the day I started Nicky on his way into the world. I know his name," said Christopher quietly, "because you more or less introduced us, the day we all met. Liza and I…we came together only that once, by the way. Liza was in distress. There had been deaths—a man called Higg, and also some of her relatives…"

"I don't want to hear. Don't tell me. It's as well you're leaving," said Peter. "If you'd tried to stay, I would have gone to your bishop myself and told him what you've done. Even if I had to go to London to find him. I'd have made him listen!"

"You need not worry. I'll be away from here tomorrow and I go of my own free will. I am sorry, Master Lanyon, for the hurt I have dealt you. I shall never see Liza again, though I shall remember her in my prayers."

"I would rather you didn't."

"Master Lanyon, *please*…if you can forgive her, do so. She's worth forgiving."

"That I know. You may leave her with me in safety."

"And Nicky?"

"Just pack your belongings and go away from here and save your soul. Nicky isn't your concern any more than Liza is. Good day."

Liza, hearing Peter's voice outside her door, hesitated before unbolting it, but after all, the moment had to come. She could not stay here forever. Already she had stopped crying, because even tears ran out in the end. She had lain, unwashed and weeping, for days on end, only nibbling at the food that Quentin brought her, but sooner or later something would have to change, sooner or later this dreadful catastrophe must be resolved in some fashion, though she couldn't imagine what. Peter's request for admittance was the signal that the time of change had arrived.

She was afraid of him, though, and as he came into the room, he looked bigger and darker than she had ever known him and his face was hard as she had never seen it before. She quailed. Peter, studying her, saw the fear in her eyes. He didn't like to see it. She was still Liza.

Quietly he said, "It's time to come out, Liza. We can't go on like this for the rest of our lives."

"But what is to happen?" Liza was so frightened that she had to push the words out as though they were swimming against a tide. "Your father wants me to go back to Dunster, I know. I've heard him shouting it! But my family might not take me in. I suppose I shall have to go to the nuns at St. Catherine's, as my mother did."

The thought was intolerable. At the time of her marriage she wouldn't have believed it, but Allerbrook, now, was home. It was *home*. To be cast out of one's home was one of the most bitter things in the world. How had her mother been able just to abandon hers?

"Do you want to leave?" Peter asked.

"No! Of course not! Oh, if only it hadn't happened! We… Christopher and me…we'd only met to talk, as friends. That was all. There was just that one time, years and years ago…"

"Maybe it was just once and maybe not…."

"It *was!*"

"He's going away. He'd decided to do that even before I turned up at Dunster Castle and told him to leave Somerset or I'd make him."

"Make him? How?"

"I meant to use the threat of reporting him to his bishop. Though as the bishop's attending the royal council just now, I'd have had to chase him to London. But there's no need. Your Christopher is leaving Dunster and going to the north. He's out of your life, and that's the end of it. As for us, Liza, stay here if you want to. We've had many good years together and I don't want everything falling apart, no, I don't."

"What does your father say to that?"

"My father," said Peter sharply, "will accept what I decide. This time it's my business, not his, and I will be a man and not a boy."

"Yes. I see." A faint hope had awakened in her. Peter's face was still strange to her, though—expressionless, remote. She was still afraid. "But...Nicky?" she ventured.

"Nicky's home is here and I will help him to...to find a calling to suit him. I have loved Nicky. I still do, in a way. But he can't inherit Allerbrook or any other Lanyon property, not now."

"Are you revenging yourself on me through Nicky?" Liza asked miserably.

"No. It isn't revenge. It's simply that...he is not a Lanyon. Is he?"

"He has lived all his life as a Lanyon. He must feel like one," said Liza. "Have you told him? Does he know?"

"Not yet. Father and I are going to a lawyer in Dulverton tomorrow to make sure that our new wills are properly worded and sign them with witnesses. There must be no mistakes. Once that's done, I'll tell him. And now..." He stood up, holding out his hand to her. "Come. There's work to do. There always is, on a farm."

"All right," said Walter Sweetwater to the physician he had fetched, personally, from Dulverton. "I can see by your face what you think. I suppose I already know it."

"He's under forty and he's strong. There is hope. But..." The physician, himself an ageing man with a straggly white beard and legs which felt stiff after riding ten miles over the moor, at speed, with Walter Sweetwater urging him on all the way, let the sentence die away, unfinished.

"He only took a chill after falling into a stream," said Walter, almost pleadingly. "He told me he had been thrown from his horse, but I could see he had been in a fight. His face was marked as only fists could mark it. In the end he admitted it. But he's had fights and fallen into streams before."

"Not when his body was still full of bad humours from a battle wound," said the physician. "And the wound has worsened since the fight, as your daughter-in-law says." He looked back toward the door of Baldwin's bedchamber, which was half open. Catherine was there, sitting at the bedside. They were speaking quietly so that she wouldn't overhear, but there was no need to worry about Baldwin overhearing. He was asleep, breathing harshly through a chest which sounded as though it were full of liquid.

"The wound probably opened again during the fight," Walter said.

"I daresay. A chill on top of that, from riding home in wet clothes, perhaps some impurity in the water of the stream—as a physician I have seen such things before. I have told Mistress Sweetwater how to make my special draught for fighting fever. But…"

Again, the sentence died away.

"He is the best of sons," said Walter bitterly. "But always a hothead. When I got him to tell the truth, well, the fight he was in—he started it. It was on a narrow bridge. Another man, someone he doesn't like, was halfway across, coming the other way, and instead of waiting for him my son ordered him to go back. It would have meant backing the pony a long way. The other man was entitled to refuse, and he did and Baldwin insisted on fighting him for right of way and tried to throw him over into the water. But in the struggle it was Baldwin who went over."

"Yes, I see. And with that wound still giving trouble…well, keep him warm and try to induce a sweat. There is poison in his blood, a black and evil earth humour, but sweat may bring it out. Though…"

"I know," said Walter. "Send for a priest. My grandson has already gone to get Father Matthew."

When the physician had left, Walter went back to Baldwin. Catherine looked around. Her kitten face was very pale. "It was such a foolish thing. An argument about precedence on a silly bridge!" She let out a sudden sob, as much of anger as distress. "What a stupid thing to die for!"

"He may not die. He's strong," said Walter, but there was little hope in his voice. "I dislike the Lanyons so much," he said, "that once I'd have been in sympathy with Baldwin simply because of that, but now—I'm getting old, my dear. It is a stupid thing and it's his own fault. I know."

Nicky sat in his window seat, as he had done the night he ran away to follow the man he thought was his father to Bosworth. He was waiting for the house to sink into slumber. He had laid his plans more carefully this time, as he now knew that when he ran off on that occasion, his mother had heard the harness-room door close. Sunset's bridle and saddle were already hidden under a bush in a corner of the ponies' paddock. No one would hear anything this time, indeed they wouldn't. He was taking Sunset, not the chestnut pony Ned Crowham had lent him. Peter, who had never forgiven Ned for forcing him to change sides, had not returned the chestnut to the Crowham manor house but had sold it and given Nicky the money. Nicky therefore had funds and he was taking those as well.

He had made a fool of himself, of course; thrown away his dignity. He shouldn't have screamed and raged like that when his father…no, Master Peter Lanyon…chose to honour a Sunday morning by telling him that he was no longer the heir to Aller-brook. The news had taken him by surprise. In fact, he had never really thought about being grown-up and living on after his father and grandfather were gone, and inheriting all that they had owned, except for a dowry for Quentin.

But once it was explained, then he knew how much he cared for Allerbrook and how much he felt that he belonged here. It was cruel to do this to him, cruel to blame him for what his mother had done. He had said that, shrieked it almost, flung himself at Father—no, Master Lanyon—tried to cling to him, tried to *make* things go back to where they were, when this man was truly his father and he was the son of the house and...

Master Lanyon had detached his grasping hands, not roughly, but firmly. He had said something about helping Nicky to find another future life, even made suggestions about it. Would Nicky like to learn to weave properly, or be apprenticed to Herbert Dyer, or to a merchant? Nicky, sickened and furious, had turned away and run crying out of the room.

No, not dignified. He was old enough to behave better. His world had fallen apart, but he shouldn't have fallen to pieces himself. At his age, he knew, the dead king, Richard III, had had a man's work to do, raising arms for his brother. It was time for Nicky, too, to become a man. He would need help, and yes, he would have to find a new future, but the Lanyons would have nothing to do with it.

His real father couldn't help him. He was a priest and he'd gone to the north of England, so his mother had said. But Nicky still had a real family, after all—his mother's folk in Dunster. He didn't understand how his mother could have broken her marriage vows, but she was still his mother; the affection she had given him all through the years was still a warmth in his memory, which was more than could be said for his grandfather's harshness. And after all, whatever else she had done, she had given him life.

That much he did understand. Working it out, painfully, through sleepless nights, he had recognised that he was glad to be alive and could hardly, therefore, turn in fury on those responsible for his existence. That would be unjust, and he knew injustice when he saw it. Grandfa—Richard Lanyon—had demonstrated it for him, all too plainly.

The house was silent now. Father Matthew had made sure that he could read and write competently and he had penned a letter in which he explained why he was going and where. He laid it on his bed and weighed it down with an empty candlestick. He picked up his cloak and a bundle of belongings he had made ready, and tiptoed to the door. Letting himself out, he made his way noiselessly down the stairs, into the hall, and unbolted the outer door. The dogs in the kitchen sensed him and he heard them stir, but they knew his smell and didn't bark.

Like a shadow he slipped away from the house and into the pony paddock. There had been some rain during the day, but the tack he had left under the bush had been protected and was dry. Sunset greeted him with a snort but came to hand willingly enough. Nicky saddled him and mounted. The sky was clear, as it had been the first time he ran away, and once again there was a moon, though only half of one. But it was enough.

He turned his back on home, and rode away.

CHAPTER THIRTY-FIVE

A SENSE OF ABSENCE

Tommy Weaver was an early riser. On this shining late September morning, which had a faint smell of frost in the air, he was out of bed at first light and hurrying downstairs in dressing robe and slippers to heat some shaving water, while Susannah still slept. Having roused the fire and set the water pot on the trivet, he said good-morning to the maidservants who by then were coming downstairs, too, and went to unbolt the front door.

Sitting on the doorstep, a riding cloak huddled around him against the early chill, was his nephew, Nicky Lanyon from Allerbrook.

"*Nicky!* What on earth…?"

Nicky stood up, shivering. "Can I come in, Uncle Tommy?"

"Of course." Tommy stood back. "But what are you doing here—when did you come? And why? What's happened?"

"I've run away," said Nicky, stepping into the main room as

Tommy closed the door after them. "No, that's wrong." He turned to face his uncle and Tommy saw that he was at the stage of growth when a boy's body begins to elongate, to stretch toward manhood, and the contours of his face begin to settle. He had always thought of Nicky as Liza's little boy, but this youth had ridden with an army and been held prisoner. His boyhood had been left behind at Bosworth. "I didn't run away," said Nicky. "I chose to leave, and it's not the same thing. But I need shelter somewhere and time to think, so I came here, to my mother's family. Will you let me stay, until I can decide what to do next?"

"Of course we'll let you stay, but why did you run…leave home? What's amiss there?"

There was a silence. Then Nicky said, "It'll upset you, Uncle Tommy, if I tell it all. Maybe I'd better not. I was the son of the house and should have inherited Allerbrook and all that goes with it, but I've been cut out of Master Lanyon's will. But it's not my fault. I've done nothing wrong, I promise. Please can we let it go at that?"

"No, we can't—don't talk nonsense!" Tommy barked. "Now, look here…oh, for the love of heaven, look at you, you're frozen. Sit down. *Sit,* I said. Don't stand in the middle of the floor like a tombstone in a churchyard! Wait." He strode through the door to the kitchen and after a few moments reappeared with a tankard of ale, a chunk of bread, a knife and a pot of honey on a tray, while behind him a maidservant ran up the stairs, calling Susannah's name.

"They're frying some bacon. They'll bring it in a minute." He pushed Nicky into a settle and pulled a table within his reach. "Get some food inside you. My wife'll be down in a minute and

I'm going to fetch Cousin Laurence. Whatever it is you're scared of saying is a boil that needs lancing. I can see that, if you can't. He'll help."

Leaving Nicky to his breakfast, he went across the road at a run, still in his robe and slippers, to pound on the door of the opposite house. He returned once more within a very short time, with both Laurence and Elena. They, too, were early risers and he had found them up and dressed, though Elena's grey hair was only roughly combed and she hadn't put her coif on, and both of them were startled and bewildered by what he had to tell them.

Susannah, also bareheaded, though she had pulled on a gown and overgown, was with Nicky when they arrived, talking to him while he ate. The bacon had been brought and he was obviously ravenous. He rose to greet his cousins, but Laurence told him to sit down again and finish eating.

"Then tell us what's brought you here. It must have been something serious to bring you riding through the night."

With Laurence's arrival, family authority had come into the room. Tommy looked at him gratefully and even Nicky seemed steadied by his elder cousin's presence, though when he had gulped his final mouthful, his first words were, "I can't explain properly. None of it makes sense. I can't stay at Allerbrook and I don't know what to do. I don't want to *say* things."

"I think there are things you will have to say," said Laurence calmly. "For one thing, Tommy says your father has disinherited you but it isn't your fault. Whose fault is it, then?"

"Nicky," said Susannah, "if you've done something to make your father angry, or he thinks you have…well, whatever it was, try to tell us about it. Please. Has it been a…a mistake? I can't believe you've done anything as dreadful as all that."

"I didn't do *anything*. It wasn't like that." The food had made him feel warmer, but the presence all around him of his elders, though reassuring in one way, was also thrusting him back toward his childhood. He had begun to feel like a little boy again, and worse than that, a little boy close to tears. The night ride had been not only cold, but frightening.

He hadn't felt like that the night he ran off to join his father on the way to war, because then he had ridden across open moorland, in bright moonlight. This time the moon was waning and rose late, and the last part of the ride had in any case been through the woods above the village of Timberscombe, farther up the Avill Valley than Dunster was.

No moonlight came through the dark trees that met above his head and although he kept telling himself not to be afraid, that there was nothing to fear, every gruesome tale he had heard in his childhood came back to him. On dark nights, ghosts and witches and demons might be abroad. Anything might be lurking in the shadows to either side. He had felt sick with the long-drawn-out dread by the time he came at last across the packhorse bridge and into the safety of the sleeping village. And after that, after turning the pony into the Weavers' paddock and leaving the tack in the shelter they had built there for the animals, and walking back to their house, he had had to sit on the cold doorstep for what seemed like an eternity.

"I'm sorry," he said. "I'm tired. I rode nearly all night. The pony's in your field, Uncle Tommy. It was still night and I didn't want to wake anyone up, so I sat on the step till morning."

"*Nicky!*" said Tommy protestingly.

"Is it a girl? Have you got a girl with child, even at your age?" asked Laurence.

"Oh, surely not!" Elena put a hand over her mouth.

"No, I haven't!"

"Nicky," Laurence said, "you must tell us! Someone else in your family will if you don't. One of us will ride out there and ask!"

Nicky gave in. "Father…Master Lanyon…says I'm not his son and Mother's been shut up in one of our spare rooms, crying all the time. Quentin took food to her. She's come out now, but she walks about like a ghost, not speaking. Not even to me, though when she sees me, she starts to cry again. And hardly anyone ever speaks to her. Master Lanyon says my real father's someone called Christopher Clerk—"

"Christopher Clerk?" said Laurence. "Him!"

"Yes. Coming home from the war, we came on him and Mother together, sitting in a hollow on the moor, and I look just like him and so I'm not a Lanyon and I can't inherit Allerbrook and…I don't want people to know about my mother. I didn't want to tell you!"

"Oh, dear God!" said Tommy.

Susannah, practical and acute, said, "You can rely on us for one thing. We'll keep your secret. Now that we know what really happened. Won't we?" She looked appealingly at the others, who nodded.

"We'll never tell anyone," said Laurence. "You came here because you weren't happy at Allerbrook. We'll say that. Your grandfather's a hard man. Anyone who's met him knows it. Don't worry."

That same night, in the candlelit sickroom at Sweetwater House, Walter and Catherine tried to quieten Baldwin as he tossed and struggled to breathe, and then saw him lapse into silence and coma and the harsh rattle of approaching death. In the unsteady light Walter's eyes met Catherine's across the bed. "I think I should wake John."

Catherine picked up Baldwin's hand and then the tears began to run, silently, down her face. "There's no life in his hand," she said. "He can't feel me. Baldwin, I'm here. Can you hear me? It's your Kitten!"

Walter left the room, but met John just outside the door, out of his own bed already, a cloak thrown around him. "I just woke and felt as if…"

"Yes. He's going, I think. Come in."

Others followed him, wakened, it seemed, by the same instinct which had roused John: the steward Denis Sawyer, Catherine's maid, Amy. They gathered at the bedside. After a time, the painful breathing grew very faint and there came a gap so long that for a moment they thought it had stopped. Then came another gasp for air and Catherine thought wildly, "I'm still married. I'm still Baldwin's wife. My husband is still alive."

Baldwin, loud, arrogant Baldwin, had not always been an easy man to live with, but he had never ill-used her. They had lived their parallel lives, meeting at board and bed and on social occasions; otherwise keeping to their own worlds. Baldwin had his horses, his hawks, his hounds and his weapons; Catherine oversaw the household, plied her needle and tended her herb garden. She had been restful; he had been protective. It had worked.

The worst criticism he had ever made of her was when he remarked once or twice that it was unlucky that she had had a difficult time bearing John and never thereafter conceived again. Even then, he qualified it, every time, by adding that John was healthy; no one could say she hadn't done her duty and provided an heir. She had been content as his wife.

Some minutes later, she knew that she had become a widow.

"Well, he can't stop here," said Aunt Cecy flatly, sitting very upright despite her eighty-two years and behaving as though she were in charge of this family conclave in the big room at the Weavers' house. "It b'ain't decent."

"It's not for you to say!" snapped Laurence. "If it's for anyone, it's for Tommy and me. None of this is the boy's fault. He's Liza's son and there's no doubt about that!"

"Yes, and what's Liza? A strumpet! She tried to run off with that man when she was a girl and now it seems she's had him after all, and Nicky's the result. Bad blood will out, my boy!"

"Since I'm over seventy, I'm not going to be called a boy by you or anyone else," said Laurence, turning red as he always did when he was angry. "Nicky's a boy, though, poor lad, and he's brave in his way and he's Liza's son, no matter who fathered him. Tommy, what do you say?"

"I agree. I don't want to see Liza ever again, but Nicky himself is a different matter. Susannah agrees—don't you, Susannah? And what about you, Cousin Elena?"

"Nicky's not to blame, but I'd rather not see Liza again either," said Susannah. "She might be bad company for our Joanna."

"I've always felt a bit sorry for Liza," Elena remarked. "Seems to me that maybe she and Christopher Clerk really loved each other. He might have found a way to free himself from the church or else, well, there's many a priest has a comely house-keeper, or an arrangement with a woman somewhere, and many a priest that has nieces or nephews, so-called, and everyone knows they're really his, but no one comments. Maybe we should have let her go."

"Never!" said Tommy, outraged. "This is a respectable family. We'd never tolerate such a thing. We gave her a decent marriage to a decent man and she should have been grateful."

"And once you're wed, you're wed," said Aunt Cecy. "Tommy's right. What's she got to complain of, I'd like to know? Living in a fine house now, b'ain't she, highly respected and all the rest of it? Yet she goes and behaves like this! I call her a strumpet and I don't want that boy of hers here. Besides, what use is he? *He'll* never be any good on a loom."

"That," remarked Laurence's son Joss, who was among the most gifted weavers in the family, "is true enough. Put Nicky in front of a loom and...well..."

They all nodded and, in some cases, sighed. The mayhem that Nicky could wreak on even the simplest piece of weaving suggested not so much ineptitude as some kind of perverse imagination.

"No, he'll never make a weaver," said Laurence. "But he's old enough to be apprenticed to a trade. We just have to find one where he won't cause muddle and confusion. Where is he now?"

"At the field, looking at his pony," said Elena.

"He's an active lad," said Tommy. "There's a merchant I know in Lynmouth—he takes cheeses and iron and leather goods abroad and imports things like silk and brocade and foreign wines and dyestuffs. Brings in dyes for Herbert Dyer—that's how I met him. Once when I was in Lynmouth I went into an alehouse, and there they were. If he's willing to take on an extra apprentice, that might suit Nicky."

"What's his name?" Laurence asked.

"Owen ap Idwal. He's a Welshman, but he married a

Lynmouth girl and settled there so as she could be near her kin. He sails with his ship sometimes, does his own selling and buying. Nicky might get a chance to travel and I somehow fancy he'd like that."

"He's got to be settled somewhere," Susannah said. "He mustn't be turned out to wander. But I think it's best if he doesn't stay here."

"It would be encouraging wantonness, to take him in," said Cecy stiffly. "But find him an apprenticeship, by all means. And there's no need to ask him what he wants. He ought to be glad of anything."

Several members of the Weaver tribe exchanged secret glances. Aunt Cecy would never grasp that she wasn't the head of the household. They had learned to see the comic side of it.

To have Blue Lyn saddled and take him out for exercise was all that Walter Sweetwater could now do for Baldwin. The house was full of weeping, but there was a dreadful sense of absence, too. Baldwin's hectoring voice was so very much not there; far more so than if he were merely hunting or hawking or even gone to a war.

It always seemed unnatural for a child to go before a parent, though it was common enough. Agnes and Baldwin had not been the only children that Mary had borne him. There had been two other little boys, both dead of childhood illnesses before their fourth birthdays. Baldwin, though, had thrived, had lived to manhood, married and had a son, had ridden to battle and come back alive. He shouldn't have died of a mere chill and a wound that ought to have healed—was healing, until he got into the fight, which reopened the wound, and fell into the river, which gave him the chill.

Now he was being washed and laid out by the womenfolk and his father couldn't bear to stay indoors and Blue Lyn was fretting in his stall. Baldwin would have wanted someone to exercise him.

The horse, sidling and restless, needed a good gallop on the moors to take the itch out of his hooves, but to begin with, Walter guided him toward the fields of the home farm to the west of Clicket, a little patchwork of meadow and barley fields like a patterned coverlet, lying smoothly over a couple of low hills and stroked by some gigantic hand down into the deep crease between them.

Walter was making for the meadow where his sheep, which had been brought off the moor for the winter, were now grazing. The flock would have to be moved in a day or two. Edward Searle had told him that sheep should never stay on the same pasture long enough to hear the Sunday church bells ring twice. The pasture would grow rank with their droppings if they did. Out on the moor, they usually moved themselves.

"Folk think they'm foolish things, sheep," Searle had said, "but that's just because they're creatures of the flock and like to be together. It looks as if they just do what the sheep alongside is doing, and can't think for themselves, but you'd be surprised, once you get to know 'un. It's a wonder to me, just as much now as it ever was, that when I've had to separate lambs from their mothers awhile, as we do at shearing, and then turn the little ones back into the flock again, the way lambs and dams know each other. To us, the ewes all look alike and the lambs all look alike, and sound alike, too, but *they* know. It's a marvel, that's what it is."

Edward Searle had understood and loved his woolly charges and in the end had died among them. His heart had stopped when he was out in a meadow with them, wanting to look at a ewe that he said seemed sickly. His son Toby had found him, just lying there in the grass, quite quiet and peaceful. Toby was a skilled shepherd, too, not quite as tall and impressive as his father, but shaped in a similar mould all the same and devoted to his work, and his eldest son Edmund, who was grown up now and worked with his father, followed the same pattern.

It had been something of a joke with Baldwin that when Toby married, the bride he brought home from nearby Withypool had pale curly hair, a bleating little voice and yellow-brown eyes very much like those of a sheep. Baldwin had said things. Baldwin had a broad, not to say crude, sense of humour....

And now Baldwin's father, trotting Blue Lyn along the path beside the sheep meadow, found his eyes stinging. He would have sold his soul at that moment to hear Baldwin laughing in his loud way at one of his own rude jokes.

What roused him from his sorrow was actually the sound of noisily bleating sheep, and as he came in sight of their meadow he saw what had happened. There was a bramble bush at the far end of it, and one of the ewes had got her fleece caught in the thorns. The rest were gathered around her in an anxious semicircle, bleating in sympathy. Spurring Blue Lyn to a canter, he hurried to the gate, pulled up and dismounted. Tying his horse's reins to the gatepost, he went in and made for the scene of disaster.

Which really was a disaster. He had seen it happen before. Sheep clearly did have sense and feeling enough to be concerned if one of the flock was in trouble, but why in the world they didn't have sense enough not to try conclusions with bramble bushes in the first place, he could never understand. Edward Searle had overestimated their intelligence in some ways. There were some ripe blackberries on the bush and the ewe had probably tried to get at them, but didn't these creatures *know* they had fleecy coats that caught on thorns?

He was wearing gloves, since the day, though clear, was not especially warm, but they weren't very thick. This, thought Walter as he began an attempt at rescue, was going to be difficult. It would have helped if the ewe had cooperated, but she was already frightened and when he took hold of her, she began to struggle, entangling herself more thoroughly than ever and kicking him hard on the knee. The oaths he let out did nothing to calm her. He tried to get a prickly branch out of the wool on her shoulder and as he had feared, the thorns went straight through his glove and drew blood, causing him to swear again.

"Need help?" enquired a voice from beyond the hedgerow that separated the pasture from the lane. Walter, still half-crouched in order to hold on to the ewe, glanced around but could see only a brown woollen cap and part of a forehead above the bushes.

"I'd be glad of it!" he called, and heard whoever it was encourage his horse into a canter, going along to the gate. A moment later the newcomer was running back through the field to join him and another pair of hands, not gloved but strong and leathery from outdoor work, were there beside his, bravely tackling the brambles. "If you'll hold her still, sir, I think I can get this branch loose…."

"Here." Belatedly, Walter remembered that as usual, he was carrying a dagger. He pulled it out. "Cut the fleece free where it's caught the worst. Keep still, you damned stupid animal! I think she thinks I've come to turn her into cutlets. So I will, my girl, if you kick me again!"

The other sheep had drawn off to a little distance but were still watching, from time to time emitting anxious baas. Walter, who now had both hands free for the task, gripped the ewe so that she could no longer struggle while his unexpected helper eased some of the prickly stems away and sliced through the fleece where there seemed no chance of disentanglement.

At last they both stepped back, to let the freed ewe bound past them and rejoin her friends, who greeted her with a different note in their bleating, of welcome and relief, before they all flowed away in a woolly stream, which slowed down as it got out into the field, spread apart and stopped to graze.

"My thanks." Walter turned to look at his companion, whom he now recognised. "Good God! Peter Lanyon! What brought you past here?"

"I was up on the moor, looking at our pony herd, and I came back this way, meaning to take a tankard in the Hart before I went home. Er…Master Sweetwater, my farmhand Alfred was in Clicket early this morning." Peter spoke cautiously. "He went to see Father Matthew. He's to marry soon. Father Matthew told him about your son and when he came back, he told me. I am very sorry for your loss. Please believe me."

"Baldwin said it was you he fought and you who shoved him over the bridge into the water."

"Yes." The monosyllable was quiet but not apologetic. "Do you know exactly what happened on that bridge, Master Sweetwater?"

"I know what Baldwin told me." Walter's eyes were like dull pewter.

"And what, exactly, was that?"

"He challenged your right of way. He admitted that it *was* your right of way. But if only you'd backed your pony as he asked!"

"He didn't ask. He ordered. I was nearly across that bridge. When I wouldn't back, he challenged me to fight and I took the challenge. Would you have backed, Master Sweetwater?"

Walter stared at him, shoulders tense with dislike, and then let them sag. "No. I would not. I can't like you, Peter Lanyon, though I must thank you for your help just now, but I am not a dishonest man. It's true. In your place, I suppose I would have done as you did."

"It ended with Baldwin going over the parapet into the river, but only because he tried to push me over first. I fought back, but I was only saved because my...my boy Nicky was there and ran to me and caught hold of my feet." It was painful to speak of Nicky. "I went down," Peter said, "and helped your son out of the water. I told him to go home and get dry. I have heard now that he had a wound from Bosworth, which opened in the struggle—the White Hart is a cauldron of gossip—but I didn't know of it then. I am sorry it happened, but I didn't try to kill him, or want to."

There was a silence. Then Peter said, "After Bosworth, I heard of two westcountrymen, a father and son, hanged at Henry Tudor's orders because they had been at King Richard's side when he fell. I wondered at first if they were Baldwin and his son. When I heard that it wasn't so, I was glad. I wouldn't have wanted such a thing to happen to them."

"Baldwin was a fool to pick a fight when he was injured. I know. So do you. You haven't said it, but I can see you thinking it."

"If you say so, Master Sweetwater. But when I offer my con-dolences, I mean them."

"If I'd realised straightaway that it was you just now, I'd have told you to go to perdition and leave me to deal with my own sheep."

"And I'd have ignored that and come to help anyway. For the sake of the sheep," said Peter.

"Bloody Lanyons. Always a thorn in our sides, like bramble in a sheep's fleece."

"I sometimes wish," said Peter, "that we could just be neighbours. Will it offend you if I am in the churchyard when Baldwin is buried? I would mean it respectfully, but I won't come if you object."

"I won't object. Just don't be noticeable," said Walter. He sounded tired and Peter, looking at him, saw that the lines in his face told the same story. "I grow weary of feuds," Walter said. "And people clack their tongues in the White Hart and laugh about us. Baldwin will be buried on Wednesday morning, the twenty-eighth. It will give time for me to send word to his sister. She may wish to come. Just about everyone for miles will be there. The Lanyons may as well join in. If your father allows!"

"I shan't ask his permission," said Peter.

Peter had left his pony tied to the other end of the gate where Walter had left his. They walked stiffly back together, loosed their mounts, nodded to each other, got back into their saddles and parted. Peter, forgetting about the tankard of ale, rode home, thinking.

He did indeed feel sorry for Walter's bereavement and he knew why. Last night Nicky had left home, although this time he had also left a note and they knew where he had gone. Richard had forbidden anyone to go after him and with sorrow, both Peter and Liza had agreed that perhaps this was best. But it was the reason Peter had saddled Plume and taken to the moor this morning. Nicky had been his son for so long, had saved him at the bridge and yet had had to be rejected. Now he had rejected Peter in turn. Nicky was lost and it was a dreadful thing to lose a son. The sense of the boy's absence hurt so much.

CHAPTER THIRTY-SIX

EXTRAORDINARY CHANGES

Quentin Lanyon loved her family. It came naturally to her. Her parents and brother were dear to her and if her grandfather was dictatorial he was nevertheless still her grandfather and it was normal for people to love their grandparents. It did not occur to her to question these things.

One day, she supposed, she would have a husband and children and would love them, as well. Beneath all this, like the hidden foundations of a house, was the assumption that all her family members loved each other.

This foundation had occasionally shuddered—for instance when Grandfather was harsh with Nicky—but always, hitherto, peace had been restored in the end. She had never envisaged a state of affairs where love would cease altogether, where the family would be split into factions, with her mother ostracised and tearful and her brother no longer a member of the family at all. It was beyond her comprehension.

At the beginning, when Liza had shut herself into a spare bed-chamber and Quentin had looked after her, Liza, sitting tearfully up when her daughter brought food to her for the second time, had wiped her eyes and made an attempt to explain.

"Have they told you everything, Quentin? Do you know what's happened, about Nicky and all?"

"Yes. I overheard some of it, anyway." Quentin spoke awkwardly, unsure what her mother expected her to say.

"I wish I could make you—or someone—understand. I care so much for your father. But Christopher—Nicky's real father is called Christopher—well, I met him before I was married and, well, it may happen to you one day and then you'll know. No one it hasn't happened to can *ever* know. You meet a man and he isn't specially handsome or clever or wealthy or…or anything that makes him different from a thousand others, but you look at him and the world turns upside down and it never turns back again."

A girlhood memory came back to Liza as she spoke, something she rarely thought about now, though when Quentin was a child, she had told her about it. "Do you remember, when you were about twelve, one January night I pointed out the constellation of Orion to you? That magnificent pattern, stamped on the sky?"

"Yes. You said you'd marvelled at it when you were a little girl yourself. But…" Quentin was now more puzzled than ever.

"Well, sometimes a man can stamp his image into your mind like that, and there it is, for always, blazing and beautiful. It's like being put under enchantment, only it isn't enchantment, it's love, and if it's real, it doesn't die. We should have married, though if we had…"

Quentin, trying none too successfully to understand what Liza was talking about, felt embarrassed by these confidences. They matched nothing in her experience and besides, it was as though she were the one with authority and her mother a pleading child, and that wasn't natural. But the hollowed pallor of her mother's face would have touched far harder hearts than hers. She put her arms around Liza, who said, "If we had married, you would never have come into being and I'm glad you did. Nothing's simple. But years ago—fourteen or so—I met Christopher again and once, just once, we gave way. And then Nicky was born."

"But the other day…?" Quentin prompted, puckering her brow, wanting to understand, although it was like trying to make sense of a very unfamiliar dialect.

"The other day we met in a dell on the moor, just to talk, to sit side by side as friends do. It was the second time we'd done so." Liza paused, finding herself unable to describe the quality of those two companionable meetings. She and Christopher had indeed done nothing but sit together and talk, of everyday things. He had told her of his work at the castle; a marriage service he had conducted recently at which the groom had got his responses muddled; and how he and the new Mistress Hilton had between them persuaded the steward to have the castle completely cleaned—"spring-cleaned, except that it was summer"—from battlements to basement.

She had talked to him of the farm and the cows, telling him how, since ceasing to be Sweetwater tenants, they had acquired a bull of their own which had chased Hodge twice, and how they had once more replaced their ram, this time with a crossbred animal which had the superb fleece of his predecessor but not the enormous horns and outsize skull.

She could not find words for the quality of those conversations, the comfort of them, the pleasure of talking so easily, without the hint of fear which her father-in-law always inspired in her and without the distortion which was slight but always there with Peter because they had not chosen each other and would, left to themselves, have both chosen differently. All she could say was, "When people grow older, Quentin, that's how it is. Just to sit and talk is enough. All the rest is in the past and long ago. Except…"

"Except that there's Nicky?" said Quentin, still puzzling it out.

"Yes, there's Nicky. And your father caught us, sitting in a dell, and Nicky—I've always known it—is Christopher all over again. There's no mistaking it, not when you see the two of them together."

Here at least was something she could grasp. "If only," said Quentin passionately, "Father hadn't taken that sheep path. If only you hadn't been right *in* his path!"

"Then no one would ever have known. I'd have taken my secret to my grave with me, darling, and who would have been harmed? Your father would have gone on thinking he had a son, and Nicky, one day, would have had Allerbrook and what would it matter?"

"Grandfather says it matters." Quentin's voice was not accusing, only bewildered. "He keeps on saying it, and thumping tables with his fist. He keeps saying that Nicky isn't a Lanyon and has no right to Allerbrook."

"Has he said that in Nicky's hearing?" Liza's voice broke, once more, into a sob. "Oh, poor Nicky!"

"Not yet, but I think he's going to. Father says I'm not to warn Nicky—they'll tell him themselves. It isn't fair," said Quentin roundly. "Lanyon or not, the farms have to be looked after by someone and why can't people just leave things alone and be happy?"

"No, it isn't fair, but that's the way it is." Tears slipped from Liza's eyes, quietly but relentlessly. "I don't know what's going to happen to me, darling. I may have to go away, go to St. Catherine's like my mother did. I don't want to go. It's strange. When I first came here, I thought I'd never get used to it, never call Allerbrook my home, but it's home now, has been for years and…and it'll break my heart if I have to leave it. Only…"

"If you go away, to Dunster or St. Catherine's or anywhere else, I'll go with you!"

"You're a dear girl, Quentin," said Liza. "The only one not to pass judgement on me."

Quentin shook her head, not in denial, but because she didn't know how to explain that she couldn't pass judgement because she didn't understand what it was she would be judging. She could not imagine being so enchanted by a man that the world turned upside down. All she could do was believe that it had happened to her mother, because her mother, whom she loved and trusted, had said so.

"I'm very glad you were born," said Liza, attempting once more to dry her eyes, "and I'm sorry to be burdening you with all this."

"You're my mother," said Quentin. "And that's that."

Only that wasn't that, because that phrase suggested finality, a settling of a problem, and the problem didn't look like ever being settled. Nicky had indeed been cruelly disinherited and although Liza had now emerged from the spare room, she crept about the house like a shadow and no one except Quentin spoke to her much beyond necessity. Betsy pursed her lips and turned away whenever Liza entered the kitchen and Ellen imitated her. Richard literally pretended that she wasn't there, even when she was handing him his dinner. His temper was very short these days, and he seemed to become crimson and breathless when provoked.

Peter did try sometimes to talk to his wife, but his voice was always stiff, as though he were forcing himself. They were sharing a bedchamber again, but Quentin knew that one of them was sleeping in a truckle bed. And now, this morning, they had found Nicky's letter and knew that he had gone. Liza, mouth trembling, said, "I hope my family will help him. He's only thirteen."

Richard said, "It's just as well. He's none of mine and I'm glad to see the back of him. I hope he doesn't try to come back, because if he does, I won't have it."

"I don't agree," said Peter. "He's only a lad. We've been his family since he was born and…"

His father brushed him aside. "He's got a family, a real one. I mean the Weavers and he's had sense enough to go to them. If any neighbours get nosy, we'll just tell them he preferred the Weavers to us and left at his own wish. The Shearers aren't that nosy, anyway," he added, swinging the conversation determinedly away from Nicky. "That was a surprise! Who'd have thought Martha would reappear with her sheep-shearing husband and apply for the tenancy when her dad died? I hear she leads old Tilly a miserable life. Revenge for being used as a maidservant when she was young, I suppose."

From then on, it seemed that Nicky's name was not to be

mentioned in the house. Richard cut anyone short who spoke it in his hearing. The news that Baldwin Sweetwater was dead, probably because of the encounter with her father on the bridge, was just one more wretchedness.

Now, helping her mother to sweep old rushes out of the hall before strewing fresh ones, in Quentin's sore heart something new had taken root—a sturdy little seedling of rebellion. The atmosphere in the house was so turgid with rage and misery that it could almost have been cut into slices with a cheese knife. The rest of her family seemed ready to live like this forever, but Quentin was not. The Quentin who had once kicked and cried in a vain defence of Nicky, had pleaded for his right to inherit Allerbrook, was pleading and kicking and crying again, inside her mind. Something must be done. She didn't yet know what, but *something*…

Liza, listlessly sweeping, seemed to lose heart. She stopped, leaned her broom against the wall, and said, "I must tell Betsy what to make for dinner. Your father likes mutton ham so we could have that, and finish the stew we had at supper yesterday…. Your grandfather hates waste…."

She was constantly making offerings of food, trying to make the angry men of the house less angry by giving them the things they liked best to eat. Quentin could have wept for her. Liza went toward the kitchen and Quentin, putting her own broom aside, followed, just in time to hear Liza explaining that the stew should be finished at dinner today, and hear Betsy reply, "Yes'm," and then, mouth primmed, turn her back and continue stirring a bowl of batter with a wooden spoon.

"I can't bear it," said Liza. *"I can't bear it!"*

"And what might that be, ma'am?" Betsy enquired in a mumbling voice and still with her back to Liza.

"This. You. As though I were a leper. Sometimes I think I'll slip out one night, as Nicky did, only I'll go to the barrow on the ridge, or maybe to the barrows on Winsford Hill. It's higher and colder there. I'll lie down in the night chill and the dew and let myself die. They say there are ghosts at the barrows. I'll be one of them then, and maybe they'll be kinder to me than you are!"

"Well, would 'ee now?" Betsy still wouldn't turn to her. "Add one mortal sin to another, would 'ee? Well, well, no surprise in that, I suppose."

"Oh, Betsy! How can you—after all these years?"

There was a sob in Liza's voice, and with that, the seedling of rebellion in Quentin shot up to full height in the space of half a second and burst into furious bloom. Darting forward, she seized Betsy's arm and swung her around. The wooden spoon scattered yellow drops in all directions. "Don't turn your back on my mother and sneer at her like that, you smug, self-righteous old *prune!*"

"What?" Betsy spluttered.

"You heard what I said! You watch your manners or I'll make you!"

Ellen, tending a pot at the fire, turned around and gaped while Betsy, outraged, flourished the spoon menacingly. "You watch your own manners, my wench. I don't talk pretty to trollops and—"

"It's *my mother* you're talking about!"

"Trollop I said and trollop I meant! Passing off a bastard as the son of the house—"

"Mistress Lanyon," said Quentin savagely, "is *still* my mother. As for Nicky, that happened fourteen years ago and for all those fourteen years you've worked for my mother and she's the same

woman now that she was all that time! Don't you dare call her a trollop again!"

"I'll call 'un what I like and I won't talk to—"

"Why not? You used to talk to Father Bernard and he was supposed to have had a son. You talk to my grandfather and I know all about him and Deb Archer, because Kat told me about them. You talked to Deb, too, apparently! So you'll treat my mother with respect and—"

"You should be ashamed! Standing up for a trollop—"

Quentin lifted her right hand and administered a box on the ear which sent Betsy staggering. She threw her spoon down, clutched at her ear and began to howl. "Quentin, don't!" Liza gasped. "Betsy's over seventy. You mustn't do that!"

"Why not?" Quentin screamed. "I'm sick to my stomach of living like this…you creeping about, afraid of everyone…people glaring and saying things or else *not* saying things…Betsy making holier-than-thou faces and turning away from you…I hate you, Betsy, you self-satisfied old besom, how dare you, how dare you? And don't you look at me like that or I'll hit you again! I won't have this…this feeling in the house, I won't! Nicky's been driven out but I'm not going to be driven out, and nor is my mother if I can help it and I'll stand up for her if I choose!"

"Quentin, Quentin…!" Liza was astounded. It was as though her sweet daughter, whose temperament hitherto had seemed perfectly in tune with her apple-blossom complexion, had undergone an extraordinary change into a wildcat.

"Come, Mother," said Quentin, turning to her. "Let's go back and finish the rushes. And you two, Betsy and Ellen, you can just do as you've been told. Mutton ham and stew for dinner and see that it's a good dinner and serve it up with pleasant faces. If that batter's for honeycakes, we'll expect them at supper, also served with a smile, do you hear?"

"Yes, I wouldn't mind seeing some pleasant faces myself," said Peter, walking into the kitchen. "I'm astonished, Quentin," he said. "I never thought my girl was such a termagant." To her surprise, he smiled at her. "In these difficult days, Quentin, I've felt better every time I've looked at you and heard your gentle voice. And now, when all of a sudden it isn't gentle, you've made me feel better still! Thank the saints you're here."

He hadn't looked at Liza. His eyes were on his daughter. "I can't hold it against you that you love your mother. It's right and proper, I suppose. I came to tell you, and you, Liza—" he turned to her at last, quite calmly "—that we all have an invitation. To Baldwin Sweetwater's funeral."

The change in the air was noticeable when dinner was eaten. Betsy and Ellen, while Quentin's dark eyes watched them with an ominous glitter, made approximately ordinary conversation. Liza, warmed by her daughter's championship, talked a little, too, instead of eating in silence with her eyes on her platter, as she had done since she left the spare room. Peter made reasonably normal replies.

Richard was the one who resisted most strongly. "I hear you've been throwing your weight about, young Quentin. Wouldn't be getting a bit full of yourself, would you, maid? Perhaps it's time we got you married."

"I will be happy to marry any suitable man you find for me, Grandfather," said Quentin. Her tone was one of sweet compliance. "But," she added, still in the same honeyed voice, "I couldn't go further than a betrothal until I felt sure that my mother was safe."

"What do you mean, *safe?* Has anyone hurt her? Though you don't mind hurting our Betsy, I hear."

"There's more than one kind of hurt," said Quentin. "When I know my mother is happy and…and…valued, and when I know that Nicky is all right, too…"

"Nicky's name isn't to be mentioned under this roof. He's no grandson of mine and I'll thank you to forget he ever breathed."

"Nicky is my brother," said Quentin. "I couldn't forget him if I tried. I will marry as you choose, but, as I said, only when I know that both my mother *and Nicky* are well and happy."

"Speak to me like that again, girl, and you'll be sorry."

"Lay a finger on her, Father, and *you'll* be sorry," said Peter, and Liza looked at him with gratitude, while Ellen, ignoring Betsy's attempt to frown at her, smiled. Suddenly the battle lines were redrawn. Liza had acquired supporters. Only Richard and Betsy now were ranged against her. They were ranged against Quentin, too, which Liza hated to see, but Quentin herself was obviously unmoved by it.

"I seem to be outnumbered," said Richard. "It's a sad day."

"If it's wrong to love my mother and my brother," said Quentin, "I'll confess the sin to Father Matthew next Sunday."

"You'll have a clever answer once too often one day," said Richard, "when your doting father isn't here to protect you!"

Peter, changing the subject with an air of determination, said, "Are you coming to Baldwin Sweetwater's funeral, Father?"

"No, I'm not. I wouldn't go to any burial of theirs except to dance on the grave," said Richard unpleasantly. "You go, if you want, you and Liza and Quentin. You'll feel awkward and so you should!"

★ ★ ★

Autumn was coming. The nights had grown cold and the day of Baldwin Sweetwater's funeral was overcast, with cloud flowing in from the west and a whisper of rain on the wind. The gathering in the church and then in the churchyard was well wrapped up against the weather.

It was a big gathering, however. Most of the village of Clicket was there, and all the tenant farmers were represented. It was easy enough for the Lanyons, who did indeed feel awkward, to lose themselves in the crowd. They stood back as the coffin was carried to the waiting grave, with Father Matthew leading the way. Six men of the Sweetwater household, including Denis Sawyer, were Baldwin's bearers. The Sweetwaters themselves walked behind: Walter, bent shouldered as no one had ever seen him before, Catherine swathed in a black cloak and holding the arm of her son, John, Agnes Northcote and her husband, Giles, pacing side by side.

John attracted some attention, since he was now nineteen and an only son, but not yet betrothed. There had been approaches made by and to the Sweetwaters, but none of the girls had pleased him enough, or his parents either, and now the growing rumours of the new King Henry's intentions toward his predecessor's supporters had made offers dry up. But something must surely be settled soon, all the same. It was time. Speculation about John had featured in the White Hart lately and it was featuring again, even here at his father's funeral.

The coffin had reached the grave and was being lowered into the earth and Father Matthew had begun the words of the committal. Only those close by could hear him, because the wind blew his words away, but they all knew what he was saying.

The Lanyons found themselves nearby, edged there by chance in the crowd. Catherine, releasing John's arm, had moved toward Walter and spoken to him, and Walter, bending his head toward her, had replied. They seemed to be trying to comfort each other. John had drawn apart. Quentin found herself suddenly very sorry for him. He looked lonely and very miserable. She knew him by sight, though she had never spoken to him. All the Lanyons said that Baldwin had been an unpleasant man, but his immediate family had apparently cared about him.

Quentin wondered sympathetically how she would feel if it were her father in that coffin, and then, on impulse, she moved forward, slipping between the people just in front of her, until she reached John Sweetwater's side. He glanced around at her, and looking into his face, she said quietly, "I am so sorry. It must be a sad thing to lose your father."

"He died in his bed, and shriven," John said. "It could have been worse. But thank you for your kind words. Who are you, by the way?"

"Quentin Lanyon."

"Oh. Peter Lanyon's daughter?"

"Yes." It occurred to Quentin that John no doubt knew all about the encounter on the packhorse bridge, but even though Baldwin's death had been largely his own fault, his son might not accept that. Perhaps she had been unwise to come up to him like this and speak to him. "I—I'm sorry," she said again. "I mean… I'm a Lanyon…." She looked away.

"It's all right." John's voice was harsh. "No one would blame *you,* anyway."

"Please…" Quentin would have liked to turn and run, but with the coffin ropes just being drawn up and Walter going forward now to toss a clod of earth onto the lid, and people all around with heads bowed in prayer, she couldn't. "We're all sorry," she whispered.

John was still studying her. Taking courage again, she once more turned to look at him. She saw that he was not quite a typical Sweetwater. He had the burly build, but his hair was dark instead of brown, and though it was wiry, it wasn't bushy. Also, instead of the chilly grey Sweetwater eyes, he had good-natured blue ones. Timidly she smiled at him. She meant it as concilia-tion, an assurance that even though she was a Lanyon she really did feel for him. She had no idea how her smile lightened her face, and made her dark eyes sparkle.

Unwillingly at first, and then more openly, John smiled back.

You meet a man and he isn't especially handsome or clever or wealthy or…or anything that makes him different from a thousand others, but you look at him and the world turns upside down and it never turns back again. It's like being put under enchantment, only it isn't enchant-ment, it's love, and if it's real, it doesn't die.

That was what her mother had said and now it had happened to her, as well. So this was what it was like—this yawning ache, this wish to *know* this young man, to seek out and become ac-quainted with every corner of his mind, understand his every thought and touch every last inch of his body. Yes, of his body. She wanted carnal knowledge of him. Father Matthew sometimes spoke of carnality in his Sunday homilies, warning his flock against it, even within marriage. Father Matthew was wrong! She wanted to slide her fingers through that dark wiry hair, press herself against John Sweetwater and investigate every curving muscle, bury her nose against his skin and inhale his scent; open to him and let him come into her and be one with her. *This* was what it was like.

His smile was fleeting, though it had remarkable charm. She could not tell whether it meant that he felt as she did, and she doubted it. He was unhappy; she had said something kind; he had perhaps noticed that she was young and nice-looking. He probably considered that her father had killed his. In any case, Lanyons and Sweetwaters were traditional enemies and no doubt he looked on Lanyons as socially beneath him. She could only let her soul be seen in her eyes, and hope, and pray, and yearn.

CHAPTER THIRTY-SEVEN ✦

PROPOSAL

"It was none of my doing!" Herbert Dyer was defensive and indignant. In his sixties, with his beard now grey, he was not as bluff and self-confident as he had been. These days, he rarely went to meet incoming ships, because long hours in the saddle, or out in a coastal vessel amid the wind and spray, now wearied him. However, Richard Lanyon, though at sixty-five he, too, showed signs of age, was still capable of being intimidating when he was angry. He was angry now.

"And I don't believe it was Simon's either, intentionally," Herbert almost gabbled. "It was an error, just a mistake. We do have customers who want cloth dyed with that costly scarlet that's made from a sort of insect in some far-off eastern country. Lady Elizabeth Luttrell, for instance. Now that she's back in Dunster Castle, there's been an order from her. She wants velvet that colour for her son's bed hangings. Simon makes out the bills, but it's a tedious task and it's never been his favourite. I daresay he was tired and just accidentally went on charging the same rate when he finished a bill for someone who ordered the expensive dye and started on bills for people who'd had less costly colours. And *I'm* tired of you poking into my business and looking for trouble!" he added with an attempt at aggression.

"I daresay you are. But I've done it regularly for years and you know why. You've a lot to lose, let me remind you," Richard said, taking Herbert's arm and steering him farther across the drying yard, to make sure that no one in the workshop could hear them. There were no flapping cloths to get in their way on this November day; it was too cold for outdoor drying. Cloth had to be hung inside the workshop. "You've a reputation," said Richard, "for good work and honesty. Why gamble with it?"

"I didn't, and nor did Simon."

"I think he did, whether you knew it or not. Like father, like son."

"Simon's a fine man. I was so thankful when he came back safe from Bosworth and—"

"May you go on feeling thankful for him. Now listen, Dyer, this is the first time you've slipped in all these years and I'm not vindictive. But if it happens again, I'll set the Watchet constable on you. I mean it. This set of bills hasn't been sent out yet. The ones with the overcharging must be made out again, correctly. You understand?"

Herbert looked at him. "I could kill you sometimes, Lanyon. I've often wanted to, when again and again you come prowling and prying into things that ought to be private to me and Simon."

"You'd have been publicly disgraced long ago if I hadn't," said Richard coolly. "You won't want to house me tonight," he added. "I'm going home by way of Dulverton, so I'll leave now and stay the night at Cleeve Abbey. It's in the right direction."

"I see," said Simon Dyer grimly to his father. "Everyone else does it now and again. It makes up for the bad payers. But we mustn't. *We've* got to be as virtuous as angels in a world where honest profits never make a man rich. That fellow Lanyon is the worst, nosiest interferer that was ever born."

"I hate him," said Herbert morosely. "I hate all the Lanyons, but mostly him. I reckon his son and Liza were his pawns when they came here prying that time, that's all. Richard's the one who's stood over me all these years, and it's Richard I blame for destroying my marriage. Margaret was a good woman and I could have made her happy, if I'd had the chance. I'd do Master Lanyon a bad turn any time."

Cleeve Abbey made its guests comfortable in an austere fashion. The guest house had neither wall hangings nor floor rushes, but the straw-filled pallets were clean. Similarly, the food, though plain, was plentiful. Richard ate and slept satisfactorily, made a donation to the abbey funds in the morning, had an interesting discussion with the abbot about sheep breeding and then started out for Dulverton, a long ride and a long route home, but Liza had asked him to visit Dulverton to buy some salt and a supply of candles.

The weather was cold and the moors misty, but the monks rose early and so did their guests. It was still only noon when he trotted Patches into the busy little town, where the clatter of looms was as persistent as it was in Dunster. Like Dunster, it had a cloth exclusive to itself.

It also had a town crier. As he rode toward Fore Street, its principal thoroughfare, he heard the jangling bell and the powerful voice of the crier announcing a proclamation. Touching his heels to Patches's sides, he caught up with the tail end of the crowd of townspeople who were following the bell toward the church. They all halted as the crier reached the churchyard gate and stood there, once more ringing his bell, until he was sure he had assembled the best possible audience.

Then he made his announcement.

Richard had to put a hand hard against his mouth in order to keep from laughing. Oh yes, this was news indeed. It was the best joke he'd ever heard. Thank God Ned Crowham had made Peter change sides at Bosworth.

He dined in Dulverton and bought good supplies of salt and candles, hiring a mule to carry them. It was coming up to the time of year when they would need candles in the evening and soon, too, they would be slaughtering pigs and salting the bacon. As he rode on home, going slowly because of the mule (pack animals were always a hindrance, which was why he hadn't taken a pack pony with him from home), he thought about the town crier's news. Halfway home, an interesting idea came into his head. He couldn't, straightaway, be quite sure about it. Perhaps it would be too expensive—or perhaps his family might object so strongly that they would stand shoulder to shoulder and actually defy him. But it was certainly an idea. That would put those arrogant Sweetwaters in their place, once and for all, and it was time that young Quentin learned that young women ought to know their place, too, and not spring like mad things to the defence of faithless wives.

★ ★ ★

So this was love, thought Quentin. This was what it felt like to be enthralled by a man. Enthralled. Placed in thralldom. Placed under tyranny. That side of it was something her mother hadn't mentioned.

John Sweetwater haunted her. He walked invisibly by her side wherever she went. The image of him standing alone at his father's graveside, and his face and his smile when she spoke to him were as vivid in her mind as though the printer William Caxton had used her brain as a sheet of paper. They hung in the air between her and the real world. They were probably in her dreams, except that she usually forgot her dreams in the morning.

Hitherto, she had been an industrious girl, helping in the house, caring for cows and poultry, spinning and weaving. Now, although winter was setting in, bringing heavy mists, or else cold winds that hissed across the heather and made the dry bracken rustle, she suddenly began to make excuses to walk or ride on the moor or go down to Clicket.

Finding the excuses wasn't difficult. Liza, as though trying in some way to make reparation for her past, had taken to being charitable. Down in Clicket, Deb Archer's former maid Allie was now a widow and in need. Her only son had gone to sea and Allie made out as best she could, keeping geese and chickens and growing vegetables. Liza sometimes made gifts to her of bacon or butter.

Sometimes, too, she sent small gifts to Tilly Lowe at what was now the Shearers' farm. In old age, Tilly had become pathetic, bullied by Martha and Martha's husband, Andrew, and sometimes by their sharp-featured fourteen-year-old-son, Philip, as well. They were a hardworking family, but impatient and parsimonious and grudged giving houseroom to Tilly, who was lame and trembly but struggled to justify her dragged-out existence by shelling peas and twirling a spindle.

"All three of them shout at her and I've seen her crying over it," Liza said indignantly when Richard protested that she was giving away too much. "And I'm sure they don't give her enough to eat. Now, you take these oatcakes to her, Quentin, and this flask of elderflower wine, and see the others aren't by when you give them to her. They'll grab the things for themselves if they get a chance."

Liza, often busy and no longer comfortable on a pony or as fond of walking as she used to be, frequently asked Quentin to be her messenger, and Quentin, these days, was more than willing to go. She went with eyes wide open, scanning the world around her for glimpses of John Sweetwater. Quite simply, she yearned to see him again, if only from a distance.

Now and then, she was lucky. Once she saw him out on the moor, cantering along on a fine black horse with bridle and scalloped reins of crimson, and carrying a goshawk on his arm. Once, visiting Allie in Clicket, she saw him ride through the street and turn in through the archway to the Sweetwater stable yard. They were glimpses to treasure, to add to her tiny store of mental pictures of him.

She had nothing else. She dared not seek anything further. She ached to be with him, to talk to him, but was afraid to search him out. He would not understand. Even if he responded, it would probably not be in the right way. She was not very old, but she wasn't foolish. When young men like John Sweetwater talked of love to girls like Quentin Lanyon, they did not talk of marriage, and Quentin knew it.

She must yearn alone, and endure, and hope for a miracle. And try not to be glad that after all she had not been betrothed to poor Eddie Hannacombe, because that meant being glad that Eddie was dead, and that would be very wrong.

The third time she encountered John Sweetwater was again in Clicket, when she was taking more gifts for Allie. "A length of green cloth this time, and a ham," Liza said, packing the basket. "She doesn't get much chance of eating meat and last time you went, you said when you came back that her gown was patched. There's cloth enough here for a new one."

Quentin had delivered the presents to a very thankful Allie, had stayed for a while to help sort some of the eggs from Allie's hens, and then said goodbye. As she stepped out again, she saw John riding past. This time he saw her, too, recognised her and smiled. Overcome, Quentin bobbed, smiled back, and felt herself turn scarlet. John, appearing not to notice this, bowed slightly toward her, lifted his black velvet cap about half an inch off his head before putting it back and then trotted on toward his home.

Quentin was left with hammering heart, wild exhilaration at having this new, precious vision of him and fury against herself for behaving like a wantwit, going red and giving him a silly, timid smile when she should have been dignified, given him a polite nod and a gracious, friendly smile as a great lady, an equal of his, would do.

John, riding back to the stable, was amused. She was a pretty thing, that Lanyon wench, and kindhearted. It was a pity that he couldn't pursue the acquaintance, but he didn't want to start up the feud between the families again. It seemed to have faded now, a very odd result of his father's death, considering the circumstances, but this was evidently the way that Grandfather Walter wanted it. The old quarrel would certainly be stirred up, though, if he seduced a Lanyon girl. No. Better leave her alone.

He rode into the stable yard, and found the grooms rubbing down two strange horses. "Have guests arrived?" he asked, swinging a leg over the saddle cantle.

"Royal messengers." One of the grooms left his task and came over to him. It was John's custom to see to his horse himself, but this time the reins were firmly taken from him. "They're with your grandfather now, sir. You may be wanted."

John raised his brows, but took the hint and went in. Denis Sawyer met him in the door to the great hall. "I'm glad to see you back, sir. There's grave trouble. Your mother's beside herself and your grandfather's well nigh in tears."

"What in the world...?" Snatching off his cap, John hastened through the entrance vestibule and into the hall. Walter was in his usual chair by the hearth. The fire crackled cheerfully and the hall was quite warm, but Walter was huddled and shivering, as though he had been stricken by winter, while Catherine was walking in distracted circles, wringing her hands. Other servants, including Catherine's maid Amy, were in the hall, too, standing in clusters, many of the women sobbing.

Also present and apparently quite unmoved by the anguish all around them were two dignified men, dressed alike, in practical dark clothes. One of them turned as John came in, and he saw the red dragon of Henry Tudor embroidered on the man's doublet.

"Who is this?" said the man, as though this were not John's own home and John himself the son of the house.

"My grandson," said Walter. "Whose inheritance you have come to steal. John!"

"What is it? What's happening?"

"They're going to take our lands away!" said Catherine on a wail. "The king sent them! We fought for King Richard, but they say it was treason and they're going to take the Sweetwater property! There'll be nothing left but my dower lands! They're letting us keep those, but we used two farms to make up Agnes's dowry!"

"So that's just the two farms in Devon left," observed Sawyer. "Both with tenants. One lot of tenants and their rents must go to make room for our household."

"Yes. It's true," said Walter. His ageing fingers gripped the arms of his chair and his knuckles showed white. "We've to be out in a week. Our estate will be sold to feed the royal treasury. The sale is being proclaimed now, today, in Dulverton, in Dunster, in Exford, in Minehead, in Porlock and Lynton and Lynmouth—everywhere! We're ruined."

"Well, I'm sorry for them," said Quentin across the supper table.

Liza looked at her anxiously, and wished her daughter wouldn't be so downright. It might make Richard angry. Richard had not forgiven Quentin for trying to protect her. He showed it every day, in half a dozen ways—by ignoring his granddaughter, or ordering her about as though she were a slave, or snapping at her for absurdly small reasons: a dish set down with a very slight rattle, a draught when she opened a door, a tear in his hose that she hadn't mended even though he hadn't told her it was there.

And today, all day, he'd been in a very curious mood. She had observed it because pouring rain had kept them all engaged on indoor jobs. He was withdrawn, thoughtful, and she had once or twice heard him humming to himself as though he were thinking of something pleasant; yet she had also caught him glancing at her and at Quentin in a way that worried her. It was hard to define, but it looked like triumph. As though he were planning something that he would like and they wouldn't. It would be better, she felt, if Quentin didn't provoke him now.

And Quentin had managed to do just that. Richard was glowering at her. "You're a fool, girl. You're sorry for everyone. You used to be sorry for Nicky when he asked for a hiding and I gave him one, and you'd probably be sorry for a felon at the end of a rope even if he'd driven your sheep flock away in the night, stolen your purse and had his way with *you*. Too softhearted for your own good, that's you, my girl."

"I was glad myself when I knew that the Sweetwaters weren't going to be hanged by Henry Tudor," Peter remarked.

"I daresay. Just because I don't want them dead doesn't mean I want them prosperous. Betsy, give me another fried trout. Plenty to go round, now that Alfred's moved in with his in-laws in Clicket. Don't know where Hodge got them from, but I'd wager it was out of a stream on Sweetwater land. It usually is. I wonder what Walter Sweetwater's eating for supper? I doubt he'll notice the taste, whatever it is. I'm a happy man tonight. Oh, that was a grand moment in Dulverton when I heard the crier give out that the Sweetwater lands were being put up for sale."

"They've been given so little time to leave!" said Quentin. "Imagine how we'd feel!"

"Will you hold your tongue, Quentin? No one wants to know what you think. Fact is," said Richard, slightly diverted by this interesting topic, "we're lucky it *wasn't* us. Peter here fought for Lancaster at Bosworth, by mistake, so to speak, but anyhow, there he was, on the winning side. The Sweetwaters fought for the house of York. This new king, Henry, he's dating his reign from the day before Bosworth. Sharp practice if ever I heard it, but I gather he likes money," said Richard.

For a few moments they ate trout in near silence. Only near silence, because oddly enough, between mouthfuls, Richard seemed to be humming softly to himself again. Liza watched him covertly and nervously. There was something in the wind, most certainly there was, but what?

Then Richard, having mopped up the last of the fish juice with bread, swallowed it, wiped his mouth with the back of his hand and declared, "I've got something to say. I've been thinking it over for a while now and I reckon it can be done, and it's high time Quentin here was married. I've settled on the man."

There was a staggered silence, until Peter said, "Just a moment. I am Quentin's father and—"

"And I'm *your* father and the head of this house. Just be quiet and listen," Richard barked.

Liza looked at Quentin, whose eyes were terrified. Under the table she reached out and took her daughter's hand. Everyone waited for Richard to go on.

"I'll have to make a few enquiries," Richard said. "The dowry's important. It's the heart of the matter, as it happens. First thing I've got to do is buy up the Sweetwater lands."

"The...*what?*" said Peter, flabbergasted.

"When I heard the announcement in Dulverton," said his father, unheeding, "there was a name given, an official of some sort, who's in charge of selling them off. Can't remember offhand what that name was but it should be easy enough to find out. I reckon we can do it. Sell off the land we bought with the proceeds of the stone quarry..."

"*My* stone quarry," said Peter sharply.

"…and maybe some of the farmland that goes with the quarry as well—not the quarry itself, of course—and very likely it would come to enough, with a bit added from our savings. I've been at your abacus, Liza, when you weren't looking."

His household stared at him, goggle-eyed. Quentin's fingers tightened on Liza's.

"But why buy the Sweetwater lands?" said Peter. "If we're going to give a dowry to Quentin—and we will have to one day, I agree there—why not just give her the farms you're talking about selling? Oh." He snorted. "To upset the Sweetwaters, I suppose, by getting hold of what used to be theirs. I see."

Richard gave him a complacent glance. "Quite. We really can do it. You always thought that building this house would bankrupt us, boy, but look how we're flourishing now! It didn't drain us the way marrying Agnes Sweetwater to a Northcote-Carew crossbreed drained *her* family. And after they'd wrung out a dowry for her, they hoped Agnes's in-laws would put Baldwin forward to be Sheriff of Somerset or Devon or something of that sort, but it never happened. She took the husband they bought for her and that was that. How do I know? Folk talk, in the White Hart and every other tavern and at every market."

Liza said, "And who is the man?"

Richard smiled. "John Sweetwater. And then we hand the family back their land, or some of it anyway as Quentin's portion. Coals of fire on their arrogant heads. Oh, how I'll enjoy their faces, trying to smile at the wedding feast."

"No!" Letting go of Quentin, Liza shot to her feet and her protest came out in a shriek. "You can't do this! I won't see Quentin sacrificed, thrown off, thrust into that family—*that* family…. Well, I hope they won't accept her. I hope they'll say no…"

"Sit down, Liza! Stop screeching! I reckon they'll say yes," said Richard. "They love their land and they'll want it back, at any price they can afford, and they can probably afford young John. Besides, what will they lose? He'll get a nice-looking wife and a family in time, I hope. It'll be a good enough bargain from their point of view."

"Yes, and what kind of life would Quentin have among them? Do you think they'd be kind to her—a Lanyon in their midst?" shouted Liza, still on her feet.

"Maybe not, but it's no more than she deserves, the way she's behaved."

"No!" Liza was crimson with fury. "Head of the house or not, you *can't do this!*"

"No, by God, he can't! You're right, Liza!" Peter roared. "I won't stand for it, do you hear, Father? You've gone too far this time. Quentin isn't going to marry John Sweetwater and that's the end of it!"

"Just a moment," said Quentin.

They turned to her, all of them. The fear had gone from her eyes. She was quite calm and indeed, smiling slightly. "I seem to remember," said Quentin, "not long ago, promising to marry any suitable man you found for me, Grandfather. I suppose that Master Sweetwater is suitable—at least he comes of a well-bred family. I only want to be sure that my mother will be well treated. Please say that she will. And then, if you so order it, I'll gladly marry John Sweetwater. If he'll have me."

Liza's mouth opened again, but this time no words came out. Peter clutched at his hair. "Quentin, you don't know what you're saying! You needn't fear for your mother, that I'll promise anyway. You don't have to marry a Sweetwater to buy her safety. You *can't* marry a Sweetwater! Not you! You're the best thing that ever came into this house! There have been times…so *many* times, when I don't know what I might have done, except that every time I looked at you or heard your voice, I felt calmer, more reasonable. I could bear things. And I want you to be happy!"

Richard, however, had thrown back his head and burst out laughing.

PART FOUR

RECONSTRUCTION
1487–1504

CHAPTER THIRTY-EIGHT

SETTLED IN LIFE

To Quentin, the birth of Johnny, as they nicknamed tiny John to distinguish him from his father, was a wonder and a revelation. It was as though she had been waiting, all her days, for the moment when her very own child was put into her arms, perfect, bawling, a little, adorable, dependent being for whom it would be her privilege to love and care.

Unlike her mother, she had quickened at once and Johnny had arrived swiftly and easily, on New Year's Day, 1487.

Much more swiftly and much more easily than her parents' consent to the marriage had been won, certainly. For Richard's scheme, tossed across that supper table, had torn the family apart nearly as thoroughly as the discovery of Nicky's true parentage. It had even torn people apart within themselves.

Peter's outrage across the supper dishes had gone on and on. He had thundered repeatedly that they would be stripping themselves of land, virtually giving it away to the Sweetwaters, and for what? For *what?* How could a Lanyon hope to be happy, married to a Sweetwater? He pounded the table so that platters jumped and beakers spilled and only by getting hurriedly onto her feet and leaning on the table with all her weight had Liza stopped him from overturning it in his fury.

While all the time her grandfather Richard had laughed, saying that after all, Quentin was a granddaughter to be proud of, a real Lanyon. "She's wiped my eye properly. But it won't get you out of it, young Quentin. You'll keep your word and go through with this. Understand?"

"Yes, Grandfather. I understand," said Quentin demurely.

Whereupon Peter had burst out again, this time so wildly that Quentin, aghast, turned white and began to cry, which caused him, briefly, to check himself.

Until Richard turned to Quentin and said, "You mean it, do you? If I can get their land and house and their agreement, you'll wed John Sweetwater and carry some of their property back to them, a gift from us, the Lanyons they have so much despised?"

"Yes, Grandfather," said Quentin, shakily, which he misinterpreted as fear of the marriage rather than distress at her father's rage. "I will. I mean it. I will do as you bid."

Whereupon Peter lost his temper again and crashed out of the house, and on returning, refused to speak to his father.

Meanwhile, Quentin, well aware that from her grandfather's point of view, marrying her to John Sweetwater was retribution for defending her mother, had decided to be circumspect. But that evening, in a private conversation with her parents in their bedchamber, she told them that at Baldwin's funeral she had met

THE HOUSE OF LANYON

and spoken to John Sweetwater and liked him. And was perfectly prepared to marry him.

"And it would please Grandfather so much, though I think perhaps we shouldn't tell him that John and I have met and that I took to him," she said, drawing her parents deftly into a conspiracy against Richard.

Peter flung up his hands, exclaimed that women were impossible, and left the room. Shortly afterward, he could be heard furiously chopping firewood. Her mother, scanning Quentin's face, said, "There's more than you've told me, isn't there? I don't, I can't, like the thought of this, but you already care for this young man, I think."

"Yes," said Quentin. "Yes, I do."

"*That* way? The way that…I told you about?"

There was a silence. Then Quentin said, "Yes. That way."

"I always swore," said Liza, "that if you fell in love like that, I'd try to help you. I know how it feels. But I never guessed the man would be a Sweetwater."

"I think John isn't quite like the other Sweetwaters. Mother, I mean it. I really want to marry him and I don't think he *dis*likes me."

She knew nothing of the stormy arguments that followed, between her parents, out of her hearing, when Peter declared that his entire family appeared to have taken leave of their senses, and her mother said that the plan had its good points; that if anyone could win the Sweetwaters over, Quentin could, and since the girl was willing, well, it would at least keep Richard sweet. To which Peter more than once replied that he didn't want to keep his father sweet; he felt more like killing him.

What finally overcame Peter's resistance was partly the fact that

Richard, though still chilly toward Liza, now became very pleasant toward Quentin, which was certainly a blessed change. Along with this was a weird but increasingly strong feeling that young as she was, Quentin knew what she was doing.

"Very well," Peter said at last, having summoned her once more to his and Liza's room. "I think you're crazy, all of you, but if you really want this marriage, Quentin, then all right. I agree! Although," he added, "I still hope my father changes his mind."

Richard didn't change his mind. Richard, like a charging bull with head lowered and nostrils snorting, plunged straight ahead. He went to Dulverton to discover the name of the right man to contact and then to Dunster, where he found a messenger in the shape of one of the young Weavers. Peter, wearily, gave consent to the sale or exchange of those items of property which had his name on the deeds. An urgent letter went to London and a deal was struck.

His grace King Henry VII is pleased to accept the lands listed in your letter in simple exchange for the house known as Sweetwater House, in the parish of Clicket in Somerset, the village known as Clicket and the following Somerset farmlands of the Sweetwater estate....

The big joke, said Richard, chortling and fairly shining with satisfaction, was that the Lanyons could never have managed any of this but for the generosity, years ago, of the man who became Richard III. Perhaps it would be as well if King Henry never found that out!

After that, he prepared another letter, this time for Walter Sweetwater, who had mournfully taken his family to stay with Agnes and Giles Northcote until he could eject the tenants from one of Catherine's dower farms. Sweetwater House was empty except for Denis Sawyer and a couple of servants who remained as caretakers. Sawyer was the messenger this time. He was a long time returning, and when he did, came straight to Allerbrook.

"There was a fine to-do," he said dispassionately, sitting in the Allerbrook hall with a tankard of cider in his hand. Denis Sawyer was not emotionally attached to the Sweetwaters, and the uproar caused by Richard's missive seemed to amuse him. "I'm sorry I was so long over it, but Master Sweetwater's got possession of one of the dower farms and he'd left Mistress Agnes's home to move in. Quick work! I had to follow him and his family there. It's too small for them, considering what they're used to. They have to live as their tenants did—no hall or solar, just one big kitchen that counts as their main room, and a tiny parlour that's hardly used because they have to work. They don't have many farmhands, and in the house Mistress Catherine's only got one girl and a handyman to help her, so she's busy with the cooking pots most of the day and Master John has to see to the animals. They all came into the kitchen to talk over that letter, though."

Sawyer grinned and held out his tankard as Liza offered him a refill from a jug. "Master Walter can't get used to the lack of space. There he was, striding about and clutching at his temples and bumping into things and tripping over people's feet and wanting to know what Master John was about, courting a Lanyon girl on the quiet and had he got her with child—was that what this was all about?

"And there was Master John saying no, he hadn't, and wouldn't, but she was a pretty maid and things had been better lately between the Lanyons and the Sweetwaters, hadn't they? Master John said a man could do a lot worse than marry Quentin Lanyon and there was no denying that it would put them all back in Clicket where they belonged and the tenants they'd thrown out so as they could move into this hen coop of a place would be able to come back. And they needed the rent...."

"Is the answer yes or no?" snapped Richard.

"Oh, it's yes," said Sawyer. "Master Walter might curse and swear and say that things being better was just on the surface and so on, but…"

Here he paused, thinking it better not to quote Walter's comments that the Lanyons weren't gentry and had always hated the Sweetwaters and even if Peter wasn't to blame for Baldwin's tragedy, he, Walter, would still be happy enough to do Richard Lanyon down and Richard would probably push him, Walter, over a bridge or off a cliff if he got the chance and he wouldn't sell his son to a Lanyon even to get his own property back.

"Mistress Catherine cried," he said, "and said that if John liked the girl and she was willing, and it would get them all home into the bargain, how could he *think* of turning the proposal down, and then Master John said he was going to marry the lass anyhow. He fancied her and he wanted to get the family property back, and he didn't need any man's consent…at one point they were all shouting—or crying, in the lady's case—at the same time. I never knew a pack of strolling players make a noisier scene."

"But what if Master Walter makes her life a misery, if she goes to live at Sweetwater House and he's there!" said Liza, her brow furrowed with worry. "She's obedient enough—" Liza had well understood that it would be better not to reveal Quentin's secret passion "—and I can see that the idea has advantages. It's a good marriage in its way. Only, Master Walter still resents us, at heart!"

Quentin, however, said, "If John and I can't live with him, we'll have to find somewhere else. But perhaps he'll get to like me, when he's used to me. I'm not afraid of him."

Peter, by then, had given in, because his entire family seemed ranged against him. "But if it goes wrong," he said to Quentin, "if you're miserable, you just come home again. We'll protect you. If it goes awry, we'll get you out of it, if we have to bribe the Pope for an annulment!"

The wedding took place the following March, and was conducted by Father Matthew at the parish church (since even Richard had recognised that it would be tactless to insist on celebrating it in the chapel at Allerbrook House). It was hardly a merry occasion. Walter scowled all the time and Liza, though dry-eyed, couldn't smile, while Peter refused to attend at all. It was Richard who placed Quentin's hand in that of her bridegroom.

There was an awkwardness, too, when the couple were at last alone. Until they were brought together at St. Anne's in Clicket to make their vows, Quentin and John had in fact exchanged very few words and never in private. They had spoken to each other at the graveside, and they had had brief conversations when John and his grandfather came to Allerbrook for the betrothal, and after that, on two occasions, when John visited her and they had made a little conversation. Always, someone else had been present. As she stood beside him in front of Father Matthew, his nearness made her heart turn somersaults, and yet he was virtually a stranger to her.

Throughout the wedding feast, though they sat next to each other, and during the dancing later on, which they had to open, John made only a few conventional remarks to her. "Will you have some more meat? I'll beckon the page." "Your dress is very fine. Pale pink looks well on you." "It's time to start the dancing." He smiled at her now and then and she smiled back, but she was too nervous to initiate any conversation of her own. Now that it was too late, she was saying to herself, *If I'd said no, and been strong about it, my parents would have backed me up, and between us, we might have withstood my grandfather. But I agreed. Of my own free will, I agreed. What have I done?*

When, at last, they lay uneasily side by side in the darkness of a curtained bed in Sweetwater House, however, she took herself in hand. The basic good sense which she had inherited from Liza, albeit alongside the contradictory ability to fall headlong into love at five minutes' notice and stay there for life, told her that she had no choice. She had made this bed herself and had better set about making it comfortable, or at least not complain if it wasn't.

She cleared her throat and then said gently, "This marriage was my grandfather's idea, but I was content with it. I wanted to give you back your own, or as much as I could. I know you haven't got quite all of it since we've kept Rixons Farm, but you've got Hannacombes and Shearers back, and Clicket and your home farm and this house and at least you're home again. I was so very sorry about...about everything. And I liked you. Just being sorry couldn't help you on its own."

For a long moment there was no response from him and her skin seemed to freeze. Then he rolled over and she felt his arm move across her. "You are kind and pretty. If only property and...and...the way our two families have wrangled all these years wasn't mixed up with it...."

"But could we ever have been married at all, unless property and...and the old quarrels...were mixed up with it?" said Quentin in a down-to-earth fashion.

There was another lengthy silence. Eventually, she added, "I will do all I can to see you don't regret it. Can we not put the old quarrels into the past?"

He laughed a little. Then he said, "Talking of quarrels—tell me, why did your brother leave Allerbrook? Was that over a dispute of some sort? All Clicket was buzzing about that, but no one ever had an answer."

Quentin decided to keep to the story Richard had insisted upon, and for the sake of trying to make interesting conversation, invented some extra details. "Yes, there was a dispute. Nicky didn't like the life of the farm. Getting up at first light and always being out of doors even in the freezing cold or the rain—it didn't suit him, and my father and grandfather were angry."

"Oh, I see. Not a typical farmer's son, then?"

"Well, no," said Quentin, sensing a covert jeer at her family's social standing but sensing, too, that John did not realise it was a jeer at all, still less that it was also a jeer at her. "He will make his way," she said. "I expect one day he'll be richer than any of us."

"Well," John said, "I have to admit that my family is richer now than it was when we all woke up this morning. But we haven't quite ratified the treaty yet, have we? I suppose it's time we did."

He rolled himself on top of her. There in the curtained darkness, nature spoke to them. By morning they had invented pet names for each other. Tentatively, quietly, a genuine friendship had begun.

At breakfast, Quentin greeted Catherine and Walter with courteous affection, and then there was a pause, while she looked shyly from one to the other, and waited for an answer. She had been well aware that yesterday, in church, Walter had glowered all the time. Later on, surrounded by wedding guests, he and Mistress Catherine had made an effort, had gone through the motions of courtesy and uttered suitable words of well-wishing, but how far had they meant them? Today she would find out just how welcome they intended to make her.

Catherine gave her a small, cautious smile. Walter stared at her, cleared his throat and then, for a few moments, was silent.

The wedding feast had been held at Sweetwater House instead of at the bride's home in the usual way. Walter wanted it so because somehow, to have it at Allerbrook would be an extra Lanyon triumph. The Lanyons agreed, for a reason they didn't mention to Walter, which was that Peter had objected violently to the idea of holding the wedding celebrations under the Lanyon roof. So Sweetwater House it had to be, which was nearer St. Anne's church, anyway.

On the way back from the church to the house, Liza Lanyon had come to Walter's side.

"Master Sweetwater, may I speak to you?"

He scarcely knew her, but she was now his grandson's mother-in-law and social proprieties sometimes had the strength of fetters. He could hardly say anything other than "Yes, of course."

Liza, with a hand placed on his arm, brought them both to a halt so that she could stand facing him. Pleasant brown eyes looked into his.

"I expect," said Liza quietly, "that this marriage isn't altogether to your taste. But somehow or other, Quentin has become enamoured of your son. Master Sweetwater, Quentin is a good girl and will make a good wife, if you will…if you will give her a chance. Whatever you feel about the Lanyons, please be kind to Quentin. Please."

She did not, as Richard would have done, add that if he were not kind, he would have the Lanyons to deal with. There was no threat in her face or voice, only appeal.

"Mistress Lanyon," said Walter, "I am not a knight, but I could have been, had I gone to war and won my spurs on the field as my father did. I still try to follow the knightly code of behaviour. I do not pursue feuds with women."

Sir Humphrey Sweetwater, knight or not, would probably have set out to make Quentin's life wretched and not thought twice about it, but Sir Humphrey had died at Towton a quarter of a century ago.

"If your daughter fills her place as she should," he said, "she will have nothing to fear from me, and my daughter-in-law Catherine has a very sweet temper. Quentin will be quite safe with us."

"Thank you," said Liza, and gave him the smile which had long ago captivated a red-haired young deacon.

Now he sat in the hall he had been able to come home to only because of this dark-eyed Lanyon interloper, and saw that the timid smile she was offering him was her mother's smile all over again. He drew a deep breath and said gruffly, "I give you good morning." And then, "I hope you will be happy with us. Be seated." He had to drag the words out of himself, but drag them he did.

"What should I do today?" Quentin asked. "I've brought my spinning wheel with me. It's in the baggage we sent here yesterday."

"You can send it back to Allerbrook!" said Walter. He almost snapped, but not quite. "You're a lady now," he said, more gently.

"Sweetwater ladies don't spin and weave. They see to the herb garden, instruct the maids and the cooks, maybe make marchpane fancies. Or they embroider. Mistress Catherine here is making covers for settle cushions. Perhaps she'll let you help with that. Eh, Catherine?"

"Yes, by all means," said Catherine, and, since she had now been in effect given permission to smile properly, did so.

Inch by inch, over the next few weeks, Quentin created for herself a niche in the household, and blew on the small fire of affection she and John had kindled on their wedding night, until it grew into a bright blaze. When she declared that she thought she was with child, Catherine embraced her, and Walter, after a hesitant moment, gave her a kiss and said, "You must take care of yourself, my dear."

The battle was won. The first fruits of victory were made apparent on the day when, about to set out hunting, Walter remarked quite jovially that if they took a deer today, they'd send some venison to Allerbrook, seeing that the Lanyons were family now.

And when, triumphantly, she presented them with Johnny, it seemed that the peace treaty between the Lanyons and the Sweetwaters was not only ratified but renewed. Life from now on, Quentin thought joyously, would be a sunlit, happy upland, like the moors on an August day, when the heather and the gorse were out and the larks were singing.

"We're not much worse off for giving Quentin her dowry." Richard, having led Liza and Peter into the hall because he said he wanted to show them something, stood in midfloor, rubbing his hands together in pleasure. "We kept Rixons for ourselves and now we've got all of the rent the Hudds pay us. And we still have the quarry. Very satisfactory. I think we'll have this plain old panelling ripped out at last and something better put in. We talked of that before, didn't we, but then the war came and we never got round to it. Let's get round to it now. There's a fashion these days for Tudor roses. They'd look handsome."

"Tudor roses?" asked Liza.

"Yes. King Henry's married King Edward's daughter Elizabeth and that's Lancaster marrying York. The white rose and the red rose have come together. The Tudor rose is half white and half red. We could have roses carved into the panelling and then coloured. I've spoken to the carpenter in Clicket already, when I was in the village yesterday. He'll come tomorrow to measure up. He's got a good wood-carver working with him these days. New panelling, good seasoned oak, with a Tudor rose in the middle of each panel, painted red and white. That's what I'll have in here, and new carved fronts for those window seats, too—more Tudor roses, to match."

"He hasn't asked me what I think," said Peter, addressing the roof beams. "He's just decided on his own. Again. And if anyone *should* ask me what I think, I think it's pointless and a waste of money. Whatever you say, Father, it'll take time to rebuild our savings. It's as well the quarry is still flourishing! I don't want to see more good gold and silver being spent on this house. From the start, it was pointless and a waste of money!"

"Nonsense!" Richard barked.

"We're *farmers*! It's land we should value, not Tudor roses in the panelling! And if we'd never built this place, we'd still be on the old terms with our neighbours. They think we think we're above them now! The Shearers almost look the other way when they come across us—Liza's charity to Tilly only matters to Tilly—and one of the Hudd boys took his cap off to me in Clicket the other day. I don't like it. It's embarrassing."

"Well, *I* like it," said Richard. "Take heart, boy. When we can afford it, you can decide what to have in the way of stained glass for the chapel. That'll be next." Peter's disgusted expression seemed to amuse him. "Then we'll have the tapestries I recall you once went all poetical about. It's odd," he added thoughtfully. "If the Sweetwaters hadn't gone hunting the day of my father's funeral and crashed into the procession, it's quite possible I'd never have built this house at all. How very strange."

"It might not have happened either if the stag had run in a different direction," Peter retorted.

Life as an apprentice with Owen ap Idwal in Lynmouth actually suited Nicky Lanyon very well. He had not forgiven his family for casting him out; he would never forgive them, as long as he lived. But nevertheless, it was a fact that life with Owen ap Idwal was more exciting than life at Allerbrook and about a thousand times more exciting than sitting at a loom in a weaving shed at Dunster.

For one thing, it didn't mean staying in Lynmouth all the time. The town at the foot of the towering cliffs was very small, and from its sister town of Lynton at the top of the same cliffs it looked as though the great walls of rock were crowding its thatched and slate cottages into the harbour. But the harbour and the ships that came and went were the heart of the place. And as Nicky soon discovered, Owen ap Idwal sometimes came and went with them, on his own ship, the *Fulmar,* and so on occasion did the boys he was training in his trade. Before Nicky had been with him for a year and a half, he had travelled to Venice and back twice.

Owen ap Idwal himself was short, dark and possessed of a crackling energy. He normally went up the creaky stairs in his house two at a time, leaped from the *Fulmar*'s deck to the quay and back again instead of stepping sedately, bolted his food, tossed drink down his gullet rather than savouring any of it, and unpacked goods at full speed, slashing wrappings away with the sharp knife he always carried, and cursing in Welsh if the knife didn't cut through them at the first slash.

Sometimes he cursed the boys as well, or even cuffed them, but there was no ill humour in it and to Nicky, after his grand-father's attentions, these occasional clouts were nothing at all. The ones handed out to the boys, the maids and her young daughter by Owen's thin, busy and short-tempered wife, Constance, were harder. Their two eldest daughters were married and gone and their son acted as the captain of the *Fulmar,* but their youngest girl, Gwyneth, who was only ten ("She came as a surprise," Owen had once said jovially) was still at home and there were two maidservants. The maidservants claimed that Constance was capable of being in half a dozen places at once and always for the purpose of finding that someone had done something wrong.

"One speck of dust on a girt old tabletop or one crumb on the floor, or else you stop mopping or beating eggs just for half a minute to chatty, like any maidens might, and there she be, all of a sudden, when you thought she was up in the attic annoying the rats!" they said.

Neither hated her, though, and Gwyneth loved her, because Constance, in her busy-brusque way, could also be kind at times and she was good to the maids if one of them were hurt or ill or needed time off for some right and proper reason, such as visiting genuinely sick parents, or courting.

"A wench has to have her chance with the lads," she would say quite tolerantly, and it was said that she and Owen had given very good wedding gifts to previous maidservants who had married.

The goods that Owen handled were interesting, too, though the cheeses he carried for export had such a powerful smell that the first time Nicky sailed with his employer, the nausea that plagued him on the first day had more to do with the reek from the hold that plagued him on the first day than did the motion of the ship.

But he liked handling the soft, cured hides: calfskin, deerskin, pigskin and the stout leather made from adult cattle. He admired the ready-made leather boots and gloves, fringed and embroidered, which Owen also took abroad, and was fascinated by the variety of things that could be made from iron.

"It's good iron, lad," Owen told him. "There's a mine or two near here, so there's not much cost for transport. I get things made by a blacksmith in Lynton." Sometimes he took Nicky and the other three youths he was training up to Lynton to watch the smith creating fire irons and rakes, bread ovens and ploughshares, hammers, chisels, currycombs, nails and buckets and chains.

Life at sea, once he had got over the sickness and learned how to sleep in a hammock and to believe that however wet and cold one got in bad weather, seawater wouldn't give him a chill, appealed to Nicky, too. He was an active boy and on his very first voyage learned how to manage the sails as well as any sailor.

Venice, the city which seemed to grow out of the very sea, amazed and enthralled him, and the goods he found himself handling on the way home gave him new cause for wonder. There were bales of gleaming silk, kegs of spices, which unlike the cheeses smelt aromatic and exciting, and earthenware jars of dyestuffs from lands so far away that they were to him little more than legends.

For all his resentment against his family, he would have said he was well settled in life. He would finish his years with Owen ap Idwal and then, he hoped, work for a similar merchant, for pay, until such time as he could set himself up in business. The Weavers had said they would help.

He was seventeen, well grown, that day in the late summer of 1489 when, returning with Owen from another voyage to Venice, he stepped onto the quay at Lynmouth and found himself face-to-face with Herbert Dyer.

CHAPTER THIRTY-NINE

TAVERN TALK

Nicky stopped short. He couldn't recall the name of the bearded elderly man with the good clothes and the square build, but he felt he had seen him somewhere before.

"Surely I know you, sir?" he said. "Are you here to see Owen ap Idwal?"

"Yes, I am. My son engaged him to bring dyestuffs in for me and word reached me that the *Fulmar* had been sighted. I had a fancy to be here to meet her when she made her home port. I've not ridden to Lynmouth for years, but suddenly thought I'd do it once more, before my limbs entirely seize up with age. And yes, I think we have met somewhere before, but I can't remember where. What's your name?"

"Nicky Lanyon, sir."

"Nicky Lanyon! So this is where you went! I heard that you'd left Allerbrook. The Weavers told me. I am Herbert Dyer."

"Oh! Yes, of course. I should have known you at once! I am sorry."

"Well, you haven't seen me since you were a boy. We met a few times at the Weavers' house in Dunster, when you came there as a lad, with your father. You've been travelling on this ship?"

"I'm apprenticed to Master Owen, sir. The Weavers arranged it. I visit them now and then, but obviously not at the same times as yourself. I haven't been there at all lately."

"There have been changes. Lady Elizabeth Luttrell and her son Hugh are back in the castle and Hugh Luttrell's been getting both Dunster and Minehead harbours dredged out. One day, your master's ship may tie up at Dunster quay. Does Master Owen suit you?"

"He would say it matters more if I suit him! But yes, it's a chance to see the world. We've just come back from Venice."

"The Weavers said you'd been thrown out after a family dispute, though they didn't say what sort of dispute."

"It wasn't a pretty business, sir," said Nicky awkwardly. If the Weavers had kept the truth from Dyer, then he wasn't going to reveal it. His mother was still his mother. It was and always had been Richard Lanyon he blamed for his exile. Dyer put a hand on his shoulder.

"I'll ask no questions. I know Master Richard is a hasty man and domineering, if you don't mind me criticising your family."

"No, I don't mind," said Nicky, pugnaciously enough to send Master Dyer's eyebrows rising toward his hairline. Nicky was himself surprised to realise how deep the wound of separation from his home and family had gone. This chance meeting had touched the scar and made it sore again. He would not now go back to live at Allerbrook for any consideration, yet he sometimes thought, *I'd like to visit, see my mother again. I miss her. Only, I can't face the thought of seeing Richard Lanyon.*

"Master Owen is below, sir," he said. "Shall I take you to him? You will want to examine your goods, I take it."

"Yes, and pay for them. Then I must organise their transport— by boat to Watchet and then packhorse to Washford, it'll be, as usual."

"I know all the boatmen here. Do you use the same ones each time? I can arrange the transport for you."

"Can you? Well, I'd be grateful. After that, perhaps we could have a drink together in a tavern, if your master will allow."

"Yes, he lets his older apprentices go to taverns." Nicky wasn't sure that he wanted to drink with this man from the past, whose conversation had already made him homesick, but it wouldn't do to refuse an invitation from one of Owen's clients. "Thank you, sir."

Dyer smiled. *A lad with something against Richard Lanyon.* He had responded by instinct to that pugnacious note in Nicky's voice. A young man who had reason to resent Richard Lanyon was someone with whom Herbert Dyer would probably get on well. "I'll take pleasure in buying you some ale, if Master Owen agrees," he said. "The Harbour Inn will do."

The Harbour Inn was a low-ceilinged cavern, badly lit, in which the sawdust on the cobbled floor wasn't changed often enough. However, the ale and cider were good, and in cold weather there was always a good fire in the hearth. When Nicky and Herbert went in, they found it crowded. Two other ships had arrived on the same tide as the *Fulmar,* and many of their crew, having furled the sails, unloaded the cargo and scrubbed the decks, were now taking their ease in the inn.

There were a number of locals, too. Nicky and Herbert squeezed between two benches full of men who smelt of fish and seemed to be discussing a mackerel catch, and found themselves a double settle close to a bald individual with tufts of greying hair over his ears, who had a small table and a stool to himself, possibly because he didn't merely smell but positively reeked of goat. Herbert gave their order to a serving girl, and then turned to Nicky.

"Tell me about Venice. That's a fine adventure for a boy brought up at Allerbrook and never going farther afield than Dunster."

A little while later, when the girl had brought their ale and the level in the tankards was going down, Herbert said interestedly, "If you don't want to tell me what went amiss between you and your family, well, as I said, I won't question you. The Weavers were obviously willing to help you and I'd trust their judgement. I suppose you fell out with your grandfather. You needn't tell me whether I'm right or not, only I know him!"

"Well, that was more or less the way of it, Master Dyer. I don't want to go back to the farm. I just feel I was done out of something that was properly mine," Nicky said.

"Didn't your father stand up for you?"

"No," said Nicky shortly, thinking that, odd as it seemed, he still thought of Peter Lanyon as his father and Richard as his grandfather and probably always would, however much he loathed those two self-righteous grown men who had victimised him, a boy of only thirteen, for something that was no fault of his.

"Overborne, I suppose. Well, as I said, he's a harsh man, is Richard Lanyon." Herbert shook a disapproving head. "His father was the same! Has it come out in you, I wonder? You don't have Lanyon looks, but maybe one day you'll be a merchant and rule your household like a tyrant king."

"I hope not, sir," said Nicky. "I value my own freedom. I'd try not to bully others out of theirs. If I'd stayed, I'd have had to marry where I was told, while now, when I meet a girl I like as I hope I will one day, I can please myself."

"If you'd stayed you probably would have had to marry to order," Herbert agreed. Their tankards were empty and, picking them up, he waved them at the girl, signalling for refills. "Did you know that before your father was wedded to your mother, he wanted to marry a girl from this very port but wasn't allowed to?"

"No—did he? A girl from Lynmouth? I never heard that."

The girl brought a jug and gave them more ale, for which Dyer paid, ignoring Nicky's attempt to do so. "It's true enough," he said, "though that time your grandfather may well have had the right of it, because I heard that the girl ran off with someone else anyway. She wouldn't have been a sound, decent wife like your mother."

"No," said Nicky, keeping his voice neutral. "Obviously not."

"As a matter of fact," said Dyer, enjoying himself, "it seems the wench was pleasing—hair like a pale gold mist, Richard Lanyon told me, or something of that kind. Marion Locke—that was her name. He even had a notion—he let this out to me once—that he might marry her instead and wipe his son's eye well and truly."

"He *didn't!*" Nicky, in the act of lifting his tankard, thumped it back onto the table. "Oh, no! He *couldn't!* That's outrageous!"

Herbert Dyer looked at him. *Good God. I shoot a longshaft into the air and phutt! It hits the target dead centre. I've had the weapon I need in my hand all these years and never knew it.*

"Well, he did. I don't suppose Peter Lanyon knows, to this day, though. I'd love to see his face if anyone ever told him. I don't somehow feel it's something he'd forgive, even after so long and even if the girl did run off. In his place, I wouldn't forgive it."

"My grandfather…" Nicky began.

"Will get his deserts one day, I've no doubt of it." *There, that'll do. The seed is planted. Best not overdo it.*

"He always wants to look bigger, more important than he is," Nicky said, ruminating. "That's why he built that great big house that I won't now inherit. And he does domineer over people, yes. I wonder if that's why the girl ran away! Perhaps she couldn't bear the thought of being married to him. Maybe her family thought it would be a good idea and were urging her to it. I wonder if she ever came back to them?"

"I don't think he ever approached them," said Herbert. "From what he told me, she ran off too soon."

"He shows off," Nicky grumbled. "He never used to ride moor ponies, you know. He liked horses that stuck in people's minds. When I left, he had a showy piebald…."

"Patches. And before that, another piebald called Magpie."

"When I was very small, I saw the horse he had before Magpie—Splash it was called. It was old by then, out at grass," Nicky said. "It was the weirdest-looking animal I ever saw—a sort of dapple grey, but the dapples were a very dark grey and there were some very big ones, and they ran into each other and overlapped as though the horse had had ink splashed on its hide. I've never seen another horse like it."

Unexpectedly, the goat-scented man with the tufts over his ears suddenly turned toward them. "Here! Do you mind me speakin' to 'ee? I couldn't help hearin' 'ee and I thought to myself, I did, that's a funny thing. That's a very funny thing, that is."

"What is?" asked Herbert, slightly annoyed by the interruption and making an effort not to hold his nose as the rank odour on the other man's clothes wafted toward him.

"Talkin' about a 'orse that looked like it had dark grey splashes all over it. I saw one like that once, but only the once, and I'm thinking, would it be the same 'orse? It were hereabouts, years back. Well, I say hereabouts. It were in that there Valley of the Rocks, up atop there, nigh to Lynton."

"When would that have been?" Nicky asked, not very interested but polite to an older man out of habit.

"Ah. Long time back. I were only a lad of fifteen, herding my goats in the valley, I was. I'm well on the wrong side of forty now. Don't know what, exactly. Never keep count of time, I don't."

"I suppose Master Lanyon could have been there for some reason or other," said Herbert. "Why shouldn't he be?"

"Ah, but he were with a wench! Pretty thing, too. I had good long-sight in them days." The goat-scented one sighed. "Didn't I hear you say summat just now about a girl with hair like a pale gold mist and him thinkin' of weddin' her? Could have been the same wench. Like a cloud round her head it were, catching the sun in glints. Sort of thing a lad like me would look at, and none of it kept decent under a coif. And the way of walking she had...aaarh!"

His audience regarded him with dislike but also with increasing interest. "And they were in the Valley of Rocks together?" Nicky said.

"Yes. Came in on the horse, with the girl behind him. There

were a dog, too, black-and-white. Never seen any of 'em afore, I hadn't. They got down and left horse and dog nigh the valley entrance and walked on. Argifyin', by the look of it. She jerked away from 'un at one point and she were shakin' her head, but he yanked her back and started walkin' her up that path round Castle Rock. You know it?"

"No," said Herbert Dyer, but Nicky said, "I know it. We go up there sometimes, me and the other apprentices, on sunny days when we've got some time off. It's fun to climb about up there."

"Well, she didn't think it fun, by the look of it," their informant said. "They'd started up the path when all of a sudden he swings round and gets hold of her arms. Looked like a proper disagreement, it did."

"And then?" asked Nicky.

The goatherd shrugged. "I didn't see no more. I thought it were all a bit funny, but I had me goats to see to. There was one limpin' like and I wanted to catch 'un and see what was wrong and anyhow, just about then a girt mist started rollin' in from the sea. Cleared a bit later, it did, just as I finished seein' to the goat. I went down to my old hut to eat a bite out of the cold and I see the 'orse and dog was gone. They'd come down and taken 'em, I s'pose. I remembered, after, 'cos the 'orse was that queer-coloured and I'd have liked to know what the man and the girl were quarrelling over, but I were only a lad myself. I never told no one, not until now."

"What are you drinking?" asked Nicky, leaning across Herbert for the purpose. "Can we get you another?"

"Cider, it be. Don't mind if I do. Like I said," said the goatherd, clearly taking pleasure in his audience, "I never told no one. But I thought about it, many a time. Leaves pictures in the mind, that sort of thing does. Queer-lookin' 'orse, and that girl with all that there pale hair and the way she moved…that were come-hither if ever I saw it. Aarh!"

The last syllable was positively lascivious. Nicky caught Herbert's eye and they exchanged speaking looks, but nevertheless, Herbert signalled to the serving girl and requested a pint of cider. The goatherd raised his existing tankard and drained it in an appreciative toast to them, and then startled them by changing his tone of voice completely.

"It was queer, that's what it was. That's why I never spoke of it. It were like a sort of dream, not real somehow and…well, it gave me a sort of funny feeling. Like it wouldn't be lucky to talk about it. I were only a lad and there were something about that day, an' those two quarrelling and that there mist drifting round—it must of caught them up there. Felt weird. That mist even scared me a bit, swirling round so as I could hardly see my feet. It were a queer sort of day altogether, see?"

"Yes," said Nicky as the cider arrived and Nicky, this time, succeeded in paying for it. "Yes, I do."

Later, as they emerged into the sunlit afternoon, Herbert remarked, "What an odd story that was. I wonder if he really did see your father's sweetheart quarrelling with your grandfather?"

"Not improbable, if he meant to separate her from my father. He went to see her, maybe."

"In the Valley of the Rocks instead of in Lynmouth?" Thoughtfully Herbert stroked his beard. It was unlikely that there was anything more in this than a chance meeting and a fleeting argument, long ago. Maybe Richard actually had proposed to the girl, been turned down and preferred not to say so, to pretend instead that he'd never had a chance to ask her. That fitted the Richard that Herbert Dyer knew.

"Have you ever seen your Allerbrook family since you left?" he asked.

"No. I don't think they'd want to see me, either."

"It's time you tried to make it up," Dyer said. "You're a young man now with a future and a trade. You won't be going there to beg. You've proved you can make your way in the world without them. It's time you went home and showed them! Your mother would like to see you, of that I'm sure—so well-grown as you are. Why don't you go?"

Nicky paused uncertainly, looking toward the quay and the *Fulmar*. "I suppose I want to, in a way, but…"

"You should. Well, think about it. We'd better part company here. I've a long ride home and I don't go fast, not at my age. I've left my horse at a stables." He clasped Nicky's hand in farewell. "If you do go, and happen to mention this odd tale we've heard, best not mention my name, if you can help it. But in your place, I must say I'd be curious. I'd want to see Richard Lanyon's face if I asked him about it."

He nodded and walked away, well pleased with himself. The seed might well have fallen on stony ground but on the other hand, Nicky was young, which usually meant indiscreet, and he was still angry. The thought of asking his grandfather upsetting questions and giving his father upsetting information might well appeal to him as much as it appealed to Herbert Dyer.

CHAPTER FORTY

KICKING A PEBBLE

T he day that was to end in chaos began gently, with a grey cloud spilling soft drizzle over the moors and hiding Dunkery from view, until the gathering power of the August sun lifted the vapours away, and the sunlight sparkled on a well-washed landscape.

"Nice drop of rain," Richard said with satisfaction, encountering Liza in the farmyard as they both returned from tasks outside. "Now, if only God sends us dry weather when it comes to the harvest, we'll do well. How's Primrose doing, Liza? You've been working hard on her."

"I've taken her to the pasture now," Liza said. "That teat is working now. I kept at it and kept at it and I think she's going to be quite all right. I must go and see to the bread."

She went indoors to help Ellen. Richard watched her go, thinking that most households would have packed her off to a nunnery but that it was just as well that he and Peter hadn't. When it came to things like difficult lambings and cows with mastitis, and making bread, she was incomparable.

And all the more these days, for Betsy was gone, carried off the previous winter by a sudden chill and lung congestion, and neither Ellen nor the two other maids who now helped her could match Liza's skills. Oh well, time brought changes of all kinds. Word had come from Dunster the year before that Laurence and Aunt Cecy, too, had passed away, Aunt Cecy very quietly in her bed one night, Laurence with mysterious pains and bowel bleeding, and then a sudden collapse. Nothing stayed the same forever. Not people and not even righteous indignation.

Liza, if asked, would have agreed that the unhappy relationship between herself and the Lanyon menfolk had changed, though it had been slow, and didn't even now go very deep.

Quentin's outburst had begun the process of reconciliation and Liza, thereafter, had fairly toiled at it. It was not a matter of forgiving or forgetting; only of raising a new edifice on the ruins of the old one. She knew she must never transgress again, by even the faintest degree, by as much as a single wistful reference to Nicky or by ever mentioning Christopher's name or by any unexplained absence for as much as half an hour. Buildings raised on top of rubble were never quite solid.

Throughout the past four years, though she and Peter had at length begun once more to share a bed, they had never coupled, but a new partnership had gradually been forged as they talked to each other of everyday, necessary matters to do with the work of Allerbrook. They had not stood side by side as parents at Quentin's marriage because Peter refused to attend it, but they had been there as grandparents at the christening of her son.

Betsy had never quite thawed, but Betsy was gone and Ellen, more impressionable and more concerned, in any case, with her forthcoming marriage to the cowman from Rixons, had been willing to make friends again. In fact, Liza sometimes suspected that Ellen was secretly rather excited by the wild romance in Liza's past.

If only, Liza sometimes thought, she could sometimes hear news of Nicky. No messages ever came to her from the Weavers, though they had let Peter know that he had indeed gone to them and later, that he had been apprenticed to a Lynmouth merchant. Peter had told her that much. But that was all. They had not mentioned Nicky again even to Peter and certainly not to her. Her family had cut her off. Unless Nicky himself one day contacted her, he was lost. She prayed that he was happy, but was afraid to speak his name and could not, therefore, ask Peter to find out for her.

Meanwhile, the morning had turned bright, and there were loaves to shape and put in the bread oven, and a capon to put on the spit for dinner. Phoebe and Hodge's small son would come to the farmhouse soon to turn it. Phoebe and Hodge believed in training their children to be useful early in life and they had already begun showing their four-year-old daughter how a spinning wheel worked.

She was in the kitchen, sorting eggs into dozens and putting them into small baskets, ready for Clicket market, when she heard Pewter, the young dog they had recently acquired, barking loudly and then Ellen, who had been out in the yard fetching water, came to say that Master Nicky had ridden in.

"Nicky!"

"Yes, ma'm. All the way from Lynmouth. Oh—here he is!"

And there indeed he was, her Nicky, a young man now, hair

as red as fire, chestnut eyes glowing, coming toward her to greet her with a hug.

"I've got permission from my master. I said it was time I visited you. I hired a nag in Lynton and started out early. The nag," said Nicky, "is lazy and slow but it's got me here. It didn't even shy when that lurcher you've got in the yard started baying."

"Pewter's new. He doesn't know you. We've got two new sheepdogs, too, Hunter and Trim. They're out with Peter and his father now—they're moving some sheep. Alfred's about somewhere."

"He's seeing to the horse. I passed Sweetwater House on the way here. Odd to think of Quentin living there. The Weavers let me know about her marriage. Is all well with her?"

"Yes, it seems that it is. The match is turning out well," said Liza. "And I'm as thankful as I can be, let me tell you. I say so in my prayers."

"I can believe it." He held her at arm's length and looked at her, smiling, glad to see her at last. He had felt unaccountably nervous on the ride. After all, he was the victim, who had been thrown out though he was innocent of any wrongdoing. If he met with any rudeness from the men who had disowned him and cast him forth, well, he had something to say that might well cause them to turn on each other. He carried it like a concealed knife. He might use it or he might not, but they had more to fear from him than he from them. He hoped they had been treating Liza well. "Am I welcome?" he asked.

"Of course you are! Come into the hall," said Liza, happily abandoning the eggs. "Ellen, bring some cider!"

She led the way to the hall. Nicky followed, frowning a little. His mother looked older, he thought, and thinner, too. Just what kind of life had she had since he left?

The question received a reply within the next two minutes, for just as Ellen came in with the cider, Richard and Peter returned for dinner. Nicky, accepting his tankard, raised his head as he heard the voices of the men who had for thirteen years been his father and his grandfather. Ellen had put down her tray and hurried out to tell them of his arrival. He could hear her explaining. Then the two of them came into the hall. Peter looked merely anxious. But Richard's face was cold and it was he who spoke first.

"And what are you doing here? We thought we were rid of you for good, you young cuckoo! If you've come to ask to be taken back…!"

"Oh…!" said Liza, shrinking. All trace of nervousness left Nicky at once and anger took over. He stepped in front of Richard and stood facing him.

"You have no right to speak to me like that. I never did you wrong, and now, let me tell you, I need nothing from you."

"Really?" said Richard.

"Yes, really! I am apprenticed to a merchant seaman in Lynmouth and in time, the Weavers are willing to help me set up for myself. I have a future, and I call myself happy. I've been to Venice three times now. I'm here to see my mother, nothing more. A reasonable thing for a son to do, don't you think?"

"Your mother doesn't need to be reminded of you and nor do we!" said Richard. "I thought we were rid of you for good!"

"Father, please!" said Peter. "Nicky is blameless and I have feeling for him, if you have not. I was glad of you, Nicky, that day on the packhorse bridge. Father, it's hardly a sin for him to want to see Liza. Let us be hospitable as we would be to any guest! I would like Nicky to join us for dinner."

Liza, evidently taking courage from this, said, "There's plenty of food. I'd like him to eat with us, too."

"Very well," said Richard. "This once. But let it be understood, young man—you chose to walk out on us and as far as I'm concerned, you're not welcome to walk back. So it's only this once."

Fury clenched in Nicky's guts. *So that's how it is! On the way up the combe I thought about the things Dyer and I heard from that goatherd in Lynmouth, but I thought I'd see what kind of welcome you gave me before I decided whether to mention them or not. Well, I've made my mind up now!*

Liza smiled at him and without a word fetched out the best pewter dishes and the silver salt which the Crowhams, long ago, had sent in celebration of the newly built hall. Richard scowled but made no comment.

Nicky, prudently, filled his stomach first, while answering his mother's questions about life with Owen ap Idwal, and the voyages he had made on the *Fulmar*. Peter and Richard were silent, neither interrupting nor attempting to join in. Ellen and Alfred and the two young maids, who were all at the table as well, were clearly conscious of family tension, and were also quiet. The gladness with which Liza had greeted him was now dimmed, like sunlight through a grimy window. She was herself aware of it. She could not properly enjoy his company, with Richard's disapproval filling the air like a disagreeable smell. Nicky sensed it, too, and knew that his mother dreaded Richard's anger. Oh yes, she had been allowed to stay, but she had not been forgiven. Not by Richard Lanyon, anyway. It hardened his heart still further.

When his mother ran out of questions and his stomach was safely laden with capon and raisin pudding, he turned to Richard.

VALERIE ANAND

"I heard the oddest bit of gossip the other day. Did you once think of getting married again, Master Lanyon? To a girl called Marion Locke, only she ran off with someone else instead?"

"Who told you that? They have it wrong, anyway," said Liza. "That was Peter, before he and I were betrothed. The girl you almost married was called Marion, wasn't she, Peter?"

"Yes. Marion Locke. That's right. But…" Richard had turned dusky crimson and Peter was looking at him curiously. "What's the matter, Father? It's just a bit of garbled gossip. I can't think how Nicky got hold of it."

"It was something I heard in a tavern. I believe this Marion Locke lived in Lynmouth," said Nicky, keeping it vague and re-membering that Herbert Dyer did not want his name men-tioned.

Richard, however, was already thinking about Herbert, and with loathing. *I let it out to that man Dyer and he talked, God curse him. He does business in Lynmouth at times. I might have known! She still haunts me. I think she gets into my soul and takes over my tongue. I still dream of her at times. She's using Nicky. I feel hot and my heart is pounding. Why did this…this little human accident have to come here and…?*

"I'm angry, that's all!" he barked. "Don't stare at me like that, boy! I don't like being gossiped about, and garbled gossip's worst of all!"

"But there was more than that," said Nicky, wrinkling his brow in a thoughtful frown. "The girl had cloudy yellow hair, hadn't she?"

"Yes, but what of it?" Richard snapped. "I saw her once, when I called on her parents to put a stop to the business of her and Peter. That's how I know."

"But at the time, you had a very odd-looking horse, called

Splash. I saw him myself, when I was a tiny boy and he was a very old horse, out at grass," Nicky said. "I was talking to a man in a Lynmouth tavern…"

"About me?" demanded Richard.

"Why not? I talk to whoever I like about whatever I like," said Nicky. "I'm not your grandson now, remember? I spoke of this girl Marion and I spoke of Splash and what he looked like and a fellow sitting nearby overheard me. He said that once, when he was a boy herding goats in the Valley of the Rocks, he saw a horseman come into the valley on a horse just like Splash, with odd-looking splodgy dapples, running into each other. He'd never seen a horse with a coat like that before and never saw another after. The man had a girl behind him, and she had hair like a pale gold cloud.

"He was almost poetic," said Nicky, enjoying his erstwhile grandfather's suffused face and glassy eyes. "They got down and left the horse—and a black-and-white dog—at the valley mouth and walked on to Castle Rock. I know the valley, so I know where he meant. They were quarrelling."

There was a silence. Then Richard said, "What's this rigmarole?" in a quiet voice which was somehow more alarming than when he was shouting.

Peter, however, was frowning. "I remember Splash and I never saw another horse like that, either. And Marion's hair…*did* you ever meet her in the Valley of the Rocks, Father? God's elbow, you surely didn't…." Richard's face now was purple, and Peter's eyes were widening. "It can't be true. You *didn't* have ideas of courting her for yourself! Did you?"

"Of course not! This is all a tarradiddle. I can't think…"

"Nicky," said Liza, distressed, "did you make this up because you are still angry at being disowned?"

"No, Mother. What I've said is what I heard. Truly."

"He's lying!" shouted Richard. "He's…!" There were beads of perspiration on his forehead. He stopped, gasping for breath, and half came to his feet, clutching at the edge of the table. Then he let go with one hand and jammed his palm against his chest. "I…"

He couldn't get any more words out. He staggered and fell, and might have pulled the table over except that Alfred and Nicky grabbed hold of it in time, and Richard's fingers lost their grip. Just as Liza sprang up and rushed around the table to help him, he crashed to the floor.

"Father-in-law!" Liza dropped to her knees beside him. "What's the matter? Oh, someone help me sit him up! What's *wrong?*"

Nicky was on his feet, too, appalled. It was as though he had kicked a pebble, and sent a landslide roaring down a hillside. Ellen and Peter had joined his mother at Richard's side and were lifting him into a sitting position, resting his back against the nearest wall.

"Can you not stand, Master Lanyon?" Ellen asked in concern. Richard, still pressing his hand to his chest, only shook his head. Sweat poured down his engorged face and his eyes were terrified. They sought Peter's and he struggled to speak but could only make gobbling sounds. Blobs of spittle appeared on his mouth.

"I'm here, Father. Take it slowly."

Somehow, Richard dragged a breath into his body and used it to force words out. "Not…slowly. No…time. Going to die. Priest."

"You're not going to die. People don't just die, like that, over dinner," said Liza in resolutely cheerful tones. "Take deep breaths."

"Going to *die.* Got to…get shriven. Can't die…with such a sin on me. Can't…"

"Father Matthew do say anyone can hear a confession if there b'ain't no priest handy," said Alfred. "Heard him tell us that, one Sunday. Master Lanyon, you ease your mind now, and then you'll likely feel better. Just to me, if you like, not bein' family. Might be easier."

"Doesn't matter…shan't be here to worry…aaah!" It was a moan of pain and he hunched forward, holding his chest as though he thought it might break apart. "Got to say…she wants me to say…she won't go away till I do…be waiting for me…"

"Who?" asked Alfred. "Who, Master Lanyon? Who is she?"

"Marion."

"Marion?" Peter burst out. "What are you saying, Father?"

"Wanted her…for me. Wanted…make her your stepmother." An awful rictus on Richard's face appeared to be a kind of grin. "Met her…in the valley. Walked her up Castle Rock. Asked her to…marry me…she wouldn't. Quarrel. Mist blowing in. Didn't mean it." His voice was fainter, as though his strength was going. "Caught hold of her. She broke away. Couldn't see…cliff edge. She…"

"She went off Castle Rock?" said Peter in a low voice. "Is that what you're saying? You…you killed her?"

"Accident. Didn't mean…" His voice gave out and his head fell back. He slid down the wall and let go of his chest, to strike feebly at the air with two clenched fists, before he slumped into unconsciousness. They shook him, shouted at him. Then Liza snatched a little silver spice tray out of the Crowham salt and held it in front of his lips. No mist appeared on it. He was no longer breathing.

Alfred, shaking his head, tested for a pulse in Richard's neck and sat back on his heels. "He's gone." He looked up at Peter. "I'm that sorry, sir."

"Sorry?" said Peter. "You may well be. I'm not. I can't believe…oh, no, *I can't believe…!*" He sprang to his feet and stood there, staring down at his father's body. "Oh, carry him to his room. Put him on his bed! Alfred, Nicky, just do it! I won't touch him! I'd sooner touch pitch…or eat muck from the midden!"

"Peter…" Liza went to him and put a timid hand on his arm, but he shook her off.

"All my life," he said, addressing not Liza but the hall in general, the table, the roof beams, the red-and-white Tudor roses on the panelling, the leaded windows, the rushes on the floor, "*all my life* I've given in to him. All my life he's been the one who says. I'm fifty years old and he still called me *boy!* He wanted a big house—I had to see our substance wasted on it. To get the substance to begin with, I was to marry for money while he indulged himself with the girl I wanted!"

"Peter!" wailed Liza.

"And when she wouldn't play his game," he shouted, "he killed her! He bloody well killed her and let me think she'd run off with another man! Let everyone think it!"

He flung away from them all in a frenzy of released rage, hammering a Tudor rose with a fist, kicking another on a window chest and shouting, shouting in repetitive fury.

"*All my life* he's had his way, never mine, never mine! He's despoiled our property for this house, like an old stag lying in a cornfield, crushing what he's lying on and eating everything within reach. Like the Sweetwaters riding across crops when they chase the same old stag! I was the one rewarded on a battlefield, but he took my reward from me and used it to suit himself. *We'll do this with it, we'll do that.* As though it were his! Always saying he's right, he knows best, he's the only one who should have a say! Calling me *boy* when I was a grown man and never a word of thanks when I looked after Allerbrook while he was away fighting—never a single word of praise! And all the time, all the time, he *killed Marion Locke!*"

"*Peter!*" Liza protested. "*Peter!* It was all long long ago and—"

"She'll never be long long ago for me. I loved her. *I loved her!*"

"And I loved Christopher Clerk!" Liza shrieked. "And now I see why! He wasn't a Lanyon!"

If anything could seize his attention, that would, but he didn't even seem to hear. "I hate this house! It's built on her bones! I'd like to burn it down! I will burn it down!" Peter bellowed, and would have made straight for the kitchen, where there was a fire, except that Liza got to the kitchen door first and stood with her arms spread wide, and Nicky and Alfred returned at that moment from laying Richard on his bed.

"I see," said Peter, glaring at his wife. "I'm still not to have my own way. Not ever, even at my age. No say in my own daughter's marriage, no say when money was cast away to build this house, or when land was cast away to the Sweetwaters! I thought I had a son once, but then I found I didn't even have that!"

"Peter, stop this, stop it!"

"Master Lanyon...Father...I still think of you as that...please don't. I never thought...I never expected..." Nicky was pale with horror.

"If he weren't dead, I'd like to kill him. I'd like to kill myself! I want to tear this place to pieces!" And once again he was hurling himself around the room, kicking and punching at the panels and the window seats.

"Nicky," said Liza frantically, "there's only one person I know of who can quieten Peter down when he's angry, and that's Quentin. He cares more for her than for anyone else in the world. She's at Sweetwater House…."

"I know. Shall I fetch her?"

"If you can. Get your horse and ride down the combe as fast as you can manage. Be careful bringing her back—she's expecting again and not far off her time. But don't lose time either. Go, Nicky, go!"

CHAPTER FORTY-ONE

A DUTY TO LIVE

N icky's hireling resented being dragged away from the manger Alfred had filled for him, and he tried to bite, but Nicky saddled him, mounted and drove him ruthlessly down the track through the combe, reaching Sweet-water House in a matter of minutes. Once there, his demands to see his sister were so peremptory and loud that Quentin herself, slow-moving now with the bulk of her second baby, heard him shouting in the courtyard, looked out of the solar window and came down to meet him.

"There's no time to lose." Nicky had not even dismounted. "Your grandfather's collapsed and your father's running mad and your mother thinks only you can calm him. It's serious! It's *urgent*. Quick, get up on this horse. Use the mounting block. Sit sideways behind me and I'll get us back to Allerbrook as fast as is safe. Come *on!* I'll explain as we go!"

"What's all this? Who are you? Where are you taking Quentin?" John ran from the house, with Walter, who these days was getting very rheumaticky, hurrying after him as best he could.

"He's my brother, there's trouble at Allerbrook, they need me to help," said Quentin rapidly. She hadn't seen Nicky for years and couldn't think where he had sprung from, but his frantic voice and the appeal in his eyes were enough. She was already perching sideways on the hireling's back, and was still finishing her explanation over her shoulder as Nicky urged the horse back to the archway.

"But you can't—" John was running alongside. "You mustn't…"

"I can. I must. Follow me if you like! We might be glad of you!" said Quentin, a new, decisive Quentin, one whom John had never seen before, and with that she was gone. The horse, his nose once more pointing to the manger from which he had been so summarily dragged, began for once to pull, and Nicky actually had to check him, so as not to jolt Quentin too much.

"What's wrong at Allerbrook?" Quentin demanded as they made for the combe. "How did you come to be there? I'm glad to see you, but…"

"Listen and I'll tell you."

By the time he had enlightened her and answered her astounded questions, they were at the top of the combe and turning toward the house. Hearing cries and thumpings, he risked a trot to get them quickly into the yard, where he pulled up sharply, while the horse, with good reason, whinnied and sidled.

Everyone except Peter was out in the yard. Ellen and the other two maids were clinging together, terrified. The dogs, all three of them, were running about, barking and yelping. Alfred was at the top of the porch steps, pounding on the door of the hall, while Liza, banging on a window and trying to see through it although it was so high that even on tiptoe she could only just peer over the sill, was screaming for Peter to let them in. And ominously, frighteningly, there was a seeping of smoke from the edges of the door, and the smell of it was in the air.

"He's in there!" Liza cried as Nicky jumped down and turned to help Quentin off. "He's setting fire to the hall and he's shut himself inside! He kicked Alfred from behind and threw him, *threw* him out of the door, and then he picked Ellen up and tossed her after Alfred like a…a piece of rubbish, and then pushed me and the other girls out, too, and Richard's dead and he's upstairs on his bed…!"

"The inner doors! From the kitchen, the workroom! The upstairs door to the spare bedrooms! What about those?" Nicky demanded.

"No use! He's bolted them all. I saw him! I could just about see! Even the upstairs door! I saw him run upstairs and do it. We can't get in!"

"Then find me something to break the front door down! Alfred! Hurry! Hurry! Anything!"

"Ah!" said Alfred, and abandoning his efforts with his fists, ran for the shed where the tools were kept, reappearing a second later with a gigantic hammer in one hand and an axe in the other, which he thrust at Nicky. "This any good?"

"Yes. Go for the hinges!" yelled Nicky. "Ellen, Quentin, get that horse away before it hurts itself or someone else!"

Ellen had pulled herself together and gone to help Quentin with the frightened horse. The two of them led it away toward the pony field, while Nicky and Alfred struggled with the door.

It was not intended to withstand such treatment and yielded quite quickly, breaking away from its hinges and falling inward. Smoke billowed out, and behind it there was fire, which flared up at the inrush of air, licking up the panelling and dancing along the floor where the rushes had been kindled, bursting into a blaze where Peter had piled wooden furniture to help it along. Peter himself, soot stained and livid, tried to attack them, but Liza, shrieking for the maids to help as well, joined in and between them all, they were a match for him.

"And no man kicks me from behind and gets away with it, not even you, Master," said Alfred grimly, grasping one of Peter's arms and helping to drag him out to safety.

"But the house, the house!" Liza screamed as flame ran across the rushes, pursuing them.

"It won't burn that easy, not all that good stone," Alfred said. "Get buckets, quick, Mistress, while we lock this madman up! And get these here dogs out from under my feet!" The lurcher, Pewter, seemed to think that Alfred was attacking Peter and had planted himself in front of them, barking furiously.

"Oh, Father, whatever is the matter with you?" Quentin and Ellen reappeared and at the sight of Peter struggling against his captors, Quentin cried out in distress. She also made haste to get hold of Pewter's collar, which brought her in front of her father. Seeing her seemed to bring Peter partly to his senses.

"Why are you here, Quentin? You're almost at your time! Nicky, if you did this…!"

"I sent him, you fool, because there's a faint chance you might listen to her!" Liza shouted. "You won't listen to anyone else! Ellen, take that dog from Quentin and shut it in somewhere! And the others!"

Ellen came running to deal with the dogs. Liza was already hauling a bucket from the well. Peter tried to break free from his captors, but they wrestled him to the shed where, long ago, Liza had seen her first pig carcase stripped of its bristles, thrust him inside and bolted the door. "Here!" said Liza, pushing the bucket at them as they ran back to her, and clattering a second one into the well.

Hoofbeats announced the arrival of reinforcements. After no more than a few minutes of distracted argument, John and Walter Sweetwater had saddled up and followed. They came headlong into the yard and pulled up, the horses sliding on their haunches. John leaped and Walter slithered to the ground, both exclaiming, "What the devil's happening here?"

"Where's my wife?" John shouted. "Quentin, put that bucket down! Have you gone clean out of your head?"

"God's teeth, John, the house is on fire!"

Hard behind them, attracted in from the fields by the sound of shouting, came Hodge, on foot, grasping a billhook. John and Walter, whose horses were edging nervously from the smell of smoke, promptly threw their reins at him, and with a shrug and a bewildered shake of the head, he led them away to add to those in the pony field.

Ellen, having shut the dogs into the tool store and sped back to join the firefighters, was too distracted to see the two new arrivals as anything but merely two new pairs of hands. She thrust a full bucket straight at Walter.

"What's this? What's this? What are you giving me this for?"

"She thought you might be thirsty! Oh, go and throw it on the fire!" shouted Liza. Walter's mouth opened in astonishment, but he suddenly grasped the need and bore the bucket to the hall as fast as he could limp. John seized Quentin, pulled her into the gateway, sat her down with her back against the gatepost, ordered her curtly to stay there and not move, and then joined in.

Alfred had been right to say that the hall would not burn easily. The panels and the floor were of seasoned oak, nearly as hard as iron, and there were still no tapestries. The pile of benches and stools, with cushions thrown in, was ablaze in midfloor, but there was no shortage of buckets, which were always needed for carrying food and water to stabled animals or getting bristles off pigs. With nine of them at the task, once Hodge had rejoined them, the flames were put out. There were dark stains on the walls and floor and window chests and a few on the roof beams and much of the furniture was lost, but the hall was still there and the damage could be repaired.

At the end of it all, Quentin rose and went to the door of her father's makeshift prison and talked to him through it. Presently, she came to the hall where the others were all busy pulling the piled furnishings apart and prowling about with buckets, looking for signs of smouldering, to say that she thought it would be safe to let him out.

"I knew you would manage him," Liza said thankfully. "He was beyond me, or I wouldn't have sent Nicky for you. If you're sure it's safe, set him free and bring him into the house. But only if you're sure."

Quentin, warily, went back to the shed. "Father? Are you all right? Please be all right. I'm so worried about you."

"There's no need to worry. There's nothing wrong with me."

"If I let you out, you won't…do anything dreadful again, will you? Please promise."

"No, I won't. I'm in my right mind now. Don't be afraid, my girl."

Quentin drew back the bolts and Peter emerged. He was trembling and looked sick. "Oh, my poor Quentin! What have I done? I think I was possessed."

His rage had gone out, like the fire. Quentin, talking gently to him, led him into the house and across the hall to the parlour. The others, still working, looked away. In the parlour she coaxed him to sit down, and a moment later Liza and Nicky joined them.

"Ellen will get us some cider," Liza said. "We've all got dry throats. The fire's out, though. Everything is going to be all right."

She said it calmly and even felt that it was true, though in his rage, Peter had uttered things which would be hard to forget. It had been wounding to hear his declaration of love for the unknown Marion, but in a way, it had eased her own bad conscience. If he had truly, all along, felt for Marion what she had felt for Christopher, then it was no wonder that they had never, quite, been able to form the bond a married couple should, and just how virtuous would Peter have stayed if Marion had been still alive and had one day come back to him?

The Sweetwaters, sooty, water-splashed and sweating, had finished in the hall and came in carrying full tankards and followed by Ellen with a trayload of more. John and Walter both looked angry.

"Just what did you think you were doing, Nicky Lanyon," John demanded, "dragging Quentin away up here, in her condition, into the middle of this?"

"Her father was in such a state. He'd learned something... something that upset him very badly," said Liza. "He wanted to set fire to the hall. Well, he did! Quentin's the only person we thought could quieten him." She looked around. "Quentin, you...where's she gone?"

"She was here beside me and then she suddenly went out," said Peter dully. "Just now."

"Ellen, go and find her!" Liza commanded.

Ellen set down her tray and disappeared. She was back in a very short time, her face frightened. "Mistress Lanyon...Master Sweetwater...I think the baby's on the way. She'm walkin' about in the kitchen but I think she did ought to be upstairs, in a bedchamber. I—"

"But it's early!" John shouted. "It's two weeks too soon!"

Peter and Nicky both sprang up.

"If anything happens to her..." Peter looked horrified.

Nicky, shakily, said, "We needed her here, but perhaps it was too much for her..." and then sat down again, his face stricken.

"You went because I sent you, Nicky," said Liza. "I'm sorry I had to send for her." She turned to Peter and her voice was pitiless. "It was all I could think of, with the house about to burn down and hers the only voice you were likely to heed. If anything goes wrong now, it will be partly my fault, but mostly yours!"

"Yes, his," said Walter savagely, and pointed a quivering forefinger at Peter. "And if my son's wife dies, I will kill him."

"Blessed Mother, intercede for her!" pleaded Ellen tearfully, down on her knees beside Quentin's bed. "Dear Lord, wilt thou not bring forth that which thou hast formed?" It was the fourth time she had uttered the ancient prayer for women in travail. The only response was another moan from Quentin and Ellen's tears flowed faster. "Ellen!" Liza said desperately. "Get up! More hot water, more cloths to wring out in it, more chicken broth and make haste."

"It's gone on too long, Mother." Quentin, weak and exhausted from twenty-four hours of constant pain without result, clutched at Liza's hand for comfort and then cried feebly as the anguish rose again. "I'm going to die. I just wish it could be over."

"You're *not* going to die," said Liza. "*Ellen! Broth!* And water and cloths!"

"I've got the chicken broth." John and Walter had ridden headlong back to Clicket, and an hour after that, John had reappeared with his mother. Catherine Sweetwater had taken charge in the Allerbrook kitchen. She had come into the room carrying a bowl. Ellen, still sobbing, got to her feet and passed her in the doorway. "At least those two maids of yours had the sense to start making the broth straightaway," Catherine said. "Now, what's all this about dying?"

"I'm going to," said Quentin, exhausted. "Can't manage it. Can't make it come."

"You've got to do it, and you've got to live. It's your duty," said Liza, wiping her daughter's wet forehead and smoothing back the soaked brown hair which had been plastered across it. "Because if you don't, your grandfather-in-law swears he'll kill your father. John didn't argue, either. Quentin, my darling girl, listen, it's up to you now!"

It's up to me. Her mother had no idea, Quentin thought as another pain twisted her guts into knots, what that phrase meant. It always seemed to be up to her. She had had to fight for her mother after Bosworth—make Betsy behave, get her father and grandfather to soften their anger. She had been the only one who really fought for Nicky. She had done that twice. She hadn't succeeded, but no one else had as much as tried.

She had eventually reconciled her father—more or less—to her marriage; within that marriage, much as she loved John Sweetwater, she had had to work to call forth an answering love from him, to make terms with Walter. And she had been the one Liza sent for in desperation when her own father was overset and dangerous. Now she must live when it would be much easier and more comfortable to die, because if she didn't, all hell would break loose all over again. Walter Sweetwater would renew the old feud, this time with lethal intent.

Sometimes she thought she had spent her whole life trying to coax other people to be reasonable. Now here it was again. She must live, or else. She was tired of it. Let them get on with it.

"No," she said wearily. "I'm going to die. I want to. I can't fight anymore."

"Rubbish, of course you can. Don't you dare give up now," said Catherine. "There are a few things we haven't tried yet. Mistress Lanyon, is there any pepper in the house?"

"I can't go on. I can't. Whoever's made threats, whatever they've said, I can't do anything about it!" Quentin wailed. "Why am I supposed to try? Why must it be me who has to stop people killing each other? Why do I have to be called because Father's trying to destroy the house? Why must it fall on me? No, I don't mean that, exactly, but…"

"Come. If you can make jokes, you're not dying," said Catherine, presenting her daughter-in-law with a spoonful of broth.

"Not making a joke. Just a mistake," said Quentin, and then, seeing that however accidental, it had indeed been a joke, unexpectedly laughed. The laugh collided with a violent contraction and turned into a cry, but as Catherine Sweetwater remarked afterward, laughter could be as good as a noseful of pepper and a few hearty sneezes for getting things to move. Five minutes later Ellen returned with the hot water and the cloths to find that a very small but very noisy girl-child was in Liza's arms and Quentin, however tired, was still very much alive.

"Elizabeth," said John Sweetwater. "We settled, if the babe were a girl, that she should be Elizabeth, for you, Mistress Lanyon, and for our queen, Elizabeth of York. It's a good Yorkist name," he added with a glinting smile full of such charm that Liza, for the first time, understood why Quentin had so improbably fallen in love with this young man. "But Quentin? You are sure she will come through?"

"Quentin is sitting up and taking broth," said Liza. "I'm rather sorry that Master Walter didn't come back with you from Sweetwater House. I would like a few words with your grandfather, John. Quentin will come through. In a few moments you can see her and your daughter. When you go home, tell Master Walter that we will hear no more talk of revenge and murder!"

"He may not have meant it," said John.

"I rather think he did," Liza told him. "Though I'd have done all in my power to stop him. I'd have made the parish constable arrest him for disturbing the peace with threats if I had to. One thing our new King Henry has done is introduce a little more law into the land."

There was a brief, tense silence. John Sweetwater's face darkened and in that moment he was wholly a Sweetwater, with as much arrogance in his eyes and the tilt of his chin as there had ever been in Sir Humphrey's.

"My late father, Baldwin Sweetwater," said John, "did not think that women should interfere in men's business."

"If Master Peter Lanyon were harmed, do you really think either Quentin or I would agree that it was nothing to do with us? That our bereavement wasn't our business? Come, come, Son-in-law," said Liza, and then, realising that she sounded exactly like her own parents, "Let us have a little common sense!"

Again there was a moment of tautness during which Liza's attempt to be reasonable strove in midair with the time-ingrained pride and the violent traditions of the Sweetwaters. She held John's eyes and almost held her breath, as well.

And then he laughed. "Quentin would think her father's death, or mine, come to that, was very much her business and I expect she'd say so. She's strong-minded, is Quentin. I saw it when she answered your call and got up behind Nicky without a second's hesitation. I pray she'll never take such a risk again."

Peter had taken no part in their exchange. He had a stunned air, as though too much had happened too rapidly for him to take in. He looked around him, at the damaged hall. "I can't believe I caused this. And I still can hardly believe that my father—"

"The burial will be tomorrow," said Liza, cutting him short. It would be better, she felt, if they didn't discuss the transgressions of Richard Lanyon. She had already told the rest of the household that whatever they had heard at that horrible dinner table had better be forgotten.

John remarked, "I think the stonework here will always carry those dark stains, but surely the woodwork can be restored?"

"Yes. It will be. I'll see to it," Peter said rather shortly, turning to him at last.

A silence fell. There might well, in the future, be a good many silences, Liza thought. There would be times when for this or that reason, conversation would veer in dangerous directions and have to stop, or change course. Walter Sweetwater and the Lanyon family would hardly be able to look each other in the face for a very long time, while both she and Peter had said things to each other which could never be forgotten but should never be mentioned again, either.

She'll never be long long ago for me. I loved her. I loved her!

And I loved Christopher Clerk and now I see why! He wasn't a Lanyon!

No. Let those dreadful, truthful, telling phrases be lost in time and silence. They must not be repeated. Nor must the scorn in *I sent him, you fool, because there's a faint chance you might listen to her! You won't listen to anyone else!*

There was one thing she must ask him, though. "Peter…"

"Yes?"

"Nicky is outside just now, attending to his horse. He'll go back to Lynmouth after the funeral. I would like it if he could visit me again, now and then. He is my son, after all." She held his eyes steadily as she spoke.

Here was another of those difficult pauses, in which the thirteen years during which Peter had believed Nicky to be his own son, and the moment when Nicky saved him from Baldwin, came to the minds of both Peter and Liza, though in John's presence they could not possibly be mentioned.

Peter was also having thoughts of his own which he knew it would be best not to utter. *I'm free now. I hated my father the day I tried to burn this house down, but now I need not even hate him. I'm even free of that. He can't control me anymore, and as for Marion…I suppose he's paid for her now.*

And because his father was gone, Peter need no longer deny those thirteen years of affection between Nicky and himself, an affection which had been strong enough to make Peter change sides at Bosworth, and bring Nicky running to his aid during the fight on the bridge. In a calm voice, he said, "But of course I'm agreeable. Naturally Nicky may visit."

John glanced at the two of them and looked as though he wanted to ask questions, but did not. The reason Nicky had left home would remain forever a Lanyon secret.

Catherine appeared at the door. "John, you can see your wife and daughter now."

CHAPTER FORTY-TWO

TOKEN

"Nicky! I'm so pleased to see you. It's been over a year!" Liza's voice was crackly now, like her weathered old skin or the creak in her joints when she moved. She was close on seventy, and felt it.

Nicky, on the other hand, was thirty-two and in his prime, a successful young merchant who had married the daughter of his former employer and now lived in Lynmouth with Gwyneth and their two little sons and had lately acquired a ship of his own.

He did not know, as he stood in the hall at Allerbrook looking at the panelling and window chests and Tudor roses, all of them carefully restored long since, that even now, when his mother was old, the sight of him made her inside turn over because he looked so like Christopher Clerk. He saw, however, that she was—as always—delighted that he had come visiting, and he gave her Christopher's tough grin, which was more of a reward than he dreamed.

"I had a good ride over the moor," he said. "Your crops are ripening well, though I think you've had deer in the barley again. You'd better have a word with the Sweetwaters' harbourer and see if he can't set the hounds on the miscreants."

"Yes, I'll tell Peter. How are your family?"

"All well—now. Gwyneth is as lively and merry as her father still is. The boys have had measles, but they've come through safely. They're good lads most of the time," said Nicky, "and even when they're not, I don't beat them. They both take after me and they might not forgive me."

There was a brief silence, one of the silences that Liza had foreseen when Richard died and Quentin's daughter was born. Nicky had never forgiven Richard for his beatings or for casting him off, and look what had come of that long bitterness. After a moment she said, "Did you call on the Sweetwaters as you usually do, and see Quentin?"

"Yes. I found her in the dairy with Elizabeth, making clotted cream. The Sweetwaters have never quite succeeded in turning our Quentin into a lady," said Nicky, grinning again. "Johnny told me that last year, at harvest time, she made him arm himself with a scythe and go out reaping with the rest of the parish!"

"I know. We had him here, taking his place in the line across the field. Her husband doesn't mind," Liza said. "John claims that his grandfather Walter was very interested in his sheep and used to go about sometimes with Edward Searle. He's happy enough to see his son and daughter learning to be practical. Walter approved, too—Catherine told me. Peter and I never spoke to him again, nor he to us, after the day of the fire until the day he died, but he valued Quentin. It was for her sake that he threatened Peter! It was all very complicated. Well, the old feud died with him."

"Thank God it died. Can I have another look at Quentin's window in the chapel?"

They went to the chapel together. It was not large, but like the rest of the house, it had been enhanced during the fifteen years since the fire, at Peter's expense. The day he made up his mind to embark on improvements for the hall and the chapel had been one of the rare occasions when an area of silence, hitherto as pristine as untrodden snow, had acquired just a few footprints.

"I've been thinking, Liza. You know, I'm quite proud of our house now. Father was right. We didn't end up dressed in rags and begging for alms in Clicket or Dulverton, did we?" He had never before made even an oblique reference to the day he had tried to burn down the house and even now, Liza silently noticed, Marion's name was not mentioned. It never would be. "We've prospered well after all," Peter said, "and I find I have land enough to content me. There are a few things I'd like to add…."

So tapestries now adorned the hall and the sun made coloured patterns on the floor of the little chapel when it shone through the stained glass of the windows Peter had installed. The first to be put in was known as Quentin's window.

"It's a thank-you to her," Peter had said. It showed an angel, whose face bore a certain resemblance to that of his daughter, standing before a building with arms outspread, denying entrance to a man who held a flaring torch aloft.

"That was a terrible day," Nicky said as they stood together, looking at it. "When the fire happened, I mean."

"Yes. Yes it was. Nicky, do you want to see Peter? He's out with the sheep—he's sixty-five but as able to get about as ever he was. He'd be sorry if he missed you. He likes to see you these days."

"Poor Peter. I still sometimes want to call him Father, you know. Now I'm grown up myself, I can see what a muddle he must have been in."

"He was. He'd loved you as a son for thirteen years and he wanted you to go on being his son and when he found that you weren't, he didn't know what to do with the love," Liza said, and then looked astonished. "I've known that for years and never put it into words before. Fancy that!"

"I'll see him—of course I will. But I want to give you something first, privately. Beside Quentin's window is as good a place as any. I think she understands you and even understands about…"

"She does." He had paused, but Liza, making a cautious footprint or two on another stretch of silent snow, finished his thought for him. "She fell in love with John just as I did, long ago, with your father."

"Here," said Nicky, and drew a small packet from inside his doublet. "I sailed north recently, to collect a consignment of copper for my first voyage abroad in my own ship. Which is lying in Dunster at the moment, by the way. The Luttrells are maintaining the harbour very well. But while I was in the north, I made some enquiries. I've seen my real father."

"You've seen Christopher! He's still alive?"

"Yes, though he's frail. I knew that he'd gone to the north. You told me that, back then, when we first found out…about everything."

"I remember. Peter told me and I spoke of it to you, before you left home."

"I've thought for years that I'd like to find him, if it wasn't too late. I'd only seen him once, and hardly under ideal circumstances. I did find him, but I think I was only just in time. He said himself that he didn't think he'd got much longer. He's still a priest, though he has a younger priest with him who does most of the work of the parish. They have a church in a Yorkshire village. He was happy to see me, very happy, and pleased to have news of both me and you. He gave me something for you. Here. Better not say he sent it, perhaps. If Peter asks, say it was a present from me. He won't mind that. My fa…I mean, Christopher said that as the end of his life couldn't be far away, he wanted you to have this, as a token of his lifelong prayers for you."

She took the packet and opened it. And then looked at what it had contained, marvelling, holding it in one palm and turning it over with her other hand.

It was a patterned silver ring.

AUTHOR'S NOTE 🪢

The origins of this book lie far back in time. It was, I think, the year 1959, and I was only about twenty-two on the day when, during a morning ride in Somerset, on the edge of Exmoor, I turned my horse onto a path halfway up the side of a narrow valley, with pine trees growing up from its floor.

I hadn't been there before. Later I learned that the pines were on average 150 feet high and were among the tallest trees in Great Britain. On that morning they almost made me giddy. The path was level, roughly, with their halfway point. When I looked down, my eyes followed their slim trunks to the ferny ground far below. When I looked up, I could see them stretching far above me, tapering toward the sky. It was staggering. It was also exhilarating; another splendid thing I had discovered about a district which had fascinated me since I saw it first at the age of eleven.

I was not yet a writer, but I knew I would be one day. On that morning, looking at those pines, I knew that I wanted, intended, was determined, one day, to write a book with Exmoor and its surroundings as a setting.

It was many many years before the right opportunity and the right theme presented themselves. And then, one day, long after I really had become a novelist, my agent telephoned me and said he knew I had always wanted to write a novel based on Exmoor. Well, it looked as though the chance had come. There was a publisher who was interested in a historical novel with an English regional setting.

The House of Lanyon is the result. Nearly every place it mentions is real, except for Allerbrook and Clicket. These, like the characters, are fictional. There is no such house as Allerbrook; indeed, there is no manor house of that type anywhere on Exmoor. Where I have placed both village and house there is in reality nothing but moorland and isolated farms.

The name of Clicket is genuine. At one time there really was a hamlet called Clicket on the outskirts of Exmoor. It was however a very small community, nothing at all like the prosperous village I have described in the book, and it wasn't in the same place. I believe it was abandoned sometime in the nineteenth century. It seemed a pleasant idea to use a genuine Exmoor name, that's all.

To save Exmoor enthusiasts the trouble of noting references to places like Dulverton, Withypool and the River Barle, getting out their Landranger maps and trying to work out where Clicket ought to be, I will tell them that it is approximately (I won't be too specific) between three and five miles west of Tarr Steps, the curious granite slab bridge across the Barle. Allerbrook House is a mile away from it, high up in a combe which is also fictional. I have simply and ruthlessly planted village, house and combe where I wanted them to be. Writers of fiction do that kind of thing.

Oddly enough, there is no reference in the book to a valley with tall pine trees in it, but the memory of that morning's ride was with me all the time as I wrote *The House of Lanyon*. I have loved writing it. I hope it will give pleasure to readers, too.

Valerie Anand
November 2006